Frances

Mental Health —Psychiatric Nursing

Editorial Board

Mental Health — Psychiatric Nursing

A Continuum of Care

A WILEY MEDICAL PUBLICATION

JOHN WILEY & SONS

New York • Chichester • Brisbane • Toronto • Singapore

Library of Congress Cataloging in Publication Data:

Psychiatric-mental health nursing.

  Includes bibliographies and index.
  1. Psychiatric nursing. I. Norris, Joan (Joan F.)
[DNLM: 1. Psychiatric Nursing. WY 160 P97203]
RC440.P736 1987   610.73′68   86-24229
ISBN 0-471-09957-0

Printed in the United States of America

10 9 8 7 6 5 4 3 2 1

Contributors

Linda S. Beeber, R.N., M.A.
Assistant Professor
Syracuse University
College of Nursing
Doctoral Student
University of Rochester
School of Nursing
Rochester, New York

Carole P. Bonds, M.S.N., R.N.
Assistant Professor
College of Nursing
University of Florida
Private Practice
Advanced Registered Nurse Practitioner in
    Psychiatric/Mental Health Nursing
Gainesville, Florida

**Barbara Gross Braverman, M.S.N., R.N.,
    C.S.**
Instructor of Psychiatry/Clinical Nurse
    Specialist
Medical College of Pennsylvania
Philadelphia, Pennsylvania

Susan I. Cullen, M.S.N., R.N., C.S.
Manager of Hospital Based Psychiatry
Harvard Community Health Plan
Boston, Massachusetts

Diane M. Dodendorf, Ph.D.
Assistant Professor, Department of Family
    Practice
School of Medicine
Creighton University
Omaha, Nebraska

Patricia Mayer Ehrhart, M.S.N., R.N.
Assistant Professor
Psychiatric/Mental Health Nursing
Creighton University
Clinical Specialist
St. Joseph Center for Mental Health
Omaha, Nebraska

David Anthony Forrester, Ph.D., R.N.
Associate Professor
Lienhard School of Nursing
Pace University
New York, New York

Formerly Assistant Professor
Acute Care Department
College of Nursing
Rutgers, The State University
Newark, New Jersey

Barbara Geach, M.S.N., D.N.Sc.
Assistant Professor, Department of Nursing
Lehman College of C.U.N.Y.
Bronx, New York

Karolyn Lusson Godbey, M.S.N., R.N., A.R.N.P.
Assistant Professor
University of Florida
College of Nursing
Gainesville, Florida

Kathryn Govaerts, Ph.D., R.N.
Pediatric Psychologist
Children's Medical Center
Tulsa, Oklahoma

Amy Marie Haddad, M.S.N., R.N.
Assistant Professor
School of Pharmacy and Allied Health
Creighton University
Clinical Consultant
American HomeCare
Omaha, Nebraska

Peggy L. Jensen-Hawkins, M.S.N., R.N.
Faculty, Department of Nursing
Nebraska Wesleyan University
Lincoln, Nebraska

Mary Ellen Kronberg, M.S.N., R.N.
Captain, Nurse Corps, U.S. Air Force
Miami, Florida

Mary Kunes-Connell, M.S.N., R.N.
Assistant Professor and Coordinator
Psychiatric/Mental Health Nursing
Creighton University
Omaha, Nebraska

Amy L. Longo, B.S.N., J.D.
Partner in the Law Firm of
Ellick & Jones
Omaha, Nebraska

Barbara L. MacDermott, M.S., R.N.
Associate Professor
Syracuse University
College of Nursing
Syracuse, New York

Daniel P. Murphy, Ph.D.
Associate Professor of Psychology
Creighton University
Omaha, Nebraska

Geraldine Renschler Newton, M.S.N., R.N.
Doctoral Student in Counseling Psychology
University of Nebraska
Lincoln, Nebraska
Formerly Assistant Professor
Creighton University School of Nursing
Omaha, Nebraska

Joan Norris, Ph.D., R.N.
Associate Professor
Graduate Nurse Education
Creighton University
Omaha, Nebraska

Mary Lou Haberman Orchard, M.S.N., R.N.
Psychiatric Consultation Nurse
St. Luke's Hospital
Fargo, North Dakota

Linda R. Phillips, Ph.D., R.N.
Associate Professor
University of Arizona
College of Nursing
Tucson, Arizona

Cordelia C. Robinson, Ph.D., R.N.
Meyer Children's Rehabilitation Institute
University of Nebraska Medical Center
Omaha, Nebraska

Mary Patricia Ryan, Ph.D., R.N.
Associate Professor
Mental Health Nursing, Niehoff School of
   Nursing
Loyola University
Chicago, Illinois
Kennedy Fellow in Medical Ethics
Cambridge, Massachusetts

Kathryn Murphy Schinker, M.S.
Director of the Shelter
Residential Facility for Abused Women
United Catholic Social Services
Omaha, Nebraska

Stephanie Stockard, M.S.N., R.N.
Nurse Therapist, Private Practice
Formerly, Coordinator and Assistant Professor
   of Psychiatric/Mental Health Nursing
Creighton University
Omaha, Nebraska

Odessie G. Taylor, Ph.D., R.N.
Graduate Nurse Education
School of Nursing
Creighton University
Omaha, Nebraska

Gordon Vogt, M.S.N., R.N.
Associate Chief, Nursing Service for Education
John L. McClellan, VAMC
Little Rock, Arizona

Consultant/Reviewer

Nancy Flinn Deitchman, R.N., M.S.
Formerly Assistant Professor
University of Colorado, Health Sciences Center
School of Nursing
Denver, Colorado
Director of Inservice Education
Mount Airy Psychiatric Center
Denver, Colorado

Preface

Psychiatric-mental health nursing textbooks have grown in size and scope and have become increasingly more sophisticated and comprehensive. Advanced practice and its knowledge base have grown concurrently, adding to the available concepts, information, and expectations for a comprehensive textbook. Nursing has grown as a profession and the body of knowledge available to be applied in clinical practice has expanded for both the generalist (entry-level professional) and the clinical specialist (master's prepared and qualified in therapy and community programming).

The editors believe that nursing as a discipline has progressed to the point that all relevant knowledge specific to an area of practice cannot and should not be compressed into a single volume that becomes all things to all people in that practice area. The purpose of this textbook is to provide comprehensive information and guidelines applicable to the generalist level of professional nursing practice. Selection of content and approach is consistent with the ANA *Standards of Psychiatric-Mental Health Nursing Practice*. The student and the entry level professional nurse both need a clear understanding of the role, pertinent knowledge, and functions of the generalist as a guide to nursing assessment, diagnosis, care planning, and evaluation. The generalist is prepared to provide preventive mental health care and health promotion for individuals and families and health restoration care for clients with psychiatric conditions.

The steps of nursing process are used as organizers throughout the book, as are the levels of prevention appropriate to the nursing care focus. Both nursing diagnoses and DSM-III terminology are incorporated in pertinent chapters.

In the interest of clarity for the reader, several decisions have been made. The authors recognize the increasing numbers of men in nursing and the presence of both male and female clients. However, the limitations of the language present some cumbersome and confusing tasks in the use of nonsexist language, which is used whenever possible. In instances that tax readability or clarity, the traditional she as nurse and he as client are adopted with apologies.

The traditional term, psychiatric-mental health nursing, is used throughout this book because it reflects common usage in nursing and in the standards of practice of the professional organization. The title of the book, however, and its organization have been purposefully selected to reflect and emphasize the distinct and independent role of the generalist nurse in promotion and maintenance of mental health in both general hospital and community settings. For this reason, two distinct units are organized around the developmental and situational challenges of living. Two additional units address the collaborative role of nursing in caring for clients in the interdisciplinary psychiatric care setting. Because of this ordering and because the editors believe in the fundamental importance of mental health promotion at the generalist level, this book is titled Mental Health-Psychiatric Nursing—A Continuum of Care.

The generalist must be prepared to provide a continuum of care to clients and families at various stages of the life cycle and in various practice settings such as the pediatric outpatient clinic, the general hospital, the psychiatric unit, the home, and the community. The principles of providing mental health promotion and support differ somewhat in focus and content from those involved in provision of psychiatric nursing care. These aspects may be taught together in a traditional course in psychiatric-mental nursing or presented separately at different points in an integrated curriculum. The editors chose to present these concepts distinctly. The chapters have been organized to differentiate normal developmental challenges and issues from content pertinent to disorders that may arise at particular stages of life. See, for instance, the unit on lifespan development with individual chapters for specific ages/stages and concepts. These chapters are clearly differentiated from later chapters which focus on psychiatric disorders that may occur in childhood, adolescence, or in the older population.

Some unique features of the book include a chapter on attachment, a chapter on anxiety which addresses both prevention and nursing intervention for aggressive and assaultive behavior, and a chapter that incorporates research utilization models and quality assurance for the generalist level of practice. Particular attention has been addressed to specific psychosocial problems which are more likely to occur in practice settings outside the traditional psychiatric unit but which call for the extensive application of psychiatric-mental health principles and knowledge in providing care. The units on developmental crises, life events, and dysfunctional life-styles address issues pertinent to pediatric, medical-surgical, and community practice with clients who may be physically ill, in mourning, mentally retarded, dependent upon alcohol and drugs, or victims of neglect or abuse.

The authors present this textbook in the hope that it will serve to clarify the generalist practice level so that students and practicing nurses can better apply comprehensive principles of psychiatric-mental health nursing across varied settings, providing a continuum of care.

JOAN NORRIS

Omaha, Nebraska
February, 1987

Acknowledgments

The editors wish to express their appreciation and gratitude to the many people who made publication of this book possible: (1) the many contributing authors who gave of their time and content expertise, (2) the secretarial and word processing staff of Creighton University's School of Nursing who worked on the manuscripts in their many revisions, (3) the publishing staff of John Wiley & Sons, and (4) Bernice Heller—our developmental editor whose wit, wisdom, and patience were essential in completing this text.

Special thank-yous are given to families and friends who provided support and encouragement throughout the lengthy process of the book's development from idea to prospectus through rough drafts and galley proofs. Mary Ellen Kronberg is recognized for her participation on the editorial board from the beginning of this process until she left to relocate in Florida—her ideas and enthusiastic assistance were highly valued.

Contents

Detailed Contents

Mental Health —Psychiatric Nursing

PART ONE

Theoretical Basis for Psychiatric-Mental Health Nursing

To know oneself and to respect the rights, dignity, and uniqueness of others is the basis of human understanding.

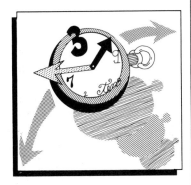

1

Theoretical Models of Personality and Behavior

Joan Norris

Learning Objectives

Upon completion of this chapter, the reader will be able to:

1. Identify key aspects of various theoretical viewpoints concerning personality and behavior.

2. Synthesize basic concepts derived from these views in understanding behavior.

3. Analyze components of selected nursing theoretical models in relation to person, environment, health, and nursing.

4. Select nursing implications from the various theoretical viewpoints for assessment and intervention.

In the behavioral sciences, unlike the physical sciences, there is no single theory that is universally accepted and accurately predictive in relationship to human behavior. Instead, several viewpoints, which emphasize particular influences on personality and development, are prevalent. Mental health professionals, including nurses, may adhere to one or another or, more likely, adopt aspects of several in an eclectic approach.

Because human behavior is so complex and subject to multiple influences, the theoretical viewpoints can be compared to the parable of three blind men trying to describe an elephant. One, feeling the leg, said, "An elephant is like a tree." Another, grasping the trunk, exclaimed, "Elephants are like big snakes." The third, holding the tail, perceived, "An elephant is like a rope." Theorists of human behavior similarly tend to describe parts of the whole as they focus, for example, on internal influences or external stimuli or interpersonal and social factors. This multiplicity of theories clearly indicates that there is no single comprehensive and universally accepted theory of personality and behavior.

Major viewpoints include the psychodynamic, behavioral, existential, and systems models. Within each of these larger categories are many related theories. Psychodynamic models may be intrapersonal (internally focused, e.g., Freud) or interpersonal (emphasizing interactive processes as Sullivan did), and may include cultural and environmental emphasis (such as Erikson's view). Behavioral approaches focus on the contingencies or occurrences that tend to shape behavior through selective reinforcement. Watson, Pavlov, and Skinner are well-known advocates of stimulus-response views. Systems views build on Lewin's and Von Bertalanffy's theories in emphasizing the variety of external factors (social-environmental forces) influencing and interacting with behavior. Systems views have also contributed to several models of family and group process that focus on interactive components of communication and behavioral patterns.

Each viewpoint shares some common assumptions about human behavior with several others but also differs in some significant aspects. For instance, psychodynamic and existential views depict man as actively shaping his own behavior through perception, interpretation, and action. Behaviorists tend to view man as passive or acted upon by his environment. Systems theorists depict processes in which man is both active and acted upon. Crisis theorists (Lindemann, Caplan)

can be described as comprehensive in that they merge the influences of perception, experience, and social system support as factors in behavioral outcomes to which people respond as they cope with the challenges of living.

These broad theories are supplemented by the work of others in studying specific factors such as motivation or psychobiology. Nursing theory is included here because of its initial contributions to the focus on man, environment, and health. These various theoretical perspectives may differ as to (1) what constitutes mental health or illness and (2) what causes or influences behavior. Models of therapy based on these views are addressed in Chapter 2, with their implications for nursing.

It is not possible to include all relevant theoretical perspectives in a single chapter. The disciplines of psychiatry, psychology, sociology, and nursing are continually refining and expanding the theoretical basis for practice. For these reasons, it is important to remain theoretically open and to become a student of human behavior in order to expand one's effectiveness in nursing practice. Human behavior is, after all, a primary focus in defining and promoting health in any area of nursing.

☐ *Psychodynamic Theories*

INTRAPERSONAL THEORIES
Freud

No discussion of psychological theory can begin without reference to Freud—the scientist, physician, philosopher, and founder of modern psychiatry who profoundly influenced twentieth-century thought. His early topographic model of the mind in 1899 introduced the "systems" or concepts of the conscious mind, the preconscious (beyond conscious awareness but accessible), and the unconscious. In 1923, he publicized his structural perspective, which described the concepts of id, ego, and superego, and reduced the earlier systems to descriptive terms for consciousness.

The id is made up of unconscious drives, fantasies, and impulses and is governed by the pleasure principle—seeking pleasure and avoiding pain. Biological drives or tensions arise in the id and enter consciousness only if acceptable to the ego. The characteristic mode of thought is the primary process. Primary process thinking is wishful, illogical, emotional, symbolic, and does not differentiate between a memory image and objective perception. There is no sense of time, and past or present may be intertwined. An example of primary process thought is a mirage—the parched traveler sees an oasis that does not exist in reality. Other examples are sensory images such as visions or voices that are not reality based and that may occur under severe stress such as panic-level anxiety or withdrawal from drugs or alcohol. Freud also believed that dreams were related to primary process thought and wish fulfillment.

The ego develops on the basis of experience, identification, and learning as the person interacts with the environment and learns conscious, rational approaches to meeting biological needs. The ego is governed by the reality principle and is able to distinguish between subjective perceptions and memory and objective reality. Secondary process thought is characteristic of the ego and involves thought, rationality, and the ability to problem solve. The functions of the ego include: (1) mediation of conflicting demands between the id and the superego (roughly, the conscience); (2) adapting inner urges to the constraints of external reality and morality; (3) reality testing; and (4) directing and stimulating the processes of thought, perception, memory, and physical activity. The ego has inherent potentials, which are developed through environmental interactions, growth, and learning.

The superego, according to Freud, develops out of the ego on the basis of assimilation and identification with parental and social moral codes. The ego ideal is the positive component of the superego, which represents the individual's perceptions of goodness. The conscience, on the other hand, is the internalized representation of badness and guilt. These components are learned through approval or rewards and punishments. The superego enforces morality by applying rewards or punishment to the ego and does not necessarily distinguish between thought and action. Thus the ego may experience guilt or punishment for thoughts as well as for actions. The system of rewards and punishment available to the superego includes both psychological and physical factors such as feelings of satisfaction or guilt and occurrences such as illness (e.g., tension headaches) or accidents. The id, the ego, and the superego are not separate or actual phenomena but represent an interaction of processes that influence psychic energy, tension relief, needs and, consequently, behavior.

Anxiety plays a key role in personality development and function. Freud felt that there were three major sources of anxiety: external threats, internal urges (id), and internal conscience (superego). The anxious person, however, is generally not aware of the true source or sources of the anxiety. Anxiety serves as a signal to the ego to ward off danger. Overwhelming anxiety, which cannot be managed effectively and so must be repressed, constitutes a traumatic event and does not promote social learning—hence one may remain fixated at an immature level in regard to the traumatic issue.

For example, a young child may be subjected to physical or sexual abuse by a parent. In order to maintain parental love and protection and cope with the anxiety associated with the event, the child may repress awareness. Even though the anxiety and related feelings have gone from conscious awareness, the trauma continues. It will unconsciously influence the child's perceptions of others and his subsequent behavior. In this way, future relationships suggestive of frightening themes such as intimacy or powerlessness are affected by early events beyond the person's awareness. Therapy may assist the person to gradually accept and integrate the experience so that it no longer exerts a powerful unconscious influence. Freud described the goal of psychoanalysis as "where id is, let ego be."

Personality development involves increasing one's ego strength and level of personal differentiation. Influencing conditions include maturation (the natural sequence of reaching developmental potential), external frustrations, internal conflicts, personal inadequacies, and anxiety. Mental mechanisms (see Table 1-1) serve to protect and defend the ego against anxiety and maintain a state of equilibrium. These defense mechanisms are commonplace and do not become problematic unless they fail in their protective role or become maladaptive by distorting the individual's ability to perceive and respond to reality appropriately. For instance, it is a rare person who has never rationalized his actions to make them appear more favorable or displaced his anger onto a "safer" person or object than the true source. However, the man or woman who projects unwanted sexual or aggressive impulses onto others and then lives in constant tension and isolation because of the resultant fears has adopted a maladaptive solution (a symptom of mental illness). Mental mechanisms are generally considered to be unconscious but may exist on a continuum from conscious to unconscious (Wallace,

TABLE 1-1 Mental Mechanisms

Mechanism	Definition	Example
Sublimation	Redirection of energy from a forbidden object to a substitute	Forbidden sexual or aggressive impulses may be expressed artistically in poetry or art
Repression	Threatening thoughts are forced out of consciousness	A person may "honestly" say, "I never get angry"
Reaction formation	Adopting an attitude that is directly opposite to an unacceptable urge in order to control and unconsciously defend against it	Becoming zealously puritanical about sex as a defense against sexual thoughts and urges
Intellectualization	Overusing cognitive-mental activities to avoid feelings	Excessive analysis of the motivations of self and others in order to ward off feelings of anger toward others
Regression	Returning to behavior characteristic of earlier stages of development in the presence of current stress	Competent adults may become dependent and demanding when ill or anxious
Displacement	Rechanneling a feeling from one object to another (generally a safer object on which to release feelings)	Criticizing a friend; kicking the dog when actually angry with a teacher or employer
Undoing	A "magical" attempt to wipe out the damage done by one's actions or unexpressed negative wishes	Lady MacBeth's handwashing after the king's murder; a child who misbehaves and then says, "Good Daddy" to avoid punishment
Denial	Refusal to acknowledge painful objective reality	A client may initially refuse to accept the surgeon's diagnosis of cancer
Introjection	An object's image is incorporated into the self, and related feelings are directed toward this assimilated object/image; similar to the process of identification	Parental values are assimilated in superego development; loss of a loved object may result in the feelings of anger (at being abandoned) being turned inward against the self
Isolation	Separation of thoughts from feelings in regard to a traumatic event	A man may be able to recall details of his wife's death but experience no feelings—"Just numb." Later he may find himself weeping unexplicably over a dead animal by the roadside

TABLE 1-1 (continued)

Mechanism	Definition	Example
Splitting	Separating the representation and related feelings of goodness and badness as if a person were actually two separate people	An abused child reponds to the "good" mother who feeds him and the "bad" mother who beats him as if she were two different mothers; common in early childhood but should not occur in the preadolescent or older age groups
Projection	Attributing one's own unacceptable thoughts and feelings to others	My own murderous impulses may be converted into the fear that others wish to kill me
Rationalization	Providing a justification or logical reason for an act that was not reasonable or logical	Compulsive behavior may be explained as justifiable—"I must wash my hands whenever I touch anything—the world is full of germs"
Suppression	Consciously making an effort to forget an idea or feeling	"I won't give in to that thought"; "I'll think about it tomorrow"

1983). Most of these mechanisms occur in everyday life (e.g., sublimation of blocked drives; intellectualization or rationalization of behavior). Others may be indicative of serious problems in adaptation such as the need to distort reality through patterns of denial or projection and the need to isolate thoughts from feelings.

■ **Point of Emphasis**

Everyone uses defense mechanisms. Maladaptive use is characterized by rigid patterns that profoundly distort reality.

Freud's definition of mental health was simple, involving the ability of the person to love and to work. Formulated in the negative sense, this would be the absence of conflicts or fixations that would inhibit psychological development in the areas of understanding and mastering one's environment and relating to other people. The major observations and theory formulations of freudian analysis are derived from his work with patients who were experiencing "neuroses" (anxiety related disorders).

Ego Analysts

These intrapersonal concepts were more fully developed by the neofreudians and the ego analysts such as Horney, Hartmann, and Erikson as they expanded on the functions of the ego and on the effects of external influences upon ego development. Karen Horney and Erik Erikson described the developmental pressures of culture and environment. The "ego analysts" such as Anna Freud, Heinz Hartmann, and David Rapaport have extended and developed freudian theory to include the direct study of normal behavior and to view it from a more complex perspective than instinctive drive motivation. Analyzing learned behaviors in terms of the ego and its functions resulted in an emphasis on thoughts and conscious attention. Additional determinants of behavior were seen to include unconscious motives, developmental sequence and experiences, psychological energy, habitually learned behavior patterns, situational events and influences, and the mutual influences of man and society interacting (Rapaport and Gill, 1959). The ego was seen as existing and operating separately from the id and the environment, permitting delay, thought, and consideration of the consequences before initiating behavior. Although Freud tended to view the early childhood years as dominant in personality development, Erikson (1964) delineated the importance of the social context in modifying behavior throughout life. Loevinger (1976), a contemporary psychologist, is researching and developing a theory that views ego development as a master trait. (See Table 1-2.) The ego analysts' contributions in establishing development, thought, choice, and consequences as potential influences on behavior underscore the importance of Piaget's work in determining the developmental sequence and nature of particular cognitive structures. Cognitive development influences one's perception and mode of thinking and is in turn influenced by life experiences.

> ■ **Point of Emphasis**
>
> *The ego analysts contributed a focus on development, thought, choice, and perceived consequences as influences on behavior.*

Whether, like Freud, one views development as proceeding out of the id, to the ego and the superego or, like the ego analysts, views these as independent processes evolving in infancy, the superego (self-evaluating thought processes) includes ideals, moral demands, self-criticism and self-punishment. Further development of this moral dimension of thought was influenced by Piaget's work, and has been described by Kohlberg. Table 1-2 includes a comparison of the developmental perspectives of Freud (psychosexual), Erikson (psychosocial), Loevinger (ego as "master trait"), Piaget (cognitive), and Kohlberg (moral).

Jung

Personality, according to Jung, is basically shaped by the attitudes that influence the relationship of each person to reality. Personality development is movement toward wholeness and integration of the real self as a goal. The individualizing aspects of Jung's attitudes and personality types incorporate the influence of cul-

TABLE 1-2 Intrapersonal Views of Development

Freud (Focus of Psychosexual Gratification)	Erikson (Psychosocial Issues)	Loevinger[a] (Ego Trait and Interpersonal Style)	Piaget (Cognitive Structure)	Kohlberg[a] (Moral Reasoning Basis)
Oral	Trust vs. mistrust (basic security)	Presocial/symbiotic impulsive (dependent)	Sensorimotor	Fear of punishment
Anal	Autonomy vs. shame and doubt	Self-protective (manipulative)	Preconceptual	Bargaining (to gain rewards or avoid punishment)
Phallic (Oedipal)	Initiative vs. guilt	Conformist (superficial goodness)	Preoperational (intuitive)	Seeking good relations and family approval
Latent	Industry vs. inferiority	Self-aware (helping)	Concrete operations	Obedience to law and order
Genital	Identity vs. identity diffusion	Conscientious (responsible-mutual concern)	Formal operations (abstract thought and awareness of multiple interrelationships)	Concern with individual rights and legal contract
	Intimacy vs. isolation	Individualistic (dependence conflicts)		Concern with consistent ethical principles
	Generativity vs. stagnation	Autonomous (interdependence)		
	Integrity vs. despair	Integrated (valuing unique individuality)		

[a] Loevinger and Kohlberg particularly do not adhere to age-related stages, focusing instead on individual development through the designated stages. Note that both Loevinger's and Kohlberg's stages are related to cognitive development also.

ture, time, and personal traits in describing the uniqueness of a man or a woman within the larger universal aspects of humanity. Jung's structure of consciousness synthesizes thought, feeling, sensation, and intuition, while his description of the general attitudes of introversion vs. extroversion depict whether the individual is primarily oriented to the demands of the environment or subjectively focused internally.

Adaptation, according to Jung, involves the person's tendency to develop those aspects of self that are already overdeveloped. Thus one who is highly rational may regard the feeling component of the self as inferior and fail to consciously acknowledge it. Dreams may be the only way of realizing these unconscious aspects of the self. Based on cultural expectations, men have traditionally developed the dimensions of thought and sensation (perceiving) while women have developed the dimensions of feeling and intuition. According to Jung, at approximately midlife the undeveloped aspects of the self will struggle to be recognized and integrated into the personality. The research of adult developmental theorists such as Levinson and Neugarten describes developmental crises or transitions in which men and women may become more like each other and less like the cultural norms as they age—women developing assertiveness and sometimes career interests in midlife or men becoming gentler and more family oriented. Jung (1970) suggests that roughly the first 40 or so years of life are focused on adapting to reality (e.g., "worldly success") and the later years are characterized by readiness to question and develop a personal philosophy (a more internal, spiritual focus).

Adler

Adler's subjectivist view of behavior emphasized cognition, believing that behavior could best be explained by knowledge of the individual's values, ideas, perception, and interests. "Truth" to Adler was clearly a matter of the individual's subjective perception, which is created out of symbolic representations of external events. This truth may be more or less accurate depending on the person's need to alter the event in order to better cope with it. All behavior was believed to be directed toward particular fictional consequences or goals, and habitual thought patterns were believed to be organized around a general goal or life-style. Thus a sensitive observer who carefully and empathically explored the subjective meaning of the per-

son's behavior and the consequences of generalized responses could determine the hidden meaning of behavior.

Adler did not view this subjective, cognitive focus as existing in isolation. He acknowledged that behavior occurs in a social context and developed some general concepts (e.g., inferiority feelings and compensatory strivings for superiority) while firmly adhering to a belief that each person is unique and must be understood from his own unique and subjective perspective. Adler assumed that all humans experience deep feelings of inferiority, particularly in the context of childhood when they are naturally smaller, less powerful, and less adept than significant others. Problems consequently assume much larger proportions. Adler considers inferiority feelings to be universal and a part of normal experience. They are perceived as painful and thus serve as motivators for behavior as persons strive to overcome both situational challenges and their own feelings of inadequacy.

Adler clearly delineated the importance of the family in the social development of children, noting that either rejection or overindulgence could be detrimental. He further suggested that the child's ordinal position in the family could influence subsequent attitudes and problems. The oldest may perceive the birth of younger children as a displacement. He may fear further displacements and, because of his family position as oldest, must carry additional responsibilities for leadership of the children and be much more sensitive to the demands of parental and other authorities. The second child is born into a different family than the first and may find competition from both older and younger children. Parents may have tempered their expectations or may find themselves with diminished energy to enforce their demands, so authority is less imposing. Number two has to try harder for attention but may often perceive the older child's position as number one as unattainable. This may result in rebellion, nonconformity, or a defeatist attitude. The youngest child, "the baby," is never displaced by the birth of another and may have an adoring circle of parents and older siblings who pamper and admire him. Asking and always receiving may diminish opportunities to build one's own competencies and sense of mastery—fostering the feeling of being lovable but incompetent. An only child may be hampered in interpersonal learning by the absence of everyday negotiations with siblings and may come to expect indulgence from others. All of these attitudes may potentially become significant aspects in the generalized behavior pattern that Adler referred to as life-style. Individuals develop fictional objectives and aspirations at an early age. These are designed to compensate for feelings of inferiority, and later behavior tends to be uniquely unified and organized around these fictional goals. Through social interaction, the individual also learns to benefit others and to reinforce his own sense of social value. This life-style or patterned behavior is not readily apparent to the person who creates and experiences it since it is never verbalized or consciously organized (Ford and Urban, 1963).

The concept of life-style is similar to that of life script as described in Transactional Analysis (which is discussed later in this chapter). The ego states of parent, adult, and child are also roughly analogous to the id, ego, and superego. Particular "safeguarding tendencies" or defensive traits described by Adler also have some analogies to several situations described in Berne's *Games People Play*. This theoretical similarity illustrates the development of the theoretical perspectives on a continuum of simple to a more complex intrapersonal focus. Early intrapersonal theorists influenced those who came after (e.g., interpersonal theorists). Adler can be variously described as a phenomenologist, an individual psychologist, and a social psychologist. Many of his contributions were adopted and enlarged upon by contemporary theorists, and the term "inferiority complex" has become a commonplace used by even laymen in attempts to explain behavior.

Adler's description of mental health (derived from his concept of disorder or neurosis) could be stated as the absence of excessive feelings of inadequacy and distress and the presence of realistic, attainable goals, concern for others, realistic perception of events, and adequate social skills. Ansbacher describes this as the ability to relate to others equally and cooperatively (1956).

Client Centered

Carl Rogers' view, like Adler's, is phenomenological—focused on the individual's subjective experience, thoughts, and feelings. Man, in Rogers' view, is innately good. Any negative behaviors are the result of inappropriate learning. Awareness is composed of internal symbolic responses (e.g., visceral changes, emotions, memories) to the perception of external events. Behavior is motivated and directed by "the urge to expand, extend,

develop, mature" (Rogers 1970:351). His view of man as maintaining and enhancing self is consistent with that of Maslow (1968) who similarly described behavioral motivators as a hierarchy of needs, physical through self-actualization. Individuals are seen as evaluating their own behavior in terms of its positive or actualizing tendencies. The concept of self evolves at an early age from awareness of personal attributes (I am pretty, I am smart), and thoughts relating to others (I am popular, I am kind), or events (I am good at math). These self-thoughts are organized into a consistent whole so that a change in one aspect has the potential to alter the entire self-concept. New consistent images are incorporated while those incongruent with the whole may be ignored. The sense of self is an ongoing process which can be modified and expanded. The most open, flexible views of self will thus be most open to growth and experiencing. The child who is loved and receives consistent acceptance and approval from others (this does not negate limits on behavior) learns self-regard and may choose behavior on the basis of its inherent enhancing potential. In this way innate and learned sequences complement each other, and self-evaluation becomes a primary motivator. Behaviors that elicit positive consequences will be learned and those with negative consequences will be avoided as learning becomes personally and socially satisfying.

Rogers' fully functioning person will develop awareness of all of his or her responses as they occur, and accurate self-evaluative thoughts will be congruent with behavior since the person can freely acknowledge both. Behavior can be freely selected on the basis of personal satisfaction and developmental direction not dictated by others.

■ Point of Emphasis

Intrapersonal viewpoint assumptions include the view of man as a unique individual, subject to various influences or determinants of behavior. These influences may be basic physiological drives or tensions (needs), pleasure seeking or the avoidance of pain, developmental phase or sequence, unconscious motivation, and social expectations or demands. All behavior is viewed as meaningful and purposeful although the individual may not be consciously aware of either its full meaning or its purpose. Thus dreams, slips of the tongue, and accidents may be influenced by the individual's internal psychic processes.

Social skills will be effective and based on awareness of the consequences of one's actions on others. Mental health, to summarize Rogers, is consistent with a positive self-concept, openness to awareness and experience, and congruence between what one is and what one would like to be.

An essential factor in mental health is the functioning of the ego—its level of maturity and the quality of its functioning as it performs the tasks of mediating between the id and the superego and between the person and external reality. "Ego strength" is the ability of the ego to manage anxiety and to maintain ego functions under various degrees of internal and external stress. The process of ego development is a key component of personality and mental health. This development has been variously described by Freud, Erikson, and Loevinger, among others. Positive outcomes in relationship to developmental task sequences result in traits or ego strengths that sustain the individual and enhance coping capacities under stress.

Individual behavior can be understood best from the person's unique perspective or subjective experience. Mental health can be described as holistic, optimal functioning with behavior characterized by conscious choice rather than unconscious determinants, accurate perceptions of reality, and the ability to relate to and have concern for others.

INTERPERSONAL VIEWPOINTS

Interpersonal Theory

Interpersonal theories focus primarily on the interactive aspects of behavior and development. As previously detailed, the intrapersonal views developed from a narrow focus on the internal processes of the individual (Freud) to an expanded view of the effects of culture (Erikson) and the family climate (Adler, Rogers) on personality and development. On this continuum of increasingly interactive processes, Harry Stack Sullivan's interpersonal theory clearly emphasizes interpersonal behaviors as central to personality development. He disagreed with Freud's view that behavior was internally motivated, seeing it instead as situationally produced.

Basic assumptions of Sullivan's viewpoint are that (1) patterns of events occurring interpersonally tend to produce relatively stable response patterns called dynamisms; (2) anxiety is elicited interpersonally and becomes a central motivator for behavior as individuals seek to avoid tension and experience security and satisfaction; and (3) development is described as the processes involved as innate responses interact with maturation and learning in an interpersonal context. Personality is viewed as the relatively enduring pattern of interpersonal relationships that characterize an individual's life.

Significant ways or modes of experiencing identified by Sullivan can be compared with Freud's description of primary and secondary process thinking. The prototaxic mode is primitive and undifferentiated, and focuses on sensory perceptions (e.g., an inability to distinguish between an object and a memory image, as in a vision of one's mother which is perceived as "real," though the person knows that the mother is dead). The parataxic mode differentiates pattern and time sequence of events but is unable to logically determine accurate cause and effect relationships (e.g., believing that one's hostile thoughts have caused another's illness or misfortune). Parataxic thought is focused subjectively on internal perceptions and consequently distorts reality. The syntactic mode is logical and differentiates cause and effect in a relatively objective view of events. This more sophisticated mode of experience is made possible by the development of language with the subsequent ability to "talk over" occurrences, either internally (thinking, analyzing) or with others and to obtain, via consensual validation, others' viewpoints. Sullivan recognized the importance of both verbal and nonverbal communication in interpersonal exchanges and described anxiety as the "destructive commonplace" in everyday living that explains interpersonal problems.

Behavior is seen by Sullivan as organized around two primary goals: physiological need satisfaction and security or anxiety relief. Physiological tensions of various intensity arise (e.g., thirst, hunger, sexual urges) and motivate behavior to reduce tension. Reducing tension leads to satisfaction in a way similar to the intrapersonal theory concept of drive reduction. Prolonged deprivation may lead to an apathetic state as when one ceases to feel hunger after a long period of starvation. Perception of tensions (anxiety) motivates behaviors to achieve security. If tensions are temporarily or persistently unrelieved, they can interfere with behaviors needed to achieve satisfaction. Individuals learn to manage these need conflicts through security operations (defenses) such as sublimation or selective inattention.

TABLE 1-3 Sullivan: Interpersonal Development

Phase (Approximate Age Span)	Achievement Marking Shift to Next Phase	Developmental Tasks	Goal to be Attained
Infancy (0–2 yrs.)	From birth to articulate speech development	Beginning to recall and discriminate objects Approach behaviors to satisfy needs Beginnings of self-system and personifications of "good" and "bad" mothers	Security: trusting that significant others will provide need gratification
Childhood (preschool)	From articulate speech to development of interactive patterns of play with peers	Developing motor and language skills Fusing of "good" and "bad" personification of others into an integrated view acknowledging both components Beginnings of logical thought and consensual validation	Acquisition of social skills and social norms (beginning of delayed gratification) in order to meet acquired needs for tenderness, playmates, and recognition
Juvenile (6–9 yrs.)	From peer interaction to establishing an intimate same-sex friendship	Acquisition of major social patterns Control of focal awareness Avoidance and management of anxiety Cooperates-accommodates behavior to needs of others and learns to cope with competition and social rejection	Development of cooperative interaction; ability to concentrate on a task
Pre-adolescence (9–12 yrs.)	From intimate same-sex friendship to onset of puberty and interest in the opposite sex	Development of patterns of intimacy in a close friendship Ability to think in terms of "we" Sharing and consensual validation permit modifications in the self-system-correction of prior distortions Coping with experience of loneliness	Development of collaborative interaction Modification of self-system on basis of peer validation and sharing
Early adolescence (12–15 yrs.)	Onset of puberty and heterosexual interest up to patterned behavior established in dating and love relationships	Intertwining of earlier interpersonal patterns with opposite sex relationships Overcoming fears and avoidance of genital sexuality based on ignorance and misinformation Resolving conflicts among issues such as (1) insecurity vs. desire for opposite sex interaction (2) exploitive lust vs. interpersonal sharing Integrating genital needs into interpersonal patterns	Managing issues of physical sexuality and establishing comfortable patterns of interpersonal interaction with the opposite sex
Late adolescence (16–21 yrs.)	Semistable patterns of sexual relationship up to establishing an intimate love relationship with another (adulthood)	Mastery of information processing/problem-solving skills Establishing stable and satisfying patterns of sexual and interpersonal relationships	Synthesis of stable effective behavior patterns in problem solving and intimate relationships

Inattention as described by Sullivan is an active process by which the person fails to perceive or respond to internal or external events. Selective inattention was Sullivan's term for an active process that defended against interpersonal anxiety.

Emotion is described as the *felt* aspect of tensions. Sullivan believed that innate emotions such as fear, rage, and disgust are present in infancy and that other feelings such as anger and shame are developed through learning.

In addition to the basic innate needs, acquired or secondary needs such as those for tenderness, friendship, and intimacy are learned interpersonally. Behavior acquires complexity with maturation and learning as (1) the individual develops the ability to integrate contradictory personifications of the "good mother" who nurtures and the "bad mother" who is tense and irritable into a representation of a mother who is at times either or both of these and (2) develops a variety of dynamisms or interpersonal response patterns. Table 1-3 depicts Sullivan's phases of development.

As the self system develops, the individual conceptualizes: the "good me" which is satisfying, the "bad me" which is anxiety provoking, and the "not me" which is so anxiety provoking that security operations such as inattention must be used. Sullivan believes this self system is relatively resistant to change because opportunities for different learning tend to be avoided (since they lead to anxiety). Behavior may become "fixed" indicating a failure to master some developmental task. This failure, for example the absence of a close friend in one's youth with whom to share values, ideas, and validate perceptions, may leave the person more vulnerable to social isolation and less likely to have childhood misperceptions corrected, thus affecting future social relationships. Sullivan's view of a mentally healthy person would include having a realistic view of both the self and external reality, which is not distorted by anxiety-laden past experiences or by selective inattention.

Transactional Analysis

Transactional Analysis (TA) as developed by Eric Berne (1978) and others is a more recent viewpoint which focuses on aspects of individual personality (ego states), transactions (interpersonal interactions), ulterior transactional patterns (games), and repetitive, compulsive scenarios enacted throughout life (scripts). The concepts and interactions are readily illustrated and understood, so that this viewpoint is popular with the public as well as with the therapists who use it.

Like Freud in his view of the id, ego, and superego, Berne described structural components consisting of the child, the adult, and parent ego states. Unlike Freud, adherents of TA do not focus on the unconscious but instead look at patterns that are clearly observable in the individual's daily verbal and nonverbal behavior. For example: a cooly analytical (adult) mathematician at work in a laboratory may become a highly competitive, impulsive, and gleefully aggressive (child) tennis player and later on the way home assume a finger-pointing, judgmental posture (parent) when another driver cuts into his traffic lane. Generally depicted as three circles, these ego states are then used to illustrate interpersonal interactions or transactions. The child state (C) is the earliest to develop and is characterized by spontaneity, impulsiveness, natural expression of feelings, curiosity, and other childlike traits such as the ability to play, have fun, and enjoy life. In addition to these assets, though, there may remain a legacy of childhood experiences such as feeling small, fearful, and helpless. The next state to develop is the parent (P), based on childhood experiences and observations of one's own parents. The parent state contains both nurturing, care-taking behaviors and critical judgments. The adult ego state (A) is factual, unemotional, and concerned with thought and analysis.

Transactions, or interactions between two people (see Figure 1-1), are described as complementary when the stimulus and the response are appropriate and naturally follow one another's expectations based on healthy relationships. An example of a complementary adult-to-adult transaction would be that of one adult asking another for the time and receiving correct information. An example of a complementary parent-to-child interaction is that of a sick child being cared for by the adult. Communication is promoted and facilitated by complementary transactions. Blocked and painfully disrupted communication can occur as a result of crossed transactions that arouse an unexpected ego state. A husband may inquire (adult-to-adult) "What's for dinner?" on arriving home. If his wife has had a frustrating day at the office, he may receive an angry response (unexpected child-to-parent) such as "The air conditioner's broken, the dog is sick—and you ask me what's for dinner. You're always blaming me when things don't get done." In order for communication to be reestablished, one of the parties

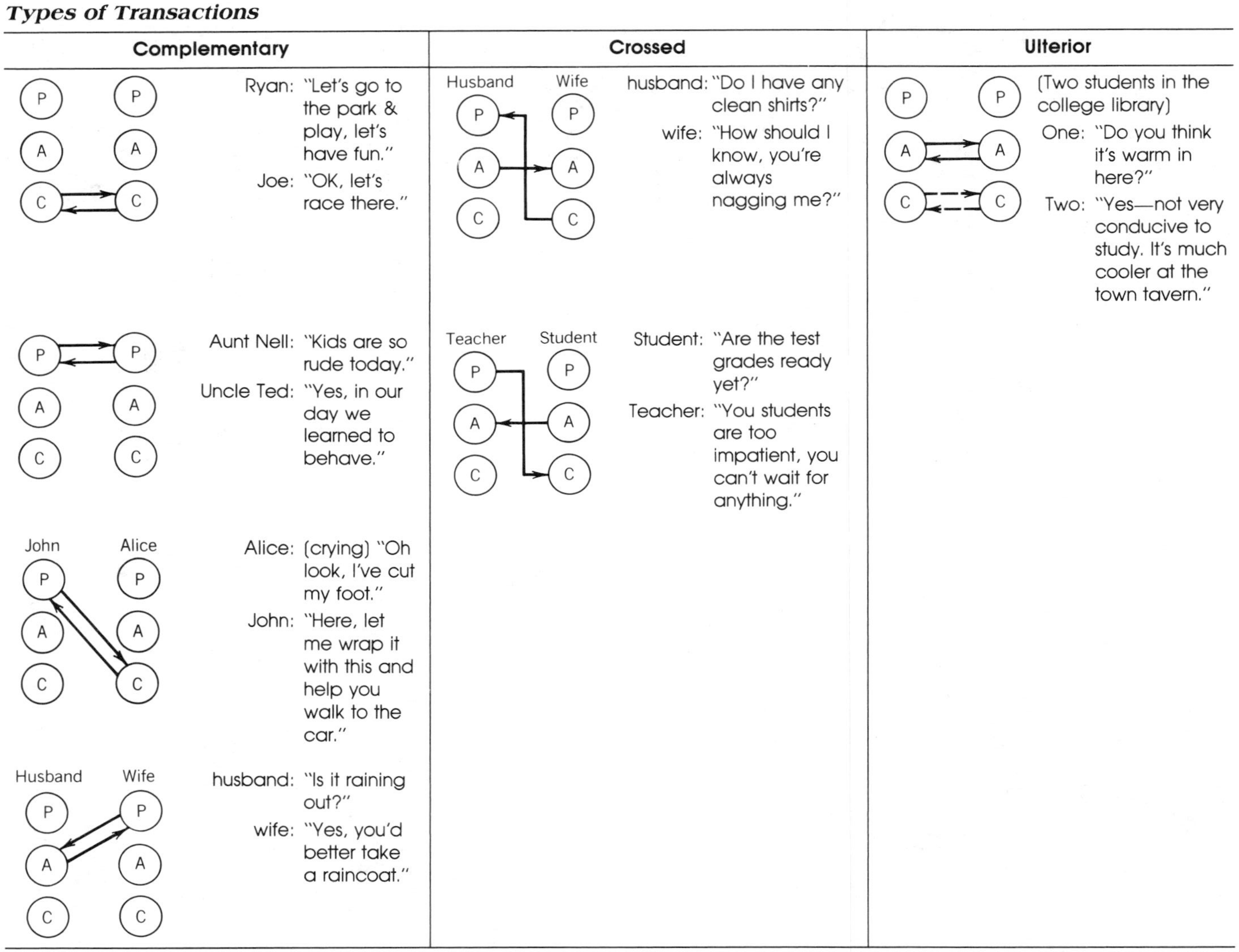

Types of Transactions

Complementary	Crossed	Ulterior

Complementary

Ryan: "Let's go to the park & play, let's have fun."

Joe: "OK, let's race there."

Aunt Nell: "Kids are so rude today."

Uncle Ted: "Yes, in our day we learned to behave."

Alice: (crying) "Oh look, I've cut my foot."

John: "Here, let me wrap it with this and help you walk to the car."

husband: "Is it raining out?"

wife: "Yes, you'd better take a raincoat."

Crossed

husband: "Do I have any clean shirts?"

wife: "How should I know, you're always nagging me?"

Student: "Are the test grades ready yet?"

Teacher: "You students are too impatient, you can't wait for anything."

Ulterior

(Two students in the college library)

One: "Do you think it's warm in here?"

Two: "Yes—not very conducive to study. It's much cooler at the town tavern."

Figure 1-1 *Types of transactions.*

in the crossed transaction must adopt a different ego state. In the illustration given, the husband might assume the role of nurturing parent with a comment such as, "I'm sorry you had such a bad day, honey—let's go out to eat." Or the wife, after lashing out, might assume the adult ego state offering an objective comment such as, "Here I am taking it out on you—and you didn't even know about any of the things that happened to me today."

Ulterior transactions simultaneously involve more than two ego states and provide the basis for "games" (manipulative, covert transactions designed to produce a particular effect or "pay off"). "Reverse psychology" is an example of an ulterior transaction in which one person's adult ego state addresses (ostensibly) the adult state of another while a component of the message is covertly directed to the other's child ego state as a manipulative ploy. For example, two sisters wish to wear the same dress to an event. The owner of the dress is trying it on and asks (adult) "How does it look?" Her sister replies, "It's a pretty color. But don't you think that the stripes make you look hippy?" Overtly this exchange was adult-to-adult. If the owner responded "Perhaps, but it is the most attractive dress I own," the exchange would remain adult-to-adult. However, if this is a successful ulterior transaction, it would address the owner's child ego state, eliciting a comment such as, "Oh, I don't want to look fat—I'll have to wear something else." Other ulterior transactions may involve four ego states. Overtly adult messages such as "Would you like to see my stamp collection?" may be ulterior flirtation messages (child-to-child) and recognized as such when the respondent accepts the invitation replying, "Oh yes, I've always been interested in stamps,"—when sexual attraction is actually what is shared.

Like Adler's concept of generalized attitudes and behaviors that constitute a life-style, Berne conceived of life scripts, which originate in childhood experiences and influence daily interactions. Scripts are predetermined role interactions that move toward a particular climax. They may be dull, happy, or tragic, and may contain elements of both individual and cultural themes, which are played out in day-to-day interactions. Themes may represent happy scripts (like the story of Cinderella in which goodness and hard work are rewarded happily ever after, or the cowboy legend in which the quiet "good guy" triumphs over evil). Scripts also may be used to reinforce defensive positions such as (1) avoidance of responsibility

for self-development ("I would be educated/successful if it weren't for———." The blame might be put on aging parents, spouse, children, or "bad breaks."), (2) projecting blame and responsibility (by refusing to make one's own decisions someone else can be held responsible when anything goes wrong), and (3) other attitudes and behavior patterns that repetitiously serve to protect the individual from responsibility, self-growth, and the accompanying anxiety.

Berne's view of mental health would emphasize individual autonomy or self-directedness, and is manifested by the abilities to (1) perceive clearly and uniquely, (2) freely and spontaneously express the full range of emotions without "game playing," and (3) relate intimately and candidly to others in a "here and now" context. This involves being responsible for one's own actions and feelings and choosing one's own destiny.

> **■ Point of Emphasis**
>
> *Interpersonal assumptions, while not ignoring individual dynamics, emphasize the interactive nature of social learning and the significance of human communication, both verbal and nonverbal. Communication may be used either to reveal or to conceal. Revealing oneself involves taking responsibility and risks. Early childhood attitudes and patterns adopted to defend against anxiety can be modified by subsequent interpersonal interactions or transactions which lead to social learning and behavior change.*

☐ Existentialism

Based in the philosophical movement initiated by the writings of Kierkegaard and the phenomenological approach popularized by Heidegger, the existentialists emphasize a holistic view of man as being self-aware and possessing the freedom to choose among alternatives in order to develop his own potential. The language of this viewpoint is somewhat difficult and frequently punctuated with hyphens (e.g., being-in-the-world) because it attempts to depict man as an interactive force, not merely a subjective being reacting to external, objective events but a participant in all events, who is both acted upon by and who acts upon the world. The importance of events, experiences, thoughts, and emotions in directing behavior is mediated by subjective perspectives (self-awareness) and the freedom to choose.

Primary emphasis is placed on being. May states that man's innate attributes of awareness or consciousness of self and the freedom to choose among behavioral options permit him to create both himself and his worlds (Ford and Urban, 1963). This freedom then carries with it a responsibility for what one becomes in the development or nondevelopment of innate potential. Like Sullivan, the existentialists believe that for man to be truly human he must engage in social interaction. Language and self-awareness develop and are modified on the basis of this interaction (being-with) and if authentically (spontaneously and honestly) shared and experienced, one's sense of identity grows.

Non-being, the threat of social isolation and, ultimately, of death, leads to existential anxiety, a feeling of dread. As people lose the strong and unquestioning faith of their ancestors, as wars and economic disasters tax their hope for the future, a philosophy may be sought that will define purpose and meaning in a person's life. Existentialism focuses on the individual's striving for meaning and purpose in being while also confronting the inevitable—non-being (Ford and Urban, 1963:445–6).

Because the individual is selective in response to a variety of interactive events, a pattern or lifestyle emerges which is characteristic of the individual's way of experiencing or relating to the world. This pattern is referred to as one's mode of being-in-the-world. *Umwelt* is a mode in which behavior is governed by biological drives and responses and aimed at achieving basic satisfaction. This is similar to the Freudian view of man. *Mitwelt* is a mode of interpersonal interaction (encounter) in which one relates authentically in a mutual interchange of here-and-now thoughts and feelings. This mode of being-with-others, similar to Sullivan's interactive view, significantly contributes to self-growth, understanding, and personal identity. *Eigenwelt* is that aspect of the self that experiences the world and chooses, based on unique personal meanings, the mode of being-in-itself. There is emphasis on self-awareness, self-actualization, and the responsibility of creating one's self. The person may strive to remain anonymous and to avoid making choices for which he could be held responsible but, in existential terms, this refusal to actively choose is a choice in itself (Ford and Urban, 1963:454–460).

Experiencing is unique to the individual and involves more than his thoughts; it also involves the sensations and feelings that occur as he interacts with the external world. A simple object like an ice-cream cone can be thought of abstractly as a concept or an idea, while the actuality of an ice-cream cone involves sensations and feelings. Sensations might include coldness, smoothness, sweetness, wetness, stickiness, or messiness. The individual's feelings about ice cream may range from a sense of childish delight to a sense of guilt and shame if the ice cream is thought to be fattening and eating it is thought to be an act of gluttony.

Experiencing also occurs in the context of time and space. The individual may react to an event on the basis of past experiences, future goals, or both. The time perspective may vary with age and events. Childhood memories of waiting for a special day illustrate how slowly time can move, while the elderly often remark how the years fly by and how 20 years can seem like "only yesterday." Spacially, people can feel "ten feet tall' or belittled; empty or bursting with joy. All of these perceptions blend into the unique and personalized meaning and purpose of behavior.

EXISTENTIAL ASSUMPTIONS

Jean Paul Sarte said, "Man is free. The coward makes himself heroic." Existentialism emphasizes the freedom and the responsibility that each individual has to choose his or her actions and, in so doing, to actively effect changes in self and world. External events and anxiety are recognized as having the potential to limit, but not do away with, choices.

■ Point of Emphasis

Self-concept is seen as deriving from interpersonal relationships on the basis of each person's needs for inclusion, control, and affection. Schultz describes joy as the fulfillment of the individual's potential (1967:119). This attainment depends upon the development of bodily functioning, knowledge, and experience; interpersonal relatedness (encounter); and relationships with one's culture and social institutions.

The mentally healthy person might be viewed existentially as someone who seeks personal growth and meaning in life, responds fully and with self-awareness to experience, and courageously shares one's self with others. The person can involve self in others without illusions and despite the inevitable disappointments in life.

The encounter movement focuses on experiencing and genuinely relating to others. May described social courage as necessary because man must confront basic fears of abandonment on the one hand and loss of autonomy on the other in order to fully respond to other human beings.

☐ Behavioral Viewpoints

Since Pavlov's classical conditioning experiment in which a neutral stimulus—a bell—was paired with food, and which provoked salivation (by the dog) in the presence of the neutral stimulus alone, there has been interest in stimulus-response views of human behavior. These views in general differ from the former theories in that human behavior is regarded passively as a response to environmental stimuli and reinforcement contingencies. Only Freud tended to view man so passively, with his emphasis on unconscious motivation.

B. F. Skinner (1965) developed the concept of operant conditioning, by which behavior can be shaped through reinforcement. The value of Skinner's techniques has been demonstrated in animal research, programmed learning, and behavior modification programs in both clinical and classroom settings. Wolpe's (1958) reciprocal inhibition or counter-conditioning techniques built on the principles of classical conditioning by pairing incompatible or antagonistic responses for the purpose of extinguishing undesirable behaviors. Dollard and Miller's (1950) viewpoint incorporated both subjective and objective responses in a theory of learned behavior disorders.

In general, behavioral theory addresses two major events: the acquisition of behaviors (conditioning) and the extinction of undesirable behaviors (counter conditioning). Each view addresses these aspects in varied ways.

OPERANT CONDITIONING

Reinforcers are events that immediately follow a specific behavioral response and modify the likelihood that the behavior will occur again. They may be natural drive reducers (eating reduces the bodily tensions of hunger) or secondary reinforcers (certain rewards have learned values—money is not intrinsically pleasurable but people value it because they have learned that they can purchase desired things with it). Positive reinforcers are rewards—they add something pleasant such as a treat or the approval of someone whose opinion is valued (a gold star on a child's perfect spelling paper, a bonus for superior productivity at work, or a hug from Dad for "being a good kid"). Negative reinforcers are equally rewarding because they remove something unpleasant or painful from the person's environment. They may include drive reduction (such as eating to remove the unpleasant sensation of hunger) or avoidance responses (e.g., staying home from school by pleading sickness to avoid taking a mathematics test one is sure to fail, drinking to forget one's troubles). Both positive and negative reinforcers increase the likelihood that the behavior that preceded the reinforcer will be repeated.

Behaviors that are not reinforced will decrease in frequency. This process is called extinction. For example, a child who craves attention may misbehave and be disruptive in school. If the teacher is able to control the situation so that the disruptive behavior is ignored by both classmates and teacher (even scolding may be reinforcing since it brings attention), then the behavior should diminish. In the early stages of the extinction process as reinforcement is withheld the disruptive behavior may actually increase as the child attempts to elicit the attention previously received. If reinforcement continues to be withheld, the undesirable behavior should diminish until extinction occurs. It is effective to pair positive reinforcement of desired behaviors (e.g., studying, remaining in a chair doing work) with the withholding of reinforcement of undesirable behavior.

Punishment is not considered a reliable form of behavior modification since it has variable effects. For instance, a child who is spanked for aggressive behavior (hitting other children) may conform on the basis of negative reinforcement (reduced hitting of other children in order to avoid the aversive consequence of being spanked—fear of pain) or may learn to fear the person who administers the spanking and avoid him in particular situations while actually increasing aggressive behaviors in other settings. In the latter case, the child may even equate hitting with power—an idea given emphasis by each spanking.

Scheduling of reinforcers is an important aspect of behavioral modification. Immediate feedback is more effective in altering behavior than delayed reinforcement. Rewarding every response results in faster acquisition of the behavior rewarded; however, a variable, intermittent schedule of reinforcement is more resistant to extinction.

Contingency management stresses assessment of the learner in order to identify desirable behaviors for reinforcement and undesirable behaviors for extinction, along with a careful evaluation of the nature of the reinforcers operating in the environment. The simple concept of reinforcement becomes much more complex when the environment must be taken into consideration. The schoolteacher who attempts to ignore disruptive behavior and reward appropriate behavior in a fourth grader may be unsuccessful, either because of inappropriate selection and scheduling of rewards or because the attention of the peer group is sufficiently rewarding to maintain the disruptive behavior despite the teacher's attempts to ignore it. Similarly the mother who slips a cookie into a child's mouth to stop his crying behavior (providing negative reinforcement to the mother by stopping the annoying crying) is actually providing positive reinforcement for the child's crying by rewarding it.

Principles of contingency management include methods for shaping and for extinguishing behavior. New behaviors may be established by the following process:

1. Identify and specify the desired behavioral outcome (e.g., communicate the goal or objective).
2. Assess for the presence of related or similar behaviors and the frequency of their occurrence.
3. Select the appropriate reinforcers and schedule of reinforcement.
4. Manage the environment and implement the planned program (initially, reinforcers may be given for "approximate" behaviors to encourage efforts toward the desired behavior—this is called shaping behavior).
5. Evaluate the frequency and stability of the new behavior.

Disagreeable behaviors may be extinguished by depriving them of reinforcement as follows:

1. Make a baseline recording of the average number of times the undesirable behavior (for example, being disruptive in school) occurs in a given time frame.
2. Identify the reinforcers for the undesirable behavior, for example (a) the laughter and attention of friends who sit nearby, and (b) avoidance of class assignments by being disruptive and being sent to the principal.
3. Institute a program for removing reinforcers of disruptive behavior (e.g., change seating arrangements to decrease chances of peer reinforcement for "acting up," ignore the disruptive behavior and establish a requirement that all class assignments be completed before the students leave school each day).
4. Give attention and other forms of reinforcement for desirable behavior.
5. Evaluate behavior change by means of comparison to the baseline (Joyce and Weil, 1980).

An additional technique sometimes used by behavioral therapists to decondition anxiety responses is "flooding." This approach confronts the client with strong and prolonged exposure to the anxiety-producing stimulus (e.g., a client with a phobia—an irrational fear—of elevators is kept in an elevator until the panic level anxiety is no longer sustained and the client gradually becomes comfortable in the confined space).

Behavioral approaches also can be taught so that individuals may learn to manage their own environment and reinforcers, and thus become more effective in such activities as study habits, weight control, and reduction of smoking.

COUNTER CONDITIONING

Wolpe's concept of reciprocal inhibition asserts that learned anxiety responses and habits can be altered if new, antagonistic responses can be developed in the presence of the stimulus cues. Each time the new behavior is practiced, the bond between the old stimulus and the undesired response is weakened. These antagonistic responses may be muscle relaxation exercises, deep breathing techniques, assertiveness, or other behaviors that desensitize anxiety through pairing more adaptive behavior with stimulus cues. Systematic desensitization to anxiety involves practicing the new techniques in the presence of an increasing hierarchy of the anxiety-provoking stimuli until the anxiety responses are extinguished. Related techniques have been used in assertiveness training, visualization techniques (such as the Simonton method of adjunct cancer therapy), and biofeedback.

The process of desensitization might involve the following:

1. Determining if the problem is appropriate and the client is capable of mastering visualization and relaxation procedures.
2. Developing the hierarchy of anxiety-eliciting scenes/items (for example, first a picture of the feared situation, then exposure to the situation at a distance, then closer contact, and so on).
3. Practicing relaxation and visualization techniques.
4. Having the client relax and presenting the lowest ranked anxiety elicitor; then encouraging positive imagery and relaxation as coping strategies.
5. Gradually increasing the intensity of anxiety-eliciting stimuli as the client masters each successfully until desensitization occurs.

Assumptions of behavioral theory are that (1) behavior is elicited in response to external variables in the environment and (2) behavior is observable and identifiable, and can be modified through controlling the contingencies of reinforcement. The emphasis is on the here-and-now.

Some behavioral theorists accept the psychodynamic view of behavior, but their focus is on current behavior, not past events and their perception—although earlier events may be explored to discover more information about the connections between the stimuli and reinforcers. Behaviorists may differ in their view of conscious will as a factor in behavior. Some (e.g., Skinner; Dollard and Miller) believe that behavior occurs relatively automatically in response to stimuli and reinforcement. Others believe that individuals can learn to manage their own contingencies of reinforcement and thus take an active role in changing their own behavior through assertiveness training and habit modification.

☐ Systems Theory

Systems theory represents an even more complex and interactive focus on the components of human behavior. Rather than viewing the individual as the central active influence on events or, conversely, considering the environment to be the determining factor in individual behavior, systems theory focuses on the interaction of the components. General systems theory, which was originated by Von Bertalanffy (1968), is highly abstract and can be applied to such diverse fields of interest as mathematics, physics, physiology, sociology, and nursing (e.g., the theoretical models of Roy and King).

Generally stated, a system is comprised of subsystems which interact on the basis of common concerns or purposes. A family system can be composed of parental, sibling, and extended kin subsystems. A political system may be composed of various subsystems such as the major political parties, special interest groups, and elected representatives serving in specific local, regional, and national governing bodies.

PROPERTIES OF SYSTEMS

Systems can be described in terms of characteristic properties such as structure, function, boundaries, and feedback mechanisms. They may be considered as open or closed depending upon whether there is an open exchange of matter, energy, and information between the system and the environment. For instance, the human body can be described as an open system that has a specific anatomical structure, various organs that perform particular physiological functions, a skin that delineates the boundaries between the internal and external environments, and various feedback mechanisms (e.g., the autonomic nervous system, temperature regulation mechanisms) that regulate internal adjustments (adaptation) in response to changes in either the internal or the external environment. These changes can be any number of things from an internal infectious process to external alterations in food supply, temperature, or social networks.

Structure

Structure refers to the definition of relationships in a system and can generally be depicted in the form of a chart or a figure. The structure of the human body can be demonstrated by figures or models illustrating various subsystems such as bone linkages and muscle groups (the musculoskeletal system) or the relationships between the heart and lungs in oxygenating blood (the cardiopulmonary system). A family may be patriarchal in structure: an illustration of the relationships would show the father as head of the family with mother in a subordinate role in charge of the children. A more egalitarian (democratic) structure might depict the couple as a partnership relationship with the children in dependent roles. As the children grow toward adulthood, the structure may change (accommodate, adapt) to admit them to full partnership in family decision making. Business organizations such as factories, hospitals, and educational systems also have structures which are generally shown in organizational charts. These charts indicate lines of authority and responsibility from executive levels through middle management to workers. Healthy structures should be flexible enough to respond to internal and external changes. For instance, family structures may need to adapt to the loss of a member (divorce, death, "empty nest") or the addition of a new member (e.g., birth of a child or an aging parent who is no longer able to live independently). Organizations such as hospitals may need to change aspects of their structure to adapt. For example, more seriously ill clients and shorter hospital stays (because of changes in reimbursement procedures) may make it necessary to add a clinical specialist or discharge-planning nurse to assure quality care.

Function

Subsystems perform various functions or tasks which meet the needs and purposes of the system and thereby help to maintain its stability. For example, one of the functions of the family is to socialize children to the expectations of the larger social systems (culture, society). This is done through informal teaching and example. Families also function as health educators and caregivers when members are ill. The affective function of the family includes providing a sense of love and belonging which contributes to members' security, identity, and ability to relate to others. Families must cope with everyday stresses and problems of living. These stresses may arise within the family (e.g., illness or conflicts between members) or from the external environment (e.g., an economic crisis or a natural disaster). These functions are carried out through various roles assigned to family members. Successful coping depends to a great extent on the ability of the family to identify and use resources, to adapt role assignments appropriately, and to use suitable mechanisms for managing stress, anxiety, and other emotions. For instance, the presence of a terminally ill child will require numerous adaptations as caretaking activities by the mother diminish her time and

energy available for other functions. If another family member is not able to assume some of the functions of caretaking and/or provide assistance in the affective, nurturing function, this illness could have long-term detrimental effects on family members.

Boundaries

The permeability of a system is assessed based on how open or closed the system is. A system may regulate its boundaries to control the level of exchange with the external environment. Living systems are in constant interaction with the environment as humans obtain food, convert resources to shelter and energy, use air and water, return waste products, and alter the environment in various other ways. Systems occur in hierarchies (subsystems are incorporated in larger subsystems and systems). Communication systems and subsystems may include family interaction patterns, interactions between the family and larger social institutions, the communication media, and many others. A closed system will deteriorate, losing organization and structure in the process of entropy. Whitley (1983) uses the example of a decomposing body in a closed coffin to illustrate entropy. A family in crisis must be open to exchanging information and resources with the environment in order to cope. A closed family system is not likely to be able to avail itself of external sources of assistance which could promote effective adaptation (mastering the crisis).

Feedback

Adjustment processes that serve to maintain the system in a steady state or state of self-regulation are referred to as feedback mechanisms. These processes do not permit the system to fluctuate widely. The central nervous system has self-regulatory mechanisms that moderate between the sympathetic and parasympathetic functions in an attempt to maintain homeostasis or an acceptable state of physiological balance. The feedback process occurs when part of the output of a system is returned in a circular way (to reenter the system as input) and can then influence the functions of the system. Positive feedback is defined as moving the system away from homeostasis or steady state and toward growth and change. (Therapy may alter dysfunctional family dynamics, permitting more effective interactions to take place.) Negative feedback, on the other hand, serves to main-

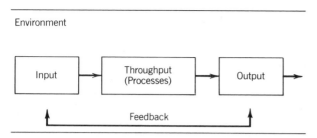

Figure 1-2 *Structural model of a system. Environment includes numerous other subsystems and systems.*

tain the system in a steady state. (A nurse who provides supportive reassurance that a family is coping effectively with particular parenting tasks, is reinforcing the current parenting patterns.)

The preceding terms are overly simplified because systems terminology is complex and abstract. A more precise understanding of this view can be obtained from other sources on systems theory. Two additional key concepts are those of unity and nonsummativity. A system is holistic and greater than the sum of its parts. The human being, for example, is far more than the bones, tissues, and fluids that comprise the body.

Systems are self-regulating and capable of growth and change. Knowledge of a system requires observation of interactive processes (rather than linear cause and effect). A conflict or change in any part or subsystem will bring about conflicts or changes in other parts of the system. In the case of linear cause and effect if "a" causes "b" then "a" must be altered to change "b," while if "a" and "b" are interactive components, either "a" or "b" may be altered to bring about a change in the other.

A family may be used as an example of systems interactions. A mother, father, and teenager are the members. The father and teenager have frequent conflicts over family rules. The teenager seeks to ally with the mother and gain her support against the father (which leads to mother-father conflict). Some theorists would conclude that the teenager is the cause of the family conflicts and that something in the teenager must be changed to restore the family to homeostasis. In a systems view, however, the interactive processes would be noted (i.e., the dynamics of the conflicts would be explored). Following exploration of the dynamics, the family conflict may be resolved by (1) a change in the way the rules are applied by the father, (2) an acceptance of the rules by the teenager, (3) a refusal by the mother to become embroiled in the

conflict, and/or (4) a renegotiation of the rules by the entire family. The focus is on the interactive nature of the system as a whole, not on any one individual's behavior.

Systems theory also sees human systems as open, freely exchanging matter, energy, and information with the environment. These concepts of interaction and environmental exchange expand awareness of the forces influencing human behavior. Lewin (1951) has conceptualized these forces as various positive and negative vectors in his force field analysis. These vectors are driving (motivating) factors and restraining (avoidance) factors in the change process. This force field becomes important if one wishes to alter any system (family, group, or other).

SOCIAL APPLICATION

Satir notes that we all live in multiple relationship patterns which influence self-concept and identity (1967). She further indicates that the impact of systems theory since the 1950s has been a result of the recognition that personal growth is a change process which is in turn an outgrowth of interpersonal transaction. Group dynamics theory, family dynamics theory, role theory, and organizational management theory have all been strongly influenced by systems views. Jones (1982) describes varying degrees of system emphasis in family theories. In the structural-functional focus, the family is examined as a social system in relationship to other institutions such as religion, schools, and government, and emphasis is placed on family patterns and functions such as family tasks and health-care utilization. Interactional family theory, on the other hand, focuses on individual units and their interactions (e.g., roles and norms enacted in the family).

Analysis of group and community interactions has significant contributions to make to one's awareness of structural, functional, and interactive system components. Hamilton (1983) notes the importance of this focus to community nursing. For example, nurses are accustomed to looking to the community for resources to assist the client. If the resources are lacking or inadequate for significant groups of the population, the nurse needs to be able to assess and influence the process of change at the agency or community level. To assess the structural components involves identifying which persons or positions actually have the power to bring about desirable changes. A functional analysis identifies roles and tasks that keep the current system operating in the status quo. The plight of the chronically mentally ill in the community may be used as an example. When a chronically ill person with aftercare needs is released after psychiatric hospitalization he is frequently given only the name and address of a community mental health center for referral. The person quite commonly ignores the referral, stops taking antipsychotic drugs, and may exist as a homeless wanderer in the city. The community mental health center, if it views its function as offering mental health services to those who seek them, never sees these people, and the fiction of aftercare service availability is maintained even though these wanderers are repeatedly admitted to inpatient services. The problem is that the mental health system does not meet the needs of this special population. Linkages need to be built to foster trust and utilization of community-based services, and the services need to be adapted to the needs of the specific population.

☐ *Nursing Theory and Models*

The models of personality and behavior and their associated philosophies that have been discussed have influenced many nursing theorists. Psychodynamic, behavioral, existential, and systems concepts can be recognized in adapted forms in several nursing models.

Concepts central to nursing, that have been identified and refined by Yura and Torres (1975) and Fawcett (1978) and are commonly addressed in conceptual frameworks for nursing education and practice, are (1) man or person, as a holistic being and recipient of nursing services, (2) society or environment as an influence on the health status of persons, (3) health and illness as a focus for nursing action, and (4) nursing as a unique focus of action directed toward the person as a recipient of nursing services. Flaskerud and Halloran (1980) note that "there is consensus among nurses on the importance of these concepts."

VIEW OF PERSON

A person is consistently viewed as holistic by nursing theorists. Biological, psychological, and social factors are specifically addressed in the models of Henderson (1966), Orem (1980), and Roy (1974). The basic attitudes of nursing toward man are well described by Wiedenbach (1964).

She views people as possessing dignity, worth, autonomy, and unique individuality. The person is viewed as striving for self-direction and independence and as having needs for stimulation, achievement, and a positive self-concept. An individual's behavior and judgment represent the best that he or she is capable of at the time. This nonjudgmental acceptance of the person is shared by other nursing theorists.

Personal development is addressed from a pattern viewpoint by Rogers' (1970) theory of unitary man. The life process is conceived of as unidirectional and the sum of one's life experiences. One cannot go backwards to undo past events. These events then become interwoven and serve as influences upon the person's overall life pattern and organization. Johnson (Riehl and Roy, 1980) describes the person as a behavioral system comprised of eight subsystems: the ingestive, eliminative, restorative, sexual, dependency, aggressive, protective and achievement subsystems.

Interactive views of person reflect interpersonal theory and stress awareness of the significance of interpersonal processes on behavior, learning, and growth. Both Peplau (1952) and Orlando (1961) emphasize the nurse-patient relationship as an interpersonal process directed toward client goals; they add that both participants may learn and grow as a result of the relationship.

The human being is viewed as an open, living system by Roy (1974). Open systems exchange matter, energy, and information, permitting individuals to adapt to changes in their internal and external environments. These changes may occur in biological, psychological, or social modalities; nevertheless, they influence the total person and other components of the interactive system, such as the family.

VIEW OF THE ENVIRONMENT

Nightingale's *Notes on Nursing* addresses the importance of the environment as an influential and supportive factor in promoting health and healing. Primary emphasis in her time was on the physical environment, although other aspects were considered. The environment as a social context and as a factor that could support, influence, or limit the individual has also been discussed by nursing theorists such as Levine and Wiedenbach.

Systems views emphasize man's interaction with the environment as constant, integrated, mutually dynamic, adaptive, and changing. Both King (1981) and Roy (1974) stress adaptation processes in the system as an individual interacts holistically in physiological, psychological (self-concept), and social (roles) modalities.

HEALTH AND ILLNESS

Nursing theorists do not address mental health as a separate entity because of their holistic perspective. Views of health focus on the ability to function independently (Henderson, Orem), a state of wholeness or integrity (Orem, Roy), and adaptation to internal and external stressors (Roy, King). King (1971) further views health as a dynamic state in the life cycle, which includes continuous adaptation to achieve maximum potential for daily living. Illness has been variously described as a maladaptation or disruption in needs (Roy, Orlando).

NURSING

Nursing is viewed as an interactive process that stresses collaborative problem identification and goal setting (Peplau, Orlando, King). The focus of nursing care is to assist clients to adapt and meet their basic biological and psychosocial needs (Roy, King, Henderson) in aspects that they cannot manage independently (Orem).

Johnson describes the primary focus of medicine as being on the pathologic or disease processes that are occurring. Nurses assist the person to cope with the stress and threat of illness, being concerned with the person rather than the disease (Riehl and Roy, 1980). In this view, nursing serves as an external resource to promote client adaptation by providing protection, nurturance, and stimulation. Protection involves safeguarding the client from hazards or threats and intervening when the client is unable to cope for himself. Nurturance supports the client's healthy, adaptive behaviors. Stimulation refers to activities that motivate and encourage new behaviors and maintain an adequate level of incentive to deter regression. These concepts have relevance for all nurses and are applicable in psychiatric-mental health practice.

■ Enrichment Activities

DISCUSSION QUESTIONS

1. Describe some examples of healthy or normal uses of defense mechanisms commonly seen in everyday life.

2. Discuss how various theorists see anxiety and related defenses affecting learning and personality development (e.g., intra- and interpersonal views vs. behaviorists).

3. Reviewing the various aspects of development depicted in Tables 1-2 and 1-3, identify some common beliefs and tendencies about development as a process.

4. Compare Freud's primary and secondary process thought patterns with Sullivan's prototaxic, parataxic, and syntactic modes of thought.

5. Place the nursing theorists discussed into the intrapersonal, interpersonal, behavioral, existential, and systems categories used in this chapter.

SELF-TEST—MATCHING OF THEORISTS AND VIEWS

1. Intrapersonal   ____ ____ ____ ____
2. Interpersonal   ____
   theory
3. Transactional   ____
   Analysis
4. Existentialism   ____ ____ ____
5. Behaviorism   ____ ____ ____
6. Systems   ____

A. Freud	H. Jung
B. Sullivan	I. Dollard and
C. Von Bertalanffy	Miller
D. Adler	J. Kierkegaard
E. Berne	K. Wolpe
F. May	L. Heidegger
G. Skinner	M. Erikson

■ Recommended Readings

The following books are recommended for enhancing basic understanding of the theoretical viewpoints. They are mainly secondary sources that summarize the contributions of a particular theorist. The primary sources listed under the references are excellent for in-depth understanding of particular theories of interest.

George, Julia. *Nursing theories: The base for professional practice.* Englewood Cliffs, NJ: Prentice-Hall, 1985. Compares nursing theories with each other and on various aspects of the nursing process. An excellent overview of nursing theory.

Hall, Calvin. *A primer of Freudian psychology.* New York: Mentor, 1979. Easy-to-read paperback summarizes key concepts of Freud's theory.

Harris, Thomas. *I'm OK—you're OK.* New York: Avon, 1969. Easy-to-read, comprehensible discussion of Transactional Analysis; illustrates analysis of communication and scripts and gives clear examples of the concepts.

Laing, R.D. *Knots.* New York: Pantheon Books, 1970. This small book of poetry illustrates some of the "knotty" issues of human interaction from the perspective of a controversial contemporary phenomenologist.

Skinner, B.F. *About behaviorism.* New York: Alfred Knopf, 1974. Skinner's discussion and defense of behaviorism's philosophy and methods is written in a clear and readable manner.

■ *References*

Ansbacher, H., and Ansbacher, R. *The individual psychology of Alfred Adler.* New York: Basic Books, 1956.

Barton, A. *Three worlds of therapy—Freud, Jung & Rogers.* Palo Alto, CA: National Press Books, 1974.

Berne, E. *Games people play—The psychology of human relationships.* New York: Grove Press. Ballantine, 1978.

Bertrand, A.L. *Social organization: A general system and role theory perspective.* Philadelphia: F.A. Davis, 1972.

Clements, I., and Roberts, F. (eds.). *Family health—A theoretical approach to nursing care.* New York: Wiley Medical, 1983.

Dollard, J., and Miller, N.E. *Personality and psychotherapy: An analysis in terms of learning, thinking and culture.* New York: McGraw-Hill, 1950.

Erikson, E. *Childhood and society.* New York: Norton, 2nd ed., 1964.

Fawcett, J. The what of theory development. In *Theory development: What, why and how.* New York: National League for Nursing, 1978:17–33.

Flaskerud, J., and Halloran, E. Areas of agreement in nursing theory development. *Advances in nursing science,* 3, 1 (October 1980):1–7.

Ford, D.H., and Urban, H.B. *Systems of psychotherapy: A comparative study.* New York: John Wiley & Sons, 1963.

Freud, Anna. *The ego and the mechanisms of defense* (*Writings of Anna Freud,* Vol. 2). New York: International Universities Press, 1967.

Freud, Sigmund. *Complete psychological works: Standard edition.* (J. Strachey, ed.). New York: Norton, 1976.

Friedman, M. *Family nursing—theory and assessment.* Norwalk, CT: Appleton-Century-Crofts, 1981.

Hamilton, P. Community nursing diagnosis. In *Advances in nursing science* (P. Chin, ed.). 5, 3 (April 1983):21–36.

Harris, Thomas. *I'm OK—you're OK.* New York: Avon, 1982.

Hartmann, Heinz. *Essays on ego psychology.* New York: International Universities Press, 1964.

Henderson, Virginia. *The nature of nursing.* New York: Macmillan Co., 1966.

Jacobi, J. *The psychology of C.G. Jung.* New Haven: Yale University Press, 1973.

Janosik, E., and Miller, J. Theories of family development. In *Family health care,* 2d ed. (Hymovich, D., and Barnard, M., (eds.) Vol. 1. New York: McGraw-Hill, 1979:3–16.

Jones, M., and Jongeward, D. *Born to win.* New York: New American Library, A Signet Book, 1971.

Jones, Susan, and Dimond, M. Family theory and family therapy models: Comparative review and implications for nursing practice. *Journal of psychiatric nursing and mental health services,* 20, 10 (October 1982):12–19.

Joyce, B., and Weil, M. Behavioral models of teaching. In *Models of teaching,* 2d ed. Englewood Cliffs, NJ: Prentice-Hall, 1980:326–454.

Jung, C.G. *The development of the personality.* In Adler et al. (eds.) *Collected Works* 2d ed. Vol. 17. Princeton University Press, 1970.

King, Imogene. *A theory for nursing—systems, concepts, process.* New York: John Wiley & Sons, 1981.

Kohlberg, L. *Essays on moral development.* New York: Harper & Row, 1983.

Levinson, Daniel, *The seasons of a man's life.* New York: Alfred Knopf, 1978.

Lewin, K. *Field theory in social science.* New York: Harper & Row, 1951.

Loevinger, Jane. *Ego development: Conception and theories.* San Francisco: Jossey-Bass, 1976.

Maslow, Abraham. *Toward a psychology of being,* 2d ed. Princeton: Van Nostrand Reinhold Co., 1968.

Neugarten, B. (ed.). *Middle age and aging.* Chicago: University of Chicago Press, 1968.

Nightingale, Florence. *Notes on nursing.* New York: Dover, 1969.

Orem, Dorothy. *Nursing: Concepts of practice,* 2d ed. New York: McGraw-Hill, 1980.

Orlando, Ida. *The dynamic nurse-patient relationship: Function, process and principle.* New York: Putnam's, 1961.

Peplau, Hildegard. *Interpersonal relations in nursing.* New York: Putnam's, 1952.

Piaget, J., and Inhelder, R. *The psychology of the child.* New York: Basic Books, 1969.

Rapaport, D., and Gill, M. The points of view and assumptions of metapsychology. *International Journal of Psychoanalysis*, 40, 1959:153–161.

Riehl, J., and Roy, C. *Conceptual models for nursing practice.* 2d ed. New York: Appleton-Century-Crofts, 1980.

Rogers, C.R. *Client centered therapy,* Boston: Houghton Mifflin, 1951.

Rogers, C.R. *On becoming a person: A therapist's view of psychotherapy.* Boston: Houghton Mifflin, 1970.

Rogers, Martha. *The theoretical basis of nursing.* Philadelphia: F.A. Davis, 1970.

Roy, Callista. "The Roy Adaptation Model." In *Conceptual models for nursing practice* (Riehl, J., and Roy, C., eds.). New York: Appleton-Century-Crofts, 1974.

Satir, Virginia. *Conjoint family therapy.* rev. ed., Palo Alto, CA: Science and Behavior Books, 1967.

Schultz, W. *FIRO: A three dimensional theory of interpersonal behavior.* New York: Holt, Rinehart & Winston, 1958.

Schultz, W. *Joy: Expanding human awareness.* New York: Grove Press, 1967.

Skinner, B.F. *Science and human behavior.* New York: Free Press, 1965.

Sullivan, H.S. *The interpersonal theory of psychiatry* (Perry and Gawel, eds.). New York: Norton, 1968.

Von Bertalanffy, Ludwig. *General systems theory.* New York: Braziller, 1968.

Wallace, Edwin. *Dynamic psychiatry in theory and practice.* Philadelphia: Lea and Febiger, 1983.

Whall, Ann. Congruence between existing theories of family functioning and nursing theories. *Advances in nursing science*, 3, 1 (October 1980):59–67.

Whitley, M. Administrative use of systems analysis to troubleshoot a problematic work situation. *Journal of psychosocial nursing and mental health services*, 21, 2 (February 1983):25–29.

Wiedenbach, Ernestine. *Clinical nursing, a helping art.* New York: Springer, 1964.

Wolpe, J. *Psychotherapy by reciprocal inhibition.* Stanford: Stanford University Press, 1958.

Young, C. Family systems model. In (Clements, I., and Buchanan, D., eds.). *Family Therapy—A nursing perspective.* New York: John Wiley & Sons, 1982.

Yura, H., and Torres, G. *Today's conceptual frameworks within baccalaureate nursing programs.* NLN Publication no. 15-1558, New York: National League for Nursing, 1975.

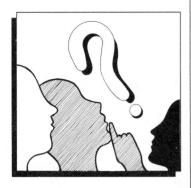

2

Models of Psychotherapeutic Intervention and Nursing Implications

Joan Norris

Learning Objectives

Upon completion of this chapter, the reader will be able to:

1. Contrast the goals and expectations of therapist and client for various models of psychotherapy and psychiatric treatment.

2. Describe information basic to understanding the use and assumptions of the various models and relate this information to nursing implications for collaborating as a member of the interdisciplinary mental health team.

3. Discuss considerations in choosing a therapist and treatment approach.

4. Identify basic assumptions and approaches in defining the role and functions of nursing.

5. Delineate levels of psychiatric-mental health nursing practice.

6. Identify psychosocial nursing functions related to levels of prevention in the mental health field.

The picture of psychotherapy that generally first comes to the public mind is that of the analyst facing away from the client, who is reclining on a couch. This image is based on the psychoanalytic model, which is only rarely in use today because of the length and expense involved in this treatment and the relative scarcity of practitioners. However the variety of treatment approaches now followed, and the diverse disciplines offering psychiatric and mental health services are a source of confusion to many members of the general public and the health professions alike. The prospective consumer may choose among analysts, psychiatrists, clinical psychologists, guidance counselors, psychiatric social workers, pastoral counselors, and psychiatric nurse clinical specialists. The choice becomes even more complex because any of these practitioners can choose from various theoretical perspectives, only some of which were touched upon in Chapter 1. Each of these aspects affects the roles and expectations of the therapist-client relationship.

Consumers may ask which of the disciplines or therapy models is most appropriate to their unique values and situation. Are all of these equally effective in promoting personal growth; diminishing the disintegration of a psychotic episode; reducing unrealistic debilitating fears; enhancing personal and family relationships? When a person sees a therapist, will the focus be on the past or the present; thoughts or emotions; ventilation of feelings; change in behavior?

The nurse may understandably be unsure when called upon to interpret the variety of mental health services available to consumers. In the psychiatric setting, the nurse's awareness of the focus and goals of the primary therapist permits greater effectiveness in supporting clients and collaborating in their care. For instance, should the nurse provide unlimited opportunities for exploration and ventilation of feelings or, on the other hand, attempt to actively involve the client in the social milieu and in problem-solving relationships within it? To some extent these kinds of decisions can be made independently by the nurse, but a collaborative approach promotes consistency and effectiveness through a goal focus which is mutually derived by client, therapist, and staff nurse.

For example, if Mrs. Brown experiences a deep depression at age 48, she may receive any of the following forms of therapy, among others, depending upon the approach selected: (1) antidepressant drugs prescribed by her family physician or a psychiatrist, (2) career/leisure counseling and referral to a women's group by a developmentally or socially focused therapist who views the problem as a "midlife crisis" related to the "empty nest" syndrome, (3) exploration of the psychodynamic meanings attached to menopause and aging which are based in her early experiences, or (4) a combination of these.

In option (1), Mrs. Brown's nurse could facilitate the antidepressant drug approach through medication teaching and assisting Mrs. Brown to problem solve and engage in activities of daily living. The nurse may never come in contact with Mrs. Brown in option (2) unless both happen to be members of the same women's group. The psychodynamic approach in option (3) would involve nursing intervention only if Mrs. Brown were hospitalized. In a therapeutic environment, a less threatening setting than home or work, Mrs. Brown still needs "real world" role models, appropriate reinforcers, and opportunities to interact and to make decisions at her current functional capability level. Although the therapy session is a place for intense exploration and expression of feelings, it would exhaust and diffuse the client's efforts if this intensity were to be maintained throughout the day with a variety of staff members. The staff needs to differentiate the therapist's focus from the milieu or environmental focus. (See Chapter 14 on therapeutic milieu.) Managing the milieu to promote health and healing has been a unique focus of nursing since Florence Nightingale first defined this aspect of the profession.

Depending on their education and experience, nurses bring their own unique and holistic perspective to a variety of roles such as therapist, liaison, and consultant. The primary focus of this chapter which expands on and is based in the theoretical assumptions addressed in Chapter 1, is models of therapeutic intervention.

□ Models of Therapy

Therapeutic approaches include psychoanalysis, a wide range of forms of psychotherapy (including brief therapy and crisis intervention), and the medical model. Each is examined from the standpoints of preparation and assumptions of the therapist, client goals, and conditions for which the model is most appropriate. Nursing models are also discussed in relation to psychiatric mental health nursing.

PSYCHOANALYSIS

Psychoanalysis is based in the approach popularized by Freud in which the client is instructed to lie on a couch, with the analyst out of direct view, and to free associate, that is, to discuss whatever thoughts or images come to mind. The analyst is a person with advanced training in psychiatry or clinical psychology and has undergone a personal psychoanalysis as part of the training and supervision process.

The goal of psychoanalytic treatment is to assist the client to overcome the resistances to conscious awareness and understanding which serve to maintain unconscious motivation of behavior and repression of aspects of the person's personality and experience. The focus of attention is the effect that early (i.e., childhood) experiences have in the continuation and repetition of current ineffective behavior patterns.

> ### ■ Point of Emphasis
>
> *Psychoanalysis emphasizes development of insight.*

Concepts and assumptions involved in the psychoanalytic method address the role of therapist and the process of treatment. The analyst assumes the role of dispassionate observer. The client reacts to the analyst in this neutral setting based on past fantasies and experiences with significant others. These reactions are called transference. The therapist must be careful not to become overly involved or to distort the client's communication based on the analyst's own prior significant interactions (countertransference). Interpretations by the analyst may vary from observations of nonverbal expression (e.g., "You're smiling but you're telling me that your father was harsh and unreliable.") to more complex patterns of behavior (e.g., "Every time you mention your father, you have a particular smile which I've also seen when you were angry with something I've said. . . . Is that what you learned from your mother when you described her as smiling through her tears?"). The interpretations are carefully selected to guide the client to personal awareness, self-understanding, and conscious (as opposed to unconscious) control of behavior.

This analytical view of mental illness is originally based in Freud's description of neurosis.

He, like most analysts, did not view the major psychoses as appropriate to this form of treatment. Freida Fromm Reichman and some others disagree with this view and have reported effective analytic treatment of schizophrenia. The neurosis as described by Freud is based in the experience of extreme anxiety and the inability to discharge the consequent tensions effectively through emotional catharsis or motor behavior (e.g., tears, escape, or aggressive actions). This leads to future situations in which recall of the occurrence or related experiences may recreate the intensity of the original negative emotions. Ford and Urban (1973:151) describe Freud's view of neurosis as similar to that of classical conditioning. For example, a middle-aged woman with a strict moral upbringing may find herself sexually attracted to her teenage son's friend. These feelings are so abhorrent to her that they cannot be acknowledged and must be repressed. Subsequent visits of her son's friend to their home or even casual meetings with any of her son's friends may evoke severe symptoms of anxiety, although the actual cause for the intensely anxious response is beyond her awareness. The current psychiatric terminology replaces neurosis with the more specific terms of anxiety, factitious, and somatoform disorders identified in the Diagnostic and Statistical Manual (DSM III) of the American Psychiatric Association, a nomenclature system for mental disorders.

Stimulus generalization may lead to extension of symptoms to coincidental and unrelated events. Traumatic events are perceived as conflict based, the experience of two opposing forces such as strong urges (e.g., sexual or hostile) which are condemned by the morality of the superego. Repression occurs, and only the learned responses that were originally associated with the event remain, such as palpitations and shortness of breath or a sense of partial paralysis. In the example given earlier, generalization may lead to acute anxiety attacks whenever the woman leaves the house or whenever anyone comes to visit any family members. This stimulus generalization can create a situation that is socially disabling.

The *effectiveness of psychoanalysis* has not been consistently demonstrated. Research has not shown it to be statistically superior to other treatment modes or to no treatment at all. Individuals for whom analysis has been effective report a freeing of energy for more effective living and a significant growth in personal awareness and creativity. Analysis requires a significant commitment of time and money on the part of the client since the course of treatment involves 1 to 3 or more hours per week for over 1 year or (more likely) many years. The client must also be verbally articulate and self-aware or at least open to becoming so.

The nurse will rarely come in contact with clients in analysis since most are treated as outpatients unless they require a period of hospitalization or the nurse works in a setting where long-term residential treatment and psychoanalysis are practiced.

In the case of the hospitalized client who is undergoing analysis, the role of the nurse is not to prolong the therapeutic hour throughout the day but instead to promote a therapeutic milieu. (See Chapter 14.) Collaboration between the analyst and nursing staff will identify any particular approaches pertinent to the client's current status. For instance, when a client experiences a period of heightened anxiety in response to dealing with painful issues in therapy, increased security and support from the environment may be required. Later the emphasis may need to be shifted to help the client distinguish between the analyst's focus on catharsis (expression of feelings) and the demands of social situations for which a degree of restraint and attention to the needs of others is necessary for effective interaction. In an analytically focused practice setting, the nurse will anticipate a very high degree of value and involvement placed on personal awareness for staff members. Personal analysis may be advocated to enhance the nurse's self-awareness and therapeutic skills.

Psychotherapy

Psychotherapy is a general term that includes various theoretical approaches, and may involve individual, family, and/or group settings for purposes of treatment. It is based on techniques to explore a client's experiences and perspective so that the therapist may offer understanding, support, and assistance in making decisions that will reduce the amount of pain and distress in the client's life. These techniques may be used in one-to-one therapeutic sessions, in family and group therapy, or in a combination of them. Although various theoretical perspectives may be used by a therapist, there are two main approaches, the psychodynamic and the behavioral. Various types of these models are discussed and significant components identified in Tables 2-1 and 2-2. Family

and group approaches may enhance basic therapy by giving the therapist an opportunity to directly observe client interactions with others and providing a realistic context for dynamic interaction.

Although many of the assumptions and theoretical perspectives of psychotherapy may be similar to those of analysis, the duration tends to be limited to the attainment of specific goals and, although expensive, the total cost is usually less than for analysis. Most psychotherapists meet their clients face to face, rather than having the client lie on a couch. Contracted times and goals are negotiated in initial assessment interviews. While insight (self-understanding) is most valued in psychoanalysis, psychotherapists may emphasize either insight or behavior change, or both. Therapists may be psychiatrists, clinical psychologists, psychiatric social workers, clinical specialists in psychiatric nursing, pastoral counselors, guidance counselors, or activity therapists. A therapist may also have unique and specialized role functions particular to a discipline such as psychological testing by the psychologist, prescription of somatic and pharmacotherapies by the psychiatrist (who is an M.D.), or the environmental focus of the nurse. All of these disciplines assume that a graduate degree has been attained and that there has been a supervised therapy practicum as a basic preparation for the practice of therapy, although the types of degrees and the duration of the practicum may vary widely. In some settings where there are financial constraints, staff members with lesser qualifications may receive informal, on-the-job training and be assigned to some therapist functions. This is fairly common but not a recommended practice.

Assumptions and roles of therapists will vary depending on the theoretical viewpoints selected. A Rogerian therapist would facilitate the personal growth and self-exploration of a client through nondirective counseling techniques. A Gestalt model would direct the therapist to become very active in confronting nonverbal and verbal cues to the client's conflicts although the ultimate goals would not differ from the Rogerian's. On the other hand, the behaviorist would contract with the client for specific behavior changes such as habit control or the reduction of specific avoidance behaviors based in irrational fears.

The *effectiveness* of psychotherapy depends on numerous variables, including the skill of the therapist and the motivation and preferences of the client. Although research studies have been minimal and inconclusive, it appears that behav-

TABLE 2-1 Models of Psychodynamic Therapy

Therapy	View of Client Problem	Approach	Strategies	Goal
Client centered (Carl Rogers)	Being out of touch with one's own values and experiential world leads to a blocked life	Nondirective counseling (goal is developing self-awareness)	Genuineness Unconditional positive regard Empathic understanding	Expands self-awareness Acceptance of experiential self
Freudian analysis	Unconscious processes dictate behavior based on repetition of early conflicts and trauma	Classic psychoanalysis (goal is insight)	Free association Overcoming resistance Analysis of transference phenomena	Insight which leads to conscious behavior control
Jungian analysis	Difficulty in recognizing and integrating opposite aspects of the self (e.g., masculine or feminine attributes) previously repressed	Modified analytic approach (active mutual effort at unfolding and synthesizing the client's life via symbolism)	Emotional reliving Support for self-acceptance and integration of unconscious attributes Analysis of dreams and fantasies Other techniques as appropriate to client need (e.g., catharsis, active imagining)	Insight Development of neglected aspects of the self
Adlerian therapy	Faulty response patterns developed to safeguard the client from the burden of own excessive feelings of inferiority	Modification of analytic approach (individual subjectivistic focus which includes exploration of life-style and goals)	Empathy Intuitive guessing Assigning "homework" tasks Analyzing/explaining faulty behavior patterns Promoting more effective social behavior	Insight Change in social behavior
Transactional Analysis (Eric Berne)	Games are fixed interaction patterns which serve to reinforce unhealthy life scripts or positions	Didactic understanding and confrontation in individual or group settings	Structural analysis of ego status and transactions, script analysis and game analysis	Specifically contracted with the client—generally the ability to relate spontaneously and openly
Psychodrama (S. Moreno)	Need to work through problematic relationships and events	Enactments of significant relationships and events in a group setting	Role play enactment Role reversal and enactment Alter-ego support Discussion	Insight Catharsis
Interpersonal therapy (Sullivan)	Distortions in development and reality perceptions based on avoidance of overwhelming anxiety	Active participation of therapist and client in an interpersonal exchange. Both participants share perceptions/observations of the client	Shared observations Consensual validation Managing interpersonal anxiety	Realistic view of self and environment no longer distorted by anxiety
Gestalt (Perls)	Failure to experience all aspects of the self	Encounter focus on self-awareness in a here-and-now context	Confrontation Dialogue with opposing viewpoint (e.g., empty chair) Bodily awareness	Insight Self-awareness and acceptance
Reality therapy (Glasser)	Self-defeating behaviors keep client from reaching goals	Identity formulation based on loving, self-esteem, and responsible behavior	Focus on behaviors Exploration of more effective actions Present orientation	Goal identification and developing capacity for caring relationships
Rational emotive (Ellis)	Failure to assume responsibility (in the existential sense) for one's feelings and actions	Cognitive orientation emphasizing self-acceptance and new behavior	Confrontation Action orientation which encourages risk taking and trying out new behaviors	Self-acceptance and behavior change

TABLE 2-2 Behavior Modification Techniques

Approach	Strategies	Goals
Training (based on operant conditioning)	Clarify objectives and theory Modeling/demonstration Simulation practice Feedback Transfer training	Communication effectiveness Increased assertiveness Develop self-awareness
Contingency management (based on operant conditioning)	Stimulus identification Behavioral response recording Reinforcement Feedback/evaluation	Behavior change Programmed instruction
Stress management (counter-conditioning)	Response substitution (relaxation)/positive reconditioning Reciprocal inhibition (biofeedback monitoring to provide reinforcement of desired physiological responses)	Mastery of relaxation Decreasing physiological arousal
Flooding (counter-conditioning)	Continuous exposure to the feared stimulus Panic-level anxiety cannot be sustained and eventually subsides resulting in tolerance of the stimulus	Working through phobic avoidance
Desensitization (counter-conditioning)	Reciprocal inhibition Response substitution	Mastery of relaxation responses Progressively increased tolerance of anxiety-evoking stimuli
Token economy (operant conditioning in group setting)	Communicate expectations and reward behavior Record and provide secondary reinforcers; conversion of tokens to primary reinforcers Facilitate transfer of skills to new situations	Reestablish social skills Improve activities of daily living (ADL) performance

ioral methods are somewhat superior to insight-oriented therapy in meeting specific client goals for habit control, reduction of phobic behaviors, sexual dysfunctions, and management of stress-related physical symptoms via biofeedback and relaxation techniques.

It is important to note that in habit control, behavior changes that bring about short-term

■ Point of Emphasis

Behavioral approaches emphasize behavior change.

outcomes must generally be accompanied by maintenance strategies to achieve long-term effectiveness. Insight-oriented methods are more appropriate to client goals relating to personal growth, interpersonal awareness, and interaction.

Pardes and Pincus (1981:18–19) cite the results of various research studies in concluding that numerous models of psychotherapy are superior to no treatment in the achievement of therapeutic results. A summary of comparative studies (Smith, et al., 1980) found that psychotherapy groups demonstrated greater improvement in 90 percent of the research cited than did the untreated control groups. This does not suggest that therapy is uniformly beneficial. Strupp and others (1977) noted that inappropriate use of techniques and some attributes of therapists may result in negative side effects for particular kinds of clients.

Wilson (1981) noted that behavioral techniques may call for variations in scheduling of sessions in order to prolong the client's exposure time during flooding or desensitization, or to cluster the frequency of sessions when attempting to establish habit control (in substance abuse of food, alcohol, drugs) or to decrease sexual dysfunctions. Therapy sessions may include a few intensive day-long sessions or weekends.

Brief Therapy

Brief therapy is defined by Budman as therapy confined to 25 or fewer sessions (1981:1). Other authors may define brief therapy as involving more sessions over a longer duration such as up to 1 year. In any case, brief therapy, which allows access of a greater number of clients to mental health therapy (Pardes and Pincus, 1981), is the customary practice in most contemporary American outpatient treatment settings. This trend has occurred in response to escalating costs, acceptance of limited goals in therapy, and the recognition that insight-oriented therapy over a prolonged time may not be appropriate to the aims and values of many people. For instance, many cultures do not encourage open expression of intimate thoughts and feelings, preferring instead a more time-limited and action-oriented approach.

Greater eclecticism in the use of theoretical concepts has also resulted in a greater variety of therapeutic approaches used by any given practitioner while at the same time leading to similarity among therapists in general. For example, the recognition that behavioral approaches are quite effective in altering the symptoms of phobic disorders has led to their incorporation in treatment by therapists whose general orientation may be psychodynamic rather than behavioral. Current emphasis on the recognition of stress factors in physical conditions and the need for a more holistic treatment focus has contributed to the in-

> ### ■ Point of Emphasis
> *Brief therapy emphasizes achievement of specific client goals in less than 1 year of treatment.*

corporation of both brief and long-term psychotherapy in the treatment of psychological factors affecting physiological disorders such as cancer.

Comparisons of brief and long-term psychotherapies indicate no differences between them in the type or level of therapist preparation. Because of the time-limited focus, some key aspects of treatment become emphasized in brief therapy. The initial assessment accomplished in the first one to three sessions must define the core issues and link the problem for which the client seeks help empathically with past patterns or themes, such as, chronic low self-esteem and the behaviors developed to defend against it (Mann, 1981:33). The therapist actively seeks to manage anxiety about the treatment process, develop trust, and build hope. Transference may or may not be a focus of therapy depending on the therapist's theoretical orientation. Dynamic, behavioral, and cognitive models of therapy are all commonly used in brief therapy.

Crisis Intervention

The interests of Lindemann and Caplan following World War II in the preventive aspects of community psychiatry and mental health led to the formulation of crisis intervention theory and methods. Crisis in this framework is viewed as a period of upset or disorganization as a person confronts a challenging event (a hazardous situation or developmental phase). The potential outcome of this brief period (4 to 6 weeks) of disequilibrium, tension, and challenge may be positive or negative in terms of the person's future mental health as new adaptive coping strategies must be learned or maladaptive patterns incorporated.

Crisis intervention seeks to capitalize on the heightened motivation of the individual in crisis for learning new behavior. The focus may be generic or individual. The generic approach concentrates on the disruptive event and the necessary related coping tasks. Caplan saw this approach as useful to all nurses, clergy, and indigenous community workers, among others, in expanding the preventive and supportive mental health services of the general community. The individual approach to crisis intervention focuses on the person's unique perceptions and processes involved in adapting to the precipitating crisis. Since this approach emphasizes dynamic aspects of the individual, it is practiced by mental health professionals (therapists) and generally only if the generic approach was ineffective. Intervention is directed toward the client's attaining an intellectual understanding of the personal meaning of the crisis, identifying feelings and expressing them to reduce tension, exploring alternative coping mechanisms, and, if social losses have occurred, encouraging expansion of social contacts. Anticipatory guidance is a crisis technique that facilitates transfer of new learning and coping strategies to future potential crises (Aguillera and Messick, 1982).

In crisis intervention, the therapist-client relationship is mutually active and collaborative, with an emphasis on solving current problems. Sessions generally number up to six, and the goal is resolution of the immediate crisis. Because crisis intervention is applicable to all levels and settings of nursing practice, Chapter 22 is devoted to this model.

THE MEDICAL MODEL

The medical model has been the dominant perspective in psychiatric-mental health treatment throughout most of the twentieth century. It has also been severely criticized for its disease orientation and the use of various treatments for which risks often outbalanced benefits (e.g., insulin therapy, prefrontal lobotomy, and the indiscriminate use of electroshock therapy in the 1940s and 1950s). By definition, the psychiatrist is a medical doctor who has additional training in psychiatry. The training of the physician focuses on: (1) identification of syndromes and diseases to enhance clinical approaches and research effectiveness, (2) the search for biological factors associated with the etiology of mental illnesses, particularly the psychoses, and (3) the use of somatic and pharmacological agents in the treatment of clients (e.g., psychotropic drugs and selective use of electroconvulsive therapy).

DSM III Classification

The first effort to develop a comprehensive and reliable classification system of psychiatric disorders was made in 1952 (DSMI). The third edition of this manual, prepared by the American Psychiatric Association, was published in 1980. The DSM III, which is compatible with the International Classification of Diseases (ICD9) as developed by the World Health Organization, consists of three axes constituting the diagnostic categories (see Appendix B) and two additional axes useful in clinical research, treatment planning, and prognosis:

1. Clinical syndromes (mental disorders) and additional conditions not related to a mental disorder (such as an adjustment disorder).
2. Personality and developmental disorders.
3. Physical conditions and disorders that may coexist (e.g., diabetes, cerebral aneurysm).
4. Severity of psychosocial stressors related to onset (rated from none evident to catastrophic).
5. Highest level of adaptive functioning reached in the past year (rated from superior to grossly impaired).

The use of medical diagnoses (a disease model) has been criticized by those within and outside of the medical profession. Many critics have objected to the client passivity implied by assigning behavior patterns (e.g., antisocial life-styles or overindulgence in chemical substances such as sedatives, opiates, or stimulants) to disease categories rather than defining them as ethical-moral problems. Others point out the likelihood of labeling and stereotyping "schizophrenics" and "neurotics" rather than responding to clients as people with unique personal perspectives and needs. Although this is not necessarily a direct outcome of diagnosis, it is important for individuals and professional groups to be aware of these issues to avoid dehumanizing their clients. Defenders of the medical model point to the progress made in improving diagnostic reliability and descriptiveness. In conditions where so little is known about the causes and interrelationships involved, the importance of consistency in naming and describing the problem and its relevance to all forms of research is evident. For instance, can specific physical brain changes and neurohormonal dysfunctions be demonstrated in clients diagnosed as schizophrenic? What relationship do these dysfunctions or changes (if any) have to the symptoms and outcomes of the disorder? Based on this knowledge are improved treatments possible?

Nurses have the opportunity to use these diagnostic terms either to the benefit or the detriment of a client. If diagnoses are used as a cue to further assessment and for consideration of possible client needs while the nurse adheres to the concept of the client as a unique, holistic being worthy of respect and dignity—the client benefits.

If, on the other hand, the diagnosis is used to label, to decrease hope, to distance nurse and client—then both the diagnosis and the client have been abused. Accurate, consistent guidelines for diagnosis of client problems contribute to the success of research into causes and treatment.

Medical Model Treatment Options

The extent of psychiatrists' use of the medical model depends on individual orientation. At one extreme is the trained analyst who rarely, if ever, uses drugs, hospitalization, or somatic treatment. Drugs are avoided whenever possible because they are viewed as reducing the motivational anxiety to work through the conflicts and resistances in therapy. Hospitalization might be used only for very short-term emergency needs for an acutely suicidal or grossly disorganized client. At the other end of the spectrum is the "medical model" practitioner. Mental illness, like physical illness, is believed by this psychiatrist to be basically biological in origin although the etiological factors are seen as varying widely from biochemical or nutritional disturbances, through brain and central nervous system dysfunctions, to less clearly delineated traits or vulnerabilities passed on by genetic and sociointeractive means. Hospitalization may be used to provide care and security when the client is acutely ill and psychotropic drugs are the primary means of treatment. Electroshock therapy may be considered for resistant depression or (rarely) other specific conditions. The psychiatrist's visits during hospitalizaton of the client would emphasize assessments of therapeutic drugs' effects/side effects, and encouragement of compliance with the medication regimen (and sometimes with hospital activities). Although not held out as a "cure," psychotropic drugs may be described in terms similar to the use of insulin for the diabetic, particularly for clients diagnosed as suffering from schizophrenia or major/affective psychoses. Group and milieu approaches may be considered but are not always highly valued since the problem is viewed as being beyond the client's control or ability to effect changes.

The majority of psychiatrists cluster at various points between these two polar opposites. Psychodynamic and behavioral approaches are used in addition to and in combination with drugs and somatic therapy. The choice of strategy will depend on the client's age, condition, diagnosis, and other factors. Medical intervention is necessary in the psychoses and in organically based mental disorders. It is not always possible to determine a psychiatrist's orientation by merely observing his approach during client hospitalization. Many who use either long-term or brief supportive therapy approaches on an outpatient basis will emphasize milieu therapy and psychotropic drugs when a client is in need of hospitalization until the client is more accessible to psychotherapy.

Nurses have particular responsibilities in regard to the promotion of a therapeutic milieu and in support of pharmacotherapy. Enhancing the effectiveness and safety of psychotropic drugs involves knowledge, assessing for therapeutic and side effects, teaching, and promoting compliance.

☐ Choosing a Therapist

The person who seeks therapy is very likely experiencing several kinds of concerns in addition to the problem for which treatment is sought. Fear of the unknown, confusion as to the treatment approaches available, the common belief that one ought to be able to solve one's own problems, financial concerns, fear of change, the stigma of mental illness, and issues of trust and confidence are all potentially involved in the decision to seek therapy (Bulbrook, 1980:51–3). Family members may also experience concerns, whether they are verbalized or not. Will they be coerced into or excluded from the treatment process? Will they be blamed for the problem? If the client changes, how will significant others be affected? Does the family have sufficient resources to cope with the financial and emotional costs involved? Will the benefits outweigh the costs? The nurse who discusses with a potential client or family the decision to seek therapy and select a therapist needs to be aware of these underlying issues, many of which will not always be addressed directly.

Considerations in the choice of a particular treatment approach include the nature of the problem, the particular values and preferences of the potential client, and issues of cost and reimbursement. If the condition in question has an organic basis or component such as behavioral changes induced by chemical exposure, circulatory changes to the brain, acutely psychotic conditions which will likely require medication or hospitalization, or addictive problems requiring detoxification, then the medical model approach is most appropriate for evaluation of the physical problems and related treatment. Once the physical condition is stabilized, referral to another type of therapy (e.g., a substance abuse treatment program) may be accomplished. The psychiatrist may be located by requesting a referral or list of recommended names from the client's family physician or from the local medical society. If the problem revolves around family relationships, then a therapist from any of the disciplines who specializes in family therapy may be the best choice. In addition to medical and psychological associations, family service agencies are good sources of referral. The devoutly religious person who is experiencing problems in coping with life events such as illness, poverty, or life changes may prefer to consult his minister or a selected pastoral counselor of the chosen faith. Most clergy are trained (or can refer to another member of the clergy who is trained) in pastoral counseling to deal with these kinds of issues of daily living. Various psychotherapists are prepared to deal with developmental adjustment problems, anxiety disorders, and problems in living. Their services can be obtained from community mental health centers, local professional organizations, and family service organizations. Sexual dysfunctions are best treated by a sex therapist. The state medical and psychological associations have referral lists available.

A client's social, cultural, or economic values may profoundly influence the acceptability of certain types of treatment. For instance, an Asian client may be more comfortable expressing personal distress in somatic symptoms rather than talking about feelings. A medical doctor or nurse might be more acceptable to this person than a psychologist or social worker. Action-oriented people may prefer behavioral approaches. Crisis services offered by a community mental health center or similar agency are likely to be most effective with clients experiencing recent acute disruptions, while the articulate, psychologically minded, upper-middle-class person might prefer to invest time and effort in psychodynamic therapy.

Costs vary appreciably and are a significant factor to most people. Those clients covered by third-party reimbursement plans such as Medicare or private insurance need to investigate their coverage and the stipulations and limitations for reimbursement. Those without mental health coverage may contact community mental health centers and family or community service agencies, most of which provide low cost services based on ability to pay.

General considerations for informing consumers include providing assurances of confidentiality in the client-therapist relationship and the awareness that they should use the first interview with any therapist to address any particular areas of concern. Many people need to be made aware, for instance, that it violates federal policy for any prospective employers to inquire about prior treatment for mental health problems. They also need to be assisted to recognize that seeking help is not a weakness but an opportunity to develop further strengths.

☐ *Nursing*

Nursing also has a particular model or approach to intervention which applies to psychiatric-mental health nursing regardless of the practice setting. Central components of this model are the nurse-client interactive relationship, environmental management, and the nursing process.

NURSE-CLIENT INTERACTION

Nursing is first of all an interactive process involving mutuality, collaboration, and problem-solving activities. This has been addressed by several nursing theorists (Levine, 1973; Peplau, 1952; Wiedenbach, 1964; Orlando, 1961, and King, 1981). The client is not a passive recipient of care (unless the level of consciousness is impaired) but an active participant in its planning and implementation. This is particularly significant to psychiatric-mental health nursing since change requires motivation and activity on the part of the client. The nurse's tools in promoting this interactive process are communication and the nurse-client relationship. Both of these tools demand self-awareness and observation skills.

ENVIRONMENTAL MANAGEMENT

Flaskerud and Halloran assert that nursing theories agree that "Nurses manage the interaction between the patient and the environment to promote healing or health" (1980:1). They further describe nursing actions such as assessment, regulation, modification, evaluation, and communication which contribute to environmental management. Nightingale originally defined this focus for nursing, and it continues relatively unchallenged as one of nursing's unique perspectives. A variety of nursing theorists including Roy, Rogers, Johnson, and Newman clearly identify the environment as a point of intervention.

In the mental health field, this environmental focus is reinforced by the concurrent developments in community psychiatry, therapeutic community, family theory, and milieu therapy. The nurse uses knowledge of the environment and systems theory in interactions as a role model, participant, advocate, socializer, and supporter. Systems theory illustrates the interactive nature of behavioral influences in maintaining or disrupting patterns of behavior. The psychiatric unit can become a social microcosm where behavior can be identified, evaluated, and altered in a social context. Family processes may be observed and more adaptive interactions promoted. The physical, family, and sociocultural contexts of the client become key components for assessment and intervention.

The roles of nurses in promoting a therapeutic environment merit further discussion. Humans are capable of imitative or social learning. Role modeling healthy behaviors in the interpersonal context of staff and client relationships becomes a significant aspect of care and treatment. Participation in interpersonal relationships provides opportunities in everyday situations for modeling communication skills, giving and receiving feedback, mutual respect, and collaborative problem solving. This approach is also related to the concepts of advocacy and social support by the nurse.

> ### ■ Point of Emphasis
>
> *Nurses provide a therapeutic environment by serving as advocates and role models, by offering social support, and by engaging clients in collaborative solving of here-and-now problems of daily living.*

Donahue discusses advocacy as the foundation for nursing intervention—a dynamic process which is consistently directed toward the welfare of the client. Advocacy calls for activity and commitment in asserting this purpose, whether the nurse is involved in behavior with the client that conveys respect for his individuality and autonomy or is required to engage in activities on the client's behalf (Bulechek and McClosky, 1985).

The nurse models social skills to assist clients who may be shy, awkward, or withdrawn to become more comfortable and adept in social situations.

The role of supporter is viewed in the broad context of social supports which encompass aspects of man's needs for belonging, nurturance, companionship, and the mutual give-and-take of close relationships. Gardner describes the nurse's presence in the existential sense as physically "being there" and psychologically "being with" clients to meet their health care needs. This can be manifested cognitively by communicating empathy or understanding of the client's experience; affectively through demonstrating genuineness, trust, and positive regard; and behaviorally by being available to help (Bulechek and McCloskey, 1985). Table 2-3 compares the environmental focus of the nurse with the therapist's approach for selected client problems.

NURSING PROCESS

Nursing process is the identified organizational methodology for nursing thought and action. It is analogous to the scientific method and the problem-solving process and generally includes the steps of assessment, nursing diagnosis or problem identification, intervention or implementation, and evaluation (Yura and Walsh, 1973; Bower, 1982; Mitchell, 1973). (See Chapter 7.)

Nursing can be viewed as an interpersonal process which actively involves the client in maintaining or restoring health. King defines health as "a dynamic state in an organism's life cycle which implies continual adaptation to environmental stressors through optimum resource utilization in order to achieve maximum potential in daily living" (1971:24). The recipient of nursing care may be a person, family, group, or community. Nursing process involves assessment, diagnosis, intervention and evaluation of clients in all settings and at all levels of prevention: (1) primary prevention which strives to remove potential hazards before they change health status, (2) secondary prevention which strives to identify and treat health problems at an early stage to minimize chronicity, and (3) tertiary prevention which seeks to rehabilitate the client and restore him to an optimal level of function.

Examples of primary prevention include mental health teaching, wellness promotion, and efforts to eradicate community stressors such as pollution, unemployment, absence of family support

TABLE 2-3 Comparison of Therapist Approach and Nursing Focus for Selected Client Problems

Client Problem	Therapist Approach	Nursing-Therapeutic Environment Focus
Alterations in socialization		
Lack of social skills (due to withdrawal and/or social isolation)	Supportive therapy May prescribe group involvement	Role model effective social behavior Use opportunities to teach and develop skills in daily interactions
Inability to respond effectively to interpersonal cues (e.g., aggressive or timid responses or inability to read cues)	Assertiveness training Sensitivity training	Provide feedback and support for skill development Evaluate progress with client
Impaired verbal communication (due to acute schizophrenic episode)	Supportive therapy Antipsychotic drugs	Listen and attempt to validate meaning Encourage clarity Provide feedback and support on communication efforts
Alterations in self-concept		
Disturbances in body image (due to psychosis)	Supportive therapy Antipsychotic drugs	Reality orientation, reassurance, emotional support
Self-esteem disturbance (due to severe losses)	Supportive therapy Insight-oriented therapy Cognitive therapy Antidepressant drugs	Promote gradual increases in decision making and environmental involvement to promote success experiences Identify and reinforce client strengths
Anxiety (severe levels)	Insight oriented therapy Antianxiety drugs	Recognition of anxiety Identification of precursers to anxiety Collaborative problem solving Coping attempts Evaluative feedback and further practice
Ineffective family coping	Family therapy	Family education and support

services, or the exploitation of particular minority groups. Secondary prevention is accomplished through screening and referral services as nurses come in contact with at-risk populations throughout the community. Tertiary prevention encompasses a variety of rehabilitation efforts designed to rebuild or restore problem-solving and social competence, sense of self-esteem and confidence, and skills in self-care, everyday living, and interpersonal relationships.

Because nursing is both holistic and an interpersonal process, assessment and intervention may focus on any or all of the following: (1) the client, (2) the family and environment, and (3) the nurse. The first two categories have been addressed, the third merits further discussion. As a participant in the nurse-client relationship, an interpersonal/interactive process, the nurse needs to develop self-awareness. Several nursing theorists including King and Peplau have discussed the importance of the nurse's beliefs, attitudes, assumptions, communication skills, and actions on the client, the interaction, and the nurse's own professional growth. Psychiatric-mental health nursing has been a primary contributor to an awareness of these realities, and their importance applies to all settings of practice.

■ Enrichment Activities

DISCUSSION QUESTIONS

1. Since all of us, to some extent or another, experience problems in living, examine your opinions about seeking psychotherapy. What approaches to therapy are most consistent with your personal beliefs and values? Under what circumstance would you seek therapy?

2. A friend or family member approaches you to inquire about whether they should consult their pastor, a psychologist, or their family physician about the unusual behavior being exhibited by an elderly member of the family. What kinds of information would help you to respond? What knowledge about the assumptions and approaches taken by psychologists, pastoral counselors, and medical doctors would be important in making this decision?

3. Compare the assumptions and approaches of nursing, medical-model psychiatry, and behavioral psychology in regard to:
   a. Views of man
   b. Views of mental health and illness
   c. Mental health treatment focus
   d. Roles of the client and practitioner in the treatment process

4. Discuss what is meant by "the medical model." What contributions and criticisms are appropriate to this model?

LEARNING ACTIVITIES

1. Compare the responses of various members of the mental health team to the following questions in regard to the same client. (E.g., ask the attending psychiatrist, social worker, assigned staff nurse, and an activity therapist.)
   a. What is the most important goal you've identified for this client's care?
   b. What interventions are most important to this goal?
   c. What do you expect the client to do to meet this goal?
   d. What other members of the health team are important to this goal?

2. Role play a discussion with a friend who is experiencing anxiety and depression following the breakup of a long relationship. The friend feels that professional help is needed but doesn't know where to turn or what to expect in the process of seeking help.

3. In your clinical care of an assigned client, identify which of your planned interventions can be classified as (1) caring for client needs until the client can care for self, (2) altering the environment to promote health, and (3) assisting the client in collaborative, goal-directed activity. What conditions based on (a) client health status or (b) your own assumptions determined interventions for each category? Did you select appropriately when considering client preference, need and level of independence?

■ Recommended Readings

Bulbrook, Mary Jo (ed.). *Development of therapeutic skills*. Boston: Little, Brown, & Co. 1980. This book is written for the advanced student preparing to become a therapist but also provides the basic nursing student or practitioner with a philosophical understanding of therapy from the perspectives of the consumer and various therapists.

Budman, S. (ed.). *Forms of brief therapy*. New York: Guilford Press, 1981. Contributors describe the methods and relative effectiveness of various approaches to brief therapy, the most widely practiced approach to mental health treatment in current use.

Balint, M., Ornstein, P.H., and Balint, E. *Focal psychotherapy*. London: Tavistock, 1972. A reconstruction of actual therapy with a paranoid client by Balint from his notes. The covers a brief therapy series with comments about aims, impressions, and afterthoughts of each session and gives the reader the opportunity to view the therapeutic process through the therapist's eyes.

■ References

Aguillera, D., and Messick, J. *Crisis intervention theory and methodology*. St. Louis: Mosby, 1982.

American Psychiatric Association. *DSM III diagnostic and statistical manual of mental disorders*. 3d ed. Washington, D.C.: American Psychiatric Association, 1980.

Barton, A. *Three worlds of therapy—Freud, Jung and Rogers*. Palo Alto, CA: National Press Books, 1974.

Bower, F.L. *The process of planning nursing care— Nursing practice models*. St. Louis: Mosby, 1982.

Budman, Simon (ed.). *Forms of brief therapy.* New York: Guilford Press, 1981.

Bulbrook, M.J. (ed.). *Development of therapeutic skills.* Boston: Little, Brown & Co., 1980.

Bulechek, G., and McCloskey, J. *Nursing interventions—Treatments for nursing diagnosis.* Philadelphia: Saunders, 1985.

Caplan, Gerald. *Principles of preventive psychiatry.* New York: Basic Books, 1964.

Clements, I., and Buchanan, D. (eds.). *Family therapy—a nursing perspective.* New York: John Wiley & Sons, 1982.

Curtis, H.C. Psychoanalysis: A basic model of psychotherapy. *The psychiatric hospital,* 14, 4, 1983:188–191.

Ellis, A., and Harper, R. *A guide to rational living.* Englewood Cliffs, NJ: Prentice-Hall, 1961.

Flaskerud, J., and Halloran, E. Areas of agreement in nursing theory development. *Advances in nursing science,* 3, 1 (October 1980):1–7.

Ford, D., and Urban, H. *Systems of psychotherapy—a comparative study.* New York: John Wiley & Sons, 1963.

George, Julia. *Nursing theories the base for professional practice.* Englewood Cliffs, NJ: Prentice-Hall, 1985.

Glasser, W. *Reality therapy: A new approach to psychiatry.* New York: Harper & Row, 1975.

Gordon, Marjory. *Manual of nursing diagnosis.* New York: McGraw-Hill, 1985.

Havens, L. Toward a general theory of therapy. *The Psychiatric Hospital,* 14, 4, 1983:213–217.

King, Imogene. *Toward a theory of nursing: general concepts of human behavior.* New York: John Wiley & Sons, 1971.

King, Imogene. *A theory of nursing—Systems, concepts, process.* New York: John Wiley & Sons, 1981.

Lancaster, J. *Community mental health nursing an ecological perspective.* St. Louis: Mosby, 1980.

Levine, Myra. *Introduction to clinical nursing,* 2d ed. Philadelphia: F.A. Davis, 1973.

Little, D., and Carnevelli, D. *Nursing care planning,* Philadelphia: Lippincott, 1976.

Loomis, M., and Horsley, J. *Interpersonal change—a behavioral approach to nursing practice.* New York: McGraw-Hill, 1974.

Mann, James. The core of time-limited psychotherapy: Time and the central issue. In *Forms of brief therapy* (Budman S., ed.). New York: Guilford Press, 1981: 25–43.

Mitchell, P.H. *Concepts basic to nursing.* New York: McGraw-Hill, 1973.

Nightingale, Florence. *Notes on nursing.* New York: Dover, 1969.

Orlando, Ida. *The dynamic nurse patient relationship: Function, process and principles.* New York: G. Putnam's Sons, 1961.

Pardes, H., and Pincus, H. Brief therapy in the context of national mental health issues. In *Forms of brief therapy* (Budman S., ed.). New York: Guilford Press, 1981:7–21.

Peplau, H. *Interpersonal relations in nursing,* New York: G. Putnam's Sons, 1952.

Perls, Fredrick. *Gestalt therapy verbatim.* New York: Bantam, 1971.

Rogers, Carl. *Client centered therapy,* Boston: Houghton Mifflin, 1951.

Rogers, Martha. *The theoretical basis of nursing.* Philadelphia: F.A. Davis, 1970.

Roy, Callista. *Introduction to nursing: An adaptation model.* Englewood Cliffs, NJ: Prentice-Hall, 1976.

Smith, M.L., Glass, G., and Miller, T. *The benefits of psychotherapy.* Baltimore: John Hopkins Press, 1980.

Stanton, M. Nursing theories and the nursing process. In *Nursing theories the base for professional practice* (George, J., ed.). Englewood Cliffs, NJ: Prentice-Hall, 1980:213–217.

Strupp, H.H.., Hadley, S.W., and Gomes-Schwartz, G. *Psychotherapy for better or worse: The problem of negative effects in psychotherapy.* New York: Jason Aronson, 1977.

Wallace, Edwin. *Dynamic psychiatry in theory and practice.* Philadelphia: Lea and Febiger, 1983.

Wiedenbach, Ernestine. *Clinical nursing a helping art.* New York: Springer, 1964.

Wilson, G.T. Behavior therapy as a short term therapeutic approach. In *Forms of brief therapy* (Budman, S., ed.). New York: Guilford Press, 1981:131–166.

Yura, H., and Walsh, M. *The nursing process: Assessing, planning, implementing and evaluating,* 2d ed. New York: Appleton-Century-Crofts, 1973.

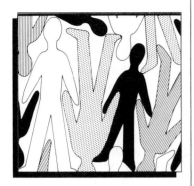

3

Cultural and Socioeconomic Dimensions of Mental Health

Kathryn Govaerts

Learning Objectives

Upon completion of this chapter, the reader will be able to:

1. Formulate a definition of multicultural nursing.

2. Discuss Leininger's and Kluckhohn's theoretical contributions to the area of multicultural nursing.

3. Describe cultural or socioeconomic characteristics for each group discussed that may necessitate a modification of the nursing care plan designed for a member of that cultural group.

4. Recognize possible limitations of existing assessment instruments and norms when evaluating minority clients.

5. Apply the *Model for Multicultural Nursing* to an individual client.

Nurses acknowledge that the biological, psychological, and social aspects of the client must all be considered in planning care. Cultural affiliation, however, is frequently relegated to the "nice to know" instead of the "necessary to know" category of data. Because culturally transmitted values and beliefs are at the very core of life choices, their contributions cannot be overstated. An awareness of the client's cultural heritage is, therefore, fundamental to nursing care in any setting, whether in exotic places, urban centers, or rural communities.

This chapter stresses the value to both the nurse and the client of including a cultural component in the nursing plan. Theoretical contributions by Madeline Leininger and Florence Kluckhohn demonstrate the importance of culturally based observations. Brief, general sketches of four American minority groups are provided as a springboard for further study. A model using the nursing process and emphasizing cultural components is presented.

☐ *Definitions*

Culture in its broadest sense includes all human deeds. It provides the guidelines for the individual's living activities such as work, rites of passage, courtship, marriage, and child rearing. Culture sets the norms for such group activities as socializing, governing, waging war, or winning peace. Beliefs about health, illness, language, and economic status are determined by the culture in which they are found. Art, music, drama, dance, and worship are important components of culture. The cultural collage gives a group its identity and distinctive place among others.

A narrower definition of culture is a people's way of life. It may refer to a large group (e.g., the American people) or a small tribe (e.g., the Maasi of East Africa). Culture is learned from the group socializers—parents, teachers, peers, or elders—who stress key beliefs that are essential to the existence and identity of the group. The ancient Egyptians' lifetime preparation for the journey to the afterlife, and the Maasi's reverence for their age groups, are examples of culturally determined values that contribute to a group's identity.

Social-economic status (SES) is the rank in a societal group determined by the amount of material assets the individual possesses. These include the tangible wealth of money and property recognized as valuable by the particular cultural group. SES is also determined by intangibles such as power, position, prestige, and freedom from the society's menial work. *Poverty* is a term describing a group's lowest level in the socioeconomic strata.

Anthropology is the study of humans that combines the scientific and humanistic approaches to describe the origin and development of races, customs, and beliefs. *Anthropologists* study people's biological, social, and behavioral development and adaptation to a wide variety of environments.

Minority literally means less than half of the whole, but it has come to refer to a societal group that differs from the dominant one. There may be racial minorities whose physical characteristics vary from the dominant group. Ethnic minorities may be dissimilar in certain cultural practices such as dress, language, life-style, or religion. Religious minorities may be unique in their choice of a deity and rituals of worship. Minority status can be assigned by gender, age, or socioeconomic class as well. It is important to note that at times the minority group may have greater numbers but retains its minority status because it has less power than the dominant group.

☐ *Theoretical Contributions*

Recognizing humans as biopsychosocial beings, nurses have long attempted to give care that responds to all three dimensions. Since the 1950s Dr. Madeline Leininger, a nurse-anthropologist using the anthropological and scientific-humanistic approaches, has emphasized the importance of considering the cultural dimension. During the 1960s cross-cultural nursing gained recognition as a legitimate area of nursing education. Dr. Leininger (1977) stresses the value of a systematic and comparative study of all world cultures in regard to health-illness beliefs, values, and behaviors.

The value of the anthropological approach has pertinence to the student of cross-cultural nursing because of its identification and study of people's successful and unsuccessful adaptation to physical, biological, social, and cultural environments. Anthropological study seeks to identify and clarify values, to discuss methods of assimilating and adapting to neighboring groups, and to delineate patterns of behavior. Anthropological studies may also reveal biological variations. Physical properties such as the characteristics of ear wax; the numbers of apocrine glands; and eye, ear, and nose structure have unique cultural distributions. The knowledge about susceptibility to certain conditions such as sickle cell anemia and increased keloid formation in members of the Negro race is important information gained through anthropological investigations. To give culturally appropriate and competent care, the nurse should actively seek authoritative information about various groups through such courses as anthropology and cross-cultural nursing.

Florence Kluckhohn's work on value orientations (1976) suggests dimensions that may be used to describe cultural variations. An awareness of the dimensions will sensitize the nurse to client behaviors and statements that provide important assessment data and suggest areas of inquiry throughout the nurse-patient interaction. The dimensions include: (1) concept of humanity, (2) ideas about humans' relationship to nature, (3) time perspective, (4) activity orientation, (5) decision-making patterns, and (6) importance of possessions (Kluckhohn, 1976).

A cultural group may view the human character as intrinsically good, basically evil, neutral, or perfectable. A client who believes man is intrinsically good thinks there is little need for strict discipline since humans want to do the best. The Rogerian theory of psychotherapy is an example of such an orientation. In contrast, one who believes humans are basically evil will insist on constant vigilance, tight behavioral controls, and punishment for infractions of the rules. Guilt figures prominently in this schema, which is illustrated by Freudian psychoanalytic theory. One who sees humans as perfectable holds to the idea that man can and will learn to adapt and change. Cognitive and behavioral psychological theories are predicated on this view of human nature.

The concept of humans' relationship to nature varies from a belief at one extreme that man dominates nature and at the other, is dominated. Man and nature in balance would be found near the midpoint. The client who sees man subjugating nature depends on science and technology for solutions to most problems. Such a stance contrasts with the more fatalistic, nature-dominant view that denies humans any power to influence events in their lives. Nature and man in harmony is suggested by ecological concern, preventive health care, and the Asian view of Yin and Yang.

A culture frequently adopts a time perspective which may be past, present, or future in orientation. Those with a past orientation value and rely on tradition; the elderly are revered. Present orientation if focused on "today." Resources are used as they become available in the "eat, drink and be merry for tomorrow we may die" mode. A group that holds a future orientation understands today's discomforts and strivings as worthwhile for later development. Saving money, pursuing education, and planning for tomorrow are all highly valued.

Activity orientation describes the sense of self as being, becoming, or doing, The client with a being orientation lives in the present and savors the moment—a philosophy exemplified in Gestalt psychotherapies. The becoming orientation focuses on self-development and self-actualization. The humanist psychotherapies of Carl Rogers and Abraham Maslow are based on the strong human propensity for self-actualization. The doing orientation focuses on the individual's behavior and accomplishments, one example of which is seen in the Puritan work ethic.

The pattern of decision making preferred by a culture may range from an individual's taking responsibility for the decision to decisions being made in a collateral or lineal fashion. The individual decision maker takes full responsibility for both the decision and its consequences and hence is often subject to greater stress when making a choice. Collateral decision making involves discussion of the problem's pros and cons with the family and perhaps even the community. Suggestions are welcomed, and conclusions are frequently reached by consensus. Lineal decision making is based on a hierarchy with authority vested in traditional roles. For example, certain family decisions regarding marriage, employment, and use of resources may be made by the father while most of the decisions about child care and family health will be made by the mother. A lineal decision maker prefers to be told what to do and when and how to do it when entering the health care system. However, the difficulties that one of high status in a particular group may have accepting directions from one of perceived lower status quickly become apparent.

The importance of possessions in a culture may vary along a continuum with a spiritual focus at one extreme and a materialistic one at the other. The client with a strongly spiritual focus does not value material possessions and frequently lives a very spartan existence. This contrasts with the ultramaterialistic orientation that prizes the accumulation of wealth and goods. Theoretically it is possible to attain a satisfactory balance between the two extremes in which one's own needs are met while demonstrating a concern for the unmet needs of others.

In applying the value orientation dimensions to client care it is important to be cognizant of the culture's dominant values—by listening to client comments, observing client behaviors, and asking appropriate, culturally based questions in the context of the nurse-patient relationship. It is also important to remember that cultures have accepted, in fact desired, ranges within the value structure. Such variation is to be differentiated from cultural deviance which is condemned by the group.

■ *Point of Emphasis*

The hypothesis about a client's value orientation must be built on as many pieces of data as possible.

PROFILES OF FOUR MINORITY GROUPS

Planning, implementing, and evaluating mental health care for the client whose cultural heritage differs from the nurse's requires an extra measure of effort. First the nurse must be aware of what her own cultural values are and how they interact with those of the client. Above all the nurse must guard against an ethnocentric point of view that pronounces her culture superior. Second, the nurse must actively seek authoritative information about the client's cultural values and preferences. While the most obvious source of such data is the client, further information may be gained from other members of the cultural group. The bicultural nurse is a rich source of information in planning for culturally relevant mental health care. Formal study of the culture in anthropology and transcultural nursing courses is also extremely useful, and a great deal can be learned from an appreciation of a culture's art, drama, dance, literature, and music. Finally, the value of seeking an understanding of the client's cultural background is not limited to any particular nurse-client combination. Cultural data are equally valuable for the dominant group-minority dyad, as for the minority-minority pair.

The following vignettes are intended to provide a starting point for the exploration of the cultural variables found in four American minority groups.

The Asian American

Asian Americans immigrated primarily from China, Japan, Korea, the Philippine Islands, and Vietnam and tend to be geographically concentrated in Hawaii, California, and New York. The Chinese began to arrive in America in significant numbers in the 1840s. The immigrants accepted less desirable work and hence were not perceived as economic competitors. However, with the discovery of California gold, the Chinese became active in the gold fields and soon became the target of much anti-Chinese sentiment and violence. The anti-Chinese movement climaxed with the passage of the Chinese Exclusion Act of 1882 which prohibited Chinese immigration until 1892. That year the act was renewed, and in 1912 it was made permanent. The restrictions on immigration were frequently circumvented, but not without great sacrifice and family disruption (Kitano, 1969).

In the 1890s Japanese immigrants began arriving to work in American industries. However, their previous experience led them to seek agricultural work whenever possible—sound knowledge of farming coupled with great determination to do well made many Japanese highly successful farmers and gardeners. The repression and violence that had earlier been directed toward the Chinese was now redirected toward the Japanese leading the government to enter into a "gentleman's agreement" with Japan limiting immigration to America. In 1913 California passed the Alien Land Law which prohibited land ownership by noncitizens. Sue (1981) states that the "discrimination and prejudice toward the Japanese were most blatantly evident in the World War II incarceration of 110,000 Japanese Americans into concentration camps. The effects of this atrocity perpetrated against the Japanese, and its humiliating effects are still very much evident today in the suspiciousness that many Asians have for the American mainstream." In many respects the story of Filipinos, Koreans, and Southeast Asian refugees has varied little from the theme of exploitation and harassment (Sue, 1981).

The Asian American experiences several problems in daily living that are directly attributable to a cultural heritage. While the Asian values emotional restraint and allegiance to familial authority, the dominant American culture encourages the display of emotions and honors individuality. The Asian American is also readily identified by physical appearance and manner of speech which has led to stereotyping and discriminatory practices (Sue, 1981).

However, the Asian American's interaction with the dominant culture has been qualitatively different from that of other minority groups in at least four ways (Kitano and Matsushima, 1981). First, much of Asian immigration has been voluntary, with the possible exception of that by the recent Southeast Asian refugees. Second, the Asian groups have maintained their cultural identity in the new environment (except for the Japanese Americans who during World War II internment were forced to abandon Japanese ways). Third, the Asian immigrant has maintained strong bonds to the country of origin. Finally, most Asian Americans have successfully remained independent of federal government subsidy.

Although the Asian American groups are separate and distinctive, they do share some values and beliefs, a knowledge of which will prove useful in caring for these clients. According to Asian tradition a holistic view of humans is essential; body and spirit are one. Man's ideal state is a harmonious balance with nature. The family is the paramount social unit, with the father its undisputed head and vertical family relationships. Communication tends to originate with one of higher status—those of lower status are expected to speak only when spoken to. The family holds certain expectations for its members. Elders and ancestors are accorded great reverence. The son's first duty is to be a worthy son. Women are to be subservient and tend to the homemaking tasks that give comfort to the husband. The rules for the smooth functioning of the family are known and rigidly practiced. Self-control, restraint, and humility are taught early. Discipline is strict and administered by the father. Because individualism is subjugated in favor of the group, all efforts are directed at conducting one's life in ways that bring honor to the family unit. Most attempts at problem solving take place within the family group, and decisions are usually the result of family consensus. Privacy and confidentiality regarding intrafamilial communications are important, and there is great reluctance to discuss family affairs with outsiders.

Research by Sue and Sue (1971) and by Marsella, Kinzie, and Gordon (1971) indicates that physical complaints are more acceptable than psychological ones. Mental illness may be described in physiological terms (Dahl, 1983). Because of the stigma attached to mental illness, the patient may not reach the attention of the health care system until the symptoms are well advanced, and the family's tolerance is exhausted (Schlesinger, 1981).

The Asian client would prefer situations in which role expectations are clear and consistent with his cultural values. It may be difficult, for example, for an elderly male Asian client to comply with requests from a young female nurse; important directives may have to come from recognized authority figures. The Asian client will prefer interaction with the nurse in which privacy and confidentialty are assured and will be more comfortable with a communication style that allows for conversation about general topics before approaching the more personal and sensitive areas. Cultural norms may make the client reluctant to reveal personal data or to participate in group settings.

The Black American

Slavery left its indisputable mark on American history. Referring to the Black American, Sue states, "Few ethnic or racial minorities in American society have been so thoroughly blocked from having a constructive identity group formation, have been pressed to trust whites more than themselves, have had a value system imposed on them that so totally and forcefully undermined their self-esteem and their very existence" (Sue, 1981). Slavery brought Blacks to America against their will and then justified their oppression by promulgating ideas of Black genetic, mental, and moral inferiority while touting white superiority. Slavery essentially destroyed the family, the central unit of Black society. Following the Civil War, the great majority of slaves were illiterate, which provided a legal reason for separate schools, teachers, and curricula. The United States Constitution itself stated that the Black was to be counted as $3/5$ of a man and was taxable as property. Health care facilities carefully segregated black and white clients. There is abundant evidence of harsh treatment and highly inaccurate diagnoses of Blacks by health professionals and of the inappropriate care received as a result. By the 1950s there was evidence of a subtle shift to a more helping stance by the mental health professions caring for the Black client, and by the 1960s, with the civil rights movement gaining momentum, mental health care attempted to be more sensitive to the Black American's needs.

Black culture is highly heterogeneous with regional, socioeconomic, and individual differences, but all Blacks share historical and participational identities (Gordon, 1964). A shared history and some behavioral similarities can be identified as points of departure for further study. Black culture is people- rather than thing-oriented (Sue, 1981), and the family is clearly a focal point. While the mother is revered and frequently initiates communications chains, the final decision often comes from the father. The stereotype of a matriarchal society probably originated during slave days when family units were destroyed by separation of the salable males. Also, today more single families are headed by Black females than by white females (Gordon, 1979). The Black family includes a broad kin network whose opinions are valued and whose assistance is sought (Hayes and Mendel, 1973). There is a strong appreciation for generational boundaries and the acceptable behaviors of each. The Black family deemphasizes gender stereotypes. There is a tendency to avoid blaming mental illness on childhood events but to see present problems as being the result of situational and environmental variables (Sue, 1981). Religion traditionally plays a significant part in the daily life of the Black family, and a strong faith in God and a belief that He is concerned about each individual is instilled early.

The Black person places a great deal of importance on the nonverbal elements of communication. Verbal patterns may differ from those familiar to the non-Black nurse. For example, the words used may be the same, but the idiosyncratic meanings may be illusive. Neither eye contact nor nodding and smiling is essential to indicate the Black client is paying attention (Sue, 1981).

For the Black client, seeking assistance for physical problems is more acceptable than seeking psychological aid, and it is admirable to be able to cope alone with psychological dilemmas (Block, 1981). For this reason presenting physical complaints may really represent a masked request for psychological help. If help is requested openly, it comes from within the family system. Difficulties are more likely to be described by life examples than by lengthy psychological introspection. Problem solving tends to be action oriented so that the Black client may become impatient if he believes that nothing is actually happening to alleviate the problem at hand

(Block, 1981). When caring for the depressed Black client, it is helpful to know that while the usual affective changes of anorexia, insomnia, fatigue, and crying will be present, the Black client is more likely to be agitated and self-destructive (Poussaint, 1972). Awareness of the high national statistics for violent death of Black adolescents by accidents, homicide, and suicide is important in planning their care.

In caring for the Black client, it is imperative to recognize and acknowledge the issues surrounding race. It is the area in which the client's experience takes place, and to believe that color is not a factor is to deny a significant part of the person's being. At the opposite end of the continuum, care must be taken to avoid assigning all problems a racial origin. Further, the nurse must be careful to avoid making cultural generalizations based on experience gained in a personal relationship with one Black person or from the media alone.

The Native American

Anthropological evidence indicates that Native Americans settled the North American continent some 40,000 years ago, giving this group the distinction of being the country's oldest inhabitants. The decline of American Indian societies may be dated to the arrival of explorers, hunters, and trappers who introduced trade, disease, and alcohol. The Native Americans were frequently exploited by those seeking economic gain, and the United States government assumed little responsibility for fair treatment of the Indians. In fact, the government has a history of broken treaties, relocation marches, and severe punishment for those who tried to resist federal mandates.

The term American Indian describes hundreds of tribes in rural, urban, and reservation settings. The United States Bureau of Indian Affairs (BIA) recognizes 478 tribes, and there are many other groups who identify themselves as Indian but are not officially recognized as such (Trimble, 1981). Unlike other American minority groups, the American Indian has been given a legal definition. The BIA says that a Native American is one whose Indian blood quantum is at least one-fourth (Trimble, 1981). However, there are broad tribal variations on this qualifier. To be sure, the criterion of percentage of Indian ancestry is an inadequate measure that fails to consider the strength of the individual's allegiance to a Native American heritage. Also unlike the Asian, Black American, and Hispanic, the Native American is not always distinguishable by surname, physical appearance, or manner of speech. Therefore, a cultural assessment may be overlooked.

Byrde (1972) has attempted to contrast Native American and Anglo values, an effort that is valuable in sensitizing the mental health caregiver to values and beliefs that the client may hold. On Kluckhohn's time dimension, the Native American is present oriented. Today is to be savored in the belief that there will be time to complete unfinished tasks tomorrow. Tradition and elders are revered, and a client may be reluctant to disagree with one considered to have higher status. Therefore some clients may not overtly disagree with the nurse but neither will they comply with treatment regimens. The Indian seeks to live in harmony with nature, leaving things in their natural form and respecting animals as equals. Illness of any type is thought of as a disharmony with nature. The Native American places tribal and family concerns before self-interest; children are a gift to be enjoyed and shared with others. Generosity with possessions is honored. One acquires possessions to share them just as nature shares her abundance with all. Humility and cooperation are virtues.

Communication first requires being a perceptive listener to the message conveyed in words, in body language, and in silence. Too much talking may arouse suspicions. Communication style preference suggests that the best way to understand the Native American begins with careful listening. This listening may take place in many settings such as Indian homes, reservation cultural centers, and social gatherings. Indians dislike being stared at, so it is to be expected that the client will avert his eyes during conversation.

The Native American takes pride in being self-directed, a fact that the nurse must consider in collaborating with the client about his care. The Indian will appreciate a display of faith in his capabilities as well as brief, succinct suggestions for needed changes.

The realities of many Native American's lives all too frequently stand in stark contrast to the foregoing ideal cultural values. Suicides among southwestern and northwestern Indian tribes were studied by Santora and Starkey (1982). These authors found that completed suicides stem from social-cultural forces as well as intrapsychic ones. The data suggest that most suicide victims are "young single men who are in conflict with values, work, or significant others" (Santora & Starkey, 1982). Alcohol was involved in the majority of cases. An understanding of the individual's values and the dissonance produced by the conflict with the values of the dominant culture would be relevant to the nurse planning mental health care.

The American Indian child is another segment of the population demanding greater attention and resources from the mental health professions. There is evidence that, with the exception of children aged 5 to 9, the Native American child is at greater risk for suicide than is the non-Indian counterpart. By late adolescence, Indian girls are the group at highest risk for entering mental health treatment, and Indian adolescents demonstrate by nearly four times a greater risk for suicide than does the non-Indian adolescent. There are many social and environmental contributors to this unfortunate situation. Many Indian children must attend boarding schools, resulting in the lack of parental and extended family support. The social disorganization that accompanies the desperate poverty with which many Native Americans must cope is another important factor (Beiser and Attneave, 1982).

The Hispanic American

The word Hispanic designates people whose ancestors claimed Spain as their homeland. Spanish remains the preferred language and the Roman Catholic church the dominant religious institution of this minority group. Ruiz (1981) states that Hispanics, more than any other minority group, have retained their native language. For this reason the bicultural-bilingual Hispanic nurse has special contributions to make to the mental health team. There are several Hispanic subgroups that tend to be concentrated in certain geographic regions. For example, the Chicano, whose ancestors were Spanish immigrants arriving in the 1500s and native Mexican Indians, are concentrated in the southwestern part of the United States. Puerto Ricans live in greatest numbers in Connecticut, New Jersey, and New York. Florida has the highest population of Cubans. In a review of descriptive studies, Ruiz (1981) reveals that when compared to the general population, Hispanics more frequently are undereducated, low-income, blue-collar workers or unemployed urban dwellers.

Delgado (1983) describes the Hispanic value orientations using Kluckhohn's formulation. The

Hispanic is more present oriented and consequently prefers an immediate intervention for problems. The present-time orientation complements an activity preference for doing as exemplified by observable accomplishments. The Hispanic tends to see people as being subjugated by nature, which leads to a belief in metaphysical causes and cures for certain illnesses. Interpersonal relationships are based on a hierarchy and therefore tend to be lineal. The hierarchy places elders at the top with men ahead of women and children. Religious leaders, family heads, and certain community leaders are the authority figures whose advice once requested will most likely be followed.

Hispanic tradition is complex with family structure and sex roles being especially important (Padilla, 1981). Family includes the nuclear family and the extended family, as well as formalized kinship relationships. Because the family is of prime importance, the individual strives to behave in ways that bring it honor. The family is a haven that provides emotional and material support to its members. To seek help beyond its boundaries is a negative reflection of its functioning. Hispanic children are highly valued, and elders and family heads are treated with deference.

The Hispanic family has clearly defined gender roles for its members. Young men are given greater independence at an earlier age than young women and are expected to be achievers in the community. Tamez (1981) describes Hispanic sex roles and reports that the father/husband is the family head and community representative. Any misdeed of a family member reflects upon the father's authority. The mother/wife is responsible for the care of her husband, children, and home but the stereotype of passive subservience is inaccurate. The Hispanic family is child oriented, and gender roles are taught early. Parental relationships with young children are close and warm. However, the father tends to become more reserved with adolescents and young adults. The mother is expected to remain close to the children even after they have established their own homes.

The word *machismo* is frequently associated with the Hispanic male. What is less commonly described in the female analogue *hembra* (Tamez, 1981). The *machismo-hembra* combination represents reciprocal and complementary roles. Tamez describes some empirical observations of the characteristics of *machismo*. Positive attributions include being a competent provider, gentle to one's wife and children, and a responsible citizen. *Machismo* or *macho* also exemplifies masculine power and virility. The negative extremes of *machismo* are the exploitation of power, self-centeredness, and the use of violence.

Padilla (1981) describes another dimension that differentiates the Hispanic from the non-Hispanic client. *Personalismo* is a word that describes the Hispanic's preference for personalized attention when dealing with social institutions. For the Hispanic client handshakes and embraces are the norm, and less formal relations are preferred (Delgado, 1983). The Hispanic client can tolerate smaller social distance when interacting with another (Padilla, 1981). Eye contact is not necessary to insure the attention and should not be forced. Ruiz and Casas (1981) believe the Hispanic client prefers to deal with one problem and one solution at a time. Whenever possible it is most productive to use concrete rather than abstract requests (Delgado, 1983). Delgado also stresses the Hispanic's preference for being actively involved in his own care and the value of involving important family and community supports whenever possible.

■ Point of Emphasis

In multicultural nursing, effective interactions will integrate a knowledge about the client's dominant cultural values with his uniquely individual variations.

Minority Status by Virtue of Socioeconomic Status

It was suggested earlier that minority status may be conferred by reason of social-economic class and gender. The problems a client experiences that are directly attributable to a lack of money need to be included in a nursing assessment. It must be made clear that membership in the dominant group does not guarantee a comfortable standard of living any more than membership in the minority guarantees poverty-level existence. Nevertheless, a disproportionate number of minority members do fall at or below poverty levels.

Socioeconomic status has significant ramifications for the individual in the mental health system, as reported in the classic study by Hollingshead and Redlich (1958). The authors' study of the relationship of mental illness to social stratification supported the hypothesis that the prevalence of mental illness was significantly related to social class. The lower class had proportionately higher numbers of mentally ill than would be predicted by its representation in the total population. Social class was also shown to influence the type of psychiatric diagnoses made. The lower class had a proportionately higher incidence of psychotic disorders. Social class also greatly influenced the type of treatment received. Higher-class clients were more likely to receive psychotherapy and be treated by private practitioners.

Wills and Langner (1980) cite several studies describing variables that contribute to mental illness in the lower social-economic classes. Included are factors such as pervasive insecurity and uncertainty caused by a continual lack of money, a greater number of unsatisfactory and broken marriages, and a shortage of social supports. Measurable decreases in levels of self-esteem correlate with decrease in social class (Ilfeld, 1978).

Information on socioeconomic status has implications for the nurse planning care. Many useful interventions may be work related. The increased need for social support in the way of marriage and family counseling is an important consideration when planning holistically for a lower SES client. Alfred Adler's notion that the mentally ill are more accurately described as being discouraged has real applicability to the impoverished client. The caregiver must be aware of the potential values conflict with the middle-class work ethic. The nurse must examine personal ideas of getting, being, and remaining poor, and attempt to discriminate between her stereotypic thinking and the daily problems with which the poor must cope.

Minority Status by Virtue of Gender

Minority status by virtue of gender presents important considerations for the nurse who desires to see the changes accomplished in the treatment setting transferred to the world in which the client must function. Many of the issues facing female clients are also pertinent for female nurses who are practitioners in a predominantly female profession.

Women's generally unequal social and economic status is common knowledge. Women earn less money than their male counterparts in similar positions. Further, they are often clustered in occupations offering low pay and low prestige. There are innumerable problems associated with being a working woman. Seven of ten women on the job are faced with the probability of sexual harrassment (Gordon, 1980). Child care is seldom easily procured, and it is expensive. Many women are forced to work because of economic need, yet they are expected to maintain the same homemaking and child care standards with minimum support.

There are inconsistent standards by which women are judged to be mentally ill or healthy. A study by Broverman (1970) demonstrated that characteristics of a healthy adult woman as described by a group of psychotherapists more closely resembled those of a less healthy adult man. Further, when describing a genderless, healthy adult, the description was closer to that of the healthy man. Women tend to be overrepresented as clients in community and private mental health centers as well as in- and outpatient facilities, with the exception of Veterans Administration hospitals where women patients are almost nonexistent (Russo and Sobel, 1981). Women are the recipients of the majority of all psychotropic medications prescribed in the United States.

Socialization of women has led many to believe that they may gain status best through a dependent stance and a successful husband. The paradox in this belief is pointed out in work by Grove and Geerken (1977) that identifies the highest rate of mental illness as occurring in married women. The prevalence of domestic violence that results in physical and psychological abuse to a disproportionate number of females must also be recognized. Women tend to outlive their husbands, and constitute over 4/5 of the elderly population (65 and older) who live in poverty (U.S. Bureau of the Census, 1977). It is not surprising that depression, probably the most common mental illness in the United States, occurs twice as often in females as in males.

Those involved in the mental health care of women can greatly enhance the efficacy of care by familiarizing themselves with and applying the feminist philosophy. The nurse must acknowledge the feminist movement in the context of its historical significance. Goals of the psychiatric-mental health nurse will include increasing the female client's awareness of her potential to be autonomous and the limitations imposed by archaic sex roles. Treatment will focus on fostering the woman's belief in herself and increased autonomy as she becomes a discriminating consumer of mental health services.

☐ *Assessment of Diverse Cultural Groups*

The physical assessment of the minority client requires a sensitivity to findings that may be different from a textbook description but are entirely within normal limits for the particular group. In assessment of psychological norms, similar considerations apply. Psychological tests all too often were standardized on majority clients who probably have had more testing experience than minority members. There are other impediments to successful testing of the minority client. Language can be a barrier. The client's general use of words or phrases may be sufficiently different from the way they are used in the test resulting in erroneous responses. If English is the client's second language, or his reading level is low, it will be difficult to obtain valid test results. The tests may make use of culturally irrelevant situations and examples. Geometric shapes are familiar to the middle-class American, but are they relevant to the reservation-reared Indian or the Vietnamese immigrant?

The testing situation itself could create a problem. The examination procedure may involve prolonged interaction with a dominant group examiner who is perceived as threatening or indifferent. This creates sufficient anxiety to confound the results. In some cases scores may indicate maladjustment to the standardizing group, but this may be a completely erroneous representation of adjustment to the cultural subgroup. Valid test interpretation cannot proceed without knowledge about the cultural background of the client. Thus, the nurse must be wary of accepting reports based on universal standards, and must place the client's responses and test profiles in a cultural context. For example, did the client answer to be polite? Do the responses represent an attempt to emulate the dominant group or do they reflect the client's own cultural expectations?

Although standardized testing may be an obstacle to some minority clients, observation without cultural awareness is not the answer. Interviews and examination by a culturally ignorant nurse will lead to interpretation according to stereotypes, personal prejudices, and incorrect assumptions that can be extremely detrimental to the client.

☐ *Applying the Nursing Process to Multicultural Nursing*

By nature of its comprehensive approach to problem solving the nursing process lends itself well to the variations required by a unique cultural background. This process is illustrated in Model for Multicultural Nursing (Figure 3-1). Although each of the 13 steps in the diagram will be considered individually, in actual practice the cultural data are used in an integrated fashion.

ASSESSMENT ☐ The client-mental health nurse relationship is a dynamic one that is influenced by both parties. The first step in such an interaction is to create an atmosphere that will foster trust and build rapport. Because creating such a relationship may proceed slowly and with difficulty, a sincere effort to respect the values and preferences of the client must be put forth by the nurse. Simultaneously, the nurse must be aware of her own cultural heritage and how it may conflict with or complement that of the client. The nurse understands the impact that membership in a particular cultural group has both on the relationship and the client's receptivity to nursing interventions. It is important to remember that groups have room for variations in values and behaviors and that some spread on the cultural continuum is to be expected. While the client shares many characteristics with his cultural group, there are also many attributes that are unique to him. The nurse, therefore, must seek to know the client both as a group member and as a separate person.

The assessment process for the recent immigrant begins with understanding the client's reasons for relocating. For the involuntary immigrant the first step in planning care may well be an assessment of the grieving process, recognizing the losses incurred by leaving country, family, and friends. It is necessary to complete mourning the old before attachment to the new can commence. Recent immigrants may experience culture shock when they find that their previously successful social coping mechanisms are not work-

---

■ *Point of Emphasis*

Results of psychological testing must be integrated with a knowledge of the client's cultural heritage.

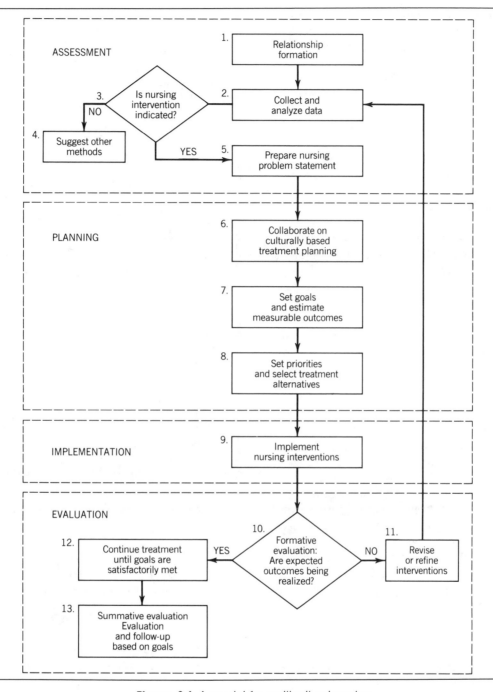

Figure 3-1 *A model for multicultural nursing.*

ing. This can result in a sense of confusion, disorientation, and despair that can erroneously be perceived as a more severe form of mental illness.

Once the client-nurse relationship is established, the next step is to obtain more specific information about the client's culture, basic values, and expectations. The nurse can begin by formulating a profile of the client's value orienta-

tions in several ways. Membership in a specific cultural group may suggest some starting points for inquiry. More particularly, the client's behavior and statements will begin to reveal the value orientations held. In addition to an awareness of the preferred values of the group and the specific behavior and comments by the client, the nurse may elicit more information by sensitive questions that allow the client to express personal preferences in a nonjudgmental atmosphere. The nurse will gather such data over time, being careful not to jump to unwarranted conclusions based on minimal information. Some possible questions for the values suggested by Kluckhohn's work are found in Table 3-1.

In addition to the more global information derived from value orientations, assessment will also include client-specific knowledge. For example, the language of first and second choice will be identified. The communication content found in gestures and nonverbal behaviors will be utilized.

Significant ceremonies, rituals, and customs play an important part in the initial assessment. Information about these events will give ideas regarding compatibility of the nursing care plan with cultural preferences and taboos. It becomes possible to avoid interactions that would be culturally offensive as well as to draw upon compatible cultural beliefs to enhance the success of the treatment.

As data about the client's values orientation are collected, trends will begin to emerge. Figure 3-2 is a pictorial display of two such trends and conveys a great deal of information at a glance. It is fair to say that Client A sees humans as basically good and trustworthy. He sees man coexisting with nature and adheres to a time orientation that is past focused. Therefore, Client A is likely to respect traditional beliefs, values, and role assignments. The client sees himself as striving to become a total person—a state not yet achieved. This client prefers a decision-making style that involves collaboration with significant family members and perhaps community representatives. Client A tends to devalue accumulating possessions but does not eschew them completely. What statements can be made about Client B?

A knowledge of folk healers and their traditional healing roles may be used to bridge some of the gap between the health care systems. Information about cultural causes and cures of illness gives clues for the most productive direction treatment should follow. Many folk explanations of illness are holistic in nature and incorporate both natural and supernatural causes and physical and psychological cures. To focus on only one of the aspects would be an unsatisfactory solution for a client with this orientation. One example of a holistic explanation of health and illness is the Hispanic belief that mental and physical health

TABLE 3-1 Assessing the Client's Value Orientations

The view held of humanity

1. If you could advise someone on the best way to rear a child, what would you say? How does this compare to the way in which you were reared?
2. What should be done about children who cause problems for their parents, teachers, or peers?
3. What should be done about adults who cause others problems?
4. Why do you think people become mentally ill? Physically ill?
5. What characteristics do you admire most in others?

Ideas about man's relationship to nature

1. Tell me about ways you and members of your family (a) stay healthy and/or (b) treat an illness.
2. When you become ill, what do you do first?

Time perspective

1. What are your plans for tomorrow? Next week? Six months? Next year? In five years?
2. When do you seek medical care?

Activity orientation

1. How would you describe yourself?
2. How do you think important others would describe you?
3. When you must solve a problem, what way(s) work best for you?
4. At the end of your life, how do you hope to be remembered?

Decision-making patterns

1. When a member of your family needs assistance, who decides what to do?
2. When important decisions must be made about allocating family resources, who makes them?
3. Who is responsible for passing on family traditions?

The importance of possessions

1. If you could give someone your most valued possession, who would that person be and what would you share?
2. What do you cherish most of all in life?
3. If you received a large sum of money, what would you do with it?

Adapted from Norris J., Kunes-Connell M., and Hartley R. Assessment Suggestions for applying Kluckhohn's scheme of value orientations.

requires a balance of warm and cold in all aspects of life. Many cultures have equivalents of the "evil eye" or powerful curses. Regardless of the efficacy of Western medicine, one believing himself to be the victim of an irreversible curse may be doomed

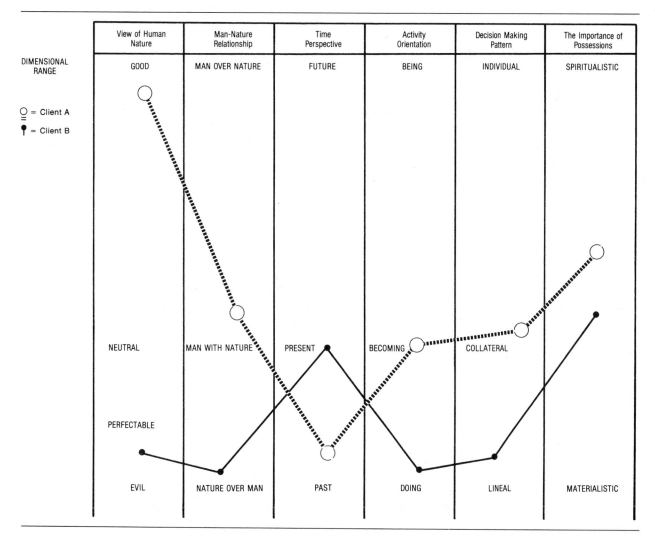

Figure 3-2 *Values dimension.*

unless the proper cultural cleansing ceremony can be performed.

The significance of family is another important area to be explored. For many groups the family is the prime support system, and to seek help beyond its boundaries is seen as a failure of the family unit. Actively involving the relatives acknowledges the client's cultural heritage and prepares for reentry into the family system once treatment is terminated. A knowledge of the importance of the extended family system and hierarchical structure is important information to predict the likelihood of compliance with the treatment regimen. For some, enlisting the assistance of a non-family member such as a revered elder or a religious leader may well be necessary to complete the treatment program. It is important to know something about how the

client views the nurse and what role expectations the client believes must be assumed to participate in the mental health system.

Finally, no assessment is complete without recognition of client strengths. No one is without some area of personal distinction, and acknowledging these positive client attributes is a powerful part of relationship formation.

During the nurse's assessment process, she will identify areas where more information is needed. The motivation to read, ask questions, and seek authoritative consultation will contribute to the validity of the assessment. The patience to make repeated observations of client behaviors and to place them in a cultural context will be very valuable in avoiding erroneous impressions that in turn could lead to ineffective treatment decisions. During all of the assessment process, the nurse's unconditional acceptance of the client, individually and as a member of the cultural group, must be genuinely and candidly communicated.

Self-Assessment □ Throughout the interactions with the minority client, the nurse makes a simultaneous self-assessment of personal ideas about the cultural group and is encouraged to make a conscious effort to name prejudices and stereotypic ideas that membership in a particular group implies. The nurse's willingness to seek consultation to clarify and resolve areas of misinformation will lead to personal and professional growth.

Problem Identification □ With the initial culturally based assessment made, the appropriateness of nursing interventions must be decided (Step 3). If the situation can be handled best by another discipline or agency, a referral is the intervention of choice (Step 4). If the analysis indicates the appropriateness of nursing interventions, the nursing problem statement is formulated making its cultural context clear (Step 5). Assessment is an ongoing process and pertinent information will continue to be added.

PLANNING □ Step 6 includes a deliberate attempt to collaborate with the client to include cultural components in the plan of care. When ceremonies, rituals, and customs are not specifically contraindicated by the prescribed treatment, they can be incorporated into the nursing plan. Religious observations and requirements should be considered. Willingness to withhold breakfast and early morning medications until after a visit from the priest is an indication that the client is seen in a holistic way. The diet may need some revision. For example, the Moslem prohibition against pork, the vegetarian's elimination of meat, and the Jewish requirement of kosher food must all be considered in planning. Planning includes attention to communication abilities. If an interpreter is needed, the nurse must ask for a translation of both words and meaning. The bilingual, bicultural interpreter is a definite asset.

When the assessment reveals that family and community are significant influences, their contributions are elicited. Perhaps the family could be encouraged to bring in traditional food or plan for ceremonies or religious observations. Some cultural groups such as Native Americans do not mind family members' being present in actual therapeutic sessions. Dress is another important element. For the ambulatory client, keeping personal clothing, significant items, or jewelry can provide security about one's identity in an alien setting.

The nursing care goals and estimates of measurable outcomes will be formulated in Step 7. The goals that are chosen will, in collaboration with the client, demonstrate an understanding of cultural roles and context. An explicit goal is essential for making probability statements for and evaluation of nursing outcomes. No culture is without goals based on its core values. The art of goal setting requires that: (1) the nurse know what the core cultural values are; and that (2) she use those values in planning for the client's health care.

In Step 8 treatment alternatives and their probabilities for success are studied in the cultural context. Priorities are selected and more culturally based information obtained about the acceptability of and likelihood for success of the nursing interventions. Expected outcomes will be known and measurable, and will include both behavioral and time components.

INTERVENTION IMPLEMENTATION □ Ideally, by Step 9 the relationship between nurse and client will be firmly grounded on a collaborative foundation. The nurse's credibility and sincerity are established, and the client's expectations for success are raised. The nurse continues to be aware of the client's perception of his difficulties as he shows an increasing understanding of the treatment, goals, and evaluation process. During the entire experience the nurse will be in an excellent position to be a client advocate to other members of the interdisciplinary team. Data about significant cultural values, the importance of cermonies, religious observations, food, or dress will be shared with others to enlist their cooperation in attending to the cultural needs of the client. In some instances the nurse will be required to intercede with administrators when the cultural aspects of the plan conflict with established institutional policies.

EVALUATION □ Evaluation is based on the expected outcomes defined (Step 7) when interventions were decided upon (Step 8). The nurse will make use of both formative and summative types of evaluation. Formative evaluation (Step 10) includes decisions about the degree to which the outcomes are being achieved. Such assessments are made at relatively close intervals throughout the treatment process. Summative evaluation takes place at the close of treatment and makes an assessment of the efficacy of care based on the designated goals.

In addition to formative and summative evaluation, evaluation of various patient domains is also in order. Included are the psychomotor or activity, cognitive or thinking, and affective or feeling domains.

Psychomotor evaluation will note changes in motor activity. For example, the pacing found in high anxiety states may be quieted, or the previously depressed client may appear more animated. Participation in the therapeutic milieu within the cultural parameters defined during the assessment process may be observed. For instance, an American Indian would not be expected to display the same amount of self-disclosure in the group setting as some of the Caucasian participants. Revealing family problems may not be appropriate for the Asian or Black client. Thus the degree of involvement is evaluated in both the therapeutic and the cultural context.

Cognitive evaluation includes an assessment of the client's level of understanding that integrates the cultural and nursing points of view regarding the present illness. There is no value judgment of the one best view but rather an appreciation of its usefulness in the more expanded world in which the client will live. Cognitive evaluation also appraises the extent to which the client understands further treatment requirements regarding medication, return visits, and health maintenance behaviors.

Affective evaluation assesses the feeling level variables. The sense of confidence in the therapeutic milieu, agency, and the nurse as a helping person is an affective measurement to be considered. The client's willingness to take risks working toward increased mental and physical health as described in the cultural context is another affective component. The goal is to maintain the cultural identity that is most productive and satisfying for the individual.

The nurse will ask how well the expected outcomes are being realized by considering the multiple evaluative aspects of formative and summative evaluation, paying attention to the psychomotor, cognitive, and affective domains. If the outcomes are not being realized, the nurse will diagnose where the breakdown is occurring (Step 11). To do so, additional data collection and analysis may be required and steps in the nursing process rethought with additional information. If the evaluation reveals that the outcomes are indeed being realized, the plan continues to be im-

Case Study

As discussed, the Model for Multicultural Nursing presents a way to incorporate cultural data into the nursing care plan. Lack of such information can have far-reaching and damaging effects as illustrated by the following case history. Joey, a Native American, was eight years old when he was referred to a children's psychiatric hospital because of "aggressive and unmanageable behavior and communication difficulties" at his boarding school. While he was living at home the previous year, his school attendance had been very sporadic so there was no useful school history to compare with the present.

On admission Joey was all that the advance publicity had promised. He was a fighter from the first minute, and the staff had minimal success making their wishes known. Because the nurse responsible for Joey's care believed she needed some important data that could be provided only by a family member, she and a social worker paid a visit to Joey's grandmother's home. It was located a long way from the nearest town on rutted roads and across fields, the two professionals followed such instructions as "left at the broken post and right at the cow's skull." The aged grandmother was initially frightened by her two visitors, but once assured that they came on Joey's behalf she gave invaluable information about her grandson. Both parents had died before Joey was three, and the grandmother had loved and cared for him in her home where the tribal language was predominant. While she provided a loving home, it was a primitive one without running water, electricity, or floors. Joey's attendance at school had been sporadic, and his grandmother instructed him in the ways of his people. When it became apparent that more consistent schooling was needed, Joey had begged his grandmother to hide him so he would not have to leave her alone. He was convinced that in his absence she would become sick and would die.

It became apparent the Joey's "communication difficulties" were in part the result of a lack of a working knowledge of English. His aggressive behavior was reframed as a child's attempt to cope with his great fear that his beloved grandmother would die unless he misbehaved enough to be sent home. The nurse asked the grandmother to choose something that could be taken back to Joey, and she selected a headband which was to become Joey's hallmark. The grandmother also described Joey's typical diet and his favorite foods. Consultation with Native American professionals at the hospital contributed additional useful data as the nursing care plan took form.

plemented as designed (Step 12). When treatment goals are satisfactorily met from both the nurse's and the client's points of view, the client will be ready to exit the system. Summative evaluation (Step 13) is now useful to summarize the encounter and identify both areas of strength and potential pitfalls in the plan. Follow-up goals emphasizing health maintenance behaviors are also included.

While Joey's story may be extreme, it is based on fact and exemplifies the need to seek out cultural information. Without such data Joey would have continued to be seen as aggressive and unmanageable. Certainly several other institutions' attempts to fit him into the white child's mold had failed and only escalated his outbursts. It was the nurse's desire to understand Joey's behavior in its cultural context that was the first step in reaching an extremely troubled boy. The psychiatric-mental health nurse is in a key position to originate and coordinate culturally based care that will create an environment in which the client may successfully learn skills that will foster the ability to live life to the fullest.

■ Enrichment Activities

You have been assigned to be Joey's primary nurse. Using the *Model for Multicultural Nursing*, formulate a nursing care plan for Joey.

DISCUSSION QUESTIONS

Assessment

Step 1: Relationship formation

Step 2: Collect and analyze data

> What is the traditional relationship of your cultural group to that of your client's?
>
> How will you introduce yourself? What nonverbal behaviors will be important?
>
> What culturally based social conventions will be especially important to observe?
>
> How will you capture Joey's interest and cooperation?
>
> Some of your preliminary observations include the fact that Joey is eating very little of what he is served. He has taken

none of the prescribed medication and was uncooperative during the admission laboratory procedures. Joey has refused to take a tub bath, and is reported to be awake every time the night nurse enters his room. After five days at school, the teacher reports that Joey is aggressive when approached by other children and does not respond to her instructions.

> What provisions will you make for communicating, since Joey's primary language is not English?
>
> What hypotheses can you make regarding Joey's beliefs about health? Illness?
>
> Will you involve others from Joey's family and/or community in his care? Who will they be? What do you hope each one can contribute to Joey's care?
>
> What other sources of information can you utilize to increase your fund of knowledge about Joey's cultural and social-economic group?
>
> What are your personal biases as you interact with Joey and members of his family and community?
>
> What strengths does Joey have that can be utilized in this situation?
>
> How would a values orientation profile like the one in Figure 3-2 look for Joey?

Step 3: Are nursing interventions indicated for Joey?

Step 4: If NO . . .

> What referrals/suggestions can be made? Support your decision with data. What is next for Joey?

Step 5: If YES . . .

> What nursing problem statements can you make regarding Joey's situation?

Planning

Step 6: Collaborate on a culturally based treatment plan

> What rituals, taboos, and/or ceremonies will be considered when planning for Joey's hospital stay?
>
> What considerations can be made concerning food, dress, and religious services for Joey?

Are you and Joey communicating accurately? If not, what plans do you have to increase the accuracy of your exchanges?

Step 7: Set goals and estimate measurable outcomes

Write the nursing goals and name possible outcomes for each one.

Step 8: Set goal priorities and select treatment alternatives

Name possible cultural and social-economic interferences and enhancers for each goal.

Implementation

Step 9: Implement nursing interventions

Describe the steps by which you will implement the selected nursing interventions for Joey.

Describe your role as Joey's advocate to other members of the treatment team and the administration.

Evaluation

Formative. During the next three months you observe that Joey has gained eight pounds, his hair is glossy, and his skin smooth and clear. Joey sleeps approximately six hours per night but is still awaking before the other children do. His hygiene is appropriate for his age. In school, Joey's overall performance is about what the average child would accomplish during the second grade, fourth month. Joey has to be reminded to remain in his seat approximately four times per school period as opposed to fifteen when he first began attending school. He is able to concentrate on his school work as long as 10 minutes at a time. His admission "on task behavior" was 3 to 4 minutes. In general, Joey does not initiate contact with members of the staff, but he does respond when people seek him out.

Step 10: Are expected outcomes being realized? Which ones are not?

Step 11: If No . . .

Explore possible reasons for each and revise or refine those outcomes that are currently unsatisfactory.

Evaluate Joey's psychomotor, cognitive, and affective domains. How does each compare to admission levels? Is the change indicative of positive growth or merely of passive compliance?

Step 12: If positive growth is indicated . . .

What behaviors are necessary for the continuation of progress toward the desired nursing goals by Joey? By you?

Summative. Following 9 months of hospital treatment, Joey's weight is within the normal range for his age and height. His general physical health and hygiene are good. He is sleeping an average of 7 hours per night. In school, his performance resembles that of the average third grader in the fourth month. His aggressive outbursts average three per week and are principally verbal. Joey is able to work at his desk on a specific task at intervals that are slightly shorter than his classmates.

Joey seems eager to spend time with you. In fact, extra time with you in the play yard is an incentive to keep his room in presentable condition. Joey has not shared his ideas about either the past or future but keeps his conversations rather straightforward and here and now.

During the final 2 weeks of Joey's stay, you observe that he seems more restless than usual, he is concentrating less on his school work, and is waking 3 hours earlier in the morning. Joey's appetite has decreased, but he has lost no weight. When you invited him to go to the play area, Joey declined.

While you are helping Joey pack his belongings for his dismissal, he presents you with a gift he has made and asks if you will write him a letter when he is home.

Step 13: Evaluation and follow-up based on the nursing goals

Following Joey's dismissal, write a summary of the nursing care plan and identify areas of strength and potential pitfalls.

What health maintenance behaviors do you suggest for Joey?

What are your views of Joey's cultural group? How do they compare to your ideas at the outset of Joey's hospitalization?

■ *Recommended Readings*

Kluckhohn, F. Dominant and variant value orientations. In *Transcultural nursing: a book of readings* (Brink, F., ed.). Englewood Cliffs, NJ: Prentice-Hall, 1976, 63–81. This chapter provides a comprehensive explanation of Kluckhohn's dominant and variant value orientations and makes application of these values to various groups.

Leininger, M. Cultural diversities of health and nursing care. *Nursing clinics of North America.* 12,1 (March 1977) 5–17. Dr. Leininger's article is based on the premise that nursing service falls short of being comprehensive if the cultural background of the client is overlooked. She carefully defines transcultural nursing and explores the meaning and significance of cultural diversity. The article concludes with descriptions of common pitfalls in cross-cultural interactions.

Sue, D.W. *Counseling the culturally different: Theory and practice.* New York: John Wiley & Sons, 1981. This book first prepares the reader by an introduction to the pertinent issues and concepts in cross-cultural counseling. A second section describes interactions with four specific minority groups written by experts in each area. Part three presents excerpts from actual cross-cultural exchanges.

■ *References*

Beiser, M, and Attneave, C. Mental disorders among native American children; rates and risk periods for entering treatment. *American journal of psychiatry*, 139, 2 (February 1982) 193–198.

Block, C.B. Black Americans and the cross-cultural counseling and psychotherapy experience. In *Cross-cultural counseling and psychotherapy* (Marsella, A.J., and Pedersen, P.B., eds.). New York: Pergamon Press, 1981.

Broverman, I.K., Broverman, D.M., Clarkson, F.E., Rosenkrantz, P.S., and Vogel, S.R. Sex role stereotypes and clinical judgements of mental health. *Journal of consulting and clinical psychology*, 34, 1, 1970:1–7.

Byrde, J.F. *Indian students and guidance.* Boston: Houghton Mifflin, 1972.

Dahl, J. Transcultural communication on depression with Chinese nurses and physicians. *Journal of psychosocial nursing and mental health services*, 21, 2 (February 1983).

Delgado, M. Hispanic natural support systems: Implications for mental health services. *Journal of psychosocial nursing and mental health services*, 21, 4 (April 1983).

Gordon, M. *Assimilation in American life.* New York: Oxford University Press, 1964.

Gordon, N.M. Institutional response: The federal income tax system. In *The subtle resolution: Woman at work* (Smith, R.E., ed.). Washington, D.C.: Urban Institute, 1979.

Gordon, S.Y. Occupational hazards include sexual harrassment. *Jobs watch*, 1, 2, 1980:12–13.

Grove, W.R., and Geerken, M.D. The effects of children and employment on the mental health of married men and women. *Social forces*, 56, 1977:66–76.

Hayes, H.C., and Mendel, C.H. Extended kinship relations in Black and white families. *Journal of marriage and the family*, 35, 1973:51–56.

Hollingshead, A., and Redlich, F. *Social class and mental illness.* New York: John Wiley & Sons, 1958.

Ilfeld, F.W., Jr. Psychological status of community residents along major demographic dimensions. *Archives of general psychiatry*, 35, 1978:716–724.

Kitano, H. *Japanese-Americans: The evolution of a subculture.* Englewood Cliffs, NJ: Prentice-Hall, 1969.

Kitano, H., and Matsushima, N. Counseling Asian Americans. In *Counseling across cultures* (Pedersen, P.P., Draguns, J.G., Lonner, W.J., and Trimble, J.E., eds.). Honolulu: The University Press of Hawaii, 1981.

Kluckhohn, F. Dominant and variant value orientations. In *Transcultural nursing: A book of readings* (Brink, F., ed.). Englewood Cliffs, NJ: Prentice-Hall, 1976:63–81.

Leininger, M. Cultural diversities of health and nursing care. *Nursing clinics of North American*, 12, 1 (March 1977) 5–17.

Marsella, A.J., Kinzie, D., and Gordon P. Depression patterns among American college students of Caucasian, Chinese, and Japanese ancestry. Paper presented at conference on Culture and Mental Health in Asia and the Pacific, Honolulu, Hawaii, March 1971.

Norris, J., Kunes-Connell, M., and Hartly, R. Kluckhohn's schema of value orientations: assessment suggestions. Manuscript, Creighton University, Omaha, Nebraska, 1983.

Padilla, A.M. Pluralistic counseling and psychotherapy for Hispanic Americans. In *Cross-cultural counseling and psychotherapy* (Marsella, A.J. and Pedersen, P.B., ed.). New York: Pergamon Press, 1981.

Poussaint, A.F. *Why Blacks kill Blacks.* New York: Emerson Hall, 1972.

Ruiz, R.A. Cultural and historical perspectives in counseling Hispanics. In *Counseling the culturally different: Theory and practice* (Sue, D.W., ed.). New York: John Wiley & Sons, 1981.

Ruiz, R.A., and Casas, J.M. Culturally relevant and behavioristic counseling for Chicano college students. In *Counseling across cultures* (Pedersen, P.P., Draguns, J.G., Lonner, W.J., and Trimble, J.E., eds.). Honolulu: The University Press of Hawaii, 1981.

Russo, N., and Sobel, S. Sex differences in the utilization of mental health facilities. *Professional psychology,* 12, 1, 1981:7–19.

Santora, D., and Starkey, P. Research studies in American Indian suicides. *Journal of psychosocial nursing and mental health services,* 20, 8, August 1982.

Schlesinger, R. Cross cultural psychiatry: The applicability of western Anglo psychiatry to Asian Americans of Chinese and Japanese ethnicity. *Journal of psychosocial nursing and mental health services,* 19, 9, September 1981.

Sue, D.W. *Counseling the culturally different: theory and practice.* New York: John Wiley & Sons, 1981.

Sue S. and Sue D.W. The reflection of culture conflict in the psychological problems of Chinese and Japanese students. Paper presented at the American Psychological Association Convention, Honolulu, 1971.

Tamez, E.G. Familism, machismo and child rearing practices among Mexican Americans. *Journal of psychosocial nursing and mental health services,* 18, 9, September, 1981.

Trimble, J.E. Value differentials and their importance in counseling American Indians. In *Counseling across cultures* (Pedersen, P.P., Draguns, J.G., Lonner, W.J., and Trimble, J.E., eds.). Honolulu: The University Press of Hawaii, 1981.

U.S. Bureau of the Census. Current population reports: characteristics of the population below the poverty level, 1975. Washington, D.C.: U.S. Government Printing Office, 1977.

Wills, T.A., and Langner, T.S. SES and stress. In *Handbook on stress and anxiety* (Kutash, I.L., Schlesinger, L.B., and Associates, eds.). San Francisco: Jossey-Bass, 1980.

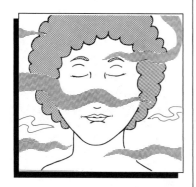

4

Self-Awareness: Basis for Personal Development and Practice

Karolyn Lusson Godbey

Learning Objectives

Upon completion of this chapter, the reader will be able to:

1. Define self and self-awareness.

2. Define three components of self.

3. Describe at least one method of cognitively increasing self-awareness.

4. Describe at least one method of affectively increasing self-awareness.

5. Describe one method for clarifying beliefs, attitudes, and values.

6. List three reasons for the necessity of developing self-awareness before empathy.

7. Describe five components of empathy.

8. List three consequences of empathy for the client.

Nursing is a health-related helping profession, and nurses are among the helpers who provide a service to clients. This service is centered on the nurse-client relationship, which is the basic building block of nursing. These two persons bring a full set of experiences, perceptions, and expectations to the relationship, and both sets influence the course of the relationship. Nurses traditionally have centered their attention on the client's influence on the interaction as if their own person was like a blank piece of paper, to be written on by the client, or a mirror meant only to reflect the client's values and behavior. Nurses may believe that their desire to help and care for the client is sufficient and that they need have no other concern about their own part in the nurse-client relationship. But this is not true. The nurse brings her own set of expectations, values, perceptions, and ways of relating to each nurse-client relationship and thus influences that relationship. She does not leave her beliefs and feelings at the nurses' station—they are present in the client's room with her whether she realizes it or not. Buber believed so strongly in the mutual relationship between two people that he had this to say about the basic word of I-You: "When one says You, the I of the word pair I-You is said, too" (Buber, 1970).

It seems significant that *nurse* is always the first word in the phrase "nurse-client or nurse-patient relationship." The nurse needs to be aware of the impact of her own feelings and values on the nurse-client relationship, and must provide for her own personal development *before* she can provide therapeutic care to her clients. She needs to give at least as much attention to her personal development as she does to the development of her technical skill, because the therapeutic tool most available and most valuable to her is herself.

The nurse can have a positive or a negative effect on the client's well-being. To develop a positive relationship, the nurse needs not only to be aware of her own thoughts, feelings, and values but also to have empathy for those of the client (Jourard, 1971; Rogers, 1980; Truax and Carkhuff, 1967). For example, in order to understand the client's state as a whole person, the nurse needs to gather information from his verbal self-disclosure as well as from the physical examination. If the nurse is empathic, the client is more likely to feel free to disclose personal information (Jourard, 1971). The positive value of an empathic mental health caregiver in helping a client maximize his potential is well established. Clients who feel cared about by their caregivers are more likely to get well. Numerous studies have shown that empathy is clearly related to positive client outcome. The evidence indicates that the more sensitively understanding the helper is, the more likely the client is to experience constructive learning and change (Bergin and Strupp, 1972; Kurtz and Grummon, 1972; Rogers, 1980; Truax and Carkhuff, 1967).

Nurses provide most of the direct client contact, especially in the hospital setting where they have round-the-clock responsibility for client care. How well nurses are able to care for and empathize with others depends on how much they know and care about themselves (Jourard, 1971). Krikorian and Paulanka (1982) found that increased self-awareness led to behavioral changes in student nurses, with consequent improvement in the quality of the patient care they provided during a psychiatric-mental health nursing rotation.

■ Point of Emphasis

Being aware of personal thoughts, feelings, beliefs, and values is a necessary step toward developing empathy for clients.

The purposes of this chapter are to help the student nurse understand the importance of and the relationship between self-awareness and empathy in the nurse-client relationship, to increase her self-awareness, and to increase her ability to experience empathy for her clients.

☐ Self-Awareness for Personal Development

DEFINITION OF SELF-AWARENESS

Self-awareness refers to having knowledge of self and entails working to bring the unconscious parts of self into consciousness.

Conscious attributes are those attributes of which one is aware. Consciousness is a prerequisite for using cognitive and affective processes for adapting to and making use of the environment. Unconscious attributes, those of which one is unaware, may sometimes be brought into awareness by turning one's attention to them. Thoughts that are stored in memory are examples of unconscious thoughts (thoughts not in awareness) that can be made conscious (brought into awareness) by turning attention to them. Conscious thoughts and feelings directly influence behavior and interactions with others. Unconscious thoughts and feelings influence behavior indirectly and may even be more powerful than conscious thoughts and feelings because they influence without self-knowledge and without control or self-regulation. For example, the nurse who is aware that the practice of abortion is in conflict with her beliefs can choose to work in an area, such as an orthopedic unit, where she is unlikely to encounter clients seeking abortions. Or, when confronted with a client who is about to have an abortion, she can suggest that another nurse care for the client, or can consciously separate her own beliefs from those of the client and attempt to listen to the client's description of her feelings and needs. The nurse who is unaware that abortion is in conflict with her beliefs will not make a conscious decision about her behavior and is more likely to behave in a way that is detrimental to the client. She may avoid the client completely or may tell her how "bad" she is for seeking an abortion.

To become self-aware the nurse must look at her own behavior and question the motivation for that behavior. If she examines feelings evoked by the prospect of changing that behavior, she may have some clues to the unconscious motivation. If the nurse can begin to examine the feelings she has when she thinks about caring for a client, she can begin to recognize her own values. Bringing these values into consciousness is the first step toward changing them. Thus, the process of self-awareness strives to bring into consciousness thoughts, feelings, beliefs, and values that have been unconscious. Self-awareness is the process of looking at one's own thoughts, feelings, beliefs, values, abilities, and behaviors in relation to past, present, and even future environment in an open and honest way. This means that the person has to acknowledge some of the feelings and thoughts that may have been denied and kept hidden over a period of years. It involves the need to look beyond the superficial explanation for behavior. In a word, self-awareness requires introspection— looking inside oneself as openly and honestly as possible.

DEFINITION OF SELF

The self refers to the totality of the person at any given moment, including both conscious and un-

conscious attributes. It is one's concept of identity as distinguished from other people and objects in the external world. It is also the esteem in which one holds oneself at any given time.

Self-concept and self-esteem evolve throughout life. They are constantly developing, emerging, and changing. They can be influenced by others and can be modified and changed by the person himself. For example, a girl who was told, as she was growing up, that she was not smart enough to succeed in college would probably develop a concept of herself that would include the belief that she was not smart. If she entered college, earned above-average grades, and received feedback from her instructors that she was intellectually capable, she could evaluate the discrepancy between her self-concept and the new feedback from her environment. She would then have the means to change her self-concept. A positive self-concept and high self-esteem enhance the ability to explore oneself in depth. Negative self-concept and low self-esteem inhibit the ability to develop self-awareness.

COMPONENT OF SELF

Man is a complex being. The psychological components of self are (1) the cognitive processes of thought, perception, and memory, (2) affect (feelings), and (3) beliefs, attitudes, and values. Each of these has both conscious and unconscious components that can be examined in various ways.

Cognition

As stated above, the cognitive processes include thought, perception, and memory. To think is to exercise mental faculties to form ideas, opinions, and beliefs, and to arrive at conclusions. It is a process of reasoning that implies a logical sequence of ideas, starting with what is known or assumed and advancing to a conclusion through inferences. Thought involves reflection—a turning back to a subject. Thought also involves the use of language with which to conceptualize ideas. Perception refers to the mental grasp of objects, situations, people, and so on in the environment, through the five senses of hearing, sight, touch, taste, and smell. Memory is the power or process of recalling what has been learned and retained. Thought, perception, and memory work together. Through perception new data are gathered from and about the world, through memory ideas are recalled, and through thought perceptions are conceptualized and analyzed.

Frequently cognition is confused with feeling. We say, "I think I am angry" when we mean, "I feel angry." Thought is involved in deciding what to study, and what dose of a medication to give, for example. Thoughts and perceptions can be consciously controlled or changed; they are subject to rational, logical processes. It is through cognition that the concept of the conscious and the unconscious, and the value of self-awareness can be understood.

Self-awareness can be fostered through rational thought processes. The nurse can apply the processes to herself as follows. The first step is to recognize your thoughts, beliefs, values, and feelings—listen to yourself. The second step is to examine your behavior and its consequences to yourself and to others. Is your behavior congruent with what you say you believe and feel? Do you receive the responses from others that you expect? What effect do you have on others? The third step is to accept yourself as you are, without judging yourself or your behavior as either "good" or "bad." Examine, instead, the reasons for your beliefs, values, and behaviors. Then you are free to decide if you are satisfied with yourself or if there are aspects you wish to change.

■ Point of Emphasis

Steps to self-awareness through rational thought processes:

1. *Identify your thoughts, feelings, beliefs, and values.*
2. *Examine your behavior and its consequences.*
3. *Accept responsibility for who you are and want to be.*

Assertiveness training can help to develop self-awareness by encouraging examination of personal behavior. One aspect that seems particularly helpful is the concept of "I-stands." Taking an I-stand requires that the person take responsibility for his own thoughts or feelings. Instead of saying "You make me angry," say "I am angry." Frequently when a nursing student is asked how she is feeling toward a client, she will reply in the following vein: "Well, you just get angry when he refuses to talk." (In context, "you" means "I.") Listen to yourself and others throughout one day and

count the number of times that you hear the pronouns *you* or *they* used when the person (you included!) means *I* (Alberti and Emmons, 1978).

If you discover aspects of yourself that you would like to change, thought-stopping and reframing are among the cognitive approaches that could be used to alter thinking patterns. Knowles discusses "thought-stopping"—the conscious effort of interrupting an unwanted thought and replacing it with a wanted thought (Howe, et al., 1984). For example, if your message to yourself is that you will not be able to finish an assignment on time, each time you have that thought you will interrupt it and tell yourself that you *will* be able to complete the assignment on time. Bandler and Grinder (1979, 1982), who teach neurolinguistic programming, describe its basis in *reframing*, a process in which an event is placed in a new frame so that it can be viewed in a different way. If you change the significance of an experience, your response to it will change. For example, suppose that you always plan to start writing assigned papers well ahead of the due date but never actually begin writing until a week or two before they are due. You always manage to turn the completed assignments in on time and earn an above-average grade. In spite of this, you spend much time berating yourself for not starting to work on the assignments sooner, telling yourself that you are disorganized and that you procrastinate. Reframing your response to this situation, you remind yourself that you do turn assignments in on time and do earn an above-average grade; therefore you know exactly how much time you need to complete assignments, you are well organized and do not spend unnecessary time working on the assignments. Thus reframing brings increased self-esteem and greater enjoyment of the time that is available both before and during the preparation of the assignments.

Thoughts and perceptions influence and are influenced by feelings, and are accompanied by feelings. In working toward self-awareness, thoughts and feelings must be distinguished.

Affect

Affect means feelings. Feelings may be painful, warning of a need or a threat, or they may be pleasurable, signaling satisfaction or relaxation. Feelings may be aroused quickly or develop slowly. They may be short-lived or of long duration. Feelings strongly influence thought and perception and, consequently, behavior. Feelings are not subject to rational thought processes. We can think about feelings, identify their sources, and consciously try to ignore them; yet feelings are not the creation of thought. Feelings are responses, and if ignored or denied they are not directly expressed but are expressed indirectly, either in immediate or subsequent behavior, or in physical symptoms such as headaches or gastrointestinal problems.

Feelings are neither right nor wrong, good nor bad; they simply *are*. Often we are told, "You shouldn't feel that way!" But feelings are not easily controlled. We continue to have the feelings we have been told not to have and think we should not have. The result often is a sense of guilt. Feelings need to be acknowledged, accepted, and understood rather than judged.

All feelings are acceptable; it is the behavior that results from the feelings that needs to be controlled. For example, to feel anger when you are fired is acceptable; to act out that feeling by hitting the boss is destructive and unacceptable.

> ### ■ Point of Emphasis
> *All feelings are acceptable; the behavior resulting from feelings is what must be controlled.*

To develop awareness of your feelings, you begin by identifying what your feelings are in a given situation. Listen to what others tell you. They may notice some signs of affect, such as a sad expression, of which you are unaware. Body language offers clues. For example, if the muscles of your neck and shoulder are tense, you may be feeling anger or anxiety even though you are not consciously aware of this. Relaxation techniques can be used to develop your self-awareness. These techniques teach you to "listen" to your body. A simplified version of one method of relaxation is presented here:

1. Sit in a comfortable position in a quiet place.
2. Close your eyes; put your hands at your sides.
3. Do not cross your legs.
4. Breathe deeply and slowly.
5. Tighten and relax the muscles, beginning at the top of your head. Continue tightening and relaxing, down to your toes.
6. Pay attention to the feelings and sensations you experience.
7. Try to "empty" your mind as much as possible, but give attention to those thoughts and feelings you do have, without dwelling on them.

Beliefs, Attitudes, and Values

Beliefs, attitudes, and values are thoughts that generally have strong feeling and judgment components attached to them. Since they are a combination of thought and feeling and since they influence behavior, sometimes directly and sometimes in very subtle ways, they are discussed separately from thoughts and feelings.

Beliefs are ideas that a person accepts as true and in which the person places faith and confidence. One may believe in God, that the medical profession wants to help people, that people are basically good, that money equals security, or that water pollution needs to be stopped.

Attitudes are similar to beliefs. Attitudes refer to a disposition or opinion toward ideas or issues—a person who believes that the medical profession wants to help others will have a positive attitude toward health professionals.

Values are ideas or issues that are important, are appreciated, or hold a position of high worth, and are usually ranked in an order of importance. For example, belief in the goodness of people might be of more importance to a person than belief in the usefulness of vitamin supplements and would be ranked higher.

Beliefs, attitudes, and values influence behavior. For example, a common belief about psychiatric clients is that they are dangerous, retarded, or hopeless. People who hold these beliefs will feel that treatment is hopeless, may fear for their own safety, and may avoid psychiatric clients. Or a person who values productivity might believe that anyone who really wanted to work could find a job; that person's attitude toward a family on welfare would be negative and would interfere with a helping relationship.

> ### ■ Point of Emphasis
> *The nurse's beliefs, attitudes, and values profoundly, and often unconsciously, affect the care she gives to clients.*

Children generally accept the values of their parents or parent-figures. Adolescents are exposed to the broader world and values of others such as teachers and peers. Those values may sometimes be in conflict with those of parents, which may cause confusion or uncertainty. It is usual, however, for a person to accept the values of adults without questioning until faced with an experience that forces those values into conscious awareness. The outcome is either a willingness to examine personal values or a refusal of that alternative and a continual acceptance of the parental values. Since decisions and actions are based on beliefs and values, uncertainty about values leads to uncertainty and confusion when important decisions must be made; for example, to leave school, to take extreme measures for a terminally ill client, or to report a nurse who is using illegal drugs.

It is helpful to have identified and ranked values before being faced with decisions. Raths (in Simon, et al.) considers the process of developing values to be more important than their actual content. The content will be different for each person and will probably change over time for each person, whereas the process may remain constant.

According to Raths, seven subprocesses are involved in the process of developing values:

prizing one's beliefs and behaviors
   1. Prizing and cherishing
   2. Publicly affirming, when appropriate
choosing one's beliefs and behaviors
   3. Choosing from alternatives
   4. Choosing after consideration of consequences
   5. Choosing freely
acting on one's beliefs
   6. Acting
   7. Acting with a pattern, consistency and repetition*

An exercise that may help the student clarify her personal values is to develop a values grid (Figure 4-1). In this grid, the student lists issues that are of value to her, such as her position on abortion or drunk drivers. She then asks herself

ISSUE	1	2	3	4	5	6	7
1.							
2.							
3.							
4.							
5.							
Etc.							

Figure 4-1 *Values grid. From Values clarification: A Handbook of practical strategies for teachers and students,* by Sidney Simon, Leland Howe, and Howard Kirschenbaum. Copyright 1972 by Hart Publishing Company, Inc.

the following seven questions about each issue listed and marks her response in the corresponding box on the grid:

1. Are you proud of your position?
2. Have you publicly affirmed your position?
3. Having you chosen your position from alternatives?
4. Have you chosen your position after thoughtful consideration of the pros, cons, and consequences?
5. Have you chosen your position freely? (Were you influenced by others?)
6. Have you acted on or done anything about your belief?
7. Have you acted with repetition or with consistency on this issue?*

Values that often are accepted without question frequently can be recognized in statements containing the words "should," "shouldn't," "good," and "bad." These words imply a value judgment. If the student finds herself using these words, she might identify the value that has been assigned to the thought, situation, or behavior, then use the foregoing list of questions to examine the process by which she reached that value.

The nurse will frequently care for clients whose beliefs, attitudes, and values are different

---

* From *VALUES CLARIFICATION: A Handbook of Practical Strategies for Teachers and Students* by Sidney Simon, Leland Howe, and Howard Kirschenbaum, copyright 1972 Hart Publishing Company, Inc., p. 19.

---

* Adapted from Simon, Howe, and Kirschenbaum, 1972, p. 36.

from hers, and it is important that she not force her personal beliefs, attitudes, and values on the client. However, if the nurse has not clarified her values, she might unknowingly impose them by, for example, making decisions that would be "right" for her but not necessarily "right" for the client. If she believes that abortion is "wrong," and is giving care to a client seeking an abortion, she might not consider the implications for the client and discourage or refuse her request. Just as important as clarifying values is a willingness to reexamine them in light of the possibly conflicting values of someone else.

PERSONAL NEEDS

As a consequence of developing self-awareness, the nurse becomes able to identify her own needs. When those needs are satisfied, she has energy to invest in others, particularly her clients. A nurse who has not met her personal needs may notice signs of stress in herself. If these needs continue to go unmet, they may interfere with both personal and professional relationships. For example, the nurse may attempt to fulfill those unmet needs through the client. Trying to meet the need to be needed through the client may encourage him to be dependent and discourage self-care, thereby lowering his self-esteem.

Personal needs include rest, food, exercise, recreation/pleasure, love/companionship, safety, and feeling valued. Early indications that personal needs are not being met may take the form of physical, affective, and/or cognitive stress. Physically, there may be muscle tension, headaches, nausea, diarrhea, and ulcers. Affective signs of stress may include a feeling of irritableness, or crying easily and frequently without appropriate cause. Cognitively, there may be preoccupation, forgetfulness, or an inability to concentrate.

The nurse should assess her personal needs, how she has met those needs in the past, and how she is currently meeting them. If she perceives that some needs are not being met, she must develop ways to fulfill them.

The one pitfall on the path to self-awareness is the idea that a person can know all there is to know about himself. The self is continually changing and unfolding. Becoming self-aware is a lifelong process—sometimes pleasurable; sometimes painful; always exciting, freeing, and unfinished. Kahlil Gibran (1923, 54–55) expresses this truth eloquently:

The hidden well-spring of your soul must needs rise and run murmuring to the sea;
And the treasure of your infinite depths would be revealed to your eyes.
But let there be no scales to weigh your known treasure;
And seek not the depths of your knowledge with staff or sounding line.
For self is a sea boundless and measureless.

Say not, "I have found the truth," but rather, "I have found a truth."
Say not, "I have found the path of the soul."
Say rather, "I have met the soul walking upon my path."
For the soul walks upon all paths.
The soul walks not upon a line, neither does it grow like a reed.
*The soul unfolds itself, like a lotus of countless petals.**

☐ Self-awareness in Professional Practice

Empathy, the capacity to perceive the moods and feelings of another person, is an essential aspect of the therapeutic relationship with the client (Berning and Berning, 1980; Carkhuff, 1970; Pareek, 1980; Rogers, 1980), and its significance in that relationship has been the subject of several studies (Forsyth, 1979; Hardin and Halaris, 1983; Kalish, 1971, 1973; Kunst-Wilson et al., 1981; Stetler, 1977). Rogers (1980) says: "A high degree of empathy in a relationship is possibly *the* most potent factor in bringing about change and learning." Empathy is critical in *every* nurse-client relationship—not only in the psychiatric-mental health setting. The capacity for empathy and its realization in interactions with each client is a unique contribution that nursing makes to health care.

■ Point of Emphasis

Empathy, the ability to perceive the moods and feelings of others, is the most potent factor in bringing about change and learning in clients.

---

* Reprinted from THE PROPHET, by Kahlil Gibran, by permission of Alfred A. Knopf, Inc. © 1923 by Kahlil Gibran and renewed 1951 by Administrators C.T.A. of Kahlil Gibran Estate, and Mary G. Gibran.

SELF-AWARENESS AS A BASIS FOR EMPATHY

Empathy can be taught (Kalish, 1971; Kirk and Thomas, 1982). But it is important that the student nurse not learn simply how to make reflective statements—empathy is more than that. Empathy involves feelings, and before the nurse can perceive the feelings of others, she must be aware of her own. In their study of counselors, Alcorn and Torney (1982) found that the level of self-awareness was directly and positively related to the counselor's ability to empathize with clients.

There are several reasons why self-awareness is necessary for the development of empathy. First, if a nurse understands herself, this helps her to understand how others might feel in a given situation. Being aware of one's own thoughts and feelings enables one to understand those thoughts and feelings in others. Second, if a nurse is not aware of her own thoughts and feelings, but denies or hides them from herself, she will not be able to acknowledge the same feelings and thoughts in others, because acknowledging them in others could be painful or threatening to her. Consider, for example, a situation in which a student nurse's parents are considering divorce. Since it is very painful for her to think of her family's disintegration, she denies that the divorce will occur and refuses to think about it. A client she is working with wants to divorce his wife. Every time the client brings up the subject of divorce it evokes discomforting feelings in the student about her parents, and she changes the subject. The student cannot help the client with his problem because she has not dealt with her own feelings. Finally, being aware of personal feelings helps the nurse to separate her feelings from those of the client. The nurse who cannot separate her own feelings from the client's may assume that the client's feelings are her own and thus feel personally threatened and as confused and upset as the client. In a therapeutic relationship, it is necessary both to understand the client and to be totally separate from him.

EMPATHY IN NURSING

As applied to nursing, empathy is the process whereby the nurse experiences the feelings and experiences of another person as if they were her own—but only *as if*. It includes communicating, validating, and clarifying that feeling with the other person. It also involves nonjudgmental acceptance of the other's feelings and experiences (Rogers, 1980; Forsyth, 1980).

The process of empathy involves several components in its continuing development.

Awareness

The nurse needs to actively listen to what the client is saying—not only listen to the words themselves, but understand and appreciate the feelings attached to the words. The nurse observes the client's posture, expression, and gestures. She then imagines herself in the client's place, saying those same words. What feelings would she be likely to have if she were the client? Awareness involves sensitivity to expressed changes in the client's feelings—feelings and meanings of which he is scarcely aware—without trying to uncover the client's totally unconscious feelings, since this would be extremely threatening to him (Rogers, 1980). In empathic awareness the nurse does not interpret the client's feelings, but rather, tries to experience them as the client is experiencing them.

Awareness of the client's current feelings requires that the nurse concentrate on the "here and now" experience. All of her energy must be focused on what the client is experiencing at that moment in time. The experience may change from moment to moment.

Objectivity

As the nurse tries to understand how the client is feeling, she avoids taking on those feelings herself. A nurse who takes on the client's feelings as her own will be unable to help him understand or handle those feelings. As Forsyth has put it: "To become subjectively involved in the feelings of another puts one in the position of needing help also" (Forsyth, 1980).

When objectivity is lost, the nurse has become sympathetic. She is experiencing the same feelings as the client and is unable to help him develop his own self-awareness because she has lost sight of her own.

Acceptance

To empathize "means that for the time being, you lay aside your own views and values in order to enter another's world without prejudice" (Rogers, 1980). The nurse needs to accept the client's feelings and experiences without judging them by her own values if she is really to experience his feelings as he is experiencing them. The ability to accept without judging is closely linked with the ability to maintain objectivity. If the nurse loses objectivity and takes the client's feelings as her own then she is sure to place her own values on them.

Validation

The only person who truly knows what he is feeling and experiencing is the person himself. To validate her perceptions of the client's feelings, the nurse needs to receive feedback from him (Margulies, 1984). It is the feedback between nurse and client that makes empathy an I-you relationship between two people rather than an internal process within the nurse alone.

Clarification

The final component of empathy is the clarification, with the client, of the accuracy of perceptions. In this step, the nurse is guided by the client's feedback. On the basis of feedback she can adjust her sense of the client's feelings, so that she is able to understand his feelings more accurately.

> ■ **Point of Emphasis**
>
> *Empathy is a continuing process that requires awareness, objectivity, acceptance, validation, and clarification.*

An empathic nurse perceptively points to the "felt meaning" that the client is currently experiencing in order to help him "focus on that meaning and carry it further to its full and uninhibited experiencing" (Rogers, 1980). As the nurse validates and clarifies her perception of the client's feelings, the client "tries them on to see if they fit." For example, during a conversation between Lisa (nurse) and John (client), John made some negative remarks about his wife. After trying to identify how John was feeling, Lisa said, "It sounds as though you are angry at your wife." John considered her statement and replied, doubtfully, "No, I don't think I'm angry. That doesn't seem quite right." Lisa said, "Perhaps you're disappointed." John replied quickly, "Yes, that's it! I am disappointed that she doesn't seem to care

about me." John was then able to continue exploring his feelings toward his wife.

Achieving empathy is a matter of degree. The nurse can attain a certain level of understanding but will probably never achieve total empathic understanding of the client. The purpose of validating and clarifying perceptions with the client is to achieve the highest level of empathic understanding possible.

Outcomes of Empathic Relationships

For the client, an empathic relationship brings positive benefits. First, the client feels understood by the nurse, rather than alienated; he no longer feels completely alone. Being connected with or understood by another person is a need and desire of all human beings. Second, if the nurse is empathic, the client feels valued, cared for, and accepted as a worthwhile person. This helps him to begin to value and accept himself. He thinks, "If the nurse accepts me, perhaps I'm not so bad after all. I trust her opinion so maybe I'm worth caring about. Maybe I could care for myself." The client becomes free to perceive and experience himself more fully, and to develop his own self-awareness. As he perceives new aspects of himself, he becomes able to change his self-concept. In turn, as the self-concept changes, the client's behavior changes to match the new self-concept. This is the therapeutic process.

> ■ **Point of Emphasis**
>
> *The outcomes of empathy are that the client can feel less alone, more valued, and free to grow and change.*

■ Enrichment Activities

DISCUSSION QUESTIONS

1. Think about the last time you talked with someone whom you felt really understood how you were feeling and thinking (empathized with you). What were the behaviors exhibited by that person that conveyed empathy to you?

2. What beliefs, values, and/or attitudes do you have that make it difficult for you to accept other people as they are? Do your parents have the same beliefs, values, and/or attitudes?

3. What beliefs, values, and/or attitudes do you have that facilitate your acceptance of other people as they are? Do your parents have the same beliefs, values, and/or attitudes?

4. Do you believe that you must have your own needs met before you can meet the needs of others? Why or why not?

LEARNING ACTIVITIES

Obtain a relaxation audiocassette tape; some of these have verbal directions for relaxation and are aimed at a specific behavior or feeling, such as increasing self-esteem, decreasing smoking or overeating, relieving tension, or improving sleep patterns. Listen to the tape twice a day.

Sources include, but are not limited to:

The Gotach Center for Health 7051 Poole Jones Road P.O. Box 606 Frederick, Maryland 21701	Well Spring 4619 East Cactus Road Phoenix, Arizona 85032

Local record stores will carry records and audiocassette tapes of environmental sounds, such as the ocean, a lagoon, a meadow, a thunderstorm, or a cricket symphony. Verbal directions or instructions for relaxation are not usually included.

This activity could help the student develop affective self-awareness. It could familiarize a student with relaxation techniques that she could subsequently use with appropriate clients.

To increase empathy for clients with physical disabilities, pair up with a friend or classmate whom you trust and who can act as your guide. For 24 hours assume a physical disability, such as blindness (wear eye patches), muteness (do not talk), paralysis (use a wheelchair), or fractured limbs (use crutches, slings, or canes). You must appear in public at least one time during the 24-hour period. Report back to your clinical group concerning your experiences and feelings.

This activity could help the student develop awareness for feelings and experiences of others and thus increase her ability to empathize.

■ Recommended Readings

Clark, Carolyn Chambers. *Assertive skills for nurses.* Wakefield, MA: Contemporary Publishing, 1978.
Focuses on developing assertive skills in the work setting. Designed for individual or group use, based on modular format. Utilizes many work situations and may help student develop assertive behaviors in professional situations.

Hardin, Sally Bosz, and Halaris, Ann Lyons. Nonverbal communication of patients and high and low empathy nurses. *Journal of psychosocial nursing and mental health services,* 21, 1, 1983:14–20. Presents results of research study to identify nonverbal behaviors (posture and gestures) of five psychiatric nurses rated by clients as having high or low empathy. May help student identify nonverbal behaviors indicative of empathy toward clients. Student could validate findings of this study in work with clients.

Kiersey, David, and Bates, Marilyn. *Please understand me.* DelMar, CA: Prometheus Nemesis Books, 1978. Presents different ways people have of viewing and approaching world around them. Based on Carl Jung's theory of personality development as developed by Isabel Myers in the Myers-Briggs Type Indicator. Presents mini-assessment similar to the Myers-Briggs Type Indicator and explanations of the 16 types identified by Myers and Briggs. This is a very positive, nonpathology oriented approach to helping people understand themselves and others. Could help student develop personal self-awareness.

Kunst-Wilson, William; Carpenter, Linda; Poser, Ann; Venohr, Ingridic; and Kushner, Kenneth. Empathic perceptions of nursing students: Self-reported and actual ability. *Research in nursing and health,* 4, 1981:283–293. Presents research study to identify difference in empathy level based on educational level plus the self-reported difficulty of student nurses to identify and handle specific feelings in self and others. Subjects were 66 undergraduate and 50 graduate students. Ranks feelings students had difficulty detecting and handling in self and others. Could help students identify own level of ability to detect and handle specific feelings, and identify the use of research in nursing.

Rogers, Carl R. *A way of being.* Boston: Houghton Mifflin, 1980. Collected papers and speeches by Dr. Carl Rogers, recounting his own personal development and the development of his philosoophy of interpersonal relationships. Could provide the student with a more in-depth understanding of the theory and concepts of self-awareness and empathy presented in this chapter.

■ References

Alberti, R.E., and Emmons, M.L. *Your perfect right: A guide to assertive behavior.* San Luis Obispo, CA: Impact Publishers, 1978.
Alcorn, L.M., and Torney, D.J. Counselor cognitive

complexity of self-reported emotional experience as a predictor of accurate empathic understanding. *Journal of counseling psychology, 29,* 5, 1982:534–537.

Bandler, R., and Grinder, J. *Frogs into princes: Neuro-linguistic programming.* Moab, UT: Real People Press, 1979.

Bandler, R., and Grinder, J. *Reframing: Neuro-linguistic programming and the transformation of meaning.* Moab, UT: Real People Press, 1982.

Bergin, A.E., and Strupp, H.H. *Changing frontiers in the science of psychotherapy.* Chicago: Aldine-Atherton, 1972.

Berning, W., and Berning, S. Becoming a husband and wife social worker team. In Bulbrook, M.J., (ed.). *Development of therapeutic skills.* Boston: Little, Brown & Co., 1980, 37–49.

Buber, Martin. *I and thou.* Translated by Walter Kaufmann. New York: Charles Scribner's Sons, 1970.

Carkhuff, R.R. *Helping and human relations.* New York: Holt, Reinhart & Winston, 1970.

Forsyth, G.L. Exploration of empathy in nurse-client interaction. *Advances in nursing science,* 1979:53–61.

Forsyth, G.L. Analysis of the concept of empathy: Illustration of one approach. *Advances in nursing science,* 2, 2, 1980:33–42.

Gibran, K. *The prophet.* New York: Alfred Knopf, 1923.

Hardin, S.B., and Halaris, A.L. Nonverbal communication of patients and high and low empathy nurses. *Journal of psychosocial nursing and mental health services,* 21, 1, 1983:14–20.

Howe, J., Dickason, E.J., Jones, D.A., and Snider, M.J. *The handbook of nursing.* New York: John Wiley & Sons, 1984.

Jourard, S.M. *The transparent self.* New York: D. Van Nostrand Company, 1971.

Kalish, B.J. An experiment in the development of empathy in nursing students. *Nursing research,* 20, 3, 1971:202–211.

Kalish, B.J. What is empathy? *American journal of nursing,* 73, 9, 1973:1548–1552.

Kirk, W.G., and Thomas, A.H. A brief in-service training strategy to increase levels of empathy of psychiatric nursing personnel. *Journal of psychiatric treatment and evaluation,* 4, 1982:177–179.

Krikorian, D.A., and Paulanka, B.J. Self-awareness—The key to a successful nurse-patient relationship? *Journal of psychosocial nursing and mental health services,* 20, 6, 1982:19–21.

Kurtz, R.R., and Grummon, D.L. Different approaches to the measurement of therapist empathy and their relationship to therapy outcomes. *Journal of consulting and clinical psychology,* 39, 1, 1972:106–115.

Kunst-Wilson, W., Carpenter, L., Poser, A., Venohr, I., and Kushner, K. Empathic perceptions of nursing students: Self-reported and actual ability. *Research in nursing and health,* 4, 1981:283–293.

Margulies, A. Toward empathy: The uses of wonder. *American journal of psychiatry,* 141, 9, 1984:1025–1033.

Pareek, U. Empathy: The critical variable in helping professions. *The Indian journal of social work,* 40, 4, 1980:417–434.

Rogers, C.R. *A way of being.* Boston: Houghton Mifflin, 1980.

Schoffstall, C. Concerns of student nurses prior to psychiatric nursing experience: An assessment and intervention technique. *Journal of psychosocial nursing and mental health services,* 19, 11, 1981:11–14.

Simon, S.B., Howe, L.W., and Kirschenbaum, H. *Values clarification: A handbook of practical strategies for teachers and students.* New York: Hart Publishing Company, Inc., 1972.

Stetler, C.B. Relationship of perceived empathy to nurses' communication. *Nursing research,* 26, 6, 1977:432–438.

Truax, C.B., and Carkhuff, R.R. *Toward effective counseling and psychotherapy: Training and practice.* Chicago: Aldine-Atherton, 1967.

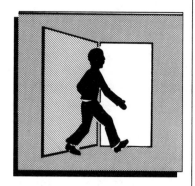

5

Client Rights and Psychiatric Nursing Practice

Amy L. Longo

Learning Objectives

Upon completion of this chapter, the reader will be able to:

1. Distinguish a voluntary admission to a psychiatric hospital from an involuntary admission.

2. Define guardianship and conservatorship.

3. Identify legal rights of the mentally ill client and recognize the legal basis for those rights.

4. Apply legal principles in implementing and evaluating nursing care.

The legal system of the United States has a tremendous impact on psychiatric care, particularly with respect to the long-term institutional care of the mentally ill and mentally retarded. The rights of the mentally ill are protected through a system of checks and balances, and their care and treatment are governed by specific laws and through interpretation of the rights afforded by the constitution.

☐ *Legal Aspects*

The body of law that is essential to all citizens of the United States is the United States Constitution. For purposes of our study the Bill of Rights, which is afforded to citizens of each state through the Fourteenth Amendment, has the greatest impact on the care of the mentally ill because the court has ruled that these fundamental rights must be preserved in treatment situations (*O'Connor* v. *Donaldson*, 1975). Each state also has a constitution which applies to persons within its borders.

WRITTEN LAWS

Federal statutes enacted by the United States Congress and regulations implementing those statutes may affect care and treatment of the mentally ill. For example, the statutes and regulations of the Health and Human Services Department regarding human experimentation affect research projects with mentally ill subjects. Alcohol and drug abuse programs are regulated by federal laws.

Each state legislature enacts its own statutes, many of which are implemented by state rules and regulations. State laws govern many aspects of treatment of the institutionalized client.

COMMON LAW

Common law is determined by custom and precedence; it evolves as present public policy requires. Many legal issues affecting care of clients will not be specifically controlled by a constitutional or statutory provision. In such a situation a court of law will look at previous custom and formulate its rationale based on how the particular issue has been resolved in earlier cases.

THE ROLE OF THE COURT

There are federal and state courts and the ultimate court in the judicial system, the United States Supreme Court. Courts interpret the written laws when there is a question about their meaning, constitutionality, or applicability in a particular case. In the absence of written law the courts interpret the common law as tempered by present public policy. Courts make decisions on a case-by-case basis.

WELFARE OF THE MENTALLY ILL

The states have the primary responsibility for the safety and welfare of persons within their borders. They derive this authority through two state powers, *parens patriae* power and police power. *Parens patriae*, or paternalistic, power is the power of the state to care for those unable to care for themselves. Police power is the power of the state to take the necessary action to control the conduct of persons who present a danger to the safety and welfare of others within the state (Matter of Guardianship of Eberhardy, 1980). Through the use of their *parens patriae* and police powers the states have a profound influence on the care and treatment of their mentally ill residents.

ENTRANCE INTO THE HEALTH CARE SYSTEM

Many clients voluntarily enter the mental health system. A person alone or with the guidance of family may request treatment. This treatment may be at a private office or clinic. Generally the legal relationship created between the client and caregiver would be governed by an agreement or contract between the individual seeking treatment and the provider. The rights and responsibilities of each would be controlled by their agreement. The client can terminate the relationship at any time.

The client may be admitted to a psychiatric hospital voluntarily upon the advice of a psychiatrist. Like a client admitted to a general hospital, the person voluntarily admitted to a psychiatric hospital agrees to admission under the terms and conditions set by the hospital, and he may leave of his own will with or without medical authorization for dismissal.

A state can order a person to be hospitalized for treatment through exercise of either its *parens patriae* power or its police power. As was established in the case of *Addington* v. *Texas* (1979), the individual can face a civil commitment or a criminal commitment if he has committed a crime. The discussion of commitment in this chapter is limited to those mentally ill persons not accused of a crime who are civilly committed for psychiatric treatment.

☐ *Civil Commitment*

Unless the state is exercising one of its legitimate powers in protecting the safety and welfare of its residents, it cannot interfere with the freedom of a mentally ill person. The United States Constitution guarantees certain basic rights, contained in the Bill of Rights, to the citizens of the various states. While a civil commitment is not imprisonment (indeed, nurses concerned with the health, care, and treatment of the mentally ill find the comparison of hospitalization to imprisonment offensive), it results in an involuntary curtailment of an individual's liberty. Before a state can deprive a person of liberty, the Fourteenth Amendment requires the state to afford the person due process of law. The meaning of "due process" is often elusive; however, in terms of an involuntary commitment it implies that the state cannot deprive a person of liberty without a legitimate reason and without giving a person the opportunity to present his side of the matter before being confined for psychiatric treatment.

Each of the fifty states has statutes governing civil commitments. Table 5-1 illustrates the variation in definitions in selected states for incompetent and dangerously mentally ill persons. While each state's statutes may vary as to the standards for evaluating whether an individual needs involuntary treatment, the actual procedures for commitment, the standard of proof for commitment, and the method of release, there are general principles applicable to all states.

DEFINITION OF BEHAVIOR NECESSITATING COMMITMENT

To comply with due process there must be a standard for judging behavior requiring commitment of an individual. In addition to a finding of mental illness, there must be a finding that the individual is dangerous to himself or others.

■ Point of Emphasis

Proof of mental illness alone is not sufficient for involuntary commitment.

THE COMMITMENT PROCESS

Generally, anyone who is in a position to observe that a person presents a danger can initiate the commitment process. The state, either through a court or specially appointed body (e.g., a board of mental health), decides whether a person should be committed. If there is reason to believe that someone poses such a danger that immediate confinement is necessary, that person may be detained for a limited number of hours prior to a hearing. Likewise, if a voluntarily hospitalized client seeks release but the health professionals caring for him consider commitment necessary, he may be detained in the hospital for a limited number of hours so that a civil commitment may be initiated.

If a commitment is initiated a certain constitutional procedural due process must be followed before the person is committed:

1. The person must receive notice of the time and place of hearings on the commitment.
2. The person has the right to have an attorney. If a person has no money, the state must have available means for the individual to obtain legal representation.
3. The person subject to commitment has the right to present witnesses on his behalf and to cross-examine the state's witnesses.
4. At the minimum, the state must prove by clear and convincing evidence that the person is in need of commitment (*Addington* v. *Texas*, 1979). This standard of proof is greater than the standard in most civil cases but less than the standard in criminal cases.

Once a person is found to be in need of involuntary commitment, the state can order hospitalization, supervise the treatment plan, and determine when discharge may take place. Civil commitment statutes also provide for emergencies. If a person is believed to exhibit behavior indicative of needing commitment and is likely to cause harm before a commitment hearing can be held, the person may be hospitalized prior to commitment hearing.

The United States Supreme Court has upheld a statute allowing a parent to admit a minor to a state mental institution even though the minor does not consent to treatment, provided that a physician representing the institution certifies the minor's need for treatment. The parent is assumed to have the best interest of the child in

TABLE 5-1 Selected Definitions of Incompetent Person vs. Dangerously Mentally Ill Person

Incompetent Person	Dangerously Mentally Ill Person
New York: If he is incompetent to manage himself or his affairs by reason of age, drunkenness, mental illness, or other cause, or is a patient, as hereinafter defined, who is unable adequately to conduct his personal or business affairs. N.Y. Mental Hygiene Law 78.1 (McKinney)	Substantial risk of physical harm to himself as manifested by threats of or attempts of suicide or serious bodily harm or other conduct demonstrating that he is dangerous to himself; or A substantial risk of physical harm to other persons as manifested by homicidal or other violent behavior by which others are placed in reasonable fear of serious physical harm. N.Y. Mental Hygiene Law 9.37 (McKinney)
New Mexico: "Incapacitated person" means any person who is impaired by reason of mental illness, mental deficiency, physical illness or disability, advanced age, chronic use of drugs, chronic intoxication or other cause, except minority, to the extent that he lacks sufficient understanding or capacity to make or communicate responsible decisions concerning his person or management of his affairs. N.M. Stat. Ann. 45-5-101 (1979)	"Likelihood of serious harm to oneself" means that it is more likely than not that in the near future the person will attempt to commit suicide or will cause serious bodily harm to himself by violent or other self-destructive means including but not limited to grave passive neglect as evidenced by behavior causing, attempting, or threatening the infliction of serious bodily harm to himself; "Likelihood of serious harm to others" means that it is more likely than not that in the near future the person will inflict serious, unjustified bodily harm on another person or commit a criminal sexual offense as evidenced by behavior causing, attempting, or threatening such harm, which behavior gives rise to a reasonable fear of such harm from said person. N.M. Stat. Ann. 43-1-2, M (1979)
Nebraska: "Incapacitated person" means any person who is impaired by reason of mental illness, mental deficiency, physical illness or disability, advanced age, chronic intoxication, or other cause except minority to the extent that he lacks sufficient understanding or capacity to make or communicate responsible decisions concerning his person. Neb. Rev. Stat. 30-2601 (1), as amended.	Mentally ill dangerous person shall mean any mentally ill person or alcoholic person who presents: A substantial risk of serious harm to another person or persons within the near future, as manifested by evidence of recent violent acts or threats of violence or by placing others in reasonable fear of such harm; or A substantial risk of serious harm to himself within the near future, as manifested by evidence of recent attempts at, or threats of, suicide or serious bodily harm, or evidence of inability to provide for his bassic human needs, including food, clothing, shelter, essential medical care, or personal safety. Neb. Rev. Stat. 83-1009, as amended.

mind. While the Court recognized that some parents abuse their children, it also held that the state has a sufficient procedure for guarding the minor's best interests. *Parham* v. *J.R.* (1979) defines the due process that must be afforded the minor when a parent seeks commitment.

NURSE'S INVOLVEMENT

A nurse has highly skilled assessment capı-bilities and through observations and interactions with the client assesses his condition. The nurse makes judgments based upon those assessments and intervenes for the client's safety and health. If the client refuses hospitalization, the nurse may be placed in the difficult position of having to initiate a commitment proceeding.

Through the professional relationship, the nurse or another mental health professional may identify a client's need for hospitalization and may have to work with the family and other health care professionals to seek civil commitment. It is important to give some thought to the delicate position of the nurse in the commitment process. Although the nurse and client generally have the same goal, in commitment their goals may be conflicting. The client obviously is refusing treatment (or the commitment would be unnecessary), while the nurse's assessment of what is necessary for the client's welfare results in actions opposing the client's wishes. The nurse may be called to testify as a witness at a commitment hearing. Usually a nurse's testimony at a commitment hearing is excluded from any nurse-client communication privilege created by certain state laws; therefore, in most situations the nurse can testify openly about her observations of an individual's behavior.

The accompanying vignettes illustrate the distinction between a client who may have symptoms of mental illness and a client who may have symptoms of mental illness and also exhibits dangerous behavior.

Vignette

Nurse Ann Smith is the nurse for J.H., who regularly comes into the neighborhood health clinic for treatment. J.H. is being treated for a manic depressive disorder. He repeatedly describes to the nurse his two past suicide attempts. On two occasions he took 10 aspirin tablets. Other than nausea and vomiting, he suffered no serious effects. On occasion he tells the nurse about his plans to kill a famous person. Although he is vague, he has described a person who fits the description of a famous cartoon character. On an outpatient basis J.H. has not made good progress toward recovery. Along with his psychiatrist, Nurse Smith has encouraged him to seek hospital treatment but he persistently refuses. His sister, who has not seen J.H. since he has been ill, is visiting and is appalled at J.H.'s condition. During the visit J.H. throws a plate at his sister, who then files a petition for J.H.'s involuntary commitment.

Question for Consideration

Does the state have the authority to compel J.H.'s hospitalization?

J. H. may be exhibiting symptoms of mental illness, but it is unlikely that there is sufficient proof that he is dangerously mentally ill. Therefore involuntary commitment would be inappropriate.

Vignette

Nurse Jones is the nurse in charge of an admitting unit of a state psychiatric hospital. A county welfare worker brings a young mother in for admission. The mother evidently has been sitting in her bedroom crying for four days, leaving her five-year-old son in charge of children two years old and three years old. The five-year-old has a large bruise across his face. The whereabouts of the father is unknown. The children have been placed in a temporary home. Prior to arriving at the hospital the young mother had not spoken to the social worker. She now is objecting strongly to hospitalization. Nurse Jones has observed no dangerous behavior and is yet unable to assess her mental condition.

Questions for Consideration

1. Can the nurse proceed to admit the mother to the hospital against her will? What rights does the mother have?

Usually the commitment statutes provide that a client may be held by a hospital for a certain interval of time if there is reason to believe that the client is in need of involuntary treatment. The mother may be held temporarily, even if she demands her release. The mother has the right to have someone represent her interests, and the nurse who is responsible for the mother's care should listen to her and contact any persons the client wants to know of her whereabouts.

2. If the patient persists in demanding release and the nurse permits her to leave, is the nurse responsible for any injury that could occur to the mother or her family if she were released?

If the client is dismissed before her potential to cause harm to herself or others is evaluated, the nurse possibly could be found liable for any subsequent injury to the mother or to her children.

Vignette

Nurse O'Reilly is working the evening shift. J.T., a voluntary admission on the unit, is suffering from the delusion that he is a prophet sent into the world to rid it of all prostitutes. His plan for carrying out his mission is becoming detailed and precise. Last night he attacked a female patient but was subdued before harming her. The nurse now believes J.T. is dangerous. He comes to the nurse and says he is signing out.

Questions for Consideration

1. Does the nurse have to let him leave?

A voluntary client may be held if there is reason to believe that he may be dangerously mentally ill; however, involuntary commitment proceedings should be initiated.

2. Is the nurse responsible for the safety of anyone besides the client?

If the client, through the lack of supervision by the nursing staff, injures someone, a nurse could be found liable for the injury. The treatment of this client should be planned to allow for the protection of the client, other clients, and the staff.

Any hospital that receives involuntary clients should have a policy relating to civil commitment. Nurses should be alerted as to how a person has been admitted to the hospital and should be aware of the principal requirements of the particular state's commitment laws. Specific guidelines should be developed for admission, treatment, and dismissal of the involuntarily committed client. The nurse should realize that the individual who has been involuntarily committed may still pos-

sess the ability to make decisions and judgments relating to care, finances, and property.

■ Point of Emphasis

The nurse must be alert to the circumstances of the client's admission and the legal requirements of care, while safeguarding client rights and dignity.

☐ Guardianship

A mentally ill person may not exhibit behavior sufficiently dangerous to require involuntary commitment yet may lack the ability to understand and care for himself. Upon petition, a court may appoint a guardian for an incompetent or incapacitated person. The guardian assumes responsibility for the care and welfare of the individual, who then becomes the guardian's ward. The following situation demonstrates when a guardianship may be appropriate.

Vignette

Nurse Ponti works at a mental health center. One of the clients is a 60-year-old widower who is depressed. He lives alone. His children are grown and working successfully out of state. His condition has declined lately, and he often roams the downtown streets carrying on long animated conversations with his dead wife about his work and their children, and he is seen rummaging through trash cans. His grooming and housekeeping have deteriorated. The nurse feels he would benefit from hospitalization, but he refuses to go. His oldest son is visiting and seeks the nurse's advice.

Question for Consideration

Should the nurse recommend involuntary commitment?

Involuntary commitment is appropriate only if the client is dangerous to himself or others. This situation may require a guardianship proceeding. A court-appointed guardian may take actions necessary to protect the client.

For a guardian to be appointed, there must be a finding that a person is incapacitated. The specific definition of an incompetent or incapacitated person may differ from state to state, however it generally means a person who, through physical or mental disability, lacks sufficient understanding or capacity to make responsible decisions about himself (*May* v. *Leneau*, 1980). Unless a person is judged incompetent, the law presumes he is competent. In practice, nurses are sometimes faced with a dilemma when certain persons not declared incompetent by a court lack the ability to make knowing and understanding decisions about their care.

In the case of an incompetent client who does not have a court-appointed guardian, the next of kin, when available, may have to participate in treatment decisions. If a client lacks the ability to make decisions about care, health professionals cannot automatically treat without consulting someone whose judgment may be substituted for that of the incompetent person.

Just because a person has been declared incompetent, he is not stripped of personal rights. In fact, the law has created guardianship in order to protect the legal rights and welfare of people who lack the ability to do so on their own. In planning an incompetent client's care the nurse should keep the guardian informed and also consult the guardian concerning the ward's treatment and welfare.

CONSERVATORSHIP

In many states there is a distinction between a person who has the legal responsibility for the physical needs of another (guardian) and a person who has the legal responsibility for another's finances (conservator). Because of age or disability, a person may no longer wish to or have the ability to handle finances. Under these circumstances, a conservator may be appointed (*In re Schock*, 1973). A person under a conservatorship does not necessarily lack the ability to make decisions about care and treatment.

☐ The Rights of the Mentally Ill Client

The rights of the mentally ill client have been carved out in many states by statute. Other rights have been defined by the courts. Through continued court challenges the rights of the mentally ill and the mentally retarded are being expanded and clarified. The guide for client rights remains the Bill of Rights of the United States Constitution (see Table 5-2).

LIBERTY INTERESTS

Freedom from Unnecessary Confinement

A mentally ill client has the right to be free from state-ordered confinement if capable of living outside an institution and not posing a threat of danger to himself or others (*O'Connor* v. *Donaldson*, 1975).

The Right to Personal Security and Freedom from Undue Bodily Restraint

The involuntarily committed person has the right to personal security and freedom from bodily restraint. However, these rights must be balanced by considerations of danger to himself and others. If the treating physician has ordered restraints, the nurses who care for the client must closely monitor the need for restraints to protect the client from harm to himself or others. If restraints are needed in an emergency to prevent injury, they should be used as a safety measure (*Youngberg* v. *Romeo*, 1982).

The Right to Treatment

At a minimum, involuntary clients are entitled to that treatment necessary to protect their liberty interests. For example, if a client is self-abusive, he is entitled to that treatment that protects him from injury (*Clites* v. *State*, 1982).

Courts have recognized that the client who is involuntarily committed to an institution is entitled to treatment designed to restore him to health, at least to the extent of allowing him to recover to his optimum level of function (*Wyatt* v. *Stickney*, 1972). The rights of the mentally ill have expanded because of recognition by both courts and legislatures that the mentally ill who are confined for treatment are entitled to that treatment necessary to increase their potential to be free from confinement.

The Right to Informed Consent to Treatment

A competent adult person cannot be treated without giving voluntary consent to treatment. To consent to treatment, a person must be capable of

---

TABLE 5-2 *The Bill of Rights From the Constitution of the United States*

First Amendment

Congress shall make no law respecting an establishment of religion, or prohibiting the free exercise thereof; or abridging the freedom of speech, or of the press; or the right of the people peaceably to assemble, and to petition the government for a redress of grievances.

Second Amendment

A well regulated militia, being necessary to the security of a free state, the right of the people to keep and bear arms, shall not be infringed.

Third Amendment

No soldier shall, in time of peace be quartered in any house, without the consent of the owner, nor in time of war, but in a manner to be prescribed by law.

Fourth Amendment

The right of the people to be secure in their persons, houses, papers, and effects, against unreasonable searches and seizures, shall not be violated, and no warrants shall issue, but upon probable cause, supported by oath or affirmation, and particularly describing the place to be searched, and the persons or things to be seized.

Fifth Amendment

No person shall be held to answer for a capital, or otherwise infamous crime, unless on a presentment or indictment of a Grand Jury, except in cases arising in land or naval forces, or in the militia, when in actual service in time of war or public danger; nor shall any person be subject for the same offense to be twice put in jeopardy of life or limb; nor shall be compelled in any criminal case to be witness against himself, nor be deprived of life, liberty, or property, without due process of law; nor shall private property be taken for public use, without just compensation.

Sixth Amendment

In all criminal prosecutions, the accused shall enjoy the right to a speedy and public trial, by an impartial jury of the state and district wherein the crime shall have been committed, which district shall have been previously ascertained by law, and to be informed of the nature and cause of the accusation; to be confronted with the witnesses against him; to have compulsory process for obtaining witnesses in his favor; and to have the assistance of counsel for his defense.

Seventh Amendment

In suits at common law, where the value in controversy shall exceed twenty dollars, the right of trial by jury shall be preserved, and no fact tried by a jury, shall be otherwise reexamined in any court of the United States, than according to the rules of the common law.

Eighth Amendment

Excessive bail shall not be required, nor excessive fines imposed, nor cruel and unusual punishments inflicted.

Ninth Amendment

The enumeration in the Constitution, of certain rights, shall not be construed to deny or disparage others retained by the people.

Tenth Amendment

The powers not delegated to the United States by the Constitution, nor prohibited by it to the states, are reserved to the states respectively, or to the people.

Due Process Clause of the Fourteenth Amendment

Section 1.

All persons born or naturalized in the United States, and subject to the jurisdiction thereof, are citizens of the United States and of the state wherein they reside. No state shall make or enforce any law which shall abridge the privileges or immunities of citizens of the United States; nor shall any state deprive any person of life, liberty, or property, without due process of law; nor deny to any person within its jurisdiction the equal protection of the laws.

---

knowing and understanding the nature of the treatment.

Truman v. *Thomas* (1980), discussed informed consent and established that before consenting to treatment a client should know the following:

1. Diagnosis
2. Proposed treatment
3. Risks and side effects of proposed treatment
4. Alternative treatments

After being fully informed and voluntarily consenting to treatment, the client's consent remains valid unless he either withdraws the consent or there is a change in the circumstances affecting the consent which may indicate that the treatment is no longer appropriate.

Mental illness does not negate a person's ability to know and understand the nature of the proposed treatment and to voluntarily consent to treatment. A mentally ill person can withdraw consent just as any other client can. Because certain psychiatric admissions are involuntary, particular care should be given as to whether or not a client is voluntarily accepting treatment. The more intrusive the treatment, the more care should be exerted in providing sufficient information and assessing the client's ability to know and understand that information.

SPECIAL CONDITIONS

Psychosurgery is intrusive and the results are permanent. Because of its nature, at least one court has held that an involuntary client is not capable of giving voluntary consent to experimental psychosurgery (*Kaimonitz* v. *Michigan Department of Mental Health*, 1973). Some states have specific statutes regarding informed consent to psychosurgery (e.g., the 1982 California Code). Special care should be taken to ensure that the client has been fully informed, that he fully understands the nature of the surgical procedure, and that the consent is voluntary. The various aspects of consent should be documented in writing in a client's chart.

Electroconvulsive therapy is another treatment that is considered intrusive. Some states have therefore enacted specific procedures for obtaining and documenting informed consent for this type of therapy (e.g., California Code, 1982).

If a particular behavior modification program infringes on client's rights as defined by the Constitution, statutes, or court cases, particular care should be taken to obtain the person's consent and voluntary participation in the program. For example if a behavior modification program calls for time out (seclusion) when a client behaves in a particular manner, unless the client consents to the seclusion program, his liberty interests may be violated.

DECISION MAKING FOR A CLIENT WHO HAS BEEN ADJUDICATED INCOMPETENT

If a mentally ill person has been declared incompetent, the court-appointed guardian may consent to treatment on the client's behalf. As discussed earlier, in the absence of a court determination of incompetence, a person is presumed competent. However, if, in the nurse's professional judgment, she believes that the client is not capable of giving an informed consent, some action should be taken to obtain a substitute consent. As a practical matter the nurse would consult the family. However, hospital policy may not allow the client's family

to consent to treatments, particularly treatments of an intrusive nature. In those situations a guardian may have to be appointed to consent on the client's behalf.

Conflict between the consent to treatment by the guardian and the refusal of the client to receive treatment may require a court order if no emergency is present (Guardianship of Roe, Massachusetts, 1981).

Right to Refuse Treatment

Just as a competent adult can consent to treatment, a competent adult can refuse treatment. The standards for an informed refusal to treatment are similar to those for an informed consent. However, adherence to informed refusal of treatment may be subjected to even more serious scrutiny than consent to treatment because of the consequences of refusal of treatment.

To make an informed refusal, the competent adult capable of making a voluntary knowing and understanding decision must receive an explanation of the diagnosis, the proposed treatment, the risks and consequences of the treatment, alternative treatments, and the risks and consequences of refusing treatment (*Lane* v. *Candura*, 1978).

Incompetent Client. Recently courts have grappled with the issues surrounding the rights of the incompetent client to refuse treatment. Courts often are reluctant to allow a guardian to refuse treatment on behalf of the ward. However, in the case of the terminally ill incompetent adult, courts will allow the guardian to refuse treatment for the incompetent adult (*In re Quinlan*, New Jersey, 1976).

Minor Client. In the case of minors, courts have not allowed parents to refuse life-saving treatment on behalf of their minor children (Custody of a Minor, Massachusetts, 1978), however in the case of a terminally ill child whose death is imminent the court may permit the parents to refuse treatment on the child's behalf.

In the hospital setting a nurse cannot take refusals lightly. Particularly when refusing treatment involves a harmful result for the client, the nurse should seek guidance from hospital administration before deciding whether or not the treatment decision of a client, or one acting for the client, should be honored.

Right to Refuse Psychiatric Treatment

The general rule that a competent adult has the right to refuse treatment applies to the competent adult in the psychiatric setting as well. Failure to identify the applicability of this legal right in the psychiatric setting has resulted in numerous court challenges to forced treatment. Courts are still in the process of defining the breadth and scope of this right, however, certain general principles have emerged. The right to refuse treatment is not an absolute right; rather, it is qualified by the facts and circumstances in each case (*Rennie* v. *Klein*, 1981; *Rogers* v. *Okin*, 1979; *Mills* v. *Rogers*, 1982).

1. In an emergency, when there is an imminent threat to the safety of the client, staff, or other clients, necessary treatment may be given to control the emergency even if the client resists treatment.

2. An involuntary client is still capable of consenting or refusing to consent to treatment. However, an involuntary, though competent, client possesses only a qualified right to refuse treatment. Generally the state commitment statutes define the limits of the involuntary client's right to refuse treatment. If treatment is necessary to prevent injury or to prevent the involuntary client's condition from worsening, usually involuntary treatment will be permitted provided it is the least intrusive treatment under the circumstances and there is a method of evaluating the need for the proposed treatment.

3. If a client has been declared incompetent by the court, the appointed guardian must consent to treatment. However, if a conflict arises between the guardian and ward regarding treatment, some states may require a judicial review of the treatment decision before the incompetent person receives forced treatment.

If a voluntary client refuses treatment, he can be discharged unless the discharge would pose a danger to him or to other persons. If danger is a factor, then civil commitment should be considered. Assessing when forced treatment may be indicated is often a difficult task.

Vignette

Mr. W. is a tall, heavy young man who is threatening the nurse with his fist, which has a coat hanger wrapped around it.

Questions for Consideration

1. Would this situation be an emergency?

If Mr. W.'s behavior is of such a nature that harm to the nurse is imminent, the situation would involve an emergency.

2. Would his conduct permit his seclusion without his consent?

Some form of removal from the present environment would be justified so that the client can regain control and harm can be avoided.

Vignette

Ms. H., an involuntary client, has a capacity for violence and "out of control" behavior. The nursing staff has decided to institute a seclusion program to control her behavior. She has been placed in seclusion, and the plan is to continue seclusion until she is able to maintain appropriate behavior. A time schedule is set up. Ms. H. resists the seclusion at all stages of the plan.

Questions for Consideration

1. Can the staff allow Ms. H.'s seclusion at any stage of the plan?

If danger is imminent involuntary seclusion would be permissible.

2. If Ms. H.'s behavior is not out of control but is still inappropriate can the staff continue the seclusion plan against her wishes?

When Ms. H. is not dangerous to others and refuses the seclusion plan, some form of hospital review according to procedures for forced treatment should take place before she is involuntarily secluded against her will.

Vignette

Mr. L., an involuntary client, is refusing his medication, which was initially required to control abrupt disruptive episodes of violence. He now is interacting calmly within the hospital community but persistently refuses any maintenance medication. From his past history the hospital fears that if he continues to refuse the medication, his condition will deteriorate to an uncontrollable level.

Questions for Consideration

1. Under the circumstances should the staff force medication?

Mr. L.'s medication should be continued only after his care is reviewed and it is determined that giving medication would be the least intrusive treatment.

2. Is there a definite yes or no answer to this question?

There may be no definite answer to Mr. L.'s situation because the deterioration may be to such an extent that forced treatment is necessary.

3. Would the answer be different if he were a voluntary client?

If a voluntary client refuses treatment, he can probably leave the hospital provided no involuntry commitment has been initiated.

The Right to Privacy

Every client seeking treatment for mental illness has an expectation that records of treatment and other communications with physicians, nurses, and other health care professionals will remain confidential. Before information may be released to any third party (including insurance companies and employers), the client must give permission for release. Federal regulations exert strict controls over release of any information regarding clients in alcohol and drug abuse programs.

As with other rights, the individual's right to privacy must be balanced against the interests of the public. This balancing has resulted in exceptions to the client's right to privacy. If there is reason to believe that an injury is the result of a criminal act, or abuse of children, the mentally retarded, or the elderly, the nurse has a duty to report information to the appropriate authorities (Child Abuse Reporting Statutes, e.g. Utah Code, 1978). Each hospital should have a policy to describe how disclosure of this information should be handled. More recently, courts have found that if a client is dangerous and has communicated that he wants to harm someone, the health profes-

sional has a duty to warn that person of any foreseeable danger (*Tarasoff* v. *Regents of University of California*, 1977; *Brady* v. *Hopper*, 1983). Involuntary commitment of the client would perhaps avoid the problem of how to appropriately warn his intended victim. However, when it is not possible to obtain commitment of the dangerous person, the health professional must take steps to warn the threatened individual. Hospital or clinic policies for releasing information should be carefully designed to balance client confidentiality with the duty to warn and to seek the best method of warning third parties of the danger.

Other Rights of the Mentally Ill

1. The right to manage their own affairs.
2. The right to marry and divorce.
3. The right to vote.
4. The right to visitation and telephone calls.
5. The right to send and receive mail.
6. The right to medical treatment for physical ailments.
7. The right to their own clothing and laundering.
8. The right to religious worship.
9. The right to be free from forced labor involving the operation and maintenance of the hospital.
10. The right to a clean living environment.
11. The right to nutritional meals.
12. The right to seek a writ of habeas corpus. Habeas corpus is a legal procedure that allows an imprisoned person or person held in a mental institution to show to a court that he is illegally detained (*Wyatt* v. *Stickney*, 1972).

☐ The Nurse's Role in Meeting Legal Standards

Up to this point consideration has been given to how the individual becomes involved in the mental health system and the rights of the individual within the system. While these are very important legal aspects of mental health care, they generally are considerations which involve institutional policies and procedures. The individual nurse plays a role in the implementation of legally acceptable practices related to the mentally ill, but in most situations, the institution and not the nurse will be responsible for complying with the legal standards discussed.

The individual nurse's conduct with respect to care and treatment of the psychiatric client will be evaluated by nursing malpractice standards. A nurse having special skills and expertise is held to a high legal standard of care. Her conduct is measured under the principles of malpractice. In evaluating nursing care four elements are considered:

1. *Duty.* The nurse has a duty to the clients assigned to her care. In meeting this duty, the nurse must perform according to the professional standard of care for psychiatric nurses, which must conform to standards of care set by statute, nursing organizations, and individual psychiatric nurses. (See Appendix A for Standards of Psychiatric and Mental Health Nursing Practice.)

2. *Breach of duty.* Failure to care for a client according to the nursing standard results in a breach of the nurse's duty to the client.

3. *Injury.* The client is injured.

4. *Proximate causation.* The nurse's breach of duty is the direct cause of the injury.

The question remains, How can a nurse be protected from liability? There is no guaranteed or foolproof method of avoiding legal liability. However, there are certain basic ways, which might seem obvious, to limit one's exposure to legal liability.

First, communicate with the client, the physician, and all other significant persons in the treatment of the client. Both verbal and written communication should be complete and accurate.

Second, know the hospital or agency policies and procedures and follow them. If there is not a policy to cover a particular situation, take action to have the policy developed.

Third, if a doctor's order or a client's request is unclear, seek clarification before, not after, acting upon it.

Fourth, if unable to handle the work assignment alone, seek assistance from the appropriate persons (e.g., a nursing supervisor).

Fifth, if an error is made, notify the physician and other pertinent staff so that action can be taken to avoid or minimize injury to the client.

Sixth, when there is no right or wrong way to treat the client, assess the situation with consideration of what is in the client's best interest.

Vignette

Mr. S. is newly admitted to the unit. After 30 years in the management of a large company, he has been laid off. At home he has been despondent, unable to eat or sleep, and indifferent to his welfare. On admission he seems pleasant and cooperative; however, his doctor has ordered suicide precautions. The hospital suicide precautions specifically state that a client can leave the unit only if attended by a hospital care provider. Mr. S. seeks permission to go to the chapel. The unit is busy and there is no one free to accompany him; his condition seems stable so the nurse allows him to go unattended. The time is 10:00 A.M. At the change of shift the nurse realizes he is not on the unit. A search is initiated. He is found at the bottom of a stairwell.

Questions for Consideration

1. Is the nurse liable for Mr. S.'s death?

In this situation the nurse may be liable for negligent supervision of the client. She had a duty to protect the client. Although in the nurse's initial judgment, the client seemed cheerful, the physician had ordered suicide precautions; the nurse failed to follow the hospital suicide precautions or to hold Mr. S. on the unit to assess his mental status. Also, the nurse did not check for his safe return within a reasonable time. More than likely, a reasonably prudent nurse would assess the client's condition, follow the medical orders, and adhere to hospital policy for suicide precautions. Therefore, this nurse violated the standard of care and breached her duty to the patient. Her breach of duty could be proved to be the direct cause of Mr. S.'s death.

2. Who else would be liable?

The hospital would also be liable for the nurse's actions.

3. How could the result have been avoided?

As the employer, the hospital may be liable for failure to provide sufficient staff to cover a busy unit.

In contrast, an actual case held that when a physician ordered that a client be allowed to leave the unit and the client has exhibited no suicidal tendencies, the staff is not liable for negligent supervision in the event the client commits suicide (*Payne* v. *Milwaukee Sanitarium*, 1977).

Vignette

Ms. X. is receiving high doses of chlorpromazine (Thorazine). She has not refused the medication because she very much wants to do whatever is necessary to maintain her health. However, she has begun to complain of uncontrollable mouth movements. The nurse has observed the mouth movements, charts the observations, and reports them to the doctor. After her treatment is reviewed and discussed with Ms. X., the doctor decides that this is a side effect from the Thorazine, but feels that her need for the drug outweighs the seriousness of the side effect. Together with the doctor, the nurse decides to note increasing side effects, but continues to administer the drug. The client is informed of this plan. Eventually the client suffers from irreversible tardive dyskinesia before the drug is discontinued. She sues the nurse and the doctor.

Questions for Consideration

Is the nurse exposed to liability for malpractice?

In this situation, although the client suffered a permanent injury, it is not probable that the nurse would be negligent. The nurse owed a duty to the client. A judgment was made that the client's need for the drug outweighed the side effects. The nurse observed the side effects and reported them. If expert witnesses testify that the judgment made by the nurse was that of a reasonably prudent nurse, it is unlikely that she would be found to have breached her duty to her client. The possible issue which could lead to liability for someone, whether nurse or doctor, would be whether the patient continued receiving the drug without being fully informed that she may have permanent side effects from it. If she continued with the drug, not realizing the side effects, she may have a claim. Therefore documentation of client teaching and the client's consent to continue receiving the drug could be very important in establishing that Mrs. X consented to continued treatment.

The psychiatric nurse plays an important role in providing care that complies with legal standards. The nursing staff should design and implement policies and procedures for admission, treatment, and discharge of clients that do not interfere with a client's rights.

The Care Plan. The care plan should be carefully designed for each individual client. When possible a nurse should allow the client to participate in the formulation of the plan, which should focus on treatment that least restricts the individual. As the client's condition changes the treatment plan should be modified.

Documentation. Treatment, care, and assessment should be carefully recorded. Documentation should include the client's understanding of the treatment. If a client is treated involuntarily, the decision-making process in administering forced treatment should be carefully documented. The nurse should maintain a complete and accurate record of nurse-client interactions, observations, and interventions.

Discharge. A client voluntarily admitted to a hospital may be discharged with or against medical advice. If a voluntarily admitted client poses a danger to himself or others, the nurse should have a working knowledge of the state's law for holding a client so that the dangerous person will not be released until commitment proceedings are initiated. If the client is not dangerous, he may leave even against medical advice. However, the nurse should spend time with the client discussing the discharge and should document the circumstances of discharge.

■ Enrichment Activities

DISCUSSION QUESTIONS

1. James Smith is a 75-year-old widower. His family is becoming increasingly concerned about his suspicious behavior. He refuses to leave his apartment, and has had the gas and electricity shut off (even though it's the middle of a cold winter) because he believes others will use these power sources to harm him while he sleeps. As far as anyone can tell, he has little food in the apartment and refuses all offers of

food brought in. His appearance indicates that he has lost weight. Would Mr. Smith be an appropriate candidate for involuntary psychiatric admission? Why or why not?

2. Your one-to-one client was voluntarily admitted yesterday expressing the concern that she was afraid of killing her children. Today she tells you that was all a mistake, and she needs to return home or she is afraid she will lose her job and her husband. She asks you to call a taxi, saying, "I signed myself in and I can sign myself out." What are your responsibilities (as a student or staff nurse) in this situation? What is the best way of dealing with this situation?

3. Ellen Green is diagnosed as having chronic schizophrenia. Her behavior is regressed and inappropriate, characterized by bizarre singing and posturing. Chlorpromazine (Thorazine) has always been effective in improving her behavior, but she is reluctant to take it, stating, "It makes my mouth all dry and the voices get blurry." She refuses the oral medication. The physician's order reads "Thorazine 100 mg. orally or 25 mg. IM q6h." Is the nurse justified in administering the dose ordered by forced injection? What is the rationale for the decision? What factors were considered? What other steps would be advisable?

4. If you were a member of a quality assurance committee, what criteria would you develop to assure that client rights are protected during hospitalization? What kinds (and from what sources) of data would you gather during a nursing audit to use these criteria to evaluate the quality of care in your institution?

5. With reference to the client rights discussed in this chapter, evaluate a psychiatric inpatient or mental health residential care setting in your community in regard to these rights.

SITUATIONS FOR ROLE PLAY

In groups of three or four, have selected members enact the nurse role and the client role. The other members serve as observers and provide information and suggestions to the member enacting the nurse role. Be sure to include strengths as well as areas for improvement. Remember also that one of the main benefits of role play is an opportunity to experience and discuss the feelings of the participants and to thus increase empathetic understanding.

1. Penny Adams was voluntarily admitted several days ago. When the nurse arrives at 3 P.M., Penny is angry and threatening to sign out because of an incident in a group session this afternoon when two other clients confronted her with avoidance of activity and interaction on the unit. Her recent history includes several suicide attempts in conjunction with drug and alcohol abuse. Her children are in a foster home because of a court finding of neglect. The nurse believes she will resume drug abuse and attempt suicide if released. This is an unlocked unit and the physician and supervisor must be contacted to arrange a transfer to a locked unit. In the meantime, Penny is throwing her clothes into a suitcase and planning to walk out.

2. John Doe is very withdrawn and apathetic. He is quite suspicious of others' attempts to interact and, if encouraged to spend time in the community rooms, feigns sleep to avoid socializing. He is beginning to feel somewhat comfortable with one nurse who is attempting to involve Mr. Doe in planning his care.

■ Recommended Readings

Barton, W., and Sanborn, C. (eds.). *Law and the mental health professions*. New York: International Universities Press, Inc., 1978. Legal and mental health experts examine significant topics such as informed consent, confidentiality, competency, client rights, and the concept of dangerousness.

Bullough, Bonnie. *The law and the expanding nursing role*, 2d ed. New York: Appleton-Century-Crofts, 1980. Covers evolving legal applications, political action, the historical context of the law, and specific legal ramifications of expanded roles in nursing.

Chodoff, P. The case for involuntary hospitalization of the mentally ill. *American journal of psychiatry*, 133, 1976:496. Discusses the concept of dangerousness and three views of involuntary hospitalization.

Daughtery, L.B. Assessing the attitudes of psychiatric aides toward a patients' rights. *Hospital and community psychiatry*, 29,4, 1978:225–229. Valuable information regarding the attitudes of psychiatric staff toward clients and malpractice.

Fiesta, Janine. *The law and liability—a guide for nurses*. New York: Wiley Medical, 1983. Presents basic comprehensive information on the nurse and the law.

Kittrie, N. *The right to be different*. Baltimore: Johns Hopkins University Press, 1971. For the nurse who wishes to explore some of the controversies between humanism and legal practicality in areas of criminal law which touch aspects such as delinquency, addiction, and antisocial behavior.

Shapiro, M. Legislating the control of behavior control: Autonomy and coercive use of organic therapies. *Southern California Law Review*, 47:237–356, 1982. Legal discussion of the controversy about banning electroshock therapy in California.

Stein, L., and Test, M. (eds.). *Alternatives to mental hospital treatment.* New York: Plenum, 1978. Explorations of options other than psychiatric hospitalization; these become important alternatives in the context of the legal requirement that care be provided in the least restrictive environment.

■ *References*

Note: The references for this chapter are listed alphabetically according to the names of the litigants in the significant case law or according to the law or topic title listed in state or national statutes. The sources listed are found in reference materials contained in law libraries, not general libraries.

Addington v. Texas. 441 S. Ct. 418 (1979).

Anderson (State ex rel) v. U.S. Veterans Hospital. 268 *Minn.* 213, 128 N.W., 2d, 710.

Brady v. Hopper. District Court of Colorado. 570 *F. Supp.*, 1333, 1983.

Cal. Admin. Code, §§ 5326. 6 and 7 (1982).

Child Abuse Reporting Statute. *Utah code ann.* § 78-36-2 (1978).

Clites v. State of Iowa. 322 N.W. 2d 917, (1982).

Custody of a Minor—Massachusetts. 379 N.E. 2d 1053, (1978).

Eberhardy (Matter of Guardianship) Wisconsin. 97 *Wis.* 2d 539 (1980); 294 N.W. 2d 540 (1980).

Goldblatt v. Hempstead. U.S. Supreme Court. 369 S. Ct. 590 (1969).

Human Experimentation Regulations. Health and Human Services Regulations in *Code of Federal Regulations*, Vol. 45, Part 46.

Incompetent Recording Statute. Reporting of abuse of children, incompetent or disabled persons. *Nebraska Revised Statutes*, § 28-711, 1982.

Kaimonitz v. Michigan Department of Mental Health. *Law Week*, 42:2069, 1973.

Lane v. Candura. Massachusetts Appellate Court. 376 N.E. 2d 1232 (1978).

May v. Leneau. 99 *Mich. App.* 209 (1980); 297 N.W. 2d 882 (1980).

Mellies v. National Heritage Inc. 6 *Kan. App.* 2d 910 (1981).

O'Connor v. Donaldson. U.S. Supreme Court. 422 S. Ct. 563 (1975).

Parham v. J.R. Supreme Court. 422 S. Ct. 584 (1979).

Payne v. Milwaukee Sanitarium Foundation, Inc. 81 *Wis.* 2d 264 (1977); 260 N.W. 2d 386.

People v. McQuillan. 392 *Mich.* 511; 221 N.W. 2d 569.

In re Quinlan New Jersey Court. 355 A. 2d 647 (1976).

Rennie v. Klein. 462 *F. Supp.* 1131; 653 F. 2d 836 (1981); *vacated*, 102 S. Ct. 3506 (1982).

Roe (Guardianship of) Massachusetts Court. 421 N.E. 2d 40 (1981).

Rogers v. Okin. District Court of Massachusetts. 478 *F. Supp.* 1342 (1979); *aff'd in part, rev'd in part*, 634 F. 2d 650 (1980).

In re Schock, Iowa Court. 211 N.W. 2d 327 (1973).

Tarasoff v. Regents of University of California. California Appellate Court. 141 Cal. 92 (1977).

Truman v. Thomas. 165 Cal. 308 (1980).

Wyatt v. Stickney. Middle District of Alabama. 344 *F. Supp.* 373 (1972).

Youngberg v. Romeo. 102 *S. Ct.* 2452 (1982).

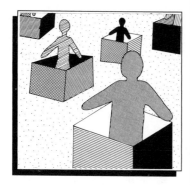

6

Ethical Issues

Mary Patricia Ryan

LEARNING OBJECTIVES

Upon completion of this chapter, the reader will be able to:

1. Recognize the duties and obligations that a nurse has according to the nursing codes.

2. Identify two ethical theories that commonly are used as a basis for critical ethical analysis.

3. Demonstrate an understanding of the ethical concepts that are important in psychiatric-mental health nursing.

4. Critically analyze cases by means of a critical ethical analysis model.

5. Value the patient as a human being who has rights by virtue of being human.

It has become increasingly apparent that considerations about ethics occupy an ever-expanding role in those health care areas that employ high technology equipment and methods in the fight against disease and death. In the mental health area, "high tech" is not very often invoked, and this may lead to the complacent attitude that ethical dilemmas are rare or nonexistent here. This could not be farther from the truth! The mental health-psychiatric nurse should be aware not only of the issues that arise in the care of mentally ill persons but also of the obligations that the caregiver should honor. In many states, mental health codes legally obligate the professional caregiver to recognize a person's rights. However, before the nurse considers the legal interpretation of rights, she needs to be aware of a moral code she should be following. Respect for a person as a human being and all of the rights to which he is entitled by reason of person falls within the realm of ethics: confidentiality, right to information, right to decide, right to refuse treatment, right to receive treatment, and justice are among the rights to which mentally ill persons are entitled.

There are special problems that arise when the competence of the mentally ill person is questionable. In some situations, the person may be competent to make decisions; in others, he may not be. The issue of competence places a moral burden on the nurse to determine when and what the mentally ill person can decide.

Historically, the mentally ill have been treated as though they had no rights, and indeed were to be feared. They were detained in institutions well away from the cities; abandoned, many times, by their families; cared for by people who often lacked the professional skills and commitment to help them to improve; and occasionally ignored by researchers involved in the quest for new drugs and treatment techniques in other areas of health care.

Only in the last half of the present century has a concerted effort been made by investigators to develop drugs to help control the behavior of the mentally ill. Although these drugs have been instrumental in relieving suffering, their use has generated ethical issues because of conflict over the person's right to decide whether or not to receive them. Such therapies as electroshock and psychosurgery have also raised ethical issues all along the way—for the sick person, the family, the professionals administering the treatment, and the public.

Even today, some stigma attaches to the mentally ill person, and when so diagnosed, the person can no longer assume that his human rights will be honored. He may be looked upon with fear, or as incompetent. A physical illness that resolves is soon forgotten, whereas the label of mental illness follows the person through life.

☐ Professional Codes

Professional codes are important guides to behavior for health workers. In the U.S., the American

---

TABLE 6-1 Code for Nurses. American Nurses' Association[a]

1. The nurse provides services with respect for human dignity and the uniqueness of the client unrestricted by considerations of social or economic status, personal attributes, or the nature of health problems.

2. The nurse safeguards the client's right to privacy by judiciously protecting information of a confidential nature.

3. The nurse acts to safeguard the client and the public when health care and safety are affected by the incompetent, unethical, or illegal practice of any person.

4. The nurse assumes responsibility and accountability for individual nursing judgments and actions.

5. The nurse maintains competence in nursing.

6. The nurse exercises informed judgment and uses individual competence and qualifications as criteria in seeking consultation, accepting responsibilities, and delegating nursing activities to others.

7. The nurse participates in activities that contribute to the ongoing development of the profession's body of knowledge.

8. The nurse participates in the profession's efforts to implement and improve standards of nursing.

9. The nurse participates in the profession's efforts to establish and maintain conditions of employment conducive to high quality nursing care.

10. The nurse participates in the profession's efforts to protect the public from misinformation and misrepresentation and to maintain the integrity of nursing.

11. The nurse collaborates with members of the health professions and other citizens in promoting community and national efforts to meet the needs of the public.

[a] Reprinted by permission of the American Nurses' Association. *Code for Nurses with Interpretive Statements*. Kansas City, MO: American Nurses' Association, 1985.

TABLE 6-2 *Code for Nurses: Ethical Concepts Applied to Nursing. International Council of Nurses*[a]

The fundamental responsibility of the nurse is fourfold: to promote health, to prevent illness, to restore health and to alleviate suffering.

The need for nursing is universal. Inherent in nursing is respect for life, dignity and rights of man. It is unrestricted by consideration of nationality, race, creed, colour, age, sex, politics or social status.

Nurses render health services to the individual, the family and the community and coordinate their services with those of related groups.

Nurses and People

The nurse's primary responsibility is to those people who require nursing care.

The nurse, in providing care, promotes an environment in which the values, customs and spiritual beliefs of the individual are respected.

The nurse holds in confidence personal information and uses judgement in sharing this information.

Nurses and Practice

The nurse carries personal responsibility for nursing practice and for maintaining competence by continual learning.

The nurse maintains the highest standards of nursing care possible within the reality of specific situation.

The nurse uses judgement in relation to individual competence when accepting and delegating responsibilities.

The nurse when acting in a professional capacity should at all times maintain standards of personal conduct which reflect credit upon the profession.

Nurses and Society

The nurse shares with other citizens the responsibility for initiating and supporting action to meet the health and social needs of the public.

Nurses and Co-Workers

The nurse sustains a cooperative relationship with co-workers in nursing and other fields.

The nurse takes appropriate action to safeguard the individual when his care is endangered by a co-worker or any other person.

Nurses and the Profession

The nurse plays the major role in determining and implementing desirable standards of nursing practice and nursing education.

The nurse is active in developing a core of professional knowledge.

The nurse, acting through the professional organization, participates in establishing and maintaining equitable social and economic working conditions in nursing.

---

[a] Reprinted by permission of the International Council of Nurses, 1985.

Nurses' Association (ANA) formulated its code in 1950, and revised it in 1976 with very few changes (Table 6-1). The accompanying interpretive statements have been amended several times since 1950, and at this writing are being revised by the ANA Committee on Ethics. It is important that the professional nurse be well acquainted with the Code for Nurses because it is the basis for judgments about unethical behavior on her part. The 1982 ANA Standards of Psychiatric and Mental Health Nursing Practice (see Appendix A) describe the duties and obligations of the mental health psychiatric nurse. The International Council of Nurses (ICN) adopted the International Code of Nursing Ethics in 1953, and in 1965 replaced it with the Code for Nurses, which is the official document of the International Council of Nurses (Table 6-2).

□ VALUES

Some mental health professionals contend that neither the therapist's nor the client's personal values have a place in the therapeutic process. They argue that the client comes to the therapist with one or more identified problems and the only duty of the therapist is to help the client to resolve the problems. However, they would probably admit that each client does have religious, moral, and cultural values; and that these must be understood for diagnostic purposes. Beyond that, "values-neutral" therapists believe that the therapist has no right to impose her own values on the client or indeed even to explore or examine the client's values. Much of this reluctance is an outgrowth of the behaviorist movement that contends that behavior change alone is important. If a behavior needs to be reinforced or extinguished, the coach (therapist/trainer) may reward or punish that particular behavior so that it appears more and more frequently, or less and less frequently. Behaviorists consider the person's "inner life" to be unimportant. The emergence of the desirable behavior or the extinction of the undesirable behavior is the therapeutic goal. The behaviorist does not enter into the process except to confer reward or punishment. The client is seen as acting alone in his reaction to the impersonal reward or punishment.

Behaviorism reached its peak in the 1960s and has been incorporated into the therapeutic approaches of many mental health professionals, including nurses. Most professionals do not use behaviorist techniques in their pure form, though the values-neutral (or values-free) stand of earlier behaviorists is still accepted. This may cause confusion or a block in therapy. Because of the behaviorists' belief that no values, neither those of the therapist nor those of the client, enter into therapy sessions, values are not often discussed. There persists the myth that values are safely tucked away during a therapy session. Frequently a nurse reports being appalled by a certain story told by a client; yet when questioned, she states that she listened to the client's recital and offered no response whatever—indeed, she did not even question the client about his feelings.

Should values enter into a nurse's relationship with a client? Is a values-neutral posture humanly possible? How do clients' values enter into the nurse-patient relationship? What should be done by the nurse about the client's values? These questions are discussed in the following sections.

WHAT IS A VALUE?

A value is a perception of worth that an individual (or a group of individuals) places on an object, an idea, or an attitude. This worthiness leads the individual to make *ought* or *should* demands on himself in relation to the value and to suffer discomfort when these demands are not met. Uustal (1978) states that values are general guides to behavior or standards of conduct which a person endorses and tries to live up to or to maintain. Values also provide a frame of reference through which a person integrates, explains, and appraises new ideas, events, and personal relationships (Uustal, 1978). Values are not directly apprehended, but are inferred from the person's verbal and nonverbal behavior. They are one part of the unique personality within a person's innermost being, as demonstrated by the act of choice (Fagothey, 1976). A person is not born having values—they are acquired through explanation, moralizing, modeling, reward or punishment, identification with a person or group, or through manipulation. They derive as a part of family life and are reinforced by school, religious, and peer influences.

VALUES FORMATION AND MATURATION

Freud's doctrine of the superego reflected his dedicated attempt to discover the childhood roots of what in the adult would be called the conscience and a system of values. Freud also exposed the irrational beginnings of the superego which a person would like to consider one of the most rational features of adult life.

Piaget's studies (1932) of moral judgments in children support the foregoing picture of early irrationality. The young child cannot fully grasp the meaning of moral values, which therefore are interpreted in a literal way that often is widely at variance with adult intentions. Values are accepted by young children with some duress; they are misinterpreted, taken over by identification, rejected in the negativism stage, and become a bone of contention in contests between parents and children.

Piaget traced the evolution of the child's moral judgment between the seventh and fifteenth years. He showed a movement from a literal belief in rules to an attitude of relativity. Young children lent to the rules a nearly independent physical existence, whereas older children developed an attitude of relativity in which rules were perceived in relation to the social purposes they were designed to serve. Piaget found that the growth trend could not be simply considered as a maturing of the intellect. It depended on the child's experience in social interactions which enabled him to see for himself the consequences of rules and their violation (Piaget, 1932).

The growth trend continues in the adult as the values are humanized. In adulthood, the person increasingly discovers the human meaning of values and their relation to the meaning of social purposes. The person also increasingly brings in his personal experiences and motives in affirming and promoting a value system.

Overall, the trend from early childhood is to move from absolute received values to a personally constructed value system (White, 1966). However, the above progression of moral development might not occur if the person's intellect becomes impaired by disease, injury, social isolation, or any other grave assault.

VALUES CLARIFICATION

Values clarification theory (Raths, et al., 1966; Simon, 1972; Uustal, 1978) offers an approach that attempts to help individuals sort through, analyze, and set priorities of their own values. Barry (1982) states that values clarification tries to help people begin to act in a way that is consistent with their own values. Values clarification is concerned primarily with the process of valuing. According to Raths (1966), there are three elements (choosing, prizing, and acting), that comprise seven steps involved in clarifying values:

1. Choosing
   Choosing freely
   Selecting from alternatives
   Choosing after consideration of the consequences of each alternative
2. Prizing
   Being proud of and happy with the choice
   Being willing to affirm the choice publicly
3. Acting
   Making the choice part of one's behavior
   Repeating the choice

Everyone would agree that a value should be freely chosen. Children learn to accept the values of their family until the time that they begin to explore other alternatives. The need to choose among alternatives is believed to be a great contributor to adolescent turmoil. Adolescents or young adults may move from one peer group to another, accepting the group's values and trying to live up to them, only to find these values not useful in meeting their personal goals. The adolescent or young adult then may experience a growing sense of uncertainty, frustration, and confusion. Some may seek professional help for the discomfort they are experiencing.

If the individual has completed the first three steps successfully, then movement is made to prizing a value. A sense of contentment and happiness is experienced in this step, and the person is ready to proclaim the chosen value publicly. It may be announced to a family member, friends, or to strangers, as at a meeting or in the classroom. The value is first prized by the self and then shared with others.

The process of valuing is not complete unless there is action. The person's behavior must indicate that there has been a shift from insight to behavior. What is the purpose of choosing and prizing unless one does something about that which is valued? Hence, the final step involves acting consistently upon a value. For example, if a person says that good health is valued but makes no effort to promote his own health, others

will begin to question whether he actually does value good health.

APPLICATION OF VALUES TO PSYCHIATRIC-MENTAL HEALTH NURSING

Personal Values

Not only must the nurse working in the mental health area be aware of her own values; she must also have experienced the process of values clarification so that her personal values are recognized as such. If the nurse does not do this, there is a danger that her values will unconsciously guide not only her own behavior but also that of the client. It is only with deliberate values clarification that the client will be able to begin the process of acting in ways consistent with his chosen goals.

Professional Values

The psychiatric-mental health nurse has at least three guides: the ANA Code for Nurses (Table 6.1), the ICN Code for Nurses: Ethical Concepts Applied to Nursing (Table 6.2), and the ANA Standards of Psychiatric and Mental Health Nursing Practice (Appendix A). These reflect the values that have been endorsed by the nursing profession to serve as standards guiding the conduct of its members. However, values do not exist in a vacuum—they are a reflection and an expansion of earlier learned personal standards. If a professional nurse has only a conceived idea about how to act and has not internalized professional as well as personal values, little pride and satisfaction will develop and commitment to the profession will be lacking. Instead, there may be anger, apathy, and destructiveness because the nurse has failed to see that professional acts are experienced by the self. Personal and professional values of responsibility and competence propel action carried out by the self. Satisfaction follows if the action is consonant with the values.

☐ General Considerations About Ethics

Ethics is the study of the nature of morals, as well as the rules or standards that govern the conduct of the members of a profession. From the many ethical theories that have been proposed, a person can select the ethical framework that most closely fits his personal value system. Two of the most prominent theories are discussed below.

UTILITARIANISM

The theory of utilitarianism is both teleological and consequentialist and is associated with the phrase "the greatest good for the greatest number." Teleological refers to the goal-oriented nature of the theory; consequentialist means that the rightness or wrongness of an act is judged based on the consequences of the act. John Stuart Mill believed that the rightness or wrongness of any act is decided by its consequences, more specifically, on whether its consequences are best for the whole. "What is best for the whole" brings about the greatest happiness or the least suffering for the largest number of people. Guided by this tenet as the single moral principle by which rightness and wrongness can be identified and judged, utilitarians assert that one ought to produce the greatest possible balance of good (happiness) over evil (unhappiness or displeasure).

The utilitarian theory is prevalent today. It functions in decision making about welfare programs, Medicare and Medicaid benefits, and in other areas of public interest that involve expenditures for public health. As applied to health care, utilitarianism influences the risk-benefit ratio involved in such decision making. Medical experimentation is said to be justified on the ground that administering possibly risky therapies to a limited number of subjects has the potential of conferring great benefit on many more numbers of people at some later time.

The theory of utilitarianism poses problems, however. The question "Who should be treated?" is answered by the statement "Those who stand to benefit most from the treatment." Those who have benefited then should contribute most to ensure the greatest benefit for the whole (Dyck, 1977, 58). On this basis, many of those with whom health care professionals work would be prevented from receiving care. The dying, mentally ill, developmentally delayed, chronically ill, and seriously ill would be much less likely to benefit that those whose disorders are minor, whose conditions might benefit from elective surgery, and the like. Most health care professionals give priority to those whose need is greatest and who are most likely to survive.

A second problem posed by the utilitarian theory is that it is future-oriented. As has been noted, its efficacy is evaluated based on the consequences of a particular action. Past and present do not play a part in decision making, and neither promises nor gratitude nor ramifications of the act are involved.

DEONTOLOGY

Deontology, or formalism, is an ethical theory that focuses on duties and obligations based on rules and principles. Contrary to the utilitarian view, Deontologists believe that they are not merely agents who initiate acts for desirable ends, but are also responders to the claims of others. Their responsibilities to others are more varied and also more specific than the responsibility to promote good. The principles that guide deontological theory are autonomy, beneficence, nonmaleficence, and justice.

Autonomy is considered with respect for persons in its many aspects: confidentiality/privacy, right to information, right to decide for or against treatment, and competence. Beneficence focuses on doing good for others, while the closely related principle of nonmaleficence encompasses refraining from both doing intentional harm and the risk of doing harm. According to Beauchamp and Childress (1979, 99–100), the duty of nonmaleficence not only prohibits intentional harm—except in special circumstances—but also requires that the agent be thoughtful and act with care. These authors state that harm or risk may be unintentional; the person—the agent—may be totally unaware of any possible risks, as well as free of any intention to do harm. The element of either omission or commission may be present. The principle of justice has to do with labeling issues which affect allocation of scarce resources and fairness of opportunity. Society assigns labels to some human conditions more readily than to others; the labels may influence not only health care decisions but access to health care as well. Labels such as aged, poor, retarded, insane, black, may become the determinants of what goods or services a person shall receive.

☐ Ethical Concepts

RESPECT FOR PERSONS

Perhaps the most important of all ethical concepts in health care is that of respect for persons. It is central to the opening statement of the ANA Code for Nurses. Immanuel Kant, the "father of deontology," believed that there was only one "categorical imperative"—the single principle upon which he based his ethical theory. Kant believed that one must always act in ways that respect each human being (including oneself) as a creature having thoughts, plans, goals, aspirations, and hopes. That is, every person should be treated as a rational creature. Stated in reverse, it is impermissible to fail to treat all human beings as rational creatures (Donagan, 1977, 59–66).

Although many mental health clients may not appear to be rational much of the time, they possess the potential for rationality. It is this potential (which may be temporarily absent) that determines whether or not the client will be treated with respect. Respect for a client demands that he be treated as an "end"—not as a means or instrument of someone else's will.

INFORMED CONSENT

Informed consent has evolved as a result of more rigid research criteria and various rights movements, including mental health client rights. The need for informed consent in conducting research became very clear during the Nuremberg Trials following World War II, out of which grew the Nuremberg Code. The first principle of the code is helpful in conceptualizing informed consent as it applies to health care:

> The voluntary consent of the subject is absolutely essential. This means that the person involved should have legal capacity to give consent; should be so situated as to be able to exercise free power of choice, without the intervention of any element of force, fraud, deceit, duress, overreaching, or other ulterior form of constraint or coercion; and should have sufficient knowledge and comprehension of the subject matter involved as to enable him to make an understanding and enlightened decision. The latter element requires that before the acceptance of an affirmative action decision by the experimental subject there should be made known to him the nature, duration, and purpose of the experiment; the method and means by which it is to be conducted; all inconveniences and hazards reasonably to be expected; and the effects upon his health or person which may possibly come from his participation in the experiment. (Nuremberg Code, Rule 1., 1949)

By and large, professional health care codes of ethics stress self-determination by clients and

require that informed consent be obtained before any significant therapeutic or research procedures are undertaken. Alexander Capron (1974) states that the primary function of informed consent is to protect individual autonomy. According to Beauchamp and Childress (1979), autonomy is fostered in at least two ways: first, at the relationship level, and second, at the societal level. At the first level autonomy is protected because the client has the right to make decisions affecting his life, though the health professional may possess more information and may have had more training. Mill (1974) suggests that at the second level, autonomy is protected by mechanisms society has created whose purpose is to protect individual thought and initiative. According to Mill, the interests of both society and the individual are thereby enhanced.

Many health care professionals are not in complete agreement with the concept of informed consent, which ensures that the client will be afforded the right to make decisions about his health care. Dealing with clients who are not consistently rational or with those who are not ever rational gives rise to a serious problem: How can the health care professional carry out the obligation of informed consent with such clients?

Beauchamp and Childress (1979) have identified four elements that are central to informed consent. The *information elements* are disclosure of information, and comprehension of information. The *consent elements* are voluntary consent and competence to consent. Because competence must be present so that the other three elements can be assessed, it is discussed first.

Competence

The concept of competence is complex. It is not a moral issue but a factual matter best determined by trained professionals. The professional will have certain responsibilities toward the client based on the finding (or its lack) of competence. A judgment about competence is a preparation for making a moral judgment but not in itself a moral judgment. Beauchamp and Childress (1979) have found that competence and incompetence are often assessed on the basis of diverse and even inconsistent theories about comprehension, rationality, freedom, physiological state, and others. Realistically, however, judgments as to incompetence often apply to only a limited range of decision making. These authors further state that persons who are judged to be legally incompetent may, nevertheless, be competent to conduct most of their personal affairs, and vice versa. A person's ability to make decisions may vary over time: he may, simultaneously, be competent to make certain decisions but incompetent to make others. Beauchamp and Childress find that the notions of limited competence and intermittent competence are useful because they require a statement about the decisions a person can make, while avoiding the false dichotomy of competence vs. incompetence. Following these guidelines would preserve maximum autonomy and justify intervention only in those areas where the client's competence is clearly questionable (1979, 67–68).

Examples of intermittent competence are often seen in clients with schizophrenia. During acute episodes, a client may be admitted to a mental health facility because he is unable to meet the most basic needs for survival. Many times, the client is so absorbed in hearing "voices" that it is impossible for the professional to include him in decision-making. Before a decision is made, however, the client should be assessed for ability to participate in its formation. Many clients can make decisions about food preferences, participation in activities, or with whom they will interact. The client should be allowed to make all the decisions possible. As treatment progresses, the clients can participate more fully in decisions about himself. He may not be competent in one or two areas of decision-making, for example, in the matter of finances, and it is in such areas that a guardian may be needed. An important point to remember is that a schizophrenic client, during acute exacerbations of the illness, may not be capable of participating in decisions about his care, but during stable periods, can make most personal decisions if allowed to do so.

The determination of competence standards is problematic. As regards health care, a de facto determination is made, based on various theories. In a court of law, a de juris determination is made, based on case law. The result of these differences is that there is not total agreement between civil and criminal courts. A reasonable statement incorporating several standards is the following:

> A person is competent if and only if that person can make decisions based on rational reasons . . . this standard entails that a person must be able to understand a therapy or research procedure, must be able to weigh its risks and benefits, and must be able to make a decision in the light of such knowledge and through such abilities, even if the person

chooses not to utilize the information. (Beauchamp and Childress, 1979, 69)

Disclosure of Information

Controversy and resistance surround the element of disclosure of information. Three standards have emerged from legal and ethical sources: (1) what is operative in the biomedical professions, (2) what a reasonable person would want to know, and (3) what individual clients or subjects of research want to know (Beauchamp and Childress, 1979, 71). At one time it was usual to follow the first standard in determining how much information should be disclosed to clients and research subjects; more recently, the second standard has prevailed. What a reasonable person should know includes the following elements (which adhere to the third standard):

1. The procedures to be followed if the proposed course of treatment is pursued;
2. The likely results of the proposed treatment;
3. The attendant discomforts and risks as well as the expected benefits of the proposed treatment;
4. The possible alternatives to the proposed treatment along with a report of their risks and benefits; and
5. The likely results if the client remains untreated.

(Muyskens, 1982, 118)

The client cannot make an informed choice unless the professional shares information about results, risks, benefits, and alternatives. It might not be possible in every case to provide all of the aforementioned information. If every fact is not known to the health professional the goal of complete disclosure is not obtainable. It is possible, however, to disclose all information relevant to a particular situation and to let the client know that further information is available to him if he asks for it. The most important point for the health professional to keep in mind is that the reasonable person is a composite—a microcosm—of society. If this is not done, and the focus is on the individual client, the net result of the disclosure could be highly subjective; also the information could be speculative rather than factual.

There is much work to be done in the realm of client and family teaching about the person's psychiatric illness. Materials are available to help the professionals explain the illness to client and family. Lay organizations have available printed materials, and many of their members are willing to share experiences with those who are confronting a psychiatric illness for the first time. Mental health professionals should accept leadership for imparting information to the client, family, and to support groups.

Another area where a lack of information is evident is the actual treatment. Client ignorance about prescribed medications is widespread. Many clients do not know, or can't remember, the name of the drug or drugs they take. Nor do they know the dose, the drug's purpose, its side effects, or complications. They may have been informed but have forgotten. The professional needs to keep in mind the client's intermittently impaired cognitive state as well as the family's anxiety level at the time the treatment information is given.

Information Comprehension

If the health professional lacks confidence in the client's ability to understand, she may fail to make a real effort to offer all of the information the client needs to make an informed choice. A client may be unable to comprehend the most basic explanation—yet often this becomes an excuse for the nurse to bypass the obligation to give understandable information. If the nurse realizes that the client may not have understood the information, as the client advocate she must challenge whoever discloses the information. If the client appears competent to understand, the nurse has a duty to see that he receives and understands applicable information. This is seldom an easy task. The nurse must remember that the standard is that which applies to a reasonable person. In working with clients, she should strive to develop appropriate contexts in which both the delivery and the receipt of information will be enhanced.

Voluntariness

The informed consent element of voluntariness centers on the client's ability to choose his own goals from among the available ones without being unduly influenced or coerced. Undue influence occurs when one person puts forth an overly persuasive argument or promises a reward that is highly desired. Coercion arises when a person actually threatens or manipulates the situation in order to influence another person's choice. Coercion and undue influence are points on a continuum, rather than discrete entities. For example, it is difficult to establish whether a mentally ill client has freely chosen to be admitted, has been unduly influenced, or has been coerced into being admitted "voluntarily."

Influence is not necessarily coercive or undue: most persons are influenced in everyday living by persuasive arguments or are swayed by a respected family member or community leader. On the other hand, many professionals may threaten to stop the therapy if the client does not agree to a decision that the professional deems desirable.

CONFIDENTIALITY

From the time when the Hippocratic Oath was enunciated, confidentiality as regards nurse-client interactions has been paramount.

The second statement of the ANA code is: "The nurse safeguards the client's right to privacy by judiciously protecting information of a confidential nature" (Table 6-1). Two points in the interpretive statements accompanying the ANA Code are important here. The first is that the interpretive statements clarify the nurse's duty regarding disclosure to the health care team:

> It is an accepted standard of nursing practice that data about the health status of clients be accessible, communicated, and recorded . . . . When knowledge gained in confidence is relevant or essential to others involved in planning or implementing the client's care, professional judgment is used in sharing it. Only information pertinent to a client's treatment and welfare is disclosed and only to those directly concerned with the client's care. Interpretive Statement 2.1, American Nurses' Association, 1976)

The second concerns disclosure to those not involved in the client's care:

> The right of privacy is an inalienable right of all persons, and the nurse has a clear obligation to safeguard any confidential information about the client acquired from any source. The nurse-client relationship is built on trust. This relationship could be destroyed and the client's welfare and reputation jeopardized by injudicious disclosure of information provided in confidence. Since the concept of confidentiality has legal as well as ethical implications, an inappropriate breach of confidentiality may also expose the nurse to liability. (Interpretive Statement 2.3, American Nurses' Association, 1976)

It is particularly important in psychiatric-mental health nursing that the nurse respect confidentiality. The nurse gains access to feelings, thoughts, values, and sentiments that may never have been shared before. These innermost confidences come from the self of the client; privacy requires that he maintain control of such information, including access to it by other persons.

PATERNALISM

The Oxford dictionary defines paternalism as: "The principle and practice of paternal administration; government as by a father; the claim or attempt to supply the needs or to regulate the life of a nation or a community in the same way a father does those of his children." Beauchamp and Childress (1979) remind us that when health professionals see themselves in the father role, they must presuppose two characteristics of fatherhood: (1) the father has the interests of his children at heart, and (2) he makes all or at least some decisions relating to his children's welfare rather than letting them make these decisions.

Paternalism has come to play an important part in many health professionals' activities. Because of their strong need and desire for help, some clients seem to be quite willing to give up all of their autonomy, if that is what it takes to get relief; but for others, autonomy is not something they will give up willingly. The inequality of power in the relationship between client and nurse puts the client at a definite disadvantage, so that his bargaining power may be significantly weakened.

The mental health-psychiatric nurse has the obligation to protect client autonomy as much as possible, resorting to paternalism only when this is essential.

Illness may prevent the client from making informed decisions, and the nurse must therefore strike a balance between client values and goals, and the "reasonable person" yardstick. Fortunately, teamwork is widely practiced in the mental health area, affording a check on paternalistic decisions made when the client is capable of making his own decisions.

Effective discharge planning requires that safeguards against paternalism be built into the procedures. The team can meet and explore the possible placements available to the client upon his discharge. Unless his preferences are taken into account, and he participates in the selection process as much as possible, his autonomy will be violated—even though it is difficult to allow a client total autonomy in the context of limited resources. The nurse has a large role to play in en-

suring client participation because she may have the most information about client preferences.

BENEFIT/RISK RATIO

The nurse must keep constantly in mind the importance of beneficence and nonmaleficence. The nonmaleficence principle is seen by most ethicists as having precedence over beneficence, however, it has been a long-standing tradition for health care professionals, especially physicians, to cite beneficence as the main reason for recommending a certain treatment. Harm was usually not perceived as having great importance in day-to-day matters. But as technology has begun to play a more important role, it is now becoming clear that harm is a possible end result of treatment.

Benefits and risks are looked at together, so that both client and professional will have some idea of the outcome before treatment is started. The following discussion of specific therapies point to the need to weigh benefits and risks and to discuss them with the client, family, and other members of the team.

Psychotropic Drugs

Psychotropic drugs are widely prescribed in most health care areas. Some of these drugs are addicting and must be supervised and dispensed with utmost care. Others may give rise to irreversible complications. A detailed discussion of psychotropic drugs is given in Chapter 15.

Electroconvulsive Therapy (ECT)

ECT was at one time commonly used in treating the mentally ill because it was considered capable of temporarily altering behavior destructive to others or to the client. Some mental health professionals disputed the claim that the changes were temporary and feared that the treatment caused a loss of brain cells. Because of this, and because painful limb fractures sometimes followed the seizures caused by this therapy, ECT fell into relative disuse. In recent years the administration of ECT has been improved to the point that complications and pain have been largely eliminated. The client is informed about the nature of the procedure and is prepared as for a surgical procedure.

Controversy remains over whether brain cells are destroyed by ECT. Until the evidence is clear-cut one way or the other, the client should be informed of the possibility of memory loss from the procedure.

Psychosurgery

Lobotomy was a fairly common procedure in years past. Though this surgery is far less frequent today, controversy remains over its use. Fromer (1981, 242) states: "The problem with psychosurgery lies in the abrogation of the liberty of individuals and in the protection of their personhood while significant aspects of their behavior are changed." In the absence of clear assurances that the person's self will not be sacrificed in the interest of controlling his behavior, controversy over the use of lobotomy will continue.

Right to Refuse Treatment

It was long believed that only health care professionals, in particular psychiatrists, could determine what was best for the client; only in recent years has this "right" been challenged.

According to Reiser, mental illness clouds the picture in several ways:

> Two questions arise: 1) Is the problem one in which the patient can weigh certain kinds of alternatives rationally despite his mental illness? and 2) How does one judge whether the behaviors contemplated are actually harmful to the patient or others? In both instances, our medical ability to make accurate judgments is limited by current knowledge. These limits require us to ask another question: When considerable doubt exists on either or both counts, where ought we chance error—on overzealous therapy that invades rights of patients or on premature withdrawal that causes injury? (1980, 331)

The mental health code in many states allows treatments to be given if the client is a danger to himself or to others. Care must be taken that the assessment of *danger to self or others* is not made capriciously and is documented in writing in the client record. Reiser states that if the patient refuses the proposed treatment and there is clear evidence that the proposed therapy holds substantial promise of improving the condition, the psychiatrists should seek court authorization to intervene therapeutically against the wishes of the patient. Reiser further states that if the treatment can do little to fundamentally change a prognosis and the client is rational, he has the right to refuse treatment (1980, 331).

Vignettes

Identify the specific ethical concepts violated in each.

M., a 25-year-old white man, was admitted to the acute ward with a diagnosis of major depression. At admission, M. states to the psychiatrist that he does not want to receive any medication. After the psychiatrist tries to persuade M. to change his mind, the subject is dropped. Mr. M. is given a vitamin supplement because of a history of alcohol abuse. About 1 week after admission, he finds out from the nurse that he is getting a tricyclic drug.

P., a 21-year-old black woman, is admitted to the acute ward of the state hospital with a diagnosis of schizophrenia. Four weeks later, she is asked if she will agree to be transferred to an intermediate ward in the same hospital for further treatment. Miss P. is disappointed because she looked forward to going home soon. She delayed making the decision. One day she met her care coordinator in the hallway. He told her that she was going to go to the intermediate ward even if he had to drag her there by her hair. He was laughing as he said this.

W., a 59-year-old white woman, was admitted to the acute ward with a diagnosis of major recurrent depression. She told her student nurse that she had a secret she'd like to share but that she didn't want anyone else to know. The student was in a bind because the client had not seemed to be responding to the attempts to build a trusting relationship, and the student feared that if she refused to keep the secret, their relationship would be damaged.

J., a 19-year-old hispanic woman, is admitted to the acute ward with a diagnosis of catatonic schizophrenia. Her family brought her to the hospital. It was found that her second pregnancy was close to term. Shortly after her arrival labor started. Since there is no obstetrical unit in the hospital, her nurse accompanies Ms. J. to the medical center next door. The psychiatric nurse notes that Miss J. is immediately restrained, even though she is not hallucinating and is trying to cooperate. The admitting obstetrical nurse appears to be frightened. The psychiatric nurse has to return to the hospital.

JUSTICE

Issues of labeling and allocation of scarce resources are involved in discussions of justice.

Labeling

Certain groups in society have been assigned labels that suggest some weakness or inferior status. Such labels may determine the sort of care a client will receive. For example, the retarded, the physically handicapped, the aged, the poor, minorities, and prisoners acquire labels that encourage others to look upon them with disfavor. Potter (1977) holds that social justice demands that all are to be treated equally unless some relevant difference can be brought forward to support unequal distribution of benefits or burdens. Potter further contends that labels are justified only when they are likely to benefit those in need of special care. It is clear that further steps are necessary to ensure that mentally ill clients will not be restricted in obtaining care appropriate to their total needs. Mental health care professionals can play a leadership role in efforts to remove all restrictive labels.

Allocation of Scarce Resources

A problem related to labeling is the allocation of health care resources. Specifically, the health needs of a group of clients may be ignored because of the chronic nature of their illness, with the consequent costs of long-term treatment. Nurses can help the public to become aware of the inequities of insurance coverage—if coverage for a chronic physical illness is compared with that for a chronic mental illness, in most instances the discrepancy is enormous.

☐ Critical Ethical Analysis

Many models have been proposed for the working through of an ethical dilemma (Aroskar, 1980; Curtin, 1978; Murphy and Murphy, 1976; Thomasma, 1978). There are similarities among all of them. One model, that of Curtin, is discussed to acquaint the reader with a method for addressing ethical issues of psychiatric-mental health nursing.

Curtin proposes a model for critical ethical analysis (Figure 6-1) that a nurse might use in a specific situation, but cautions (1978, 12) that it is merely a tool and that "it can no more guarantee infallibility than it can dictate action." The model consists of:

Background Information. Facts that have a direct bearing on the situation must be identified and organized so that the decision maker(s) can get a clear picture of the problem.

Ethical Components. Ethical components include: individual freedom versus safety for society; treatment versus nontreatment; confidentiality versus safety of others; benefit from specific drugs or surgical procedures versus harm.

Ethical Agents. All of the persons who are involved in the situation should be identified. In questions of mental health, these persons are the client and most likely one or more of the following persons or agencies: psychiatrist(s), nurse(s), social worker, psychologist, psychiatric technician(s), family, social agencies in the community, police officer(s), court.

Options. The decision maker(s) must explore all possible options and accept or reject them according to the actual or potential results each action could or would produce, bearing in mind their duties and responsibilities.

Application of Principles. The decision

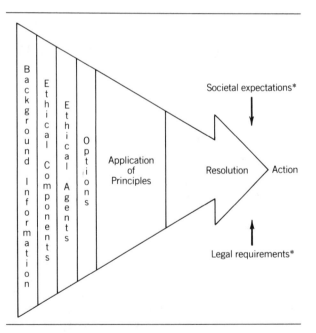

Figure 6-1 *Curtin's schematic of a proposed decision-making model (1978). Reprint permission granted by author and publisher, 1986. Credit Nursing Forum Vol. XVII, No. 1, 1978.*

---

* These extrinsic factors may sway the resolution of the conflict one way or another. But one must not confuse the notions of what is legal (or expected) with what is good, right or proper—they may or may not coincide.

maker(s) examine what (if any) principles are involved in the action. For example, in deontology the objective is to act *correctly* according to a moral principle regardless of the consequences. In utilitarianism, an action *per se* is neither right nor wrong. It becomes right when it produces the greatest happiness or the least harm to the greatest number.

Resolution. After examining the background information, identifying the ethical components and ethical agents, discussing all of the actual and potential options, and, applying the principles involved in the specific situation, the decision makers should be prepared to determine a course of action. The client, of course should be the ultimate decision maker. If the client is not competent, the nurse as a member of the team may participate in ethical decision making. It is for this reason that the nurse must develop skill in using a model.

■ Enrichment Activities

DISCUSSION QUESTIONS

The cases that follow are presented to afford the reader a basis for discussing with others what should and could be done to resolve the ethical issue presented. Use the model presented in this chapter or one which is already known. It is suggested that the cases be discussed in clinical conference to help the nurse gain confidence in recognizing and expressing her ethical duties and obligations to clients.

Application of the Theory

Background Information: B. is a 35-year-old black male being readmitted to an acute ward. He has received a diagnosis of paranoid schizophrenia and is having auditory and visual hallucinations. Mr. B. responds best to phenothiazines but these drugs were stopped because of the potential for tardive dyskinesia. The new drug prescribed is not controlling Mr. B.'s symptoms, and he cannot understand why the previous medication has been discontinued.

Identification of Ethical Components: Mr. B. believes that the first medicine helped him, and he preferred it to the new medication. The psychiatrist and the nurses are reluctant to prescribe and administer the phenothiazine because of the possibility of tardive dyskinesia, which is irreversible.

Ethical Agents: Mr. B., the client; the psychiatrist who prescribed the drug; the nurses who care for Mr. B. and who reported the symptoms to the psychiatrist.

Identification of Options: (1) The psychiatrist can have Mr. B. continue on the present medication and ignore his request. Mr. B. will probably be angry. (2) The psychiatrist can prescribe the phenothiazine again and risk the consequences to the client. The client will be pleased, the nurses will probably be angry; the psychiatrist will probably be worried. (3) The psychiatrist can have the client continue on the present medication and ask the nurses to instruct him about the possible harm to him if he were to have the phenothiazine. The psychiatrist will be relieved; the nurses will be relieved; the client may or may not be pleased.

Application of Principles: The principles of autonomy, beneficence, and nonmaleficence are all involved. The client is denied the freedom to choose the medication he prefers. The professionals believe that the principle of doing no harm (nonmaleficence) takes precedence over doing good (beneficence).

Resolution: The third option was chosen. The professionals were relieved. The client was upset at first but he came to appreciate the wisdom of the decision.

■ References

American Nurses Association. *Code for nurses with interpretive statements.* Kansas City, MO: American Nurses Association, 1976.

Aroskar, M.A. Anatomy of an ethical dilemma: the practice. *American journal of nursing*, 80, 1980: 661–663.

Barry, V. *Moral aspects of health care.* Belmont, CA: Wadsworth, 1982.

Beauchamp, T.L., and Childress, J.F. *Principles of biomedical ethics.* New York: Oxford University Press, 1979.

Capron, A. Informed consent in catastrophic disease and treatment. *University of Pennsylvania law review*, 123, 1974: 364–376.

Curtin, L.L. A proposed model for critical ethical analysis. *Nursing forum*, 17, 1978:12–17.

Donagan, A. *The theory of morality.* Chicago: The University of Chicago Press, 1977.

Dyck, A.J. *On human care: An introduction to ethics.* Nashville: Abingdon, 1977.

Fagothey, A. *Right and reason*. St. Louis: Mosby Company, 1976.

Fromer, M.J. *Ethical issues in health care*. St. Louis: Mosby Company, 1981.

International Council of Nurses. *Code for nurses: Ethical concepts applied to nursing*, 1943.

Mill, J.S. *On liberty*. New York: New American Library, 1974.

Murphy, M.A., and Murphy, J. Making ethical decisions systematically. *Nursing '76*, 5, 1976: 13–14.

Muyskens, J.L. *Moral problems in nursing: A philosophical investigation*. Totowa, NJ: Rowman and Littlefield, 1982.

The Nuremberg Code. In *Trials of war criminals before the Nuremberg military tribunals under Control Council Law No. 10*, 1949. Washington, D.C.: U.S. Government Printing Office.

Piaget, J. *The moral judgment of the child*. New York: Harcourt, Brace and World, 1932.

Potter, R.B. Labeling the mentally retarded: The just allocation of therapy. In *Ethics in medicine* (Reiser, S.J., Dyck, A.J., and Curran, W.) Cambridge, MA: MIT Press, 1977.

Raths, L., Simon, S., and Merrill, H. *Values and teaching*. Columbus, OH: Charles E. Merrill Books, 1966.

Reiser, S.J. Refusing treatment for mental illness: historical and ethical dimensions. *American journal of psychiatry*, 137, 3, 1980: 329–331.

The shorter Oxford English dictionary. 3d ed. S.V. "paternalism."

Simon B. *Values clarification: A handbook of practical strategies for teachers and students*. New York: Hart Publishing, 1972.

Thomasma, D.C. Training in medical ethics: an ethical workup. *Forum in medicine*, 12 (December, 1978).

Uustal, D.B. Values clarification in nursing: application to practice. *American journal of nursing*, 78, 12, 1978:2058–2063.

White, R.W. *Lives in progress: A study of the natural growth of a personality*. New York: Holt, Rinehart & Winston, 1966.

PART TWO

Professional Skills in Psychiatric-Mental Health Nursing

The tools of psychiatric-mental health nursing are not products of technology but of the nurse's very being, the self. Caring is the essence. The client may be an individual, a family, or a group in need of health care.

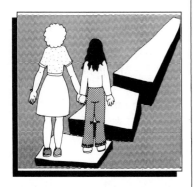

7

The Nursing Process

Joan Norris

Learning Objectives

Upon completion of this chapter, the reader will be able to:

1. Describe the components of the nursing process.

2. Identify the content and process of nursing assessment and nursing diagnosis.

3. Delineate significant aspects of nursing intervention including goal setting, planning, and implementation of care.

4. Recall steps of the evaluation process.

5. Incorporate knowledge of the standards of psychiatric mental health nursing practice into the nursing process at the generalist level.

The nursing process is the underlying scheme that provides order and direction to nursing care (Stanton, 1980:12). This process is based on the scientific method and the problem-solving process, which provide a systematic organization for nursing thought and action. Nurses generally agree on the steps included in this process as those of assessment, intervention or implementation, and evaluation. Assessment incorporates data collection and analysis which leads to a statement of the client problems—the nursing diagnosis. Intervention includes goal identification, planning, and implementation through nursing actions. Evaluation determines the progress made toward the goals and reexamines the entire process for needed modifications.

This process is applicable to all settings for nursing practice and is certainly not unique to psychiatric-mental health nursing. The Standards of Psychiatric and Mental Health Nursing Practice (See Appendix A) provide direction and guidance in determining quality of care. It is important to remember that although the nursing process is essentially the same whether used for a client who is undergoing a major illness or one who is experiencing a crisis of self-esteem, there are subtle complexities and broad areas of ambiguity that can make the process more difficult in the psychosocial domain. It is also essential to recall that for every client both the physical and psychosocial domains are present. There are no disembodied psyches in the mental health center, and certainly in the general hospital, both the new mother and the client diagnosed with cancer will have various thoughts, fears, and a wide array of emotions based in their unique situations.

The following discussion is designed to clarify relationships and techniques useful at various steps of the nursing process as carried out by the generalist in psychiatric-mental health nursing. Its application is appropriate to patients in psychiatric units, general hospitals, and community settings.

☐ *Assessment*

DATA COLLECTION

Data collection is systematic and comprehensive. The total value of the nursing process depends upon the quality of the data collected. Omission and inaccuracies result in misdiagnosis and in-

appropriate care since the usefulness of any plan of care is dependent on its relevance to the client's actual problems.

There are a variety of useful organizers to aid in planning assessments. These include functional areas of health assessment (Gordon, 1982), basic human needs (Maslow, 1954), and others which similarly incorporate aspects of physical, mental, and emotional needs; development; and functioning. A comprehensive database should be established initially and updated regularly and whenever significantly new data occur such as a change in a client's physical or emotional status. The family is included in assessment as a unit itself and as a source of additional information about the client. The client's cultural beliefs are assessed as a means of understanding the spiritual, religious, and philosophical aspects of his life. These become significant in identifying individual strengths and resources as well as being considerations in planning coping and change strategies. Community resources, influences, and interactions are also assessed.

> **■ *Point of Emphasis***
>
> *Data collected must be accurate, comprehensive, organized, and updated regularly.*

ASSESSMENT SKILLS

Observation and communication skills are basic to the assessment process. Whether the nurse is performing a formal assessment interview, interacting informally in social and health care situations, or making a variety of naturalistic observations, client data are being obtained. It is important to accurately record the data in a descriptive manner so that the information can be made available to others.

RECORDING

Changes in emotional status and behavior occur slowly and gradually. Without a clearly recorded baseline of descriptive data, progress is difficult to monitor. Common errors in recording assessment data include the use of vague generalities, emphasizing trivial details rather than vital descriptions, and omitting key nonverbal and social data. Compare the two examples of narrative in Tables 7-1 and 7-2. Both describe the same client

---

TABLE 7-1 Vague, Meaningless Narrative Data

Admission Assessment Notes

This middle-aged woman was admitted accompanied by three others. She is expensively dressed and wearing furs. She declined the admission interview and is sitting quietly on the sunporch watching TV with four other clients.

Her husband says she is depressed and doesn't take care of herself anymore. Vital signs and appearance are normal.

---

and activities but only one gives a picture of the client's actual status on the day of admission.

SOURCES OF DATA

The primary source of data is the client—his non-verbal behavior and appearance, his subjective statements recorded in his own words, and the nurse's observations of his interactions with other people and the environment. The client needs to know that he has rights and responsibilities and a significant role in planning his health care. The client who denies illness and resists treatment may refuse initially to collaborate in this process.

TABLE 7-2 Descriptive Narrative Data

Mrs. X is a 48-year-old woman of Irish-American descent who was admitted the evening of May 2 accompanied by her husband, eldest son, and the family lawyer. She is wearing attractive clothing that is somewhat large for her. Her hair is oily and unkempt in appearance, and a noticeable body odor is present. When asked why she was being admitted she said "Ask them" in a flat monotone, and walked down to the sunporch. She seated herself apart from the group in front of the TV, and sits without moving or showing facial expression.

The husband states she has been depressed for three or four weeks: "Not eating, not sleeping, not taking care of herself." Her son expresses concern because she recently made a new will and has commented that "it won't be much longer now" and "the sadness and pain will be over soon." They report she was previously hospitalized for "menopausal depression" two years ago and recently became depressed again following her daughter's marriage and move out of town. According to her husband and son, she leaves the house lately only to attend church on Sunday.

She is pale, tall, and slender with dry, flaking skin and oily dark hair. BP is 140/90, P 100, R20, Ht 5'6", Wt 100#. No visible bruises or abnormalities. Eyes are red rimmed and puffy. Expression is flat and sad. Shoulders are slumped and gait is very slow.

The nurse still has a wealth of behavioral data accessible based on appearance, interactions, mood, activities, and conversation (or lack of it) on various topics, and can include the client in the process as soon as he is ready.

Additional secondary sources (such as family, friends, health professionals who have worked with the client) can provide data that clarify or extend the database and give varied perspectives. The richest sources of data are observable everyday client interactions since we bring ourselves and our ways of being and relating with us wherever we are and whatever we do. Any observant eye will detect clues to problems. If the nurse is unfamiliar with the client's religion, culture, neighborhood, or ethnic group, she needs to become a student of the culture. The client can explain his belief system and compare it to the beliefs of his family and group. Indigenous workers are lay members of the client's culture or group who can assist the nurse to develop sensitivity to the values that are demonstrated in cultural behaviors. Indigenous workers interpret the culture and can also provide information on community problems, attitudes, and available resources.

For a complete discussion of neurological and psychosocial assessment see Chapter 10. Recall the components of the physical assessment from appropriate texts and apply them consistently for a comprehensive assessment.

ANALYSIS OF DATA

Once data have been accumulated in an organized manner they are reviewed to discover significant facts, findings, and relationships that have particular relevance to the nurse-client relationship and to identify actual or potential client problems. Initial impressions or inferences are drawn based on the available data. These may be as vague as "client seems reluctant to share information in this area" or as specific as "complaints of muscle weakness and serum K+ of 3.0 indicate hypokalemia." Analysis involves applying both knowledge and powers of perception. The nurse may notice that the client tends to avoid social contact and conversation, the family may describe the client as a "loner" who has few friends, and the client may describe an absence of any social contacts since becoming unemployed. Relating these three pieces of client data to a basic knowledge of the universal human need for human contact and a sense of belonging, the nurse is able to identify a problem of social isolation.

VALIDATION

Validation is an important aspect of problem identification and is a confirmation of the nursing diagnosis through other sources. The best sources of validation are the client and the family. Phrasing the problem in their own terms and asking for verification is the clearest form of validation. For example, "Have you been feeling alone and isolated since losing your job? It sounds as if you didn't socialize much outside of work and now you rarely see anyone." If the client agrees with this statement, the problem of social isolation has been validated. Other means of validating an analysis include application of theoretical concepts and consensual agreement by another staff member. Textbooks document man's need for social interaction and other staff members can contribute their perceptions as to whether the client appears to them to demonstrate the problem behavior.

Some client problems in psychiatric nursing particularly require theoretical and consensual validation by other staff members. The grandiose and delusional client would not be able to acknowledge the underlying lack of security and self-esteem which created the need to present himself as a supernatural figure. However the nurse's understanding of the underlying cause is vital to planning effective intervention.

■ Point of Emphasis

Validation is vital in confirming identified problems and can be accomplished with the client and others.

☐ Nursing Diagnosis

The nursing diagnosis conventionally includes a description of (1) the client problem or potential problem, (2) the cause or related influencing factors, and (3) the resulting signs or symptoms exhibited by the client. This is referred to as formulating the problem in PES format: problem, etiology, and symptoms (Gordon, 1982).

Not all client problems are appropriate to a nursing diagnosis. Gordon limits nursing diagnosis to problems "which nurses by virtue of their education and experience are capable and licensed to treat" (1982:3). Appendicitis, emphysema, cancer, and schizophrenia are medical—not nursing—diagnoses. Each of these medical problems does, however, have related human responses which nurses can diagnose and treat—such as

pain; impaired gas exchange; and nutritional, coping, and self-care deficits.

The list of nursing diagnoses currently approved for research and revision by the National Conference Group is presented in Table 7-3. Each diagnosis also has a definition, defining characteristics (signs/symptoms), and a listing of known etiological factors which can be found in Gordon's *Manual of Nursing Diagnosis* (1982).

Whether the nursing diagnosis is stated in the conference group's terminology or in the more general or individualized terms of the nurse, the diagnosis is the clearly stated problem for nursing intervention which is firmly based in assessment of the client. The client's problem list should be reviewed and updated with resolved problems noted and any newly identified problems added.

☐ Intervention

PRIORITY SETTING

Once the nursing diagnoses are established, priorities must be set according to immediacy of client needs. Readiness and timing for intervention are equally important in planning care. Coordination of the interventions among the interdisciplinary health team is also vital. Theoretical principles and nursing judgments are an important part of these processes. Life-threatening problems are afforded primary priority. These may include suicidal impulses, refusal to eat due to suspicion or guilt feelings, impulsiveness with the potential for injury, or overactivity to the point of exhaustion. Priority setting is also influenced by the client's perception of the problem and readiness to work toward a particular goal.

The nurse may identify underlying dynamics or related problems which must be resolved first before other problems can be dealt with. For example, the nurse who wishes to expand the interpersonal comfort and social network of a suspicious or very withdrawn client must first promote and achieve a sense of trust and security in one or two selected relationships. The nurse also recognizes that mutual goal setting with the client is basic if actual behavior change is to be possible and that goals must be within the client's current ability level.

☐ Planning

Planning should involve the client, significant members of the health team, and the client's fam-

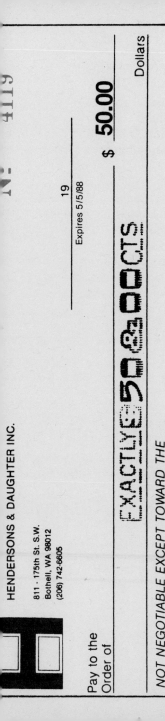

N° 4119

HENDERSONS & DAUGHTER INC.

811 - 175th St. S.W.
Bothell, WA 98012
(206) 742-6605

Pay to the
Order of

19 _____

Expires 5/5/88

EXACTLY 50 & 00 CTS

$ **50.00**

Dollars

AUTHORIZED REPRESENTATIVE

*NOT NEGOTIABLE EXCEPT TOWARD THE
PURCHASE OF HENDERSONS & DAUGHTER
SECURITY DOORS OR WINDOWS. ONLY ONE
CHECK PER DOOR OR EACH $800 WORTH
OF WINDOWS.*

TABLE 7-3 Nursing Diagnoses[a]

Health Perception-Health Management Pattern
Health Management Deficit, Total
Health Management Deficit (Specify)
Infection, Potential for
Physical Injury, Potential for
Noncompliance (Specify)
Noncompliance, Potential (Specify)
Poisoning, Potential for
Suffocation, Potential for

Nutritional-Metabolic Pattern
Decubitus Ulcer
Fluid Volume Deficit Potential
Fluid Volume Deficit (Actual) (1)
Fluid Volume Deficit (Actual) (2)
Nutrition, Alteration in: Potential for More than Body
    Requirements, or Potential Obesity
Nutrition, Alteration in: More than Body Requirements, or
    Exogenous Obesity
Nutrition, Alteration in: Less than Body Requirements, or
    Nutritional Deficit (Specify)
Skin Integrity, Potential Impairment of, or Potential Skin
    Breakdown
Skin Integrity, Impaired

Elimination Pattern
Alteration in Bowel Elimination: Constipation or
    Intermittent Constipation Pattern
Alteration in Bowel Elimination: Diarrhea
Alteration in Bowel Elimination: Incontinence or Bowel
    Incontinence
Urinary Elimination Pattern, Altered
Urinary Elimination, Impairment of: Incontinence
Urinary Elimination, Impairment of: Retention
Stress Incontinence

Activity-Exercise Pattern
Activity Tolerance, Decreased (Specify level)
Airway Clearance, Ineffective
Breathing Pattern, Ineffective
Cardiac Output, Alteration in: Decreased
Diversional Activity Deficit
Gas Exchange, Impaired
Home Maintenance, Impaired (Mild, Moderate, Severe,
    Potential, Chronic)
Joint Contractures, Potential
Mobility, Impaired Physical (Specify level)
Self-Care Deficit, Total (Specify level)
Self-Bathing–Hygiene Deficit (Specify level)
Self-Dressing–Grooming Deficit (Specify level)
Self-Feeding Deficit (Specify level)
Self-Toileting Deficit (Specify level)
Tissue Perfusion, Chronic Alteration in

Cognitive-Perceptual Pattern
Cognitive Impairment, Potential
Comfort, Alteration in: Pain
Pain Self-Management Deficit
Knowledge Deficit (Specify)
Sensory Deficit (Specify), Uncompensated
Sensory-Perceptual Alterations: Input Deficit or Sensory
    Deprivation
Sensory-Perceptual Alterations: Input Excess or Sensory
    Overload
Short-term Memory Deficit, Uncompensated
Though Processes, Impaired

Sleep-Rest Pattern
Sleep-Pattern Disturbance

Self-Perception–Self-Concept Pattern
Anticipatory Anxiety (Mild, Moderate, Severe)
Anxiety, Mild
Anxiety, Moderate
Anxiety, Severe (Panic)
Body Image Disturbance
Depression, Reactive (Situational)
Fear (Specify focus)
Personal Identity Confusion
Self-Esteem Disturbance

Role-Relationship Pattern
Grieving, Anticipatory
Grieving, Dysfunctional
Independence-Dependence Conflict, Unresolved
Parenting, Alteration in
Parenting, Potential Alteration in
Social Isolation
Socialization, Alterations in
Translocation Syndrome
Verbal Communication, Impaired
Violence, Potential for

Sexuality-Reproductive Pattern
Rape Trauma Syndrome
Rape Trauma Syndrome: Compound Reaction
Rape Trauma Syndrome: Silent Reaction
Sexual Dysfunction

Coping-Stress Tolerance Pattern
Coping, Family: Potential for Growth
Coping, Ineffective Family: Disabling
Coping, Ineffective Family: Compromised
Coping, Ineffective (Individual)

Value-Belief Pattern
Spiritual Distress (Distress of Human Spirit)

[a] Reprinted with permission from Gordon, M. *Manual of Nusing Diagnosis.* Published by McGraw-Hill, © 1982.

ily or support system. A coordinated effort makes it much easier for the client to assist in his own treatment. The community nurse communicates and coordinates with others involved in client care and, when necessary, may call for a joint planning meeting. In the hospital setting, primary health team members involved in the client's care meet to develop the comprehensive treatment plan.

The planned interventions should be clearly and specifically recorded so that all members of the health team can readily understand and follow the approaches agreed upon. Accountability for specific aspects of care should be identified by name (e.g., leisure counseling by Ann Smith, RT; dismissal and aftercare coordination by Jim Kinney, MSW, and K.C. Irving, RN).

The interventions themselves are based on sound principles of nursing and behavioral science. They include the content of the planned intervention (for instance, for a former carpenter, promote a sense of mastery and competence by involving him in a leadership role in a group woodworking project in OT) and also the process of relationship-focused aspects of care. The latter are the most difficult to plan since they involve the use of spontaneous interpersonal situations to promote social learning. General approaches or guidelines can be stated in the care plan such as "promote open expression of feelings and needs" or "encourage inhibition of impulsive and aggressive responses to anger such as yelling, kicking, and pounding on objects." The nurse will, however, have to operationalize these guidelines as the situation permits, for example, by saying to the physically aggressive client when he begins to pound on the table: "I feel intimidated when you do that and I can't listen to what you're saying. . . . Please take a minute to become calm so we can talk." Other examples of process intervention include being respectful and trustworthy (which promotes relationship building) and commenting on the relationship itself, i.e., "We seem to be getting more comfortable with each other. What do you think?"

☐ *Implementation*

Implementation involves actual nursing actions of at least three different forms according to Stanton (George, 1980). First, the nurse may assume responsibility for the client's needs until he is able to assume independent responsibility. This might include dressing and feeding clients who are immobilized by guilt and depression or disorganized by confused thoughts and bizarre misperceptions. It may require reducing choices to a few in order to promote the client's ability to make decisions despite a high anxiety level and lack of self-confidence.

The second form of action involves manipulating the environment to promote health (e.g., meeting safety needs, providing security against impulsive actions, reducing stressful stimuli, and focusing social interactions on interpersonal learning and testing new behaviors). Examples

include maintaining suicidal precautions for the depressed client and using interpersonal situations in the milieu to encourage the passive client to develop and try out assertiveness skills.

The third action is helping the person toward some goal. The nurse and client collaborate to share information, promote coping skills, or solve a problem. For example, in the working phase of the nurse-client relationship, mutual collaboration promotes problem-solving activities and personal growth on the part of the client.

During the implementation phase, the nurse continues to assess the client as to whether new problems are developing and whether progress is being made toward goals. As short-term goals are met, such as those that relate to basic physical and safety needs, new long-term goals are established. Timing is an important element in the sequence of planning care. The nurse observes whether the client appears ready to meet more complex environmental demands. For instance, the depressed person who was unable to perform self-care actions may become more alert and responsive, suggesting that independent actions may be appropriately expected. The withdrawn client who begins to trust a staff member may be introduced into new relationships with the trusted person's help.

The generalist in nursing will provide comprehensive care supportive of the client by identifying and reinforcing healthy behaviors and assisting the client to modify dysfunctional responses. The range of interventions required calls upon the nurse's skills in communication, relationship building, and physical and psychosocial assessment. Knowledge of behavioral concepts such as anxiety, loss, grief, crisis, and the dynamics and treatment of specific psychiatric disorders will guide nursing intervention. Nursing implications will be developed for care based on knowledge of any prescribed pharmacotherapy and somatic therapies. The ability to perform self-care and identify needed support systems are vital components of intervention planning for individuals and families being returned to or maintained in the community.

☐ *Evaluation*

Evaluation requires data collection pertinent to the outcome criteria identified for each goal. The evaluative data are compared with the baseline data and the criteria for the goal to determine the progress to date (if any) toward goal achievement. If all goals have been met this is the final stage of the nursing process.

For the unmet goals, reevaluation of the entire nursing process is required. Is the data base adequate and accurate? Is the diagnosis appropriately formulated? Is the goal pertinent and are the outcome criteria relevant? Are the interventions based on sound principles and appropriately adapted to the specific client? Have the interventions been implemented consistently and carried out as planned? Changes are made as needed throughout the care plan, and the revisions are communicated to other staff members for implementation and further evaluation. Tables 7-4 and 7-5 illustrate interactions between the nursing process and the nurse-client relationship for assessment, intervention, and evaluation.

■ *Enrichment Activities*

DISCUSSION QUESTIONS

1. How may the steps of the nursing process be applied to any problem-solving situation?

2. What are the strengths and weaknesses of using a predetermined problem list such as that used in Gordon (1982) *Manual of Nursing Diagnosis*?

TABLE 7-5 Intervention and Evaluation: Interactions Between Nursing Process and Nurse-Client Relationship

Intervention		Relationship
Care and nurturance that meet needs of disorganized clients	promotes →	Trust in the orientation phase
Planning and goal setting	← promotes	Initiating collaborative goal setting and exploration of alternatives in working phase
Individualizing	promotes →	Recognition of client's uniqueness and developing empathy for the client
Implementation	promotes →	Collaborative behavior testing and feedback in the working phase; process interventions using the interpersonal environment
Evaluation Data collection for goal criteria	← promotes →	Shared discussion of goal progress in termination phase

---

3. Compare and contrast the goal-setting process in relation to physical, emotional, and behavioral problems. When is it important to have direct client validation of the problem? What goals require client motivation for achievement? How does the nurse effectively involve the client in validating problems and setting goals?

LEARNING ACTIVITIES

1. From a hypothetical client data base, identify a problem list individually. Compare problem lists indentified by different members of the group and then discuss the value of consistency in defining client problems.

2. Recall the nursing process completed on your last client. Identify which of the problems were validated and by what method.

3. Exchange care plans with another student and suggest improvements. Are the interventions comprehensive and individualized? Do they

---

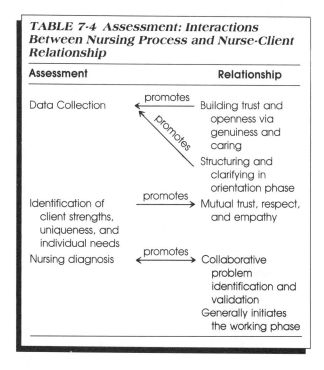

TABLE 7-4 Assessment: Interactions Between Nursing Process and Nurse-Client Relationship

Assessment		Relationship
Data Collection	← promotes / promotes ↘	Building trust and openness via genuiness and caring / Structuring and clarifying in orientation phase
Identification of client strengths, uniqueness, and individual needs	promotes →	Mutual trust, respect, and empathy
Nursing diagnosis	← promotes →	Collaborative problem identification and validation / Generally initiates the working phase

clearly relate to the problem and goal? Are they specific and clear enough that the nurse on night shift would know exactly what to do?

4. Develop a long-term client goal. Then derive short-term goals that lead step by step to the long-term goal. Write criteria for goal evaluation for each short-term goal and set realistic timetables.

Following this, discuss how this process promotes more effective evaluation and also helps to prevent nurses from overlooking progress made (no matter how small) when working with complex long-term goals for behavior change. Discuss how this can assist the nurse in recognizing and encouraging client progress.

■ Recommended Readings

Bower, F.L. *The process of planning nursing care: Nursing practice models.* St. Louis: Mosby Company, 1982. Teaches the steps of the nursing process and uses case histories to assist application and learning.

Carpenito, L.J. (ed.). *Nursing diagnosis: Application to clinical practice.* Philadelphia: Lippincott, 1983. Discusses the value and use of a diagnostic taxonomy for nursing. The nursing process is well described and specific applications related to the individual diagnoses are made.

Kim, M., McFarland, G., and McLane, A. *Pocket guide to nursing diagnoses.* St. Louis: Mosby Company, 1984. A handy reference that contains the nursing diagnoses, etiologic factors, and defining characteristics that have been approved for further research by the National Conference Group. Prototype care plans for anxiety and grieving are of particular interest to psychiatric-mental health nurses, pp. 100–129.

■ References

American Nurses Association. *Standards of psychiatric and mental health nursing practice.* 1982.

Bower, F.L. *The process of planning nursing care—A model for practice.* St. Louis: Mosby Company, 1977.

Bower, F.L. *The process of planning nursing care: Nursing practice models.* St. Louis: Mosby Company, 1982.

George, Julia. *Nursing theories—The base for professional practice.* Englewood Cliffs, NJ: Prentice-Hall, 1980.

Gordon, Marjory. *Manual of nursing diagnosis.* New York: McGraw-Hill, 1982.

Little, D., and Carnevali, D. *Nursing care planning.* Philadelphia: Lippincott, 1976.

Maslow, A.H. *Motivation and personality.* New York: Harper & Row, 1954.

Mitchell, P.H. *Concepts basic to nursing.* New York: McGraw-Hill, 1973.

Peplau, H. *Interpersonal relations in nursing.* New York: G. Putnam's Sons, 1952.

Stanton M. Nursing theories and the nursing process. In *Nursing theories: The base for professional practice.* (George, J. ed.). Englewood Cliffs, NJ: Prentice-Hall, 1980:213–17.

Yura, H., and Walsh, M. *The nursing process—Assessing, planning, implementing and evaluating,* 2d ed. New York: Appleton-Century-Crofts, 1973.

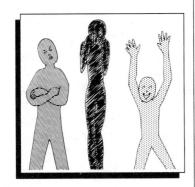

8

Communication

Joan Norris

Learning Objectives

Upon completion of this chapter, the reader will be able to:

1. Define communication as a process.

2. Identify the importance of communication skills to nursing practice in general and to psychiatric-mental health nursing.

3. Describe several theoretical viewpoints on the communication process.

4. Apply communication skills to nursing assessments.

5. Identify problems in communicating that occur in self and clients.

6. Apply specific skills of empathy, recognition of strengths, and stimulating goal-directed activity to client intervention strategies.

7. Consider various approaches including feedback, consultation, and supervision to develop communication skill.

8. Recall strategies for evaluating progress in improving communication in self and others.

☐ *Definition*

Simply defined, communication is a complex process of exchanging verbal and nonverbal messages and interpreting their meaning. Both senders and recipients of messages are influenced in this process by internal values, expectations, thoughts, feelings, and concerns. Both participants also rely on external cues such as voice tone, body language, facial expression, and gestures in their efforts to interpret meaning. Communication consists of content—the informational component of the exchange—and metacommunication—aspects that influence the relationship between the communicators and suggest how meaning can be inferred. For example, Mary joins two friends who have been invited to a party given by a mutual acquaintance. The hostess greets Mary by saying "What a surprise, do come in." The content of this message conveys surprise and an invitation to enter. Metacommunication processes will nonverbally convey the relationship and feeling components of the message. This may be delight at the unexpected pleasure of Mary's company or polite dismay and controlled anger that Mary's friends brought a disliked and unwelcome guest with them.

Interpreting meaning is a very complex activity because even people who share the same language and culture may attribute different meanings to a statement. For example, such a slang phrase as "He's 'bad'" may mean he's attractive, to the teenager; or may mean evil ("Get the shotgun, George, she's not going out with that boy!") to the teenager's parents. When sex therapists and plumbers speak of coupling, they are speaking of very different kinds of activities. Very different types of "peace-keeping activities" are intended when advocated by either the military or nuclear-freeze activists.

Compounding this lack of consensus on the meaning of common terms is the difficulty people have in making subjective judgments about nonverbal components. Nonverbal aspects are generally believed to be more accurate guides to feeling and meaning than the message content, and are even more likely to be influenced by the internal processes of both the recipient and the sender. This can lead to distortion and misunderstanding. When Al tells Ellen "Don't get uptight about it," is he offering reassurance or accusing her of generally overreacting to situations? Both Al's intent and Ellen's perception are the result of internal, individual factors and both will serve

as additional stimuli in the exchange and interpretation of messages. Cultural differences can further complicate exchange of information and meaning because participants may hold different values and expectations for the communication process itself as well as the topics under discussion. For example, the present time focus of American Indians, an outcome of their values and way of life, leads them to attend to immediate needs of friends and family rather than to planned schedules or deadlines. The white middle class in America strongly values punctuality and the work ethic, perceiving the Indian, who may frequently be late for work or miss appointments, as lazy and shiftless.

☐ *Significance to Nursing*

Nursing is an interactive process involving the nurse and individual clients or groups of clients, mutually collaborating, to meet health-related goals. Communicating with clients is essential at every step of this process as nurses collect data, identify and validate problems, set goals, foster problem-solving activities, and evaluate their effectiveness in meeting goals.

Although nurses have acknowledged the importance of communication to their practice by incorporating it into nursing conceptual frameworks for education and theory development in the discipline, the results have not been impressive. Research has demonstrated that nurses generally do not rate high on communication skills necessary for therapeutic effectiveness (Pluckhan, 1978; Friedrich et al., 1985). The latter further note that data by Truax and Millis (unpublished study, 1971) found nurses and factory supervisors to score lowest among 13 occupations on empathy, warmth, and genuineness.

This skill deficit may develop on the basis of several influencing factors. Students and practicing nurses may devalue the importance of communication in relation to the scientific and technological aspects of nursing. They may feel that they have been communicating all of their lives and need no educational assistance with "old, established skills"; they may actively resist any attempts to change their customary ways of interacting. Educators may present facts about communication without providing opportunities to practice, obtain feedback, and correct techniques. The pace of institutional practice may lead nurses to state that there are so many tasks to accomplish that there is no time to talk to clients. All of these factors have some degree of basis in reality; nevertheless, if nurses are to be accountable for the quality of their practice, then they must also be accountable for the effectiveness of their communication skills.

■ Point of Emphasis

Skilled communication is essential in collecting comprehensive and accurate data, in providing care and comfort to clients, and in engaging in the nursing roles of teacher and counselor for health maintenance, promotion, and restoration.

The nurse-client relationship in psychiatric-mental health nursing is particularly dependent upon the communication skill of the nurse. As the nurse interacts with individuals, groups, and families she serves as a role model and teacher of interpersonal and communication skills; she uses these skills to assist clients to formulate problems and engage in problem-solving activities; and she communicates in various ways her respect for clients, her attitude of hope that they can become more effective in daily living, and a recognition of their unique strengths and potential. To accomplish these functions effectively, the nurse must recognize the importance of interpersonal communication, make a commitment to regularly monitor and develop these skills throughout her professional life, and master a basic understand-

ing of specific goals in the communication process and the techniques and skills that assist in attaining these goals. Several authors have recommended that communication skills be learned in an orderly developmental sequence, with opportunities for practice and feedback (Egan, 1982; Friedrich, et al., 1985; Norris, 1986).

This chapter presents initial theoretical perspectives on the interviewing and helping process, then organizes specific skills and processes in relation to the steps of nursing process. Skills of empathy and focusing may be used in interviewing and assessment, and questioning and clarification are useful in problem solving. However, particular phases of the communication process emphasize specific skills and techniques. Learning the predominant skills and sequencing of the communication process is helpful in organizing the content and activities even though all aspects of the process may be called upon in any particular situation.

☐ *Theoretical Knowledge*

SOCIAL VS. THERAPEUTIC FOCUS

Initially it is helpful to point out some differences between social and professional communications. Not all of the social learning which takes place informally in communicating from infancy through adulthood applies in the professional or therapeutic relationship. Some of these differences are summarized in Table 8-1.

TABLE 8-1 Professional-Therapeutic vs. General-Social Communication

	General-Social	Professional-Therapeutic
Relationship	**Two-way focus**	**Client centered**
Time structuring	Varies to include pastime activities, task focus or intimately relating (in selected instances). In general most activities are characterized by pastime or task activity.	Varies from emphasis on task activities to relating openly.
Self-disclosure	Mutual exchange at various levels	Selective to promote client-centered goals
Duration	Open ended	Time limited
Goals	Self-determined by each participant	Mutually determined by client health needs

Relationship and Time Structuring Influences

In a social relationship, there is give and take. Each participant expects to initiate activity and receive benefits as well as to make some accommodation to the other person's needs. In planning for a professional-therapeutic relationship, the professional has a responsibility, because of specialized knowledge, to direct the communication to a degree that will promote the client's needs. This means that the nurse identifies communication goals and selected approaches to meeting these goals for the interaction. This need not imply that the nurse rigidly controls all of the communication in any given interaction, but it does require that she formulate goals for what is to be accomplished in communication just as goals and plans are formulated to exercise weakened muscles or to assess for new or ongoing physical problems.

In the acute care unit, the nurse recognizes that a communication goal to assess the concerns of the client who is recovering from a myocardial infarction is as important to long-term client recovery as assessments of vital signs are to monitoring immediate physiological processes. Poor nursing care results if either is omitted. The nurse who engages in the social chit-chat pattern, which is characteristic of two strangers passing time while temporarily spending 20 minutes together, may meet the client's expectations for superficial exchanges in the dentist's or doctor's waiting room but has not met nursing expectations for professional care. This importance of distinguishing between social and therapeutic patterns is often overlooked. Psychosocial needs must be assessed first in order to determine those needs. This requires goal-directed communication. Then a social amenity or chit-chat pattern may be appropriate if and only if the client has no more pressing needs or has demonstrated a strong insistence on a superficial level of interaction, or needs role modeling and practice in superficial social skills (e.g., a chronically mentally ill client who needs to become more socially adept). Most likely, a more therapeutic approach will be called for.

Time-structuring activities have been described by Berne (1972) as follows:

1. Withdrawal or avoidance. This includes taking refuge in tasks or activities such as reading a newspaper or a book so that others are discouraged from initiating or pursuing communication.

2. Rituals. These predictable exchanges recognize the presence of others without conveying information or affect. ("Hi, how are you?" "Fine, how are you?")

3. Work or task activities. These exchanges focus on external realities and getting instrumental activities accomplished by requesting or giving information and directions.

4. Pastimes. Less rigid than rituals, these exchanges center around superficial or nonpersonal information. (They consist of social chit-chat such as "How many children do you have?" "What are their names?" "My aunt's name was Helen, too." "What does your husband do?" "Plumbers are so in demand these days." "Do you think it will rain?" "Who do you think will win the pennant?") Many times nurses amass a body of superficial facts using this pattern while overlooking the fact that they have not given the client an opportunity to discuss real feelings and concerns. The purpose of this form of social exchange is to kill time in a friendly way without being involved.

5. Games. A means of avoiding honestly relating through use of repetitious patterns of interaction in order to obtain a particular "payoff"—which may be distancing others or exploiting their weaknesses. ("Why don't you" . . . ? "Yes, but. . ." is a game in which the nurse may offer numerous suggestions that the client refuses with numerous excuses. Both can pretend to have engaged in problem solving while each actually perceived the problem as being hopeless.)

6. Intimacy or openly relating. This is characterized by genuine, nonexploitive, mutual exchange which can be focused in a social relationship (intimate friendships or loving relationships) or in a professional-helping relationship in which the nurse engages the client at the level of exploring and experiencing him as a unique person.

Self-disclosure

Revealing ourselves to others is generally a gradual process which occurs through mutual give and take in social relationships. In the professional or helping relationship, the focus of interaction is maintained on client needs, and the topic of conversation is redirected as needed to maintain that focus. There are times when the conversation strays and focuses on the nurse, either because the client is operating with conventional social expectations, is unsure of the nurse's acceptance, or is uncomfortable with the level of focusing on self. The client may directly inquire about the nurse's personal life, beliefs, or feelings. In confronting this issue, the nurse needs to address the relationship-enhancing aspect of self-disclosure while keeping the focus on the client and his needs. An abrupt redirection, as in the following example, can be threatening to the client. Nurse: "What kinds of feelings are you having about your hysterectomy now that you're ready to go home?" Client: "I'm not sure. . . ." (Hesitantly) "Are you married?" Nurse: "Why do you ask?" Client: "Oh, no reason—just curious." A better approach could recognize the implied concern behind the question rather than focusing only on the factual question. The nurse might respond "yes" or "no" and add "I'm wondering if you are concerned about whether I could possibly understand what your feelings are like." In other situations, the client may ask the nurse's response to a particular situation: "How would you have felt about that?" or "What would you have done if you'd been in my shoes?" The client is not really asking for the "right way" to have acted or responded in that situation; if, however, the nurse responds directly by describing her feelings or opinions, she may be perceived as conveying "the right way" to think or feel.

Goals and Duration

In a social relationship the duration and goals (e.g., friendship, mutual assistance, love) are based on the individual needs and preferences of each participant. The professional relationship focuses on the health needs of the client, so mutually agreed-upon goals determine the duration of the relationship. A verbal contract may define the purpose and responsibilities of nurse and client. (Refer to Chapter 9 for a discussion of contracting in the introductory phase of the one-to-one relationship.)

King's View of Nursing

Imogene King (1981) has developed a theory that focuses on goal identification and attainment in nursing. She describes individuals as open systems who engage in dynamic interactions between individuals (the personal self), groups (in-

terpersonal systems), and society (social systems). Nursing is viewed as an interactive process with the client, involving sharing of information, perceptions, and values in order to mutually establish goals that will maintain, promote, or restore health and to plan approaches to attain those goals.

Nurse-client interactions may be influenced by a variety of factors including the subjective perceptions, goals, needs, and values of either of the participants. These two individuals meet in the health-care situation and react to each other on the basis of the role expectations that each holds. For example, a client who views his role as that of a passive receiver of care (who will be cured through medication) will experience role confusion and/or conflict when the nurse attempts to engage him in active problem solving. His expectations of the nurse role may include activities such as giving medications, recording vital signs, or being friendly and supportive, not mental health education or counseling. The expectation that he is to take an active part in defining and resolving his own problem is also in conflict with his concept of the client role. In order to effectively attain health-care goals in this situation, client and nurse must engage in transactions or interactive processes which they begin by making each other aware of subjective perceptions or expectations through exchanging information and values. Participants react to each other in this exchange, identifying disturbances (problems) and negotiating role expectations until common areas of agreement permit mutual goal setting and exploration of various means to goal attainment. Figure 8-1 illustrates the interactive nature of the influences of perception and communication in the process of transaction.

King further notes that nurses perform their

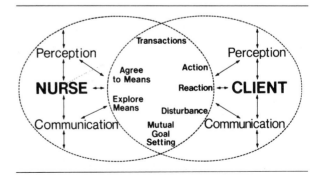

Figure 8-1 King's model of goal attainment (From King, Imogene, A theory of nursing: Systems, concepts, and process, p. 157. © 1981, John Wiley & Sons, Inc. Reprinted with permission.)

role functions in an interpersonal field. This necessitates a basic attitude of caring and respect for the client, a recognition of the importance of verifying (validating) perceptions, evaluating client readiness for learning or problem solving, and searching for meaning in the client's behavior. This dynamic process of interaction has the potential to result in satisfaction and personal growth on the part of both participants in the relationship as self-awareness and coping abilities develop.

> **■ Point of Emphasis**
>
> *King's theory of goal attainment stresses the importance of communication in nurse-client interactions to resolve differences in role expectations, validate perceptions, and engage in mutual goal setting and exploration of the means to achieve these goals.*

COMMUNICATION THEORY

The therapeutic communication process in general serves two broad purposes: (1) promoting greater self-awareness, and (2) enhancing self-disclosure with its associated benefits of increased self-acceptance and closeness to others. This process can take place in therapeutic exchanges on a one-to-one or group basis. The Johari window (Figure 8-2) illustrates dimensions of the self as known to the person and as known to others. The public self includes those aspects that are freely acknowledged to oneself and to others. The semi-public self incorporates aspects of the self that are

	Known to Self	Unknown to Self
Known to others	1 Public self	2 Semi-public Self (blind area)
Unknown to others	3 Private self	4 Inner (unconscious) self

Figure 8-2 *The Johari Window. From Joseph Luft. Group processes: An introduction to group dynamics. © 1970. Reproduced by permission of Mayfield Publishing Company.*

evident to others but that one conceals from oneself (for instance, a woman who is very ambitious may be blind to this aspect of herself because she believes it is unfeminine to be career oriented and competitive; a man may be unable to recognize and express anger even though others are aware of the physiological symptoms and hear the angry voice tone). The private self includes those aspects that a person knows about himself but withholds sharing with others until sufficient trust has been established—revealing self carries risks of losing the other's admiration and approval. The inner self includes unconscious aspects which may become accessible only after one's defenses become less strong. Most aspects of the unconscious remain unknown. During therapeutic encounters in private or in groups, clients receive feedback about themselves from others. This may include observations of nonverbal responses, perceptions of strengths, and ways of relating. This increases one's self-awareness by reducing the aspects of the semipublic self—those "blindspots" of which the person lacked prior awareness. The person also gradually risks increasing levels of disclosure of the private self. As these disclosures are accepted, the person experiences a sense of closeness to others and increasing self-acceptance. This model describes the process by which the therapeutic benefits of communication (counseling and therapy) occur.

Carl Rogers

Carl Rogers' (1951, 1961) view of the therapeutic relationship describes the attitudes that the therapist (or nurse) must convey if the communication process is to promote the client's ability to make healthy changes. These attitudes denote respect for the individual dignity and worth of the client and are manifested in (1) a sense of unconditional positive regard—through which the client comes to experience self-acceptance; (2) nonpossessive warmth—which provides a sense of being cared for without any demands being made on the client (the client is not there to serve the ego needs of the therapist or nurse); and (3) empathic understanding—which involves the sharing of observations about how the client's perspective appears to another person and a reflection and summation of the client's thoughts and feelings, and unique meaning to the client from the other's understanding. This is consistently done in a nonthreatening, gentle, and supportive fashion, which permits the client to feel understood and accepted. These three concepts are not easy to implement, and require a great deal of personal awareness. Therapists and nurses are human. Frequently they feel impatient (e.g., If the client would only try harder and do better, he would be "fixed." This sentiment may be coupled with a sense of pressure that the client *must* progress in order to demonstrate that the therapist or assigned nurse is competent.) These pressures, if not confronted by the nurse before the interaction, convey negative feelings to clients and destroy the conditions that Rogers describes as necessary for therapeutic change. This is why it is important for the nurse to assess herself during the communication process.

Transactional Analysis

Transactional Analysis (TA) was introduced in Chapter 1 as a theoretical viewpoint that discussed the analysis of several aspects of interpersonal behavior such as ego states, transactions (communication), life scripts, and games. Analysis of interpersonal transactions is discussed further here because of the contribution this model makes to understanding and evaluating communication. As King noted in her model of goal attainment, people have expectations in interpersonal situations. Personal expectations influence both the senders and the receivers of messages. Berne (1972) developed a means of diagramming these expectations, values, and attitudes through the ego state representations of parent (P), adult (A), and child (C).

The parent (P) ego state can be either nurturant or judgmental and carries the accumulated values learned from parents and social institutions. It is recognized by others on the basis of both the verbal content of the message (often "shoulds," "should nots," or other directive statements delivered for the other person's "own good"). Nonverbally, we identify finger pointing and expressions of approval/disapproval as indicators of the parent ego state. The sender of messages may be variously perceived when interacting from the parent ego state. For example, if the receiver is feeling small, dependent, and helpless and is responding from the child ego state, then the directive message is complementary.

> (P) (EMPLOYER): Just finish what you're doing now and then go home and go to bed—you're tired.
>
> (C) (SECRETARY): Oh, thank you, I am so tired I could cry.

This can be diagrammed as follows to indicate a complementary transaction. The ego states and expectations complement each other.

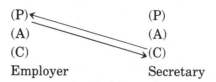

On the other hand, if the secretary is feeling confident and has planned to work late to "clear the desk" to begin a new project the next day or to permit scheduling some compensatory time off for personal reasons, the response will be different. The secretary in this case is operating objectively and autonomously from the adult ego state.

> (P) (EMPLOYER): Just finish what you're doing now and then go home and go to bed—you're tired.
>
> (A) (SECRETARY): I'm not tired. I want to finish these things so I can come in later tomorrow. I've arranged for Ellen to cover my desk so I can attend a parent-teacher conference.
>
> (P) (EMPLOYER): Married women shouldn't try to work and be mothers if they don't have to. They can't do a good job on either one if they're always tired and running here and there.

This can be diagrammed as a crossed transaction since the expectations are not complementary. The secretary sees herself as a competent adult who is meeting her responsibilities. She is certain to resent the unsolicited advice ("shoulds") that was offered by the employer.

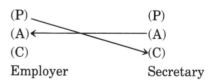

The adult (A) is the factual, objective, information-processing ego state. This state facilitates problem analysis, decision making, and professional or collaborative relationships. The secretary in the example would be wise not to impulsively lash out at her employer nor to dissolve into tears. Both of these are characteristic of the child ego state, which would restore the complementary nature of the transaction but in a way that confirmed the employer's negative expectations ("My secretary is really overly emotional—she's tired and cranky. As I said, mothers shouldn't work too. I'll need to be alert for more signs of pressure and inefficiency.") Instead, the secretary may use a very objective question requiring a factual answer in order to encourage the employer to respond from the adult ego state. In response to the employer's final comment that "married women shouldn't try to work. . . . They can't do a good job on either one. . .," the secretary may choose to respond objectively "Is my job performance acceptable, Mr. Smith? I wouldn't want to let my home responsibilities interfere with my work." Assuming that her secretarial responsibilities were consistently well performed, Mr. Smith is likely to respond "Oh yes, I didn't mean you weren't doing a good job—you just looked tired to me. I only wanted to give you a break." In this way, a potential conflict which arose by a crossed transaction is defused by influencing the conversation in the direction of an adult-to-adult transaction.

Another type of apparently adult-to-adult transaction has an underlying meaning which the receiver is to read. This ulterior type of transaction is adult-to-adult in content and structure but nonverbal cues such as a nudge, wink, or twinkle of the eye convey that it is to be responded to on the child level with a feeling component. The message may be a thinly veiled flirtation, an invitation to "play hooky," or a droll or sarcastic comment about another person. An ulterior transaction (e.g., flirtation) can be diagrammed on two levels as follows:

> AL: (with a wink) Would you like to come up and see my etchings?
> SUE: (Knowing smile) I would, I'm very interested in the arts.

(P)   (P)
(A)⟵══════⟶(A)
(C)⟵--------⟶(C)

The child (C) ego state is observable in manifestations of spontaneity, impulsiveness, and emotional expressiveness. Emotional displays from joyful giggles to temper tantrums are recognized as manifestations of the "child" in each of us. Indeed, some of the best times that adults have are occasions when they "let their child out to play." On the other hand, most people have also experienced the frail vulnerability and anxiety of the child ego state when confronted by a demanding, critical superior and a task which at the moment seems impossible.

In summary, Transactional Analysis does not simply judge a particular type of interaction as being good or bad. For instance, not all complementary transactions are "good"; and one may choose to use a crossed transaction in order to try to engage another's adult ego state for a more objective discussion. Nor is adult-to-adult always the best transaction since there are situations in which parent-to-child or child-to-child transactions are most appropriate. Examples follow.

> MOTHER (to 3-year-old): Don't run into the street. (P) → (C)
> ONE FRIEND TO ANOTHER, WITH A GRIN: Have you heard the latest gorilla joke? (C) → (C)
> NURSE TO CLIENT WHO IS TENSE: Turn over and let me give you a relaxing backrub. (P) → (C)

Figure 8-3 reviews examples of transactions from Chapter 1

■ Point of Emphasis

Transactional Analysis provides a way of analyzing some of the expectations of participants in interactions. By diagramming the ego states involved in the messages, one can identify complementary, crossed, or ulterior transactions. In addition to an analysis of the transactions, the goals of the participants should also be evaluated in relation to the situation.

Nurses will find TA to be a useful skill to develop for self-evaluation and awareness in looking at both the overall interaction patterns which may be consistently employed (e.g., overuse of a particular ego state or inability to use a particular ego state when appropriate) and in analyzing the exchanges in a given set of transactions for complementarity, appropriateness, and goal effectiveness.

Carkhuff's Helping Model

Carkhuff (1980) has developed a model of helping that describes helping skills of attending, responding, personalizing meaning, and initiating activity to meet client goals of self-exploration, self-understanding, and action to solve problems. Attending includes physical and verbal behaviors which communicate attention and involvement to the client. In addition to communicating one's

Types of Transactions

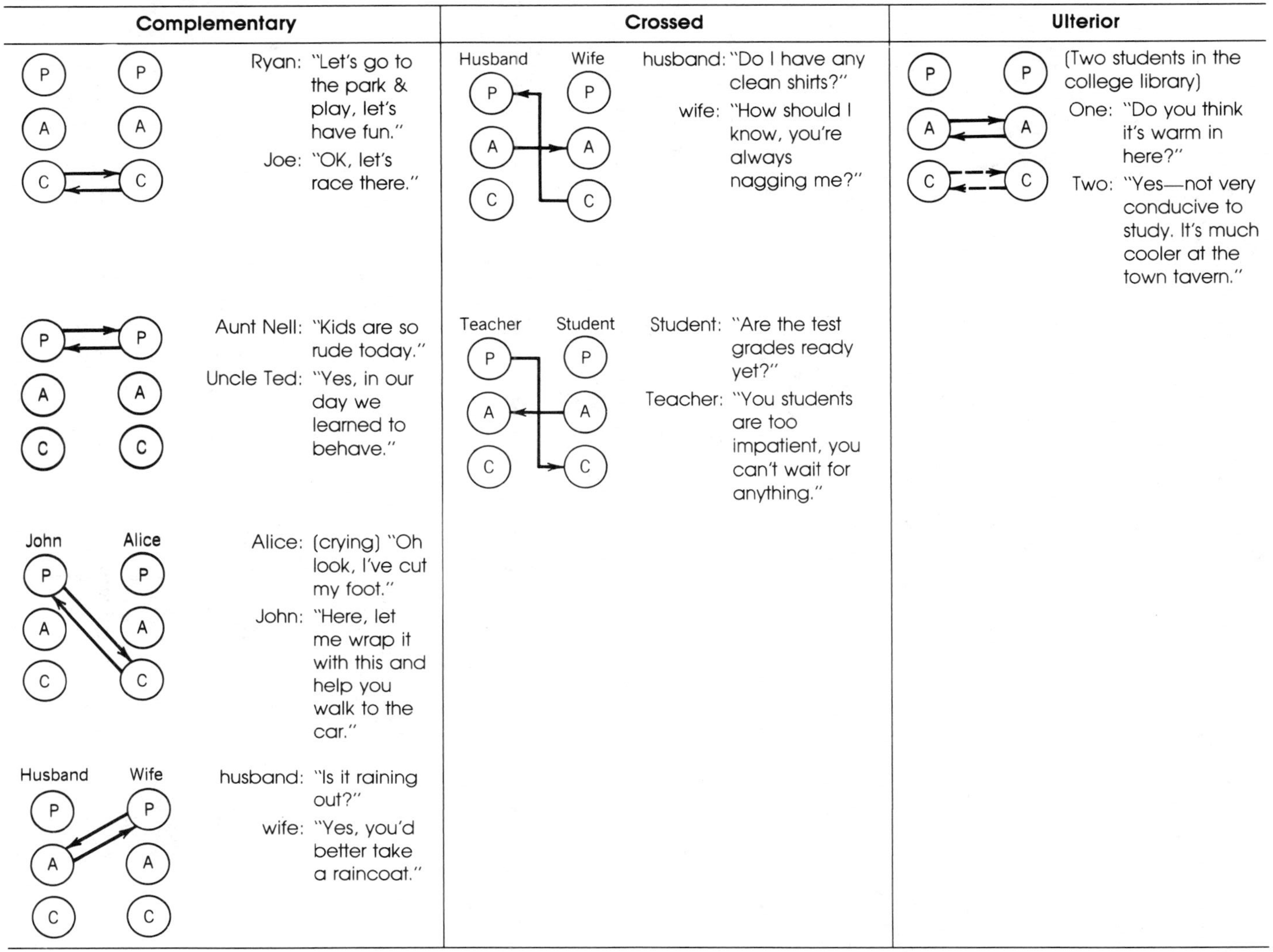

Figure 8-3 Types of transactions.

own involvement, it is also helpful to encourage client communication and participation by discussing the potential benefits. For instance, the psychiatric nurse may describe the benefits of a helping relationship to a client as "getting to know and understand yourself better." Another aspect of attending focuses on the environment to facilitate communication. This involves attending to seating arrangements, comfort factors, and minimizing distractors. Personal aspects of attending include body language, nonverbal communication, and positioning to demonstrate the nurse's attention and interest in the client.

When truly attending, nurses hear what clients say and see their nonverbal cues. This makes it possible to share these observations in order to enhance the other person's self-awareness. Observing incongruence (discrepancy between aspects of the self such as feelings, thoughts, energy level, and behaviors) permits the nurse to share these observations if the client is ready to confront them. It is not helpful to confront clients with threatening topics which may be perceived as harmful or rejected defensively. Timing requires careful consideration of client readiness to look at previously concealed aspects of the self. A relatively nonthreatening example of sharing an observation of incongruence, which is appropriate to any stage of the nurse-client relationship, follows.

> POSTPARTUM CLIENT: (tentatively) Good morning, are you my nurse today?
>
> NURSE: Yes, please call me Alice. How are you feeling this morning?
>
> CLIENT: I'm fine (sighs—eyes are downcast, voice tone is shaky as if client is anxious or on the verge of tears).
>
> NURSE (comes closer and sits down to give full attention): You say you're fine but you don't sound as if you're fine. Can you tell me more about what you're feeling?

On the other hand, a confrontation that points toward discrepancies between client goals and self-defeating behaviors must be withheld until several conditions are met: (1) Nurse and client have established a trusting, working relationship (refer to Chapter 9); (2) The client is ready to deal with aspects of behavior without perceiving this information as a negative appraisal of the self; and (3) The nurse is able to formulate the shared observation in a helping, caring way that does not threaten client self-esteem.

Listening requires that one suspend personal judgments in the helping situation. This means that the nurse does not give approval or disapproval or advice about solutions; rather, she learns from the client how particular events and actions influenced him. This permits the nurse to understand events from the client's perspective rather than her own values and judgment. Listening also involves attending to themes and gaps (things not spoken about) in the client's communication. Themes are recognizable concepts that run across various aspects of life in the client's conversation. A client may discuss how his parents "run my life," his boss "never listens to my suggestions," and "no one seems to care what happens to me." A common theme of powerlessness characterizes these examples as the client describes his feelings of being unable to exert control in home, work, and personal aspects of his life.

Responding to both content and feeling levels of client communication permits one to validate and convey understanding of the communication and expand the client's self-awareness. This involves empathy—an attempt to perceive the client's experience and feelings from the client's unique perspective or to "walk in his shoes" for the moment. Responding to feelings may include reflecting the feelings expressed, asking for feelings, or reflecting feelings implied by client statements. The nurse responds to both positive and negative feelings. It is important to try to capture the level of intensity of the client's feeling in the helping response so that feelings are not minimized or distorted. For example, when someone says "I'm really down today" a response of "not feeling very chipper" seems too little while "hopeless and depressed" is too intense to reflect the stated feeling level.

By responding to the situation and feeling, the nurse can identify the particular meaning to the individual and be empathic. In similar situations, two people who are promoted may respond very differently; one predominantly with pride and pleasure, the other with great anxiety about the new position. In either case, an accurate and empathic response will recognize and validate their feelings, promote a sense of being understood, and enhance the relationship between the two people in the interaction. Empathy also personalizes the meaning of the individual's experience and helps in looking at where the person is in comparison with his preferred state—working toward goal setting. Goals will generally evolve from themes that recur in various discussions and that reflect the person's desire to move toward some preferred state. Once the goal is articulated in mutually understandable terms, the stage of initiating is possible.

Initiating does not mean solving the client's problems or giving advice; it does, however, involve action and direction on the part of the helper. First the helpee must be assisted to make the desired goal concrete and attainable. Just as in the nursing process, this involves setting measurable criteria. The helper may ask the helpee "How will we know when your goal is met?" The goal must also be attainable by the individual, that is, stated in terms of behavior over which he has control. For instance, a goal of increasing personal assertiveness should not be measured by whether other people concede one's point of view but by whether one has increased effective use of specific assertive behaviors in daily interaction. This increases the likelihood that others will respond positively but does not place one's own success or failure in terms of people over whom one has no control.

Involving the helpee in planning a sequence of actions to meet the goal requires mutually generating several approaches, having the helpee select those most likely to be effective for him in his current situation, and agreeing to begin to try out the necessary new behaviors. The helper then asks for feedback on the progress made as the helpee tries the new behaviors, and gives reinforcement, encourages persistence in continuing to work toward the goal, and assists in exploring alternatives to approaches that are ineffective for the client. Setting short-term goals in this sequence generally helps in providing achievement milestones and reinforcement of progress made.

■ Point of Emphasis

Carkhuff's helping model describes helper skills of attending and responding which lead to mutual exploration, personalizing, and understanding of the helpee's goal. This permits the helper to encourage initiating steps to operationalize goals and mutually plan a sequence of helpee actions to meet the goal.

Listening and Interviewing Skills

Ivey and Gluckstern (1976, 1982, 1983) have further developed the work of Rogers and Carkhuff to make it more readily taught in several ways that emphasize attending and empathy in a culturally appropriate manner, interviewing, and helping or influencing skills.

Attending Skills

Attending refers to the active process of listening to another and observing nonverbal responses. In this process the nurse looks for changes in the client's usual pattern of eye contact, assumes a body posture which is relaxed and looks open to others (e.g., leaning forward, arms not crossed), pays attention to tone of voice and the rate and fluency of speech (for both helpee and self), and stays with the topic instead of interrupting or changing the subject by nervously pursuing irrelevant facts (playing "twenty questions") or selectively not following client leads in areas of helper discomfort. It is particularly important to note and respect the client's cultural patterns in eye contact, personal distance, and time focus behaviors. For example, the American Indian perceives direct eye contact as disrespectful. Some cultures place little emphasis on punctuality, valuing instead the needs and priorities of the moment. A hispanic client may expect some social conversation to indicate the nurse's interest in the person and his family (see Chapter 3).

Only when we make a serious effort to listen and observe another during interaction (instead of thinking about out next question or making assumptions about the possible problem) is it possible to recognize how little we truly attend to each other in everyday communication. Most individuals can readily identify instances in which they were talking to someone who was not really listening. Attending demonstrates real interest and encourages the client to talk.

Opening Discussion. Broadly focused openers or questions are preferable to introduce the main topic or to permit the client to select the focus for discussion. For instance, the nurse who wishes to do an assessment of the client's family would best begin by saying "Tell me about your family." Other examples of broad openers include: "Describe what a typical day is like for you" (lifestyle assessment opening) and "Tell me about your work." The nurse who wishes to use a broad opening when meeting a client in a one-to-one relationship might ask "What things would you like to talk about today?" The broad focus of these statements encourages the client to tell his story in his own words. This generally leads to getting better information than if the nurse had asked a series of closed or specific questions (e.g., "Are you married?" "How many children do you have?"). The closed question, however, is very valuable for clarifying or obtaining specific information (e.g., "Was this before or after your first hospitalization?" "How long does the pain last?" "Does resting make it better?").

Clarification of Content. Encouraging cues to the client to continue talking (nodding, saying "Umhmm, go on" . . .) and the use of a paraphrase of the client's key comments serve to promote further discussion and exploration of the topic. If the nurse is uncertain or confused by what the client is saying, she may wish to ask him for examples (e.g., "You say you felt 'funny' at work, can you give me an example of your work situation and what things were happening at that time?"). She may ask for further explanation ("What do you mean when you say you feel 'funny'?") and may ask specific clarifying questions ("How many times has this happened?"). It is also important that the nurse not make assumptions about the client's vaguely stated problems without validating their accuracy. If the nurse assumes that a reference to "ugly feelings" means feeling unattractive, when the client is actually referring to violent impulses, she will distort a key problem. Equally important is the clarity and concreteness of the nurse's own statements and questions. Clear communications enhance the client's ability to understand and respond accurately and also provide role modeling to assist his own efforts at being more effective in communication.

Response to Feelings. Assisting the client to focus on feelings may involve assisting him to identify the feelings associated with a particular situation. This can be accomplished by directly inquiring about feelings (e.g., "How did that make you feel?" or "What were you feeling then?") or by reflecting the feelings that are implied by the situation described and the voice tone and body language used in the description. For instance, "You sound angry to me when you talk about that." Or "I would've been angry if that had happened to me. How did you feel?" If the client has identified the feeling component, the nurse can encourage further exploration by reflecting it back to the client "You were feeling really lonely" and using encouragers such as "Tell me more about that." Careful exploration of the emotional component of experience is important to the

client's self-awareness and the nurse's understanding of his overall problem. Too frequently, nurses deal with tasks and overlook emotional aspects. Some clients may need to talk about feeling powerless and out of control while in severe pain as much as they need the palliative measures of medication. Discussing the client's feelings about chronic illness and being on long-term medication is a key component of promoting compliance, as important as teaching basic information, whether the client is a diabetic who needs to follow a certain diet and receive insulin or a schizophrenic who requires an antipsychotic drug and long-term follow up in a community agency.

Summary and Validation. At the end of an involved discussion of a particular issue or problem and at the end of an interview, it is helpful to summarize the content and feelings discussed for the client so that he may consider its accuracy and completeness. This gives both nurse and client a better understanding of the situation. This summary statement includes a paraphrased description of the major content aspects of the problem or issue, the feelings identified, and any themes that characterize the emotional experience. The nurse may end an interview with a summary such as: "You've been saying that for the past year you've had more and more difficulty relating to people at home and at work. You've felt isolated and fearful and at times have even thought of quitting your job and leaving home but you know that would make the fear and isolation even worse. Is that a correct summary of our talk today?" If the nurse has accurately understood and reflected the content, feelings, and meaning of the client's statements, she has responded with empathy.

■ *Point of Emphasis*

The basic listening sequence provides skills of interviewing which are used by professional counselors, social workers, and nurses to identify problems, to validate understanding, and to convey empathy to the client (Ivey, 1982). These skills are essential in assessment and are basic to any helping interaction.

Helping Skills

Once the goal has been validated and specific, desirable outcomes have been decided, the nurse

**TABLE 8-2 Directive and Nondirective Illustrations
Initiating Client Problem Solving**

Nondirective	Directive
N: "The last we met, you decided on a goal of becoming more assertive. You were going to give some thought to how you'd like to go about building this skill." (Summarizes client's key statements.)	N: Yesterday, after the assertiveness presentation, you said you'd like to work on those skills when we met today."
	C: "Yes I really need to be more assertive at work."
C: "Well, first I need to get some idea of what I'd like to say and how to say it."	N: "We can do some role play to practice what you learned yesterday."
	C: "That might help."
N: "You'd like to discuss some situations and try out ideas of what a good assertive response might be, is that right?" (Paraphrasing and validating.)	N: "All right. First, describe for me a specific situation at work in which you'd like to be more assertive. Be sure to give me enough information so I'll know what kinds of things to say to you when I'm acting as the other person in that situation." (Providing structure and directions.)

may need to use additional skills in order to guide and promote client problem solving and action. Ivey (1983) refers to these as influencing skills which include directives, logical consequences, self-disclosure, feedback, interpretation, suggestions, and confrontation. Therapists and counselors may use the full range of these skills or selectively apply only a few, depending upon their theoretical viewpoint. The following discussion emphasizes a modification of these skills which is appropriate for use in generalized helping situations that the nurse experiences when assisting clients to cope with life tasks and problems such as parenting, resolving interpersonal conflict, grief, and illness. These skills are more directive but do not involve advising the client how to solve his problems; instead, they give direction and assistance in going about the work of problem solving and adopting new behaviors.

Initiating Problem-Solving Activity. Initiating activities or giving direction assists the client to begin to work on the task in an organized way. In a nondirective approach the nurse might ask "What would you like to talk about today?" or "How would you like to go about working on this problem?" In a directive approach, the nurse would establish an overall approach to the activities for the interaction, such as "Today I'd like to have you brainstorm some alternative approaches to the problem you're having and then we'll go back over each one in our later discussions." Further examples of directive and nondirective approaches are illustrated in Table 8-2. The decision to use a directive (structured) or non-

directive (open-ended) approach will be influenced by factors such as the client's preference and need for structure in initiating activities and the nature of the client's goals. For instance, a depressed and hesitant client may need a fair amount of structure in order to identify and plan a concrete activity for an off-ward pass. It would be important to keep this activity clearcut and attainable to ensure success. Structuring the activity may increase the likelihood of success. On the other hand, a nondirective approach would be most appropriate in working with a client on his goal of increasing independent decision making and learning the skills to do this.

Nursing care goals such as performing assessments, client teaching, and the evaluation of its effectiveness are best accomplished using a directive approach if client readiness has been adequately assessed. It would be inappropriate to rely on the client to initiate a request for information about discharge planning. It is the nurse's responsibility to plan and initiate these activities, allowing, of course, for client needs and preferences to be incorporated. When taking a directive approach, clarity becomes important.

Often, inexperienced helpers confuse nondirective communication with vague communication and directive communication with giving advice about how others should solve their problems. The purpose of a nondirective approach in initiating problem solving is to give the client control over defining not only the outcomes but the method and speed at which he will work toward them. A directive approach uses the nurse's knowledge of problem-solving activities to help

TABLE 8-3 Examples of Vagueness vs. Clarity

Vague Statements	Clear Statements
"What are you like?"	"Describe yourself to me as if you were describing one of your friends. What are you like?"
"How are you when you're angry?"	"If you were angry with me, how would I be able to know that?"
"Let's talk about this again sometime."	"I'd like to talk more about this tomorrow when we meet again."

the client work through the steps of planning and implementing solutions to solving his problem. Vague communication leaves the client unclear about what has been said, what is to be done, and who is to decide how to go about it. It is not effective, does not contribute to a purpose, and results in confusion. See Table 8-3 for a comparison of vague and clear statements.

Another benefit of clarification is that by assisting the helpee to make his statements more clear and specific, the problem itself is often narrowed and made more specific. The following example illustrates this point.

SUE: This whole place is a zoo—they only care about themselves and don't care what happens to us.

MARY: Who do you mean by they?

SUE: The administration—the people who make the decisions around here.

MARY: Can you give me an example of a specific administrative decision that's bothering you?

SUE: You bet I can—the decision to use float personnel in the intensive care unit. It's not safe for patients or staff.

MARY: Are you aware that that was just a proposal being circulated by the policies committee to get input?

SUE: No, I heard it was a new policy.

MARY: There's a notice in the lounge that gives details on how to provide input about any concerns or questions. I believe the policy committee is having an open discussion.

SUE: Thanks for the information—I really want to go to that. I have some concerns they need to hear.

Self-disclosure. The general rule in helping is to maintain the focus on the client. Occasionally the helper may decide to share a small aspect of the self to promote open communication. This decision requires serious consideration and careful formulation of the idea or feeling to be shared. Occasional self-disclosures may add an element of immediacy to the relationship, promote a sense of the common human elements of the client's experience, or provide recognition and reinforcement for client progress. Genuineness is essential to self-disclosure, and negative feelings or judgments about the client are not appropriate for disclosure. These feelings should be addressed and resolved in supervisory conferences or peer support sessions.

A self-disclosure statement that pertains to the relationship might include either of the following:

"I'm a little confused, our discussions seem uncomfortable and guarded and I'm feeling that I don't know much more about you than when we started talking three of four sessions ago."

"I'm really pleased by our discussion today. I feel that I understand you much better as a person since we cleared up those concerns about what you expected from me."

Often clients will put the helper "on the spot" by asking "How would you feel?" in his situation. On occasion, it can convey acceptance of the client's feelings if the helper is able to genuinely say "I'd be angry, too" and then refocus on the client's experience and needs. It is important not to go into details or depth because this distracts from the client focus. It is equally important not to convey that this is the way the client "should" feel.

Focusing on Consequences. There are many times when helpers are realistically concerned about a behavior pattern or a prospective intention to act that seems self-defeating to the client. The helper does not wish to give advice or render judgments yet feels the need to do something to assist the client in exercising judgment. The helper can ask the client to describe the likely consequences that are foreseeable for self and others and can also give feedback on specific concerns about these consequences (which might be financial, legal, personal, or social). For instance, the adolescent considering dropping out of school can be asked to explore the consequences of this action on his future job opportunities and income, on his relationships with his parents and home situation, and on his current life-style.

Confrontation. This complex technique relies on the skilled observations and listening proficiency of the helper in noting areas of incongruence between verbal and nonverbal messages or between desired goals and actual behaviors. Gentle, nonjudgmental confrontation invites clients to further explore underlying issues and feelings that pose real problems in their ability to relate to others or to alter behavior in the directions that they intend. Several essential components must be addressed in deciding to undertake a confrontation.

Is the behavior within the client's control? Confronting a physiological response such as blushing because it interferes with a goal of self-confidence would not be helpful, since the blushing cannot be controlled by the client.

The confrontation should be structured in a way that does not threaten the client's self-esteem or imply that he is a "bad" person (judgmental statement). For example "You want to lose weight but find it difficult to avoid fattening foods you really like." *Not* "You're not serious about wanting to lose weight or you wouldn't be sneaking foods that aren't on your diet." A well-formulated confrontation can assist the client to explore deeper aspects of the problem. A poorly handled confrontation can increase client defenses and impede the relationship.

Giving Feedback. The most effective feedback provides positive reinforcement for client progress made. Specific concrete examples of the new and effective behaviors can be acknowledged. For example: "You showed real assertiveness yesterday when you told Nancy that it bothered you when she expected you to babysit without checking with you first. You were clear about what you wanted from her and you stuck to your point when she started making excuses."

It is also valuable to verify the client's perceptions of the feedback to make sure there is no misunderstanding and also to ascertain the client's perception of his own progress. Often others see positive changes before the client is able to identify them in himself.

■ *Point of Emphasis*

Helping skills—particularly those of initiating, confronting and giving feedback—assist client problem-solving efforts.

□ Communication and Nursing Process

ASSESSMENT □ Communication, as an interactive process, requires careful assessment of self and client. In this section, particular assessments and tools are discussed in relation to assessing various communication factors, and barriers to effective communication will be identified as they influence both client and nurse.

Client Assessment □ Individual or client-based factors that can influence the communication process include level of development, sensory functioning, articulation, and psychological influences. Age, education, and mental ability of the client influence vocabulary and understanding as well as the ability to master complex phrases and to deal with abstract concepts. It is important to keep the factors of age, education, and intelligence in mind as an initial assessment in order to avoid confusing the client by "talking over his head" or annoying him by "talking down to him."

Simple assessments of sensory status are broadly focused, gross assessments of sight and hearing. Does the client see well enough to discern changes of facial expression, read newsprint, and distinguish one person from another? Does the client hear well enough that he can accurately perceive a loudly whispered and a normally spoken phrase at a normal social distance against normal level of background noise? If not, modifications will be called for to avoid distortions of verbal messages. Does the client use particular assistive devices or techniques to promote communication? These should be clearly communicated so that their use is not neglected. Problems of articulation such as speech impediments or stuttering should be identified and particular approaches noted that assist the client to communicate better (e.g., a calm, unhurried manner generally helps the client to decrease his stuttering).

Psychological barriers to open communication may include passivity and low self-esteem, negative expectations, or inadequate skills in expressing oneself. These are generally not directly assessed but are implied from other statements and behaviors. Cues that the client is testing the nurse's acceptance level regarding certain topics may include questions such as "Are you married?" when the client is uncertain whether it is appropriate to speak of sexual concerns to a young nurse or "Have you ever known anyone who had a nervous breakdown?" if the concerns are about psychological status. If the nurse knows that common concerns are associated with a particular situation or condition, it is often possible to assist the client by commenting, for example, "Many people worry about whether this kind of surgery will affect their sexual functioning. I'm wondering if you have any questions or concerns you'd like to discuss." It is also important for nurses to recognize that "acting out" behaviors such as rebelliousness, flirtation, sexual innuendos and gestures may represent attempts to communicate concerns too threatening for the person to express directly. Aggressive and sexual behaviors may be the only avenue through which some men may initially confront their fears of losing masculinity, just as, in our culture, women may communicate sadness and caring by distributing gifts of food. To be aware of these aspects is to recognize the wide variation in personal and cultural expression of values.

Nurse Self-assessment □ Hardin and Halaris (1983) suggest that nurses who are not highly empathic may be more anxious than nurses who are able to truly "be with" the client. Initial self-assessment, then, would include one's level of anxiety and any factors that may be influencing higher levels of anxiety. Are there certain aspects of the client, the situation, or potential issues to be discussed that make the nurse uncomfortable?

Blocks to Effective Communication. Communication blocks or barriers include leading questions, "why" questions, not allowing sufficient response time, giving advice, giving approval or disapproval, interpreting, agreeing or arguing, becoming defensive, using cliches, and giving false reassurance (Davis, 1984).

Effective interviewing and helping skills focus on the client. Any approaches that detract from this focus can serve as barriers to communication. Questions that lead or direct the client's response in a particular direction do not promote real communication. More likely, they result only in a client response that tells the nurse what she wants or expects to hear. Examples of leading questions: "You're feeling better, aren't you?" "You don't need anything now, do you?" and "You don't have any thoughts of hurting yourself, do you?" Questions like those generally elicit the expected answers—they are implicit in the questions.

"Why" questions are difficult to answer if the person is not introspective or has not considered the problem in any depth. These questions also may be perceived as being judgmental: "Why can't you stick to your diet?" "Why didn't you take your medication?" As a rule, "why" questions should be avoided.

Allowing inadequate response time is a frequent occurrence when the nurse works with elderly or depressed clients who are somewhat slow to respond. A typical ineffective exchange: Nurse: "How was your weekend at home?" (brief pause) "Would you say it was better than last weekend?" (brief pause) "You looked better when you came back this Sunday."

The nurse asked two questions and finally made up her own answer without waiting for the client to respond.

Advising, agreeing, and disapproving are all forms of focusing on the helper's values rather than the client's. This alters the relationship from an adult-to-adult focus on client needs to a parent-to-child focus characterized by the helper approving or passing judgment on the client's ideas or plans. This impedes therapeutic effectiveness.

Defensiveness in response to client complaints about care given or other situations is not uncommon. A defensive response such as "You have to understand how busy the staff is" or "I don't know what goes on when I'm not here" conveys to the client that the nurse does not wish to hear about his concerns. Merely listening to what the client has to say does not mean that the nurse has responsibility for the particular situation, often the client can identify an effective way to resolve his feelings or problem if someone will hear him out.

Offering cliches and false reassurances is a polite way of stopping discussion of client concerns. "Don't worry," "Everything will turn out all right," "Things happen for the best." These are meaningless expressions which offer no help and may be untrue in specific situations. Recognizing such common communication barriers in one's own communication practice indicates a need to work on listening and responding to real concerns of clients.

Nurse Assessment Tools. Several approaches have been devised that facilitate nurse self-evaluative activities. These include audio- and videotaping, process recording, role playing, and the supervisory process used by clinical instructors and consultants. All of these methods share a common goal—providing feedback on communication. The evaluation emphasis may vary from primarily self-evaluative to greater reliance on input from others.

Devices for recording narrative interaction include audiotaping, videotaping, and making written records of either role-played communication situations or actual nurse-client interactions. Each approach has strengths and weaknesses. Videotaping provides the best opportunity to monitor both content and nonverbal messages, but the presence of the camera along with the need to have a camera operator can be very intrusive unless a special room or studio is available. Both video- and audiotaping of clients require obtaining a signed consent form from all participants with assurances of informed consent and confidentiality. In many settings, the client's physician's signature is also required. Use of audiotapes or videotapes by nurses in hypothetical role-play situations preserves accuracy of feedback while avoiding the need to obtain client consent. Two nurses can role play realistic situations and observe their responses when in the helping role.

The narrative process recording involves making a complete record of the verbal and nonverbal exchanges in a nurse-client interaction. This method protects client confidentiality and privacy by referring to the person only by initials. The difficulties of recording accurately and completely, however, make it the least reliable method. It is most distracting to write while interacting with the client, although taking only a few notes may assist later recall. It is essential to allow time immediately following the interaction for preparing a written account of the recalled observations so as to ensure accuracy. Later, the nurse can complete the evaluative aspects. Role play can also be used (without recording) with feedback provided by one's partner or a neutral observer. In the supervisory or consulting session, the nurse shares her goals and approaches with a more experienced person who assists her in identifying areas in which she may be overlooking key aspects of interaction. The purpose of this method is not to provide answers to the nurse but to assist her in exploring the nurse-client relationship and to promote her self-awareness.

Regardless of the method used to collect data, the process and content of the self-evaluation are similar. The nurse considers her own communication, verbal and nonverbal, and its effectiveness in the situation. Areas for consideration include (1) identification of therapeutic approaches followed and their influence on the client; (2) reformulation of a preferred response when an ineffective response is identified which contributes to one's range of responses and makes it likely that a more effective response will be used in the future; (3) identification of any barriers to communication, such as leading questions or use of numerous narrow questions; (4) awareness of nonverbal aspects of the interaction; and (5) evaluation of whether the initial goals set for the interaction were met. Sample process recording forms are shown in Table 8-4, A and B.

TABLE 8-4, A *Process Recording Form for Assessment of Self and of Client.*

Describe environmental factors that influence the interaction

Prior to the interaction: Describe situations or influences that may affect either nurse or client responses in the interaction. Goals for the interaction: Nurse-related goals and client goals (e.g., nurse's goal may be a psychosocial assessment and client's goal may be an increased sense of trust in the relationship.)

Verbatim Narrative	Technique and Purpose	Nurse Awareness and Evaluation of Effectiveness	Client Goal: Focus and Observations

Summary: Evaluation of goals and plan for next interaction.

TABLE 8-4, B   Process Recording for Nurse Self-Evaluation

Verbatim Narrative	Technique and Purpose	Nurse Awareness and Evaluation of Effectiveness

Family Communication Assessment □ Assessment of family communication is a more complex task than assessing one-to-one interactions. In general, it is helpful to identify patterns of interaction characteristic of the family, level of expressiveness, and the quality of the communications.

Patterns may be described as (1) a pyramid in which one or both parents communicate information in a top-down manner and other members are not seen as providing valued input; (2) a wheel in which one member is the hub or center of communication for the "spokes" or other members; and (3) the star, in which communication is a pattern of mutual exchange among all members. The last of these is generally considered most effective, since opportunities for exchange are maximized while the potential for distortion is reduced.

Satir (1967) describes functional family interaction and communication as characterized by a tolerance for errors and differentness (individuality) and the ability of members to firmly state their case, clarify and qualify messages as needed, and to ask for and be receptive to feedback. Dysfunctional communication in families is characterized by one or more of the following problems: Individuals may make assumptions about others without validating them; may speak for others ("Jean thinks so too"); may overgeneralize ("Everybody's mad at me"); may express hurt as

anger; may sulk resentfully in silence; or may engage in blaming and other self-esteem lowering behaviors. Some families avoid discussing painful topics altogether, restricting conversation to the details of daily existance (Friedman, 1981).

Problem Identification □ The nursing diagnosis of impaired communication can be further delineated as to the specific problems or dysfunctions and may be applied to the client or the family. The problem may also apply to the nurse. Regardless of the source of the problem, it is important to recognize the interactive nature of the process and the multiple approaches to intervention. Equally important is recognizing the aspects of communication that are strengths and will form the basis for effective skill development. For instance, the person who has difficulty responding to expressions of feelings may be very skillful in questioning and clarifying content. Confidence in one aspect of communication will give encouragement for additional development of separate but related sets of skills. It is important to identify the specific subcategories of problem communication so that interventions can address the particular barriers in question.

NURSING INTERVENTION □
Nurse Communication Self-Improvement □ Following careful assessment of strengths and weaknesses based on use of feedback and identification of barriers or problems, the nurse can identify specific goals for skill development. Recognition that skill improvement requires self-monitoring, practice, and feedback will assist the nurse to plan realistic approaches. Change takes time, and refining communication skills requires much practice, until they become a "second nature" component of one's communication. This is a key point. Many people abandon the effort to develop the skills after only one or two trials, feeling that the result seems forced or artificial. Skills should be practiced in a safe and nonthreatening environment, such as in role play with a friend, until they can comfortably be incorporated into practice. With greater familiarity in practicing the skills, confidence grows until finally the skill becomes an integral component of professional communication.

Client and Family Intervention □
Physical or Sensory Problems. The client with a physical problem or sensory barrier may already

have developed specific techniques to improve his ability to communicate. The nurse's first approach, then, is to inquire about how best to support his efforts and to recognize that pressure and anxiety are likely to exacerbate whatever problems exist. Remaining calm and quiet is helpful. Positioning oneself to be seen and/or heard better is helpful to the client who has visual or auditory problems. Mechanical aids and writing materials may be useful. Obtaining a referral for appropriate therapy is useful if this has not already been done.

Client Education. Preventive and remedial interventions to improve general listening and communication skills emphasize client education through specific techniques to enhance communication effectiveness. These techniques are based on the theoretical viewpoints discussed earlier in this chapter. Several approaches such as Gordon's Parent Effectiveness and Teacher Effectiveness Training and Popkin's Active Parenting share a focus on particular skills.

I messages focus on helping the individual directly state his feelings and preferences in a given situation. The skill involves avoiding "you"-oriented or blaming messages which cause others to become defensive, and instead, identifying one's own feelings in response to a particular event. For instance "I get really discouraged when I've cleaned the apartment and half an hour later it's littered with discarded clothing and dirty dishes" is more likely to promote positive action than a derogatory "you"-oriented message such as "You're just a bunch of pigs and this place looks like a sty no matter how often I pick up after you!"

Listening skills include teaching clients how to pay attention, listen for content, and identify feelings associated with the message.

Responding skills emphasize empathy and mutual respect—not blaming, belittling, or giving advice. By responding to feelings and exploring alternatives and consequences, adults and children can be helped to express feelings rather than act them out, and to make decisions in a supportive environment.

A *family council* is one means advocated for expanding open communication and democratic functioning in families. Each member has a turn "chairing" the weekly meetings, and any member can pose a problem for discussion and solution.

Family enrichment refers to communication and activities that directly support a sense of love and belonging in the family through verbal, non-verbal, serious, and playful approaches to communicating caring.

Conflict resolution skills are based on active listening and responding techniques. Using these skills, two people each present their perspective on a problem and negotiate a solution to the problem; the solution may involve a compromise (each gives up something) or a reformulation of goals in a new way that accommodates the needs of both (a win-win strategy). For example: She is bored by football, he dislikes movies, both are resentful of the little time they spend together on weekends and dislike the other's favorite pastime (movies and football respectively). After hearing each other out, they work out a compromise solution, deciding to attend a football game one weekend and a movie the next. Or, on the other hand, they may redefine their goal as each weekend promoting a shared interest that both enjoy, such as camping, hiking, and biking. Movies and football become individual activities to be pursued as each prefers but they have formulated a new shared activity based on a common goal.

EVALUATION ☐ Various feedback devices used for assessment also provide opportunities to reassess progress toward communication goals. It should be remembered that communication is a process—not a product—so skills can be developed and improved over a lifetime of interactions. One never becomes so skilled that self-awareness and skill monitoring become unnecessary. A summary Table (8-5) describes the stages of the nurse-client relationship, the nurse's goals, and key skills for goal attainment at each stage.

■ *Enrichment Activities*

DISCUSSION QUESTIONS

1. Discuss the effects of information giving vs. advice or approval giving in various nursing situations.

2. In a group, plan an effective topical outline and broadly focused introductory questions about a specific area of assessment.

3. Describe ways of assessing and monitoring personal communication skills for career development.

4. Identify community resources for individuals and/or families who wish to develop their skills in communication.

TABLE 8-5 Stages of the Interviewing and Helping Process With Key Skills

Stage or Phase	Nurse Goals and Purposes	Key Skills for Goal Attainment
Initial or introductory	Orienting client to the purpose and expectations of the relationship Establishing the contract Communicating limits of the relationship and the expected outcomes Establishing trust and rapport	Attending behaviors (eye contact, voice, posture and expression) Client observation (nonverbal appearance and behavior) Active listening and responding (questioning, verbal following, use of encouragers, restatement, summarizing, identification and reflection of feelings and meaning) Conveying warmth, genuineness, and caring

Client assessment (Introductory and working phases of nurse-client relationship)	Identifying, with the client, existing problem(s); validating the problem, its meaning, and any influencing factors
	
	Indentifying client strengths and assets which can then be integrated into problem solving and client goal attainment.
		Attending, observing, actively listening, and responding (as above). In addition: Focusing (clarifying and keeping the interaction directed):
		    on the client (summarizing feelings, values, and meaning of problem)
		    on the problem and related factors (exploring the situation, significant others, and cultural influences, validating understandings with the client)
		    on strengths (exploring from client's viewpoint, sharing nurse observations of assets demonstrated in nurse-client interactions or other context in which strengths were noted)
		Reinforcing actual accomplishments (such as completing school, holding a job, developing a sense of humor, helping others)
		Demonstrating nonjudgmental behavior and positive regard

Setting goals (working phase of nurse-client relationship)	Assisting client to define goal(s) and desirable outcomes based on the validated summary of the problem(s) and meaning	Attending, observing, actively listening and responding, and focusing (as above). In addition: Confronting (reflecting incongruencies between verbal and nonverbal messages, between client ideal and real self, between current situation and desired outcomes, and between stated goals and current behaviors)
Problem solving (working phase of nurse-client relationship)	Initiating client efforts to generate a wide variety of alternatives to select from in resolving the problem Analyzing alternative courses of action and selecting an approach	Attending, observing, actively listening, responding, focusing, and confronting. In addition: Influencing (promoting goal-directed activities), confronting inability to move or generate options and discrepancies as identified above Giving directions (e.g., tasks or homework), identifying priority values in evaluating approaches Providing information and explanations, evaluating consequences of various actions Selecting preferred course of action, summarizing, and providing feedback
Generalizing and transfer of learning (working and termination phase of nurse-client relationship)	Promoting practice and use of new behaviors or learning Encouraging future transfer of problem-solving process	All of the above. In addition: Use of approaches to promote client skill and confidence toward new behavior, willingness to practice and use new behavior, and reinforcing new behavior Practice activities such as role play rehearsal, and visualizing effective use of course of action Keeping a record of pertinent behavior and progress Assigning behaviors and reporting back Providing follow-up and support
Termination	Summarizing progress and strengths; dealing wih feelings about termination	Giving anticipatory guidance on progress to date and future applications of the process in everyday situations

Adapted from: C. Rogers (1942). *Counseling and psychotherapy*; R. Carkhuff (1980). *The Art of Helping IV*; and A. Ivey (1983). *Intentional interviewing and counseling.*

LEARNING ACTIVITIES

1. Role play (in groups of three) an interview with a depressed client, a helping session with an anxious parent, and a consultation with another nurse about one's communications with a client. Take turns in the roles of helper, helpee, and observer. The observer should observe strengths and weaknesses noted in the helper role enactment for discussion after each role play.

2. Enact a family situation such as the parents describing the father's new job which necessitates a move to another state. The children are ages 6, 10, and 14. Decide how the communication should be patterned using the triangle, the wheel, and the star models. After role playing each pattern, discuss which would be most effective in terms of facilitating communication goals to (1) inform family members of the move, (2) identify their responses to the move, and (3) provide mutual support.

3. Complete a self-evaluation of an actual or role-played interaction using one of the process recording guides (Table 8-4, A or B).

4. Role play the steps of actively listening, responding to feelings, and exploring alternatives and consequences with a partner. Have the partner give feedback on strengths and weaknesses.

5. Role play barriers/blocks to communication to gain a perspective on their effects. For instance: "Twenty questions," "Why" questions, not allowing sufficient response time, giving advice, "leading questions," disapproving, or becoming defensive. Discuss the influence these behaviors have on client feelings and perceptions.

■ Recommended Readings

Either of the following is a clearly written manual on self-development of communication skills:

Carkhuff, R. *Helping IV,* Human Resource Development Press, 1980.

Ivey, A. *Intentional interviewing and counseling,* Brooks-Cole Publishers, 1983.

Communication techniques for parents are taught by a variety of community agencies such as the schools, the YMCA, and family service agencies. Materials for two of these approaches may be obtained by reading Gordon, T. *Parent effectiveness training.* New American Library, 1970, or by viewing the 1983 videocassette programs by M. Popkin called "Active Parenting" (Active Parenting 4669 Roswell Rd, Atlanta, GA.)

Assertiveness training approaches that emphasize effective communication include those of Jakubowski and Spector in a film called *Responsible Assertion,* and a book by Fensterheim, H., and Baer, J. *Don't Say Yes When You Want to Say No.* McKay, 1975.

■ References

Berne, Eric. *What do you say after you say hello?* New York: Grove Press, 1972.

Carkhuff, Robert R. *The art of helping IV.* Amherst, MA: Human Resource Development Press, 1980.

Davis, A.J. *Listening and responding.* St. Louis: Mosby Company, 1984.

Egan, Gerard *The skilled helper.* Belmont, CA: Wadsworth, 1982.

Evans, D., Hearn, M., Uhlemann, M., and Ivey, A. *Essential interviewing—A programmed approach to effective communication.* Belmont, CA: Wadsworth, 1979.

Friedman, M. *Family nursing,* Chapter 9, Norwalk, CT: Appleton-Century-Crofts, 1981.

Friedrich, R.M., Lively, S.I., and Schacht, E. Teaching communication skills in an integrated curriculum. *Journal of nursing education,* 24, 4 (April 1985): 164–167.

Hardin, S., and Halaris, A. Nonverbal communication of patients and high and low empathy nurses. *Journal of psychiatric nursing and mental health services,* 21, 1, 1983:14–19.

Ivey, A. *Intentional interviewing and counseling.* Monterey, CA: Brooks-Cole, 1983.

Ivey, A., and Gluckstern, N. *Basic influencing skills.* North Amherst, MA: Microtraining Associates, 1976.

Ivey, A., and Gluckstern, N. (1982). *Basic attending skills,* North Amherst, MA: Microtraining Associates.

King, Imogene. *A theory for nursing: Systems, concepts, process.* New York: John Wiley & Sons, 1981.

Norris, Joan. Lecture and role play instruction for communication skills: An analysis of the influence of student attributes and teaching strategy on learning outcomes. *Journal of nursing education,* March 1986.

Pluckhan, Margaret. *Human communication: The matrix of nursing.* New York: McGraw-Hill, 1978.

Rogers, Carl. *Counseling and Psychotherapy.* Boston: Houghton Mifflin, 1942.

Rogers, Carl. *Client centered therapy,* Boston: Houghton Mifflin, 1951.

Rogers, Carl. *On becoming a person: A therapist's view of psychotherapy,* Boston: Houghton Mifflin, 1961.

Satir, Virginia. *Conjoint family therapy,* Palo Alto: Science and Behavior Books, 1967.

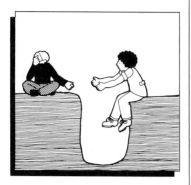

The One-to-One Relationship

Stephanie Stockard

Learning Objectives

Upon completion of this chapter, the reader will be able to:

1. Describe the one-to-one relationship as a therapeutic tool in psychiatric nursing.

2. Discuss therapeutic use of self and the importance of trust in the one-to-one relationship.

3. Describe various phases of the therapeutic relationship and ways to facilitate growth in the client.

4. Discuss common barriers to the development of a therapeutic relationship.

5. Identify the significance and occurrence of burnout, as it relates to the therapeutic relationship.

6. Describe the use of the therapeutic relationship in other nursing care settings.

The one-to-one, or therapeutic nurse-client relationship, is an interpersonal experience between a client and a nurse which is based upon and fosters a sense of caring, empathy, understanding, acceptance, connection, hope, and enabling. This relationship consists of a series of planned, goal-directed interactions, the purpose of which is to provide the client with the opportunity to understand and resolve difficulties in relations with others, with the environment, and with attitudes and beliefs about himself.

The therapeutic one-to-one relationship is a major factor in facilitating growth and change for the client. In any health care setting, the nurse seeks to establish a relationship that promotes learning and the client's ability to be self-caring. Through use of theoretical and technical knowledge and interpersonal skills, the nurse can assist individuals to deal with problems by helping them to develop new coping skills, recognize their own needs and feelings, and change unhealthy behavior to self-enhancing behavior. This chapter explains the use of the one-to-one relationship and describes essential features and dimensions of this mode of intervention.

☐ *Caring: A Framework for a Therapeutic Relationship*

Caring is the essence of the therapeutic relationship. Mayeroff (1971) states that caring for another person, in the most significant sense, involves helping that person to grow and actualize himself. Self-actualization is the process of becoming all that one is capable of being; caring from another person promotes this process. In order to care, one must understand the other's needs, and respond properly: this requires knowledge and skills. The nurse studies physical, social, and psychological sciences as well as humanities in order to better understand the client's needs. The application of theoretical knowledge and technical skills is the nurse's response to the client's needs. Caring for the client in all of its dimensions implies that the whole person is the focus of care.

Mayeroff believes that to care for someone, one must know many things, including: Who is the other? What are the person's powers and limitations? What are the person's needs? What will help the person to grow? How can I help? What are my abilities and limitations?

In the process of the therapeutic relationship the nurse seeks answers to these questions. The answers are as unique as each individual client. The sense of caring that is the essence of the therapeutic relationship includes other factors that contribute to the establishment and growth of the nurse-client relationship—empathy, understanding, acceptance, connection, hope, and enabling.

FACTORS IN THE THERAPEUTIC RELATIONSHIP

Empathy

The nurse must possess the ability to empathize—to put herself in the client's place. This ability allows her to share in the other's emotions or feelings although she may never have experienced those situations or feelings. In contrast to sympathy, which implies mutual commiseration, empathy allows the nurse to enter into the experience of another and view it from his perspective, with respect for his emotions and feelings. (See Chapter 4 for further discussion.)

> ■ *Point of Emphasis*
>
> *The ability to be empathic is dependent to a large degree upon the nurse's setting aside her personal values and beliefs while working with the client.*

The capacity to be nonjudgmental is based on the ability to empathize. *Being* nonjudgmental differs from *acting* in a nonjudgmental manner. To judge means to form an idea, opinion, or estimate about a matter. It also means to criticize or censure. The nurse is human, and it is unrealistic to believe that she will not form opinions or criticize or censure something. However, although a person is constantly forming judgments, whether consciously or unconsciously, in the therapeutic relationship it is essential that the nurse be aware of judgments she has made about the client, analyze them carefully, and assess their effect on the relationship.

The nurse then must set aside any judgments that hamper clear perception of the client as a person and must *act* in a manner that is nonjudgmental. If she is unable to relate to the client in a nonjudgmental way, empathy will not develop.

Failure to approach the relationship empathically precludes the development of rapport—the sense of harmony between client and nurse that is essential for an effective working relationship. Without empathy, understanding, a critical component of the relationship, is also inhibited.

Understanding

Understanding involves grasping or perceiving clearly and fully the nature, character or function, and problems of the client, and the relationship with the nurse. This is a difficult goal to achieve as it is questionable whether one human being can ever fully understand another. In a practical sense, however, the nurse attempts to gain an understanding of the client through the assessment portion of the nursing process. In addition to observing, collecting, analyzing, and interpreting data, the nurse attempts to understand herself, and her personal feelings and reactions toward the client.

Acceptance

The word "acceptance" has positive implications. A dictionary definition states that it is a favorable, willing reception or approval, or a belief in something; this certainly is different from the resignation or defeat that many people associate with the word. In the therapeutic relationship, "accepting the client as he is or where he is" is a frequently stated dictum. By her acceptance, the nurse demonstrates a willingness to experience the client as a unique individual within the framework of the relationship.

This does not mean that the nurse accepts the client's behavior in its totality. *Being* differs from *doing*; "who I am" differs from "what I do." At times "what I do" expresses "how I feel about myself." The client who is self-rejecting or self-destructive is not a useless or worthless being. While the nurse does not permit harmful behavior toward herself or others, she views the *person* as being separate from his behavior—and as having value.

Connection

A connection is a relationship or an association between people. Human beings depend on and are involved with each other. Their actions and reactions often follow, or are the result of, this involvement with each other. Estrangement from one's self due to self-rejection or alienation, as well as difficulties in relating to others, is frequently believed to be the basis for mental illness. Moustakas (1961) defines loneliness anxiety as resulting "from a fundamental breach between what one is and one pretends to be, a basic alienation between man and man and between man and his nature." Through the therapeutic relationship, nurse and client attempt to heal this breach.

Hope

Hope is a desire accompanied by the expectation or the sense that what is wanted will happen. In the one-to-one relationship, the nurse, through interest in the client, use of scientific knowledge and special skills, and belief that the client is capable of changing so as to achieve more satisfaction in living, instills a sense of hope in the client. Without hope, the client has no motivation to change or to believe that life is meaningful.

Enabling

"Enable" means to "make able; provide with the means, opportunity or authority to do something"; to make possible or effective. Enabling, in the one-to-one relationship, results when empathy, understanding, hope, acceptance, and connectedness are present, and when the nurse uses her special knowledge of human behavior and communication, her specific skills, and her self-awareness.

The purpose of the therapeutic relationship is to enable the client to understand and work through his personal and interpersonal problems. Enabling allows the client to be in control and to make decisions about his life, rather than to believe he is a passive, helpless victim of life.

All of these elements are present throughout the nurse-client relationship. Though there may be variation in how the nurse demonstrates them, they are critical in creating and sustaining a growth-promoting environment.

> ### ■ Point of Emphasis
>
> *Each nurse is unique and each client is unique. Because of the individuality of the participants, no two therapeutic relationships will be alike.*

In 1946 psychiatric nurses began to examine, analyze, and expand theoretical knowledge about the nurse-client relationship. In 1947, graduate programs in psychiatric nursing were introduced. Following World War II with its emotional sequelae, there arose overwhelming demands for psychiatric services. Nurses, along with other mental health professionals, began to examine therapeutic modalities such as the one-to-one nurse-client relationship, group therapy, and psychopharmacological intervention.

Many psychiatric nursing pioneers contributed to the evolution of the one-to-one relationships, but three theoretical frameworks have emerged in the last three decades.

In 1952, Hildegard Peplau's book, *Interpersonal Relations in Nursing*, was published. Although nurses in many settings had long recognized that the quality of their relationship with a client directly affected his emotional and physical health, Peplau was a pioneer in developing a theoretical framework for a therapeutic nurse-client relationship that could be applied in all nursing settings. Peplau's work was based on the psychological theories of Harry S. Sullivan, who believed that the interaction of the self with the environment was the critical factor in personality development. Peplau describes how the nurse assists the client to examine here-and-now interpersonal experiences in order to remediate or improve those competencies. Observation, description analysis, validation, testing new behavior, and integrating this new behavior into the self are the steps involved (Lego, 1980). Peplau provided inspiration for the development of many further approaches by other psychiatric nurses.

The work of June Mellow, in the late 1950s, designated nursing therapy, focuses on the intense one-to-one relationship developed between nurse and client. Two levels of therapy are involved: first, the nurse becomes an identity figure for the client; second, the relationship between the two is examined. The purpose is to provide a corrective emotional experience that promotes growth in the client (Lego, 1980).

Orlando's (1961) theoretical framework centers around the nurse's observing the client's needs or distress, assisting the client to verbalize the meaning of the behavior, and helping him to examine his sense of distress so that assistance can be offered. The nurse works collaboratively with the client and validates observations or reactions with him.

The three theories are similar in that they emphasize examination of what the client is experiencing "here and now." Also, each theory has as its outcome goal an improved ability to function in daily life. The two participants, the nurse and the client, are the most important factors in creating a therapeutic outcome. Therefore, the nurse *as a person* is equal in importance to the knowledge and skills she brings to the relationship.

☐ *The One-to-One Relationship in Various Health Care Settings*

Aspects of the nurse-client relationship may be seen in settings where the client and nurse have at least a minimum of consistent contact, such as a clinic or community health setting, or where the client is hospitalized for a length of time. In medical-surgical settings, the client's state of crisis may allow a rapid movement into the working phase because the client sees the nurse as helpful in providing care for an observable problem.

The nurse's communication skills; her understanding of human needs, anxiety, and defenses; and her ability to set goals with the client are applicable to any setting (see Figure 9-1). The holistic nature of the relationship promotes recognition that the interaction of physical and emotional factors affect the client's sense of well-being. The accompanying case study on page 139 illustrates this point.

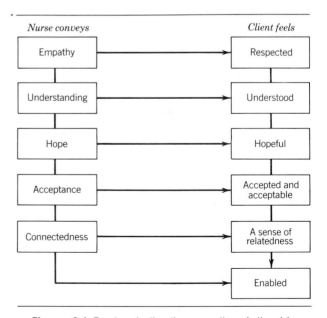

Figure 9-1 Factors in the therapeutic relationship.

Case Study

Pearl G., 52 years old, was admitted to the surgical unit for a breast biopsy. On admission, Pearl was very anxious; she paced the floor, wrung her hands, spoke rapidly, and laughed inappropriately. The nurse administered a prescribed anxiolytic and began to assess Pearl. Pearl stated that her husband, Sam, a fisherman, was at sea and she had been unable to make radio contact with him before traveling into town to the clinic, where she learned that she required prompt hospitalization. Physical assessment revealed discoloration, swelling, asymmetry, and discharge from the client's left breast, which could have indicated a well-advanced malignancy. When asked when she first noticed the lumps, Pearl replied, "Oh, a long time ago but I just didn't want to think about what it could be."

After receiving several doses of the medication, and talking with the nurse, Pearl was able to sleep, in preparation for surgery the following day. A left radical mastectomy was done; the pathologist's report confirmed the presence of metastases.

The admitting nurse was Pearl's primary nurse, and whenever possible she spent at least 15 minutes during the shift talking with her. The extensive twice-daily dressing changes gave the nurse additional time to talk with Pearl. Throughout repeated hospitalizations for purposes of radiation and chemotherapy, Pearl stayed in the same unit. She revealed that she had been married three times, and the last marriage had been her only happy one. She stated, "We're still newlyweds—we've only been married four years."

She went home when she was able, but had to be readmitted several times.

Throughout her illness, Pearl denied she was dying. Although aware of the situation, she insisted she would "fight it and win." The nurse did not challenge this denial, although the prognosis was grim: instead, she made Pearl as comfortable as possible and gave her many opportunities to verbalize her feelings. Pearl's husband, now returned from sea, spent much of his time at the hospital, and he too received emotional support from the nurse.

As she cared for Pearl, the nurse learned a great deal about her and began to understand why Pearl had delayed seeking treatment. Pearl told her that her life had been one of difficulty and heavy responsibility for family members. She felt, when she met Sam, that her "whole life" had improved and she was having a "terrifically good time." They traveled, danced, played cards, and had many friends. Now the newfound happiness she felt she had earned was threatened.

Pearl's expressed concern that her husband might be alone was the closest indication she gave the nurse that she realized she was dying. In all other respects she remained cheerful, complained rarely, and refused to give up.

The day Pearl died, the nurse had visited her in the intensive care unit. Pearl indicated she wanted her oxygen mask removed for a moment. She grinned at the nurse and whispered, "Soon as they get this stuff off me, we're going dancing, kid."

THERAPEUTIC USE OF SELF

As has been indicated, the nurse must bring certain theoretical knowledge and skills to the relationship. Her understanding of psychology, philosophy, sociology, theology, and science contributes to the sum total of her knowledge, as do the experiences of daily living, and her interpersonal relationships. All that the nurse *is* contributes to the relationship. This is the "therapeutic use of self." In this relationship, the nurse calls upon her thoughts, feelings, behaviors, knowledge, and skills to promote growth in the client. The critical element of self-awareness must be present. Reviewing research on the characteristics of the helping person, Carl Rogers (1979) concluded that attitudes and feelings of the helper are more important than particular theoretical orientations. In addition, the client's perceptions of the helper's attitudes are crucial. According to Rogers, the ability to foster growth-promoting relationships is a measure of growth within the self.

TRUST AS THE BASIS FOR RELATING

It is difficult to achieve a significant interpersonal relationship without first establishing a level of trust between the two participants. Trust may be defined as a firm belief in the honesty, integrity, reliability, or justice of a person. It implies faith, reliance upon the other, and a confidant expectation. An inability to trust others gives rise to loneliness, isolation, and anxiety. Learning to trust is the first and most important developmental task of life, according to Erikson (1963). The infant learns that the world is either a reliable place where his needs will be met in a warm, consistent fashion or that it is an indifferent, uncaring, or hostile place where people are to be mistrusted.

> ■ *Point of Emphasis*
>
> *When a person fails to develop a sense of trust, the ability to form satisfying relationships is severely compromised; the person cannot meet his needs for acceptance, belonging, and self-actualization. In extreme situations, this inability may prevent even the basic needs for food, shelter, and clothing from being met.*

Impairment in interpersonal relationships restricts communication so the person is unable to validate observations with others, receive corrective feedback, consider new ideas, and acquire broadened perspectives. This may cause rigidity of personality and inflexibility toward life; and it severely inhibits the ability to consider various alternatives in solving problems.

Ruditis (1979) lists three important features of developing trust: reliance on another, risking something valued, and attempting to achieve a desired goal.

These features may appear to be simple, but demand much of a person who has been unable to trust others. Risking the self, and leaving the self open to possible rejection or hurt by relying on another, requires tremendous strength and a large measure of confidence in the other.

To build trust, there must be a continuing interest over a period of time. Trust is not an instant result of the nurse's interest in the client. The nurse must herself be a trustworthy person. Ruditis (1979) describes ethos or intelligence, character, and good will as important qualities. Expertness and confidence in self are also pertinent. The beginning student in psychiatric nursing, although lacking expertness and confidence, may still possess ethos and the strong desire to learn new skills with which to assist the client, and thereby may develop greater self-confidence.

The client must feel that the nurse "will act in beneficial ways without attempting to control or manipulate" (Ruditis, 1979). Throughout the entire relationship, the nurse builds and reinforces a sense of trust that will enable the client to attempt new behaviors, look at new alternatives, and form more satisfying relationships. Attitudes and behaviors of the nurse that enhance trust are:

1. Respecting and recognizing the individual as a unique human being.
2. Providing information to the client about situations that affect him. This includes information about the one-to-one relationship, the roles of each participant, and other aspects of care.
3. Collaborating (when possible) with the client about goals and desired outcomes for the relationship. Negotiation about differing goals of the nurse and client may be necessary.
4. Behaving in a consistent and reliable manner toward the client (e.g., being on time, being honest, meeting regularly).
5. Accepting personal limitations and feeling comfortable with saying "I don't know."
6. Expressing, verbally or nonverbally, throughout the relationship, the belief that the client is worthwhile and capable of feeling better.
7. Providing honest, direct, constructive feedback to the client throughout the relationship. The nurse describes her observations of the client's verbal and nonverbal behavior in a noncritical manner, as it occurs.
8. Recognizing the client's strengths and efforts to change.
9. Recognizing when her own needs are interfering with meeting the client's needs.
10. Projecting warmth and genuine interest in the client.
11. Practicing congruent behavior. The nurse's verbal and nonverbal behavior should convey the same message (e.g., she should not express great concern for the client and then miss several meetings without offering an explanation).
12. Setting limits that foster growth. Limits are boundaries that assist the nurse and client to maintain respect for each other. Trust is enhanced when the nurse defines her personal limits as well as limits for the client. Limits are set on behavior that violates the rights of others, or that is self-destructive to the client. The nurse may pick up cues or sense the need for limit setting; or the client may request help in controlling himself.

Confidentiality

Confidentiality is important in achieving trust. The nurse should clearly communicate to the client who will have access to information about him and what information may be shared. Professional ethics demand that the nurse avoid discussing the client with people who have no direct professional involvement in the client's care.

In the educational setting, the student nurse may use formal clinical discussions to share learning with peers, but the client's privacy should be respected at all times. She should avoid careless conversation in the halls or cafeteria, or casual discussion with peers not involved in the client's care.

Information shared by the client that could be detrimental to his health or well-being should be reported to an appropriate person such as an instructor, staff nurse, supervisor, or the client's physician. The important point is that the client be made aware that information of this kind will be communicated only to those involved in his care. An example of how a student nurse handled the issue of confidentiality with an 18-year-old client hospitalized following a drug overdose is given below.

CLIENT: It's been pretty boring up here on this unit. I'm getting tired of being here. Hey, can you keep a secret?

NURSE: Well, any information you share with me, I do discuss with my instructor and the staff.

CLIENT: Oh, yeah. Well, I'll tell you anyway. A few of us with off-ward privileges have been going down in the evening to that hallway to the general hospital. Tom's (another client) friend has been bringing us beer. It's sort of made things more exciting.

NURSE: So, have you had any?

CLIENT: Yeah, a few.

NURSE: You're not taking any medication but several of the other fellows may have bad effects from the alcohol.

CLIENT: I didn't know that. I did know we aren't supposed to be drinking anyway.

NURSE: I am going to let the staff know because this could endanger the other clients. Also, I'm wondering why you decided to get involved in this.

In this example, the client felt uncomfortable with the drinking and wanted to let someone know about it without directly reporting it. By telling the nurse, the client knew the information would be utilized for the safety of the other clients and himself, and was in fact asking that a limit be set because he did not know how to extricate himself from the situation that was causing him a problem. The nurse would later explore with the client ways in which he might have handled his discomfort more directly with the other clients or have refused to participate.

EMOTIONAL INVOLVEMENT

In a therapeutic relationship, both parties must be emotionally involved. Both open themselves to experience another human being—and this involves risk. The client, however, risks considerably more than the nurse during this time of emotional turmoil and crisis. His vulnerability demands that the nurse be sensitive and empathic in caring for him.

There is sometimes confusion about the matter of emotional involvement. Nurses generally enter nursing for altruistic reasons—they desire to help and care for others. However, this desire to help may translate into behaviors that discount the client's strengths and abilities. Nurses may attempt to impose their personal values, beliefs, and expectations on the client. If he doesn't respond in the way that the nurse expects, the nurse may reject him and avoid being actively involved in his problems and his care.

For example, a nurse may have made every effort to make a client comfortable following surgery for removal of a malignant tumor. She may expect gratitude and be angry when the client doesn't express thanks. She has failed to recognize that the client may be so preoccupied with his personal fears and concerns that he is unable to meet her needs to have thanks expressed.

Many nurses feel overwhelmed with pity or sympathy for the client. It is true that the nurse will encounter situations that are heart-breaking. However, "smothering" the client with attention and doing for him what he can do for himself may not only impede return to wellness; it also conveys the message that the client is perceived as being helpless and incapable. This immature, growth-inhibiting involvement arises when the nurse pities the client rather than seeing his strengths and encouraging him in areas where he can be successful. This behavior tends to satisfy the nurse's needs to have control over and direct the client, rather than assist the client to function independently.

Another reaction to the client's emotional pain which is destructive to both client and nurse is detachment on the nurse's part. It may happen that although the nurse cares about the client, her sense of helplessness about his situation creates in her an attitude of detachment that protects *her* from emotional pain. To be truly helpful, the nurse must become emotionally involved in a growth-promoting, constructive sense.

☐ *Developing the Therapeutic One-to-One Relationship*

As with all human relationships, the therapeutic relationship has a beginning, a middle, and an end—each important in the success of the relationship. Moreover, the period immediately before the first interaction has importance also. There is some overlap between phases, though each phase carries its distinctive features. Throughout each phase, the nurse uses nursing process, as she assesses, identifies problems, intervenes therapeutically, and evaluates. The process is a dynamic one in that the relationship is ever-changing because the two participants are not static.

PREINTERACTION PHASE

Prefacing the actual initiation of the therapeutic relationship is the period that Doona (1979) labels the preinteraction phase. In this phase a major part of the assessment portion of the nursing process is performed. The nurse first selects a particular client and gathers information about him from available sources such as the interview (which she may or may not have conducted). Information from a thorough nursing assessment and input from other mental health professionals are usually available in the client's record or chart. The nurse may also gather information from other sources such as the physician, other staff nurses, the psychologist, and the social worker. The nurse's focus is on problems that the client is currently experiencing.

Doona (1979) emphasizes that a second important feature of this phase is an awareness by the nurse of her own thoughts, feelings, and actions before the first interaction with the client. It is helpful for the nurse to record these in a journal so that the notes can be referred to as the relationship progresses. Various common feelings and fears that the nurse may experience before interaction are described below.

Fear of Rejection

Fear of rejection arises from the possibility that the client may elect not to work with the nurse.

It is important that the nurse realize that rejection usually stems from the client's own concerns and fears about relating to others, not to the nurse as a person. The beginning student may feel either distressed or secretly relieved by this. As she examines her reactions to rejection, the nurse needs to view the rejection in context. ("How did I contribute to this situation?" "What concerns did the client have that may have caused the rejection?") The nurse may then identify the reasons for the rejection and be able to approach the client again.

Feelings of Helplessness

The nurse may feel overwhelmed by the apparent magnitude of the client's problems or by her own ineptitude or lack of experience in relating to clients with emotional problems. Nurses often feel a lack of control because the essence of the therapeutic relationship involves "being and doing with" rather than "doing to" a client in a specific bed, specific room, and with a specific physical disease. Technical skills may seem useless and the nurse may feel doubt that "use of self" will be in any way therapeutic to the client. In this situation the nurse must acknowledge her feelings of helplessness and recognize a personal need to be in control. She must honestly examine what she can offer to the relationship that will help both nurse and client to learn and to grow.

Fears of Verbal or Physical Aggression

Some clients may engender fear in the nurse through behaviors that are verbally or physically aggressive. It is important that the nurse recognize aggression as a response to fear. The client may feel threatened by the nurse or by others, and may attack them verbally or physically; he is protecting himself from emotional involvement which, in the past, has proved painful.

The student nurse may have beliefs about mental illness that reinforce the stereotype that all clients are violent. Exposure to a variety of mental health settings will help her to reexamine her prejudices and to dispel them. If a client with whom the nurse plans to establish a relationship has a history of physically assaultive behavior, careful assessment of this behavior (see Chapter 11) may clarify the reasons for this way of acting and reduce the student's fear.

Fear of Mental Illness

All too often, the beginning nurse finds examination of thoughts and feelings to be threatening in that it raises questions about her own mental health. Students in all areas of nursing frequently identify with the subjects they are studying; for instance, study of the gastrointestinal system raises concerns about ulcers, cancer, and so on. So too, the study of mental health and illness raises awareness of one's own mental health. The nurse who has experienced mental illness in her family may wish to avoid this area as a way of suppressing the feelings of pain and helplessness, anger, and frustration that this family situation had evoked. It is essential that she develop an awareness of these feelings and fears, discuss them with an instructor, colleague, or supervisor, and recognize their influence on the client-nurse relationship.

When the nurse has accomplished these two tasks—selection and beginning assessment of the client and awareness of her own thoughts, feelings, needs, and actions—then the relationship with the client may be initiated. At this time the nurse also establishes goals for the first interaction, as she will do through all subsequent interactions.

THE INTRODUCTORY PHASE

The First Meeting

The therapeutic relationship begins when the nurse and client interact for the first time. Usually the interaction is superficial to give both nurse and client time to get acquainted. After the nurse introduces herself to the client and explains her role, she should try to perceive the client's understanding of his needs. The nurse should emphasize that the purpose of the relationship is to have nurse and client work together to identify and resolve difficulties.

After the client has received any needed clarification or explanation, both make an agreement about the relationship; this covers time, days, and location of meetings. The contract may be written or verbal. The length of each meeting depends upon the needs and abilities of the client and the nurse's own time demands. For example, a client in a community mental health center outpatient clinic may agree to meet with the nurse weekly for one hour. A severely withdrawn client hospitalized on an acute care unit may be unable to make the agreement, but able to tolerate 10 minutes each hour with the nurse during her shift. At this initial encounter, client and nurse should also discuss when the relationship is to end. Establishment of the formal relationship is the first step in developing trust.

A client in crisis who is open to problem solving may rapidly move into the working relationship, in contrast to the person who has greater difficulty developing a trusting relationship and has greater impairment in relatedness.

The nurse begins to learn about the client, his lifestyle, and his current feelings and needs during this time. Reclarification and repetition are frequently necessary, as both client and nurse may have a high anxiety level at first. (Signs and symptoms of anxiety are discussed in Chapter 11.) The inexperienced nurse may become aware of certain personal behaviors that might indicate high anxiety, such as staying in the nurse's station if on an inpatient unit, avoiding the client, busying herself with paperwork or housekeeping activities, and reading every individual item on the chart before meeting the client. Or she may stay close to other staff or students, forget what both she and the client said in the initial meeting, forget the procedure or assignments (if a student), and spend a great deal of time looking things up in various references. If her anxiety level is high, she will need adequate coping skills, or may need to request the assistance of colleagues or her supervisor so that she can give attention to the client.

One student used her journal as a vehicle in which she could express and examine her feelings about the initial encounter with an 18-year-old man who had attempted suicide and who was to be her client:

> Earlier, I asked George if I could get to know him better by setting aside a time to talk each Tuesday and Thursday. He seemed pleased and said we could do this. We agreed to meet at 10:45, but the first day, he didn't show up! I felt terrible—did he forget or did he just decide it would be a waste of time? I found out later he had left the unit for psychological testing! Later we talked and I said "I hear you went for some tests" and he said "Oh yes, I would have told you if I thought they'd run past 10:45 but I didn't know what kinds of tests they'd be." I was really glad to get this cleared up!

In moving from the beginning to the working phase, a significant obstacle may be the perception each has of the other (Doona). Either nurse or client may view the other as a stereotypical example of a racial, social, economic, cultural, or religious group. The particular status, attitudes, or values either participant perceives the other to hold can block further development of the relationship. Therefore, the nurse must not only exercise honest self-appraisal about her perceptions, feelings, and beliefs, but must also try to determine how she is perceived by the client.

In a conference with her instructor, one student expressed distress that her previous five meetings with her client "seemed to go nowhere—they were so superficial!" They discussed the different economic backgrounds of the client and the nurse, based on the client's frequent comments to the student such as, "But you wouldn't know about that, would you?" when the client related something about her daily life. The student decided to explore this comment with the client and discovered that the client perceived her as a "rich kid from the university" and "too young to understand." They were able to discuss the client's perception of the nurse in a more realistic light. The student was able to explore the notion that she was like "all those university students" as well as what importance age held to the client. She acknowledged that she had not had many of the same life experiences, but that she wanted to understand these situations as they affected the client. This clarification process entailed three meetings, after which client and nurse were able to begin working together collaboratively.

Transference and Countertransference

In transference, the client views the nurse as being similar to someone who was significant in his past and relates to the nurse as if she *were* that person. This process takes place at an unconscious level—out of the client's awareness—and it exerts a strong influence on the therapeutic relationship. Transference is significant in that it sheds light upon the client's relationship with the person whom the nurse represents. Early family conflicts may be repeated with less intensity in the relationship with the nurse. The client may display extreme anxiety, illogical hostility or paranoia, clinging affection, or serious sexual or aggressive acting-out behavior.

Transference may occur in any phase of the one-to-one relationship. During the introductory phase, it may inhibit progress because nurse or client is rendered unable to view the other as a unique individual. The following case study illustrates transference.

Case Study

Karen, 28 years old, was admitted because she was depressed about her impending divorce. She had filed for divorce, but was feeling guilty and upset about her decision. She described herself as a "people pleaser" and questioned her fairness to her husband, although she felt she had done everything possible to work out their marital problems and had had little cooperation from him.

When Karen was a child, her mother was verbally critical of her and "put me down a lot." In the therapeutic relationship, Karen frequently interpreted the nurse's neutral comments as negative criticism. For example:

N: It sounds like some of your husband's behaviors were pretty hard to live with.

C: Yes, I guess I am stupid for putting up with him. I should have known when I married him he had problems.

or

N: You've tried several ways to help your husband and your marriage.

C: I probably didn't do enough—I should have done more.

Karen regarded the nurse's neutral statements as being critical. Her mother's comments often had been critical, making Karen feel stupid and inadequate. Karen was unaware that her inability to please her overly critical mother had resulted in her extreme need to please anyone she viewed as an authority—often to her detriment. In relating to the nurse, she attempted to please by agreeing with "criticisms" of herself, just as she had sought to please her mother.

Countertransference in the nurse takes the form of negative reactions towards the client—anger, impatience, resentment. What is happening is that the nurse's unconscious feelings, originating from early irrational projections and identifications in her life, are now reinforced by the client. The following case study illustrates countertransference.

Case Study

Barbara, a 23-year-old nursing student, initiated a one-to-one relationship with Delores, a 54-year-old woman with a history of severe psychotic depression. When the relationship was initiated Delores no longer demonstrated psychotic behavior in the form of hallucinations and delusions, but was withdrawn and nonverbal. Barbara spent a great deal of time sitting with Delores quietly and taking care of her physical and hygienic needs. She did not encourage Delores to become involved in activities but tended to protect her from other clients.

In conference with her instructor, Barbara's seeming overprotectiveness toward Delores was discussed. Barbara said, "She seems so fragile. I'm afraid if I push her to try harder, she'll withdraw from me more." Intellectually, Barbara could see that gentle firmness in encouraging Delores would assist her to be more independent. Barbara's fears of being rejected by Delores were discussed and Barbara agreed that she would try harder to encourage Delores.

A few days later, Barbara found herself unable to be firm with Delores about certain activities that Delores was capable of doing and became discouraged and frustrated. In talking with her instructor, she said, "You know the way I feel about Delores is a lot like the way I feel about my Great Aunt Sarah, who lived with us when I was about six. She would get these spells and everyone would tiptoe around her and try not to upset her. She'd go into her room for weeks and talk to herself and if anyone bothered her she'd scream terrible things. Sometimes I'd hear her at night prowling around the house. When I was about seven, Great Aunt Sarah died and nobody would talk about it in front of me."

In discussion with the instructor, Barbara was able to see how this past experience influenced her relationship to Delores. The differences in Delores and Great Aunt Sarah were discussed; this helped Barbara to see that her fears about Delores were actually based on her earlier fears. Barbara then was able to involve herself more therapeutically with Delores, encouraging and assisting her in self-care and involving her in interactions with other clients. Delores, in turn, responded positively to Barbara's interest and encouragement and began to speak more freely and to express some of her feelings.

■ Point of Emphasis

Difficulties arise in the therapeutic relationship when the nurse lacks an understanding of transference and countertransference. She must try to become aware that these emotional responses can occur and must examine their influence on the progress of the relationship.

Role Expectations

Both the nurse and the client may have expectations of each other that are unrealistic. Zyl and colleagues (1979) reported that clients expected directive therapy, that is, being told what to do to feel better. Nurses, however, expected clients to be self-directed in working to feel better. This difference in expectations may create difficulties. Many clients think that taking a pill or following certain precepts will somehow make them feel well. Historically, the health care system has fostered dependence in the client, and the result has been that the client feels it is up to the health professional to make him feel better, either physically or emotionally. In an extremely acute illness this may be true; in the nurse-client relationship, however, the client is viewed as an individual capable of making decisions about his life.

In similar fashion, the nurse may hold certain expectations about the client. She may assume that every client wants to feel better and may feel frustrated when a client apparently chooses to continue a life-style that is potentially hazardous to his physical or emotional health. The nurse must recognize that, although a client's particular behavior may be unrewarding, at least it is well known and familiar to him. Changing an old behavior that has become uncomfortable for the client means he must take a risk, venturing into the unknown. This gives rise to anxiety and fear, which in turn may cause feelings of helplessness and hopelessness about the changes.

Nurses may also believe clients have sufficient knowledge, information, and capability to effect change in their lives. The nurse should assess the client's desire and ability to change. The proper tools for change need to be available for the client. For example, if the client allows others to use him, he may need to practice assertiveness, in which case he needs to have information about assertiveness and assertiveness training.

> ### ■ *Point of Emphasis*
>
> *The desire to change and the tools for change must both be present, so that the client will be more willing to take the emotional risks necessary to personal growth.*

In the introductory phase the expectations of both nurse and client should be discussed and clarified. Awareness of possible misperceptions and expectations must be mutually developed so that transition to the working phase of the relationship can occur.

THE MIDDLE OR WORKING PHASE

As trust is established and distorted perceptions are recognized and dealt with, the nurse and client enter the working phase of the relationship. The nurse will be aware of a mutual sense of empathy, and each participant will view the other as a unique person.

In this stage both nurse and client are likely to feel more comfortable, and to sense their growing rapport. At this time, too, the client may test the nurse to see if the nurse's concern is genuine. For example, the client may skip a session and see if the nurse notices or pursues the incident. Agreements about the relationship may be violated by the client to see if the nurse in consistent in what has been decided between the two. The nurse should discuss the behaviors with the client and explore their meaning for him.

A limit may need to be set on a particular behavior. For instance, if a hospitalized client is consistently busy elsewhere when the agreed-upon meeting time arrives, the nurse may inform the client where she can be found and the length of time she will be available (e.g., "I'll wait 15 minutes") rather than looking for the client each time. This demonstrates the nurse's reliability and consistency, which contributes to the development of trust between nurse and client.

Although the nurse sets goals prior to each interaction with the client, it is not until trust and rapport are established that both can collaborate effectively toward meeting their mutual goals.

Boettcher (1978) states that collaboraton in establishing goals attests to the client's strengths and the right to be a participant in his care. Therefore goal setting should be a positive practice.

Goals determined by mutual negotiation and collaboration are more likely to be successfully realized.

Those needs or problems that the client perceives as meaningful afford greater motivation to change than those that only the nurse identifies. Change requires risk taking; to take a risk one must perceive possible benefit from so doing.

Of course, timing is of critical importance. The nurse needs to assess the client's physical and psychological state, and if he is in a state of extreme incapacity she must set goals for him until he is able to begin working with her.

Goals

How does one set goals? Nurses are told when to set goals, what sort of goals to set, and what is to be achieved; but the process of goal setting is less frequently explained.

A goal is a desired outcome or an aim. A person may be only vaguely aware of his goals; more often he may know what he does not want.

> ### ■ *Point of Emphasis*
>
> *The two most important elements in setting a goal are identifying a specific outcome and the steps required to reach it.*

A person who is seeking assistance because of emotional problems generally wishes to feel better, but his familiar coping behaviors have not helped him. Another person may never have learned how to solve problems, resolve conflicts, or have his needs met in a healthy way.

Once a goal is set, the most important factor in reaching the goal is the client's motivation. Motivation for change is very difficult. One can be motivated by threats (e.g., divorce, separation from loved ones) fears (e.g., going crazy, rejection, loss of material possessions) or incentives (rewards—material or emotional), or one can be motivated by an internal desire or wish. This latter type of motivation, self-motivation, is the basis for any real and lasting change. Meyer (1972) describes motivation as a desire that is "held in expectation with the belief that it will be realized."

Belief in one's self and in one's ability to change and to hope that things can be better must be created within the nurse-client relationship. The nurse, by taking an interest in the client as a unique individual and building a sense of trust, provides a stable foundation for change. The therapeutic relationship provides a safe environment in which the client can experiment with new behaviors that will contribute to an improved sense of emotional well-being. Fearing to risk, human beings fail to gain, or as Shakespeare stated: "Our doubts are traitors and make us lose the good we oft might win, by fearing to attempt."

Goal Setting

The first and most obvious step to setting a goal is to define what one wants. It is often also the most misunderstood and overlooked step. Many people set goals that are vague ("I want to be happy" [pretty, thin, handsome, and so on]). These goals are so vague that they cannot be evaluated. Moreover, the perception of the goal varies from person to person. (How rich is rich? How will I know if I'm happy?)

1. A goal must be specific. It must describe exactly what one hopes to accomplish. For example, rather than wanting to be thin, weight that can be attained is decided upon.

2. The goal must be worthwhile. The aim must be something that the client actually wants, rather than something he believes he should want or ought to feel or believe. If the outcome is not really desired by the client he may consciously or unconsciously create an environment that will frustrate its attainment.

3. Priorities should be set for each goal. For example, clients who fear causing themselves physical harm must give priority to the goal of discussing these feelings with the nurse when these arise as opposed to the goal of finding a new job. The former goal is obviously the one that takes priority.

4. A goal should be positive. For example, rather than stating "I want to stop feeling lonely and miserable," a positive goal would state "I want to get to know other people."

5. A goal should be broken down into a series of small steps or actions that will ultimately achieve the desired outcome. For example, the goal "I want to get know other people" may be broken down as: (a) Saying good morning to the man I see in the elevator each morning, (b) asking a co-worker or fellow client I don't know well to join me for coffee, and (c) joining a photography (or other) club. Small daily actions facilitate attainment of the goal.

6. Barriers to achievement of goals should be identified. Barriers may be within the self or in the environment. It is often much easier to change one's environment than one's personality, habits, or ways of thinking that have developed over many years. In fact, it is a very human tendency to blame others or the environment for problems rather than to look at one's own role in creating and perpetuating a problem. However, no human being can completely control or change the environment or others.

7. Imagination is important in designing and achieving a goal. The client should be encouraged to envisage every possible good or disastrous result of the goal. Also, encouraging the client to think about or imagine goals is an important part of breaking out of the rut of behavior that has led to the current crisis. This does not mean encouraging unrealistic beliefs or giving false reassurance; it merely provides a stimulus to look at problems from a different vantage point or to develop new ideas.

8. Achievement of goals requires persistence, patience, determination, and courage. It is much easier to revert to old, comfortable, ineffective behavior simply because it is familiar. New behaviors, and new reactions and relationships with others, introduce anxiety and fears which often accompany the unknown. Sustained effort coupled with belief in oneself is necessary for the achievement of any goal.

9. Support is essential is the fulfillment of goals. The nurse provides the client with a nonthreatening environment in which he may try out new behaviors with minimal risk. The trusting relationship allows him to receive constructive feedback through interaction with the nurse. She gives encouragement and praise when the client expands new knowledge skills and behaviors into his personal relationships. And, finally, the nurse teaches the client how to give himself the support and positive acceptance necessary to maintain belief and confidence in himself.

10. It is helpful if the collaborative goals are written, with the specific actions defined. In this way, client and nurse can evaluate the client's growth or reevaluate the goals in a definitive manner.

Failure to achieve goals may be due to any number of reasons:

1. Lack of specificity in defining goals.

   Specific: I will ask Mary to eat lunch with me.

   Nonspecific: I'd like to have Mary be my friend.

   Specific: I will take my own shower today without help.

   Nonspecific: I want to stop feeling so helpless.

   Specific: Client will be able to state one positive feeling experienced today.

   Nonspecific: Client will feel less depressed.

   Specific: Client will walk down the hall twice each day and evening shift with assistance.

   Nonspecific: Ambulate client each shift.

2. Unrealistic goal for the person's talents and skills *at that time*.

   Examples:

   Asking a severely withdrawn client to plan the next day's menu

   Assigning the job of activity director to a client in manic phase of bipolar disorder

   Expecting behaviors inappropriate for the client's developmental level

   Expecting a client who has never discussed feelings to express them

3. Failure to set priorities.

   Clients need to discuss with the nurse what is most important to them at the particular point in time. It is fruitless to redirect clients to a goal that seems unimportant when their emotional energy is concentrated elsewhere. Set priorities as follows:

   Assuring physical health and safety

   Facilitating expression of feelings and identifying emotional needs

   Assisting the client to recognize underlying needs and reasons for behavior (when client is able)

   Assisting the client to try new behaviors

4. Lack of motivation to change.

   The lack of motivation to change may be due to several factors which may operate together or singly to prevent the client from making changes. Some of these factors include:

   A sense of helplessness in which the client feels no alternatives are available

   A sense of hopelessness in which the client feels things will never be better

   Fear that a new behavior will bring negative results

   Fear that significant others may reject the client if change occurs

   Feeling no need to change despite encountering problems

   Secondary gain from others or from the mental health system—including food; shelter; kind and concerned staff; attention from family; avoidance of possible legal difficulties; avoidance of life situations that the client may find intolerable (He may regard a hospitalization, whether for physical or emotional illness, as a reprieve from the stressors in life.)

5. Lack of belief in self. The client may feel so inadequate and unable to help himself that meeting a goal seems impossible. When an individual experiences stress and conflict and is unable to cope with it, his self-esteem is diminished. The need to feel in control is universal, and if past and present life events have slowly eroded this sense of control or confidence, a person will feel unable to make choices and to act in ways that are beneficial. Among the many causes for a lack of belief in self are:

   Childhood experience of abandonment or a sense of being unloved or unwanted

   Ideas conveyed by significant others that the person is stupid, clumsy, ineffective, unlovable, and so on

   Constantly comparing self with idealized others and finding oneself wanting

   Feeling one must be perfect in every area—the best, the smartest, the most talented

   Life situations over which the person has little or no control but for which he nonetheless feels responsible (e.g., death, illness, behavior and actions of other family members)

   Conditions of society about which the individual experiences a sense of inadequacy (e.g., racism, sexism, poverty)

Doona (1979) defines nine overall goals of the nurse in the one-to-one relationship: assisting the client to deal with "here and now" problems; helping the client define or identify the problem(s); enhancing the client's understanding of his participation in life experiences as an active agent, rather than a helpless victim; helping him to deal with problems that emerge from deeper exploration of the superficial problem; creating and using various alternatives in solving problems; trying new behaviors; communicating more effectively; deriving pleasure from interaction with others; and finding meaning in illness which contributes to inner growth and actualization.

With each client the nurse seeks to personalize and develop specific goals based on those general goals.

Nursing Process

Nursing process plays a role in the one-to-one relationship. In the beginning phase the nurse assesses and identifies the client's actual and potential needs and problems. In the working phase, the nurse continues to gather data, make observations, and interpret the data. As a mutual sense of trust develops, the nurse is able to elicit more information and gain greater insight into the client. Themes—recurring ideas—begin to become evident, and they help the nurse to focus on issues of great importance to the client. (Some common themes are low self-esteem, fear of closeness, lack of control, feelings of being unloved, fear of angry feelings, and rejection and hurt.) Problems and need identification are now more personalized to the specific client; they are reassessed as new information develops and the client changes.

After the nurse has collected and analyzed the data and has formulated the problems, her interventions must be developed, preferably in collaboration with the client. The interventions, or goals, must be specific and written. As these are implemented the nurse carries out ongoing or formative evaluation of the effectiveness of the interventions. If necessary, the goals can be renegotiated with the client or reevaluated periodically to assess their value to the client at a given time. It is helpful to differentiate short-term from long-term goals.

It should be remembered that the feelings, behaviors, or situation that the client is currently experiencing did not occur suddenly. As a consequence, the client may not be able to meet the goals quickly, especially when attitudinal and behavioral changes are necessary. Long-lasting changes require time, commitment, persistence, and support.

Connectedness

During the working phase the sense of connectedness or relatedness is established with the client. Empathy, understanding, warmth, and concern that arise in the working phase create a climate that cements the bond of trust and gives the client hope. The client is now able to reveal his feelings and allow his true self to emerge in relation to the nurse. The nurse, too, is less concerned about techniques, roles, and status and is able to share knowledge and sensitivity in a productive way. Although the relationship is designed to benefit the client, every meaningful human interaction provides both participants with an opportunity for growth—thus the nurse will also reap the rewards of sharing herself with another human being.

Reminders of Termination

At the beginning of the relationship the nurse and the client had agreed upon the length of the relationship. Throughout the working phase, the nurse periodically brings up the issue of termination so that both can prepare themselves to end the relationship.

PROBLEMS THAT MAY ARISE IN THE WORKING PHASE

The nurse's work with the client may be temporarily or permanently impaired by any of several situations. These can arise when the nurse fails to use her theoretical and scientific skills, when she misuses them, or when she is lacking in them. The relationship is stymied until the nurse recognizes that an obstacle exists. She needs to institute such interventions as will overcome the barriers. On the other hand, it may be the client's responses that are the root of the problem. Several behaviors and feelings common to either client or nurse are presented below to help the nurse become more aware of these obstacles.

Problems Arising from the Client's Responses

Anger. The response of anger, as both a feeling and an action, is a frequent cause of difficulty. It is only human to respond to anger by becoming defensive and angry in return, as one feels he must protect himself from verbal or physical displays of anger. (This discussion is limited to responding to anger that is verbally expressed. Physically assaultive behavior is discussed in Chapter 11.)

Anger is a response to hurt or loss. When a person feels let down, frustrated, or emotionally wounded, the response of anger discharges the anxiety created by the unpleasant feeling of hurt. Of course, feelings in themselves are not right or wrong. Feelings are valid, and everyone is entitled to his own feelings—it is the way in which feelings are expressed that may cause the difficulty.

Expressing anger verbally, using "I" messages, such as "I am very angry," "I am very upset," "I am furious!" are healthy ways to express anger. Unfortunately, however, society frowns on such direct expressions of negative feelings, especially in women, as being "impolite." Many people either refuse to admit they are angry and simply store up their angry feelings, or project responsibility for their feelings upon someone or something else. In other words, they displace their anger.

The nurse who is confronted by an angry client may wish to react initially defensively, especially if the anger is directed at her; but anger should not be dealt with defensively. Some points to keep in mind when confronted by an angry client:

1. Anger is a reaction to hurt—don't increase the client's pain by getting angry yourself.

2. Resist the impulse to be defensive if the anger is directed at you. Be aware of your anxiety level when encountering anger.

3. Reflect verbally, recognize the client's feelings of anger, and help him develop awareness of his anger; sometimes stating your observation of nonverbal anger is helpful. "I see your fists are clenched and your face is red. You look really upset."

4. Help the client take responsibility for his feelings. Encourage him to use "I" statements. Communicate that anger is an acceptable feeling.

5. Explore with the client the reasons for the anger (e.g., disappointment, frustration). "It sounds like you felt let down by John."

6. Clarify any misunderstandings that may have led to the angry response. "What happened before the fight?" "What did you think your wife meant by that remark?"

7. If the anger is directed at you, assess the validity of the client's reason for anger, not the feeling. All feelings are valid, but the cause of the feelings may or may not be based on realistic expectations.

8. Practice or role play situations in which the client expresses anger.

9. Identify alternative ways of expressing anger, such as physical exercise, or using pillow bats or punching bags.

10. Encourage and support the client in his efforts to express his angry feelings directly to the source.

Sarcasm, withdrawal, and passive aggressive behavior are covert ways of expressing anger, and the nurse must be aware of the anger reflected in these behaviors.

c: (Shouting) I don't want to ever see your stupid face again!

n: Joan, you sound really upset! (Reflecting feeling tone)

c: Who, me? Upset? You're certainly observant. What was your first clue?

n: (Silence—maintains eye contact) (Does not respond defensively)

c: What are you sitting there for? Should I talk about my feelings? OK, here goes! You have totally destroyed my marriage with your crummy advice. I went home this weekend and my husband's filing for divorce, thanks to you!

n: Your husband's planning to divorce you? (Clarification)

c: Yes, thanks to you, Miss Smart Nurse!

n: Tell me what happened this weekend. (Clarification)

c: OK—I'll tell you. I got home and everything was fine. Then, my husband and I were talking and I "expressed my feelings" (mimicking nurse) like you told me. I told him I thought he needed counseling about his drinking. Isn't that expressing my feelings? Now he wants a divorce!

n: It sounds like you and your husband had an argument, right? (Clarification)

c: (Nods yes)

n: You told him you wanted him to get some help for his drinking and he got upset. (Clarification)

c: (Nods) That's the understatement of the year!

n: It sounds like things got pretty hot and you're

feeling surprised and scared by it all. (Reflection of feeling tone)

c: (Starting to cry) Oh—it was awful! He said terrible things to me—I'd had such high hopes for us working things out and now look! (sobs)

n: You're really hurting. (Reflection of feeling tone)

In this situation the nurse helps the client express her feelings of fear and hurt without responding defensively to name calling and blaming. Later, she would retrace the client's argument and assist her to see that telling her husband *he* had a problem is not the same as expressing her feelings about his drinking. Using the situation for learning, the nurse would also help the client see how she projected her anger onto the nurse because of her fears. Still later, role playing both the husband-wife argument and what occurred in the nurse-client relationship would clarify the client's understanding of why she became angry and how she handled the anger.

Withdrawal or Nonverbal Response.

Many clients use the response of withdrawal or silence to protect themselves from their own feelings or from relating to others. The client may be overly sensitive, suspicious, shy, unable to distinguish reality, apathetic, emotionally blunted, frightened, or lonely. He may avoid others by removing himself physically, by emotional detachment, or by lack of verbal response. Whatever the reason, it is important for the nurse to understand the meaning of such behavior.

There are several principles that the nurse must keep in mind. First, her own attitudes and actions as well as those of others must convey that the client is worthwhile and is cared for. Nursing actions that convey this attitude are: (1) recognizing the withdrawal and the events that trigger it; (2) frequently seeking the client out; (3) involving the client in daily life activities; (4) protecting the client from harming himself or others, when necessary; (5) encouraging and assisting, if necessary, good personal hygiene, nutrition, and exercise; (6) accepting hostility, rejection, and rebuff; and (7) observing carefully for symptoms of physical illness which the client might not report.

Second, the nurse must recognize that the client needs to feel that a relationship will not be harmful before she can try to involve him in it. Positive nursing actions are: (1) staying with the client even in silence; (2) consistently attempting to draw the client out without demanding a response; (3) recognizing the client's efforts to be involved even though these may be awkward and socially inept; (4) being consistent, fair, and honest; (5) treating the client appropriately for his age; (6) keeping the environment consistent and secure.

Third, the nurse must recognize that the client's feelings about himself directly influence his relationships with others. Appropriate nursing actions are: (1) providing steady encouragement and support; (2) drawing the client gradually into group activities; (3) helping the client to develop better social skills; (4) initially avoiding situations in which the client will fail, and helping him to feel ready to take new risks; (5) avoiding judgmental actions or responses.

Helplessness and Hopelessness.

Helpless behavior and hopeless feelings can combine to become a very difficult obstacle in the nurse-client relationship. Schneider (1980) defines hope as a psychic or internal commitment to life which stimulates a person to seek new experiences. Conversely, hopelessness is the sense of impossibility—life is too much to handle, and it will not change. Helplessness, a response in which outcomes are seen as uncontrollable, is a feeling that the nurse frequently encounters. The client may feel that he has tried everything in order to feel better and nothing works; in fact his efforts may frequently make matters worse. The client views himself as a victim. This view engenders "learned helplessness," or as Schneider defines it, a lack of motivation in regard to voluntary response. In helplessness, the environment is blamed. In hopelessness, the person is unable to cope, sees no change, and blames himself.

It is extremely important in this situation that the nurse convey, by words and actions, a sense of hope. She will need to take the initiative and direct the client (e.g., by ensuring adequate nutrition and physical care). She may even instruct the client to do certain things so that he may regain a sense of control over outcomes. Schneider suggests several steps for restoring a sense of hope and motivation: (1) allow as much control as possible; (2) respect the client's decisions and desires; (3) provide information to the client about his care; (4) involve family and significant others; (5) talk about the future and express hope for the client; and (6) demonstrate, in word and action, concern for the client.

> ### Vignette
>
> Donna, age 14, was admitted to the adolescent unit: she was withdrawn and uncommunicative. She lay on her bed in a fetal position, facing the wall. The nurse assigned to work with Donna began the relationship by sitting with her for 10 minutes each hour, introducing herself, and explaining her role. She would occasionally either mention superficial topics or sit silently. The next day, Donna permitted the nurse to wash her hair, although she remained downcast. Previously, she had allowed no one to touch her, even for physical care.

Intellectualization. Intellectualization as a defense protects the client from his painful emotions. He analyzes situations or offers information, but exhibits little emotional tone. Woosley (1980) asserts that the basis for this defense arises in early adolescence, when the adolescent must control his drives, try to express his emotions, and understand and integrate his new feelings. These new demands are seen as threatening; the adolescent processes the new information, but detaches the feelings aroused by them.

Detachment of feelings must be discussed with the client so that he can become aware of it. Rather than interpreting how or why the client does this, it is more helpful to encourage expression of feelings. Increasing his self-esteem enables him to feel less threatened. (See vignette, "Mr. H.").

In the working phase of the relationship, the nurse can matter-of-factly point out that the client is stating a thought or belief rather than a feeling: "Mr. H., you are telling me what you *think* about the treatment. The *feeling* I hear is discouragement," clarifies this for the client and differentiates beliefs and attitudes from feelings.

Passive Aggressive Behavior. Meeting needs and expressing anger are two functions served by passive aggressive behavior. This behavior gives rise to difficulties because, although it is passive (indirect, nonactive) it is also aggressive (creates interpersonal problems) in its outcome. Somatic complaints, pouting, procrastination, stubbornness, "forgetting," a "yes, but" response, the silent treatment, incongruent verbal and nonverbal behavior, overdependence, and helplessness are some of the many manifestations of passive aggressive behavior.

This behavior is learned early in childhood, when it developed because direct expression of needs or negative feelings was discouraged or threatening.

People may use this behavior to have their needs met; when, as a result, their interpersonal relationships become impaired, they may be considered to have a personality disorder (see Chapter 27).

In dealing with passive aggressive behavior, the nurse first observes the behavior and attempts to understand in what ways it meets the client's needs. She then discusses the behavior with the client, basing her remarks on what she has observed. Her approach is straightforward and matter-of-fact. Timing is important. She encourages the client to express his anger—keeping in mind that through it he is trying to protect his fragile self-esteem. Later, more direct ways of meeting his needs can be discussed. If it becomes necessary

> ### Vignette
>
> Mr. H., 28 years old, had been hospitalized several times because of his violent behavior toward family and business contacts. His wealthy, prominent family were embarrassed by his behavior. Mr. H. starts the session:
>
> **MR. H:** Well, all I can say is, this is my third hospitalization and it's done no good.
>
> **N:** You sound pretty frustrated today, Mr. H.
>
> **MR. H:** No, I'm not frustrated, I just think with all these drugs and all the training these doctors and nurses get I'd be cured. I'm wasting my time.
>
> **N:** You're feeling pretty discouraged about getting better.
>
> **MR. H:** No, I just think these benzodiazepines and piperazines are worthless. You pay a fortune for this place. My family can't afford this and what's the use? Anytime I've come here, I go home and it happens all over again. Don't you think these drugs are a waste of time? Psychiatry is a bunch of charlatanism—they just want your money. I never get better.
>
> **N:** It sounds like you're feeling both discouraged and angry.
>
> **MR. H:** What's the use of being angry—all it does is get me in here!

to set limits on the client's behavior, the limits should be fair, nonpunitive, and consistent.

Manipulative Behavior. Manipulation carries the negative connotation of artful or shrewd control, mangement, or influence. The nurse is likely to respond to such behavior with anger and distaste, and then to avoid the client. Yet, all humans try to influence and control situations in such a way as to meet their needs. Thus, manipulative behavior that causes problems in the therapeutic relationship must be understood as the client's attempt to satisfy some personal need. Recognizing this, the nurse is able to direct the client's activities toward healthier channels of personal satisfaction.

Manipulative behaviors include flattery, making threats, verbal abuse, feigning helplessness, provocation, pitting staff and client against each other, breaking rules, and starting rumors. An angry nurse will find such behaviors difficult to deal with. She may say, "He's just being manipulative," and avoid dealing with the situations.

It is more helpful to recognize the behavior for what it is, and, without getting into a power struggle, to state your observations to the client. Assist him to examine the anticipated outcome and what actually was gained from it. The nurse may find it necessary to set firm limits on behavior, both to protect other clients and to maintain an open and accepting attitude toward the manipulative client. (Chapter 27 discusses specific nursing interventions for dealing with such behaviors.)

Problems Arising from the Nurse's Response

There are periods in the relationship when the nurse may recognize that progress is being impeded in some way, yet may not be able to identify the source. A sense of uneasiness, a change in the client's manner, or the nurse's own manner of relating may be the clue that tells her that something is amiss. Often, it will become evident that the client is experiencing transference or that the nurse is experiencing countertransference.

The nurse must be honest with herself if she is to develop an awareness of her own feelings. A more experienced colleague, a supervisor, or an instructor can help her to explore her feelings about the client and see what is wrong. Nurses,

like all other humans, make mistakes, and sometimes it is through making mistakes that one learns. The nurse need not be perfect in order to help the client! In fact, realistic recognition of limitations and imperfections may relieve the client of the fear that one must be perfect to feel good about himself.

Feelings that nurses commonly experience are described below.

Rescue Feelings. These feelings arise when the nurse believes she alone can help the client— when the nurse feels she must protect the client from "hostile forces" such as the client's family, doctor, or employer. These feelings prevent the nurse from appreciating the client's strengths and viewing him realistically as a human being with actual and potential abilities to become self-caring. In a word, the nurse sees the client only as a victim.

Feelings of Pessimism. When it appears that the client is not making changes toward healthier ways of behaving, must be readmitted to the hospital, fails to take his medications as prescribed, or returns to his earlier self-defeating behaviors or the earlier unhealthy environment, the nurse may become discouraged and angry, and may come to feel that all the time and personal investment she has made in the client have been futile. She needs to remember that lasting change does not come easily, and that a lifetime spent in an unhealthy environment, with the associated need to adapt to it, is not quickly overcome. These feelings may be due to any of several factors: (1) The goals that were set for the client may be unrealistic; (2) the nurse may have been focusing only on the client's weaknesses and may not have been fully aware of his strenghts; (3) the nurse may be experiencing burnout (Figure 9-2); or (4) she may be taking personal responsibility for the client's behavior.

The nurse needs to reexamine the goals of the relationship and her own beliefs about potential for change. She will more readily see the strides the client has made by this type of review. In many cases, readmittance to the hospital is a sign of the client's strength, indicating that he recognizes the need for intervention and support, rather than regressing to his earlier situation.

Many seemingly insignificant events may deeply affect the client. Although he may not be able to articulate the meaning of the relationship

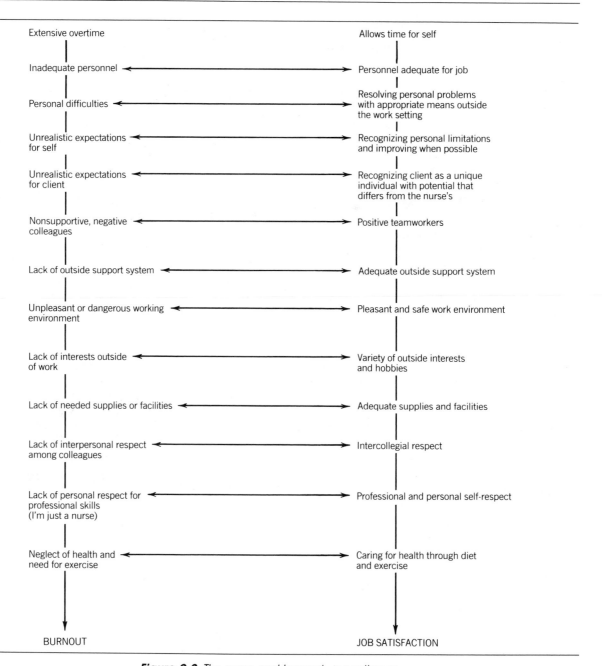

Figure 9-2 *The nurse and burnout: a continuum.*

with the nurse, it may be one of significant influence to him.

Feelings of Omniscience or Omnipotence. Often professionals believe they know more about the client's feelings and reasons for actions than he himself knows. The nurse who holds this belief impedes the potential for truly experiencing another human being. Every person is best able to evaluate his own inner feelings and reactions. Given emotional support and opportunity to ex-

plore alternatives, every person is also usually able to arrive at solutions that best suit his needs and situations. Just as each individual is unique, no single solution applies to a given problem.

Feelings of Overidentification. The nurse may strongly identify with a serious problem her client is facing. Since most of us have experienced profound feelings of many varieties, it is very likely that the nurse is capable of understanding whatever it may be that the client is feeling.

When the nurse overidentifies with the client, however, the therapeutic benefit of the relationship is lost. She stops seeing the client as a unique person, and sees him as someone "just like me." It may then be impossible for her to present to the client alternative ways of viewing the problem. Finally, the nurse may use the relationship to resolve her personal problems, at the client's expense. By thus focusing on herself and her personal needs, she is disrupting the therapeutic process.

A nurse who becomes aware that she is strongly identifying with a particular client and his problem should immediately discuss this with a more experienced colleague or instructor. It is the mark of a professional to recognize when personal feelings are interfering with delivery of therapeutic care. For example, a nurse who as a child had been physically abused may be unable to work with parents who abuse their children. Or a nurse whose parent was severely depressed or schizophrenic may find it extremely painful and difficult to engage in a relationship with a client having similar difficulties.

The nurse should not deliberately select a client who elicits such strong reactions. Of course, however, she does not always select clients. If as-signed to a client with whom she overidentifies, she should seek regular supervision from a colleague or more experienced professional. The nurse may also find it beneficial to seek counseling so that she can work through her unresolved feelings.

Painful Feelings. The sensitivity and caring requisite to the one-to-one relationship can become a source of difficulty. The suffering of another human being, and the sharing of his suffering in an intimate way, can give rise to overwhelming feelings in the nurse. She may sometimes want to say "Enough! I can't stand to hear anymore!" or may avoid the client or may emotionally withdraw to protect herself.

The client who relates to the nurse his feelings of isolation and of being unloved, and his sense of grief and loss, may arouse in her feelings of anger and helplessness, and the remembrance of similar pain. Again, sharing such feelings with a supportive colleague or supervisor allows the nurse to bear the client's painful feelings in a way that will not leave him with the sense of being engulfed in loneliness.

Behaviors that impede the therapeutic relationship are presented in Table 9-1.

TABLE 9-1 Barriers to the One-to-One Relationship that May Be Created by the Nurse

Barrier	Manifestation
Advice—Giving	Deciding on a goal for the client and directing him toward it. Does not allow client to make choices and become responsible for his own behavior.
"Confrontation" in punitive manner	The nurse vents her anger at the client under the guise of "pointing out behavior."
"Instant psychoanalysis"	Reading deep meaning into everything the client says or does.
"Pep" talks	"Encouraging" the client to get better by "getting hold of himself," "keeping a stiff upper lip" and using similar cliches. The client does not need a cheerleader.
Labeling	Dehumanizing the client by viewing him as a group of symptoms, rather than a person.
Nontherapeutic involvement	Meeting with the client socially. If he requests a phone number or address, the reasons for this should be explored, and the nature of the therapeutic relationship explained once again
Talking too much	Usually due to nurse's anxiety and her need to "make the client well."
Doing too much	Usually due to the nurse's discomfort with "just talking" with the client, and meets her needs while fostering dependence in the client.

Burnout. Dr. Christina Maslach (1976) coined the term burnout to describe a complex of emotions, attitudes, and physical symptoms that may arise in the person who works in a health care or other human services setting. It is signaled by emotional and mental exhaustion. Nurses in general, and psychiatric nurses especially, are at high risk of experiencing burnout.

Maslach described feelings and behaviors that signal burnout. Zaleznick (1977) identified five physical manifestations of organizational stress which may indicate burnout (see Table 9-2).

Other indications of burnout are increased use, or abuse, of alcohol, and marital or family problems resulting from job stress displaced onto family members.

■ *Point of Emphasis*

It is crucial to the therapeutic relationship that the nurse prevent burnout. She needs to maintain a sense of balance, since the emotional involvement inherent in the therapeutic relationship demands a great expenditure of energy.

One student expressed it in the following fashion in her clinical journal: "One thing I'm realizing is that although I look forward to coming, the listening and analyzing really drains me emotionally and results in what I call the 'scrambled brains syndrome' on clinical days."

How can the nurse replenish her energy stores, so that she feels refreshed physically and mentally, and becomes able once again to offer therapeutic care?

First, she must recognize her physical limitations. She needs to maintain physical health by getting sufficient sleep, and by eating properly and exercising regularly (Stockard, 1978). And she must attend to her own mental health. Family, friends, and other supportive persons—her support system—can help her meet her need of belonging and strengthen her self-esteem. She needs to pursue other interests or hobbies, as well as cultural and educational activities. These will give her a better perspective about herself and her clients. To state it differently, therapeutic use of self in the one-to-one relationship is enhanced by improving the self one has to offer.

Should the nurse nevertheless recognize symptoms of burnout—which often go unnoticed until pointed out by a co-worker—it is essential that she closely examine her feelings and behaviors. She has probably lost her sense of perspective and needs to take a break so she can reevaluate her personal and professional needs and goals. Positive steps include the following: (1) Taking a vacation, short leave, or "mental health" day; or

---

TABLE 9-2 Clues to Burnout

Feelings	Behaviors	Physical manifestations
Loss of concern about the client	Referring to clients in a detached or dehumanizing way (e.g., "that turkey")	Depression manifested in fatigue, poor appearance, moodiness, irritability, insomnia or hypersomnia, overeating or overdrinking, boredom
Feelings of cynicism or negativism about the client	Using derogatory labels (animals, gomers) and cliches (welfare client) malingerer)	
Feeling the client deserves his problem	Intellectualizing situations that arouse powerful emotions and thus denying those feelings	Medication and/or substance abuse: barbiturates, narcotics, tranquilizers, vitamins, amphetamines, even antibiotics
	Minimizing physical closeness to the client by avoiding eye contact, spending more time with other staff members than with clients; reducing the number of meetings with the client	Cardiovascular problems: hypertension, angina, even myocardial infarction
		Gastrointestinal disturbances including ulcers, colitis, nausea, diarrhea, constipation, most likely to develop in women who are highly educated and hold jobs of high responsibility but low authority (e.g. nurses)
	Going rigidly by the book	
	Constant griping and complaining	Respiratory problems evidenced by allergic flare-ups, colds, and chronic infections such as sore throats
	Using malicious humor and making jokes about clients	
	Escaping into paperwork	

changing jobs; (2) providing time for rest and mental relaxation, or a stimulating activity; (3) taking care of physical needs, and exercising; (4) if symptoms are severe (e.g., depression, alcohol abuse), seeking personal counseling; and (5) reexamining personal and professional goals, making a written list, and setting priorities about accomplishing them.

> **■ Point of Emphasis**
>
> *Every person knows best what activities provide relaxation and comfort for him. It is just as important to extend the same kindness, caring, and firmness with oneself as one would extend to the client.*

TERMINATION

At some time, every one experiences an inevitable loss of significant persons. Thus, the final phase of the therapeutic relationship recalls in both client and nurse the experience of loss (Sene, 1969). How one deals with loss and separation in early childhood significantly affects how one deals with them later (Nehron and Gillian, 1965).

Termination constitutes a form of loss. Campaniello (1980) lists six reasons for terminating the therapeutic relationship:

1. Symptom relief
2. Improved social functioning
3. Greater sense of identity
4. More adaptive defenses
5. Accomplishment of goals
6. Impasse in therapy that the nurse is unable to resolve

Termination elicits strong feelings in both client and nurse. The client may sense a surge of anxiety along with feelings of helplessness, loneliness, and grief (McCann, 1979). These are normal responses when trust between two people has grown. On her part, the nurse may experience feelings of loss, because she has been deeply involved in the unique life of another person. Sharing their feelings about the experience can be therapeutic, like other features of the relationship.

As the nurse facilitates the expression of these feelings, the client is helped to learn that the painful feelings associated with loss and separation are not unbearable (Koehne-Kaplan, and Levy, 1978). Nurse and client together review the entire relationship and evaluate it.

Koehne-Kaplan and Levy (1978) suggest the following technique to facilitate termination. Before the final session, the nurse asks the client to spend at least half an hour, alone and undisturbed, in a quiet place. Next she asks the client to reminisce about the relationship, and to fantasize his version of how he would like to share the final session. The nurse carries out the same steps before the final meeting. Then, at that session, the thoughts and feelings generated by the fantasized terminations are shared, and, to the extent possible, implemented.

Difficulties Associated with Termination

Nehron and Gillian (1965) list defenses characteristically found in termination, including denial, anger and hostility, projection, withdrawal, and regression. By refusing to discuss termination, the client is attempting to deny anxious and painful feelings.

Anger and hostility are client reactions that defend him from feelings of hurt. He may reject the nurse, believing that it is better to end the relationship first, rather than be—as he perceives it—rejected by the nurse. The client may withdraw by skipping sessions, being late for them, or by refusing to share his feelings. He may project his anger onto the nurse, by saying, "You're angry at me—that's why you're leaving," when, in fact, it is the client who is angry at the nurse. By regressing to earlier unhealthy behaviors the client may be unconsciously saying "Look, I'm still sick—I still need you!"

The nurse must recognize the meaning of such behaviors, and encourage the client to express his anger, hurt, and sadness rather than utilizing unhealthy behaviors. She also needs to deal with her personal feelings about the termination. Peer or instructor supervision can help her to express her feelings. Sadness, concern that the client is returning to an unchanged environment (a factor in the illness) may trouble her. This is especially true when the termination results from external reasons (e.g., discharge, client relocation, institutional factors) rather than as a planned outcome.

If either client or nurse wishes to continue the relationship outside the therapeutic involvement, this wish must be explored within the relationship. The client may want to use the relationship as a social relationship; or perhaps he has not yet come to terms with the feelings of loss engendered by termination.

■ Point of Emphasis

The nurse who wishes to continue the relationship outside is most likely meeting her personal needs, rather than the client's.

Continuing the relationship outside the formal structure generally leads to anger and rejection. The client, still viewing the nurse as a therapeutic care giver, calls on her at home or at work, still seeking the attention and support that were part of the formal relationship. The nurse may grow angry that the client is making demands upon her personal time, and may reject him. This is destructive to both participants. (See case study below).

As a rule, the conclusion of the therapeutic relationship marks the end of the nurse-client relationship. McCann (1979) suggests that an "open door" policy exist, especially in the case of children. If the client wishes occasionally to phone or mail a post card to the office or mental health center, this may be a way for him to reminisce about his positive feelings toward the nurse. In a healthy termination, the client generally will not abuse the opportunity to make a personal call. The therapist, too, may call on the client as a way of staying in touch with him. This expression of interest is pleasing to most clients.

■ Enrichment Activities

DISCUSSION QUESTIONS

1. How does the therapeutic relationship differ from a social relationship?

2. What behaviors do you believe indicate caring?

3. Describe a time when you felt lonely. How does loneliness differ from being alone or being lonesome?

4. Discuss what it means to be nonjudgemental.

Case Study

Brad, a 30-year-old student nurse, had established a one-to-one relationship with Martha, 55 years old. She had been hospitalized several times for treatment of depression and suicidal gestures. Her behavior at times was dramatic and bizarre, and she told fanciful stories about various situations. Previous medical diagnosis as well as the current diagnosis was depression, with hysterical personality disorder.

Brad was able to establish a very warm therapeutic relationship with Martha. At discharge, she asked him for his address. Although he was aware that he needed to explore the possibility that she intended to continue the relationship outside the hospital, Brad did not want to hurt her feelings, and gave her his address.

A few days later, Martha, who, as it happened, lived in Brad's neighborhood, took to standing outside his apartment house. This went on for several days. She then moved into the foyer of the apartment house where she would stand for several hours. Brad's wife, who was at home with their small children, became alarmed and mentioned the behavior to Brad. Brad talked to Martha, who told him she wanted it to be like "old times." Martha stated her outpatient therapist wasn't helping her and she wanted Brad's help.

Although he felt extremely uncomfortable, Brad talked to Martha several times. Finally, he realized that he would have to terminate the relationship. After talking with his instructor, Brad was able to recognize that by initially failing to explore Martha's request for his address, he had conveyed the impression that it was permissible for her to come by. He also realized he had failed to define the limits to the relationship by not making clear that the relationship ended over at the hospital and not allowing Martha to discuss her feelings about leaving. Finally, he recognized that Martha was pitting him against her present therapist and thus was not deriving the full benefit from her current therapy.

Brad genuinely liked Martha, but felt frustrated and trapped, and didn't want to hurt her or upset her. With his instructor's encouragement, he was able tactfully to tell Martha that she could no longer come to see him, and explained that she needed to deal with her current therapist. He told Martha he liked her, but that the therapeutic relationship was ended. Martha accepted this explanation and said she realized it was an imposition, but he had been so kind to her. The relationship ended in a friendly manner.

5. Describe a situation in which someone judged you. How did you feel?

6. Discuss the traditional concept in health care of taking responsibility for another as it applies to the client with emotional problems.

7. Is there such a thing as too much emotional involvement? What does this mean to you?

8. Discuss reasons why people fail to achieve their goals.

9. Discuss burnout. What role does it play in creating problems in the therapeutic relationship? What can the nurse do to prevent it?

LEARNING ACTIVITIES

1. Keep a diary of thoughts, feelings, and perceptions about an individual client or about self and daily activities.

2. Tape-record interactions between self and client, then transcribe and analyze these communications. Write a process record after the interaction if you do not have access to a tape recorder.

3. Reflect upon a personal experience that was painful but that ultimately promoted personal growth. What happened? Who was helpful/not helpful? What did the other person say or do? What did you learn about yourself?

4. Write a short essay on one of the following topics:

Loneliness	Sensitivity
Caring	Helping
Friendship	Loyalty
Wholeness	Kindness
Pain	Awareness

Each member of the group reads her essay and discusses its similarities to or differences from others' essays.

5. Set one goal for yourself in each of these areas:

Professional/educational	Family
Physical health	Financial
Mental/spiritual	Social

Write each goal specifically and set a date for accomplishing it. Review the goal each day and write specific activities to be done each day that will move you closer to that goal.

6. Recall a situation in which you terminated an important relationship. What were your feelings? What behaviors did you and the other person demonstrate?

7. Keep a diary of situations in which you felt hurt or depressed. Did you feel anger? How did you express or not express your anger? What behaviors did you engage in?

■ Recommended Readings

Fromm-Reichmann, F. *Principles of intensive psychotherapy*. Chicago: University of Chicago Press, 1950. This book outlines interpersonal principles of psychotherapy applicable to psychotic clients and to clients with disorders related to anxiety. It is psychoanalytically based and illustrates the importance of the relationship between therapist and client as a way of alleviating the client's difficulties through insight and dynamic changes. It is written for the advanced practitioner and requires familiarity with psychoanalytic theory.

Kanfer, F.N., and Goldstein, A.P. *Helping people change. A textbook of methods*. 2d ed. New York: Pergamon Press, 1980. A "textbook of methods" is the descriptor about this book. It gives a comprehensive view of various forms of therapeutic intervention. Written from an interdisciplinary standpoint, the book covers relationship therapy, attitude modification, cognitive change, modeling, simulation and role playing, operant and fear reduction, hypnosis, and biofeedback. Recent research and explanations of various methods make this text helpful to the beginner wishing to learn more about various methods in therapy.

Mayeroff, M. *On caring*. New York: Perennial Library, Harper & Row, 1971. Mayeroff's classic book explores the concept of care, the components of caring, and the qualities of the caring person. It is excellent reading for the nurse in any professional setting as well as for all persons, since caring is an essential part of all human relationships.

Moustakas, C. *Loneliness*. New York: Prentice-Hall, 1961. This is an absorbing personal and philosophical account of a universal human feeling. Distinguishing "aloneness," "lone-some," and "loneliness," the book explores the experience of loneliness and alienation from others. This book is excellent, providing greater understanding of the client whose emotional difficulties increase isolation as well as increasing the nurse's awareness of her own needs for connection to others.

Powell, J. *Why am I afraid to tell you who I am?* Niles, IL: Argus Communications, 1969. Powell's book provides some insights on self-awareness, personal growth, and communications. It provides basic explanations of how one can grow as a person, learn to deal with emotions, and why people use defenses. The nurse will find this book helpful to her personal growth and her understanding of why other persons relate as they do.

■ References

Anderson, M.L. Nursing interventions: What did you do that helped? *Perspectives in psychiatric care,* 21, 1983:4–8.

Boettcher, E.G. Nurse client collaboration: Dynamic equilibrium in the nursing care system. *Journal of psychiatric nursing and mental health services,* 161, 1978:7–15.

Campaniello, J.A. The process of termination. *Journal of psychiatric nursing and mental health services,* 18, 1980:29–32.

DeLeo, D., Magni, G., and Vallerini, A. Anxiety and depression in general and psychiatric nurses: A comparison. *International journal of nursing studies,* 19, 1982:173–5.

Doona, M.E. *Travelbee's intervention in psychiatric nursing.* 2d ed. Philadelphia: F.A. Davis, 1979.

Erikson, E. *Childhood and society.* 2d ed. New York: Norton, 1963.

Gibran, K. *The prophet.* New York: Alfred Knopf, 1971.

Hoeffer, B., and Murphy, S. The unfinished task: Development of nursing theory for psychiatric and mental health nursing practice. *Journal of psychiatric nursing and mental health services,* 20, 1982: 8–14.

Hughes, J. Manipulation: A negative element in care. *Journal of advanced nursing,* 5, 1980:21–29.

Koehne-Kaplan, N.S., and Levy, K.E. An approach for facilitating the passage through termination. *Journal of psychiatric nursing and mental health services,* 16, 1978:11–14.

Krikorian, D.A., and Paulanka, B.J. Self awareness—The key to a successful nurse-patient relationship? *Journal of psychiatric nursing and mental health services,* 20, 1982:19–21.

Lego, S. The one-to-one nurse patient relationship. *Perspectives in psychiatric care,* 18, 1980:67–89.

Maslach, C. Burned-out. *Human behavior,* September 1976, 16–22.

Mayeroff, M. *On caring.* New York: Harper & Row, 1971.

McCann, J. Termination of the psychotherapeutic relationship. *Journal of psychiatric nursing and mental health services,* 17, 1979:37–39.

Mellow, J. Nursing therapy as a treatment and clinical investigative approach to emotional illness. *Nursing forum,* 5, 3, 1966:64–73.

Meyer, P.J. *Dynamics of goal setting.* Waco, TX: Success Motivation Institute, 1972.

Moustakas, C.E. *Loneliness,* New York: Prentice-Hall, 1961.

Murphy, P.L., and Schultz, E.D. Passive aggressive behavior in patient and staff. *Journal of psychiatric nursing and mental health services,* 16, 1978:43–45.

Nehron, J., and Gillian, N. Separation anxiety. *American journal of nursing,* 65, 1965:109–112.

Orlando, I.J. *The dynamic nurse-patient relationship: Function, process and principles.* New York: G. Putnam's Sons, 1961.

Peplau, H. *Interpersonal relations in nursing: A conceptual frame of reference for psychodynamic nursing.* New York: G. Putnam's Sons, 1952.

Pines, A.M., and Kanner, A.D. Nurses burnout: Lack of positive conditions and presence of negative conditions as two independent sources of stress. *Journal of psychiatric nursing and mental health services,* 20, 1982:30–35.

Rogers, R. The characteristics of helping relationship. In *The nursing process: A humanistic approach* (LaMonica, E.L., ed.). Menlo Park, CA: Addison-Wesley Publishing Company, 1979.

Ruditis, S.E. Developing trust in interpersonal relationships. *Journal of psychiatric nursing and mental health services,* 17, 1979:20–23.

Sene, B. Termination in the student patient relationships. *Perspectives in psychiatric care,* 7, 1969:39–45.

Schneider, J.S. Hopelessness and helplessness. *Journal of psychiatric nursing and mental health services,* 18, 1980:12–21.

Stockard, S. *Burn out in nursing.* Workshop, 1978–1983.

Sullivan, H.S. *The interpersonal theory of psychiatry.* New York: Norton, 1953.

Woosley, D.G. A working concept of intellectualization. *Journal of psychiatric nursing and mental health services,* 18, 1980:36–39.

Zaleznick, B. Stress reactions in organizations: Syndromes, causes and consequences. *Behavioral science,* 22, 3, 1977:151–162.

Zyl, S.V., Ernst C., and Salinger, R.J. Role expectations: A significant concern for the nurse therapist. *Journal of psychiatric nursing,* 17, 1979:23–27.

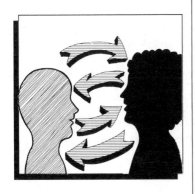

10

Psychosocial and Neurological Assessment of the Individual

Peggy L. Jensen-Hawkins and Gordon Vogt

Learning Objectives

Upon completion of this chapter, the reader will be able to:

1. Describe the purpose of a neurological assessment and relate pertinent aspects to psychosocial assessment.

2. Describe the purpose of a psychosocial assessment.

3. Discuss the assessment component of nursing process in relation to psychiatric-mental health nursing.

4. Describe the process of psychosocial nursing assessment.

Nursing assessment is the procedure by which information about a client or problem is collected systematically, purposively, and continually by an experienced professional. Interpretations (inferences) are made about the data collected, and problem or need identifications (nursing diagnoses) are formulated. Therefore, the three-step procedure for assessment is data collection, data interpretation, and problem/need identification.

Data interpretation and problem/need identification are the components that formulate nursing diagnoses. The American Nurses' Association describes diagnosis as the start by which a problem/need is objectified. This is the beginning of understanding and taking action on a situation.

This chapter discusses psychosocial and related aspects of neurological nursing assessment with the focus on the adult. However, one must remember that other basic human needs of the client must also be assessed. These include oxygenation, fluids and electrolytes, food, elimination, exercise, rest and sleep, and skin integrity. The significance of assessing all basic human needs is twofold. First, even though the client may appear outwardly healthy, the ability to attend to the tasks of daily living may be diminished because of illness. Therefore, the client may require assistance in meeting these needs. The nurse is skilled in this area. Second, in a psychiatric setting auxiliary personnel may not be skilled in assessing a person's needs other than the psychological ones. The nurse's holistic approach to client care is therefore vital. For further information on physical assessment the nurse is referred to a basic physical examination text.

Purpose of Psychosocial Nursing Assessment

Usually, the initial nursing assessment is conducted as an interview in the early face-to-face contact between the client and the nurse. Occasionally, the initial contact may be by telephone. Completing the assessment in psychiatric nursing has a twofold purpose: (1) to collect data and ascertain the client's needs or problems, and (2) to initiate the therapeutic relationship.

It is preferable, whenever possible, for the client's primary nurse to conduct the assessment. The primary nurse needs to obtain the data firsthand in order to eliminate as much interviewer bias as possible. The beginning phase of the therapeutic relationship is facilitated by conducting this interview. (The therapeutic relationship is discussed in Chapter 9.)

Purpose of Neurological Nursing Assessment

An accurate neurological assessment is a very important aspect of care. Not every client will need a complete neurological examination but it is the nurse's responsibility to be able to utilize the components of the assessment that are relevant to the client's condition. The neurological assessment will allow the nurse to: (1) observe changes in the client's condition, (2) assist the health team in determining the severity and progression of the disorder, (3) identify and possibly prevent temporary or permanent problems that may result from disorders that have disrupted normal functional activities, and (4) aid the nursing staff in developing individualized and therapeutic interventions relevant to these problems. In addition, the neurological assessment will assist the nurse in recognizing differences between functional mental disorders and organic brain dysfunctions. Organic changes may cause a variety of psychiatric syndromes and in many clients they are the presenting complaint.

Nursing Process

Nursing process is the problem-solving technique used by nurses. The purpose of nursing process is to assist the client in adaptation. This is accomplished in a systematic problem-solving approach. The steps of nursing process are assessment, nursing diagnosis, planning, implementation, and evaluation (Yura and Walsh, 1983; Marriner, 1983; Sundeen, et al., 1981).

Nursing process in psychiatric-mental health nursing is basically no different than in other specialty areas of nursing. The assessment of neurological and psychosocial aspects of the client is, however, emphasized.

DATA COLLECTION

Data collection, for purposes of this chapter, is defined as the nurse's systematic observation of objective and subjective data regarding a client or problem. However simple this may seem, it is not a simple task. Data collection requires acute awareness of what the nurse actually sees, hears, touches, and smells.

Objective data are generally nonverbal and are obtained by observation. The following is an example of selected objective data concerning a 48-year-old woman:

> Mrs. A. cried uncontrollably for 5 minutes. She did not smile once during a 1-hour interview. She showed no eye contact with the nurse during this time. Body odor was evident within an arm's length of Mrs. A. Her hair was oily and uncombed. Her clothes were baggy and ill-fitting.

Subjective data are verbal pieces of information that the nurse hears the client say. These can be recorded using quotation marks. Examples of Mrs. A.'s subjective data are as follows:

> I went to the doctor because I have lost so much weight. Instead of running tests, he sticks me in here. My husband died three months ago. What is it going to be like without him? I just don't think I can go on anymore. I haven't had a good night's sleep in weeks. I've lost 20 pounds.

Sources of Data. Data can be obtained from a variety of sources. The most significant source is the client. Obtaining corroborating or additional data from the client's significant others is also the nurse's responsibility. These sources can be family or friends, other health care professionals (e.g., referring physician or psychologist), old records, and community resources such as schools and church. To avoid breach of confidentiality, permission from the client is required before other agencies or community resources can be contacted. The nurse obtains this permission in writing from the client or guardian.

Obtaining information during an interview with family or friends may or may not take place with the client present. In order to make this determination, the nurse has to evaluate the situation. Will the client and/or family speak openly in front of each other? Will separate interviews cause undue suspicion about what is being said when one or the other is not present?

Some interviews are conducted in stages, a portion of the interview being done with the client and with family and friends separately and then a portion with them together.

Accurate Data. In collecting data, the nurse has certain responsibilities about the quality of the data. Although this holds true for data collection from clients in all settings, it has particular importance in the psychiatric setting.

The nurse wants to know that the data presented in pure form are as accurate as possible. Interpretation is much easier when the data presented can be relied on to be accurate. Unfortunately, this is not always true. Accurate information cannot be guaranteed. Variables that influence the correctness of the data obtained are the client, the interviewer, and the latter's skill. (Millon, 1984).

Client Objectivity. The client, by virtue of being a human being, is a dynamic individual who is constantly changing. The environment that surrounds the client is also changing. As the environment changes, it may influence the client. Data that were collected hours ago may no longer be accurate. The client may simply have difficulty remembering the information which leads to providing incomplete data. The client may not place any significance on some information and therefore not mention it during the assessment. The reason for the client's admission into the psychiatric health care system may affect the quality of the information. The illness may even interfere with the ability to relate factual information. These factors all affect the quality of the data that can be collected.

Interviewer Objectivity. The nurse, as the interviewer, also affects the accurateness of the data. No matter how accepting and nonjudgmental, the nurse cannot remain totally impartial. Nurses are human and, therefore, have biases and make judgments. Nurses must be aware of their biases and make a conscious effort not to have them interfere. Individuals adhering to a particular theoretical viewpoint tend to give more importance to data that reinforce that theory. The data that do not support the theory tend to be ignored (Pasmanick, et al., 1959). Then too, the interviewer may, unconsciously, fail to collect data about matters that cause personal discomfort, such as sexuality, race, spiritual aspect, and potential suicide.

Interviewer Skills. Proper use of communication skills by the experienced nurse is required. The nurse will not obtain accurate data when communication skills are not effectively utilized. Asking leading questions obtains only the information that the nurse expects to hear and not necessarily what the person wants to relate. Questions of a closed nature requiring only a one-word response do not aid in obtaining complete information. (A detailed discussion of communication can be found in Chapter 8.)

Structured versus Unstructured Assessment Interviews.

An unstructured interview is one in which there is no patterned organization developed into the questioning. A structured interview is one that is organized into a specific pattern before the interview is initiated and in which the questions are predetermined.

A semistructured interview has been found to be most effective in obtaining information from clients (Kolb and Gunderson, 1980). Questions organized in a systematic manner as opposed to a free-style approach to assessment have been found to be essential in collecting quality data. Using a standardized format that permits the freedom to explore further any pertinent information is likely to elicit comprehensive information (Saghir, 1971). No disadvantages have been found in this type of semistructuring of interviews (Cox, Rutter, and Holbook, 1981).

When developing a semistructured questionnaire the nurse must avoid double questions—such as "Have you attended school or work?"—which can be answered in the affirmative but will not clarify which part of the question is being answered. Direct questioning is often needed to elicit certain information. One-word responses are adequate for information such as dates or admissions. A semistructured approach allows freedom to explore pertinent material while avoiding ambiguous questioning. It requires effective communication skills throughout the assessment and of direct questions when advantageous.

Use of Aids.

Certain aids may facilitiate nursing assessment. A typewritten form with sample questions can be of help to the nurse to ensure inclusion of all assessment areas. However, this can lead to dependence on these questions and inhibit exploration for further information. Also, if the nurse is writing down the client's responses, his nonverbal behaviors cannot be observed. A compromise on the use of aids is recommended (Eaton, 1981). A list of sample questions as a guide, and brief note taking are advocated. When the face-to-face contact is terminated, the collected data can be completely recorded.

The need for note taking during assessments is eliminated when interviews are videotaped or tape-recorded. The disadvantages of this type of aid are the need for specific client consent, the possibility of client suspiciousness, and the need to eventually transfer all the information into writing.

Many institutions have an interview tool or guideline for nursing assessments developed for use in a semistructured format. These interview guidelines range in comprehensiveness from a few questions requesting identifying data to a thorough assessment. Whatever type of format is used, the nurse remains responsible for recording the collected data and communicating the findings to other health care professionals.

Table 10-1 is an example of a partial assessment tool that might be used. It provides sample questions for the interviewer and space for brief notation of the objective and subjective data. It also allows space for the nurse to begin interpreting the data after the interview is completed.

Data Recording.

Communicating client information is traditionally accomplished by charting. Charting can take two forms: source-oriented and problem-oriented records. Originally, charting was source oriented. In this type of record each health team member makes notations in separate sections of the chart. A narrative account of client information is given in chronological order. This type of charting does not facilitate open communication among members of an interdisciplinary health team.

Problem-oriented records (POR) have replaced source-oriented records in many hospitals and agencies. Utilization of the problem-oriented record facilitates client care since it is organized similar to the problem-solving approach. The four components of this type of record are the database, problem list, initial plans, and progress notes. The initial database includes the assessments, laboratory findings, history, physical examination, mental status examination, and psychological tests. The findings are summarized into a problem list. Initial plans are developed for each problem. Progress notes are used to follow the client's care. The recording of information is done under SOAPE, the acronym for subjective data, objective data, assessment, plan, and evaluation. Flow sheets and a discharge summary of each problem are also included in the progress notes.

Client Comfort.

The client's comfort during the assessment interview is important. A com-

TABLE 10-1 *Partial Nursing Assessment with Guideline Questions*

Assessment Guideline (Adult)	Objective Data	Subjective Data	Inferences	Problem/Need Identification
History				
Present problem Patient's perception "I am interested in knowing what is the nature of your problem, Mrs. ___?" Others' perception "Mr. ___, what do you see is the problem that Mrs. ___ is experiencing?"				
Past psychiatric history "Have you been hospitalized before?" "What was the date?" "Where? "What was the problem you experienced?" "Have you been a patient in a community mental health center?"				
Influence of chemicals "What medications are you using that a doctor has prescribed for you?" "What medications are you using that you can buy over the counter?" "What street drugs do you use?" "Do you use alcohol? beer? wine?" "Do you use coffee? tea? cola?" "When do you use this?" "How often?" "Quantity?" "How long have you used this?" "What happens before and after you use this?"				
Family history and profile (draw family diagram) I'd like to learn more about your family. Tell me about any problems that they may have had, causes of death & their ages. Mother? Father? Any stepparents? Grand parents on mother's side? Grandparents on father's side? Aunts? Uncles? Brothers? Sisters? Children?				

(*continued*)

TABLE 10-1 (continued)

Assessment Guideline (Adult)	Objective Data	Subjective Data	Inferences	Problem/Need Identification
Educational and vocational history "What is your occupation?" "I'd like to know about your work history." "How important is this job to you?" "What is your job like for you?" "What would you like to do instead of this work?" "Describe your financial status." "Have you been in the service?" "What was it like?" Psychosocial history Developmental task attainment tasks-early adulthood "Do you have a spouse?"				

fortable chair is likely to be satisfactory. The nurse arranges the room so that the client is comfortable and can be easily observed for nonverbal behavior. Blocking the only exit can be threatening to the client even when done in a nonthreatening manner. The interview is conducted in private to reduce distracting stimuli and to facilitate trust. Comfort measures such as a glass of water or a box of tissues are provided.

Time planning is essential for client comfort. A thorough nursing assessment takes about 1½ hours to complete. The client's tolerance for this time span needs to be assessed. Agitated clients may not tolerate an assessment of this length. Alternatives such as frequent breaks or a shortened schedule may be needed.

Data Collection as a Time to Experience.

The nurse does not interpret information while initially collecting data. The focus is on gathering factual, high-quality data in a semistructured manner. This time is for experiencing what and how information is conveyed, not interpreting it. The time for interpretation is after the data collection is formally completed. Data collection requires active listening and attending solely to the

material being presented. The following explains experiencing during data collection (Doona, 1981).

> Experiencing as an aspect of observation is difficult to define; it is probably akin to a mosaic structure, composed of various elements. Experiencing includes collecting data using all sense modalities, while holding interpretation of the data in abeyance. It means focusing on the individual within the total context of his setting and environment, not parts or aspects of the whole. One reacts as human to human and allows the other's personality and uniqueness to become real, on the level other than what is known about him. There is a vividness to experiencing, an immediacy and sense of confronting a real person rather than behavior we have scrutinized, categorized or dissected.

Data Interpretation.

Perceptions, assumptions, or analysis do not enter into the data collection step of nursing assessment. Rather, the second step of nursing assessment, interpretation, is the beginning of the abstract component of nursing process. This requires not guesswork or intuition but clinical judgment. The nurse takes the previously collected data, uses clinical judgment, and interprets or gives meaning to the vast amount of information that has been gathered. This step requires that the nurse compare the data that have been gathered to norms. Hence the nurse needs to understand normal growth and development. This step requires analysis, reflection, thought, and knowledge base but it is not intuitive. To judge is to draw appropriate conclusions about the situation. Interpretations cannot be considered correct in the absence of accuracy and reasoned analysis.

Problem Identification. Interpretation is data-based, individualized formulation of client problems or needs. By individualized is meant that the problem is uniquely this specific person's problem and not a standardized statement. This does not negate the use of taxonomies or classification of nursing diagnosis. Rather, it is meant to enhance their use (Lunney, 1982).

The nurse calls upon her knowledge base and clinical judgment when formulating the problem. This is not to be confused with medical diagnosis. There is no reason to keep the identified problems a secret from the client. Rather, the collaboration of both client and nurse in the interpretation stage of nursing process can help ensure client cooperation (Doona, 1981). A discussion with a client may start something like this:

> NURSE: Mrs. A., I've been thinking about what you have told me yesterday. I believe you're having a most difficult time adjusting to the loss of your husband. What do you think?

If Mrs. A. agrees that she continues to be acutely distressed and unable to cope, the problem has been validated.

STATEMENT OF THE GOAL

The establishment of goals by the nurse and client is the initial step in the planning stage. Goal setting is stating the realistic, expected outcome of the client's problem. Resolution is hoped for but is not always realistic. The nurse needs to have knowledge of theoretical concepts if the goal statement is to reflect the reality of the situation.

It is desirable to establish both short-term and long-term goals. Long-term goals can be overwhelming to the client, and several short-term goals can seem more attainable and therefore more likely to be achieved. A short-term goal for a client might be, "The client will not cause harm to herself." This goal is based on suicide prevention and is realistic. One long-term goal for this client might be, "The client will grieve appropriately for her husband, reaching acceptance of his death."

Assessment is not completed after it is done once; it has only begun. Although assessment is the focus at the beginning of the relationship, it is an ongoing process—the phases of data collection, interpretation, and goal setting are repeated throughout the therapeutic relationship. The reason for this is that not all pertinent data can be collected in the initial few hours of contact. As the client changes, grows, and begins to feel better, additional data must be obtained to reflect the changes. Psychiatric clients typically require health care longer than other clients. For this reason the nursing process can become a quite lengthy process.

☐ *Psychosocial and Neurological Assessment*

Traditionally, assessment was done by a psychiatrist who completed a history and mental status examination. The psychiatrist's goal, based on the medical model, was to form a psychiatric diagnosis. Although the psychosocial assessment still includes the history and mental status examination, various psychological and social aspects of the individual are also involved, the purpose being to identify problems, needs, strengths, and weaknesses.

Components that comprise a thorough data collection during a nursing assessment are presented below, with typical headings for organizing data. Some sample questions are included.

HISTORY

Present Problem

Initial data collection often begins with the determination of the client's presenting problem. The nurse inquires about what brought the client to seek help. The purpose is to identify the major problem and have the client describe it as accurately as possible. His perception of the problem is very important, and his own description can be helpful.

Examples of some opening questions are: "What caused you to be concerned enough to seek help?" or "I am interested in knowing the nature of your problem." A useful opening statement is: "I have (have not) had the opportunity to hear something about your problem but am interested in hearing what you have to say." Mrs. A., in the example previously given, may respond by saying, "Because I've lost weight."

The parent's or significant other's perception of the presenting problem is also obtained and recorded in his own words. This view may differ from the client's. The nurse may ask Mrs. A.'s son, "What do you see as the reason for your mother needing hospitalization?" The son may respond, "My mother is sad to the point she can't take proper care of herself."

Getting a thorough description of the presenting problem requires that the nurse learn about several specific elements: client behaviors attributed to the problem; and the duration, onset, and frequency of occurrence. The behaviors that the client attributes to the problem are identified. An example of a question the nurse might ask in attempting to determine duration is: "How much of each day do you spend feeling sad?"

It is also helpful to differentiate times of the day and situations in which the person feels better or worse. For instance by asking "Are there times of the day when you feel better than others?" "Are any things particularly associated with feeling bad?"

In some disorders, such as depression, the onset of symptoms is a differentiating factor. An example of a question the nurse might ask is, "When did you first become aware of this problem of waking up early in the morning?" or "This problem has been present for 3 months. What has brought you now to seek help?"

The client's information about how often he experiences problems can help define their magnitude. He might be asked, "How many times has this happened to you in the last week?"

Past Psychiatric History

The nurse asks specifically about any previous hospitalizations, including general admissions, and about psychiatric outpatient admissions. Factual data are obtained most easily by asking for dates and descriptions. This is one example of assessment where open-ended communication is not the best approach. Examples of questions include: "Have you been hospitalized in any psychiatric hospital before?" "What was the date of this admission?" "What was the problem you experienced that caused this hospitalization?" "Have you ever been a client in a community mental health clinic?" "What were the dates of these visits?" "What was the problem?" "Did you think the problem was resolved?" "Have the problems that you experienced in the past been similar to those you are experiencing now?"

Influence of Chemicals

The nurse needs to obtain information about certain chemicals that clients might use. Some are commonplace, and although they may seem insignificant, they are not. Consumption of any substance that may alter the client's physical or cognitive status is pertinent. (See Chapter 15 for further discussion.)

Information about the use of tobacco is needed. The question, "Do you smoke?" is not exacting enough. The client should be asked whether he smokes a pipe, cigars, or cigarettes, and whether he chews tobacco or sniffs snuff.

Drug use is assessed in five areas: (1) prescription medications ("What medications are you using that a doctor has prescribed for you?"); (2) over-the-counter medications ("What medications are you using that you can get yourself?"); (3) illicit drugs ("Do you use drugs for recreational purposes?"); (4) alcohol ("Do you consume alcohol? beer? wine?"); (5) caffeine ("Do you consume coffee? tea? colas? over-the-counter stimulants?").

The nurse ascertains what the client uses, when it is used, how often it is used, the quantity each time it is used (per day or week) how long it has been used, and what feelings or behaviors result. She also asks the client about preceding events, and about his feelings while he is using the substance. The nurse seeks specific, accurate replies. The response, "A few beers," can mean different things to different people, while "A six-pack of beer every night" cannot be misconstrued.

Family History and Profile

The nurse should take a thorough medical and psychiatric history of the family, including illnesses, cause of death, and the members' ages at the time of these events. Particular attention is given to significant psychosocial events within the family.

Figure 10-1 is a genogram, or diagram of a client's family tree. A code represents the indi-

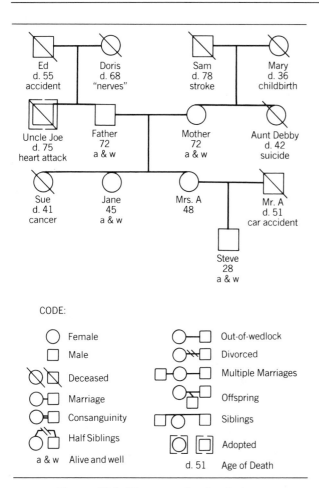

Figure 10-1. *Diagram of a family tree.*

viduals. Social workers make frequent use of genograms. The nurse may draw a genogram to construct a concise picture of the family.

■ *Point of Emphasis*

A genogram gives a straightforward pictorial history of a family. Although genetic counselors were the first to use this form of history taking, many health professionals now find the genogram to be a concise means of gathering information about several generations of a family.

School and Vocational History

Level of schooling completed, and where and when it was completed, should be discussed if appropriate. The client's reactions to school life may give useful information. He can be asked to relate his perceptions of relationships with peers and

teachers. Information about extracurricular activities and grades also affords clues. The nurse should inquire about any sudden dysfunctions the client experienced while attending school.

The client's age is significant in the school history. A young adult or a child would be asked more probing questions than other groups, simply because schooling is such an important activity during that period.

Vocational history is given greater emphasis when the client is an adult. A chronological history will help simplify the organization of the data. Information the nurse is seeking includes the client's current occupation, past jobs, and the type of work done. Is the job of importance to the person? Is it stressful? Is it what the client wants to be doing? What would the client like to do instead of that work? What is the client's financial status? Military history is sought if appropriate.

This line of questioning is meant to help determine whether there is a pattern in life-style and to learn whether there are any health hazards associated with the work. Significant findings would include factors such as that this person is unable to hold a job, has a position that is highly stressful, or works with toxic chemicals. Such findings would bear on the nursing interventions.

Psychosocial History

The purpose of the psychosocial history is to obtain information about the client's growth and development, life-style, and interpersonal relationships. Although the components of data collection previously discussed are similar to those in other fields of nursing, the data about psychosocial history are given greater emphasis when psychosocial problems are present. The data collection of psychosocial history is organized into the following areas.

Developmental Task Attainment. The purpose of this assessment is to compare and contrast the client's developmental task attainment with normal expected development. This requires thorough knowledge of normal developmental growth as described by leading theorists. (See related chapters on development.)

An assessment of developmental task attainment is made by comparing the accomplishments of the client's developmental tasks against the relevant age group. If the tasks for the current level have not been attained, the nurse assesses earlier developmental tasks to determine the level of at-

---

TABLE 10-2 Developmental Tasks through Adulthood[a]

Developmental Tasks of Early Adulthood

Selecting a mate
Learning to live with a marriage partner
Starting a family
Rearing children
Managing a home
Getting started in an occupation
Taking on civic responsibility
Finding a congenial social group

Developmental Tasks of Middle Age

Achieving adult civic and social responsibility
Establishing and maintaining an economic standard of
    living
Assisting teen-age children to become responsible and
    happy adults
Developing adult leisure time activities
Relating to one's spouse
Accepting and adjusting to the physiological changes
    of middle age
Adjusting to aging parents

Developmental Tasks of Later Maturity

Adjusting to decreasing physical strength and health
Adjusting to retirement and reduced income
Adjusting to death of spouse
Establishing an explicit affiliation with one's age group
Meeting social and civic obligations
Establishing satisfactory physical living arrangements

[a] From *Developmental Psychology* (p. 7) by E. Hurlock, 1953, New York: McGraw-Hill Book Company. Copyright 1953 by the Mc-Graw-Hill Book Company. Reprinted by permission.

---

tainment. Table 10-2 lists developmental tasks of the adult (Hurlock, 1953).

Peer and Family Relationships. The purpose of data collection in this area is to determine the quality of the client's interpersonal relationships with peers and to determine characteristics of the family system. (Chapter 12 focuses on the family system.) The genogram described earlier will help to clarify the information.

During data collection the nurse attempts to define the family's interpersonal structure. Any power struggles, competitiveness, coalitions, and alliances are assessed. Often the role of scapegoat is assigned to a family member and this person is identified. The client is asked about his perception of significant personality traits of family members. Information about education, work habits, and religious beliefs of family members can be sought. How the client lives, with whom, living arrangements, and type of dwelling are necessary data.

In addition to getting a description of the family system and home life, the nurse observes the family communication. During the initial interview when the client and family are seen together, the nurse notes who speaks to whom, the quality and clarity of messages sent from one family member to another, and presence and quality of physically demonstrated affection among family members.

Family B enters the interview room. Father sits by the door with 10-year-old son. Mother disregards an available chair next to them, and sits next to the 14-year-old daughter, the identified client. The mother kisses and hugs the daughter frequently. She reiterates, "My poor baby." When the daughter is directly questioned her mother answers for her before the girl can do so. Mother's conversation dominates the interview. The son and father whisper between themselves. The father's responses, when given, are along the lines of "I don't know anything about it," or "I can't remember." The mother contradicts most of the father's statements.

The nurse might infer that the coalitions in this family are mother-daughter and father-son. The father remains uninvolved while the mother is domineering. These inferences may lead to the identification of a problem of dysfunctional family interaction.

Specific questions should be asked about client interaction with peers and the quantity and quality of friendships. It may be helpful to ask questions such as: "Tell me about your friends." "What's friendship (or lack of friends) like for you?" "How long have you been friends?" "When did you last see this person?" A schizophrenic client may describe in great detail a person who does not exist or a friendship that occurred 10 years ago. Careful questioning will help determine if those persons are part of the client's delusional system and the extent to which they are a part of the person's present life.

Sexual History. A sexual history is pertinent. The nurse ascertains adjustment of sexuality through such questions as "At what age did you experience puberty? What feelings did you have concerning this? How frequently do you have sexual intercourse? Are you satisfied with your sexual relationships? Do you have particular concerns about sexuality?" Unsatisfying encounters or frequent multiple partners can indicate interpersonal problems. Chapter 21 discusses sexuality in greater detail.

Significant Life Stressors/Events. The purpose is to determine whether the client is unduly susceptible to certain disorders, and the degree to which stress is a factor. The client is asked to relate the important events in his life. The nurse wants to know what happened, when, to whom, and why. Additionally, how the client responded to the event is explored. When a client can identify a particularly stressful period, the nurse should ask "What else was happening in your life or in the family when that feeling began?" For example, Miss S. attributes great importance to her parents' divorce. Although the parents have both remarried, she fantasizes their reconciliation.

Customary Coping Patterns. The purpose of defining the client's coping skills is to learn which are ineffective and which are of benefit. After this determination the nurse can, in the next step of the nursing process, plan to explore new coping skills to replace those that are not effective and encourage and strengthen those that are. Identifying coping strategies may require prolonged observation of the client, as well as direct questioning: "What do you usually do when something upsets you?" "Tell me how you handle yourself when you're stressed?" "What are your strengths?" "Are you able to identify the feelings you experience?"

Support System. A support system contributes to successful adaptation to stress. Support systems can be composed of people, agencies, and/or religious beliefs. In determining the client's support system the nurse needs to learn to whom, or where, the client goes for help when unable to cope. This is important since many psychiatric clients are limited or lacking in adequate support systems. One might ask the client "Where do you turn when you need help?" Information about family, friends, and social activities is useful in this assessment.

Interest and Leisure Activities. The purpose of this line of questioning is to find out how the person spends his free time. Is the time spent productively? Does he withdraw? What are his hobbies? What motivates the client to seek out these activities? How much free time is spent doing these things? How often? When?

Cultural and Ethnic Background and Beliefs. The purpose of examining cultural and ethnic factors is to help define the client's background and values. The nurse attempts to collect data about religion and ancestry, so she can understand how this influences the client's life. (Chapter 3 goes into greater detail.)

Cerebral Function/Mental Status

Mental status assessment is concerned with general cerebral functions. Psychiatrists use the mental status examination to reach a tentative diagnosis. Nurses need to understand the components of this examination in order to understand the psychiatrist's findings, to identify client problem areas, and to plan appropriate nursing interventions. Some components such as general appearance and affect are routinely completed by nurses. An experienced and skilled nurse can conduct the entire examination. Clinical specialists in outpatient settings may have this responsibility.

Level of Consciousness. Determination of level of consciousness is the first observation to make when examining mental status, because consciousness is a basic brain function. Disorders such as tumors, abscesses, hematomas, and hydrocephalus give rise to increased intracranial pressure. Associated alterations in brain function; imbalances in fluids, electrolytes, and acid-base; and toxicity due to liver or kidney failure, or to alcohol, depressant drugs, or other drugs are other causes of increased intracranial pressure.

Level of consciousness is described in the following terms:

Alert: Oriented to person, place and time, awake, and responsive

Lethargic: Reduced wakefulness, may have periods of excitability and irritability which alternate with periods of drowsiness

Stuporous: Unresponsive to stimuli unless stimuli are very strong and are repeated

Comatose: Completely unresponsive to stimuli

A brief description of the client's behavior should be recorded. Identify the intensity of stimulation needed to arouse him. For example: Was the person's name called in a normal conversational tone or in a loud voice; was he roused by using a light touch on the arm, vigorously shaking the arm, or applying painful stimulation? Describe the client's response, including the degree and quality of movement, content and coherence of speech, and the presence of eye opening and eye contact. Finally, describe what the client does when the stimulus is removed.

General Appearance. General appearance is a good indicator of the client's overall mental status. What is his weight, height, and general body build? Is the client's physical appearance appropriate to his chronological age? Are there any physical injuries or defects? What is the general state of cleanliness (condition of skin, hair, nails, and teeth)? What is the manner of dress (style, condition, and cleanliness of clothing)? Does the client use cosmetics? If so, are they appropriate in application and appearance? Is there eye contact with the examiner? Describe the client's posture and position. Is there any muscle weakness or paralysis?

A careless, disheveled appearance may indicate self-neglect or a preoccupation with other activities. A pale, emaciated, sad appearance and messy dress may indicate depression.

Speech. Speech, in reference to mental status, pertains to the client's speech pattern. Is speech production appropriate? Are there any speech disorders? Is a pattern discernible in the topics chosen by the client?

Productivity in relation to speech refers to the quantity of words spoken; overproductive speech is characterized by an excessive number of words; underproductive, by minimal word content. The client's reaction time to the nurse's questions is noted as fast or slow. Speech disorders such as stuttering are noted. The client's replies are examined for relevance, coherence, and logic, as is his ability to organize his conversation.

The following are some characteristics of speech:

Blocking: Cessation of speech as the client loses his train of thought. The cause is usually at an unconscious level. Example: "Well, then, this person (pause) oh, what was it I was going to say?"

Mutism: Absence of speech. The mute person is physically capable of speaking but does not. Mutism is associated with a catatonic form of schizophrenia and may be seen in severe depression.

Echolalia: Verbal repetition by the client of words he hears. Example: The nurse states, "My name is Mary." The client exhibiting echolalia responds, "Mary."

Verbigeration: Repetition of the same words, sentence, or phrase several times. Example: No matter what is asked, the client responds, "This is the time. This is the time. This is the time." This is manifested primarily in the catatonic schizophrenic state.

Perseveration: Not to be confused with verbigeration, perseveration is the involuntary repetition of the answer to a previous question when answering a new question. Example: The name Mary is given regardless of what name is requested. Perseveration also describes an endlessly repeated activity. Example: A boy takes one step in and one step out of every doorway he enters, and continues to do this until he is taken by the hand out of the doorway. Perseveration is associated most frequently with brain damage but can appear in schizophrenia. Some psychologists use the term to describe an inability to shift from one task to another.

Pressured speech: An increased quantity of speech in a given time as compared to normal conversation. The speech tends to be loud, rushed, and emphatic.

Neologism: Words invented by the client, and having a special meaning to him. Example: A knot of rags carried constantly by an elderly schizophrenic woman who calls it a petaby. She asks others about their petaby, and refers to any love object as a petaby.

Looseness of association: A frequent speech characteristic in which the point of the client's conversation shifts abruptly without any apparent connection. Example: "My dog's name is Fido. We've had men fly to the moon. The police are always driving white cars."

Flight of ideas. A continuous often rapid flow of speech which jumps from topic to topic but in which there is some relationship among topics. Example: "I was so hungry, so we went to eat but the store was out of hamburger. Then this dog had an empty bowl, too. Farmers just don't work for nothing. Their gardens ain't empty I bet. If Russia would only take care of their own people and not take my food."

Circumstantiality. A disorder of association in which excessive associated ideas come to consciousness because selective suppression is reduced. The client describes every detail about the topic that is being discussed. Example: In response to a question asking what occurred this day, "Well I first rolled over onto my left side and I noticed the birds were singing but then I thought well, it might be a nice day. Then I opened one eye and could see the sun was shining. Before I rolled onto my back, I opened the other eye. Before I got out of bed I said to my husband, I said "The birds are singing." Then he said, "Oh."

Affect and Mood. Affect is the visible manifestation of feelings, while mood is the feeling tone experienced internally. Questions such as, "What feelings are you experiencing?" and "Tell me what it is you are feeling" may be asked.

Affect can change from minute to minute—from a pout to a roaring laugh if external stimuli warrant such a change. This may be called the range of emotion. Rapid and dramatic fluctuation in the range of emotion is called lability of affect. Absence of change in emotion is called flat affect. Although technically, flat can refer to any sustained affect that does not vary, it is ordinarily used to describe a dull, bleak, unresponsive, cold, remote, or uninvolved affect. Flat affect is noted in schizophrenia and in Parkinson's disease.

Appropriate affect is characterized by spontaneous nonverbal responses that match the content and feelings expressed in the verbal message. Inappropriate affect, frequently noted in psychiatric clients, is characterized by inconsistency between verbal expression of a feeling and what typically would be nonverbally expressed. Examples: A person who laughs at the funeral of a loved one; one who smiles when discussing an anger-provoking situation. Inappropriate affect is most apparent in schizophrenic disorders but can be seen in other conditions as well.

Though mood, too, may change throughout the day, most of the time there is a prevailing mood—the basic feeling that the client generally experiences. Example: The client whose prevailing mood is depression may smile occasionally in an appropriate manner, then revert to his prevailing mood of depression.

Intellectual Performance. Several simple tests can be conducted to afford a picture of the client's intellectual abilities. These tests comprise the sensorium and mental capacity portion of the mental status examination. It is a screening test to detect organic brain syndrome. Should organic brain syndrome be suspected, more thorough physical, neurological, and psychological testing would be warranted. The components of testing intellectual performance are discussed below.

Orientation: Ask questions that determine whether the client is aware of the time, the year, where he is, and who he is.

Attention span: The ability to remain at a task for an appropriate length of time differs according to age and developmental level. Direct observation of the client's attention during the interview is one indicator of attention span.

Immediate and delayed recall: By immediate recall is meant the ability to remember something that has just been said; by delayed recall, the ability to remember something after a reasonable amount of time has elapsed. The interviewer tests immediate recall by saying, "I want you to remember three words and I will ask you to repeat these to me later. The three words I want you to remember are cup, sock, and pillow. What are the three words I want you to remember?" The interview tests delayed recall by asking the client to repeat these words again, in 5 to 10 minutes. "What were the three words I asked you to remember earlier?"

Recent memory: Recent memory is tested by inquiring about something the client has experienced in the hours or days before the assessment data were collected. The examiner asks only questions whose correct responses he knows he can obtain, e.g., by validating them with a family member. A client who is unable to remember may invent plausible answers to mask his memory deficits. This is called confabulation. Questions that may be asked to test recent memory include the following: "What did you have for breakfast today?" "How long have you been in the hospital?" "What time did you get up today?" "I introduced myself earlier. What is my name?"

Remote memory: Remote memory is the ability to remember events of the more distant past. Queries such as: "Where were you born?" "When were your children born?" or "Where did you attend high school?" are typical. Recent memory loss is noticeable in organic disorders, whereas remote memory often remains intact.

Rote memory: By rote memory is meant the ability to recall mechanically without concentrated thinking. The interviewer has the client recall a series of numbers of increasing length. "I want you to repeat these numbers: "7-2-1" (response); "6-0-1-4" (response); "8-3-1-4-5" (response). This is continued until the client becomes unable to restate the numbers in the order given. The number of correctly recalled numbers becomes the database for mental status. Normally, a person is able to remember eight digits in a given order.

Counting and calculation: Arithmetic questions appropriate to the client's age test the client's ability to calculate. He can be asked to subtract 7 from 100, 7 from 93, and so on. Inability to do so may point to the presence of organic brain syndrome.

Reading and writing: Reading ability is tested by giving the person an appropriate book or other reading material and asking him to read a few lines aloud. Writing is tested by asking the client to write certain information. These tests screen for the presence of dyslexia, or may indicate the presence of a central lesion.

Comprehension: Comprehension is the ability to follow directions, involving a three-step process: understanding the material, retaining it, and repeating the content. These steps are called registration, storage, and retrieval. The person is asked to remember an address or a line of poetry. A period of 5 to 10 minutes is allowed to elapse, then the client is asked to repeat the content.

Concept formation: Tests for the ability to engage in abstract thinking can be done by asking the client the meaning of several proverbs. A test question might be, "What is the meaning of the proverb 'People who live in glass houses shouldn't throw stones'?" The reply "Glass breaks" is an example of concrete thinking. This may be indicative of organic brain syndrome or severe anxiety. Schizophrenic individuals may give concrete, elaborate, or bizarre answers. Inability to give any answer offers a clue to intellectual ability or may indicate the presence of brain damage. An answer such as "If you don't want to be criticized then don't criticize others" is an example of abstract thinking.

Tests of similarity also assess concept formation. The interviewer asks the person to describe in what way paired items are similar. The pairs are designed to be of increasing abstraction, for example:

Pen-pencil (writing utensils)

Socks-shoes (worn on the feet)

Hat-pants (clothing)

Cat-elephant (animals)

Eye-ear (senses)

Air-water (required for life)

Poem-statue (works of art)

Egg-seed (embryonic)

Fly-tree (living)

Lesions of the left hemisphere can interfere with ability to recognize similarities.

General knowledge: This refers to the client's ability to recall knowledge likely to have been learned at an age-appropriate level. Test questions such as, "Who is the president?" and "Who was the president before him?" can be asked.

After these tests have been completed the interviewer can estimate the client's level of intelligence. Psychological testing can be requested if further testing is indicated.

Thought Content. Thought content is assessed throughout the interview. Statements made spontaneously and responses to questions are examined closely by the interviewer, who seeks clues to the possible presence of certain patterns of thought, as follows:

1. Suicidal ideation or self-destructive thoughts.
2. Violence.
3. Recurring thoughts or dreams.
4. Obsessions. The client cannot control the repetition of unwanted ideas, emotions, or thoughts.
5. Superstitions.
6. Delusions. False beliefs or misjudgments of reality that are of great magnitude. Delusions of grandeur and delusions of persecution are two prominent forms of delusion.
7. Illusions or distorted perceptions of reality. Example: Itching due to dryness of skin is perceived as due to a bug crawling.
8. Worthlessness.
9. Paranoid ideas (feeling of being persecuted).
10. Ideas of reference—distorted thoughts about an event relating directly to the client. Example: Belief that the television announcer is talking directly and personally to the client, through the television.
11. Ideas of influence—distorted thoughts about an event that occurred because of the client's influence. Example: Belief that an earthquake occurred because the client did not attend church that day.

Behavior. Any observable actions that have not been described elsewhere are recorded in this section. Examples of observed action are eye contact, wringing of hands, pulling hair, or a tic.

Judgment. This refers to appropriate problem solving. Is the client able to decide on the correct approach to a problem? Is the client able to control his impulses? Is the chosen approach feasible? A question that allows the interviewer to assess the client's judgment might be this: "What would you do if you were lost in a strange city?" Sound judgment would be indicated by answers such as "Ask a policeman," or "Look for a street sign." Unsound judgment would be indicated by the response "Leave town."

Insight. By insight is meant awareness of personality characteristics or behavior patterns. In reference to the client, insight is his ability to see himself realistically and have an awareness of his illness including the surrounding circumstances. Assessment of insight can be derived from direct questioning: "What do you think has caused your depression?" "Have you noticed a change in yourself?" In psychotic states, insight is generally not present.

Perception. Perception refers to either mental or sensory perception. (Sensory perception is discussed later in this chapter.) Mental perception is the realistic interpretation of reality. Perception of an external stimulus when that stimulus is absent is called a hallucination. This is differentiated from illusion by the fact that in illusion, an external stimulus is present but it has been misinterpreted.

The nurse may see clients who have a disintegration of perception. Disintegration of perception may involve one or more of the senses—auditory, visual, tactile, olfactory, or gustatory. These misperceptions may be mild and transitory, or may be constant, giving rise to strange or even bizarre behavior. Visual and auditory hallucinations are the most common in psychiatric disorders, and auditory hallucinations are prevalent. Tactile, olfactory, and gustatory hallucinations are most often related to organic disorders. An example of disintegration of sensory perception is the situation of a client who is withdrawing from alcohol or barbiturate addiction and has vivid hallucinations.

Cranial Nerves. As discussed in the previous section on perceptions, there may be a disturbance of one of the cranial nerves, causing a sensory defect. Both physician and nurse need to make a specific assessment to determine whether the nerve is intact and functioning properly. Hysterical conversion reaction may involve one or more of the auditory, visual, tactile, or other sensory processes. Example: The client complains that he has become suddenly totally blind or that his peripheral vision has narrowed. The neurological assessment, however, indicates that the pupils react appropriately to light and no organic disturbance is present.

Sensory Perception. The sensory system carries impulses from the various areas of the body to the central nervous system, which registers and interprets them. Perceived sensations include simple touch, pain, temperature, stereognosis, two-point discrimination, and the extinction phenomenon.

Abnormal sensations that the client may perceive include: anesthesia, complete loss of the ability to perceive stimuli; hypesthesia, reduced sensory perception; hyperesthesia, increased sensory perception; paresthesia, abnormal sensation such as tingling; and dysesthesia, an abnormal sensation recognized by the client as noxious or painful.

Any of those sensations may be felt in somatoform disorders (conversion reactions). Normally, those sensations follow the distribution of a nerve. In a somatoform disorder, however, this is not the case. Example: In hysterical anesthesia, the loss of sensation may involve one extremity along a defined line, above which sensation is normal. The involved area and the degree of disturbed sensation may vary from examination to examination.

A client who is experiencing a disturbance in sensory and/or motor function is likely to experience mental changes as well. The person's concept of his body may be greatly diminished. He may lose interest in personal grooming due to a grief reaction. He may be very demanding, yet withdrawn, at the same time.

Cerebellar Function. The cerebellum controls equilibrium and muscle movement, so that normally movements are smooth, steady, and coordinated. Cerebellar dysfunction can result from several causes, including cerebellar degeneration, cerebellar tumor, and Parkinson's disease. Abnormal findings may include intention tremor, cerebellar ataxia, cerebellar nystagmus, adiadochokinesia, and cerebellar speech. An intention tremor is a rhythmic, involuntary movement of voluntary muscles which increase with voluntary activity. In cerebellar ataxia, the client must keep his legs widely apart in order to stand, and has an unsteady gait. In cerebellar nystagmus there are abnormal rhythmic movements of the eye, which may be in any plane or may be spontaneous. Adiadochokinesia is the inability to perform rapid alternating movements. Cerebellar speech or scanning speech is a disorder in which the voice is a monotone, with explosive irregularity in volume.

An abnormality in cerebellar function creates difficulties in carrying on normal activity. The client may become dependent upon others or upon mechanical devices when preparing a meal, bathing, or walking. There may be feelings of loneliness, sadness, and uselessness. If the client is a child, even play may not be a part of the normal daily routine, because he is not able to perform simple manuevers.

Motor System. Neurons carry impulses from the cerebrum to the skeletal muscles. Two motor tracts, the pyramidal and the extrapyramidal, are involved in impulse transmission. Impulses traveling along the pyramidal tract stimulate individual muscles. Those traveling along the extrapyramidal tract stimulate groups of muscles. The portion of the tracts from the cerebrum up to but not including the anterior horn motor neurons are called the upper motor neuron tracts; those including the anterior horn motor neuron to the skeletal muscles are considered the lower motor neuron tracts.

In an examination of the client's motor system, the muscle size, tone, and strength are observed. Injury to the motor system will cause specific signs and symptoms, manifested correspondingly to dysfunction in an upper motor neuron tract or in a lower motor neuron tract. Symptoms of an upper motor neuron tract disturbance are: (1) hyperreflexia below the area of disturbance; (2) pathological reflexes; (3) hypertonicity of large groups of muscles; (4) no fasciculations; (5) mild muscular atrophy; and (6) slightly below strength. Symptoms of a lower motor neuron tract disturbance are: (1) absence of reflexes below the area of disturbance; (2) no pathological reflexes; (3) hypotonicity confined to a specific group of muscles; (4) fasciculations; (5) severe muscular atrophy; and (6) absence of strength. The gait may be abnormal in an organic disturbance.

As with sensory symptoms that may be associated with a somatoform disorder, the motor disturbances may also be varied. In all of them,

TABLE 10-3 Comparison of Conversion Reaction vs. Organic Paralysis

Conversion Reaction Paralysis	Organic Paralysis
No appreciable muscle wasting	Appreciable muscle wasting
Proximal muscle paralysis is greater than paralysis of peripheral muscles	Peripheral muscle paralysis is greater than paralysis of proximal muscles
Forearm is extended	Forearm is moderately flexed
Deep tendon reflexes are present, in flaccid forms	Deep tendon reflexes are absent, in flaccid forms

function is disturbed though there is no demonstrable physiological change. Examples of motor disturbances associated with somatoform disorders include tic, tremor, and various paralyses (see Table 10-3). In the catatonic stupor of schizophrenia, the client may remain in one position for an extended length of time such as a day or even longer. Occasionally the symptoms are similar to those of parkinsonian akinesia and rigidity; the schizophrenic, however, may not react to painful stimuli.

Psychiatric clients may experience organically based seizures or psychogenic (emotionally caused) seizures, or may feign seizures to gain attention or perhaps a prescription for medication. Table 10-4 compares some differences between organic seizures and those that may be either psychogenic or feigned.

TABLE 10-4 Comparison of Physical Responses in Psychogenic vs Grand Mal Seizure

Psychogenic seizures	Grand mal seizures
Pupils normal	Pupils fixed and dilated
Respirations may be more rapid than normal	Respirations temporarily interrupted, then correspond with muscular contractions. May be stertorous
Muscular contractions irregular, random	Muscular contractions very forceful, rhythmic
May respond to painful stimulus	No response to painful stimulus
Usually not incontinent of urine	May be incontinent of urine and/or feces

Reflexes. A reflex is an involuntary response to a stimulus involving both a sensory and a motor component. Three types of reflexes may be tested: deep tendon, superficial, and pathological. Grading the strength of each reflex is done on a scale of 0 to 4+; 0 is no response, 2+ is normal, and 4+ is hyperactive with sustained clonus. In the client experiencing a conversion reaction, the reflexes are usually normal as compared with those of the client experiencing true paralysis whose reflexes are diminished or absent.

PSYCHOLOGICAL TESTING

A component of a thorough mental health assessment is psychological testing. The clinical psychologist administers the tests and reports the interpretation of the findings. The nurse's responsibility is to be informed of the test results and to incorporate the relevant information into nursing process.

One group of tests measures a person's intelligence. Frequently used intelligence tests include the Stanford-Binet test, the Wechsler Adult Intelligence Scale Revised, and the Wechsler Intelligence Scale for Children Revised. These tests are individually administered oral tests consisting of two parts; one part is a verbal test, the other, a performance test.

Another group of tests includes personality and projective tests. These are so designed that the response is necessarily determined by the client's psychopathology, mood, or personality. The client projects his inner self through the indirect approach of these tests. Some of the more frequently used personality and projective tests include: the Rorschach test, the Minnesota Multiphasic Personality Inventory (MMPI), the Sentence Completion test, the Draw-A-Person test, and the Thematic Apperception Test.

The Rorschach test involves a series of ten inkblots of varying abstract designs and colors. The client is asked to describe his thoughts or impressions about each inkblot. The clinical psychologist analyzes by a systematic approach the content of the responses to aid in evaluating the client's personality.

The Minnesota Multiphasic Personality Inventory (MMPI) is a questionnaire in which 550 statements are answered from the client's perspective as true or false. A statement is similar to the following: "I often feel as if my stomach is turning to brass. T or F." The answers are scored on several different scales. The psychologist then reports his professional opinion of the type of personality suggested by the client response pattern and the possible diagnoses.

The Sentence Completion test is a series of partial sentences that the client completes. The responses are analyzed by the psychologist. Example: "When I get mad I . . . ."

The Draw-A-Person test is an analysis of a picture of a human being that the client has been asked to draw. The interpretation is systematic and is correlated with diagnoses.

The Thematic Apperception Test (TAT) is a projective test. The client is shown a number of pictures that illustrate ambiguous situations and is asked to describe what is happening to the people in each picture. The responses are systematically evaluated by the examining psychologist. This test is particularly helpful in exploring interpersonal relationships and conflicts.

The battery of tests described above provides further information relevant to diagnosis of the client's problem and his personal characteristics. The information is useful in the planning of care appropriate to the client's behavior and his problems.

■ *Enrichment Activities*

DISCUSSION QUESTIONS

1. Discuss the importance of a physical and neurological assessment in a psychiatric setting.

2. Clients with various physiological disorders, such as Huntington's chorea or mental retardation, are often admitted to psychiatric settings. What aspects of the nursing assessment might need to be given special attention?

3. Obtain an assessment guide from a psychiatric facility. What is the importance of each item or area of questioning?

LEARNING ACTIVITY

Development of good assessment techniques requires practice and critical review of each interaction. Role play a nursing assessment with a peer. If possible, videotape the experience. Evaluate and examine the experience as to technique and content.

■ Recommended Readings

Bates, B. *A guide to physical examination.* 3d ed. Philadelphia: J.B. Lippincott, 1983. Describes the step-by-step procedure for examining a client. The neurological component is discussed thoroughly.

Dodd, J. Assessing mental status. *American Journal of Nursing*, 78, 1978:1501–1503. Describes the procedure for assessing mental status, emphasizing those components that are of interest to the nurse.

Marriner, A. *The nursing process.* 3d ed. St. Louis: Mosby Company, 1983. Describes in detail the problem-solving technique of nursing process.

Voght, G., Eslner, M., and Miller, M. *Mosby's manual of neurological care.* St. Louis: Mosby Company, 1985. A thorough manual which describes nursing care for the client with neurological problems.

■ References

Allen, R.M. *Student's Rorschach manual*, rev. ed. New York: International Universities Press, 1978.

Andreason, N.C. Thought, language, and communication disorders: I. Clinical assessment, definition of terms, and evaluation of their reliability. *Archives of general psychiatry*, 36, 1979:1315–1321.

Anthony, C.P., and Thibodeau, G.A. *Textbook of anatomy and physiology*, 11th ed. St. Louis: Mosby Company, 1983.

Bates, B. *A guide to physical examination*, 3d ed. Philadelphia: Lippincott, 1983.

Block, G.J., Nolan, J.W., and Dempsey, M.K. *Health assessment for professional nursing: A developmental approach.* New York: Appleton-Century-Crofts, 1981.

Campbell, R.J. *Psychiatric dictionary*, 5th ed. New York: Oxford University Press, 1981.

Cannel, C. Interviewing. In *The handbook of social psychology*, 2d ed., vol. 2. (Lindzey, G., and Aronson, E. eds.) Reading, MA: Addison-Wesley Publishing Company, 1968:526–596.

Carotenuto, R., and Bullock, J. *Physical assessment of the gerontologic client.* Philadelphia: F.A. Davis Co., 1981.

Conway, Barbara L. *Carini and Owen's neurological and neurosurgical nursing*, 8th ed. St. Louis: Mosby Company, 1982.

Cox, A., Hopkinson, K., and Rutter, M. Psychiatric interviewing techniques. II. Naturalistic study: eliciting factual information. *British journal of psychiatry*, 138, 1981:283–291.

Cox, A., Rutter, M., and Holbook, D. Psychiatric techniques. V. Experimental study: eliciting factual information. *British journal of psychiatry*, 138, 1981:29–37.

DeJong, R.N. *Essentials of the neurological examination*, 4th ed. Philadelphia: Smith-Kline Corp., 1979.

Dodd, J. Assessing mental status. *American journal of nursing*, 78, 1978:1501–03.

Doona, M.E. *Travelbee's intervention in psychiatric nursing*, 2d ed. Philadelphia: F.A. Davis Co., 1981.

Eaton, M.T., Peterson, M.H., and Davis, J.A. *Psychiatry*, 4th ed. Garden City, NY: Medical Examination Pub., 1981.

Gahan, K.A. Using problem-oriented records in psychiatric nursing. In *Current perspectives in psychiatric nursing: Issues and trends*, vol. 1 (Kneissl, C.R., and Wilson, H.S., eds.). St. Louis: Mosby Company, 1976:117–134.

Garrison, V., and Podell, J. Community support. Systems assessment for use in clinical interviews. *Schizophrenia bulletin* 7, 1981:101–108.

Gordon, M. *Manual of nursing diagnoses.* St. Louis: McGraw-Hill, 1985.

Granacher, R.P. The neurological examination in geriatric psychiatry. *Psychosomatics*, 22, 6, 1981:485–499.

Helzer, J.E. Standardized interviews in psychiatry. *Psychiatric development*, 1, 1983:161–178.

Henderson, S., Duncan-Jones, P., Byrne, D.G., and Scott, R. Measuring social relationships. The interview schedule for social interaction. *Psychological medicine*, 10, 1980:723–734.

Hill, M., and Humphrey, P. *Human growth and development throughout life.* New York: John Wiley & Sons, 1982.

Hillman, R.S., Goodell, B.W., Grunde, S.M., McArthur, J.R., and Moller, J.H. *Clinical skills: Interviewing, history taking and diagnosis for nurses.* New York: McGraw-Hill, 1981.

Hopkinson, K., Cox, A., and Rutter, M. Psychiatric interviewing techniques. III. Naturalistic study: eliciting feelings. *British journal of psychiatry*, 138, 1981:406–415.

Hurlock, E. *Developmental psychology.* New York: McGraw-Hill, 1953.

Johnson, J.L. Psychosocial assessment of the handicapped. *The journal of school health*, 50, 1980:252–255.

Kernberg, O.H. Structural interviewing. *The psychiatric clinics of North America*, 4, Edited by M.H. Stone. 1981:169–195.

Kim, M.J., and Moritz, D.A. (eds.). *Classification of nursing diagnosis: Proceedings of the third and fourth national conferences.* New York: McGraw-Hill, 1982.

Kolb, J.E., and Gunderson, J.G. Diagnosing borderline clients with a semistructured interview. *Archives of general psychiatry*, 37, 1980:37–41.

LaMonica, E. *The nursing process: A humanistic ap-*

proach. Menlo Park, CA: Addison-Wesley Publishing Company, 1979.

Larkin, P.D., and Backer, B.A. *Problem-oriented nursing assessment*. New York: McGraw-Hill, 1977.

Lucas, M.J., and Folstein, M.F. Nursing assessment of mental disorders on a general medical unit. *Journal of psychiatric nursing*, 18, 1980:31–33.

Lunney, M. Nursing diagnosis: refining the system. *American journal of nursing*, 82, 1982:456–459.

Malasanos, L., Barkauskas, V., Moss, M., and Stoltenberg-Allen, K. *Health assessment*. St. Louis: Mosby Company, 1981.

Margolin, C.B. Assessment of psychiatric clients, *Journal of emergency nursing*, 4, 1980:30–33.

Marks, P.A., Seeman, W., and Haller, D.L. *The actuarial use of the MMPI with adolescents and adults*. Baltimore: The Williams and Wilkins Co., 1974.

Marriner, A. *The nursing process*. 3d ed. St. Louis: Mosby Company, 1983.

Michaels, R.M., and Sevitt, M. The patient and the first psychiatric interview. *British journal of psychiatry*, 132, 1978:288–292.

Millon, T. *Abnormal behavior and personality, a biosocial learning approach*. Philadelphia: W.B. Saunders Co., 1984.

Navin, H.L., and Wilson, J.A. Caffeine consumption and sleep disturbance in acutely ill psychiatric inpatient. *Journal of psychiatric nursing*, 18, 1980:37–42.

Pasamanick, B., Dinitz, S., and Lefton, M. Psychiatric orientation and its relation to diagnosis and treatments in a mental hospital. *American journal of psychiatry*, 116, 1959:172–182.

Rarick, L. Motor development: Its growing knowledge base. *Journal of physical education and recreation*, 51, 1980:26–27, 56–61.

Rudy, E.B., and Gray, R. *Handbook of health assessment*, Bowie, MD: Robert J. Brady Co., 1981.

Rutter, M., and Cox, A. Psychiatric interviewing techniques: I. Methods and measures. *British journal of psychiatry*, 138, 1981:273–282.

Ryback, R., Fowler, D.R., and Longabaugh, J.R. *The problem-oriented record in psychiatry and mental health care*. 2d ed. New York: Grune & Stratton, 1981.

Saghir, M. A comparison of some aspects of structured and unstructured psychiatric interviews. *American journal of psychiatry*, 128, 1971:180–184.

Schell, P.L., and Campbell, A.T. POMR—not just another way to chart. *Nursing outlook*, 20, 1971:510–514.

Sharla, P., and Kapur, R.L. The burden on the family of a psychiatric client: Development of an interview schedule. *British journal of psychiatry*, 138, 1981:332–335.

Simons, DeLane. *Classification scheme for client problems in community health nursing*. U.S. Department of Health and Human Services, Publication No. HRA 80-16, 1980.

Smitherman, C. *Nursing actions for health promotion*. Philadelphia: F.A. Davis Co., 1981.

Spitzer, R.L., Fleiss, J.L., Burdock, E.I., and Hardesty, A.S. The mental status schedule: rational, reliability, and validity. *Comprehensive psychiatry*, 5, 1964:384–395.

Stanley, B. Evaluation of treatment goals; the use of goal attainment scaling. *Journal of advanced nursing*, 9, 1984:351–356.

Sundeen, S.J., Stuart, G.W., Rankin, E.D., and Cohen, S.D. *Nurse-patient interaction*, 2d ed. St. Louis: Mosby Company, 1981.

Taylor, J.W., and Ballenger, S. *Neurological dysfunctions and nursing intervention*. New York: McGraw-Hill, 1980.

Tsuang, M.T., Woolson, R.F., and Simpson, J.C. The Iowa structured psychiatric interview. Rationale, reliability, and validity. *Acta psychiatrica Scandinavia supplementum*, 283, 1980:62.

Wells, C.E., and Duncan, G.W. *Neurology for psychiatrists*, Philadelphia: F.A. Davis Co., 1980.

Whall, A.L. Nursing theory and the assessment of families. *Journal of psychiatric nursing*, 19, 1981:30–36.

Wolber, G. A practical approach to the psychological evaluation of elderly clients. *Perceptual and motor skills*, 51, 1980:499–505.

Yura, H., and Walsh, M. *Human needs three & the nursing process*. New York: Appleton-Century-Crofts, 1983.

Yurick, A.G., Robb, S.S., Spier, B.E., and Ebert, N.J. *The aged person and the nursing process*, 2d ed. New York: Appleton-Century-Crofts, 1984.

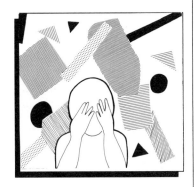

11

Preventing and Coping with Aggressive and Assaultive Behaviors

Carole P. Bonds

Learning Objectives

Upon completion of this chapter, the reader will be able to:

1. List symptoms that indicate increased potential for violence.

2. Develop increased self-awareness about working with aggressive or assaultive clients.

3. Consider and plan three levels of intervention for clients displaying increased potential for violence.

4. List categories of individuals felt to have increased potential for violence.

5. Plan quality nursing care for clients displaying various levels of increased potential for violence, or actual violence.

6. Differentiate between the need for seclusion and for restraints.

7. Define and discuss the concept of least restrictive alternative.

The relative paucity of textbook discussions of aggressive and assaultive behaviors of clients suggests that nurses as health professionals might prefer to think they will not have to deal with such behaviors. How much better, however, to be aware that the potential for violence does exist in psychiatric settings and to describe techniques that can reduce the potential and minimize the consequences of violent, aggressive behavior.

Perhaps the memory of measures used in the past to control violent behaviors makes nurses more hesitant to address this need in the contemporary setting. In the nineteenth century it was not unusual for clients to be manacled to walls for a period of months, or even years. There was very little, if any, distinction between measures used with criminals and those used with the mentally ill. In some cases, moreover, the criminals were treated more humanely.

Certainly great progress has been made in the care of the mentally ill. With the advent of psychotropic medications (in certain instances referred to as chemical restraints) the reliance on indiscriminate use of mechanical restraints was considerably reduced. Even before such medications became available, however, progress had been made in developing more humane treatment methods. Pioneers like Dorothea Dix were at the forefront in this fight for improved care.

Yet, despite the progress that has been made, there are times when the psychiatric nurse will be confronted with a client who is behaving in an aggressive or assaultive manner. This chapter looks at measures to prevent aggression and assault or to cope with these behaviors when they do occur.

☐ *Theoretical Perspectives*

There are a number of theories about the cause of aggression. Some of these perspectives regard aggression as an innate characteristic in every individual, or an instinctual drive. Others view aggression as a learned response to stressors or a result of person-environment interactions. Still other perspectives attempt to integrate the innate and the learned aspects. The following section reviews some of these various perspectives.

PSYCHOANALYTIC THEORY

Freud (1932) felt that aggression was instinctual. Initially, he viewed aggression as an aspect of the sexual instinct but in later years came to view it as separate. He theorized that this instinct, which he called thanatos or the death drive, struggled against eros, the life-drive. Eros is expressed through one's sexuality. Adler (1964) also viewed aggression as instinctual but theorized that it was an attempt to master inferiority.

DRIVE THEORY

Dollard and his associates (1939) viewed aggression as arising from frustration over failure to achieve a desired goal. Anxiety and anger result from this frustration which then leads to aggression. While they believed that this type of response was innate, they also thought that it could be inhibited.

SOCIAL LEARNING THEORY

Bandura (1973) felt that aggressive behavior was learned through social interactions. That is, the individual can learn aggressive behaviors from having observed aggressiveness in others, or from self-trial ("trying out") of such behavior. According to that theory, such behavior is rewarded or reinforced in some way from the social environment, and is also instigated by interaction with the social environment. Thus, when the aggressive behavior is rewarded or reinforced, it is likely to be continued.

INTEGRATED MODEL

Boettcher (1983) proposed an integrated theoretical model for nursing whose purpose was to prevent violent behavior. Need theory was the foundation for Boettcher's model, and it was based on the premise that any individual has an innate potential for violence. She stated, "Violence is a powerful way to communicate and is one of the most immediate, direct, albeit destructive, ways of communicating an intense human need. Identifying that need and addressing that need is paramount if violent behavior is to be prevented."

SELYE'S STRESS-ADAPTATION THEORY

Selye (1956) felt that any emotion or activity requiring a response produces some degree of stress. The theory he developed is known as the stress-adaptation theory. The stressor may be either positive or negative and may be physiological, psychological, or environmental in nature. The same stressor may be perceived in various ways by different people. For example, a father may view his child's marriage as affording relief from a financial burden, while the mother may perceive the same event as portending loss of a significant role for her.

Selye described three stages, together making up what he called the general adaptation syndrome (GAS). The first stage is the alarm reaction; in this stage the individual is alerted to the stress and may feel anxiety, but problem-solving behavior is present. In the second stage, resistance, there is increased anxiety, with defensive measures being employed instead of problem solving. The third stage, exhaustion, shows increased disorganization of thought which may progress to loss of contact with reality. Death may occur if the stress level reaches the exhaustion stage and there is no relief. These stages may be correlated with various levels of anxiety, from mild to severe. It is in the later two stages that the potential for violence may be increased.

☐ *Anxiety*

Anxiety is an unexplainable feeling of discomfort or apprehension related to experiencing a threat to the self or to significant relationships. The threat is usually vague or nonspecific. It may take the form of a threat to self-esteem or to one's well-being. How the individual perceives the threat is highly significant. A threat may elicit only mild anxiety in one person; the same threat may elicit severe anxiety in another person.

Four levels of anxiety have been identified: mild (+), moderate (++), severe (+++), and panic (++++). Many of the symptoms of anxiety are present at all four levels but differ in intensity or degree, increasing at higher levels. Table 11-1 lists common symptoms of anxiety.

An important point about these anxiety levels is the individual's sensory perceptions and abilities to focus attention and learn. Hildegard Peplau (1952) has addressed these differences. She described anxiety as "an aspect of the first step in solving problems, namely, the 'felt need' leading to a concentration of resources." As anxiety increases a further narrowing of perceptions occurs which allows a smaller area of focus, the problem area. However, as anxiety increases to severe or panic levels the perceptions are narrowed to a crippling degree. "The patient sees less and takes less and less into account in considering what is

happening. His ability to observe what is happening and to make use of past experience in evaluating present events gives way to overfocalization on the discomfort itself." At higher levels of anxiety little if any learning is possible.

The level of anxiety must be assessed, because both the approach and the interventions differ for each level. The nurse needs to identify the presence of anxiety at the earliest possible level to increase the likelihood that problem solving and learning can occur.

The general approach at lower levels is to assist the client in recognizing his anxiety and in associating the feelings that precipitated the anxiety. Identifying the nature of the problem may of itself serve to reduce the anxiety. Once the problem has been identified, basic problem-solving skills can be utilized. The nurse facilitates the client's review of past successes in managing similar situations. She may also assist him in exploring new options for dealing with the problem, or finding alternative solutions. When an alternative is selected and acted on by the client, the nurse will assist him in evaluating the effectiveness of this approach.

At the higher levels of anxiety the main focus of treatment is simply to reduce the anxiety to a lower level. It is important for the nurse to stay with the client and communicate a sense of calmness and a sense of her own capability to manage the situation. She should communicate in short, concise statements since the client's ability to concentrate is impaired. Nonverbal techniques, such as walking with the client or taking long deep breaths with him, are also beneficial, as is removing the client to a quieter environment away from other stimuli. Medications such as antianx-

---

TABLE 11-1 Symptoms of Anxiety

Verbal expressions of	Increased muscle tension
Nervousness	Hand tremors
Tension	Irritability
Helplessness	Increased heart rate
Unfocused	Diaphoresis
apprehension	Dilated pupils
Hypervigilance	Pallor
Jumpiness	Cold, clammy hands
Increased startle response	Urinary frequency
Rapid speech	Dry mouth
Voice tremors	Nausea
Change in voice pitch	
Motor restlessness	

iety agents or sedatives may be indicated if relief is not obtained with other measures.

Acting-out behavior and overt expressions of anger and hostility are discussed later in this chapter. Other maladaptive responses are described elsewhere in this book.

☐ *Increased Potential for Violence*

The model in Figure 11-1 conceptualizes the potential for violence and the use of various levels of intervention. Though it may be said that any individual has a potential for violence, those with certain characteristics (as shown in the figure), are believed to have greater potential. Such clients are categorized as persons having (1) impaired thought processes, (2) ineffective coping, (3) organic impairment, (4) depression, and (5) antisocial behavior.

CATEGORIES OF INCREASED POTENTIAL

Impaired thought processes may contribute to an increase in the potential for violence. Of partic-

ular importance is to note those who are experiencing auditory hallucinations of a command nature, e.g., hearing a voice telling them to harm themselves or someone else. Hallucinations that are especially frightening to the person may also influence him to strike out in an effort to escape or protect himself from the perceived threat. Delusional thought content, especially of a paranoid nature, may also increase the likelihood of aggressive or assaultive behavior occurring. For example, if a person feels that a particular staff member is trying to poison him or otherwise harm him, the staff member may be at increased risk of being harmed.

The second category of individuals who have increased potential for violence are those with ineffective individual coping—those experiencing severe anxiety, fear, or anger. While everyone experiences these feelings at times, those who are unable to deal effectively with these feelings have greater difficulty handling their aggression. This category also includes individuals with maladaptive interactional patterns, such as those who are extremely passive or those who have learned aggressive responses from other family members. Individuals who generally display extremely passive behavior have the potential for explosive outbursts. Persons whose family members frequently

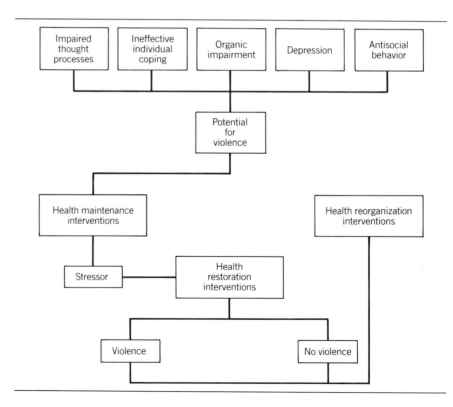

Figure 11-1. *Model: potential for violence.*

...ly to behave aggres-
...in the family gen-
...gressive re-

...ve in-
...ose ex-
...tion due
...l lobe epi-
leps...   ...ated blood
urea nit...   ...organic impairment.

Depressives ...   ...th category. In
this group, the agg...   ...ypically turned
against the self, rather t...   ...hers (see Chapter
33).

In a fifth category are those who exhibit antisocial behavior. They have very little regard for the welfare or the rights of others. Because their impulse control is also poor, these individuals are likely to be more unpredictable in their behavior.

■ Point of Emphasis

The identification of a client as belonging to a category of increased potential for violence is useful as a warning that additional data are needed in your assessment. A care plan for a high-risk individual needs increased attention to preventive measures and to continual monitoring for signs or symptoms that indicate escalating potential for violence.

Figure 11-1 illustrates the need for providing three levels of intervention that will influence whether violence occurs and the health status of the individual following the incident. The following section discusses the components of these several levels of intervention.

□ Levels of Intervention

The three levels of intervention shown in the figure have been formulated by Burgess (1978): (1) health maintenance, (2) health restoration, and (3) health reorganization. Each plays an important role.

Health maintenance interventions are those that protect or maintain health. These are primary prevention measures whose purpose is to promote positive adaptive responses. Health teaching, anticipatory guidance, assistance in ad-

justing to sociocultural situations, promotion of positive interpersonal relationships, and provision of a safe environment are examples of health maintenance interventions. These measures may be promoted regardless of the client's current health status.

The second level of intervention is health restoration or secondary prevention. When experiencing a period of health disorganization, a person has an imbalance between adaptive ability and the level of stressors being experienced. Interventions are directed toward restoring health. The type of stressor may be psychological, interpersonal, or environmental, as well as physiological.

During this phase the nurse first tries to identify the problem or imbalanced state as early as possible, to facilitate an early resolution. Once the problem has been identified, the nurse directs her efforts to promoting the client's use of his own adaptive capacities. At times it may be necessary to temporarily support, or even substitute for, the client's adaptive capacities. For example, it may be necessary to provide a respirator for a client following surgery until he is able to reestablish his own capability to provide his body with oxygen. Or to offer a manic client high calorie nutritional supplements which can be eaten while he is moving about, until he is able to sit quietly to eat a meal. The need to protect the client from further stressors during the period of disorganization is another component of the restoration phase. The nurse wants to take every possible measure to decrease the likelihood that the client will experience additional stressors while still in a disorganized state. Applying sterile techniques when changing a dressing to prevent nosocomial infection is an example of how the nurse might protect the disorganized client. Or, she might remove a client who is hallucinating to a quieter environment in order to decrease incoming stimuli.

The third level of intervention is the health reorganization phase. The nurse wants to assist the client to attain the highest health state possible for him by promoting the achievement of a new balance between adaptive ability and stressors encountered. In this way the client may attain a higher level of health than he had before the period of disorganization. For example, if he became able to learn some new coping skills and to experience success in using them, he would then have an increased repertoire from which to draw in future periods of stress. Of course it can happen that the client will not be able to return to his previous level of functioning. If, for example, a client's leg was amputated, the goal would be to make the best possible adjustment to the loss.

As indicated in Figure 11-1, the phase of health reorganization must occur whether or not there has been violence. The client needs to assimilate the experience so he can make the most positive adjustment possible.

The following sections address Burgess's three levels of intervention as they apply to preventing and coping with aggressive and assaultive behavior. The nurse will be primarily involved in dealing with these behaviors on an inpatient unit, but much of the discussion is applicable to other settings, such as community mental health centers.

PRIMARY PREVENTION

Primary intervention is certainly the most significant with regard to preventing violent behavior. At this level, measures are taken to promote positive adapative responses or to protect or maintain the client's health. If the client is not currently displaying aggressive or assaultive behavior, the nurse focuses on helping him to remain nonviolent while facilitating his use of techniques for positive adaptation to stress.

Maintaining an atmosphere on the unit that promotes a sense of safety, caring, and respect is essential. A client who feels safe, cared for, and respected is much less likely to act in an aggressive or assaultive manner. The total environment is made up of administrative policies and procedures, staffing, physical environment, and the therapeutic milieu, as well as the more tangible elements such as equipment, layout, and facilities.

Administrative Policies and Procedures

The written administrative policies and procedures on a unit generally indicate the standard of care that is expected. If these policies and procedures reflect a holistic view of the client and respect for personal rights, it is likely that they will be supported by staff on the unit.

Included in written policies and procedures should be criteria for use of seclusion and restraints. These criteria should meet standards established by both the Joint Commission on Accreditation of Hospitals (1983) and the state. Reasons about why such treatment is required

and the nursing care standards for clients secluded or restrained are part of the documentation. A monitoring system needs to be established to review incidents leading to seclusion or restraint.

A procedure for admitting clients that facilitates a positive adjustment to the unit and provides staff with needed information for assessment should also be established. The client's first 5 minutes on the unit may set the tone and color of his entire stay. He should be made to feel as comfortable as possible. Simple steps like showing him around the unit and introducing him to some of the other clients can make a big difference in how he views the experience. Recognition of the stress involved, especially in first admissions to a psychiatric unit, certainly increases the nurse's ability to empathize with the client's situation.

A comprehensive history is a part of the admission procedure. Questions that are particularly important to ask in taking the client's history are:

1. What is your usual way of dealing with frustration or anger?
2. Have you ever felt like hurting yourself or someone else?
3. Have you ever been involved in situations where you behaved violently toward other people?
4. Have you experienced violence from others?
5. Have you taken alcohol or drugs in the past 24 hours?
6. If you are hearing voices, what kinds of things are they saying to you?
7. If the client is delusional, what are the general content themes he expresses?

This information will enable the staff to plan care that may decrease the potential for violence, and to be alert to early signs of difficulty. While the following categories fall ultimately under administrative responsibilities, they are discussed individually for convenience.

Staffing

The initial selection of staff for a psychiatric unit may greatly influence the number of aggressive and assaultive incidents that occur. Personnel who have a need to control others or who frequently display verbally aggressive behavior are likely to escalate situations in which the potential for violence already exists. Staff members whose self-esteem is very fragile and easily threatened will also find it difficult to deal therapeutically with clients who are agitated and verbally abusive. In addition, staff members who have a history of violence in their own families may find it difficult to deal therapeutically with patients displaying aggressive or assaultive behavior. With increased self-awareness and training, it is possible for staff members to overcome these difficulties, but it is first necessary to become aware that the problem exists.

Staff training is another key element. During the orientation procedure, training should include various verbal and physical techniques to prevent and/or deal with aggressive and assaultive behavior. Role playing is part of the training. Opportunities also need to be provided for staff to review these procedures periodically. Some specific techniques are discussed in later sections of this chapter.

Staff's ability to develop therapeutic, trusting relationships with clients can be highly influential in decreasing the number of violent incidents. Clients frequently know when they are close to losing control of their behavior and will often communicate this to a trusted staff member. For example, a client may tell a staff person that voices are telling him to hurt his roommate, but he doesn't want to do it; he may even request extra medication and some time-out in seclusion.

The movement toward deinstitutionalization has changed the role and focus of many community hospitals. While in the past many psychiatric hospitals provided long-term care, the trend is toward short-term stays. Thus, therapeutic relationships were formerly generally of long term, and this often is no longer true. This lends importance to the need to consider the cumulative effect of several short-term hospitalizations and relationships—which can be equated with a single long-term relationship. This is an important point to consider. Even though the nurse is aware that a client is hospitalized for only a few days, the relationship begun—good or bad—will be reinforced at the next hospitalization. As mentioned earlier, a positive relationship may decrease the likelihood that a violent incident will occur.

Adequate staffing also plays a part in preventing aggressive or assaultive behavior. Neither clients nor staff feel safe on an inadequately staffed unit. Though there are standard formulas for determining the ratio of staff to clients, the administrative person responsible for staffing must have authority to exercise a degree of flexibility. A system of assigning acuity levels to clients might be an aid in making staffing decisions, as the array of client behaviors is as important as the number of clients. As an example, one may hear a staff member say "Our census is a little low, but you can feel the tension when you walk onto the unit."

Some effort should also be made to have both male and female staff on each shift. There are always likely to be some clients on the unit whose response to a male staff member will be more positive than to a female, and vice versa. If, for example, a client has had a poor relationship with his father and has experienced difficulty in dealing with men in general, he is much more likely, in a crisis situation, to respond positively to a female staff person. There is also the possibility that in an emergency situation, a physically strong person may be better able to prevent injuries to the client or staff, suggesting the wisdom of including male staff.

Physical Environment

The design of the unit has a bearing on physical safety for both clients and staff. One of the first considerations is to provide adequate space for the number of clients so that crowding is not a problem. Persons likely to exhibit violent behavior require "buffer zones," and need to be able to move about—this may be a positive coping measure for them. Access to an outdoor area is desirable, affording an area for large muscle activities and recreational diversions.

To increase safety, the unit design should be such that the unit is visible from the nursing station to the extent possible. This enables staff to note potential problems or emergencies immediately so that early intervention may be instituted.

Properly equipped seclusion rooms should be provided. Ideally, cameras are placed in these rooms to allow continuous observation of the client from nursing station monitors. Lighting should be soft, and wall colors subdued. The seclusion rooom also needs to have adequate ventilation with suitable means for heating and cooling. Care needs to be taken that there is adequate venting to the heating and cooling system.

The seclusion room should be furnished with only a mattress on the floor. Though the room may look quite stark, client safety is improved as there is little on which he could injure himself. However, if the client cannot cooperate and bangs his head or body against the wall, restraints would then be required.

A separate restraint room should be kept properly equipped at all times so that it is always ready for use when needed. There should be a hospital bed with two wrist and two ankle restraints already attached to the frame. There are several types of restraints available: leather restraints are less likely to cause the client to sweat than plastic ones, and they appear to be more durable. The use of straitjackets and full body type restraints is not recommended. These restraints restrict freedom of movement to a degree beyond that required for staff and client safety.

Also to be considered is the installation of only unbreakable or safety glass on the unit. An agitated client may intentionally break glass in order to use it as a weapon, or may accidentally break glass and injure himself or others.

Restrictions obviously should be placed on client possession of firearms or knives on the unit; care should also be taken that there is not easy access to items that could readily be used as weapons (e.g., razors, pool cues, and baseballs). Any such items that are allowed should be used only under staff supervision. The furniture should be very sturdy and not easily picked up. Lack of easy access to a weapon will most certainly decrease the likelihood of its being used. (Shakespeare commented on this in *King John* Act II, "How oft the sight of means to do ill deeds, makes ill deeds done.")

The Therapeutic Milieu

The therapeutic milieu can have a positive influence. In a therapeutic milieu there is opportunity for group efforts to enhance the client's adaptive skills. One such group might focus on passive/ assertive/aggressive behavior; another on relaxation training; and another on role playing or actual attempts to facilitate exploration of the various coping techniques.

Provision for recreational and occupational therapy activities that may channel aggression in a positive fashion is important. Activities that allow the client to use the large muscles of the body are an example.

Maintaining a schedule of activities provides external structure to client behaviors. As discussed earlier, some activities afford an appropriate way for the client to express his aggressiveness, or an opportunity for him to learn new coping skills.

Staff should be on the unit at all times, not only at the nursing station. If the nurse is more easily accessible, the client is more likely to let her know at an early stage that he is experiencing difficulty. The nurse is also in a better position to observe any early warning signs when she is closer by. Attention to administrative policies and procedures, staffing, the physical environment, and the therapeutic milieu may be very effective in reducing the potential for violence, contributing to the client's positive responses and to protection of his health status. Safety is of primary concern in preventive measures as well as when episodes of aggressive or assertive behavior occur. The nurse must consider not only the client's safety and her own, but also that of other clients and other staff.

SECONDARY PREVENTION

In planning interventions at the health restoration level it is important for the nurse to keep in mind that clients who display aggressive or assaultive behaviors are experiencing some sort of stressor or threat. This threat may be real or imagined. It may involve a threat to the physical self, to possessions, or to self-esteem. Thus, interventions that are aimed toward decreasing the threatened feelings are most likely to succeed in preventing violence.

The type of threat experienced is likely to vary somewhat according to the client's preexisting problems. For example, to a client whose thought processes are impaired to the point of paranoia, the experience of seeing two staff members talking quietly becomes a threat to his self-esteem; his interpretation may be that staff are talking about him in a derogatory manner. Or, a phone conversation may be perceived as a threat of some sort.

Early Detection of Imbalance

When an imbalance between level of stressor and adaptive ability places the client in a state of disorganization, it is essential to note the problem as early as possible. The longer the situation remains unchanged, the greater the likelihood that the imbalance will increase in magnitude and progress to violence.

The nurse's observational skills are of primary importance in developing the capability to identify early warning signals. Many of the symptoms indicating that the potential for violence is escalating can be viewed as on a continuum, in which the symptom remains the same but the variation is in degree of intensity.

Subtle or early displays of symptoms may be observed only with difficulty. If, however, the nurse is highly empathic, she may sense a client's increased tension or unbalanced state even before there are observable signs of this. She then can approach the client and help him to verbalize his concerns while the stress remains at a low level. She might say something like "You seem tense to me; is that how you are feeling?" This opens the way for further exploration.

Changes in client behavior that signal heightened stress are noted so that the nurse can determine the nature of the difficulty and devise appropriate interventions. The nurse uses the senses of sight, hearing, and touch to detect early symptoms of disorganized behavior (see Table 11-2). Her observations contribute to the assessment part of nursing process.

Promoting Adaptive Capacities

Once an imbalance or disorganized state has been determined an immediate response is most effective. The nature of the response will vary somewhat according to the level of stress being experienced at the time the imbalance is noted. For convenience, these levels are classified as early, middle, and late; they correlate to Selye's (1956) general adaptation syndrome levels of alarm, resistance, and exhaustion.

Early Stage. At this stage signs and symptoms of distress are apparent but there has been no threat or actual violence. The nurse assists the client in identifying the stressor, whenever possible. Even if the stressor cannot be immediately identified, the feeling associated with the threat usually can be determined. Enabling the client to verbalize his feelings will decrease the possibility that he will need to act them out. Most importantly, the nurse assists the client in seeking alternative coping mechanisms. A supportive, empathetic approach is needed.

Middle Stage. At this stage the observable symptoms are more pronounced and hostile or threatening comments are made. The nurse informs the client that her expectation is that he

TABLE 11-2 Nursing Observations: Increased Potential for Violence	
Sight	
Tremulousness	Clenched fists
Nail biting	Hyperventilation
Scratching	Deep sighing
Hives	Hands on hips
Flared nostrils	Angry, anxious, or fearful facial expressions
Dilated pupils	
Glaring eye contact	Exaggerated startle response
Vasomotor flushing	
Distended neck and face veins	Pounding fist
	Slamming doors
Increased perspiration	Motor restlessness, that is, pacing, foot swinging
Increased muscle tension	
	Throwing objects
Hearing	
Sighing	Hostile comments, i.e., belittling, profanity
Irritability	
Accusatory statements	Threatening statements
Threatening statements	Boasts of past injuries inflicted on others
Statements about fear of loss of control	
	Loud speech
Statements about fear of harming self or others	Demanding statements
Touch	
Increased pulse	
Increased muscle tension	
Increased perspiration	

will remain in control of his behavior. She assists him in differentiating between his thoughts and feelings and his behavior. Again, it is helpful to have the client identify his feelings and openly talk about his stress. The nurse more actively explores alternative behaviors or suggests others that would be acceptable. She encourages him to consider the consequences that he may face if he were to carry out his threat, taking care that this exploration is not perceived by the client as a threat. It is preferable to take the client to a quiet area away from others, to lessen the likelihood of further threats to his self-esteem as well as the risk of harm to others. If medication is indicated and has been ordered, she offers it to the client. At this stage the nurse uses a kind, firm, more directive approach. She sets firm limits on the client's behavior and must be prepared to respond appropriately and quickly if the client does not maintain his behavior within these acceptable limits.

Case Study

A 24-year-old white male was brought by law enforcement officers to a locked psychiatric unit. The reason for admission was that he had been verbally threatening his outpatient case worker. He had a history of previous admissions and a diagnosis of paranoid schizophrenia.

The client's face was bright red. The veins of his neck and face were extremely distended. He spoke in a loud, angry tone and continued to make verbal threats of physical harm, still directed at the outpatient worker, who was not present; "I would like to throw her on the floor and grind her head into the floor with my boot until her brains oozed out onto the floor." The statement was accompanied by stomping his foot, twisting it randomly, and punching one fist into the other hand.

It was immediately decided to postpone the usual admitting procedure. A nurse who had previously established a relationship with this client was the staff person assigned to assess whether he would require seclusion or restraint or if the situation could be handled safely without these measures. Other staff were aware of the potential for violence and carefully observed the situation from a distance.

After talking with the client for only a few minutes, the nurse determined that he was not then psychotic, but that he was very angry. She said, "I can see that you are very angry. I'd like to talk with you about what happened if you'll let me." When the client again began making verbal threats about what he wanted to do, the nurse helped him to differentiate between his feelings and his behavior, and to look at the possible consequences of such behavior. "While you felt like doing these things, you didn't do them. You were able to exercise self-control. I'm really glad because had you acted on those feelings, I'm afraid you would have ended up in jail, and I would not like to see that happen." After further discussion the nurse suggested they walk up and down the longest hall in the unit while they talked, to help him get rid of the tense feeling he was experiencing. The nurse was able to contract with the patient that he would not harm anyone on the unit, and that he was not angry with any of them.

No seclusion or restraint was necessary in safely managing this situation. The client was eventually able to discuss appropriate ways to deal with his angry feelings, and with staff support to discuss the particular problem with his outpatient worker. The client was discharged the next day, equipped with new coping skills and improved confidence in his ability to maintain self-control.

Late Stage. This is the stage in which physically aggressive behavior is either displayed or is impending (throwing objects or escalating verbal threats). A verbal approach is inadequate. Medication and/or seclusion with or without restraints must be considered. The nurse still tries to communicate with the client and gain his cooperation. Her statements to him are short and concise, informing him what his behavior should be and what is expected of him.

Tupin (1983) recommends three classes of drugs for short-term emergency use: barbiturates, antianxiety agents, and antipsychotics. Some caution is to be exercised in using antianxiety agents, as they may produce disinhibition, and aggravate the situation. Tardiff (1982) has reported that the need for emergency control measures was significantly less with chronic clients taking chlorpromazine daily as compared to clients taking other antipsychotics.

If the client refuses medication, it may be possible to administer it intramuscularly after he is restrained. However, laws vary greatly from state to state on this issue, and the nurse must familiarize herself with the laws in the state where she practices.

Medication, seclusion, and mechanical restraints are mechanisms that temporarily support or substitute for the client's adaptive capacities, to be used when the latter are temporarily inadequate.

Seclusion and Restraints. When the decision to seclude or restrain a client is made the nurse must keep in mind the legal/ethical issues, personal and client safety, and nursing care issues, as well as consider self-awareness before, during, and after the seclusion or restraining procedure.

The Joint Commission on Accreditation of Hospitals (JCAH) has established standards for seclusion and restraint (1983). They are revised every 2 years so the nurse must review current standards. Many of the standards relate to acceptable rationale and documentation criteria. A few relate to the care clients are to receive while they are restrained or secluded. There may be other standards that the nurse will be required to follow depending on the practice setting. There may be state requirements that must be followed, and many institutions have established internal standards that must be applied. The nurse assumes the responsibility to follow requirements or standards in her practice setting.

According to JCAH, acceptable criteria for use of restraint or seclusion are similar to those of many of the states to justify involuntary hospitalization of a client. One is that the patient is a danger to himself or others because of mental illness and that less restrictive intervention techniques are either not available or are inadequate. Another is that the client is seriously disrupting the therapeutic environment for others. Both of these standards leave room for interpretation, but the nurse must be careful not to broaden the interpretation to the point that the rationale is useful primarily for the convenience of staff or as a punishment method.

Whatever the rationale, it must be documented in the client's medical record. The documentation should include not only the general criteria, such as that the client was a danger to others, but also descriptions of specific behavior that led to the conclusion, such as that the client threw a chair against the wall and threatened to throw another one at a staff person. A clinical assessment might also include further subjective or objective data. The client may have verbalized his anger and at the moment may be unable to use alternative coping measures, or may lack sufficient judgment and impulse control to ensure that others are safe. Another assessment may indicate that the client reported having been told by voices to pick up the chairs and throw them. All data pertinent to the decision to restrain a client must be documented, including past history of displays of aggressive behavior. Though past history is not of itself a sufficient cause, when coupled with current behavior it will be an influencing factor.

Whenever possible the documentation also indicates the unavailability or inadequacy of less restrictive treatments. Examples might include statements such as the following:

Client refused to take offered oral medication and continued to exhibit threatening behavior.

Client refused to take 15-minute time-out in his room and continued to display threatening behavior.

Client was assessed to be so far out of control

that he could not be safely managed in a less restrictive way.

Client requested that he be placed in restraints because of command auditory hallucinations which caused him to fear a loss of control of his behavior.

The actual order for restraint or seclusion must be given by a physician, according to JCAH standards. In an emergency a designated person on the treatment team may give the order, but it must be followed with a verbal order from the physician after 1 hour. There must be a physician's written order within 24 hours, and such orders must be renewed every 24 hours. PRN restraint or a seclusion order is not acceptable.

There should be a designated person on the treatment team who daily reviews all uses of restraint and seclusion. Ideally, a committee periodically reviews these records and compiles data to discern patterns of use and relationship between use of restraints and other elements in the unit.

Bell and Palmer (1981) have reported that 15.6 percent of the subjects in their study required seclusion or restraint, while Phillips and Nasr (1983) reported that 51 percent of their clients required seclusion or restraints. Obviously, much more research needs to be done in this area.

There must be an established procedure for notifying other staff personnel when assistance is required. At times when staffing on the unit is inadequate to manage the situation, there should be an established procedure for obtaining personnel from another unit or for summoning security personnel.

Staff must be available who are adequately trained in assessing emergency situations. There is often a fine line between managing the situation without having to resort to use of restraints or seclusion and allowing the situation to get out of hand before implementing restraint procedures. At times a staff member's reluctance to use restraints may contribute to the client's or others' being injured because that person waited beyond the point where safety could be preserved.

The first staff member to become aware of an impending emergency situation should summon assistance, while other personnel remove the other clients from the area of danger. The nurse may request that they go to their rooms or move to the other side of the room. Ideally, a team of five people is available, four of whom are assigned to control the client's limbs, and one of whom unlocks the doors, administers the medication, and so on. One person, designated to assume leadership in such situations, should be the spokesperson to the client; it is too confusing for the client to try to listen to more than one person tell him what to do. That person should also assign the others to the various tasks.

Often merely a show of sufficient force to control the situation is all that is required to ease the crisis. The spokesperson tells the patient in a calm, concise manner what behavior is desired. For example: "We will not permit behavior that threatens others on the unit. I would like you to walk with us to the quiet room now so that you can have some time to regain control of your behavior." This statement is not critical of the client; it informs him what is expected of him at the time.

Many times the patient will comply, in which case seclusion alone, or with medication, may be sufficient. If the client does not comply with the request to go voluntarily, the staff group must be prepared to move quickly on the leader's signal. The client's limbs should be held near the joints so as to minimize the possibilities of injury. The client should be lifted and carried to the seclusion room as quickly as possible. Each person assigned to control a limb will need to continue to control the limb while restraints are applied. It is imperative that each member be able to trust the others to perform their assigned task adequately. If one limb is not controlled, the possibility for injury to staff will increase.

A client placed in seclusion or restraints must be searched to ensure that he has nothing on his person that could be harmful to him. The client will be unable to remove himself from anything in that room that might be dangerous—such as a fire set by a client who had matches in his pocket. The nurse cannot assume that, because it is against unit policy for clients to possess such articles, the client has nothing harmful on his person. Many times clients are put in hospital pajamas to ensure that they do not have available potentially harmful objects.

There are methods that are used when only one, two, or three staff persons are available. These are not completely safe and frequently are used temporarily to restrain the client until additional help arrives.

The methods previously discussed apply in situations where no weapon is involved. The presence of a weapon makes establishment of control much more difficult. The safety of other clients is of primary concern. The nurse communicates with the client holding the weapon from a sufficient distance so as to give him adequate body buffer zone. She tells him she is going to request that the other clients go to their rooms and close their doors, and that she does not want to see anyone get hurt. She tells the client she'd like to discuss the problem with him, but finds it difficult to listen and concentrate on what is being said while the weapon is being held. She asks him to place it on the floor and move away from it.

The nurse will have previously summoned security personnel in the manner used in her facility. If it becomes apparent that the client will not relinquish the weapon, the goal is to take the weapon from him without causing injury to client or staff. A bed mattress can be used to pin him against the wall or on the floor until the weapon can be taken. Knives, razor blades, and even guns have found their way onto psychiatric units. Pieces of broken glass, metal rods from closets or showers, and other items that may be found around a unit can also be used as weapons. Once the weapon has been removed, the client is taken to seclusion in the same manner as other clients.

The designated spokesperson should always inform the client of the reason for seclusion or restraint. She should also tell him in what manner he will be observed and how frequently. If a camera is to be used for continuous monitoring, the client should be so informed. The client should be assured that his nutritional and hygienic needs will be met even though he is in seclusion or restraints. Some indication of expected duration of seclusion and behavioral requirements for release should also be communicated to him.

The decision to use seclusion alone or with restraints is based on the clinical judgment of the designated leader. Seclusion alone is less restrictive than seclusion plus restraints, and the nurse will try to choose this method whenever it is felt to be a safe choice. The American Nurses' Association Standards of Psychiatric and Mental Health Nursing Practice (1982), Standard 5, states: "The nurse sets limits in a humane and least restrictive manner to assure safety of client and others." If the client's present mental status allows him to be cooperative enough not to injure himself or try to injure staff who would need to monitor him, then seclusion alone would be a good choice. If, however, the client is too out-of-control for his own safety, even when in seclusion, or if he presents further danger to staff, then the decision must be made to use restraints in addition to seclusion.

The number of restraints required must be decided. Initially, a client is generally restrained with either two-point or four-point restraints. Four-point restraints refer to use of the restraint cuffs on all four limbs, at wrists and ankles. With two-point restraints, one wrist and the opposite ankle are placed in the cuffs. Again, a consideration in the decision is the least restrictive alternative that will be effective in providing safety for client and staff.

When the decision is made to place the client in four-point restraints, the nurse needs to continually assess his physical and mental status. As it improves, the number of restraints may be reduced.

It is never acceptable to restrain a patient on a psychiatric unit unless he is in a locked seclusion room or is being monitored continuously by a staff person. If for some reason a client is restrained in his room or even in a chair in the dayroom, it is imperative that he be continually monitored to prevent other clients from harming him. The client is totally vulnerable when restrained and unable to defend himself from others. He is completely reliant on staff for meeting his basic needs including safety.

When applying restraints, the nurse needs to be sure they are tight enough to be effective, but not so tight that circulation is impaired. It is debatable as to what is the best position in which to place the client. Some professionals support the idea that clients should always be placed in a prone position because the risk of aspiration is diminished, as is sexual vulnerability. Those supporting the use of the supine position feel that a client's needs can be met better in this position, e.g., feeding, toileting, giving medication, and that he feels more vulnerable when he cannot see who is approaching his room. The supine position should probably be used only in facilities where the client can be constantly observed. The head of the bed should be slightly raised, or a pillow may be provided. However, if the prone position is used, a pillow should not be given as it may increase the risk of suffocation.

Care of Client in Seclusion.

When a client is in seclusion, he should be visually observed by staff personnel at least every 15 minutes. The staff person should let the client know when she is looking in on him. This practice should be followed even in facilities where there is provision for constant observation by cameras in the seclusion rooms. The staff person who observes the client at 15-minute intervals should record his behavior each time. A form that provides a list describing suitable behaviors simplifies and standardizes the process. It promotes easy access to data which can then be compiled for research in various aspects of the seclusion experience.

One reason for observing the client at regular intervals is to determine whether his status has improved sufficiently for release. Plutchik and his associates (1978) suggested viewing seclusion as a behavioral model and considering the seclusion as a "time-out." Time-outs have been shown to be most effective if their duration is approximately 30 minutes. However, in Plutchik's study the average length of seclusion was approximately 4 hours. Another study (Campbell, et al., 1982) reported an average length of stay in seclusion of 2.6 hours, with 53 percent of the clients remaining for less than 1 hour. Certainly the goal is to allow the client increased freedom as soon as he is judged clinically to be in control of his behavior to the degree that safety may be preserved. Especially when medications are given with the initiation of seclusion, the length of time required may frequently be 1 hour or less.

If the client is to remain in seclusion longer than 2 hours, an opportunity for toileting and receiving fluids should be provided every 2 hours. Toileting should also be provided on client request. At least two staff members should be available when the seclusion door is opened.

If a client remains in seclusion at a mealtime, he should be served his meal. It is preferable to use paper plates and plastic utensils, and these should be removed as soon as he has eaten. Opportunities for oral hygiene should also be provided.

In the unusual circumstance that a client would need to remain in seclusion for over 24 hours, he should have an opportunity to shower or bathe. Maintaining personal hygiene may prevent further deterioration of his mental state.

Communication with the client should continue throughout the seclusion experience. Even though the client is isolated from others, the nurse can interact therapeutically with him. He should know that the nurse is continuing to care for him and provide for his needs. She should make him aware at each 15-minute check that she is there to see how he is doing. The nurse should communicate to him that while his behavior may have been inappropriate, he is not felt to be a "bad" person and is not being punished. She should do everything possible to treat the client with dignity and respect and to communicate positive regard for him.

Caring for a client in seclusion or restraints is a psychiatric intensive care situation. The nursing care is time consuming and requires attention to details. The care plan for a client in restraints requires the same interventions as for the client in seclusion, plus some additional measures. A basic care plan is shown in Table 11-3. The one imperative thing that the nurse must keep in mind at all times is that the client is totally dependent on her.

Protecting the Client from Further Stressors

A further aspect of health restoration interventions is protecting the client from further stressors when he is disorganized or imbalanced. One way to do this is to remove a stressor. Simply turning off a television when the noise level is too high is one example. The nurse may also decrease stimuli by taking the client to a quieter area of the unit. Putting the client in seclusion is another example. Measures used to give care to the client while he is in seclusion or restraints are other examples. In this case, protecting the client from physiological stressors, such as dehydration or skin injury, is the goal.

TERTIARY PREVENTION

In the health reorganization phase the nurse promotes the achievement of a new balance between adaptive ability and stressors. If the nurse is to enable the client to achieve the highest health state possible, it is necessary that she help him incorporate his experience of loss of control or near loss of control.

Plutchik and his associates (1978) reported one of the very few research studies available on the seclusion experience from the client's point of view. Structured interviews were conducted with clients who had experienced seclusion and with a control group of clients who had not experienced seclusion. They found both differences and similarities between the two groups.

On the issue of how long a patient should be secluded, the secluded group believed 1 hour was acceptable while the nonsecluded group believed 4 hours was acceptable. There were no significant differences between the two groups in selecting from a list of behaviors those that would result in seclusion. Those behaviors reported most likely to

result in seclusion were as follows: (1) physical aggression toward staff members or other patients, (2) behavior destructive of objects or property and (3) agitated, uncontrolled behavior.

A majority of the secluded clients reported that seclusion helped them to calm down but also made them feel frustrated. About 40 percent felt seclusion had not been helpful to them.

Most of the clients did not feel the seclusion room should have an unlocked door, and did not believe that a staff member should remain with them. The clients did make some suggestions, such as providing a punching bag, music, and more comfortable furnishings.

The client needs to have the opportunity to discuss his feelings about the incident. He also needs to be encouraged to examine what occurred to see whether he can identify the events that led up to his having those feelings. If he can identify similarities between this incident and others when he experienced the same feelings, it will facilitate his beginning to learn to identify his difficulty at an earlier stage.

If the client was able to use a new alternative adaptive skill in avoiding loss of control in this incident, he needs to receive positive reinforcement. He also needs to review the way in which this new skill worked for him and how he might be able to use it again. Helping him see the value of learning new skills can be a positive outcome of a difficult situation.

The teaching of assertiveness skills may benefit most clients. Being able to honestly express feelings or needs while respecting the rights of others is commendable and desirable; being able to refuse unreasonable demands without feeling guilty is also positive. Clients who are categorized as having increased potential for violence, have a difficult time recognizing and expressing their feelings.

Angry feelings are probably the most difficult for such a client to admit and openly express in acceptable ways. Teaching him that anger is an acceptable emotion and that there are many appropriate ways to express it will reinforce his health state. Directing him toward verbally expressing his feelings and verbally problem solving will reduce his need to act out his feelings.

Relaxation techniques are helpful in dealing with periods of increased stress. Progressive relaxation, meditation, and deep breathing exercises are some examples of these techniques. Clients can be taught to utilize these skills at any time they feel stress to the degree of discomfort.

TABLE 11-3 Nursing Care of Client Who is Restrained

Nursing Diagnosis	Goal	Interventions
Potential for violence due to identified risk factors present or due to actual physical aggression	Client will refrain from harming self or others	Place client in mechanical restraints in order to provide external controls Administer prescribed medications Take vital signs prior to administration of additional medication Observe for side effects to medication Observe client's behavior every 15 minutes and record Assess mental status of client every ½ hour to evaluate whether he may be released from restraints
	Client will regain emotional control	Assist client to verbalize the precipitating stressor Provide opportunity to explain feelings experienced Indicate confidence in his ability to regain control Explore alternative response to stressor
Impaired physical mobility due to mechanical restraints	Client will mobilize limbs every 2 hours	Release restraints one at a time Instruct client in active range of motion exercises Observe for adequate mobilization of limbs If client unable to comply with instructions, provide for passive range of motion exercises
	Client will maintain skin integrity	Pad restraints if client's skin is fragile or if limbs are very thin Check limbs for adequate circulation at time of application Check skin condition under restraints every 2 hours. Reposition if indicated.
Self-care deficit, total, due to mechanical restraints	Client will drink a minimum of 2880 cc/24 hr	Offer client 240 cc of fluid every 2 hours Record intake of fluid
	Client will eat at least ⅔ of each meal served	If client's mental status permits, loosen one restraint so he may feed himself Assist client as required with opening cartons, and so on If client unable to feed self, feed him Remove tray as soon as meal completed
	Client will utilize facilities offered for elimination every 2 hours	If client's mental status permits accompany him to toilet facilities every 2 hours If mental status does not permit release from restraints for toileting, offer bedpan or urinal every 2 hours, or on request
	Client will maintain cleanliness	If client's mental status permits, escort him to shower at least once every 24 hours If client's mental status does not permit shower, provide basin of water with soap and cloth for bed bath If client's mental status permits, remove restraint so that he may bathe self If client unable to bathe self, give bed bath Change bed linens at least once every 24 hours, or at any time they are soiled

A component of the health restoration phase involves the evaluation, by both the nurse and the client, of how effective the earlier interventions were. Also, consideration needs to be given to revisions that need to be made to prevent potential for violence or actual violence in the future. The review of the incident with the client not only assists him to integrate the experience but also provides the nurse with important evaluative data.

☐ *Self-Awareness*

The nurse needs to be aware of her own feelings, thoughts, and values toward individuals who behave violently. Her attitude may hinder her ability to deal with them in a therapeutic manner. For example, a nurse who feels that anyone who threatens or displays violent behavior deserves to be punished will have a difficult time responding in a therapeutic manner. She will need to become aware of these feelings and reexamine them in order to enhance her ability to deal with these clients in a more positive way.

The nurse also needs to have self-awareness about the feelings generated by the actual encounter with an aggressive or assaultive patient. Anger, fear of harm, and fear of losing control are just some of the feelings that might be aroused. An opportunity needs to be available to discuss such feelings following each incident in which violence occurred. Lanza (1983) reported that 50 percent of staff members who were victims of assault on a psychiatric unit did not respond to 65 percent of the items related to emotional reactions. Questions arise about staff's ability, for whatever reason, to admit the feelings associated with violent interactions between staff and clients. It has been suggested that perhaps staff feel they do not have a right to react emotionally, as violent interactions are just "part of the job." Or perhaps staff fear that if they allowed themselves to openly express feelings associated with violent incidents, this might prevent their being able to function in their jobs.

It has become a universally accepted practice to hold staff meetings following suicide of a client, or self-inflicted violence by a client, in order to explore feelings associated with these incidents. There is a definite need to provide opportunities for such exploration of feelings following client-staff violence.

■ *Enrichment Activities*

DISCUSSION

1. Obtain and review standards about involuntary use of medications, seclusion, and restraints from the state in which the student nurse plans to practice. Compare the standards of various states.

2. Obtain a cassette tape of relaxation techniques to play in class for students to practice. Discuss feelings experienced. (These tapes are readily available in most bookstores.)

3. Discuss personal attitudes about clients who display aggressive and assaultive behavior.

LEARNING ACTIVITIES

1. Role-play physically restraining and lifting a struggling client. Discuss feelings aroused during this experience.

2. Role-play discussion with a client who is exhibiting symptoms of increasing potential for violence. (See Figure 11-1.)

3. Tour a psychiatric unit and identify objects in the environment that could readily be used as weapons.

■ *Supplemental Recommended Readings*

Kutash, I.L., Schlesinger, L.B., and Associates. *Handbook on stress and anxiety.* San Francisco: Jossey-Bass, 1980. Addresses both theoretical and research aspects of anxiety and stress. Several chapters cover relationship of stress or anxiety to other variables. Various treatment approaches are also discussed.

Lion, J.R., and Reid, W.H. *Assaults within psychiatric facilities.* New York: Grune & Stratton, 1983. An excellent resource that includes information about phenomenology and epidemiology issues related to violence in psychiatric settings. Considerable attention is also given to policy issues and management of violent or assaultive behavior.

May, R. *The meaning of anxiety.* New York: Norton, 1977. Explores the nature of anxiety from a number of different perspectives. Many case studies are included as examples of various concepts. Management or treatment is also addressed.

Spielberger, C.D., and Sarason, I.G. *Stress and anxiety.* Edited by P.B. Defares. Washington: Hemisphere Publishing, 1985. A compilation of papers from two

■ *References*

Adler, A. *Superiority and social interest*. Evanston, IL: Northwestern University Press, 1964.

American Nurses' Association. Standard V-C. Intervention. *Standards of psychiatric and mental health nursing practice*. Kansas City, MI: American Nurses' Association, September 1982.

Bandura A. *Aggression: A social learning analysis*. Englewood Cliffs, NJ: Prentice-Hall, 1973.

Bell, C.C., and Palmer, J.M. Procedures in a psychiatric emergency service. *Journal of the National Medical Association*, 73, 1981:835–842.

Boettcher, E.G. Preventing violent behavior: An integrated theoretical model for nursing. *Perspectives in psychiatric care*, 21, 2, 1983:54–57.

Burgess, A.W. *Nursing: Levels of health intervention*. Englewood Cliffs, NJ: Prentice-Hall, 1978.

Campbell, W., Shepherd, H., and Falconer, F. The use of seclusion. *Nursing times*, 78, 1982:1821–1825.

Dollard, J., Dobb, L.W., Miller, N.E., Mowrer, O.H., and Sears, R.R. *Frustration and aggression*. New Haven, CT: Yale University Press, 1939.

Freud, S. *The complete psychological works of Sigmund Freud*. London: Hogarth Press, 1932.

Joint Commission on Accreditation of Hospitals. *Consolidated standards manual/83 for child, adolescent,*

chiatry, 34, 1 (January 1983):44–47.

Lanza, M.L. Origins of aggression. *Journal of psychosocial nursing and mental health services*, 21, 6 (June 1983):11–16.

Maslow, A.H. *Motivation and personality*. New York: Harper & Row, 1954.

Peplau, H. *Interpersonal relations in nursing*. New York: G. Putnam's Sons, 1952.

Phillips, P., and Nasr, S.J. Seclusion and restraint and prediction of violence. *American journal of psychiatry*, 140, 2, (February 1983): 229–232.

Plutchik, R., Karasu, T.B., Conte, H.R., Siegel, B., and Jerrett, I. Toward a rationale for the seclusion process. *Journal of nervous and mental diseases*, 166, 1978:571–570.

Rigdon, I.S., and Godbey, K.L. Threats to survival. In *McGraw-Hill handbook of clinical nursing*, (Armstrong, M.E., Dickason, E.J., Howe, J., Jones, D., and Snider, M.J., eds.). New York: McGraw-Hill, 1979:1186–1198.

Selye, H. *The stress of life*. New York: McGraw-Hill, 1956.

Tardiff, K. The use of medication for assaultive patients. *Hospital and community psychiatry*, 33, 4 (April 1982):307–308.

Tupin, J.P. The violent patient: A strategy for management and diagnosis. *Hospital and community psychiatry*, 34, 1 (January 1983):37–40.

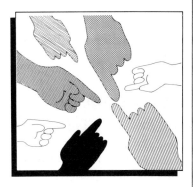

12

Family Dynamics

Susan I. Cullen, M.S.N.

Learning Objectives

Upon completion of this chapter, the reader will be able to:

1. Identify a variety of existing family forms.
2. Identify major theories of family and family therapy.
3. Identify the developmental tasks and stages of the family.
4. Describe the family as a system.
5. List some functions and dynamics of the family.
6. Identify functional and dysfunctional ways in which families relate.
7. Identify the three areas of prevention in relation to the family.
8. Discuss some specific techniques utilized in the process of family therapy.
9. Relate nursing process to intervention with the family.

Working with the family is not a new activity for nurses. What may be different today is the nurse's perception of the family as this relates to the client's care. At times the family is viewed only as an obstacle to care, but with the increased emphasis on treating the client as a total person, the family has become such an important part of the client's care that the nurse can now regard the entire family as the client.

The nurse comes into contact with families frequently, whether in a hospital, clinic, school, or other setting. Adopting a view that includes the family as the client can help increase the nurse's effectiveness whether she is treating the family as a whole or an individual member. This chapter presents a definition of family, reviews major family theories and concepts, and applies nursing process to a case example.

As in any other area of nursing, the nurse's most effective tools are her skills. The nurse should not underestimate her ability to intervene with the family. Understanding basic family theory can make every relationship with a family a health-promoting experience.

☐ *Definition of Family*

Before working with the family, the nurse needs to ask, "What is a family?" "How do I define the family? What makes this group a family?" Do you describe the family according to blood relationships, legal contracts, feelings of commitment between members? Do you see the definition as static or constantly changing? Identifying your own beliefs about the family is an important first step in giving nursing care. It is important also to be aware of how the client's own definition of his family affects you. You may find yourself surprised at the variety of definitions that exist. Acceptance of the client's definition is necessary if you are going to involve the "family."

THE 1980s FAMILY

During the past decade a popular concern has been not so much the definition of the family, but whether it is an institution that is becoming outmoded in our society. Those in the health care fields often argue that something must be done to save the family. What actually seems to be in danger of extinction is not the family itself, but merely its more traditional forms. The family of the 1980s is different from earlier families and exists in a variety of forms.

The Traditional Nuclear Family

Virginia Satir (1972) describes the traditional nuclear family as "one man and woman of the same race, religion and age, of sound mind and body, who marry during their early or middle twenties for life and are faithful to one another for life, have their own children, raise them, retire, and die." Although this description appears narrow, it has maintained popularity for some time and is still seen by many as the most desirable family form. A more current definition of the nuclear family allows for more variation. According to this newer definition, it is a family of two generations formed by a married woman and man with their children by birth or adoption. Within this family, as within all identified family forms, the functions performed by each member may vary. For example, a common structure has the father working outside the home and the mother working at home attending to the children and household tasks. Today, both mother and father are often seen working outside the home. Caretaking of the children may be shared by the couple and also shared with others outside the family such as in a day care center.

A term that has come into popularity as a result of changes in the traditional nuclear family is the extended family. The extended family is multigenerational and includes all relatives by marriage, birth, or adoption. It consists of the grandparents, aunts, uncles, nieces, nephews, cousins, brothers, sisters, and in-laws. The current trend for children to leave the homes and communities of their parents has resulted in a separation of the nuclear family from the extended family.

Alternative Nuclear Family Forms

The following forms may or may not be referred to as nuclear families, since they are variations of the traditional form of family.

The Single-Parent Family. This family consists of two generations and is made up of a mother or father and her or his children by birth or adoption. The single-parent family is increas-

ital relationship; adoptions by single adults are not unusual. A single-parent family can also be created by the death of a spouse.

The Blended Family. The blended or reconstituted family is a family of "put together parts of previously existing families" to form a new nuclear family (Satir, 1972). As with the traditional nuclear family, it is two generational. The blended family differs in form. It may be made up of a single person who marries a person with children, or of a man and a woman, both of whom have children, who marry. This couple may also have biological children—a "yours, mine, and ours" family. The composition of the child's blended family can become complex with the variety of stepbrothers, stepsisters, and stepparents that can result. How many members actually comprise this family depends on how active the divorced spouses and multiple grandparents are in the life of the blended nuclear family.

The Nuclear Dyad. This family form is one generational and made up of a married couple without children. The couple is childless because they have chosen not to have children, because they are not able to have children or to adopt them, or because the children have died. Although this family form is frequently thought of as a beginning point for the formation of the family, the numbers of nuclear dyad families are growing and it is a functioning family.

Special Family Forms

A wider array of family forms is observed if ideas about marriage and the requirement that the nuclear family is essential to the definition are put aside. These groups function as families, and this must be recognized. These families may be either one generational or multigenerational. There are two or more adults and both may or may not be of the same sex.

Commune. A commune is a group of people with intertwining husband-wife, parent-child, members, with specific rules and expectations for each member.

A commune may come into existence when people have a common goal (e.g., religious, philosophical, political) or a common need (e.g., economic, social, physical). Some examples of communes are the Israeli Kibbutzim, religious cults, residences for the elderly, and households with couples sharing resources.

The Gay Household. Perhaps as a result of the gay rights movement, gay (homosexual) couples have more openly taken up residence together. Because society hesitates to accept this family form, it remains difficult for the gay couple to either adopt children or to be given custody of children when a gay partner divorces. Some gay households consist of two people and function as the nuclear dyad discussed previously. Others may consist of more members.

The Family of the Future

As society changes, family forms will also change. A flexible definition of the family accommodates new forms as well as the more traditional ones, and gives the nurse a useful point of reference for her work with the client.

The family may be described as a group of people (two or more), usually in a shared living situation, who are united by contract (marriage, adoption), blood relationship (parent-child, sibling), or common bond (a goal, a need). The one element that is constant is that there is a family bond that ties the individuals together and encourages them to relate to one another. Table 12-1 describes four types of family bonds: biological, psychological, economic, and social. Ackerman (1958) believes that one or more of these bonds must exist in order for a group to be seen as a family.

Families also have common characteristics and functions. Understanding them helps the nurse to understand the individual family member and his response to society. The nurse is encouraged to think about how these features apply to each of the family forms previously discussed.

TABLE 12-1 Family Bonds

Bonds	Purpose	Examples
Biological	To bear offspring and perpetuate the species	Having biological children Protecting the young or disabled family from external threats
Psychological	Providing for affectional and self-image needs of the individual	Giving physical affection such as hugging and kissing Giving verbal support (e.g., "You did such a good job on that")
Economic	Providing for the material needs of the family members	Providing shelter (e.g., house or apartment) Providing clothing, food, and money
Social	Providing an environment in which the individual family members can learn to relate to each other and society at large	Teaching about rules—and consequences if they are broken Helping family members to reality-test information about themselves and their experiences

☐ Development of Family Theory

For many years the emphasis in psychiatry and mental health has been on psychoanalytic theory to provide an understanding of the individual and his development. Treatment was effected through the one-to-one relationship. The effect of the family on the individual's development as a dynamic force did not begin to be recognized until the 1940s. Although some appreciation of the importance of the family began to emerge at that time, the family as a whole was still not involved in the treatment process.

In the early 1950s a number of therapists began to work with the family, rather than with only the client. These therapists were unaware of one another's work, and the notion of family therapy rather than traditional one-to-one therapy was revolutionary. Uncertainty about the exact nature of their involvement with the whole family, as well as concern about isolation by unsympathetic colleagues, were problems that arose during this period.

Armed with results of their initial research efforts and notes based on sessions with families, family therapists by the mid '50s were starting to openly discuss and write about their work. Research and treatment at that time was focused primarily on the family's relationship to the client and its effect on the development of schizophrenia. The ideas that emerged from this work are important in the understanding of families in general.

From the mid-1950s to the early 1960s, the concept of family therapy gained momentum, and today family therapy as a legitimate, effective method of treatment is well accepted.

The focus now becomes the choice of one or more treatment approaches or theories that will be useful to the nurse. The effectiveness of her interventions lies not so much in the theory she subscribes to but in her ease and skill in applying the theory.

☐ Major Family Theories

As stated previously, a number of theories and treatment approaches have been developed. Susan Jones (1980) suggests recognition of seven major theories that have been widely disseminated and have the broadest influence in the field. These are the integrative approach, psychoanalytic approach, Bowen approach, structural approach, interactional or communication approach, social network approach, and behavioral approach (Table 12-2). Therapists may ascribe to a

TABLE 12-2 *Theories of Family*

	Theory: Integrative approach
Major theorist	Nathan Ackerman
Identified client	Individual family member and/or the family
Family as a system	No. Believed systems theory did not give sufficient recognition to individual dynamics
Pathology origin	Gives equal weight to individual dynamics and the external (family) dynamics as a cause of pathology
Family history important	Yes, believes should look at family development
Insight used in treatment	Yes
Therapist becomes part of family process	Yes. Believes development of transference relationship with the family is important for the working through of earlier, distorted family relationships
Major concepts	Social role—how the individual adapts to environmental demands, the social self
	Theory: Psychoanalytic approach
Major theorists:	Ivan Boszormenyi-Nagi, Geraldine Spark, and James Framo
Identified client	Individual family member and/or the family
Family as a system	Yes, a psychological system
Pathology origin	Emphasizes the individual member's dynamics
Family history important	Yes, to understand how relationships affected the individual's development
Insight used in treatment	Yes
Therapist becomes part of family process	Yes. Like Ackerman, focuses on the transference
Major concepts	Psychic determinism—every behavioral act of individual based on his history and past experiences Anxiety—conflict between id, ego, and superego results in anxiety
	Theory: Bowen approach
Major theorist	Murray Bowen
Identified client	Individual family member and/or the family
Family as a system	Yes. An emotional and relational system
Pathology origin	Emphasizes both individual and family dynamics
Family history important	Yes
Insight used in treatment	Yes
Therapist becomes part of family process	No. Believes that triangulation would occur
Major Concepts	Differentiation of self—the ability of an individual member to express individual feelings and thoughts, even though they are different than other members of the family Triangle as the basic emotional unit[a]—a three-person emotional unit Nuclear family process—patterns of emotional functioning in a single generation Family projection process—parental feelings and problems identified as belonging to the child Multigenerational transmission process—family projection process occurs over several generations with individuals becoming increasingly impaired Sibling position profiles—characteristics of an individual can be predicted by sibling position in family Emotional cutoff—how the individual separates from parents to start adult life. Looks at ability to renegotiate roles to establish healthy relationships Societal regression—extends the emotional system of the family to society at large. Identifies society as an emotional system as well

(continued)

TABLE 12-2 (continued)

	Theory: Structural approach
Major theorist	Salvador Minchin
Identified client	Family only
Family as a system	Yes. A transactional, structural system
Pathology origin	Emphasizes family and environmental dynamics
Family history important	No
Insight used in treatment.	No
Therapist becomes part of family process	Yes. Believes therapist must join the system to use self as a change agent
Major concepts	Systems[a]—the family is made up of interactional units interrelated to make a whole
	Subsystems[a]—the division within the family that identifies the individual's power and is the medium for teaching skills
	Structure[a]—determined by the subsystems and boundaries within the family. The functional demands that organize the way the family interacts
	Transactional patterns—determine how, when, and with whom individual family members interact
	Enmeshment—intense, excessively close contact between family members. Individual identity gets lost
	Disengaged—disconnectedness among family members. Little structure, order, or ties between family members

	Theory: The interactional or communication approach
Major theorists	Gregory Bateson, Don Jackson, Paul Watzlawick, Jay Haley, and Virginia Satir
Identified client	Family only
Family as a system	Yes. A behavioral and communicational system
Pathology origin	Emphasizes the family and environmental dynamics
Family history important	No. (Satir is exception—believes it is important)
Insight used in treatment	No
Therapist becomes part of family process	Yes. Sees joining the family system important for role as change agent
Major concepts	Double-bind*—messages in family are conflicting
	Pseudomutuality and pseudohostility*—family presents image opposite to reality
	Schism—a coalition (unity and mutual support) between parents is absent. There exists chronic discord and recurring threats of separation. Produces anxiety in children, with resulting mistrust
	Skew—harmony in marital relationship maintained by one partner being dominant and the other submissive
	Homeostasis[a]—the maintenance of harmony within the family system
	Family rules[a]—determinants of individual behavior and roles

	Theory: Social Network Approach
Major theorists	Ross Speck, Carolyn Attneave, and Uri Rueveni
Identified client	Emphasizes the family and its social network
Family as a system	Yes, interrelated to the larger social system
Pathology origin	Family and the environment. Believe that sick families are the result of a sick society
Family history important	No
Insight used in treatment	No
Therapist becomes part of family process	Yes. The therapist is to become part of the social network

(*continued*)

TABLE 12-2 *(continued)*

Major concepts	Social network—all the relationships of the family in the social setting including friends, relatives, coworkers, and so on. Treatment setting may include 15 to over 100 people
	Retribalization—the rejoining of the family with others who share their experience and history
	Network effect—the part of the process in which the group begins to work together, realizing they are part of a human cluster. A feeling of closeness and commitment develops
	Theory: Behavioral approach
Major theorist	Gerald Patterson
Identified client	Individual family member and/or family
Family as a system	Yes. A behavioral system
Pathology origin	External or family oriented only
Family history important	No
Insight used in treatment	No
Therapist becomes part of family process	Yes. Believes it necessary to act as a role model and teach family new behaviors
Major concepts	Responses and stimuli—responses are segments of behavior. Stimuli are the environmental events that trigger the behavior
	Positive reinforcer—a stimulus that encourages a behavior to continue through positive rewards
	Fading—repeating an activity a number of times, steadily decreasing the therapist's involvement
	Extinction—the withholding of positive reinforcers to cause the frequency of a behavior to decrease until it has disappeared
	Stimulus generalization—stimuli related to one behavior begin to cause a different behavior which is not directly related to the original stimuli

a Discussed more fully in the chapter text.

theory in "pure" form, adhering to specifically de-scribed concepts of an individual theory, or may follow an approach that incorporates concepts and interventions from two or more theories.

FAMILY SYSTEMS THEORY

Except for Ackerman's integrative approach to family therapy, the family's identification as a system is an important premise in all the major family theories. How each of the major theorists conceptualizes the family system varies, yet there are general characteristics that can help the nurse identify and understand family behavior.

Systems and Subsystems

General systems theory describes a system as a group of interrelated parts or units that form a whole. As applied to the family, the individual family members are those units that make up the identifiable family system. In addition, the parts or units act as one or more subsystems within the larger system. In the family system, the subsystems refer to the way in which the members align themselves with each other. For example, the parents may be a subsystem, the children another, while the males and females may be two other subsystems. Subsystems are made up of dyads (re-lationships between two members), triads (rela-tionships among three members) and larger groups which are linked by some common factor.

Membership within the subsystems is deter-mined by generational considerations, sexual identity, areas of interest, or specifically desig-nated functions. Individual family members may belong to several different subsystems at the same time. Further, family members also simultaneously belong to external systems. Figure 12-1 illustrates these relationships.

Subsystems can be easily understood if thought of as a way in which the family handles the division of labor. A subsystem is constructed in order to ensure that an important function is carried out that will maintain the overall family structure.

Interdependence of System Units

Each family member is one unit of the family system. Interdependency of family members refers to the relationship in which change in one member of the family also causes changes in the rest of the family members. Some common changes are the birth of a child, the death of a family member, marriage of a child, divorce of the parents, illness or increased health needs of a member, and role changes. For example, if a father becomes ill and is unable to continue at his job, the mother may become employed outside of the home for the first time in many years. Tension between the couple may develop due to difficulty accepting the change in roles. The children in the family begin to have more fights and to be less responsive to their parents' wishes. This family's system becomes upset due to the effects of the father's illness.

Interdependence of the individual family members is related to the concept of homeostasis. In order to remain functional, a system must maintain a balance between both internal factors and external influences. Stress and changes from within the family system and from its milieu (environment) can upset the family's balance and cause illness or dysfunctional behavior. The family strives to maintain homeostasis so that family functions can be carried out. If a family member does not behave in his usual manner, the other family members will attempt to minimize the disruption of the established protocols. The need for homeostasis can act as a deterrent to individual growth which can result from the acceptance of illness. Example: John had been constantly in trouble for some time. The difficulties became so great that he was sent to see a counselor to "straighten him out." As John became more able to talk about his feelings and use less disruptive behavior, the family became upset with his more direct expression of anger. They insisted that John had not changed in any way and was "fooling" the counselor. The family was in fact attempting to reestablish John's unhealthy behavior.

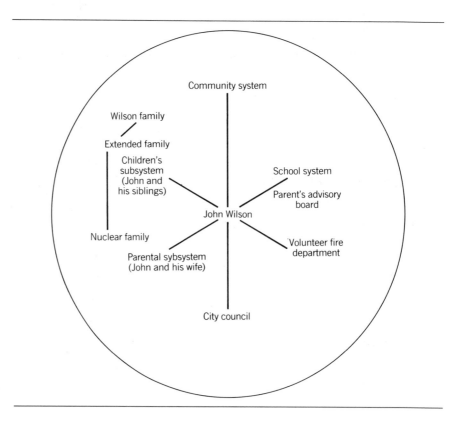

Figure 12-1 Multiple membership in systems and subsystems.

Boundaries of the System

The boundaries are defined by the rules specifying the members of a system or subsystem and the roles the members take. Boundaries can be most easily understood if thought of as lines that separate the family from the external environment, and of lines that define the subsystems within the family. Boundaries can be rigid, clear, or diffuse. Rigid boundaries are closed, so that the individuals within such a system or subsystem feel isolated and are unable to obtain support from others outside the subsystem. Diffuse boundaries lack clarity; there are overly involved or dependent relationships between members of the family system. The individual does not feel a strong sense of individual identity or family identity. Both rigid and diffuse boundaries are problematic and cause dysfunction. Clear boundaries allow for open and honest communication while promoting individual identity and responsibility. Individuals have a clear understanding of what their functions are, and can allow influence and support of others both from within the family and from the outside.

An example of the boundaries between the parent and child subsystems may serve to clarify that statement. When the boundary is rigid, if the mother becomes ill and is unable to discipline the children, an older child would not be permitted to perform that role. The discipline would not be done. If there is instead a diffuse boundary, the transition during the mother's illness may, in fact, be easier for the family. At the time of the mother's return to normal functioning, however, conflict could be anticipated between her and the older child, as well as confusion for the younger children as to whom they should be listening to when limits are needed. When boundaries are clear, the older child can assume the new role when that is needed and give it up when the need no longer is there.

Boundaries within a system also determine the system's hierarchical power structure. In most families it is the adults who have the most power, making the decisions for the family and distributing both rewards and discipline for good or unacceptable behavior. If boundaries are not clear, the parental subsystem can be ineffective. It may be unclear who has the authority in the family, or power may be inappropriately distributed. This will cause anxiety and stress in the family. For example: Terry, the 7-year-old daughter in the family, frequently made demands on her mother and requested immediate attention. Although her mother would tell Terry to wait, Terry would become more demanding, saying to her mother, "You do it now!" Rather than taking control and setting limits with Terry, she would eventually do as Terry told her to do. Terry was in control and was making the decisions for her.

Another characteristic of a system that is related to boundaries is openness or closedness. An open system means that the family is flexible, allowing new information and ideas to enter for consideration. A closed system will distort or block information in order to maintain balance. The amount of openness or closedness of each family will differ, but no family is totally open or totally closed.

Developmental Tasks

As in any other system, the family has functions to perform for the benefit of its individual members and the system as a whole. A major function of the family relates to developmental tasks. When the family promotes them successfully, independence and healthy functioning is encouraged in the individual family members. Table 12-3 describes some of the developmental tasks of the family. Although one-generational families have some of these same tasks, there are also parallels with individual development.

☐ Family Characteristics and Dynamics

Families can be placed on a continuum ranging from the functional (a high degree of health) to the dysfunctional (a high degree of illness). The nurse can distinguish the functional family from the dysfunctional family by the amount of time and energy spent in attempting to maintain homeostasis in the family system. Within the functional family a higher amount of energy can be directed to growth-promoting activities instead of maintenance activities. Regardless of where the family fits on the continuum, there are certain characteristics and dynamics in process.

FAMILY ROLES

Individual family members each have a part to play in the daily functioning of the family. The particular behavior each member uses relates to

TABLE 12-3 Family Developmental Stages and Tasks[a]

Stage	Task	Explanation
Beginning the family, the couple relationship	Intimacy vs. idealization or disillusionment	Individuals work to achieve intimacy. Involves development of a realistic perception of each other in terms of abilities and needs, learning to problem-solve and resolve conflicts and developing ways to support each other.
Childbearing and preschool years	Replenishment vs. turning inward	Family works to develop ways to nuture and support each other. Parents, as well as the more dependent children, must have emotional support. Both internal resources and supportive environment important.
School-age years	Individuation of family members vs. pseudomutual organization	Individual interests of family become primary concern. Children moving out of the family environment more independently and increasingly involved in the external systems such as school. Parents' roles changing, with children becoming less dependent.
Teenage years	Companionship vs. isolation	All family members begin to deal with separation issues. Increased sexuality of children increases family anxiety. Support for restructuring relationships important (e.g., helping children to develop peer-group friends). Parents must begin increasing their involvement with each other.
Children leaving home	Regrouping vs. binding or expulsion	Placement of children into society as adult individual members, releasing them from family of origin. Modification of family structure occurs with members leaving; often very difficult stage.
First postparental phase	Rediscovery vs. despair	Family works on renegotiation of roles between children and parents, developing an adult-to-adult relationship. Parents work to revive interest in each other to reestablish early balance that existed when they were the original nuclear dyad.
Second postparental phase	Mutual aid vs. uselessness	Occurs from the parents' retirement to death. The work is to develop a mutual aid system with other, their extended family, and the community at large. The goal is to preserve dignity and a sense of usefulness. Interlocking roles between generations important.

[a] Adapted from Rhodes, S. The developmental approach to the life cycle of the family. *Social casework*, 5, 1971:301–11.

his assigned family role. The role, or pattern of behavior, is a sequence of acts directed toward a goal. Each family member's role contributes to the functioning of the entire family.

Family Rules

The roles within the family system are governed by the family rules. Rules may be overt (clearly defined and readily apparent) or covert (not stated and hard to define). The rules define what roles will exist and what family members will perform them.

Overt Rules. Jackson (1965) states that the family operates as a rule-governed system. The overt rules are clearly available to all family members. They make each member of the family aware of the expectations for each other. An example of a well-known overt rule in our culture is that mother provides for the nurture of the children and father provides monetarily for the needs of the family. With economic and social changes, both parents in many families now work outside the home. The family must be able to renegotiate the overt rule to allow for change, or stress and anxiety will result. Father and older children may need to share more in the care of the younger children. In the healthy family, the overt rules may be renegotiated and modified to adjust to the current needs of the family.

Covert Rules. Ferreira (1963) and Bying Hall (1979) suggest a close relationship of family myths with covert rules and family roles. Ferreira defines the family myth as "a series of fairly well integrated beliefs shared by all family members, concerning each other and their mutual position in the family life, beliefs that go unchallenged by everyone involved in spite of the reality distortions which they conspicuously imply" (p. 457). In short, the family myths help define the roles for family members in a covert way. For example, a daughter may be considered to be "just like her mother was at that age." Since everyone remembers her mother as the "high strung" type when she was younger, the daughter receives the message that this is how she is to behave and think of herself. Since she is so anxious, the family accommodates her in order to avoid unnecessary stresses. The role is that she is "high strung"; the rule is "don't upset her."

Bying-Hall says that the stories that support the family myths take primarily five forms: fam-

ily yarns or tales, fables or lies, family legends, family secrets, and recalled events. Table 12-4 describes these five types of stories.

The importance of the family myth is its value for the family in maintaining homeostasis. In the healthy family, the stories are used to establish a family background and identity. The family can build a current identity on the myths. The old rules can be renegotiated and incorporated into new family rules. Healthy family myths help to fill gaps in family history. Further, they can reinforce the idea that people are sometimes fragile and capable of making errors, through the use of gentle humor. A favored story in my family is of a time my mother forgot one of the children in the small local grocery store. No harm came to the 4-year-old, and the local grocer had her busy filling a shopping basket by the time her absence was noticed.

TABLE 12-4 Family Stories

Family yarns or tales	Told with the understanding that it is permitted to fantasize to enrich the tale—the "fun" telling of family history. For example, your grandfather tells of a fish he caught that must have weighed "over 50 pounds." and took him "nearly all day" to pull in.
Fables or lies	Entirely fictional. The purpose is to fill a painful gap in the family history—such as the time a family member was absent because he was in prison.
Family legends	Generally based on an actual family event. Told through the generations to convey messages about how the family should behave and view itself. Told as truth but can contain alterations due to the constant retelling.
Family secrets	Usually available to only a "chosen few" family members; based on reality or fantasy. Difficult to identify as they are not talked about openly.
Recalled events	Based on fact as much as possible—accuracy is important. The teller will seek factual documentation such as photos and letters as a means of verifying the information. These stories are the actual building blocks of the family; they are important for healthy family functioning.

The dysfunctional family will tend to observe myths that are rigid and reinforce stereotypes. These myths are used to protect the family and do not allow for growth of the individual members. One way in which this happens is the use of myths to prove that the present will inevitably repeat the past and that it is predetermined how individuals will develop. For example, a son is told that he is so much like his father that he will "go bad" and end up in prison as his father did. The expectation of going bad can influence the son's behavior enough that he lives out the script he has been given. And when he does go to prison, the family is protected from dealing with this problem because it was in some way predetermined.

A second way in which family myths can promote illness is by eliminating parts of the family history rather than editing and integrating them. The refusal to share a part of the family history can often result in its being subtly conveyed as more terrible than it really was. Distortion of reality because of the family's difficulty in accepting it has a deleterious effect on the individual process of self-acceptance. Members of the family believe they must be protected from the truth, and an atmosphere of guilt prevails in the home.

Family roles are assigned by the family rules. However, even if the rules dictate that a family member is to assume a role, this may not occur. There may be several reasons: the expected role is not clearly defined for the individual (e.g., a new mother may not have had satisfactory role models and does not know how to mother a child), the individual is not allowed input into the role and rebels against it (e.g., a new mother did not want to have a baby and feels trapped and angry), or the individual is not allowed to fulfill the role because other family members interfere (e.g., a new mother's mother insists she knows better and takes over the job herself). If a role is to be filled by a family member and the tasks completed, it must be both clear and possible.

FAMILY THEMES

Themes are the issues involved in ongoing daily life that demand a high level of attention. Families have both positive (constructive, growth-promoting) and negative (destructive, growth-stifling) themes. Positive themes are usually focused on attainable, pleasurable activities such as children's achievements or home improvement. A message of positive worth is given to the individ-

ual members and the family. The same issues can be related to a negative theme. The difference in the message is one of failure or shortcoming, such as a child's inability to handle a new task or a parent's unfailing inattentiveness to a necessary repair in the home.

Identification of family themes is important for understanding the expectations an individual is given by the family. Also, positive themes can be reinforced and negative themes disrupted by changing the rigid, automatic responses that have been learned by the family.

The dysfunctional family usually has a number of negative themes and uses them as a way of maintaining homeostasis by holding on to the status quo. An example of this is a family who identifies a disruptive, acting-up child as the reason for their problems. The child begins to be credited for anything that goes wrong. This allows the family to avoid anxiety-producing concerns or changes in already established patterns of behavior. A theme may also involve others outside the family. For example, a family may continually talk about how they are "not like those freeloaders" who do not want to work and are on welfare. They consider themselves a hard-working family with each member pulling his own load and not expecting anything for nothing. This theme can make it difficult for individual members to ask for help when they need it.

☐ *Communication and the Family*

Communication is an interactional process that includes both the giving and the receiving of verbal and nonverbal messages. It is a primary way for family members to share their thoughts, wants, needs, and feelings. The process of communicating is a continuous and integral part of the family's daily functioning.

■ *Point of Emphasis*

Watzlawick (1967) says that all behavior is some form of communication. Since it is impossible for the individual to have no behavior, one cannot not communicate.

Individuals communicate both verbally and nonverbally. The verbal aspect is the actual words spoken, as well as the way they are phrased, their tonal quality, and their volume. The nonverbal aspect is the behavior used, such as physical posturing (e.g., standing with the hands on the hips, or shaking a clenched fist) and the facial expression (e.g., tears, frowning, smiling). In addition, family members have established relationships that are expressed when they communicate. Although what is being communicated may not be apparent to someone who is not involved in the relationship, the involved member will understand a message based on what he has learned from past experiences. As an example, Tim's mother has heard that Tim misbehaved in school. She calls Tim to come into the kitchen. When he arrives he begins to feel he wants to cry, as his mother is standing with her fists clenched on her hips and is frowning. Her voice tone and physical stance tell Tim he will get a spanking. His mother has not needed to say this directly to him.

Within the healthy family, the communication is clear and there is little confusion as to the meaning of what is said. Within the dysfunctional family there are several confusing patterns of communication which are identified as related to the development of illness of one family member or more.

DOUBLE-BIND COMMUNICATION

Double-bind communication is based on the use of the paradox, which is a double-binding message that occurs frequently in everyday conversation. Two conflicting messages are present. For example, Tom says, "You better start getting ready. It's getting late." Mary replies, "I am ready. Doesn't this look alright?" Tom then says, "Oh yeah, you look great." The first message implies that Mary should change her clothes, while the second message says that she looks good the way she is dressed.

A series of paradoxes creates the double-bind communication. Generally, double-bind communication is discussed in terms of the family that has a member with schizophrenia, although it happens in other dysfunctional families as well.

Jackson (1968) points out several factors important for double-bind communication to result in family dysfunction.

1. There must be at least two people involved, and one of these people is the victim. The victim is dependent and must struggle to understand the message.

2. This type of communication must occur over a period of time, and becomes automatic, habitual, and expected. The individual learns not to trust the verbal communication.

3. The messages are contradictory, and carry negative implications or threats. The victim can't win either way.

4. The victim sees no alternative ways of responding because of his allegiance to the family and need to remain within it. Healthy communications and relationships outside of the family are not available to the victim.

It is important to note that both conflicting messages do not have to be verbally communicated. A father may be smiling while he scolds his son for fighting at school. At the end of their discussion he may even give his son a playful punch on the arm. As the receiver of these messages, the boy does not know whether his father wants him to fight or not. His father's smile and playful punch reinforce fighting and his words say he must not fight.

COMMUNICATION ROLES

Satir (1972) says that dysfunctional families use communication to maintain harmony by helping them to avoid making changes or problem solve when there are conflicts. She identifies four important communication roles which are assigned to family members in their effort to maintain harmony.

1. *Distractor:* The family member attempts to distract and avoid conflict by shifting the focus away from the immediate problem. For example, when tension increases, one member may begin to complain of feeling ill or may bring up a different subject that is irrelevant to what is happening.

2. *Placator:* The family member reduces tension by being overly agreeable or passive with the other member or members. Peace, no matter what the cost to himself, is his motto.

3. *Blamer:* The family member changes the situation by increasing tension temporarily to force the other member or members into submission. As a result, there tends to be overreaction to situations. One way this

is done is by the member beginning to yell or cry.

4. *Computer:* The family member attempts to use logic and reasoning to handle problems, neglecting the feeling level because it does not fit well into the equation.

PSEUDOMUTUALITY AND PSEUDOHOSTILITY

Pseudomutuality is a condition of false closeness within a family. In a relationship having true complementarity or mutuality, there is a fitting together of people even though each maintains an individual identity. A couple will unite to form a common identity and work together while still maintaining individual interests and characters. An interest in maintaining the relationship and keeping harmony is balanced with an interest in sustaining individual identity. In pseudomutuality, the family strives to maintain harmony and peace at all costs. The basic message in this family is "You're going to enjoy this family if it kills you!"

Pseudohostility defines a state of chronic conflict and alienation among family members, a condition that is essentially denied by the family. The problems are seen as only minor, but individual family members are remote from each other. They will admit there is conflict but will minimize the importance of it.

Both of these conditions occur in rigid families where relationships are fixed, and do not allow for individual change. They are techniques of communication in which a family's underlying fears (e.g., separation anxiety, anger, intimacy) can be avoided.

TRIANGULATION

The dyad, two people, is the basic structure of all family forms. A large portion of human communication occurs within the dyad structure. The dyad not only communicates within itself, but communicates with its environment either through individual members or as an interrelated couple giving one message. The dyad is frequently affected by a third person. What can occur then is called triangulation.

The triangle occurs whenever another person is introduced into the dyadic relationship. The members of the triangle may be family members or may include someone outside the family. Family members may belong to more than one triangle at a time. Bowen (1966) considers the triangle a basic building block of the family's emotional system.

The triangle is understood as involving two people who have chosen to communicate with each other and meet each other's needs, and a third person who has formed a relationship with them. When there is stress between the two members of the dyad, the third person may become a means of relieving the stress. For example, when parents feel stress in their own relationship, they may find themselves in conflict with one of their own children or parents, rather than with each other. This allows them to unite and focus on the unruly child or the interfering parent and avoid conflict between themselves.

A couple that is disrupted emotionally might triangulate in a different way: one member of this dyad would form a closer, more supportive relationship with a child or parent. At the same time as this tighter bond was being formed, the stress in the relationship with the spouse could be reduced.

One important feature of the triangle in the stress situation is that there is often one person feeling left out. Also, the triangle is not always composed of a dyad and a third family member; one person might reduce tensions in the dyad by focusing on a job, hobby, lover, or other person or activity outside of the family. The triangle relationship is depicted in Figure 12-2.

The nurse can become part of the triangle relationship. When a member of the family becomes ill, the nurse may assume the uncomfortable position of the third person. For example, Mrs. Mark was given the diagnosis of cancer. Neither she nor her husband was able to talk with the other about how this affected them and their relationship. Instead, they focused on the nurse who had been caring for Mrs. Mark, and were angry and critical of her. Defensiveness on the nurse's part allowed triangulation to continue, while the real issue of the impact of Mrs. Mark's diagnosis on the couple was avoided.

SCAPEGOATING

Scapegoating is a process in which a family member becomes the object of blame for family problems or the bearer of unhappy feelings projected by other family members. Scapegoating can involve either an individual or a group. A housewife chose to take a job outside of the home even though her husband was providing a very adequate income. She was blamed for new problems

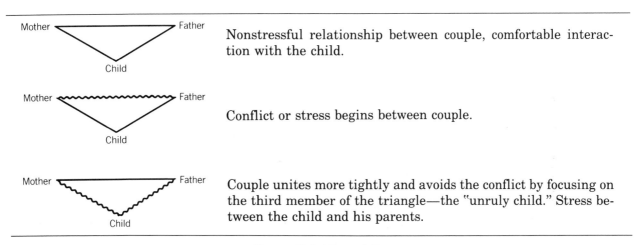

Nonstressful relationship between couple, comfortable interaction with the child.

Conflict or stress begins between couple.

Couple unites more tightly and avoids the conflict by focusing on the third member of the triangle—the "unruly child." Stress between the child and his parents.

Figure 12-2 Triangulation.

the family faced when other family members were unwilling to take on responsibilities she no longer had time for. The family became involved in counseling because of incidents of spouse abuse by the husband. The general opinion of most family members was that the abuse would not have happened if the mother had not changed her role to suit her own needs. Only one teenaged daughter was not comfortable with this interpretation, and through this daughter's insights, the family was able to redistribute functions within the family. Three important roles that occur in the scapegoating process were present: the victim or scapegoat was the mother; the persecutor role was taken by most of the other family members; the daughter served as a rescuer.

Within the family, the scapegoat is the symptom bearer for the family. The willingness of the member to assume the role varies. Sometimes the scapegoat will appear to eagerly accept the role of the problem, due to his need to remain in the family and preserve family harmony. At other times, the scapegoat will not want the role, but feels overwhelmed and unaware of having any other choices.

Understanding the concept of scapegoating is important to the nurse. The family member who either presents himself or is presented by the family for treatment often has been scapegoated. The symptoms must be viewed as the family's rather than just the individual's.

Observing and understanding the structure and functioning of the client's family is not just an interesting or academic effort for the nurse. Learning about such things as their rules, themes, myths, roles, distribution of power, and communication patterns will not only allow her to intervene more effectively in the client's illness, but can also help her understand how she is being involved in the dynamics of his family.

☐ Family Therapy

Family therapy is an approach to treating the individual by involving the entire family and treating them as a group. Family therapy became increasingly popular with the idea that the "sick" individual was the symptom bearer for the family's "sick system." The actual process of treating the family will vary according to the particular theoretical model followed by a therapist, but there are some common general principles and forms. These are identified to familiarize the nurse with the process. Nursing process is then discussed in relation to case examples.

LEVELS OF PREVENTION

As in other areas of treatment, the concept of prevention is valuable. The importance of the family in the development of the individual has been stressed throughout this chapter. The potential for health can be increased through prevention. The nurse can see a variety of ways (Table 12-5) in which she can be involved with prevention on a primary, secondary, and tertiary level.

Primary prevention is the intervention that takes place before there is an illness. The focus is on preventing illness rather than on treating one.

Secondary prevention occurs early when the illness is mild and has not proved totally disrup-

TABLE 12-5 Levels of Prevention

Level	Interventions	Goals
Primary	Family life classes in the school system Prenuptial classes for engaged couples Parenting classes for expectant or new parents Communication education courses, for example, on stress management and assertiveness skills Support groups for individuals approaching developmental changes (e.g., retirement support group) Community programs to improve living conditions (cleaning up neighborhoods or the establishment of a good neighbor program)	To assist the family in improving health and coping skills before an illness occurs—through improvement of an individual member's functioning or approaching family as a whole
Secondary	Support groups for families with handicapped or ill members (e.g., ALANON, ALA Teen, groups for parents of terminally ill children) homemaker services, emergency babysitting services for abusive parents, hostels for victims of family abuse Brief outpatient therapy and walk-in clinics	To assist the family to develop new coping and problem-solving skills to contain the effects of the stress and illness. Disruption can be kept at a minimum level
Tertiary	Family therapy done by a trained professional Long-term supportive care such as halfway houses Hospitalization of one or more family members	To assist family to cope with the illness that has proved very disruptive to family system.

tive to the family system. Intervention is directed at an identified population that is known to have a high risk for the development of an illness.

Tertiary prevention is necessary when the disruption is so severe that the family has become dysfunctional. Hospitalization of one or more members may be necessary. The goal at this time is to reestablish health.

THERAPIST QUALIFICATIONS

As the process of family therapy is very complex, a therapist should be specifically trained through formal education and supervision. With basic preparation, the nurse will be able to understand the therapeutic process and integrate family con-

cepts in the clinical setting. This knowledge can increase her effectiveness in a variety of situations, even though it does not prepare her to do formal family therapy.

SELECTION OF CLIENTS

Initially one must decide whether to treat an individual client or the entire family. Elton (1979) says that when one of the following four types of family systems is involved, working with the entire family is the appropriate choice.

1. Scapegoating families. In this family's system, one member is labeled as the sick member and carries the burden for the

family. There is no recognition by the family that they share in the problems.

2. Enmeshed families. Extreme boundary and role diffusion occur in this family. Feelings and ideas are expressed in familial terms rather than on an individual basis. Members will frequently speak for each other.

3. Paranoid-schizoid families. This family's members are also heavily overinvolved with each other. They share a mutual identity to such an extreme degree that, without the family, no self-identity for individual members is available. In short, this means the individual can know who he is only when he is a part of the family.

4. Crisis situations. When there is an identifiable stress or crisis affecting all the members of the family system, the entire family should be involved. Examples of this would be the loss of an important family member through death, or relocation of the family to another community.

Isolation of specific types of families for family therapy does not mean that this form of therapy is not helpful with other families, or that the concepts cannot be useful in individual therapy. It does provide guidelines for the therapist in selecting those families who are most likely to benefit from this approach.

PHASES OF FAMILY THERAPY

The phases of family therapy include assessment, intervention, and evaluation. Although each of these has specific techniques that can be identified, they often overlap. The phases of family therapy can be compared to nursing process. Nursing process differs in that the phase of problem identification is more clearly separated.

Client (Family) Assessment

The initial phase in treatment serves several functions. The first is to establish a contract with the family. Some basic items to be considered are: (1) who will attend the family meetings; (2) when the meetings will occur; (3) where the meetings will occur (in the family's home or the therapist's office); (4) the frequency of meetings; (5) the duration or time expectations for each session; (6) basic rules about involvement (e.g., there will be no hitting, every member will be permitted to talk, no property may be destroyed).

These guidelines may appear very simple and self-evident but need to be clearly stated so that each participant has an understanding of the expectations. This conveys the idea that rules within any system need to be understandable, and allows the therapist to model health communication and negotiation. Another important aspect to setting up a contract in this manner is related to control; the therapist is saying she can and will take control. Many dysfunctional families feel a lack of control and need to feel safe when the present status is threatened by therapy.

Another function of the assessment phase is the emphasis on gathering the baseline data on which to formulate a diagnosis and identify the specific problems needing intervention. Some of the family problems will be clearly stated by the family, and some will be identified through the therapist's observations of the family's interactions. Problems need to be separated into immediate and long term. Some specific observations should be made during the assessment phase:

1. Seating arrangements. Who sits next to whom? Does the family sit in a closed circle or are some members left on the fringes? Do members take the same seats each time or does the pattern vary?

2. Communication patterns. Who talks to whom? What is the information content of messages? Does the information vary depending on to whom the message is addressed? Is the affectional content consistent with the informational content?

3. Statements of expectations. Are rules clearly stated to family members by each other? Do the parents make clear statements of their expectations for each other and for the children?

4. Family history. What information about the extended and nuclear family histories is presented by the parents and the children? When did the couple meet; why did they get married? When were children born, and how was the decision made to have a child? Is there significant information in the family stories that are told?

The information gathered during the assessment phase of treatment can help the therapist to identify the family dynamics and characteristics that show strength or dysfunction within the family system. Based on these data, the interventions are designed.

Interventions

In family therapy, intervention must begin at the time the initial contact is made with the family. As stated earlier, the therapist models clear and goal-directed communication as a way to teach the family better ways of communicating. This is therapeutic intervention. However, the main body of intervention is based on the assessment and observations made in the initial phase. The following are some specific interventions used in treating the family.

Identification and Discussion of Specific Problems. This is done by using material presented by the family in relation to recent or present critical events. A crisis is identified clearly so that all members can understand it as a problem. Then the therapist explores each member's role in the crisis, giving feedback to each member.

The therapist works to increase the flexibility and creativity in the family's methods of problem solving. The family must be actively involved in the process through mutual sharing of information and ideas rather than through instructions given dogmatically. The more the family identifies the solutions as their own, the more committed they will be to follow through with them. Families often have felt locked into a set of behaviors, not seeing that they have alternatives. The act of finding new solutions to one problem can free them to expand their efforts to other problems.

Improving the Communication. The nonverbal and verbal means of communication among family members is identified. This is done through the therapist's feedback and the discussion of each individual's perceptions of what has been communicated. Some common problems that will occur are lack of congruency (consistency) between factual information and the information being presented, lack of congruency between the spoken message and the affectual message, and a tendency for family members to speak for each other.

Lack of congruency between factual information and presented information happens as a result of knowledgeable distortion, because of in-

adequate interpretation skills, or as a result of inaccurate recall due to passage of time or to painful emotions evoked by the facts.

Lack of congruency between the verbal and the nonverbal message often occurs when a felt emotion is not acceptable to the family member. A way the therapist may approach the contrast between these two communication patterns is by focusing on the affect or feeling level and avoiding arguments about what is right or wrong.

One member may answer questions addressed to another member rather than allowing the other member to respond, or by telling his story for him. This can be effectively handled by setting limits on the interfering person, and redirecting the question to the intended family member.

Defining and Renegotiating Family Roles. The therapist helps the family members identify the roles each assumes or is given in the family system. The feelings each one has about his role are discussed. Communication roles, task-oriented roles, and emotional roles are examined. If the roles are unacceptable or dysfunctional, the therapist takes an active part in helping the family negotiate role changes.

Defining and Renegotiating Family Rules. Attention is focused on the overt and covert rules of the family. The rules the family uses are identified and clearly stated to the family for discussion. As with the family roles, the rules are considered in terms of whether they promote health or dysfunction and whether family members feel a need to change them. The overt rules are clearly stated, (e.g., bedtime for the children is 9 o'clock), while the covert rules must be identified from the family's behavior and communication. An example of a covert rule is that only the father in this family can express anger. No other family members openly express their angry feelings.

Evaluation

In the final stages of treatment the task is to help the family identify the ways they have learned to more effectively solve problems and relate to each other, so that they can continue the growth process following therapy. An important aspect is the reinforcement of each individual member's responsibility and worth in the family system as well as to himself as an individual. Evaluation involves summarizing as well as the choosing of goals with the family. The actual termination phase of treatment begins with the evaluation process. At some point the therapist and the family decide that treatment can come to an end. In making this determination, some clues the therapist can use are:

1. Communication among family members is more open and satisfying.
2. Daily problems and conflicts are resolved with a minimal increase in tension levels. Family members are more satisfied with the outcomes.
3. Short- and long-term goals can be defined and are at a realistic level.
4. New behaviors are being internalized, eliminating some of the rigid, ritualistic behavior patterns.

By this process, family members can become more hopeful and in control of their lives. Behavior will be more growth-directed and change will be less threatening.

☐ Nursing Process and Family

Nursing process is compatible with the phases of family therapy. Differences in levels of training between the nurse with basic preparation and the family therapist should be remembered in the consideration of the case history presented, which involves long-standing and complex family problems.

ASSESSMENT

Self-Assessment

As discussed previously, positive involvement with the family by the nurse requires insight into her own ideas of the constitution and functioning of the family. If not recognized, the biases she may have can impede her assessment and intervention with the client and his family.

If she believes, for example, that all parents are loving and that family members always care about and nurture each other, it will make it difficult for her to recognize illness or dysfunctional patterns. A good understanding of how she feels about her own family is essential in keeping her own needs from interfering with the needs of the family with whom she is intervening.

Client Assessment

The assessment method outlined in the section on family therapy is a good guideline for the nurse to use in her assessment of the family. In addition, the nurse will want to obtain information about the family's relationship with the community. For example, how involved are members with individuals and groups outside the immediate family? Is the extended family available to the nuclear family for support? One other area of major importance is the appraisal of community resources available to the family in regard to material concerns and health care. Is there adequate food, clothing, and housing available? Does the family have access to facilities for its general health care?

PROBLEM IDENTIFICATION

The nursing diagnosis can be effectively applied to care of the family as well as the individual. The nurse is encouraged to apply this tool to make both the identification of problems and the appropriate interventions easily communicated to others. Examples of nursing diagnoses as applied to the family are given in Table 12-6.

TABLE 12-6 Nursing Diagnosis

A client is hospitalized for treatment of a medical or psychiatric problem. There is separation from the family, and the individual is not able to function in his usual way. The feelings of fear and anxiety are usually present when there is an illness. The following are possible diagnoses that could be made for this family.

1. Impairment in fulfilling family functions and activities as a result of separation from family.
2. Inadequate family coping as a result of anxiety about health status of individual member.
3. Inadequate communication among family members as a result of anxiety.
4. Disruption of family support system as a result of inadequate coping mechanisms of individual member.
5. Inadequate coping mechanisms of family as a result of insufficient knowledge about individual member's illness.
6. Impaired problem-solving skills as a result of denial of individual or family illness.
7. Inadequate role fulfillment as a result of fear about possible impairment from illness.

INTERVENTION AND EVALUATION

Whether in the psychiatric or the medical-surgical setting, the interventions used by the nurse are related to goals that are based on the nursing diagnosis. The evaluation will allow the nurse to determine whether the interventions are successful or if alternatives need to be implemented.

The following case study (see below) of intervention by a nurse trained in family therapy includes nursing diagnoses as well as discussion of interventions and will assist the nurse in applying nursing process to the family setting.

The discussion of this family's management covers a limited number of the interventions that were used to promote a higher level of health and function in this family system. It is meant to serve as a guide for the nurse in building her own approaches to the family. It is important to assess the degree of family dysfunction and level of intervention that is required. Many situations are best dealt with by the nurse who is already involved in the family, while others are more appropriately managed by referral to a family therapist.

EVALUATION

Evaluation is a process of summarizing and reflecting upon the effects of therapy. It is done by observing the amount of change in the family's behavior in relation to the goals that were mutually established. In addition, this time is used to help the family formulate other goals for themselves and define some ways in which they can be reached.

■ Enrichment Activities

DISCUSSION QUESTIONS

1. Explore the relationship of physical, psychological, and/or social development changes to the role changes that occur within the family.

2. Identify and explore the differences between individual therapy and family therapy in relation to the functions of the psychiatric nurse as a therapist.

3. Discuss the meaning of the term "family" in your own personal belief system and how that affects your response to nontraditional families.

4. Consider the effects of societal and/or cultural changes (e.g., separation from extended family) and their effect on family functioning.

5. Present and discuss a case example in which you interviewed the family. Identify your database, interventions, and nursing diagnosis. Evaluate these with your fellow students.

Case Study

Mr. and Mrs. W. were referred for treatment of their son to a mental health center by the school counselor. Mark was 10 years old and was having persistent behavioral problems. Mark and his parents had already been called in by the school for special conferences on a number of occasions. The focus of these conferences was on Mark's unruly behavior, for example, teasing other children, leaving his desk without permission, talking out of turn. In addition, Mark's teacher expressed concern about his marginal academic performance. She believed Mark was brighter and more capable then was reflected in his work.

After Mark was seen for an initial evaluation, the entire family was asked to come in for sessions. Mark's parents were reluctant to do so, since it was "Mark who was having the problem" and his sister Sally was "too young for something like this." Sally was 5 years of age. Agreement was finally reached and all members of the family began to attend the therapy sessions. This initiated the formation of a treatment contract and began to establish a trust relationship.

Assessment and Problem Identification □ It was noted that during the initial sessions Mark's parents sat next to each other, with Sally sitting on one of their laps or next to them. Mark generally sat isolated from them, usually across the room. Before the sessions began, the chairs were arranged in a circle with equal spacing between them. The family would move the chairs to achieve the split in seating. (Nsg. Dx.—Impaired family communication process as a result of isolation of a family member.)

A family history was taken. Mark's parents described uneventful and typical courtship, marriage, and childbearing periods of time in their lives, during which they considered theirs a happy family. They both identified the time that Mark started misbehaving as shortly after his sister was born. Mrs. W. said that Sally was always such a cute and well-behaved little girl; she thought Mark was just jealous and had developed a mean streak. It should be noted that even before the birth of Sally, Mark had been using much the same behavior but a great deal of importance had not been attached to it. Mr. W. would dismiss it as normal, saying that "Boys will be boys." The change in their perception of Mark occurred when he started hurting Sally. (Nsg. Dx.—Impaired family role function as a result of changed role expectations without adequate support from other family members.)

A family myth that became apparent through the family history was that Mark was just like his uncle, who was "bad." Mr. W. had been teased and at times physically hurt by his older brother while growing up. Mark's parents identified his behavior as a mean streak, just like his uncle's. Mark's temperament, and even physical characteristics, were compared to his uncle's. Mark was being given a message to be bad and then would be punished for displaying the expected behavior. (Nsg. Dx.—Impaired family role function resulting from double-bind communication.) Mark's differentness from the rest of his primary family was also reinforced when his parents would ask why he just couldn't be good like his sister and get along with people like the rest of the family.

The nurse noted that Mark was the scapegoat or symptom bearer for the family. Whenever a subject was discussed in which the tension for the family members increased, Mark would become increasingly disruptive by banging his chair against the wall or teasing his sister. The focus would then shift to Mark and identify him as the problem. Mr. W. to Mark, "Why can't we do anything without you making trouble?" Mark acted as the scapegoat and as the third member of a family triangle with his parents. (Nsg. Dx.—Ineffective family coping as a result of scapegoating of a family member.)

The communication patterns in Mark's family were disrupted. Mark experienced confusion about the messages he received from his parents. Two behaviors were identified that related to this. First, the verbal and affectual aspects of the message were often conflicting. For example, Mark would frequently be told by his parents that they were not angry, yet they were frowning and using angry tones while speaking to him. Second, there were many messages in which there were distortions that were presented as factual. Mr. W. would say, "Mark doesn't want to get along with

people, but prefers to fight and make trouble." It was later learned that Mark felt sad about how he got along with people but did not know how to change. (Nsg. Dx.—Ineffective communication patterns as a result of a lack of consistency in messages.)

Mark's family also had problems of the family structure. Although Mr. and Mrs. W. denied there were problems in their relationship, they frequently had conflict when they were unaware of each other's wants. In addition, if wants or needs were expressed, one of them would typically respond to the request from the other in a negative way, by pointing out how, in fact, he already had to do too much and was not getting enough in return. They were distanced from each other. Mr. W. was involved in his work and activities with his male friends, while Mrs. W. spent most of her time at home with the children. Much of the home responsibility was left to her to manage, and she in turn assigned certain responsibilities to Mark and Sally. Confusion resulted at the times when Mr. W. was more available at home. This caused changes in the established patterns and relationships. Mrs. W. and the children had settled on routines of doing the dishes and other household chores. When Mr. W. would attempt to exert parental authority and assign different duties, Mrs. W. would become defensive and angry. She would then give the children permission to do the tasks in the usual way and not as their father instructed them. Mr. W. would become angry and accuse his children and wife of not respecting him. (Nsg. Dx.—Ineffective parenting resulting from parental power struggles.)

Intervention □ Working with the W. family included a variety of interventions. The methods used were as follow:

Establishing a Trust Relationship. As stated earlier in the discussion of family therapy, the nurse models clear and goal-directed communication when setting up the contract. It is also the beginning of a trust relationship. The nurse lets the family members know what they can expect from her in the relationship, and she conveys some of her expectations for them. The contract with the W. family included who would attend, how frequently sessions would occur, and what guidelines or rules for accepted behavior applied during the meetings. The contract also helped to establish mutual goals (family-identified goals and goals identified by the nurse) for the treatment process. (These elements were covered more completely in the discussion of family therapy.)

(continued)

Important parts of the trust relationship are patience and realistic expectations. Change in the family is a difficult process.

Identification and Discussion of Family Issues.
In the W. family, Mark was identified as being the "problem." There was no insight into the difficulties between other family members and into the problems of the family structure itself. There was no recognition that other family members could be involved, in any way, in how Mark behaved. He was identified as being totally responsible. For example, Mr. W. frequently encouraged Mark's behavior even though he complained about it as well. The nurse helped Mr. W. understand this by pointing out that he encouraged Mark when he told him boys were tough and he needed to learn to take care of himself "like his old man." Mark's father "took care of Mark" when he acted up by slapping or spanking him. When Mark would copy his father's behavior and use aggression to express his upset feelings, Mr. W. would scold or hit Mark for picking on others. Reviewing this and similar behavioral cycles with Mr. W. allowed him to understand how he shared a part in the problem.

The nurse then talked with Mr. W. and Mark about other ways for Mr. W. to respond to Mark's aggressive behavior. One agreement that Mark and his father made was that Mr. W. would not hit Mark and Mark would listen to what his father had to say, instead of continuing the disruptive behavior until he was hit. These interventions achieved the goal of improving ineffective family role functions resulting from incorrect, conflicting expectations.

Another aspect of the identification of Mark as the problem related to his scapegoating by the family. Mark's mother and sister contributed to maintaining the focus of family issues on Mark. Sally would frequently exaggerate what Mark had done to her when they fought. Since an issue in this family was the inability to directly express angry feelings, Sally found a way to express them indirectly. When Mark was spanked by his mother or father, Sally was able to express her aggression by seeing Mark spanked. Mrs. W. unquestioningly accepted Sally's interpretation of an incident between her and her brother because of the "fact" that Mark was mean. After discussing this, it was agreed that if Mrs. W. did not actually see the fight, or see evidence that Mark had hit Sally, she would punish neither of them, but physically separate them for a period. This intervention helped achieve the goal of improving family coping. (Nsg. Dx.—Ineffective family coping as a result of scapegoating of a family member.)

Assisting Family Members with Communication.
As stated before, there existed inconsistencies in the W. family's communication. Mrs. W. would frequently deny she was angry even though she sat with her mouth set in a frown, her voice raised, and her fists clenched. Rather than challenging the denial, the nurse would assist Mrs. W. to explore her fears about being angry and showing anger to others. For example, "I wonder if you could tell me what you think happens when people get angry?" In addition, the nurse would ask Mrs. W. to define an angry behavior she was displaying. For example, "What do you think your fists are saying right now?"

Inconsistency was also noted between factual information and presented information. Mr. and Mrs. W. frequently distorted information in processing events that occurred between them. Distortion of the facts occurred because of defensiveness and anger. The nurse dealt with this by shifting the focus from the factual content to the emotional content. For example, "I'm not sure that who is right or wrong is most important right now. You both sound very upset and I'm wondering what you think that means about how you are feeling." The feelings could then be more clearly stated and the underlying needs of each person more clearly identified.

Both of these examples have to do with the goal of increasing the effective communication by increasing the consistency in the messages. (Nsg. Dx.—Ineffective communication patterns as a result of lack of consistency in messages.)

Assisting Family Members in Fulfilling Family Functions.
In exploring the problem of who should have the authority, it was noted that both parents had ambivalent feelings about this position. Mr. W. was, in fact, the primary disciplinarian and Mrs. W. would frequently threaten the children with what would happen when their father got home. Mr. W. said he always felt like the "bad guy" as he would get home and be expected to start "spanking on his kids." His anger at his wife for assigning him this role began to shift to Mark as he was the one most frequently identified as needing a spanking. The nurse helped Mr. and Mrs. W. to problem-solve and reach an agreement to share the discipline more. This changed Mr. W.'s role as the punisher enough to allow him to feel he could also relate to the children on a happier level. His anger toward his wife decreased, allowing him to give her more support. A more unified front was presented to the children. These interventions were intended to improve the parental functioning of Mr. and Mrs. W. (Nsg. Dx.—Ineffective parenting resulting from parental power struggles.)

LEARNING ACTIVITIES

The following are to be done by the student with a client with whom she is working. These are a few examples of exercises that can be helpful in understanding a family's interactions.

1. Identify a family myth. Ask the client about his family. Identify any stories that convey a family myth, such as: The Jones have always been of hearty stock, never needed to see a doctor. This can help give information about covert family rules.

2. Identify an overt family rule. Ask the client about what he knows is or isn't allowed in his family (e.g., no talking back to their parents by children; the time a child has to be home).

3. Have the client draw a family picture. When doing this, consider how family members are placed on the paper in relation to one another, or if they appear at all. Also, whether the members are shown doing an activity, and what the activity is. This gives information about roles and individual status within the family.

4. Identify a triangular relationship within his family. Talk with him about who is close to whom in the family. This can give information about family roles and how reinforcement is given to individuals.

5. Identify some of the family's communication patterns. Look at who talks to whom and the affect that is used when speaking to various members.

6. Identify the significant people for the client within and outside the family. Whom does the client feel emotionally close to or severely distanced from?

■ Recommended Readings

Agee, J. *A death in the family*. New York: Bantam Books, 1967. Explores the dynamics and process of a family when a member dies. Focus is on the family's experience as a basic human occurrence rather than as a pathological event. The family's experience is universal and therefore a valuable resource for the nurse.

Bartlett, K., and Nicinski, D. Family nursing: A theory that works. *Canadian Nurse*, 79, 1983:46–49. Presents clear, understandable guidelines for involvement of the nurse with families. Examples are given that are related to medical-surgical settings.

Kramer, C. *Becoming a family therapist—Developing an integrated approach to working with families*. New York: Human Science Press, 1980. Discusses the treatment process, pitfalls, treatment failures, and ways to approach them. Very readable and easily understood. Good for the beginning family therapist.

Leaderer, E., and Jackson, D. *The mirage of marriage*. New York: Norton, 1968. Discusses reasons marriages fail and how individuals can change to improve a marriage. Covers false assumptions about marriage, how to appraise the marriage relationship, elements of a satisfactory marriage. Gives clear, easily understood examples.

Miller, S., Nunnaly, E.W., and Wackman, D.B. *Alive and aware*. Minneapolis, MN: Interpersonal Communication Program, Inc., 1975. Covers relationships and communication within the couple and family. Good tool for understanding and teaching communication skills.

Walsh, W. *A primer in family therapy*. Springfield, IL: Charles C. Thomas, 1980. Analyzes several models of family therapy, allowing the reader to compare and contrast them. Good basic reference book for the beginner.

■ References

Ackerman, N. *The psychodynamics of family life*. New York: Basic Books, 1958.

Ackerman, N. *Family process*. New York: Basic Books, 1970.

Beavers, W., and Voeller, M. Family models: Comparing and contrasting the olson circumplex model with the beavers systems model. *Family process*, 22, 1983:85–98.

Bowen, M. The use of family theory in clinical practice. *Comprehensive psychiatry*, 7, 1966:345–374.

Box, S. The elucidation of a family myth. *Journal of family therapy*, 1, 1979:75–86.

Braverman, S. Family of origin as a training resource for family therapists. *Canadian journal of psychiatry*, 27, 1982:629–633.

Byng-Hall, J. Re-editing family mythology during family therapy. *Journal of family therapy*, 1, 1979:103–116.

Dare, C., and Lindsey, C. Children in family therapy. *Journal of family therapy*, 1, 1979:253–269.

Dunn, G. When the family must change too . . . each member of the family is an influencing factor in mental illness. *Nursing mirror*, 155, 1982:28–29.

Dydyk, B., French, G., Gertsman, C., and Morrison, N. Admission of whole families. *Canadian journal of psychiatry*, 27, 1982:640–643.

Elton, A. Indications for selecting family or individual therapy. *Journal of family therapy*, 1, 1979:193–207.

Ferreira, A. Family myth and homeostasis. *Archives of general psychiatry*, 9, 1963:457–63.

Ford, F. Rules: The invisible family. *Family process*, 22, 1983:135–145.

Golan, N. *Passing through transitions*. New York: Free Press, 1981.

Haley, J. *Problem solving therapy*. San Francisco: Jossey-Bass, 1976.

Haley, J., and Hoffman, L. *Techniques of family therapy*. New York: Basic Books, 1967.

Jackson, D. *Communication, family and marriage*. Palo Alto, CA: Science and Behavior, 1968.

Jenkins, H. A life cycle framework in the treatment of underorganized families. *Journal of family therapy*, 5, 1983:359–377.

Jones, S.L. *Family therapy: A comparison of approaches*. Bowie, MD: Robert J. Brady, Co., 1980.

Jones, S., and Dimond, M. Family theory and family therapy models: comparative review with implications for nursing practice. *Journal of psychosocial nursing and mental health services*, 20, 1982:12–19.

Jung, M. Directions for building family development theory. *Social casework*, 64, 1983:363–370.

Lanta, J., and Treece, N. Identity operations and family treatment. *Journal of psychosocial nursing and mental health services*, 20, 1982:20–23.

Loader, P., Kingston, W., and Stratford, J. Is there a 'psychosomatogenic' family? *Journal of family therapy*, 2, 1980:311–326.

Lyles, M.R. Myths and strengths of the black family: A historical and sociocultural contribution to family therapy. *Journal of the national medical association*, 74, 1982:1119–1123.

McNabb, R. Family function and depression. *Journal of family practice*, 16, 1983:169–170.

Minuchin, S., and Fishman, C. *Family therapy techniques*. Cambridge, MA: Harvard University Press, 1981.

Olson, D., Russell, C., and Sprenkle, D. Circumplex model of marital and family systems: VI. Theoretical update. *Family process*, 22, 1983:69–83.

Patterson, Gerald. *Families*. Champaign, IL: Research Press, 1975.

Satir, Virginia. *Conjoint family therapy*. Palo Alto, CA: Science and Behavior, 1972.

Seltzer, W., and Seltzer, M. Magic, material and myth. *Family process*, 22, 1983:3–14.

Swanson, A., and Hurley, P. Family systems: values and value conflicts. *Journal of psychosocial nursing and mental health services*, 21, 1983:24–30.

Viaro, M., and Leonard, P. Getting and giving information: Analysis of a family interview strategy. *Family process*, 22, 1983:27–42.

Watzlawick, P., Beavin, S.H., and Jackson, D.D. *Pragmatics of human communication*. New York: Norton, 1967.

Wechter, S. Separation difficulties between parents and young adults. *Social casework*, 64, 1983:97–104.

Will, D. Some techniques for working with resistant families of adolescents. *Journal of adolescents*, 6, 1983:13–26.

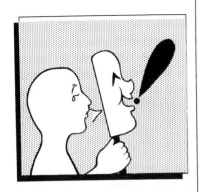

13

Group Dynamics and Leadership Interventions

Joan Norris

Learning Objectives

Upon completion of this chapter, the reader will be able to:

1. Discuss a variety of goals and levels of prevention appropriate to the nurse's use of a group approach.

2. Differentiate the goals and strategies used in various group approaches valuable to nursing practice including therapeutic groups, socialization groups, and task groups.

3. Apply knowledge of group theory in assessing group structure, stages of group process, interaction patterns, and membership roles.

4. Identify needs of the group and of individual members based on assessments of group dynamics.

5. Describe interventions that may be directed to the group as a whole and to individual members in order to promote group process and effectiveness.

6. Identify methods of evaluating group process, goal attainment, and leadership effectiveness.

7. Delineate appropriate role and preparation of the nurse in relation to leadership for various group approaches.

Group approaches can be used to enhance nursing practice and patient care in various settings to meet many diverse objectives. The functions of the nurse as educator, mental health promotor, interpersonal facilitator, socializer, problem solver, and supporter may all be implemented in groups. Nurses frequently find themselves in groups as a part of their work environment, whether the focus is planning care as a member of the health team, working on specific tasks such as policy making and planning, or facilitating groups of patients in working toward particular goals. The nurse may choose to use the benefits of a group approach in preparing clients for general aspects of surgery prior to individualized teaching, in providing guidance to parents on childbirth and child rearing, or in meeting health education needs of various ages and populations. Group support can enhance the ability of clients and significant others to cope with disability, chronic or life-threatening illness, bereavement, or other stressful events. Socialization may be a major focus of groups designed to improve skills of chronically mentally impaired patients or to decrease the loneliness and isolation of some elderly in either residential care or community settings. Nurses may also serve as organizers or resource persons to self-help groups.

Nurses who work in psychiatric settings generally serve as facilitators or coleaders of community or client government group meetings, problem-solving and small therapy groups in inpatient settings for clients and families. With increasing awareness of the needs of nurses to have basic group facilitation skills and to be comfortable with them, nursing education is providing additional theory and practice in these areas. Formerly, the nurse in generalized practice had to develop these skills through continuing education or on-the-job training.

The focus of this chapter is to provide a basic understanding of group dynamics and group leadership for nursing practice. The nurse who wishes to expand on this knowledge and practice would seek graduate level preparation as a clinical specialist in psychiatric-mental health nursing and, with additional supervised theory and training, would be qualified to practice as a cotherapist or therapist in outpatient and community settings.

☐ *Beginning Group Membership*

The initial introduction to working with a group is generally accomplished through being a member (a participant observer) in a group. This permits the beginner to experience group membership, apply theory, and observe a more experienced person in the role of leader. Initial participation in a group generates concerns and anxieties similar to those the nurse has when initiating the nurse-client relationship. (Will I be accepted? Will I say the right thing? Will I do harm?) These and other concerns often preoccupy the novice on entering a group and may inhibit participation. These uncertainties are similar to those experienced by any member beginning a group and are best dealt with by talking with the clinical instructor or group leader and remembering that the nurse, like other members of the group, has feelings and experiences to share as a person and that nonparticipation can be perceived as a barrier by other members of the group. This is not to suggest that student feelings or problems become a focus of the group (unless that is the stated group goal) but that students who actively participate in a genuine way to promote group goals and cohesiveness are better accepted in groups.

☐ *Basic Terms*

Some major concepts of group work are; group process, group dynamics, structure, goals, and leadership. *Group process and group dynamics* are general terms used somewhat interchangeably to describe the development and changes that take place in a group. Specific stages and issues are likely to arise in individual members and in the life of the group itself as it forms, interacts, and develops. *Structure* refers to the basic purpose, types of members, and expectations of groups. The term is also used as a verb to describe the ways in which leaders and members communicate their purpose and expectations to the group as a whole. A leader may choose to provide a high degree of structure in, for instance, a health education group by initially defining the exact objectives to be met, the method and content of presentation, and a format for questions and application. In another situation a leader may provide less structure (as in a coping group) with a simple statement that "in this hour each week we will talk about ways of dealing with feelings and everyday problems." This latter approach provides the group and its members the opportunity and responsibility for defining and working through the issues and problems for discussion. *Goals or objectives* for a group may vary widely from provid-

TABLE 13-1 Relationship of Curative Factors to Goals and Outcomes of Groups[a]

Objectives		Psychotherapy	Human Relations	Learning	Socialization	Task	Support
Process	Instillation of hope	X		X			X
	Universality	X	X	X	X		X
	Imparting information	X	X	XX		X	X
	Altruism	X	X	X	X		X
	Corrective family group	X					
	Developing socializing techniques	X			XX		
	Imitative behavior	X	X	X			
	Interpersonal learning	XX	XX				X
	Group cohesiveness	X	X	X	X	X	XX
	Catharsis	X					
	Existential factors	X					
	Task orientation			X		XX	
Outcomes	Maintenance	Low	Low	Low	High	Low	High
	Learning	Med	High	High	Low	Med	Med
	Behavior change	High	Med	High	Low	Med	Low

[a] Reprinted with permission from Loomis, Maxine, E. *Group Process for Nurses.* St. Louis: C. V. Mosby, 1979:42

ing information, learning more effective ways to relate to others, experiencing the sense of belonging to a group, sharing feelings and insights, or many combinations of these and other goals. *Leadership* is the quality that enables the group to interact effectively and move toward its goals. The interrelationship of these concepts will become clearer as the theory and application of nursing process in group dynamics is developed throughout the chapter. Table 13-1 depicts these relationships.

☐ *Assessment*

Assessment in groups serves the same purpose as individual assessment. It serves to focus observations and apply theoretical knowledge in identifying problems and needs of the group in order to plan appropriate interventions. This process in-

volves looking at the content discussed in the group, themes suggested by the content, and the dynamics of the interactions occurring in the group over time. Data to be collected include: (1) a description of the physical environment in which the group meets, (2) the directional flow of the conversation and variations in contributions by the participants, (3) the content and general themes of discussion, (4) nonverbal participation of members, and (5) the stage of group process as evidenced by individual members and the group as a whole.

THE PHYSICAL ENVIRONMENT

The physical setting in which a group meets affects interaction in various ways that may enhance or inhibit communication. The room in which the group meets should be of an appropriate size. A small group in a huge room may cause members to feel uncomfortable and isolated. The group may spread out, increasing the distance between members and thus decreasing interaction. A large group in too small a room leads to crowding, discomfort, and difficulty in seeing all of the members; naturally this has the same effect of decreasing participation and interaction. Comfort factors such as temperature, ventilation, and the general attractiveness of the surroundings are important in how members view the group and, if sufficiently negative to cause discomfort, may be distractions and barriers to interaction. Chairs should be arranged in a close circle so that each person can see all of the other members without having to strain or change position. The presence of a large table may promote comfort but decrease awareness of members' nonverbal actions. A sense of privacy permits members to converse freely and promotes the confidentiality so vital to open communication. The presence of smoking, beverages, or snacks, if permitted, also affects group dynamics. Some group members may be distressed by others' smoking, and eating or drinking during meetings generally promotes a social atmosphere but may distract the group from more serious interaction. This needs to be addressed in relation to the overall goals for the group. The decision to permit or discourage these activities during group may be made by the leader or by the group.

■ Point of Emphasis

Assess the setting to eliminate distracting noises, discomforts, or barriers to attention and interaction.

Although it is rare to achieve the ideal setting for group, assessment of the physical environment is essential to promote effective interaction. This is of particular importance since the physical setting has powerful effects and is the most easily changed factor in group dynamics.

GROUP MEMBERSHIP

The composition of the group has a vital relationship to structure and goals. The number of members affects the degree and depth of participation possible. A therapeutic community or self-government group may have as many as 30 or more members with all patients and staff on a unit included. In general, the recommended size for a small group is 8 to 15 for optimal involvement of all.

Larger groups limit opportunities for participation, while very small groups of three or four tend to lose their effectiveness. Staff and students should not outnumber other members of the group. Membership may be homogeneous—alike in significant factors such as age, sex, and identified problems; or it may be heterogeneous—characterized by diversity. Homogeneous groups may be unified by shared interests and problems such as womens' issues (e.g., displaced homemakers, coping with widowhood), support in chronic or debilitating illness (e.g., diabetic teens, arthritic clients, parents of retarded children), or bereavement, although members may of course differ in other respects. Heterogeneous groups constitute a social microcosm—a small cross-section of the larger population that provides richer opportunities for varied interactions and increased understanding of other people.

In planning or assessing the makeup of a group, the nurse must be alert to attributes that might cause a member to feel isolated or less a part of the group. Such characteristics might be sex, age, culture, race, economic status, or educational level. Being the only male or elderly person in a group does not necessarily create a sense of isolation, but the observer needs to be aware of the potential for the problem to occur.

STAGES OF GROUP PROCESS

The assessment of the stage of group process is more complex and involves attention to the content of group discussions, themes of content, the emotional tone of the group, and identification of the phase of development in the group (Table 13-2). These stages have been variously described and numbered. Most simply, there are three broad developmental phases: (1) the *initial* or *introductory* stage in which the issues are group membership, leadership, and purpose, (2) the *intermediate* or *working* stage characterized by group cohesiveness and goal-directed activity; and (3) the *final*, or *termination*, phase in which the issues of achievements, separation, and loss must be worked through. Some members may be in a different phase from that of the group as a whole, either because of individual factors, or because of entering the group later than others.

Initial or Introductory Phase

The initial or introductory phase in a group is characterized by uncertainty and reliance on the designated leader (or, if none is designated, a

TABLE 13-2 Stages and Issues In Group Process[a]

Phase	Schultz 1960 (Interpersonal need focus)	Bales 1955 (Task focus)	Tuckman 1965 (Group behavior focus)	Bion 1959 (Evolving ways of coping with core issues of engulfment vs. estrangement)
Initial	Inclusion (Who belongs?)	Orientation (What is the task?)	Forming (Coming together; identifying purpose of and resources in the group)	Fight vs. flight (Avoidance of conflict as a means of handling anxiety)
	Control (Who is in charge?)	Evaluation (How does the group feel about it?)	Storming (conflicts about leadership)	
Intermediate	Affection (Caring and closeness)	Control (What should we do about the task?)	Norming (Establish rules and a sense of closeness)	Dependency (On leader or group as a whole)
			Performing (Working on task or purpose)	Pairing (Subgroup formation and attraction)
Termination	Termination (Dealing with separation			

[a] *Sources:* Compiled from Schultz, W. C. *FIRO: A three-dimensional theory of human behavior,* New York: Holt, Rinehart & Winston, 1960; Bales, R. F. The equilibrium problem in small groups. In, *Small Groups* (Hare, A. P., Borgatta, E. F., and Bales, R. F., eds.). New York: Alfred Knopf, 1955; Tuckman, B. Developmental sequence in small groups. *Psychological bulletin,* 63, 1965:384–399, and Bion, W.R. *Experiences in groups,* New York: Basic Books, 1959.

search for leadership) and concerns about acceptance and belonging as a member of the group. Communication is generally directed toward the leader or dominant members. Content of the discussion is often of a tentative nature (e.g., asking questions and inquiring about goals and direction). Sharing of ideas and feelings is generally guarded and hesitant. Content themes often relate to uncertainty, direction seeking, and acceptance. The feeling tone of the group is characterized by anxiety and a desire to please. Members may assume various social roles such as that of host or hostess (making introductions and engaging in social pleasantries), organizer (inquiring of or suggesting goals or procedures for the group), or tension-reliever (making humorous remarks). As the group continues in this phase, the focus of discussion may change to individual frustrations directed toward the leader or the group, or may be less directly manifested by discussing events outside the group, or scapegoating of a particular member who becomes a focus for individual or group frustration. Other themes might include griping, power or control, mistrust, and leader-

ship as the members begin to come to grips with the difficulties of becoming an accepted member, competing for the attentions of the leader and group, and expressing their preferences for the group. The feeling tone becomes angry. Members may engage in overt verbal attacks or decrease their attempts to participate, sitting in uneasy silence. Silences may give rise to a power struggle with the leader, or members may become very anxious and attempt to fill any pause in conversation with irrelevant chatter or forced participation. Individuals may exhort the group to get down to business or come to an agreement on the goals or focus. Less direct behaviors may include complaining about the world situation, administrative issues, or other factors over which the group has little or no control. Coalitions may form among members, and subgroups develop. Nonverbal behaviors common to this stage include limited eye contact, tardiness or absence, increasing distance or pulling back from the circle, and "closed" body language. After overt expressions of anger or frustration, the group may retreat for a time to its former polite hesitance.

As the group members become more comfort-able and open with each other in working through the issues of the introductory phase, a sense of group cohesiveness and acceptance of members as individuals develops. The group reaches a sense of agreement on goals and expectations but has also grown in its ability to tolerate and accept in-dividual differences and expressions of dissent. Members are more open in expressing views and feelings. Leadership issues are resolved as group members become more confident, and sharing of leadership roles often results among one or more members of the group.

Intermediate or Working Phase

The intermediate or working phase results from the achievements of the group in working through the issues of the previous stage. Communication patterns are now more evenly distributed as mem-bers interact with each other rather than focusing on the leader. Norms for group behavior are es-tablished and accepted. Discussions now tend to be more relevant to the goals of the group and the interrelationships within it. The feeling tone var-ies with the group themes and goals but is gen-erally characterized by trust, cohesiveness, and hopefulness. Of course disruptions may occur, and not all members may be actively involved. For some people, the highest level of participation may be active listening and thoughtful consid-eration of the discussion. This can be assessed through awareness of individual attention and nonverbal cues. Behaviors observed at this stage include help seeking; problem solving; sharing of opinions, perceptions, and feelings; attempts to include others; and positive support and reinforce-ment. Members may linger after group or form friendships outside of the group.

The Stage of Termination

The stage of termination occurs when members are scheduled to leave the group or the group is to be disbanded. Separation creates anxiety and feelings of loss. Communication patterns may re-main open or may revert to earlier patterns be-cause members feel less secure and attempt to avoid painful topics. Some may regress to behav-iors exhibited earlier in group. Successful reso-lution of the termination phase involves actively working through the issues and feelings. Content themes may relate to inability to resolve prior losses, lack of confidence in ability to cope without the support of the leader and the group, and dif-ficulty in or avoidance of saying goodbye. Sadness and anxiety are common. Group members being left behind may feel envious. Behaviors demon-strated vary widely and may include avoidance (prematurely terminating attendance or attend-ing but not discussing the issue); gift giving (me-mentos or food); expressions of loss, reassurance, and support; reviewing of individual or group achievements; expressions of good wishes and hopes of retaining the sense of cohesiveness either in memory or through hope of future contacts. Nonverbal behavior may include either increased or decreased eye contact, tears, handshakes, and hugs.

COMMUNICATION PATTERNS

In assessing the communication patterns in groups, it is useful to diagram interactions. A sim-ple tool is a sketch of the group circle with mem-bers labeled by initials. Each member's comments are then depicted by arrows directed to the person addressed. A two-way arrow indicates mutual in-teraction. Lines are made heavier when addi-tional comments flow in the same direction. Ques-tions or comments directed toward the group in general are shown as an arrow pointing to the center of the circle. Diagrams may illustrate changes in patterns from the beginning to the end of a group or from one group meeting to the next. This approach assists in identifying the style of interactions, such as group reliance on the leader, domination of interaction by one or more members or a particular subgroup, or shared participation by the majority of group members. Figures 13-1 and 13-2 show typical patterns of interaction observed in the initial and intermediate stages of group process, respectively. Diagrams should not be drawn while the group is meeting but are a useful tool for recalling interaction patterns immediately following a group.

IDENTIFICATION OF NEEDS AND PROBLEMS IN GROUPS

The purpose of assessment in groups is to identify the needs of the group in terms of the stage of group process and the general needs of the group in relation to overall goals, and to recognize factors that impede group dynamics. The identification of these needs or problems permits planning and implementation of appropriate interventions.

Needs at Specific Stages

Whether spoken or unspoken, groups have particular needs based on the current stage of group process.

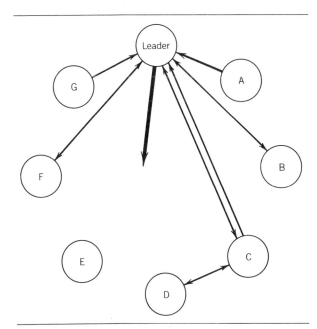

Figure 13-1 First meeting of the group shows a common communication pattern in the introductory phase of a group. The leader is the focus of the interactions as several comments (heavy arrow) are directed to the group as a whole. Several members (A, B, C, F, G) interact with the leader, E interacts with no one and only C and D interact with each other as members of the group.

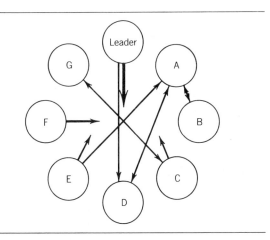

Figure 13-2 Meeting number 16. More complex and evenly distributed interaction patterns are characteristic of the working phase of a group.

1. Initial phase needs include becoming acquainted with others in the group, establishing a climate of trust and acceptance and clarifying the basic purpose and expectations (norms) for group.
2. Intermediate phase needs include elaboration and acceptance of group norms, focusing of support and feedback on problem-solving activities, summarizing, and recognition of participation and achievements.
3. Termination phase needs include dealing with feelings about separation, summarizing accomplishments, and placing these in the context of life experiences.

General Needs of Groups

Several theorists have attempted to identify the behaviors and factors that promote effectiveness in groups. Bales (1958) described two major factors: *task roles* which promote the specific work of the group and *maintenance roles* which promote group harmony and cohesiveness. Yalom (1967, 1975), with others, has investigated the curative factors that operate in groups, by interviewing successful clients and group leaders. These roles and the communication functions relevant to them, when combined with the conditions described as curative factors, provide a basis for understanding the therapeutic or basic needs of groups. They may be present in varying degrees and at various times for different types of groups. Together they form the theoretical basis for identification of group needs.

Bale's task and maintenance roles have been elaborated on by numerous theorists (Table 13-3). These functions are essential not only in group leadership, but to the group as a whole, especially as the group reaches the working phase.

Yalom's (1975) curative factors are eleven conditions that promote therapeutic effectiveness in group.

1. Instillation of hope refers to the attitude that present difficulties can be borne with the expectation of change. This may result from viewing the progress of others and the expectation that, through the support and help of the group, one can be more effective in living.

2. Universality is the sense of not being alone in one's problems. Through sharing experiences, members of the group learn that others experience similar difficulties and dilemmas.

3. Imparting information includes relating

TABLE 13-3 Task and Maintenance Roles and Functions in Groups[a]

Task Roles	Maintenance Roles	Task Roles and Maintenance Roles
Initiating activity: proposing solutions, suggesting new ideas, new definitions of the problem, new attack on the problem, or new organization of material	*Encouraging:* being friendly, warm, responsive to others, praising others and their ideas, agreeing with and accepting contributions of others	*Evaluating:* submitting group decisions or accomplishments to comparison with group standards, measuring accomplishments against goals
Seeking information: asking for clarification of suggestions, requesting additional information or facts	*Gatekeeping:* trying to make it possible for another member to make a contribution to the group by saying "We haven't heard anything from Jim yet," or suggesting limited talking time for everyone so that all will have a chance to be heard	*Diagnosing:* determining sources of difficulties, appropriate steps to take next, analyzing the main blocks to progress
Seeking opinion: looking for an expression of feeling about something from the members, seeking clarification of values, suggestions, or ideas	*Standard setting:* expressing standards for the group to use in choosing its content or procedures or in evaluating its decisions, reminding group to avoid decisions which conflict with group standards	*Testing for consensus:* tentatively asking for group opinions in order to find out whether the group is nearing consensus on a decision, sending up "trial balloons" to test group opinions
Giving information: offering facts or generalizations, relating one's own experience to the group problem to illustrate points	*Following:* going along with decisions of the group, thoughtfully accepting ideas of others, serving as audience during group discussion	*Mediating:* harmonizing, conciliating differences in points of view, making compromise solutions
Giving opinion: stating an opinion or belief concerning a suggestion or one of several suggestions, particularly concerning its value rather than its factual basis	*Expressing group feeling:* summarizing what group feeling is sensed to be, describing reactions of the group to ideas or solutions	*Relieving tension:* draining off negative feeling by jesting or pouring oil on troubled waters, putting a tense situation in wider context
Elaborating: clarifying, giving examples or developing meanings, trying to envision how a proposal might work if adopted		
Coordinating: showing relationships among various ideas or suggestions, trying to pull ideas and suggestions together, trying to draw together activities of various subgroups or members		
Summarizing: pulling together related ideas or suggestions, restating suggestions after the group has discussed them		

[a] Reprinted From: J. W. Pfeifer and J. E. Jones (Eds.), *The 1976 Annual Handbook for Group Facilitators.* San Diego, CA: University Associates, 1976. Used with permission.

health facts, coping strategies, and other related understandings basic to physical or mental health.

4. Altruism is the opportunity to be of help to others through caring, concern, support, or offering information or similar experiences.

5. Corrective emotional experience refers to the opportunity provided for transference of attitudes and behaviors learned through earlier experiences in the family to a new situation where these attitudes and behaviors can be examined, better understood, and altered in more adaptive ways. The group can be an arena in which previously learned automatic ways of interacting can be recognized and changed to more directly and effectively meet real needs.

6. Developing socialization can bring about improvement in everyday social interaction skills. This may involve learning basic social amenities on the part of the mentally retarded and the chronically mentally ill, or it may be developing self-confidence and assertiveness in relating to others on the part of individuals who experience shyness, overdependency, or overly aggressive interactive styles.

7. Imitative behavior is based in the role modeling of healthy attitudes and behaviors by the leader and other members of the group. These may be social skills, communication techniques, self-disclosure, or the validating of perceptions with others.

8. Interpersonal learning occurs as a result of constructive feedback given on the effects of one's behavior on others and a supportive atmosphere for trying out new ways of relating.

9. Cohesiveness is the sense of attraction to other members of the group and the feelings of belonging, identification, and interdependence that evolve.

10. Catharsis refers to the ability to ventilate strong feelings rather than keeping them bottled up inside. This is dependent upon a sense of trust and security in the group's acceptance of emotional expression.

11. Existential factors refer to the sharing and acceptance of the meaning and reality of human existence. This includes aware-

ness that all individuals, no matter the amount of support available to them, must choose and accept responsibility for living their own lives, and that suffering and death are inevitable parts of life.

Further, this includes the recognition that life is at times unfair; that there is no escape from some of life's pain and from death; that no matter how close one is to others, one faces life alone; that facing basic issues of life and death leads to living life more honestly and being less concerned with trivialities; and that one must take ultimate responsibility for living one's own life regardless of the guidance and support available from others.

Loomis (1979) has developed a model that depicts the relationship of the relative importance of curative factors to the goals of groups. (Table 13-1).

Problems in Groups

Related to the task and maintenance roles that facilitate group process are some individual roles that impede group cohesiveness and effectiveness (Table 13-4).

Individuals' behaviors and attitudes may block group interaction and goal-directed activities. The barriers need to be identified and understood in terms of their underlying needs or dynamics before the nurse can effectively respond or intervene. Other factors that may disrupt group interaction and progress include interferences caused by negative factors in the physical setting, conflicts between individual members, and scapegoating of a member. The introduction of a new member or members can also be expected to temporarily disrupt the group process.

□ Leadership Interventions

Interventions may be implemented by the nurse as the designated leader or co-leader of a group and by a nurse or student who is assigned to the group as a participant observer. All will intervene in various ways to facilitate group interaction and group process although the designated leader will have greater experience and responsibility.

TABLE 13-4 Blocking or Self-Serving Role Behaviors[a]

Being Aggressive: Working for status by criticizing or blaming others, showing hostility against the group or some individual, deflating the ego or status of others.

Blocking: Interfering with the progress of the group by going off on a tangent, citing personal experiences unrelated to the problem, arguing too much on a point, rejecting ideas without consideration.

Self-Confession: Using the group as a sounding board, expressing personal, nongroup-oriented feelings or points of view.

Competing: Vying with others to produce the best idea, talk the most, play the most roles, gain favor with the leader.

Seeking Sympathy: Trying to induce other group members to be sympathetic to one's problems or misfortunes, deploring one's own situation, or disparaging one's own ideas to gain support.

Special Pleading: Introducing or supporting suggestions related to one's own pet concerns or philosophies, lobbying.

"Horsing around": clowning, joking, mimicking, disrupting the work of the group

Seeking recognition: Attempting to call attention to one's self by loud or excessive talking, extreme ideas, unusual behavior.

Withdrawal: Acting indifferent or passive, resorting to excessive formality, daydreaming, doodling, whispering to others, wandering from the subject.

---

[a] Reprinted from: J. W. Pfeiffer and J. E. Jones (Eds.), *The 1976 Annual Handbook for Group Facilitators*, San Diego, CA: University Associates, 1976. Used with permission.

DECISION MAKING

Several aspects are involved in the decision to initiate and plan for a group. First of all, a need for the group must be established. This need may be identified in the potential members of the group, or in the care setting itself. The former may involve needs for information, socialization, interpersonal learning, or problem solving, all of which may be enhanced by a group setting. The care setting may also have needs that encourage consideration of group strategies such as increasing the quality and efficiency of client education offered, involving health care consumers in planning for programming, or reaching target groups for primary prevention and community service. The following aspects should be considered in the decision-making process.

1. Needs assessment: (a) Are there enough interested potential members to warrant establishment of a group? (b) Are there likely to be sufficient numbers to require planning for two or more groups?
2. Availability of resources: Is it possible to (a) recruit membership, (b) obtain a suitable setting, and (c) provide adequate leadership within the available budget?
3. Constraints: (a) Is there administrative support within the sponsoring agency for initiating the group? (b) Are there external constraining forces likely to affect the group? If either the agency administration or larger community is indifferent or hostile to the goals of the group, it is not impossible to initiate and maintain it, but the commitment required of leaders and members will be significantly greater and the chances of success greatly reduced.

The answers to these questions need to be obtained before planning for the group itself. A group approach is not appropriate for all needs and problems. Occasionally, a group setting for a particular service is selected for economic reasons; however, if not enough staff time and physical resources are available, the result is not economy but inadequacy and a waste of time for all involved. The organizers or leaders of the group should also assess their own motives for wanting to form a group in the context of the needs, resources, and constraints involved. A group that is started merely to meet the professional growth needs of the leaders (in the absence of appropriate member needs) exploits the members and is unlikely to provide either leaders or members with a satisfactory experience. Involving inappropriate members in a group to maintain adequate attendance is also counterproductive. Most importantly, if insufficient planning and resources are involved in a group effort the results may be detrimental to individual members whose needs are not being met and to future attempts at initiating groups.

PLANNING

Once the decision is made to establish a group, it becomes important to recruit and prepare members and to plan for a successful group. Potential members should be contacted well in advance to acquaint them with the purpose of and expectations for the group. This would include aspects such as meeting times, participation expected, confidentiality, fees, and a description of the benefits to be expected. Once a commitment to join is obtained, it is still helpful to provide reminders of time and place until attendance becomes regularly established. Personal contact and the attitude of the leader in clearly communicating the goals and expectations for the group are significant factors in motivating involvement.

Selection and management of the physical setting is vital in establishing a comfortable climate for group participation. This entails continual attention to preparing the setting by arriving early to place the chairs in a close circle and, in general, promoting an environment conducive to group involvement.

COLEADERSHIP ISSUES

The use of cofacilitators or cotherapists has potential benefits and disadvantages that depend primarily on the relationship and communication between the leaders. Disadvantages arise from poor planning and competitiveness, which can disrupt the group, increase factionalism among members, and diminish the effectiveness of leaders in working toward the goals of the group. Leadership rivalry may also reinforce maladaptive behavior patterns members have learned in similar situations in the family.

The advantages of using cotherapists derive from the variety of roles and perspectives that can be shared and used to enhance group work. Hellwig and Memmott (1978) have described the importance of a trusting, collaborative, open relationship between therapists, which permits them to play complementary roles, serve as observers for each other, provide healthy role modeling of interpersonal relationships (including disagreements), manage group anxiety, and support each other. This requires that time and effort be spent on building a healthy, collaborative relationship and on open discussion and evaluation of each other's approaches and their effects.

An example of this complementary process is that of one therapist providing empathy and supportive encouragement to a member who is being confronted or pushed to be more open by the other cotherapist. This provides two approaches toward the same end and diminishes the likelihood of the member feeling the need for self-defense rather than using the confrontation productively. The use of male and female cotherapists is very common in sexuality and marriage counseling because it permits greater opportunities for group members to identify with a leader and enhances opportunities for the leaders to role-model healthy interactions and open communication between the sexes. In these examples, leadership roles are equal and complementary. In other coleader situations, one therapist may assume a more active role in the group while the other serves as a process observer and facilitator. These roles should be discussed and evaluated on a continuing basis.

> ### ■ Point of Emphasis
> *Coleaders need to plan and evaluate their approaches together for teamwork and effectiveness.*

GENERAL LEADERSHIP INTERVENTIONS

General strategies for promoting group work relate to the attainment of four goals:

1. To create a social climate of caring and acceptance for members
2. To establish expectations and norms for group behavior
3. To reinforce appropriate participation and feeling-oriented discussion
4. To promote awareness of group dynamics through focusing on group process

A combination of task and maintenance role behaviors will be used by leaders in implementing these strategic goals.

Authier and Gustafson (1976) have described basic interventions that are applicable to the inpatient psychiatric setting, in which nurses frequently lead community meetings and small groups. These approaches focus on establishing a social climate and expectations for group behavior. They are particularly helpful in working with groups in which membership may be heterogeneous and frequently changing. These interventions, which concentrate on establishing norms of appropriate interaction and discussion of feeling-oriented topics of common interest, are most necessary in the early stage of group process and should be reinforced as needed throughout the life of the group.

Seat members in a close circle. If members sit outside, they should be invited into the circle so that all members may see and talk to each other.

Start and finish on time. Establishing a schedule and minimizing distracting interruptions promotes discussion. If one of the leaders or staff must arrive late or leave early, that person should role-model appropriate behavior by excusing herself and explaining the necessity of violating this norm.

Introduce new members. Acknowledging and welcoming new members promotes a climate of group acceptance.

Briefly review goals of the group. This serves to remind members of the purpose of the meeting. Established members may orient newcomers to these goals, thus promoting the factor of altruism.

Keep people in the group for the entire session. Members should be discouraged from wandering in and out of group to obtain coffee or to avoid discussing uncomfortable topics. Some members may be too hyperactive or anxious to conform to this norm; they should be evaluated to determine whether additional individual support is required or whether it would be best to defer membership in the group until the individual is better able to tolerate it.

Keep people aware. Members may be drowsy from sedation or may withdraw to avoid interaction. Gentle prodding and attempts to involve more members actively may be helpful, or the leader may wish to ask uninvolved members what they feel would help them to be more participative. Often, it is sufficient to restate the norm that members will stay involved in group.

Allow only one person to talk at a time. "Gatekeeping" interventions are needed to assure that members are heard without interruption and that the discussion does not turn into an incoherent free-for-all.

Point out the importance of sticking to the topic. This tactic promotes greater exploration and discourages confusing and superficial shifts in the discussion. Important but irrelevant issues can be noted and deferred until the current topic is completed.

Ask members to look at one another when speaking. Eye contact is important to both the sender and the receiver of the message. Members should be assisted to learn awareness of nonverbal communication.

Direct members to talk to one another. This is of particular value in the early stage of group when members may talk to and "through" the leader. Redirecting questions to the group as a whole is effective for general questions directed to the leader. Members who comment about other group members should be directed to make their questions or statements directly to that member. Talking about people not present in the group should be discouraged since their views cannot be heard.

Ask members to share common experiences and feelings. This increases participation and appreciation of universality. Members can be assisted in generalizing a topic from an individual problem. For example, if Joe is angry with a demanding boss the leader may suggest a general topic of "experiencing and coping with anger" to which all members can contribute (Authier and Gustafson, 1976). In some therapy groups, an individual's problems may be the focus of group but in most of the groups led by nurses, generalized topics are desirable to maintain the interest and involvement of all group members.

Reinforce appropriate participation. Acknowledging involvement and feeling-oriented discussion recognizes the contributions of group members and encourages further contribution by those members and others. Interventions related to this overall strategy include thanking members for their participation, summarizing the discussion and accomplishments of the group, re-marking on the productivity of the group, and making a statement that this is a place to explore feelings and problems in daily living.

Promote group awareness of the dynamics occurring. This can be accomplished in various ways, primarily by making direct, non-judgmental observations of the feeling tone, content, or interaction patterns evident in the group. These aspects are generally relevant to the stage of group process and related issues. Some examples of situations, identified stage issues, and basic process interventions follow.

Situation A: A group, having met only a few times, lapses into an uncomfortable silence after several superficial attempts to initiate conversation fail.

Stage issue: Uncertainty, groping

Process intervention: "We seem to be having difficulty getting started. I'm wondering what the group is feeling right now."

Situation B: Several members have proposed feeling-oriented topics for discussion. Two members (A and B) support each other in saying to the leader that they don't think these are appropriate topics to bring up in group now.

Stage issue: Rivalry with and dependence on leader

Process intervention: "A and B, you seem to disagree with the others about what to discuss in group; this is your group too. I want you to tell *them* what your concerns are."

Situation C: Several members (A, B, C) have shared their feelings about a situation involving them. Other members provided feedback on their perceptions and responses to A, B, and C's behavior. A, B, and C gained new perceptions of how others respond to them and appeared to appreciate this information.

Stage issue: working as a group

Process intervention: "I think the group really accomplished a lot today; A, B, and C got us started and X and Y gave them some really constructive feedback.

I sense a feeling of closeness and real communication in the group today. How did others feel about it?"

INTERVENTIONS FOR SPECIFIC PROBLEMS

People in groups frequently demonstrate attitudes or blocking behaviors that impede individual or group progress (Table 13-4). Interventions are often required to promote continued work toward goals. These interventions are best if group members contribute them but, when the need arises, the leader should intervene if others do not. Vriend and Dyer (1973) have identified the following occasions that call for specific intervention.

When a member speaks for the group as a whole by saying "We all think or feel . . ." it is an assumption that tends to discourage individual viewpoints and expression of divergent opinions. The facilitator's goal should be to encourage sharing of opinions and feelings by asking if there are any members of the group who disagree, or (if nonverbal communication of a member suggests disagreement) directing a question such as "Is that true for you?" to a specific person. This encourages the speaker to validate rather than assume, and encourages members of the group to express their individual perceptions.

If one person speaks for another by commenting "What he really means is . . ." or "I think she wants . . ." this tends to communicate that the competent "helper" can do a better job of communicating the other's thoughts or feelings than the latter can. The facilitator should focus on the individuals and their personal goals in this situation by asking, perhaps of the more passive member, if the statement was accurate and how it feels to have others interpret for you. Ultimately, the idea would be to have the passive member become more active and clear in stating his own needs and to help the helper provide more valuable assistance through asking the passive member to restate or clarify unclear statements. This reinforces the aim of individual members to formulate and work on achieving their own objectives for self-growth.

Focusing on irrelevant people or events often occurs early in a group's development, since the work of becoming a group is anxiety provoking. It is easier to complain about external forces than to involve each other in here-and-now interactions. This complaining, however, accomplishes nothing. Leadership should involve redirecting the group's focus by pointing out that very little is being accomplished by their complaining about things over which they have little control. Attention should be focused on what members can do to bring about changes in themselves or their situations.

A member who lacks self-confidence may verbally or nonverbally consistently seek the approval or acceptance of the leader or group before speaking or expressing an opinion. Pointing out this behavior when it occurs by commenting that "You seem to be asking me if your opinions are acceptable" assists the person in recognizing it. As further instances arise, other members may also point out the behavior and encourage more assertive communication.

Often, people avoid assuming responsibility for their own feelings and behavior by blaming others. "If my mother were kinder" or "If my spouse were more understanding" (then I'd be happier, or more productive, and so on). Although relationships and events are significant factors, this avoidance and blaming is self-defeating and accomplishes nothing. The facilitator's goal is to bring about hope and a sense of active choice. A comment such as: "Who really is in charge of your life?" may initiate movement in this direction.

Many people are passive and fatalistically state that they have always been shy (or lazy, or whatever) in a manner suggesting that that is how they always expect to be. Others, equally passive but optimistic, suggest that things will get better if they just wait. Both attitudes are unlikely to contribute to any changes or personal growth. The facilitator or group needs to point out that individuals do have some responsibility and control over their own lives and that positive changes rarely "just happen" through waiting. (Vriend and Dyer, 1973)

Additional Problems In Groups

Scapegoating. Because of particular characteristics of a member and related anxieties of other members, one individual may become the focus of blame for the group's anger or inability to resolve conflicts. The group leader is responsible for pointing out that all members of the group share responsibility for what happens in group, and for pointing out these dynamics. For example, the leader might comment "I don't think one member is totally responsible for the difficulties the group is experiencing. What other kinds of things are going on?"

Help-seeking and Help-rejecting. Some members present problems and ask the group for suggestions, which are then countered with various forms of "Yes, but" (reasons why the suggestions couldn't possibly work). If this becomes a pattern or takes up a great deal of group time, the leader may wish to redirect the discussion by summarizing in a way that notes that several useful suggestions have been made and that the member is of course free to use them or not, as he sees fit.

The interventions suggested are not intended as the sole "prescribed" ways of responding. Individuals develop their own facilitative styles based on personality and experience. Gentle humor, mock exaggeration, and other qualities have been used effectively within the context of leadership. The important point to keep in mind is the genuineness and respect that is communicated to the group. If the leader is a successful role model, group members will assume a greater role in intervening effectively with one another. The altruism, universality, and social learning provided create the positive outcomes of group approaches.

☐ Levels of Prevention and Mental Health Promotion

The use of group approaches is appropriate to all levels of prevention of mental illness and mental health promotion. The nurse as health educator may serve as an agent of primary prevention through group education strategies for an endless variety of populations and topics. These might include parenting skills, sexuality, coping with stress, understanding the aging process, or other community programming needs. The nurse as case finder in secondary prevention may use assessment skills in contact with groups at risk for particular problems to identify those with needs for specific referral, for example, a particularly stressed pregnant teenager who needs to be referred to a prenatal teaching group, or a severely depressed middle-aged woman who needs a group aimed at helping people adjust to divorce. The rehabilitation focus of tertiary prevention can be practiced using group strategies in a variety of settings, such as the medical hospital, psychiatric inpatient unit, outpatient clinics, or community facility, for patients experiencing a variety of conditions affecting physical and emotional well-being.

ASPECTS OF PREVENTION

Nurses using group approaches in primary and secondary prevention (in which education is the focus) will most likely emphasize the curative factors of imparting information, instilling hope, and universality. Task orientation and group cohesiveness will also facilitate goal attainment. Role modeling and demonstration may enhance imitative behavior in learners. The factor of altruism may operate if the group is encouraged to share experiences and coping strategies. Teaching strategies will most likely involve a structured presentation using appropriate visual aids or demonstration as needed. This can then be followed by discussion, questions, and practice or role-play to clarify and apply the information presented. Group skills will be vital in the follow-up discussion, in which members should be made to feel comfortable in sharing ideas, feelings, experiences, and needs for further assistance. The discussion also provides opportunities for the nurse to recognize and refer individuals who need more assistance than the group can provide (the screening or case-finding function of secondary prevention).

Tertiary prevention in the mental health field refers to helping clients to develop or rebuild social and interpersonal skills, gain support and coping skills, and develop an understanding of themselves and their behavior following an illness. This process begins in the inpatient setting and may be followed up in partial care and outpatient care in the community. Group therapist in the multidisciplinary mental health team is a generic role—a group therapist may be a psychiatrist, psychologist, nurse, social worker, or activity therapist. Basically prepared nurses in inpatient psychiatric settings are likely to serve as group leaders for community meetings and small support and coping groups. A clinical specialist in psychiatric nursing is qualified for a more independent role as primary group therapist in either inpatient or outpatient settings.

☐ Types of Therapeutic Groups

Specialized techniques of group therapy are numerous and are based on diverse theoretical approaches and diverse special needs of patient populations. A description of some commonly used group approaches, their theoretical bases, and specific applications follows.

SOCIALIZATION GROUPS

Nurses in everyday practice come in contact with a variety of patients lacking adequate socialization skills whether the cause is, for example, chronic mental illness or the physical, environmental, and socioeconomic factors that tend to isolate the elderly person from social contacts. The major emphasis in this type of group is on providing opportunities for the use or development of social skills. Reducing anxiety, which may be associated with reintroduction to social contacts, is a vital component of success. Varied activities that provide a focus for social interaction may be used including games, trips, refreshments, or discussions of common interests and current events. The leaders serve as role models and social facilitators in making introductions, identifying interests of group members, and generally making the group a pleasant social experience. Elderly patients may particularly enjoy structured opportunities for reminiscing. Bringing in articles that stimulate memories, such as old household articles or tools, may promote great storytelling.

Seasonal themes may be used to enhance participation. Filling "trick-or-treat" bags for children, making decorations for Halloween and sharing stories of the Halloweens of one's own childhood, or decorating Valentine cookies and talking about dating and courtship in youth are some examples. The chronically mentally ill person may be assisted in sharing interests or experiences through drawing pictures of favorite times or making a collage that "tells about me," and sharing these with the group. The opportunities are as diverse as the imagination of the leaders can make them. These groups generally are held weekly or monthly.

> **■ Point of Emphasis**
>
> *Leaders in socialization groups model social skills and promote socialization among members.*

SUPPORT AND COPING GROUPS

Groups emphasizing support and coping are appropriate to the majority of clients, both medical and psychiatric. These may include persons adapting to chronic or life-threatening dysfunctions, those coping with situational stresses, or psychiatric patients experiencing anxiety disorders or major psychoses. These groups tend to meet weekly; clients may attend as few as six to eight sessions, or may continue for up to a year or more as needed. Generally, support groups tend to be formed to meet a particular common need, for example: coping with grief, coping with a specific type of illness, or supporting the formerly institutionalized mentally ill in adapting to the stress of everyday living. Members are selected on the basis of these common needs or problems, although in other respects the group may be quite heterogeneous. Group cohesiveness and interdependence is a primary factor in goal attainment, although some positive transference and dependency on the leader may occur. There is no focus on dreams or unconscious processes. The content of group places emphasis on strengthening defenses, interpersonal skills, and coping abilities. Information and suggestions are freely shared.

Universality, instilling hope, and helping one another are strongly stressed. Reality testing may be also be a focus, particularly in groups of clients who have experienced thought disorders (e.g., distorted ideas, confusion, or disorientation). Group structure may be relatively loose as attendance patterns may vary, and group members' needs will be the focus for discussion.

> ### ■ Point of Emphasis
> *Support group leadership emphasizes sharing of information, feelings and coping strategies among members.*

SELF-HELP GROUPS

Self-help groups are a form of support group in which professionals are not the primary source of leadership, although they may be used as resource persons and referral agents. The oldest self-help groups, dating back to the 1930s, are Alcoholics Anonymous and Recovery Incorporated. These organizations and numerous similar groups are based on the belief that people who have experienced and overcome a problem are the best source of help for those currently struggling with that problem. Group cohesiveness, hope, and altruism are major factors. In addition to regular group attendance, members may be offered the option of calling another member in time of need. Since Alcoholics Anonymous and its related family of self-help groups (Alanon, Alateen, Alatot) have become established, other similar groups, based on the same approach, have developed, for example, Gamblers Anonymous, Overeaters Anonymous, and Parents Anonymous (for actual or potential child abusers).

Recovery Incorporated, a self-help organization that defines its membership as nervous and ex-mental patients, uses an approach based on the teachings of Dr. Abraham Low. A particular method of spotting (recognizing) and coping with anxiety is taught to members, and group meetings are geared toward teaching and reinforcing the use of this approach. Leaders are selected and trained from within the membership. Professionals may attend but are not to participate in a helping capacity.

"Make Today Count" is a more recently formed group currently approaching national scope. It was formed in the Midwest by Orville Kelly, a man diagnosed as terminally ill, to assist the dying and their significant others in coping with life in the face of terminal illness.

> ### ■ Point of Emphasis
> *Self-help leadership is generally provided by experienced lay members based on personal experiences.*

Numerous other groups are available throughout the country to meet the needs of parents with developmentally delayed children, parents of children who are terminally ill or who have died, women recovering from mastectomies, and innumerable other clients and their families coping with specific illnesses and conditions. Information about similar resources in communities can generally be obtained from community service organizations or medical centers. Professionals who wish to evaluate these services for potential referral of clients are urged by Newton (1984) to gather information on membership eligibility, type of services and approaches, referral sources, leadership, and level of acceptance by the professional community. Attending several meetings is advised in order to assess the following: (1) membership characteristics; (2) evidence of climate of acceptance, mutual assistance, and provision of accurate information in relation to health education focus, level of prevention addressed; and (3) potential problems that might threaten the effectiveness or continuation of the group (e.g., lack of funds, lack of referrals, deficiencies in leadership skills). This information will be of assistance in evaluating the overall potential effectiveness of the group and the likelihood that a specific client will feel comfortable as a member.

SPECIAL GROUP TECHNIQUES FOR THE NEEDS OF ELDERLY PATIENTS

Particular group techniques have been developed to serve the needs of the elderly. The goals of these varied approaches are: (1) reorientation to increase alertness and reduce confusion, (2) remotivation to increase awareness and stimulate involvement, and (3) reminiscence which may be used either to promote socialization (as was described earlier), or in a therapeutic sense to meet developmental needs of aging, characterized as the life review.

Reorientation groups are highly structured, brief, and repetitious. For maximum effectiveness, they are held almost daily, and the content is reinforced throughout the day. Simple introductions and the use of large, easily read name tags enhance the recollection of names by group members. Information about the date can be reinforced through commenting on the weather in relation to the season and placing the date in the context of immediate or upcoming events. Time orientation can be promoted by reviewing the upcoming day's schedule and by having an easy-to-read copy of it kept at all times in a prominent place. A "buddy system" may be followed to provide support to newer persons by those already familiar with the routine and the setting. Reorientation techniques can readily be incorporated into the day's activities, such as in an after-breakfast session in a group dining room. If tactfully and supportively handled, these approaches may meet the needs of well-oriented persons to structure and plan their day while providing orienting information to confused patients and those adapting to new surroundings.

■ Point of Emphasis
Reorientation is best characterized by brevity, clarity, and repetition of information in a well-structured environment.

Remotivation techniques focus on increasing stimulation and awareness of one's surroundings. Depending on the needs and composition of the group, it may meet weekly or more often, providing various activities that engage members in primarily sensory activities, or may involve more mentally challenging games for members who are alert and who retain good memory. Very withdrawn or apathetic persons may be awakened by basic sensory activities such as moving to music, sharing in tactile stimulation (feeling and describing familiar objects without looking at them such as sandpaper, china, velvet), or evoking memories through familiar sights, smells, or sounds (fall leaves, spring flowers, spices or sachets). Members may be encouraged to comment on any events brought to mind. "Trivia" themes may appeal to the more alert elderly. Recognition of pictures of old movie stars or famous world leaders may promote active participation. If a game format is used, it is important that there be no losers and that members not be made to feel that their memory is being tested. These techniques may be varied or combined to meet needs assessed in the group.

■ Point of Emphasis
Stimulation, variation, and direct involvement promote remotivation.

Reminiscence groups may meet weekly or less often and have names such as "Down Memory Lane" or "Good Old Days." Members are selected for their ability to participate appropriately, and the group should be fairly small (six to eight) to facilitate interaction. The goal and theoretical rationale for reminiscence is promotion of the developmental need for integrity (the sense that one's life was essentially good in the context of the opportunities and circumstances that existed). The leadership focus is to provide positive reinforcement and topics as needed. Curative aspects are primarily universality, group cohesiveness, and the existential factors. Nurses interested in initiating reminiscence groups should read Burnside (1976).

PSYCHODRAMA AND ROLE PLAY

Moreno (in Kaplan and Sadlock, 1983) describes psychodrama as a means of group therapy that maximizes self-awareness and interpersonal learning. In psychodrama, the protagonist or actor chooses to enact an important situation, past or future, as if it were presently occurring. Expressiveness and subjectivity are encouraged in the enactment in order to focus on identification of feelings and responses. This action-oriented mode of therapy may be helpful for a broad array of patients and is particularly attractive to adolescents. Other members of the group generally play supporting roles as auxiliary egos or provide a back-up commentary on the protagonist, identifying with the actor as a double. Staff and clients may play these roles. The session generally progresses from a warm-up through the dramatization and is followed by group discussion to promote the factors of universality and cohesiveness, and to assist in integrating the interpersonal learning. A therapist should serve as the director. It is also possible to adapt some of these techniques to coping, awareness, and problem-solving groups. Brief descriptions of some of these techniques follow. Psychodrama groups generally meet once or twice weekly.

Role play: enactment of a fantasy or significant event, past or future, as if it were happening in the present (the major focus of psychodrama).

Rehearsal: practicing a future event such as a job interview, personal confrontation, or other significant interaction to build confidence, practice congruence and appropriate behavior, and receive feedback from others (a form of role play).

Reenacting: replaying a particular situation (e.g., family disagreement or unit conflict) to defuse an emotional event and experience various perspectives of those involved (also a form of role play).

Exercises: trust games such as "blind walk" or being lifted in the air by the group may be used as warm-ups and may promote a sense of group cohesiveness.

Sociodrama: a more complex reenactment of a group event such as staff-patient conflict or a problem in the social environment.

Role reversal: enacting the role of a significant other, often done in combination with enactment of the original situation from the protagonist's perspective. This may be used to facilitate interracial or intergenerational understanding through adopting the role of "other." Moreno cautions that clients with weak egos (e.g., psychotic persons) can feel deeply threatened by this technique particularly in regard to actual authority figures.

Moreno believes that the self emerges from the varied roles a person plays from early childhood. The focus on self-awareness and identification of feelings is coupled with an emphasis on universality. The protagonist should never be left feeling alone in the problem situation. The leader is responsible for eliciting similar feelings and problems from the group to enhance identification and cohesiveness in the postdiscussion period as well as integrating the interpersonal learning aspects.

BEHAVIORAL APPROACHES IN GROUPS

Psychotherapists may use behavioral approaches in groups but the primary focus is individual desensitization procedures in a group setting. The therapist's approach is didactic and supportive, and the interactions occur primarily between individual patients and the therapist rather than among the members of the group. The goal is removal of distressing symptoms of anxiety.

Assertiveness training groups are led by a variety of group-prepared workers. The focus is on a didactic presentation of assertiveness concepts and practice in self-disclosure and effective, assertive communication. Relaxation techniques are often incorporated to deal with anxiety. This short-term treatment (weekly sessions for approximately 6 to 14 weeks) is directed toward learning more adaptive behaviors and the extinction of the less adaptive (in this case passive or aggressive ways of interacting).

TRAINING GROUPS

Also referred to as T-groups or sensitivity groups, training groups focus on personal growth, self-awareness, and interpersonal learning. They may develop leadership or management skills and are generally short-term. The group is the focus for experiential learning and developing increased interpersonal sensitivity. The brief nature of these groups makes real behavior change unlikely and, if the leader is not skilled and able to anticipate potential problems, their intensive nature may be detrimental to some members who are marginally adjusted.

PSYCHOANALYTIC GROUPS

A Freudian, Jungian, or Adlerian (or other school) psychoanalytic approach entails long-term (up to 3 years) therapy one or more times per week. Members will most likely be experiencing anxiety disorders or personality dysfunctions. Content of the groups is likely to involve analysis of dreams, analysis of transference behavior, past and present relationships inside the group, and significant interactions. The leader is active in confronting defenses, interpreting behavior, and sharing responses or advice. The focus may be either on individual therapy in the group setting or on group interactional therapy. The goal of therapy is increased self-awareness, interpersonal learning, and behavior change. Yalom's curative factors all apply.

COMMON PSYCHOTHERAPY GROUPS

Many therapists use one or more theoretical models in short-term (6 months to 1 year) treatment, emphasizing primarily the present. The theoretical basis may be Gestalt, Transactional Analysis, Reality Therapy, some other theoretical base, or a combination of several. The focus may vary from individual treatment in a group setting to group interaction. (See Chapter 1 for a description of the theory and content of these approaches). The majority of the curative factors would apply in these groups with the primary emphasis being interpersonal learning and behavior change. In addition to group interaction goals, the therapist will have specific outcome goals in mind for individual patients.

> ■ *Point of Emphasis*
>
> *Therapy groups seeking insight and behavior change are led by experienced psychotherapists.*

TASK GROUPS

Nurses are likely to find themselves in a variety of task-oriented groups throughout their practice. Task groups are varied in scope and complexity. A client group given the assignment of planning the recreational program for a psychiatric inpatient unit is a task group. Membership in professional or educational organizations involves work through committees with assigned tasks such as program planning, public relations, policy review. Hospitals are large organizations in which group task work plays a significant part in unit management, setting standards, and coordinating the efforts of the various hierarchies such as medical staff, hospital administration, and nursing service.

Knowledge of group dynamics and stages of group process is relevant to task-oriented groups. It is also important to keep in mind that individual members may have additional goals, sometimes called "hidden agendas," which may be different from and occasionally in conflict with the stated goals of the group. To illustrate this point, consider a group of students given the task of planning a recognition day for student achievement. May, president of the student council, is the designated leader. Representing several student groups are John, Sue, Jim, and Carol. Sue is representing unaffiliated students and feels too much attention is given to membership and offices in student organizations. She would like to see recognition limited to academic achievement. Jack believes that athletics are being overlooked in this college and wants participation in intramural sports to be acknowledged as a form of student organization activity. Carol has a research examination the next day and wants the group to come to a quick decision so she can study. May and Jim have both devoted substantial efforts to honoraries, social fraternities, and student government. They feel these activities have made a real contribution to campus life but have reduced the time available for their own study and academic achievement. The task of planning the recognition day appears to be a simple goal. The individual goals of members, however, are likely to initiate group conflict and impede work toward task attainment. This is fairly common phenomenon in task-group activity.

Influencing Factors

Tasks vary in their inherent complexity; in the amount of group cooperation and collaboration required to meet the goal; and in the quality and status of leader-member relationships. Numerous theories have addressed the issues of task-group activity and effectiveness. In general, the strengths of task groups can be stated as (1) providing more information and perspectives on the problem or task than is obtainable by an individual, (2) representing a wider range of the values at issue in task or problem resolution, and (3) increasing the level of commitment to the decisions or solutions made by the members participating in the group. Negative factors include the increased amount of time required of group, as compared with individual, decision making and the likelihood that not all members of the group will be motivated to participate actively. An additional problem that may occur is that of a pressure for consensus ("groupthink"). Group members may develop a feeling of group invulnerability; an attitude that the group is invariably good and right and outsiders wrong and evil; pressure to conform to group opinions; and a related tendency of members to censure nonconformity (Janis, 1971).

In demonstrating groupthink the members of a project group may ignore information about outsiders who have solved a particular problem satisfactorily. The member who brings the topic up may be told that the group of outsiders does not have the expertise to resolve the problem and surely their solution will be found to be unworkable. If the member persists in bringing up this issue, he may be asked to which group his loyalties and identity belong ("our group—love it or leave it"). Ignoring this information may serve to perpetuate a problem that could have been resolved by utilizing the other group's information and approach. In this instance, the cohesiveness

of the group negatively influences openness to new ideas. Leadership approaches that promote brainstorming and careful consideration of all ideas regardless of source can help to reduce the effects of groupthink.

Fiedler (1967) has developed a situational model of leadership style effectiveness in relation to task structure, group atmosphere, and leader power position. Leadership style is defined on the basis of the degree of interpersonal relationship vs. task performance orientation of the leader. Task structure is identified as routine vs. complex based on goal clarity, type of decision required, and alternative options available. Interpersonal relationship is the quality of trust, friendliness, and respect between leader and members. Fiedler's model suggests that different levels of emphasis on each of these three dimensions may be called for in particular situations.

In path-goal theory, the function of the leader is supplemental (supportive) and motivational and to a degree dependent upon the characteristics of the group members and the task environment. Leadership behavior varies according to the stage of group development and involves four dimensions:

1. Instrumental behavior—planning and providing structure and expectations

TABLE 13-5 Leadership Style and Group-Development Stages: A Path-Goal Interpretation[a]

Group-Development Stage	Leadership Style			
	Instrumental	Supportive	Participative	Achievement Oriented
Orientation	Assign tasks; clarify roles, rules, and procedures	Give support and consideration to employee needs and behavior	Consult with subordinates in plans, process, and procedures	Develop plan for task accomplishment; set challenging goals
Internal Problem Solving	Revise and strengthen rules and standards; clarify expectations	Exhibit confidence in subordinates' ability to complete the task	Develop participative climate; resolve conflict	Emphasize completion of tasks
Growth and Productivity	Develop feedback; strengthen information networks	Emphasize personal growth and development of subordinates	Develop cohesion; strengthen or elevate group performance norms	Motivate toward task accomplishment
Evaluation	Develop evaluation mechanisms; strengthen feedback; revise rules and procedures	Support group activities; accentuate group accomplishment; emphasize prestige of group	Consult on evaluation procedures; strengthen cohesion and norms	Motivate toward task accomplishment; revise and evaluate goals and plans

[a] From ORGANIZATIONAL BEHAVIOR AND PERFORMANCE by Andrew D. Szilagyi, Jr. and Marc J. Wallace. Copyright © 1980 Scott, Foresman and Company. Reprinted by permission.

2. Supportive behavior—displaying concern for members' well-being and creating a pleasant environment

3. Participative behavior—sharing and seeking information and opinions in the group, and consultation with members

4. Achievement-oriented behavior—setting goals, exhorting performance, and displaying confidence in the group's ability to meet goals (House and Mitchell, 1974)

Both the situational and path-goal models are attempts to predict leadership behaviors that will best promote task group achievements. This is an area of increasing interest and research, particularly in the management field. For a path-goal theory interpretation of leadership behavior in relation to the stage of a task group's development, see Table 13-5.

☐ *Evaluation*

Group evaluation has three important general components: leader effectiveness, group process, and individual member satisfaction and goal attainment. Each of these components has its own goals and related criteria. Individual goals for each member may be common to all in relatively homogeneous groups or very diverse in heterogeneous groups. For example, all members in a short-term assertiveness training group will share the following goals (sample criteria for evaluation are also included):

Learning techniques of effective communication (criterion: formulate "I" messages that directly communicate feelings and needs in a practice situation)

Practicing assertive behaviors in role-play situations (criterion: maintain eye contact and confident body posture, show congruence between verbal and nonverbal communication)

Learning techniques for reducing anxiety in interpersonal situations (criterion: demonstrate progressive muscle relaxation, describe use of visualizing oneself being assertive in specific situations)

Applying assertiveness in real life (criterion: report a situation in which assertiveness techniques were used and describe the outcomes in terms of own feelings and situational effects)

An individual's goals in a support group might be broadly stated as (1) coping with feelings of loneliness, anger, and depression following a divorce, and (2) developing skills and initiative to increase socialization. The criteria for evaluating goal attainment can be quite specific based on the person's perception of "how we'll know I've met my goals." These criteria might be (1) using new coping skills such as identifying angry feelings and using physical activities to relieve them instead of displacing anger at work or at home or (2) initiating social interactions daily by inviting a coworker to lunch or suggesting a trip to the movies to a neighbor. Evaluating a member's satisfaction with the group can be done through asking how effective and helpful group membership is for him or if any aspects of the group are specifically helpful; or any other open-ended approach may be used. Attendance patterns, when used in combination with other information, also provide an indication of member satisfaction.

Group goals relate to short- and long-term expectations in regard to indicators of the stages of group process and the presence of appropriate curative factors in group interaction. A log or diary kept to record significant aspects of each group meeting can provide baseline information on which to evaluate movement in terms of group process. This is particularly valuable to students and beginning group leaders. A sample form is included at the end of this chapter. Descriptive data should be recorded relevant to each of the previously discussed areas: communication patterns (see Figures 13-1 and 13-2), indicators of stage of group process, general feeling tone, content of discussion (general topics), needs demonstrated and whether they were met, and curative factors demonstrated. These elements can also be evaluated through later discussion by staff attending the group. This is valuable in planning for the next group and in gaining information about the perceived effectiveness of various interventions attempted.

Leader or facilitator effectiveness should be assessed through a self-evaluation of performance and by obtaining feedback from other staff members in the group. Attention should be focused on the leadership goals and specific behaviors identified that contributed to attainment of the goal, as follows.

1. Establishing a climate of warmth and acceptance

   Examples:

   Introduced new member and asked other

members to share in introducing themselves

Shared personal feelings of satisfaction
about the achievements that occurred in
group today

2. Clarifying Expectations
   Examples:
   Reviewed group norms at the beginning of
   the meeting

   Reminded members who arrived late that
   it was important to be on time so as not to
   disrupt discussion

3. Managing the environment
   Examples:
   Arrived in time to arrange chairs in a close
   circle

   Closed the door at the beginning of the session to minimize distractions

4. Maximizing participation
   Examples:
   Directed open-ended questions to the group
   as a whole

   Noted Mr. P.s look of disapproval and
   asked for feelings

5. Focusing interventions
   Examples:
   Redirected discussion to the topic when the
   group began to ramble

   Asked Mrs. L. to talk to Mr. S. instead of
   about him when he's present in the group.

Outline form for recording descriptive observations to be used in evaluating groups

1. Communication/interaction diagram:
2. General goals and purpose for group:
   a. Task and maintenance role behaviors:
   b. Blocking behaviors observed:
3. Stage of group process evidenced:
   (Describe observed reasons for defining at
   this stage)
   a. Content (summary of topics discussed)
   b. Themes of the discussion
   c. Accomplishments of the group (if any
      observed)
   d. Curative factors demonstrated
4. Own participation and goals/rationale for
   interventions
   a. Effectiveness of own participation in re-
      lation to goals

Own goals:
Group's goals:
   b. Evaluation of leader effectiveness:

■ Enrichment Activities

1. Participate in a group activity on a regular
   basis and observe for the behaviors in the
   group that are characteristic of the stages of
   group process.

2. Have a simulated group experience. Identify a
   hypothetical task or situation for the group and
   assign five to eight members to the group. Give
   each of these members a specific task role,
   maintenance role, or blocking role to enact during the simulated group. Assign coleaders to
   facilitate the group and a nonparticipant observer (or two) to record impressions of group
   dynamics and role behaviors. Allow ten to fifteen minutes for observer feedback and discussion following the group.

3. Think of various task groups you have participated in (e.g., in school, work, or social organizations) and consider the various roles described in Tables 13-3 and 13-4. Can you recall
   task-oriented, maintenance-oriented, and self-
   serving role behaviors that were displayed in
   the group?

4. Discuss or consider leadership strategies to
   deal with the following problems arising in a
   group.

   a. Members act bored and uninvolved, and
      there are long, uncomfortable silences. One
      of the members turns angrily to the leader
      and says: "This is our third meeting and I'm
      not getting a thing out of this—it's a rip-
      off."

   b. Two or three members of the group begin
      sitting next to each other at every session.
      They often make quiet comments to each
      other during the group discussion and, if
      they speak to the group, they turn only to
      each other for agreement or comments.

   c. A withdrawn, shy member of the group
      rarely speaks and is always ignored by oth-
      ers. Sometimes he appears to be bored or
      sleepy but you suspect he is just too non-
      assertive to feel comfortable initiating con-
      versation.

5. In a group of three to five, take materials (e.g.,
   modeling clay, finger paints, building blocks)
   and complete one unified group project in a 20-

minute time limit. Following this activity, discuss the group dynamics involved in planning and initiating the project. What roles were enacted by individual members? Were there significant behaviors that promoted or impeded group progress?

■ Recommended Readings

Sampson, E., and Marthas, M. *Group process for the helping professions.* New York: John Wiley & Sons, 1977.

Loomis, Maxine. *Group process for nurses.* St. Louis: Mosby Company, 1979. Both books are clearly written and contain appropriate information for nurses involved in group work.

■ References

Authier, Jerry, and Gustafson, Kay. Group intervention techniques: A practival guide for psychiatric team members. *Journal of psychiatric nursing and mental health services* (July 1976):19–22.

Bales, R.F. The equilibrium problem in small groups. In *Small groups* (Hare, A.P., Borgatta, E.F., and Bales, R.F., eds.). New York: Alfred Knopf, 1955.

Benne, K., and Sheats, P. Functional roles of group members. *Journal of social issues* (Spring 1948):41–49.

Bion, W.R. *Experiences in groups.* New York: Basic Books, 1959.

Blake, D.R. Group work with the institutionalized elderly. In *Psychosocial nursing care of the aged* (Burnside, Irene, ed.). New York: McGraw-Hill, 1976.

Burnside, Irene. *Nursing and the aged,* McGraw-Hill, 1976, 1981.

Chen, Martha. Applying Yalom's principles to crisis work . . . Some intriguing results. *Journal of psychiatric nursing and mental health services* (June 1978):15–17.

Clark, Carolyn Chambers. Teaching nurses group concepts: Some issues and suggestions. *Nurse educator* (January–February 1978):17–20.

Eddy, F., O'Neill, E., and Astrachan, B. Group work on a Long Term psychiatric service as conducted by nurses and aides. *Perspectives in psychiatric care,* 6, 1968:9–15.

Fiedler, Fred. *A theory of leadership effectiveness.* New York: McGraw-Hill, 1967.

Hellwig, Karen, and Memmott, Rae Jeanne. Partners in therapy: Using co-therapists' relationship in a group. *Journal of psychiatric nursing and mental health services* (April 1978):42–44.

House, R., and Mitchell, T. Path-goal theory of leadership. *Journal of contemporary business* (Autumn 1974):81–98.

Janis, Irving. Groupthink. *Psychology today* (November 1971):71–89.

Johnson, D., and Johnson, F. *Joining together: Group theory and skills.* Englewood Cliffs, NJ: Prentice-Hall, 1975.

Jones, Harvey. Psychodrama with adolescents. *Nursing times* (December 14, 1978):2052–4.

Kaplan, H.I., and Sadock, B.J. *Comprehensive group psychotherapy.* Baltimore: The Williams and Wilkins Co., 1971:72–102.

Kaplan, H.I., and Sadock, B.J. *Comprehensive group psychotherapy,* 2d ed. Baltimore: The Williams and Wilkins Co., 1983:158–166.

Loomis, Maxine. *Group process for nurses.* St. Louis: Mosby Company., 1979:1–43.

Newton, Geraldine. Self help groups: Can they help? *Journal of psychosocial nursing and mental health services,* 22, 1984:7.

Parloss, M., and Dies, R. Group psychotherapy outcome research 1966–1975. *International journal of group psychotherapy,* 27 (July 1977):281–319.

Pfeiffer, J., and Jones, J. (eds.). *The 1976 annual handbook for group facilitators.* San Diego, Cal: University Associates, 1976.

Ross, D., Uecker, et al. The impact of group and individual therapy socialization of residents in an institutional setting. *Issues in mental health nursing,* 2, 4 (June 1980):33–42.

Sampson, E.E., and Marthas, M.S. *Group process for the health professions.* New York: Wiley Medical, 1977:173–85.

Scheideman, J. Remotivation: Involvement without labels. *Journal of psychiatric nursing and mental health services* (July 1976):41–42.

Schultz, W.C. *FIRO: A three-dimensional theory of human behavior.* New York: Holt, Rinehart & Winston, 1960.

Slater, P.E. *Microcosm.* New York: John Wiley & Sons, 1966.

Smith, L. Finding your leadership style in groups. *American journal of nursing,* (July 1980):1301–1303.

Szilagyi, A., and Wallace, M. *Organizational behavior and performance,* 2d ed. Santa Monica: Goodyear, 1980.

Tuckman, B. Developmental sequence in small groups. *Psychological bulletin,* 63, 1965:384–399.

Veringa, R., and Fredlund, D. Teaching the group approach. *Nursing outlook,* 22, 1974:373–376.

Vriend, J., and Dyer, W. *Counseling effectively in groups.* Englewood Cliffs, NJ: Educational Technology Publications, 1973:168–183.

Yalom, I. *The theory and practice of group psychotherapy,* 2d ed. New York: Basic Books, 1975.

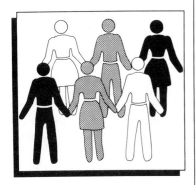

Therapeutic Environment and Therapeutic Community

Mary Kunes-Connell

Learning Objectives

Upon completion of this chapter, the reader will be able to:

1. Discuss the relationship between an individual's ego and his interpersonal and physical environment.

2. Identify the characteristics of a therapeutic community.

3. Describe the twofold role of the client in a therapeutic community.

4. Describe the role of the nurse and other professional team members in a therapeutic community.

5. Discuss the influence of the physical environment on a therapeutic community.

6. Discuss the purpose of the community meeting and client-team meeting in a therapeutic community.

7. Identify treatment modalities that can be used in a therapeutic community.

8. Identify four problems inherent in a therapeutic community.

The concept of milieu (environment, French) therapy is a reflection of the mental health professionals' view that man's behavior is modified in response to his physical, interpersonal, and cultural environment. Skinner (1979) discusses milieu therapy from a philosophical and a practical standpoint. Philosophically, milieu therapy is a belief in the interactive nature of man—that is, man develops behavioral responses as a result of his dynamic and always-changing interaction with the interpersonal and physical environment. Milieu therapy focuses on man's interaction in a therapeutic environment. A therapeutic environment is a positive atmosphere in which the client has an opportunity to develop appropriate responses to individuals and situations that he encounters. From a practical perspective, milieu therapy is a treatment mode in which personnel deliberately plan and structure the client's interpersonal and physical environment in an attempt to modify maladaptive behavioral responses while promoting more positive insights and responses. To effectively modify a client's maladaptive behavior, personnel must be comfortable in limit setting a client's inappropriate responses. To effectively promote insight, self-responsibility, and positive responses, the staff must function as role models and teachers of psychosocial skills. The treatment strategies of limit setting and teaching of psychosocial skills hold equal status in the therapeutic milieu and must be performed simultaneously (Abroms, 1969; Skinner, 1979; Visher and O'Sullivan, 1970). In the hospital environment implementation of milieu therapy is termed the "therapeutic community." In this chapter, the term milieu therapy will be used in reference to the overall ideology and philosophy of treatment while the term therapeutic community will be employed in discussion of the practical implications for practitioners.

☐ *Historical Perspective of Milieu Therapy*

Prior to the early part of the nineteenth century the emotionally disturbed person was treated as an outcast and subjected to oppressive environments. During the nineteenth century the predominant philosophy was humanism and moral treatment—the individual was viewed as good and worthwhile even in times of emotional disorder. If the individual was to be respected, then the treatment environment had to be humane.

The first formal treatment milieu advocating a humane environment for the client was the asylum, which was established to be a safe and restful environment insulated from everyday stresses. Because its focus was rest, it did not promote the active treatment characteristic of modern milieu therapy. The asylum presented many problems that diminished its effectiveness as a therapeutic milieu. It was overcrowded, underfunded, and understaffed, giving rise to an environment concerned only with custodial care. The restful treatment milieu became an institution of long-term maintenance in which the client often deteriorated.

During the twentieth century there was a shift in the focus of treatment. Freud's psychoanalytic theory transferred attention from the environment and its effects on the individual to the intrapersonal nature of the individual (the internal thoughts and emotional processes that consciously or unconsciously direct a person's outward behaviors). As medical research advanced, newer and more sophisticated somatic treatments were developed. By alleviating specific symptoms, somatic therapies focused on the behaviors of the individual rather than the alteration or restructuring of his environment. The increased emphasis on the use of somatotherapies implied that the individual was passive and could do nothing to alleviate his own problems. The individual was considered "sick" and the treatment environment reflected this view. The milieu became one of providing care to or doing for the client; it was commonly known as the medical model of treatment. The client was regarded as not having the capability to actively participate in his own treatment. A strict and rigid hierarchy emerged in which the doctor maintained almost sole control of the client's treatment environment.

The physical and interpersonal milieu, as a treatment variable, reemerged following World War II. The impact of social-psychological forces on the individual's behavior was recognized. The individual was no longer seen as passive but, rather, as an active participant in his environment. This philosophy led to the development of a form of milieu therapy known as the therapeutic community. The interpersonal, physical, and cultural environment became major variables in the hospital treatment of an individual experiencing emotional disorders. In the therapeutic community, the hospital environment was to be structured so as to simulate everyday living-learning situations in which the client would encounter common interpersonal conflicts that would require an active confrontation and adaptation of behavior (Jones, 1953). Passivity on the part of the client would give way to active participation. Treatment planned solely by the physician would give way to the sharing of treatment by all team members as well as the client.

☐ *Theoretical Framework for Milieu Therapy*

The medical model is not adequate to describe the concept of milieu therapy. Milieu therapy goes beyond mere alleviation of psychiatric symptoms; rather, it focuses on the promotion of individual growth and adaptation in a social environment. The basis of milieu therapy is the social learning model (Cummings and Cummings, 1963; Jones, 1968). This model describes the relationship between the ego, emotional disorders, and the therapeutic milieu. In order to successfully implement a therapeutic community, the nurse must have a working knowledge of the interrelationship between the individual's ego and his ability to successfully problem-solve everyday interpersonal crises.

The ego, an intricate aspect of the personality, facilitates one's ability to accurately assess and problem-solve situations that occur in one's environment. The ego involves one's thought processes, feelings, and perceptions. It is the ego that allows one to assess the everyday environment in a holistic manner and develop appropriate reality-oriented responses to this environment. The social learning model emphasizes the development of the ego and the response of the ego to the interpersonal and physical environment.

An individual's ego further develops and grows as a result of crises. A crisis is any event in the interpersonal or physical environment that causes a temporary disequilibrium in the individual's ego. This results in a temporary feeling of unpreparedness and inability to solve the problem using one's old patterns of behavior. Crisis requires a reorganization of one's thoughts, feelings, and problem-solving skills. This reorganization gives the individual new ways to deal with the problem. As the crisis is resolved, the ego grows and adapts. In this sense, a crisis could be considered a positive growth experience. In essence, the ego facilitates one's responses to the events in the environment. If conditions in the interpersonal or physical environment are destructive, the ego may be unable to reorganize effectively following a crisis, thereby fostering a continued sense of disorganization. This brings about an inability to meet and adequately relate to new situations.

According to the social learning model, the inability of the ego to appropriately develop results from an inadequate or unsafe interpersonal and physical environment. Such an environment is one that fails to: (1) foster open communication between the individual and the environment; (2) foster an atmosphere in which one can freely examine his feelings, thoughts, and behaviors; (3) properly set limits on inappropriate behavior while supporting the individual in his attempt to test new patterns of behavior; and (4) provide appropriate role models for behavior (Jones, 1968). Therefore, the hospital must provide an environment that is deliberately structured to offer positive situations (corrective emotional experiences) that require active analysis and problem solving on the part of the client. While providing these living-learning situations, the hospital must also foster a protective and supportive environment in which the client can successfully test new patterns of behavior. This hospital environment is called the therapeutic community (Campbell, 1979; Cummings and Cummings, 1963; and Jones, 1953). Figure 14-1 illustrates the influence of the social learning model on behavior development and the potential impact of this model on the development of a positive hospital environment (therapeutic community).

☐ *Therapeutic Community*

The major characteristics of a therapeutic community evolve from the social learning model. These characteristics are open communication and shared decision-making (Jones, 1953, 1976a). Often, the hospital hierarchy promotes one-way communication—communication that comes from above and extends downward. This type of communication often fosters, at least to some degree, passivity on the part of nurses and clients because these two groups are at a lower level in the hierarchy and often have little influence on the treatment plans or policies. This one-way communication closely correlates to the medical model of treatment. Two-way communication implies that every individual involved in the treatment community is given an opportunity to pro-

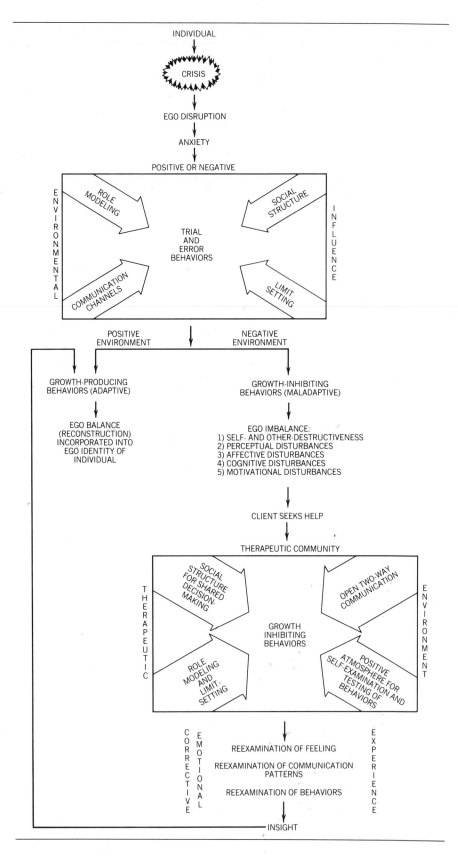

Figure 14-1 *Adaptation of social learning theory to milieu therapy.*

vide input into the happenings of the community. Open communication leads to shared decision-making, which means that everyone involved in a particular plan decides on the actions to be taken. This type of decision-making involves the democratic process and leads to a shared power among all involved in the community.

Team meetings and staff T-groups, common components of the therapeutic community, are designed to prevent or intervene in interstaff difficulties by promoting open communication between staff. The team meeting should take place on a weekly basis (Abroms, 1969) and should be attended by the immediate unit staff members. This meeting affords the opportunity to discuss overall hospital policies affecting the staff or the unit as well as on-the-ward staff or administrative problems. It is also a time for the staff to discuss delegation of paperwork, staff assignments, and lunch hour problems, and to make announcements of educational opportunities. It provides an excellent opportunity to review new studies in mental health through journal reviews or inservice activities. Staff T-groups, which should meet weekly for a 1-hour period (Abroms, 1969), serve a different purpose. The therapeutic community requires that staff work closely together, which can give rise to interpersonal conflicts among staff. These conflicts can include the development of the "my client" syndrome: each discipline develops an attitude that no one understands the client as well as it does; authority power struggles occur between staff members and between staff members and clients; and other personality conflicts occur between staff members. Because staff tensions can be easily felt by the clients, therapy will not be effective unless the conflicts are resolved. Also, unresolved staff conflicts can result in staff being unable to invest in the client because of the excessive emotional time involved in trying to deal with interstaff difficulties (Tuohey, 1978). The T-group focuses on the analysis of here-and-now interactions between staff personnel. It allows them to ventilate feelings and express problems that arise among themselves and increases staff self-awareness regarding interactions with each other. (Chapter 13 discusses T-groups in detail.)

☐ Interpersonal Environment

The therapeutic community has had a tremendous influence on nursing in recent years. Nurses'

view of clients' roles has changed, as has their view of their roles in relationship to other team members.

CLIENT ROLES AND RELATIONSHIPS

To achieve maximum effectiveness in the therapeutic community, flexibility must exist in both client and staff roles. The nurse must accept the twofold role of the client in the therapeutic community. The first is the traditional client role. Most individuals enter the hospital due to a temporary inability to cope with the stresses of their environment. This inability to cope often leads to maladaptive behavioral responses. Abroms (1969) discusses several categories of maladaptive behaviors that develop as a result of poor coping skills. These behaviors include: self- and other-destructiveness (e.g., suicide or assault), perceptual disturbances (e.g., hallucinations), affective disturbances (e.g., the client is unable to make or be responsible for decisions and behaviors and, therefore, becomes depressed), cognitive disturbances (e.g., delusions), and motivational disturbances (e.g., withdrawal) (Figure 14-1). These behaviors indicate an inability on the part of the ego to effectively assess and problem-solve crises that occur in the environment. The traditional role allows the client the freedom to ask for assistance in adapting to the environment. This role does not imply his inability to be active in his care; rather, it states that the environment is temporarily so overwhelming that he lacks the necessary skills and resources to respond appropriately.

The second role of the client is, at times, difficult for the nurse or for other professionals to accept. This role is that of an active participant. The active role stems from the belief that commitment to changing one's behavior is strengthened when one can participate in one's own care. Active participation provides the client with a sense of investment and fosters a feeling of accomplishment and success. Therefore, if the client is able to perform a certain task, let him do it. One task that can be performed in collaboration with the client is the development of his care plan. This requires meeting with the client to mutually determine priority problems, goals, and approaches. By allowing the client input, his self-esteem is strengthened and his sense of responsibility and accomplishment is enhanced. Furthermore, allowing the client to make decisions regarding his own care forces the disorganized ego to become more organized, that is, the client is supported and encouraged to appropriately assess his problems and determine the best ways to deal with them. The client is also moved toward greater ego organization as he is forced to take part in solving the problems of others on the unit.

> ### Vignette
>
> Mrs. J. is 25 years old. She has been admitted because she has been experiencing increasing feelings of depression, low self-esteem, and withdrawal. Mr. J. states that his wife has been unable to make everyday decisions about the care of the children, household, or herself to the extent of withdrawing to her room and neglecting the children and the household. She also phones Mr. J. several times a day to talk about trivial matters. Mrs. J. states that she feels incompetent to care for her family. If the personnel do not allow her to participate in her own care, they only foster her feelings of inadequacy in decision making. On the other hand, by encouraging Mrs. J. to have input into the goals and approaches, her sense of responsibility and accomplishment increases, resulting in more positive self-esteem.

Participation in the care of others and peer pressure are also powerful tools in changing behavior patterns in both self and others (Jones, 1976). The unit, as a therapeutic community, is a microcosm of the larger environment. Those living on the unit establish norms (rules) regarding acceptable and unacceptable behavior. Peers become effective in enforcing these norms, confronting individuals, and providing constructive feedback to others on how to change behaviors. Peer pressure and client participation become especially effective in the daily community meeting as clients confront and support each other at times of crisis.

Nurses and other professionals must keep in mind that clients will be at different positions along the passive-active continuum throughout hospitalization. In the case of Mrs. J., it may not be appropriate to expect her participation in either her care or the care of others immediately following admission. Her depression combined with her anxiety about hospitalization renders her relatively ineffective in making appropriate decisions, and asking for her participation would serve only to increase her feelings of inadequacy. Therefore, the first step may be to accept her passivity and provide a supportive, caring environ-

ment. As she begins to feel less anxious, the environment can then be structured to provide events that require active decision making and participation. Table 14-1 is a sample care plan for Mrs. J., employing the principles of milieu therapy on a therapeutic community.

> ### ■ Point of Emphasis
>
> *An effective therapeutic community allows the client to take an active role in his own treatment. It is the community's attempt to dispel the myth that the client is a passive recipient of care.*

NURSING ROLES AND TEAM RELATIONSHIPS

Abroms (1969) proposes two major functions of the therapeutic community—setting limits on behavior and learning psychosocial skills. These two functions coincide with the two major roles of nursing in a therapeutic community—the authority role and the therapeutic role. The nurse must be able to strike a proper balance between these two roles if she is to effectively set limits on maladaptive behaviors while concurrently promoting a more positive response to the environment. The first step in social learning is for the client to gain insight into responses that are considered inappropriate. Often the client is unaware of or has not been taught that behaviors such as assault, self-destructiveness, and excessive isolation are not proper responses to interpersonal crises and serve only as self-defeating behaviors. It becomes necessary for the nurse to limit those behaviors that do not prove to be self-enhancing. Setting limits establishes external controls on the client until he has the resources to develop inner controls over his behavior.

A second step of social learning is for the client to develop adaptive responses to the environment. The nurse must adopt the therapeutic role in order to foster the client's psychosocial skills. This requires the nurse to structure the environment so that every interaction has value in teaching the client both problem-solving and interpersonal skills. This is best accomplished through an accurate individualized assessment and implementation of treatment modalities. It is hoped that through an increased self-awareness of behavior patterns and a learning of more positive behaviors the client will take more respon-

TABLE 14-1 Sample Care Plan: Effective Use of Treatment Modalities in Milieu Therapy

Problem: Disturbance in self-concept: ineffective role performance related to feelings of failure, resulting in inability to make decisions regarding family, home, and self-care, and social isolation from family and peers.

Long-Term Goal: Mrs. J. will be able to return to the home situation capable of: (1) independently making decisions and taking actions regarding self, family, and home care; and (2) socially interacting with family and friends.

Short-Term Goal: (1) Mrs. J. will decide on and attend daily unit activities.

Intervention[a]	Rationale	Evaluation
1. Mrs. J. will be given daily expectations by the one-to-one nurse to attend three unit activities per day. a. The weekly patient/staff meeting will, initially, be used to provide Mrs. J. an agenda of the activities. In the beginning, three activities will be assigned to her. b. The expectation to attend the activities will include a supportive statement by the nurse that she does not have to verbally (actively) participate with peers or staff personnel. c. During the unit activities Mrs. J. will be assigned to a peer in order that she may ask questions about the unit or activities. d. "Positive strokes" will be given to the patient for her participation in unit activities. e. A community meeting will be established to keep the peers informed of Mrs. J.'s treatment plan and their role in "stroking" Mrs. J. for her participation and decision making on the unit.	On her initial admission to the unit, the staff recognizes the effect of the new environment and the overwhelming recent home situation on Mrs. J.'s ability to make decisions and her level of ego organization (Mrs. J. has an inability to assess and effectively problem-solve every day situations) resulting in the maladaptive behaviors of excessive dependency, decreased self-esteem, and increased social isolation from family and peers. This set of interventions recognizes the need to decrease Mrs. J.'s overwhelming anxiety and make a supportive environment for her by allowing the patient to take on the patient role in eliciting and accepting help when needed. As immediate active involvement is not expected the patient is allowed time to adapt to the new situation. However, complete isolation or withdrawal (maladaptive) is not allowed and, thus, the expectation to attend activities, at least physically, is a limit set on the maladaptive withdrawal; it paves the way for the next step of learning basic psychosocial skills of problem solving and social interactiveness.	Each goal and set of interventions will be evaluated as to: 1. Mrs. J.'s anxiety level when decision making and interacting with family and peers. 2. Mrs. J.'s dependency on others in the unit and her family to meet her needs. 3. Mrs. J.'s interaction with family and others on the unit. 4. Mrs. J.'s ability and progress in problem-solving—from simple unit decisions to complex home and family decisions.

Short-Term Goal: (2) In the daily one-to-one with the nurse Mrs. J. will freely ventilate both positive and negative feelings and concerns about her role in the home and her role in social-interpersonal relationships.

2. Initially, Mrs. J.'s one-to-one nurse will set up a special time each day for a 45-minute period to allow for ventilation of feelings and anxiety about home and social situation with friends and peers on unit. Mrs. J. will not, initially, be expected to initiate any 1:1. a. "Positive strokes" will be given for any ventilation of feelings or initiation of topics in order to decrease Mrs. J.'s sense of failure.	Same as Goal 1 and the first set of interventions	Same as Goal 1

Short-Term Goal: (3) Mrs. J. will structure each one-to-one session with the nurse to:
  a. Discuss own concerns about daily home-life decision making and social interaction with family and friends.
  b. Establish goals for returning home.
  c. Establish own interventions for successful and independent decision-making social interactions.
  d. Independently plan own therapeutic pass with family with written plan regarding social activities to be done at home and family care decisions to be made.
  e. Make one decision per day regarding her degree of participation in the daily unit activities.

(continued)

TABLE 14-1 *(continued)*

Intervention[a]	Rationale	Evaluation
3. The weekly patient/staff meeting will be designed to provide feedback to Mrs. J. regarding overall weekly unit progress in relation to the goals of decision making (without aid from personnel or peers) and social interactiveness on the unit. a. This meeting with Mrs. J. will also be used to explain that, in situations in which Mrs. J. has a choice, she will be expected to verbalize her steps in the decision-making process and make her own conclusions and take actions for herself. This approach will also be taken in the one-to-one session and will be explained to Mrs. J.	Goals and interventions 3, 4, and 5 are established as Mrs. J. can take one more step in her own staff/therapeutic/active role. Based on the evaluation of Goals 1 and 2 the staff members are able to determine whether Mrs. J. can begin to take responsibility and initiate her own treatment regimen. Group therapy, the community meeting, the one-to-one, role playing, and family conferences are the modes to promote her psychosocial skills of problem solving and social interactiveness.	Same as Goal 1

Short-Term Goal: (4) Mrs. J. will communicate her needs and concerns to her husband in family conferences.

4. The weekly patient/staff meeting will explain the purpose of various techniques directed toward aiding Mrs. J. in developing effective assertiveness within the family situations, for example, role playing, family conferences.	Same as Goal 3	Same as Goal 1

Short-Term Goal: (5) Mrs. J. will initiate and structure two small groups prior to discharge regarding:
          a. Her ability to make decisions
          b. Her ability to socially interact

5. Through the weekly patient/staff meeting and the one-to-one Mrs. J. will be given the expectation to set up and initiate the small group therapy:
  a. The community meeting will be used to inform the patients of Mrs. J.'s duties regarding small group.
  b. Mrs. J will also be given the expectation to elicit feedback from peers during activity groups about her participation and ability to make decisions on the unit.
  c. Mrs. J. will then be given the expectation to report the feedback that she receives to the small groups.
  d. Mrs. J. will also be given the expectation to inquire into the progress of one patient per week in small groups or during regular activities time.
  e. "Positive strokes" will be given as Mrs. J. initiates/participates in her own treatment plan, groups, activities, and conferences.
	Same as Goal 3	Same as Goal 1

[a] These interventions are client-oriented. Interventions (T-Groups, the unit meeting, among other interventions) used by staff members to work through their frustrations of dealing with a dependent client are not discussed in this care plan even though these are a necessary component of the successful therapeutic community. It can be seen that all of the techniques of the therapeutic community (i.e., small groups, one-to-one and community meeting, among others) can be structured to aid the client in accomplishing the goals of limit setting one's own maladaptive behaviors and developing more adaptive and successful psychosocial behaviors.

sibility for himself and his interactions with the environment. To properly provide role modeling and promote the client's sense of self-responsibility, the facilitator (nurse) must relinquish some of the authority and control traditionally held in the nurse-client relationship. The client must be allowed to make decisions regarding his own care, readiness for treatments, passes, and discharges. He must also be allowed to give input on unit matters that directly affect him (e.g., active planning, room changes). Relinquishing power and authority is often difficult for the nurse who has been socialized into the traditional hospital structure; the nurse-client authority issue can be effectively dealt with by the nurse in the staff T-groups. Figure 14-2 illustrates a sample unit schedule for a therapeutic community. The activities are designed to enable the client to problem-solve in a variety of areas of his life and develop skills enhancing his ability to function appropriately in his environment.

> ### ■ Point of Emphasis
> The nurse has a dual role in the therapeutic community—the authority role (setting limits) and the therapeutic role (modeling psychosocial skills).

The issue of authority again surfaces when discussing interstaff relationships. The medical model supports a distinct hierarchy of power within the hospital. The social model diffuses this power by advocating a more equal power sharing among the team. All members of the team collaborate in decisions about the unit, client care, and certain hospital policies. This creates an atmosphere in which holistic care is implemented. However, this is not to say that all issues are determined by group consensus. If a policy does not involve nursing, then nursing may not be included in the decision-making process. The concept of power sharing can create problems if various disciplines are unsure of their role and the relationships of the roles to each other. This can result in role confusion or role blurring.

The client and staff roles and team relationships have impact not only on providing an effective therapeutic community on a mental health unit, but also on the care provided on a medical-surgical unit. A more comprehensive and holistic approach can be taken in promoting wellness if team members have equal input into the client's care. Also, allowing the client to have some control over his own care increases the likelihood of compliance to the medical regimen because the client experiences a sense of investment in his own care. The client no longer experiences a sense of dependency and helplessness but instead has a sense of power and control.

□ Physical Environment

The physical environment has tremendous impact on one's anxiety level, violent capacities, and frustration levels, among other affective responses (Davis, 1979). The therapeutic community on the hospital unit attempts to create a safe and home-like atmosphere. Though most mental health units successfully communicate a sense of safety they also give a feeling of sterility and alienation to those living on the unit. A physically safe environment is necessary to protect clients from their own or others' destructiveness. Therefore, it is not inhumane to install safety mirrors, Plexiglass, and sturdy furniture. However, this does not imply that the unit must be prisonlike and monotonous, an environment that can be detrimental to the client's progress. Monotony has been shown to produce such psychoticlike behaviors as hallucinations, illusions, delusions, and general disorientation (Birren, 1979). This type of environment serves only to intensify the behaviors and feelings of emotionally troubled clients. Because the nursing staff and client population spend the most time on the unit, these two groups should be able to have input into its design.

Colors can produce striking effects. In a hospital environment colors must be balanced in order to promote a stimulating yet soothing atmosphere (Davis, 1979). A unit is composed of a heterogenous group of clients and, therefore, color must meet the needs of the various groups. White, a traditional color of most hospitals, is not always the most appropriate. It represents a starkness and sterility and is emotionally bland in that it neither stimulates nor soothes clients. White is also an unsuitable color when considering the type of lighting on most units. Artificial light on a white background casts glares and bizarre shadows. It has been shown to generate such somatic complaints as headaches and blurred vision. With psychotic clients, fluorescent light on a white background might cast shadows that only serve to exaggerate perceptual and thought disturbances such as hallucinations, illusions, and delusions.

Sunday	Monday	Tuesday	Wednesday	Thursday	Friday	Saturday
8:30–10:00 Breakfast / Hygiene	7:30–9:00 Breakfast / Hygiene	7:30–9:00 Breakfast / Hygiene	7:30–9:00 Breakfast / Hygiene	7:30–9:00 Breakfast / Hygiene	7:30–9:00 Breakfast / Hygiene	8:00–10:00 Breakfast / Hygiene
	9:00–10:00 Community meeting	9:00–10:00 Community meeting	9:00–10:00 Community meeting	9:00–10:00 Community meeting	9:00–10:00 Community meeting	
10–10:30 Religious services	10–10:30 Free time	10–10:30 Free time	10–10:30 Free time	10–10:30 Free time	10–10:30 Free time	10–11:00 Community meeting
10:30–11:30 Community meeting	10:30–11:30 OT / RT	10:30–11:30 Exercise hour	10:30–11:30 Women's/men's group	10:30–11:30 Exercise hour	10:30–11:30 OT / RT	
						11–12:00 Self-esteem groups
11:30–12:30 Art therapy	11:30–12:30 Case conferences with clients/one-to-one time	11:30–12:30 Self-esteem group I Assertiveness group II	11:30–12:30 Case conferences with clients/one-to-one time	11:30–12:30 Stress management group I Assertiveness group II	11:30–12:30 Case conferences with clients/one-to-one time	12:00–12:30 Free time
12:30–1:30 Lunch	12:30–1:30 Lunch	12:30–1:30 Lunch	12:30–1:30 Lunch	12:30–1:30 Lunch	12:30–1:30 Lunch	12:30–1:30 Lunch
1:30–2:00 Free time	1:30–2:00 Free time	1:30–2:00 Free time	1:30–2:00 Free time	1:30–2:00 Free time	1:30–2:00 Free time	1:30–4:00 Field trips
2:00–4:00 Visitors / Exercise and relaxation	2:00–3:00 Smaller groups (e.g., ADL, Parenting, discharge planning)	2:00–3:00 Self-esteem group II Assertiveness group I	2:00–3:00 Client council	2:00–3:00 Stress management group II Assertiveness group I	2:00–3:00 Smaller groups (e.g., ADL, parenting, discharge planning)	
	3:00–4:00 Staff T-group / Free time for clients	3:00–4:00 Small group therapy groups I and II	3:00–4:00 Team meeting—staff / Free time for clients	3:00–4:00 Small group therapy groups I and II	3:00–4:00 Music therapy	Speakers from outside agencies
4:00–5:00 Music therapy	4:00–5:00 Medication education group	4:00–5:00 Music therapy	4:00–5:00 Medication education group	4:00–5:00 Art therapy	4:00–5:00 Horticulture therapy	4:00–5:00 Health group
5:00–6:30 Dinner / Free time	5:00–6:30 Dinner / Free time	5:00–6:30 Dinner / Free time	5:00–6:30 Dinner / Free time	5:00–6:30 Dinner / Free time	5:00–6:30 Dinner / Free time	5:00–6:30 Dinner / Free time
6:30–7:30 Family group	6:30–7:30 Health group	6:30–7:30 Family group	6:30–7:30 Communication groups	6:30–7:30 Family groups	6:30–7:30 Communication groups	6:30–7:30 Exercise / Relaxation
7:30–9:00 Visitors / One-to-one time	7:30–9:00 Visitors / Movie	7:30–9:00 Visitors / Social Hour	7:30–9:00 Visitors / Table Games	7:30–9:00 Visitors / Movie	7:30–9:00 Visitors / Social hour	7:30–9:00 Visitors / Planned activity by clients

Figure 14-2 *Sample unit activity schedule for a therapeutic community.*

If the goal of a therapeutic community is to create a homelike environment, then a combination of warm and cool colors must be utilized. Various shades of blues and greens are appropriate as they tend to be soothing and relaxing. This is an important consideration since most hospitalized individuals have an increased anxiety level. Color schemes are of special significance when a unit contains a seclusion area. Some tones of peach or pink might be appropriate as these colors are calming. But a hospital environment does not have to confine itself to the use of relaxing, calming colors. There are situations in which stimulating colors, such as reds and yellows, serve a purpose. A unit housing isolative or apathetic individuals might require colors that produce a sense of stimulation and uplifting mood. It must be remembered that color schemes are important in both mental health and medical-surgical units. On a medical unit white creates an impersonal environment that serves only to increase the anxiety level and impersonal feelings already experienced by the client who enters the hospital.

Choosing proper colors should taken into account furniture and carpeting as well as walls. Furniture should be durable but comfortable. Vinyl-covered furniture gives a cold, impersonal effect, whereas heavy-duty wood frame furniture with soft padding gives a homelike atmosphere. The style of the furniture should be varied, and it should include couches, desks, soft arm chairs, and different styles and sizes of tables. Choosing appropriate furniture becomes an important function in that decisions are based not only on the design of the furniture, but on the behavior of the clients. For instance, a children's unit might require furniture that can be jumped on or thrown about without being badly damaged. Also, the furniture should be such that it can be rearranged. The environment becomes increasingly personalized when clients can rearrange the furniture to accommodate various activities and groups.

In addition to furniture, decorations are important elements in achieving a comfortable environment. Clients should be permitted to keep personal possessions on the unit, because they give the client a sense of belonging (e.g., to home, to significant others), and diminish his feeling of alienation. However, nurses need to be keenly aware about what types of articles are brought into the hospital; for example, a suicidal client may have a calendar, a transistor radio, posters, books, or plants, but articles made of glass or containing glass will be prohibited.

Art, specifically chosen for the hospital, is just as important as the personal articles. Hyman (1979) states that from the moment an individual enters the lobby until the moment he reaches the living area, art should create a pleasant environment. Bare walls lend monotony and blandness to the environment and should be avoided.

■ Point of Emphasis

The physical structure of the environment has an important impact on the therapy program of the unit. Color, furniture, and art are only a few of the variables that must be considered in providing a therapeutic environment. Lighting, room size, room shape, location of nursing stations, and design of dining areas are among other physical factors that must also be taken into consideration.

TREATMENT MODALITIES

A variety of treatment modalities are available to meet the individual needs of clients. Each is essential in providing a medium in which the client can express his feelings and successfully work through his stresses. Among the treatments that can be effectively employed to create a therapeutic milieu are: community meeting, client-team meeting, therapeutic recreation, occupational therapy, music and art therapy, horticulture therapy, social work therapy, and psychological testing.

Community Meeting

The community meeting is the essence of the therapeutic milieu. Established by Maxwell Jones (1953, 1976a, 1976b) the community meeting is broadly defined as a meeting of all clients and staff who work and live in a defined area for the purpose of providing a climate for free expression of feelings between staff members, staff members and clients, and clients. This 1-hour meeting should occur on a daily basis. As opposed to small group therapy which should consist of a maximum of 12, the community meeting can accommodate large numbers. Jones (1968, 1976a, 1976b) states that the purposes of the community meeting are to provide methods for staff and clients to: (1) examine and clarify their roles and corresponding behaviors on the unit; (2) examine and clarify hospital, unit, and group rules and norms along with the methods for rule enforcement; (3) examine in detail the problems and tensions that can occur between staff and clients or between clients; and (4) to discuss the domestic details of daily unit upkeep.

The first purpose, role examination, is vital to the success of the therapeutic community where role blurring between clients, between clients and staff, and between staff members is a constant danger. Power struggles may occur between the older and newer clients on the unit. Clients who have lived longer on the unit take on a role of authority or power over the newer clients. To prevent a possible abuse of power this authority struggle must be kept in check through the examination of client behavior by the other clients and by staff members. Staff struggles also exist due to the imposition of the traditional hierarchical structure of the medical model on the social organization of the therapeutic community. This hierarchical structure consists of medical professionals, medical students, a head nurse, staff nurses, psychiatric technicians, and student nurses, along with the allied health team. This structure sometimes makes it very difficult not to assert the power traditionally associated with the role, for example, the head nurse stepping in to make a unit decision that affects clients without obtaining client input. Role blurring frequently occurs between the nursing staff and the medical and allied health professions. Traditionally, the nurses lead group therapy; however, in the therapeutic community there is a sharing of leadership among the staff or clients. This is sometimes viewed as a relinquishment of power traditionally held by nurses. Unless the attitude toward roles and role relationships is carefully examined and clarified the community meeting will be faced with many obstacles.

The second purpose, the clarification of rules, is important because of staff and client turnover. With new staff and clients come new rules and norms along with a reiteration and reevaluation of the old ones. Unless there is a constant flow of communication about the rules for staff and clients, therapy will be inconsistent. The community meeting assures consistent communication. In some cases this daily 1-hour community meeting is insufficient for behavior examination. Groups such as children, adolescents, or acutely psychotic individuals require more immediate and more frequent feedback and may need to meet for one hour at the end of both the day and evening shifts. At this time there would be an examination of the behaviors and goals of the clients as well

as the staff's responses to the clients and their behaviors.

The third purpose is an examination of conflicts among staff and clients that are caused by living together with the same group day after day. Often, clients enter the hospital because they were unable to deal with these types of conflicts at home. The community meeting allows for the free expression and problem solving of these conflicts.

The fourth purpose, unit upkeep, can be discussed in community meeting or a client council meeting once or twice a week (Jones, 1976b). Because the community meeting often concentrates on the first three purposes, a special time must be set aside to discuss unit housekeeping. Decisions made during this time include television programs to be watched, ward responsibilities, activity planning, and the use of unit materials, among others. The client council may be composed of all the clients or a few selected by their peer group. Staff should also be represented to clarify policies as well as to provide input into unit functioning. The client council should not take the place of the community meeting.

The importance of the scheduled community meeting should be emphasized—it should not be cancelled or marred by frequent interruptions by physicians, allied health personnel, other nurses, and visitors, or by clients or staff coming and going throughout group.

Jones (1976a, 1976b) recommends that a staff review take place following each community meeting. This review, ideally, should last for 1 hour, though modification may be necessary depending on the unit, its schedule, the client population, and the need for staff supervision. The staff review follows the same principles as group meeting and might include an examination of the content of the community meeting, an analysis of the roles and role relationships in the group, thorough staff review of responses to the various clients and to the presentation of certain issues, and a review of staff skills. This examination calls for openness on the part of staff to giving and receiving feedback—the staff must be open to self-inspection. Their self-awareness is enhanced by this type of review.

The purpose of the community meeting is not to deal with the personal problems of clients. To allow them to more intensively look at their own problems apart from unit problems, the community meeting should be supplemented with a small group therapy consisting of no more than 6 to 12 clients (Jones, 1976a, 1976b).

Client-Team Meeting

The client-team meeting, which should take place weekly, is a more personalized interaction between the individual client and the team members for the purpose of reviewing care plan goals and approaches. Abroms (1969) discusses the benefit of this meeting for the client. First, it allows the client to define his problems more accurately. Most clients, on initial hospitalization, are vague about their problems, and vagueness does not lend itself to specific approaches. For example, on admission a client might state that he is hospitalized for "nerves." This type of problem cannot be specifically dealt with and serves only to increase the client's anxiety level. However, with feedback from staff, the client eventually defines his problem, for example, excessive drinking due to increasing pressures at his job. Because this problem is more clearly defined, it is more easily approached. Second, the meeting gives the client more input into choosing treatment approaches. It increases his understanding of the treatment selected, and this promotes his compliance.

Therapeutic Recreation

Therapeutic recreation is a professional discipline in which the therapist purposefully plans and controls recreational situations for individuals in order to: (1) maximize their biological, psychological, and social development, (2) provide ample opportunities for strengthening positive responses to the environment (socializing, structuring free time, and increasing self-confidence in tasks), and (3) promote more effective coping skills in anxiety-provoking situations (O'Morrow, 1976). To successfully meet this goal within the milieu, the therapist must work in cooperation with other team members and with the client in order to provide recreational services conducive to promoting overall change in his response to his environment. Assessment, goal development, interventions, and evaluation can be accomplished in the weekly client-team meeting.

Occupational Therapy

Occupational therapy's major concern is the maximization of an individual's performance in relation to his cultural, social, and work environment. This requires, on the part of the occupational therapist, a holistic approach to the assessment of the individual's sensory, cognitive, motor, and psychosocial functioning. Following the comprehensive assessment, the occupational therapist sets up purposeful, goal-oriented activities to maximize the client's capacity to respond to his environment (Mosey, 1980). These activities are individualized depending on the client's needs, and may range from individual to group tasks. As with the recreational therapist, the occupational therapist must work in conjunction with the client and other team members in order to make the goals and interventions appropriate to the client's lifestyle. Again, the client-team meeting is the major vehicle by which the occupational therapist integrates interventions with the team.

Music and Art Therapy

When verbal communication about emotions is difficult to achieve, music and art represent two alternative media through which one can freely express onself. The music therapist builds on the client's musical talent or love of music in an attempt to bring about an outward expression of feelings. This intervention is based on the premise that musical choices often accurately indicate one's emotional level. Art therapy is based on a corresponding premise. First, one's choice of images and color often reflect thought patterns and feeling tones. Second, drawing is an uninhibited yet private way by which one can express the inner self. Both art and music therapists must complete extensive training so that they can understand the interrelationship between their media, interpersonal communication, and the dynamics of emotional disorders.

Horticulture Therapy

Horticulture therapy involves the use of gardening as a form of treatment. Through gardening the therapist can facilitate the building of a client's self-esteem. If a client can successfully grow a living thing, he can begin to feel that there are elements in his own life that he can successfully manage. The client is taught that he must exert some control and responsibility if he expects to achieve his desired results. In gardening this is accomplished by making the client aware that what he does with the seeds, soil, water, and other materials will have an effect. The horticulture therapist must complete training that goes beyond gardening, and must be able to understand and apply the principles of gardening to various emotional disorders.

Social Work Therapy

The primary focus of the social worker is to determine how the physical, cultural, and sociological variables in the environment negatively affect an individual's behavior, and how they can be altered. Following this, the social worker helps the client to adapt to the environment through the use of community resources. The social worker's role is twofold—a referral source and a counselor. Counseling tasks might range from financial counseling to parenting techniques. The social worker is a vital member of the client-team meeting, keeping the staff informed about the client's relationship to his environment outside the hospital.

Psychological Testing

Psychology is not a therapy; however, it is a necessary discipline in a therapeutic milieu. The major emphasis in psychology is on an assessment of the client's mental status with possible recommendations for treatment. Through a series of interviews, tests, and observations the psychologist aids in diagnosing areas of difficulty in client functioning. Thus, the psychologist becomes an important member of the health team. Through the psychologist other team members gain insight into the client's behavior patterns and possible reasons for them. This understanding is vital if the team and the client are to set realistic goals and interventions for improvement. Without a knowledge of *affect*, the individual's organic, cognitive, emotional, sensory, and social functioning goals and interventions often become unrealistic, and the client's efforts are doomed to fail (e.g., one cannot expect abstract problem solving in a client who exhibits severe organic brain dysfunction). It is the psychologist who often brings these variables to the team's attention. It is necessary, therefore, for the psychologist to attend client-team meetings.

■ Point of Emphasis

The therapeutic community is more than a title for a unit; rather, it is an approach to treating the client experiencing emotional disorders. Through the planned structuring of the social, interpersonal, and physical environment, the therapeutic community becomes a social learning environment for clients and staff who enter it.

☐ Problems of Therapeutic Community

The therapeutic community, like other treatment modalities, is beset with numerous problems. Four problems stand out: possible lack of commitment to the team, role blurring, permissiveness and lack of responsibility, and client length of stay (Campbell, 1979; Jones, 1976b).

Staff commitment to each other and to the concept of the therapeutic community is essential for the successful functioning of the community. The social organization of the community implies that individuals work as a team to provide therapy. When commitment is absent, there is a lack of cohesiveness among the team members, culminating in different approaches by different individuals. These different approaches are not necessarily inappropriate—but the lack of commitment often leads to lack of communication among staff. There is then inconsistent limit setting and role modeling of psychosocial skills. Not only does lack of staff commitment make it difficult for the client to learn new patterns of behavior; it also encourages a corresponding lack of commitment in the clients, because a cohesive staff is needed to promote commitment among clients to work as a group. Staff commitment can be promoted through the use of staff T-groups and of client-team and team meetings, so that the staff can perceive the accomplishments that can be achieved through team effort.

Role blurring often gives rise to lack of any formal authority. Staff have a difficult time understanding who has authority in a particular situation, which can result in a laissez-faire approach by staff toward clients. This in turn often leads to excessive permissiveness and little or no limit setting (Campbell, 1979). Thus, the client has no guidelines as to appropriate versus inappropriate behavior. For certain groups this can be nontherapeutic. The impulsive individual will thrive on permissiveness (Campbell, 1979). The psychotic client cannot tolerate a too permissive environment. The reason is that in a therapeutic community, permissiveness requires that the client take responsibility for his behavior. In an acute phase of his disorder, the psychotic client cannot take responsibility for himself and set limits on his own behavior. He needs a structured, well-defined interpersonal and physical environment.

The fourth problem stems from the frequent client turnover in the hospital system. Jones

(1976b) believes that for the community meetings and other group treatment methods to be effective, there must be continuity of clients so that older clients can facilitate the orientation of newly admitted clients and role-model appropriate communication and problem-solving techniques in crisis situations. The emphasis on clients learning from each other is diminished as length of stay is shortened.

■ Enrichment Activities

DISCUSSION QUESTIONS

1. Compare and contrast various theoretical frameworks for care in relation to their usefulness in setting up a therapeutic community.

2. As you work in a therapeutic milieu:
   a. Assess the strengths of the interpersonal and physical milieu that enhance the delivery of care to the client.
   b. Assess the weaknesses of the interpersonal and physical milieu that inhibit the delivery of care to the client. Based on your assessment identify needed interventions that will maintain the therapeutic milieu for the clients.
   c. Identify the physical and interpersonal influences that enhance the needed changes. Identify the physical and interpersonal influences that may inhibit the needed changes.

LEARNING ACTIVITIES

1. Miss M. is a 23-year-old Caucasian who has entered the mental health facility complaining of feeling "blue" for the past 3 months. During this period, Miss. M. has had difficulty sleeping (insomnia), a constant feeling of fatigue, and anorexia. She has stated that she has no energy to attend her weekly exercise class or activities with friends. She also states that she would prefer to stay in her room all day. Miss M. related a difficulty in talking with people and describes herself as a "controlled" person who rarely expresses her feelings. She has been employed as an elementary school teacher for 2 years. Her contract was terminated approximately 3 months ago, and since that time Miss M. has not sought further employment.

In a group of eight, develop a comprehensive treatment plan (each person should be assigned one of the following roles: nurse, recreational therapist, occupational therapist, horticultural therapist, music therapist, art therapist, social worker, and client). This comprehensive treatment plan is taking place during the client-team meeting.

■ Recommended Readings

Cummings, John, and Cummings, Elaine. *Ego & milieu: Theory and practice of environmental therapy.* 2d ed., New York: Atherton Press, 1963. A classic work that analyzes the influence of the interpersonal and physical milieu on the development of ego. The first portion of this book centers on a workable definition of ego, by integrating the views of numerous theorists. It then views emotional disturbances as a disorganization of the ego. The second portion of the book centers around milieu and its effect on ego reorganization.

Jones, Maxwell. *The therapeutic community.* New York: Basic Books, 1953. Jones focuses specifically on the therapeutic community as an aspect of the broader concept of milieu therapy. This work integrates the theoretical principles of systems theory and social learning with the practical aspects of developing an inpatient setting resembling a self-governing community.

■ References

Abroms, Gene M. Defining milieu therapy. *Archives of general psychiatry*, 21, 1969:552–560.

Altschul, Annie. The role of professionals. *Nursing times*, 76, 1980:555–556.

Alvermann, Mary M. Toward improving geriatric care with environmental intervention emphasizing a homelike atmosphere. An environmental experience. *Journal of gerontological nursing*, 5, 3, 1979:13–17.

Birren, Faber. Human response to color and light. *Hospitals*, 53, 14, 1979:93–96.

Braff, David L., John Bachman, Ira Glick, and Reese Jones. The therapeutic community as a research ward. *Archives of general psychiatry*, 36, 1979:355–360.

Bulbrook, Mary Jo Trapp. Formal preparation of traditional psychiatric team members. In *Development of therapeutic skills*. Boston: Little, Brown & Co., 1980:247–255.

Campbell, W., The therapeutic community: A history. *Nursing times*, 75, 1979:1985–1987.

Campbell, W. The therapeutic community: Problems encountered by nurses. *Nursing times*, 75, 1979: 2038–2040.

Carser, Diane. Primary nursing in the mileu. *Journal of psychiatric nursing and mental health services*. 19, 1981:35–41.

Coltrane, Frances, and Pugh, Carol. Danger signals in staff/patient relationships in therapeutic milieu. *Journal of psychiatric nursing and mental health services*, 16, 1980: 34–36.

Cummings, John, and Cummings, Elaine. *Ego and milieu: Theory and practice of environmental therapy.* 2d ed. New York: Atherton Press, 1963.

Davis Charles, Glick, Ira, and Rosow, Irving. The architectural design of a psychotherapeutic milieu. *Hospital and community psychiatry.* 30, 7, 1979:453–460.

Devine, Barbara. Therapeutic milieu/milieu therapy: An overview. *Journal of Psychiatric nursing and mental health services*, 19, 1981:20–24.

Druck, Andrew B., The role of the psychoanalytically oriented psychotherapist within a therapeutic community. *Psychiatry*, 45, 1, 1982:45–58.

Hyman, Richard. Choosing art for your hospital: Some basic do's and dont's," *Hospitals, J.A.H.A.,* 53, 6, 1979:95–98.

Jacobs, Bernard, J., and Schweitzer, Robert. Conceptualizing structure in a day treatment program for delinquent adolescents. *American journal of orthopsychiatry.* 49, 2, 1979:246–251.

Jones, Maxwell. *The therapeutic community.* New York: Basic Books, 1953.

Jones, Maxwell. *Beyond the therapeutic community.* New Haven: Yale University Press, 1968.

Jones, Maxwell. *Maturation of the therapeutic community: An organic approach to health and mental health.* New York: Human Sciences Press. 1976a.

Jones, Maxwell. The therapeutic ccmmunity: Milieu therapy. In *Psychopathology today: Experimentation, theory and research.* 6th ed. (Sahakian, William, ed.). Itasca, MN: F.E. Peacock Publishers, Inc., 1976b.

Kynaston, Trevor. A special kind of help. *Nursing mirror*, 250, 1980:26–28.

Labarca, Judith R. Communication through art therapy. *Perspectives in psychiatric care*, 17, 3, 1979:118–122.

Lacy, Marcia. Creating a safe and supportive treatment environment. *Hospital & community psychiatry*, 32, 1, 1981:44–47.

Michel, Donald. *Music therapy: An introduction to therapy and special education through music.* Springfield, IL: Charles C. Thomas, 1976.

Miller, Thomas W., and Lee, Lily I. Quality assurance: Focus on environmental perceptions of psychiatric patients and nursing staff. *Journal of psychiatric nursing and mental health services*, 18, 1980:9–13.

Mosey, Ann Cronin. A model for occupational therapy. *Occupational therapy in mental health*, 1, 1, 1980:11–33.

Oberlander, Rachel. Beauty in a hospital aids the cure. *Hospitals, J.A.H.A.*, 53, 6, 1979:89–92.

O'Morrow, Gerald S. *Therapeutic recreation: A helping profession.* Reston, VA: Reston Publishing Company, Inc., 1976.

Rasinski, Kenneth, Rozensky, Ronald, and Pasulka, Paul. Practical implications of a theory of the 'therapeutic milieu' for psychiatric nursing practice. *Journal of psychiatric nursing and mental health services*, 18, 1980:16–20.

Russakoff, L. Mark, and Oldham, John M. The structure and technique of community meetings: The short-term unit. *Psychiatry*, 45, 1, 1982:38–43.

Skinner, Kathryn. The therapeutic milieu: Making it work. *Journal of psychiatric nursing and mental health services*, 17, 1979:38–44.

Spelfogel, Benjamin, and Modrzakowski, Malcolm. Curative factors in horticultural therapy in a hospital setting. *Hospital and community psychiatry*, 31, 8, 1980:572–573.

Touhey, Cecelia M. Influence of group process on the unit milieu. *Nursing Clinics of North America*, 13, 4, 1978:665–671.

Visher, J.S., and O'Sullivan, M. Nurse and patient responses to a study of milieu therapy. *American journal of psychiatry*, 127, 1970:451–456.

Wilmer, Harry A. Defining and understanding the therapeutic community. *Hospital and community psychiatry*, 32, 2, 1981:95–99.

Wolf, Margaret. A review of literature of milieu therapy. *Journal of psychiatric nursing and mental health services*, 15, 1977:26–32.

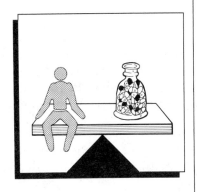

15

Pharmacotherapy: Implications for Nursing

Linda S. Beeber and Barbara L. MacDermott

Learning Objectives

Upon completion of this chapter, the reader will be able to:

1. Recognize the synergism between medication therapy and interpersonal nursing interventions with psychiatric clients.

2. Identify the most common medications within the three major classes of drugs used to treat symptoms of mental disorder.

3. Assess the client as to actual and potential health problems related to pharmacotherapy.

4. Design nursing interventions that are pharmacologically appropriate and that address the client's biopsychosocial needs.

5. Evaluate the effect of psychotropic medications on the client's state of wellness.

6. Recognize ethical and legal issues surrounding pharmacotherapy.

Psychotropic medication—preparations that "change the mind"—were introduced in the early 1950s and quickly became one of the standard forms of treatment and symptom control in psychiatric patients. Until then, psychiatric nursing was primarily custodial and was practiced almost exclusively within institutional settings. Nursing interventions included assisting the client in the activities of daily living, protecting and restraining acutely disturbed clients, and assisting with treatment such as hydrotherapy, hyperthermia, and insulin shock. Descriptions of nursing care prior to 1950 also include nursing measures such as suggestion, persuasion, and habit training. The nursing role in assisting the client toward personal change was not well developed (Peplau, 1982).

Psychotropic medications dramatically changed the treatment of clients with psychiatric problems in the following manner: (1) treatment could be given outside the institution; (2) clients' symptoms could be controlled in a more humane manner; (3) clients' symptoms could be reduced or eliminated more quickly; (4) treatment personnel could rapidly establish relationships with the client, and interpersonal treatment could begin earlier; and (5) clients experienced hope arising from a greater sense of control over their symptoms.

Generally, pharmacotherapy was a positive force for client and nurse. The high level of interactions that became possible between them catalyzed the development of a new role for nurses in the psychiatric setting. This new role was that of interpersonal change agent. The nurse could intervene in the client's maladaptive interpersonal patterns and provide opportunities for him to learn new behaviors. The nurse could apply skilled interpersonal techniques and elicit the feelings and experiences from the client in an atmosphere of trust and caring. Psychotropic medications were an important avenue to personal change through the creation of a safe treatment environment where, as symptoms decreased, the strengths of the client could emerge.

On the other hand, pharmacotherapy had these unintended negative effects on client and nurse: (1) the client's hospital stays became shorter which has had the advantage of maintaining the client as a member of the community, yet has reduced the period and the intensity of contact with key people such as the nurse, (2) nurses were drawn away from the client and into medication-related activities, (3) nurses lost faith in the power of slower, less dramatic interpersonal interventions, (4) a number of clients who took medications developed complications, some of which were irreversible and created further behavioral disruption, and (5) clients who could not or would not take medication were increasingly likely to need treatment programs beyond those that relied on pharmacotherapy.

As the treatment of psychiatric clients moved from institution to outpatient setting, the behavioral role expectations for the client changed. He was encouraged to become an active participant and collaborator in his treatment, rather than a passive recipient of care (Durel and Munjas, 1982). Caregivers, however, have resisted the client's more active participation. Frequently, the most valued behavior in clients is compliance with medication regimens. A true collaborative relationship between client and caregiver would involve resistance and requests for information by the client before he agrees to take a drug. Such behaviors, however, are often treated as problems rather than as healthy behaviors in an actively collaborating client. Resistance of caregivers to collaboration may account for clients having inadequate knowledge about pharmacotherapy, and perceiving themselves as powerless to make critical decisions about their care (Durel and Munjas, 1982). A major role for nursing is to serve as advocate for the client and then to teach the client to become his own advocate in the process of pharmacotherapy. (See the section, "Helping the Client to Collaborate in Pharmacotherapy.")

The primary function of psychotropic medication is to reduce suffering and to control symptoms while long-term behavioral change is occurring. Research continues to provide clues but not conclusions about the existence of biochemical bases of psychological dysfunction. Whereas empirical use of pharmacologic preparations promises to bring greater understanding about the nature of mental problems, their use also carries

---

■ Point of Emphasis

The goal of nursing is to ascertain that the client receives the correct medication through the least injurious route that offers the most control, for the shortest period of time necessary to alter the course of the psychiatric symptoms. Nursing intervention always addresses the interpersonal changes necessary to help the client make permanent alterations in his life pattern.

risks. The nurse views the psychiatric client as a person larger than the sum of his symptoms. Consequently, she identifies and protects existing strengths, and uses these strengths as islands from which to help the client build more adaptive behaviors. The nurse evaluates the client, contributes to decision making about medication, monitors the impact of medication upon all aspects of the client's life, and offers interpersonal learning guidance toward permanent behavioral change.

□ Note to the Student

Learning to interact effectively with clients in psychiatric settings is challenging, but stressful. Fear, worry about saying the wrong thing, and struggles to accept clients are common reactions. Although they wish to feel compassionate toward psychiatric clients, students cannot escape cultural stereotypes that portray the client as dangerous, helpless, or weak. These attitudes, combined with the absence of true "right" and "wrong" responses leave the student feeling uneasy about what to do therapeutically with the client. Students may find, however, that the nursing activities surrounding psychotropic medications are familiar to them and involve skills with which they feel comfortable. Dispensing medication, assessing health problems, and providing information to clients are interventions students may carry out while they learn to help clients change maladaptive behaviors.

This chapter is organized into four parts. Information about the drugs used to treat symptoms associated with psychiatric disorders appears first. The next two sections describe nursing interventions planned to protect and improve the client's state of health, and interpersonal interventions that enhance the effectiveness of pharmacotherapy. Selected legal and ethical issues in drug therapy with psychiatric clients appear at the end of the chapter. Since information about pharmacotherapy changes rapidly, the factual information in this chapter must be used only as reference material and all drug-related material checked against more current sources such as the *Physicians' Desk Reference* or the information insert packaged with the drug. Nursing diagnoses form the framework for the sections of the chapter that address nursing interventions; these diagnoses are based on the Fifth National Conference

on Classification of Nursing Diagnoses (Kim, et al., 1984).

Current nursing practice with psychiatric clients requires integrating beneficial effects of medication with interpersonal nursing interventions to help the client achieve long-term life-style changes. If medication is viewed as an adjunct to interpersonal change, the nurse will seek to help the client accept the drugs and will assist him in developing new ways of coping with the stresses of life.

□ *Psychotropic Medications: Essential Information*

DEFINITIONS

The following are frequently used throughout this chapter.

Antipsychotic medication. A preparation used to treat psychosis, a state of mental dysfunction resulting from a variety of causes with misperception of reality as a central feature. Other terms describing this type of medication include "neuroleptic," "phenothiazine," and "major tranquilizer." These terms are less accurate and refer to side effects and chemical classifications of these drugs.

Antidepressant medication. A preparation used to treat depression, a state of dysfunctionally saddened mood, altered thinking, and behavioral changes. Depression results from a variety of causes, some of which are related to maladaptive life patterns, and some of which seem biochemically guided.

Antimania medication. A preparation used to treat mania, a state of euphoria or heightened mood. Mania tends to be a transient state that alternates with profound depression. Evidence suggests that familial traits may be a factor in the development of mania.

Antianxiety medication. A preparation used to treat the somatic sensations of anxiety, a state of readiness for flight and mobilization which may or may not be related to a realistic threat to the person.

Dystonia. Spasm of the muscles of the jaw, tongue, trunk, legs, and neck which may occur with use of antipsychotic medication. Young men receiving high doses for the first time are especially likely to experience these spasms. Oculogyric crisis is a rapidly developing dystonia involving torticollis (twisted neck), and eyeballs rolled back and fixed. Opisthotonos is a form of dystonia involving the accessory spinal and back muscles and resulting in a marked flexion of the spinal column.

Akathisia. A side effect of antipsychotic drugs involving a state of subjective discomfort that may or may not be accompanied by restlessness. The client may appear to be unable to remain still or to sit down. The hyperactivity may resemble anxiety and agitation.

Akinesia. A side effect of antipsychotic drugs characterized by apathy, apparent laziness, and muscle weakness and fatigue. The client may fall into a chair as if terribly tired, and have difficulty gripping objects such as doorknobs and jar lids. The state is often mistaken for the withdrawal or apathy of psychosis.

Pseudoparkinsonism. A side effect of antipsychotic drugs wherein a Parkinson-like syndrome is produced with masklike face, shuffling gait, and repetitive tremor.

Tardive dyskinesia. An adverse effect of antipsychotic drugs characterized by repetitive movements of the tongue, jaw, hands, pelvis, and legs. These movements go on continuously, interrupting voluntary activities. The onset is insidious and the movements may not be noticed until the drug dose is reduced or stopped. The disorder is generally permanent once it has developed, thus making early recognition imperative.

Pigmentary retinopathy. An adverse effect of antipsychotic medications in which pigment is deposited in the retina, resulting in blindness. Symptoms include narrowing of the visual field and hemeralopia (day blindness).

Blood dyscrasias. Abnormalities of blood that may result from use of antipsychotic medications and tricyclic antidepressants. Typical manifestations include leucopenia and agranulocytosis. Fever, buccal lesions, and sore throat are important signs of the development of a dyscrasia. Elderly women are especially susceptible to development of these abnormalities.

AIMS examination (Abnormal Involuntary Movement Scale). A structured symptom-eliciting examination to detect tardive dyskinesia.

PRINCIPLES OF THERAPY

A guide to help the nurse assess whether pharmacotherapy is being carried out in the safest manner possible for the client is presented below:

1. Pharmacotherapy is an adjunct to more permanent types of change therapies. Even lithium therapy, in mania, is best accompanied by supportive individual therapy and family therapy. Clients are especially likely to see antianxiety medications as a "cure" for the discomfort of anxiety, rather than seeing anxiety as a signal that underlying problems are present.

2. Whenever multiple psychotropic medications are prescribed, the nurse should request the rationale for prescribing. A choice should be made about the central symptoms, and one correct drug for those symptoms prescribed. Exceptions to this rule are the treatment of major depression in which an antipsychotic may be used with an antidepressant, and the treatment of mania in which an antipsychotic may be used to control acute symptoms while lithium therapy is being started.

3. Psychotropic medication should be prescribed by a psychiatrist, preferably one who is experienced in medication use and who has a central role in performing other therapeutic activities with the client. Except in special circumstances, the client should see the same person for both medication prescribing and psychotherapy. Splitting these functions between the psychiatrist and another therapist always creates some degree of fragmentation and should be avoided.

4. One or two "target symptoms" should be identified before medication is begun, and retained throughout treatment so that the client's progress toward the goals of medication therapy can be assessed. A symptom that can be observed by all caretakers and by the client himself should be chosen. Symptoms that create great anxiety, for example, violence, are not appropriate, as observations will not be accurate.

5. Whenever a client who is taking a psychotropic drug reports feeling a change in his overall state, always consider whether a medication may be the cause before considering the possibility of a psychological basis.

6. At the start of medication therapy, always establish with physician and client the proposed plan for stopping the therapy. This is especially important in the treatment of initial episodes of a disorder and in the use of antianxiety drugs.

7. Never give medication to a family member to be dispensed to the client except in the presence of a diagnosed organic or developmental disorder characterized by confusion, or when the client is incompetent to self-medicate. Families should be taught to recognize dangerous effects, such as lithium toxicity, but should never make decisions about the client's medication therapy. This statement may seem contradictory to principles of family involvement applicable to other areas of nursing care. However, family systems theory views the symptomatic member as expressive of problems within the entire family. Allowing family members to give medication to the symptomatic member locks the client into the role of "sick one" and reduces motivation for the family to engage in searching out deeper sources of trouble within itself. Regardless of the form of treatment, it is the client who ultimately bears the physiological effects and risks of medication therapy.

8. The decision to give medication may be influenced by the nurse's feelings. Clients who are frightening to the nurse may receive excessive doses of medication. The nurse who interacts with a client who is much like herself must struggle to administer medication objectively. Consultation with peers or supervisors is a helpful way to eliminate biased responses to clients.

Determination of Choice and Dose

Table 15-1 follows the categories used in the Diagnostic and Statistical Manual of Mental Disorders (APA, 1980) and organizes psychotropic drugs commonly used for disorders within these categories. Variation is always possible as new uses for psychotropic medication are being tested continually.

Although prescribing medication is the function of the physician, the nurse is instrumental in choosing medication and adjusting the dose through sharing observations and opinions with the physician. The following general information is presented to be an aid in the collaborative process of choosing the drug and adjusting the dose. (The reader is encouraged to consult several of the specific texts for more information about each group of medications presented.)

Antipsychotic Medications. These are chosen depending on the physician's familiarity with the drug group, the client's history of drug use, side effects, and other factors such as potency and available forms. No one preparation of the drugs or group is presently seen as having more effectiveness or a specific effect on symptoms of psychosis. Dose is determined empirically by the client's response, a balance being struck between reduction of symptoms and presence of side effects. If adverse effects develop, an antiparkinson agent may be given, or a drug from a different group may be tried (Hahn, et al., 1982; Pirodsky, 1981).

TABLE 15-1 DSM III Categories and Psychotropic Medications

Antipsychotic Medications	**Antidepressant Medications**
DSM III Categories	DSM III Categories
Schizophrenic disorders	Major affective disorders
Paranoid Disorders	Major depression
Psychotic Disorders	Major depression with melancholia
Major depresson	Atypical depression
(Antipsychotics may be used alone or	Major depressive episode with psychosis
with tricyclic antidepressants)	(Antidepressants may be used alone or
	with antipsychotics)
Antimania Medications	**Antianxiety Medications**
DSM III Categories	DSM III Categories
Major affective disorders	Phobic disorders
Bipolar disorder	Panic disorder
	Generalized anxiety disorder
	Agoraphobia with panic attacks

Antidepressant Medications. Tricyclic and tetracyclic forms are generally the first choice among antidepressants. Some physicians test urine to determine whether the client is likely to respond to certain groups of tricyclics. These medications are adjusted according to the client's symptomatic response. A "therapeutic window"—a specific plasma level of the drug above or below which therapeutic response does not occur—seems to determine dose adjustment. Monoamine

---

TABLE 15-2 Psychotropic Medications

Medication	Dosage Range	Routes of Administration
I. Antipsychotics		
A. Phenothiazines		
Aliphatic		
Chlorpromazine (Thorazine)	50–1200 mg. daily	Oral, parenteral
Triflupromazine (Vesprin)	30–150 mg. daily	Oral, parenteral
Piperadine		
Thioridazine (Mellaril)	50–800 mg. daily	Oral
Piperazine		
Fluphenazine (Prolixin, Permitil)	2–20 mg. daily	Oral, parenteral
Fluphenazine decanoate (Prolixin decanoate)	25 mg. every 3 weeks	Parenteral
Fluphenazine enanthate (Prolixin enanthate)	25 mg. every 3 weeks	Parenteral
Perphenazine (Trilafon)	12–64 mg. daily	Oral, parenteral
Trixenoperazine (Stelazine)	5–40 mg. daily	Oral, parenteral
B. Butyrophenones		
Haloperidol (Haldol)	2–100 mg. daily	Oral, parenteral
C. Thioxanthenes		
Thiothixene (Navane)	5–60 mg. daily	Oral, parenteral
Dihydroindolones		
Molindone (Moban, Lidone)	5–225 mg. daily	Oral
E. Dibenzoxazepines		
Loxapine (Loxitane, Daxolin)	15–100 mgs. daily	Oral
II. Antidepressants and Antimania Agents		
A. Tricyclics		
Amoxapine (Ascendin)	150–400 mg. daily	Oral
Amytriptyline (Elavil, Amitril, others)	75–300 mg. daily	Oral, parenteral
Desipramine (Pertofrane, Norpramine)	75–300 mg. daily	Oral
Doxepin (Sinequan, Adapin)	75–300 mg. daily	Oral
Imipramine (Tofranil, others)	75–300 mg. daily	Oral, parenteral
Nortriptyline (Aventyl, Pamelor)	40–100 mg. daily	Oral
B. Tetracyclics		
Maprotiline (Ludiomil)	75–300 mg. daily	Oral
C. Serotonin inhibitors		
Trazadone (Desyrel)	50–300 mg. daily	Oral
D. Monoamine oxidate inhibitors		
Phenelzine (Nardil)	15–90 mg. daily	Oral
Tranylcypromine (Parnate)	10–60 mg. daily	Oral
E. Antimania agent		
Lithium (Lithane, Eskalith)	900–1800 mg. daily	Oral
III. Antianxiety Agents		
A. Benzodiazepines		
Alprazolam (Xanax)	0.75–4.0 mg daily	Oral
Chlordiazepoxide (Librium)	15–100 mg. daily	Oral, parenteral
Diazepam (Valium)	5–50 mg. daily	Oral, parenteral
Orazepam (Serax)	30–120 mg. daily	Oral
B. Propanediols		
Meprobamate (Equanil, Miltown)	1.2–1.6 grams daily	Oral

TABLE 15-3 Drugs Used to Treat Extrapyramidal Symptoms of Antipsychotic Agents

Name	Dosage Range	Forms Available
Amantadine (Symmetrel)	200–300 mg. daily	Capsules, syrup
Benztropine (Cogentin)	0.5–6.0 mg. daily	Tablets, ampules
Biperiden (Akineton)	2–8 mg. daily	Tablets, ampules
Diphenhydramine (Benadryl)	75–150 mg. daily	Capsules, enteric-coated tablets, elixir, vials
Ethopropazine (Parisidol)	50–500 mg. daily	Tablets
Procyclidine (Kemadrin)	10–20 mg. daily	Tablets
Trihexyphenidyl (Artane)	6–10 mg. daily	Tablets, elixir, sustained-release capsules

oxidase inhibitors generally carry greater risk than tricyclics, and are therefore a second choice for symptoms that do not respond to tricyclics. Dose is determined by a fixed schedule of increments and adjusted on the basis of any side effects produced (Hahn, et al., 1982; Pirodsky, 1981).

Antimania Medication. Linthium carbonate is prescribed on the basis of body weight, and the plasma level of lithium after its absorption. A blood level of 1 to 1.5 mEq/liter is desirable. Symptoms of toxicity may begin to appear when the blood level reaches between 1.5 and 2 mEq/liter (Gever, 1982).

Antianxiety Medications. Choice of medication is based upon expected duration of effects (short- or long-acting) as well as whether the medication has hypnotic or muscle-relaxing effects (Hahn, 1982).

Medications Most Frequently Prescribed

Table 15-2 lists psychotropic medications presently in use, and Table 15-3 presents drugs used to treat extrapyramidal symptoms due to antipsychotics. The available administration form is indicated, since this information is useful in the emergency treatment of dystonias.

☐ Nurse-Client Collaboration in Client Pharmacotherapy

ASSESSMENT ☐ Psychotropic drugs have the potential of altering the client's perceptions, feel-

ings, and behavior. As a result, the views of family and friends toward the client may change. Consequently, pharmacotherapy cannot be viewed in a compartmentalized way. In order to knowledgeably predict the impact of pharmacotherapy on the client as a whole person, the nurse initiates a comprehensive assessment before the physician prescribes. Information gleaned through assessment is utilized in an interdependent process between psychiatrist and nurse. The psychiatrist contributes an expert diagnosis which is validated by the nurse's observations. The physician then chooses the most beneficial drug and the nurse contributes information about the form, dose, and route most compatible with the client's needs. Together, nurse and physician develop a joint educative approach designed to relay important information to the client at a pace consistent with his ability to implement it. The nurse considers the client's probable future concerns, namely, the continuation of drug therapy at home and whether or not he will be able to self-medicate. The nurse always asks the physician to provide a specific plan by which the drug therapy will be evaluated and discontinued.

The nurse develops independent diagnoses and interventions based on a broad, health-fo-

---

■ *Point of Emphasis*

Multiple medications, doses which are below or above accepted standards, and failure to involve the client in the decision-making process are immediate reasons for the nurse to request consultation with the physician before giving the drug. Continual communication with the psychiatrist is necessary throughout the client's treatment.

TABLE 15-4 *Determining the Impact of Psychotropic Medication on Functional Health Patterns*

Health-perception-health management pattern
  History of medication-taking practices including drugs for pleasure
  Degree to which client actively tries to control own health status
  Manner in which client has collaborated with health caretakers over medication. Does he ask questions?
  Accuracy with which client has successfully complied with self-administration of medication in the past
  Delusions, misperceptions about medication ("poison," "cure")
Nutritional-metabolic pattern
  Weight (actual and desired), height
Typical intake with special note about inadequate or excessive amounts of food or fluids; specific dietary lists may be required if client is to be treated with monoamine oxidase inhibitors
  Special conditions for which nutritional or fluid intake must be monitored, e.g. pregnancy, diabetes, renal insufficiency, eating problems
Elimination patterns
  Typical pattern of elimination
  Special dietary relationships to bowel/bladder regularity. Does client eat specific foods to help elimination or drink large amounts of fluids to stay hydrated?
  Typical pattern of perspiration
  Dependence upon laxatives, vomiting or purging behaviors
Activity-exercise pattern
  Pulse, respiration; range of motion, hand grip
  Typical expenditures of energy during daily routines ("pace")
  Self-prescribed exercise routines
  Movement and coordination
  Hobbies and activities allowing sublimation which client regularly practices, especially those requiring fine motor skills, alertness, clear vision
Cognitive-perceptual pattern
  Cognitive capacity to learn technical material about medication
  Adequacy of perceptual capabilities
Sleep-rest pattern
  Typical sleep-waking pattern
  Special procedures for going to sleep or waking up
  Quality of waking function (indirectly measures quality of sleep)
Self-perception self-concept pattern
  Clarity of self-boundaries ("space"—self and others)
  Self-worth
  Status related to becoming dependent on medication
Role-relationship pattern
  Major roles assumed by client in family and society; family roles include physical maintenance, resource allocation, division of labor, socialization, reproduction and maintenance of membership, maintenance of order, and maintenance of morale
  Impact of pharmacotherapy on assumed roles
Sexuality-reproductive pattern
  Typical expression of sexual identity; impact of pharmacotherapy
  Reproductive system assessment; rule out pregnancy
  Knowledge of sexual and reproductive functions
  Knowledge of potential impact of pharmacotherapy on sexual and reproductive functions
Coping-stress tolerance pattern
  Typical defenses used for anxiety (unconscious mechanisms)
  Typical coping behaviors used during anxiety (conscious mechanisms)
  Impact of medication on use of these mechanisms
  Use of medication as a coping mechanism
Value-belief pattern
  Belief about the role of drugs in personal change
  Values about interpersonal change, interpersonal relationships
  Values about illness and being in need of treatment

cused goal that extends beyond disease and treatment to health promotion. Gordon (1982) suggests that a unified assessment of a client can be based on 11 functional health patterns (Table 15-4). These questions should be included in a total nursing assessment. A complete physical examination by the physician should precede pharmacotherapy and should include routine tests, such as blood counts, and any special tests related to the particular drug.

The necessity to do a comprehensive assessment becomes clear when one realizes that controlling symptoms is not in itself an end of treatment. Consider, for example, the situation in the vignette below.

Once a broad assessment has been done, the nurse prepares a concise list of baseline observations that provide a picture of the client before medication is begun, and are essential for diagnosing any untoward responses to the medication. The variable factors should be observed or measured in a consistent way. A schedule of observation should also be determined, especially about the variable factors for which continuing observation is necessary after the client has stopped taking medication. See Table 15-5, in which the variable factors are related to the functional health pattern categories in Table 15-4 (Gordon, 1982).

In the interest of client safety, the nurse should be especially careful to note:

1. Temperature, blood count. Changes may be a forewarning of the development of an anemia or an allergy to a drug.
2. Seizures. In a person without an identified disorder, they may indicate that the dose is too high; in a person with an identified seizure disorder, they may indicate need to adjust the dose of the seizure medication.
3. Thought and speech. Lack of clarity may indicate early lithium toxicity.
4. Coordination and movement. Alterations may show the development of tardive dyskinesia, especially if the changes follow a decrease in medication dose.

Vignette

Manya N., a young lawyer employed by a busy firm, is experiencing psychotic symptoms. Seven years earlier, when she left home to attend college, she had been treated for similar symptoms. Those symptoms had responded well to use of chlorpromazine (Thorazine). She graduated college, and successfully completed law school. Her current symptoms began shortly after she started to work in a law firm and had begun her first serious relationship with a man. She is required to be alert and quick-thinking in her job and to interact with clients as a representative of the firm. Her major source of relief from anxiety is her hobby of egg painting, an intricate art form.

During the assessment, Manya indicates that she values the medication, having used it successfully in the past, but worries that the sedation it produces will interfere with her job performance. At one point during the assessment interview, Manya sighs and states, "I guess I'll have to give up my eggs for a while." Upon further questioning by the nurse, Manya tells her that a side effect of the medication—extreme blurring of vision—had interfered with her painting hobby during the 6 months she used the drug after the first episode. The nurse praises Manya for sharing these worries and arranges to discuss these issues in a meeting with Manya, the physician, and herself.

The nursing assessment has revealed some interesting information about Manya. Because Manya had successfully completed a demanding professional education, the nurse predicts that Manya will be able to understand the significant information about the medication, and that she will probably be able to be a full partner in her treatment. The nurse does not assume, though, that Manya will be unaffected by anxiety, which may interfere with learning about medication. That Manya's symptoms have appeared during significant life events, and that she needed medication only for about 6 months after her first episode, are facts that suggest she may need medication for only a brief period now. The nurse would be certain that Manya clearly understands this pattern, and that a plan for stopping therapy is constructed at the time it is begun. The nurse also knows that Manya has certain hobbies and that she must be alert at all times in her job; she would be certain that these needs will be brought up in the conference and an appropriate choice of a less sedating medication be made. In the event the symptoms return, the nurse might plan to have Manya work with an occupational therapist with a view to taking up a hobby or recreational activity that requires coarse body movement. Manya would then possess an additional coping behavior that she could practice during pharmacotherapy.

TABLE 15-5 Baseline Observations of the Client Taking Psychotropic Medication

Nutritional-Metabolic	Activity-Exercise	Cognitive-Perceptual
Weight	BP, orthostatic (standing and lying)	Thought clarity
*Temperature	Pulse, apical/radial	Speech clarity
*Monitor CBC, WBC, differential	Coordination*ᵃ*	Vision
Skin	Movements (tongue, fingers, gross	Seizures
Mucous membranes	body)*ᵃ*	
Fluid intake (actual, thirst sensation)	Gait/posture*ᵃ*	
	Range of motion	
	Handgrip	
	Handwriting	
Elimination	**Coping-Stress**	**Sexual-Reproductive**
Urinary (specific gravity, output)	Suicidal*ᵃ*	Interest/activity
Bowel (constipation, diarrhea)	Symptom change (+/−)*ᵃ*	Physiological (erection loss,
		menstruation changes, pregnancy)
Sleep-Rest	**Target Symptom(s)**	**Specific Variables**
Pattern change		Different for each drug
Dream pattern change, nightmares		

ᵃ These variables need to be observed after medication is discontinued.

---

5. Blood pressure and pulse. Irregularities may indicate a developing problem of orthostatic compensation or a conduction disorder of the heart.

6. Suicidal behaviors. A medication may become the vehicle used in an attempt at suicide.

Once the assessment has been done and the baseline observations established, the nurse can begin to plan interventions toward the goals that have been developed with the client. The purpose of these interventions is first to protect the client, then to encourage his ability to collaborate in treatment and, ultimately, to rehabilitate him so that the use of psychotropic drugs will become unnecessary.

INTERVENTION □ Nursing interventions have four aims: (1) to protect the client from actual and potential health problems, (2) to use pharmacotherapy as a means for teaching basic health management, (3) to help the client collaborate in his treatment, and (4) to help the client use medication as a catalyst for change.

Protecting the Client from Actual and Potential Health Problems □ Protecting the client who is taking psychotropic medication begins with safety measures that ensure that the correct medication is given to the correct client. Medication procedures developed for bedridden clients, who are usually identified by bracelets bearing their own names, may differ if the psychiatric setting is an outpatient facility or an inpatient setting that emphasizes client autonomy. Before giving medication, the nurse should always learn the agency's procedure for identifying clients and should ask another staff person to identify a client if unsure about his identity. Principles and safeguards related to dispensing medication should be carefully practiced. Adequate staff should be available should it become necessary to restrain a client, so that, in an emergency situation, medication can be given as required.

Since psychiatric nursing focuses primarily on psychological factors, the client's physical symptoms may be overlooked or misinterpreted. Continual assessment of the client's physiological status is one way to ensure safe practice.

Interpersonally based interventions with a client rest upon a foundation of trust. Trust is built on a series of experiences between nurse and client characterized by open communication, consistency, and congruence between what is said and what is done. Interaction focusing on medication issues is frequent during the early stages of treatment. If these interactions are conducted toward the goal of developing trust, the client will sense an atmosphere of safety in which the nurse responds immediately to his expressions of concern.

Side effects and adverse effects occur with psychotropic drugs. A side effect is defined as a pharmacologic result different from the one primarily sought. An adverse effect is defined as a harmful effect of a medication (Martin, 1978). The nurse's primary response to the presence of a side effect is to offer comfort measures and counseling, and to make careful observations. In the case of an adverse effect, however, the nurse may need to carry out specific, immediate actions to protect the client's safety. Tables 15-6 and 15-7 clearly differentiate situations requiring supportive nursing intervention from those requiring specific immediate action.

The most common side effects (Table 15-6) associated with psychotropic drugs are anticholinergic, sedative, and cardiovascular in nature. Dry mouth is an example of a common anticholinergic effect which can be remedied by use of sugar-free fluids and lozenges. When anticholinergic and sedative side effects are combined, safety precautions are required to prevent the client from falling. Anticipatory guidance before side effects arise is helpful to the client.

> ### ■ *Point of Emphasis*
>
> *The most important principle in creating a trusting pharmacotherapeutic alliance is to believe the client when he reports experiencing a side effect, and always to respond in some fashion, such as spending time with the client and discussing the situation. If side effects are diagnosed and treated by the nurse, the client will feel that his concerns are important, and will begin to regain hope that he can be cared about by others.*

Three adverse effects that are of special concern to the nurse are tardive dyskinesia, lithium toxicity, and overdose (Table 15-7). These conditions are of special importance to the nurse because they are best prevented rather than treated, and nursing skill is a major means of prevention.

TABLE 15-6 Side Effects of Psychotherapeutic Drugs[a]

| | Phenothiazines | | | Butyrophenones | Thioxanthenes | Dihydroindolones | Dibenzoxazepines | Tricyclics/ Tetracyclics | Serotonin inhibitors | Monoamine oxidase inhibitors | Lithium | Benzodiazepines | Propanediols |
	Aliphatic	Piperadine	Piperazine										
Anticholinergic[b]	+	+	+	+	+	+	+	+	+	+		+	
Cardiovascular hypotension, usually orthostatic	+	+	+	+	+		+	+	+	+			+
ECG abnormalities	+	+	+		+	+	+	+			+		+
Endocrine:[c]	+	+	+	+	+	+	+	+			+		
decreased libido, inhibition of ejaculation	+	+	+					+		+		+	
Extrapyramidal													
akithesia	+	+	+	+	+	+	+						
pseudoparkinsonism	+	+	+	+	+	+	+						
Ophthalmologic:													
retinitis pigmentosa		+											
lenticular pigmentation	+		+	+	+								
Sedation	+	+			+		+		+	+	+	+	+
Skin													
allergic reaction	+	+	+	+	+		+	+				+	+
photosensitivity	+	+	+	+	+			+	+				
skin pigmentation	+												

[a] Frequency and severity of side effects vary widely with each drug and class. List is not inclusive. Refer to other sources for additional listings.
[b] Most common are dry mouth, blurred vision, constipation, urinary retention.
[c] Amenorrhea, galactorrhea, thyroid dysfunction, changes in blood glucose levels.

TABLE 15-7 Adverse Effects of Psychotherapeutic Drugs and Some Nursing Implications

Adverse Effect	Drug Class[a]	Nursing Implications
Hypertension/hypertensive crisis	MAOI	Teach need to avoid foods high in tyramine—caffeine, beer, aged cheese, chicken liver, chianti wine. Special diet should be started two weeks prior to first dose and continued two weeks after termination of drug therapy.
Dystonias	AP	Seek PRN order for antiparkinson medication when antipsychotic medication is begun. Investigate any altered body sensation. Teach patient and family to recognize onset and to contact nurse or physician immediately. Dose reduction and/or regular use of antiparkinson medication should be discussed with physician.
Oculogyric crisis	AP	Recognize high-risk groups. Watch for patients avoiding eye contact and other attempts to hide symptom. (See Dystonias, above, for antiparkinson medication.)
Tardive Dyskinesia	AP	Regular, periodic assessment for beginning symptoms is essential: excessive blinking and wormlike movements of tongue and lips. Use AIMS scale at least monthly, especially in high-risk populations. Investigate any repetitive movements.
Cholestatic jaundice	TCA, MAOI, AP, AA	Withhold medication and request medical evaluation.
Agranulocytosis, leukocytosis	AP, TCA, MAOI, AA, Lithium	Investigate fever, sore throat, lethargy. Monitor blood counts and seek order at least monthly. Withhold medication and request medical evaluation.
Dermatitis, urticaria	AP, AA, TCA	Withhold medication and request medical evaluation. Have emergency drug, such as epinephrine, available.
Seizures	AP, AA, TCA	With history of seizure disorder, dose increases should be gradual, along with increase in anticonvulsant dose. Be prepared to intervene should seizure occur.
Paralytic ileus	TCA	If symptoms develop, request medical evaluation.
Lithium toxicity	Lithium	Narrow therapeutic range increases likelihood of toxicity. Monitor intake and output. Watch for early signs: nausea, fine hand tremors, diarrhea, muscle weakness. Obtain order for blood levels at least monthly.
Overdose: unintentional	All	Initiate emergency measures, which may include gastric lavage and other neutralizing measures. Supportive medical and nursing treatment is initiated depending on symptoms produced. When client is discovered, reasons for overdose should be investigated.
Overdose: intentional	All	Same as unintentional overdose. Depressed patients are especially at risk.

[a] AP = antipsychotics
TCA = tricyclic antidepressants
MAOI = monoamine oxidose inhibitors
AA = antianxiety agents

Tardive Dyskinesia. This disorder, caused by the use of antipsychotic medication, is characterized by bizarre mouth movements such as lip smacking, puckering, and tongue protrusion, and uncoordinated movements in the upper and lower trunk and extremities. Table 15-8 lists areas of the body that may be involved in the client with this disorder.

Although tardive dyskinesia had been thought to result from use of these medications in high doses over along period of time, it has developed also in clients on short-term low-dose medication. The cause is presently not understood, but is thought to be an outcome of damage to nerve pathways. There is no general agreement about the reversibility of the disorder, and, as a consequence, many clients are likely to manifest bizarre behaviors and health problems. While experimental approaches to treating tardive dyskinesia are being explored, early recognition is the primary means to intervention. The Abnormal Involuntary Movement Scale (AIMS), used to assess early signs of the disorder, elicits symptoms that may be masked by normal movements.

TABLE 15-8 Common Manifestations of Tardive Dyskinesia[a]

Face
  Blinking of eyes
  Tremor of upper lip
  Pouting of lower lip; lip smacking
  Puckering, chewing, sucking mouth movements
  Pressing tongue against cheek as if holding candy in mouth
  Tongue tremor; rolling wormlike movements with mouth closed
  Lateral movement of jaw

Trunk
  Slow, twisting movements
  Front to back hip rocking
  Rhythmic to-and-fro movements of upper torso

Other
  Grunting or difficult breathing

Head
  Nodding—either rhythmic or nonrhythmic
  Overextension of neck with head bent backward
  Downward and lateral fixation of chin

Upper limbs
  Sudden abrupt wide swinging of arms
  Sudden nonrhythmic, purposeless, coarse, jerky movements of fingers and wrists (choreiform movements)
  Continuous, slow, rhythmic, wormlike movements of fingers and wrists (athetoid movements)
  A combination of athetoid and choreoathetoid movements

Lower limbs
  Crossing, uncrossing legs
  Restless legs
  Stamping movements
  Rotation or flexion of ankles
  Toe movements

---

[a] Adapted from Jewell and Chemij. Tardive dyskinesia: The involuntary movement disorder that no one really understands," *Canadian nurse* 79, 1983:20–4.

The nurse has access to the client during activities such as bathing, eating, and exercising, when certain parts of the body are visible (toes during bathing, tongue during denture cleansing), or when fatigue might elicit symptoms. A critical diagnostic cue for positive diagnosis of tardive dyskinesia is the disappearance of the movements during sleep, making nursing observation during the night an important key to early diagnosis. Any repetitive movement, particularly of the mouth or the tongue, should be followed up by a thorough examination by a physician familiar with the disorder. Administration of the drug may be stopped, in which case, the symptoms will worsen. If detected early, the movements may disappear. Since the disorder is often detected as medication is being discontinued, the client should be taught to watch for the characteristic signs. Regular assessment should continue after the medication therapy is stopped. The client should be informed about risks associated with the disorder, and should be asked to give informed consent to treatment. When the disorder is manifested, nursing interventions are aimed at decreasing the severity of the abnormal movements and reducing the associated health problems (Jewel and Chemij, 1983).

Lithium Toxicity. Lithium toxicity develops because the blood level of lithium required to control the symptoms of mania is very close to the toxic level. Imbalance in hydration or a lowering of dietary sodium can cause toxicity rapidly. Since clients experiencing manic symptoms often overexert themselves, and their fluid intake is poor, careful nursing observation and supportive care may prevent toxicity from developing (Gever, 1982; Hunn, et al., 1980). If renal effects (polyuria) are recognized early, symptomatic treatment can be given and dehydration prevented. Toxicity is detected by exacerbation in the side effects generally associated with lithium use. The tremor increases, lethargy gives way to confusion and slurring of speech, nausea is followed by frank vomiting, and diarrhea develops. Often, these symptoms are observed before a confirmatory blood test is done. If medication is withheld and fluids and dietary sodium intake are increased, detoxification will be improved and treatment can continue. It is essential that seizures and coma be prevented.

Drug Overdose. Overdose, whether intentional or unintentional, should be prevented rather than treated. Intentional overdose is often predictable, because the client's medication behavior provides warning signs. If these signs are made a part of the premedication baseline, the nurse can regularly observe for their occurrence in periods of change or stress in the client's life. For example, if a client tries to overdose whenever his parents are out of town, a careful structuring of his environment, combined with interaction with the nurse, will help him gain insight into the meaning of his action. Safety measures, such a limiting access to areas where drugs are kept, may be instituted in the hospital (Boettcher and Alderson, 1982). The possibility of unintentional overdose requires that the nurse assess the client's ability to take his medication safely. Learning experiences in self-medication should begin as soon as the client is able. These trials, under the supervision of the nurse, will reveal whether mechanical or emotional barriers to safe medication exist. Unintentional overdose often occurs because clients want to reduce their bothersome symptoms. Teaching the client about the value of interpersonal contact in relieving symptoms is a preventive measure.

Table 15-9 combines currently accepted nursing diagnoses with common side effects of psychotropic medication. A comprehensive assessment of the client may lead to many different diagnoses. Consequently, linking these nursing diagnoses to certain treatment effects is intended not to restrict the diagnostic process, but to suggest a way in which this aspect of nursing intervention arises out of the nursing process.

Teaching Basic Health Management through the Use of Pharmacotherapy

□ Generalizations of any kind are apt to be inaccurate. However, one useful generalization about clients requiring psychotropic medication is that their interpersonal relationships lack the intimacy and clarity that most people take for granted. As a consequence, the psychiatric client often does not receive information about basic health matters that is learned casually from parents and peers. While carefully assessing and monitoring the effects of the medication, the nurse is able to discuss relevant topics with the client that are not normally volunteered by him. These discussions open the door for the client, enabling him to obtain good new information about his body.

Two common problems of health maintenance in the psychiatric client are weight and exercise management, and sexual activity.

Controlling Weight. Weight gain is common with antipsychotic medication. Whether caused by drug-induced appetite increase or inactivity associated with hospitalization, the end result is an alteration in body image and a decrease in self-esteem. Since oral gratification is important as a symbolic expression of the client's need for nurturance, the nurse must see to it that he has ample nourishing food. Providing suitable low-calorie foods and encouraging the client to take an interest in a healthy eating and exercise program may build habits during recovery that the client can follow indefinitely (Harris and Eth, 1981; Conroy, et al., 1982). Long-term improvement in self-image may evolve as the client begins to sense that he has control over his appearance.

Understanding Sexuality. Information about sexual matters is often gained through discussion with peers during adolescence. The client requiring psychotropic medication typically has a social history of isolation and consequently has many distorted ideas about sexual functions. An example will illustrate. A nurse was assessing a young male client as she prepared to begin therapy with an antipsychotic known to cause ejaculatory inhibition. The nurse planned to recommend that the physician choose a different drug in light of the client's age and social needs. During the assessment, the young man suddenly made reference to his "sinful" nights. Through discussion with the client, the nurse understood that his reference was to nocturnal emissions. She indicated her willingness to pursue the discussion, and thus the young man learned for the first time that what he experienced was a normal event. Since he had never had a close friendship, he had never been able to discuss and share these experiences with another person, and consequently felt that they were pathological.

Nursing diagnoses that may be useful in organizing interventions through which the client can learn to improve his health management include the following: diversional activity, deficit; health maintenance, alteration in; knowledge deficit; nutrition, alteration in; and sexual dysfunction.

Helping the Client to Collaborate in Pharmacotherapy

□ Collaboration by a client ideally means that the client accepts the prescribed treatment and follows the suggested regimen. In a functional collaborative relationship, one might expect that the client would at times resist treatment for various reasons: he experiences uncomfortable side effects, he feels he lacks knowledge about the treatment, or he feels psychological discomfort toward both the actual treatment and the role of a person being treated. Noncompliance is often seen only as a refusal to take drugs; however, noncompliance can refer also to a client who takes too much medication or uses the medication for purposes other than those that have been prescribed. A typical example is the long-term, chronic use of antianxiety medications, in which drug-taking is used to "solve" an array of everyday problems.

Resistance to pharmacotherapy must be explored, and should be looked upon as an opportunity to develop the client's collaborative skills. Overpowering the client physically, or intimidating and threatening him wins only in the short

TABLE 15-9 Actual and Potential Health Problems with Psychotropic Medications: Nursing Diagnoses and Implications

Nursing Diagnosis	Side Effects	Drug Class[a]	Nursing Implications
Potential for injury	Orthostatic hypotension	AP TCA MAOI	Take BP 30 minutes after each dose, sitting and standing, 5 mm fall is significant. Compare with baseline BP established by taking BP sitting and standing q12h for 3 days prior to start of drug therapy. Provide supervision when walking after lying down/sitting. Teach client to dangle feet when arising. Use elastic stockings as appropriate. Apply before arising. Teach isometric exercises to be used before arising.
	Pseudoparkinsonism: altered gait	AP	Supervise ambulation. Consider use of walker for elderly client, provided this does not promote undue dependency. Provide handrails as necessary. Use hard-soled footwear. Avoid high heels and styles that dislodge from feet easily.
	Drowsiness	AP TCA AA	Collaborate with physician to seek loaded bedtime dose or to secure order for another subclass of medication if symptom persists after 2 weeks. Offer caffeine in moderation.
Impaired physical mobility	Pseudoparkinsonism	AP	Ambulate client at least 15 minutes BID. Supervise active ROM and quadriceps setting daily and perform passive ROM to joints when client is unable to do so.
	akathisia	AP	Reassure client that side effect is reversible. Seek order for antiparkinson medication. Assist physician to differentiate between side effect and worsening of pathology.
	akinesia	AP	Same as akathisia. Structure period of exercises for at least 20 minutes daily to combat low energy.
	ataxia	AP AA Lithium	Assist with ambulation as necessary.
	Muscular weakness	AA TCA MAIO Lithium	Assist with activities of daily living as necessary. Maintain joint flexibility and prevent muscle atrophy by active and passive exercise daily.
	Fine tremor	Lithium TCA	Assure client symptom is drug related. Work and leisure activities may have to be curtailed temporarily.
Sensory-perceptual alteration	Blurred vision, pigmentary retinopathy, lens opacity	AP TCA	Magnifying lens may help in reading. Encourage client to report *any* vision changes. Be alert to clues about vision difficulties (e.g., "I wonder if I need glasses"). Seek immediate evaluation of any vision change.
	Peculiar taste	TCA Lithium	Highly spiced foods/food flavorings may disguise unpleasant taste. Make certain that sodium levels are kept normal.
Alteration in nutrition	Increased appetite, weight gain	AP AA	Meet oral needs with low calorie foods, sugarless gum, increased water intake. Consult with dietitian about low calorie/weight loss diet.
	Anorexia	AP Lithium TCA	Record intake and review daily. Encourage frequent small meals. Consult with dietitian about serving favorite foods, if not contraindicated.
	Nausea	Lithium TCA AP	Same as for anorexia. Crackers, tea, chipped ice, cold carbonated beverages or cola syrup over ice may help reduce nausea.

(continued)

TABLE 15-9 (continued)

Nursing Diagnosis	Side Effects	Drug Class[a]	Nursing Implications
Sleep pattern disturbance	Insomnia	AP MAOI TCA	Establish a sleep/bedtime routine. Assignment to room farthest from nursing station/activity center may help.
	Nightmares	TCA	Comfort client who wakes and is frightened. Seek order for divided daily dose instead of bedtime dose.
	Day-night reversal	AP TCA AA	Do not allow long naps or frequent naps during day. Encourage physical exercise/activity during daytime hours.
Alteration in bowel elimination	Constipation	AA TCA AP MAOI	Encourage high fluid intake. Order diet high in bulk. Check frequency and type of bowel movements against baseline assessment daily.
	Diarrhea	Lithium TCA AP AA	Record each bowel movement. Check hydration status. May need ointment to rectal area. Over-the-counter antidiarrheal agents may be helpful if they do not interfere with absorption of medication.
Alteration in patterns of urinary elimination	Retention	AP TCA MAOI	Record time, amount, and specific gravity of each voiding. Observe for distention.
	Frequency	Lithium AP	Large volume output suggests lithium toxicity—obtain blood level. Provide easy access to bathroom/commode. Limitation of fluids may be dangerous. Provide fluids equal to fluid lost.
Alteration in oral mucous membranes	Dry mouth, decreased salivation, fungal infection	AP AA TCA MAOI	Offer low calorie fluids frequently. Have available sugar-free lozenges/gum and mouth rinses. Inspect mucous membrane of mouth daily. Seek treatment if infection noted.
Impairment of skin integrity	Photosensitivity; severe sunburn from slight exposure	AP	Limit outdoor exposure or use true sunscreen. Long sleeves and long pants recommended. Monitor ultraviolet light sources (e.g., tanning parlors). Remember that dark-skinned persons can receive sunburn.
Sexual dysfunction	Ejaculatory inhibition	AP AA TCA MAOI	Establish relationship that allows client to discuss personal issues. Pursue dose reduction or medication change. Anticipatory guidance before medication is begun.
	Altered body structure: breast enlargement (male), pseudopregnancy (female)	AP TCA	Anticipatory guidance before medication is begun. Order pregnancy test if symptoms appear. Counsel males how to dress to minimize external appearance of gynecomastia.
Self-care deficit	Pseudoparkinsonism	AP	Assist client with eating, bathing, dressing, movement (activities of daily living) as needed. Promote self-care behaviors as much as possible. Pursue dose reduction/antiparkinson agent.
	Akinesia	AP	Same as above. Support, instruct client about reversibility. Distinguish side effect from worsening of psychosis or physiologic problem.
	Akathisia	AP	Same as akinesia. Finger foods (sandwiches, carrot sticks) are helpful when client is unable to sit still long enough to eat.

[a] AP = antipsychotics
TCA = tricyclic antidepressants
MAOI = monoamine oxidose inhibitors
AA = antianxiety agents

run, and the attitude it conveys defines the client-caregiver relationship as adversarial, not as an alliance. The client who says "no" to taking medication is opening the door to collaboration, not closing off negotiations. Conversely, the client who quietly accepts medication without questioning is demonstrating a dysfunction in consumership and desperately needs nursing intervention. The following section describes the nursing diagnosis, noncompliance, from the standpoint of etiological factors and nursing intervention designed to help the client collaborate in his care.

Noncompliance, Active Refusal

Behaviors evidenced by clients include direct verbal refusal, spitting out medication, clenching teeth, and making threats.

Etiologic factors and interventions

1. *Ambivalence.* Ambivalence is the simultaneous presence of two strong, opposing feeling states. The nurse frequently encounters the client who both wants and does not want to take medication. The primary intervention is to offer medication consistently in a positive manner. Ambivalence is a state of change between extremes; helping a client accept medication is often only a matter of approaching him when he has reached the positive extreme.

2. *Suspicion and/or fear.* Interventions include (a) developing a sense of trust and making consistent contact with the client to create a feeling of familiarity, (b) choosing a mildly sedating medication (since hypervigilance is a major coping method of clients); (c) offering reassurance (e.g., "This medication is meant to help you"); (d) using direct terms such as "psychosis" even if this generates demands for further explanations (in the long run, honesty will breed trust); and (e) remaining with the client after medication has been given to ascertain that he has taken it (if he appears to be hiding it under his tongue or in his cheek, encourage him to spit it out and to talk with you about his reasons for resistance).

3. *Terror of being dependent.* The client will often express this fear by demanding to be in control, or by acting in a manner that forces others to take control. Interventions

include (a) increasing the client's control over his medication as much as possible (e.g., he might self-administer medication under supervision); (b) similarly increasing his control over other aspects of treatment; (c) setting limits on essentials and allowing control of nonessentials (e.g., "You may choose whether to take it before or after breakfast, but you must take it before 10 o'clock"); and (d) providing nonthreatening sources of nurturance (e.g., expressing interest without prying, offering additional food and drink).

4. *Operative strength that indicates the client's capacity to be a full collaborator.* An operative strength is defined as an island of healthy functioning in a client's behavior. Interventions include (a) validating and sanctioning the behavior (e.g., "It's wise to want information before you take a medication; I'll be happy to help you learn about _____ [drug]"), and (b) providing educative experiences as necessary (distinguish this need from passive noncompliance).

5. *Value conflict.* Interventions include (a) acknowledging that the nurse's valuing of medication is different from the client's; (b) helping the client identify his values about taking medication; and (c) assisting the client to make an informed choice between different values toward medication.

Noncompliance, Passive Refusal

Behaviors include forgetting, tardiness in dose-taking, letting pills remain in the mouth, making constant requests for information that does not lead to an increase in acceptance.

Etiologic Factors and Interventions

1. Any of the factors leading to active refusal (see above) may motivate passive refusal. Interventions will be similar.

2. *Low self-esteem.* This will be most noticeable in the depressed client, whose message is "I am not worthy of medication or help." The manic client will often feel the same unworthiness, but will express it in an opposite way as "I am too good to need medication." Interventions include (a) expressing consistent positive regard; (b) persistently offering the client medication; and (c) minimizing the benefits of medi-

cation (e.g., offering it in a neutral fashion, "Here is your medication") which helps the client feel less guilty about accepting it.

3. *Slowed thought and lowered motivation.* Again, this pattern will tend to occur in depressed clients and in psychotic clients who are withdrawn. Interventions include (a) remaining calm and composed in the presence of the client's slow response; (b) bringing medication to the client; and (c) consistently giving the client low-key expressions of positive regard.

4. *Anger.* Medication may become a way of expressing anger toward the nurse who represents a parental figure to the client. Interventions include (a) encouraging verbalization; (b) encouraging recognition of the meaning of refusing the medication; (c) encouraging direct expressions of anger.

5. *Manipulation.* An abused term, manipulation in the present sense refers to the attempt to have one's needs met indirectly through use of a substitute issue. Nurses frequently see the client as needing attention, when the true need is interpersonal interest and contact. Interventions include (a) setting limits on refusal if medication is essential; (b) validating the client's pattern of behavior with him; (c) helping the client understand the need behind the behavior; and (d) encouraging the client to ask to have his needs met more directly.

6. *Operative strength.* Interventions include (a) encouraging the client to be more direct about his concerns; (b) praising any attempts he makes toward being direct; and (c) encouraging education activities. Medication groups are superb for these clients since those who are more assertive can verbalize their concerns.

Noncompliance, Overuse

Behaviors include frequent requests for medication; anxiety over dose reduction; taking too much medication too often; taking medication without asking questions; and failure to report side effects, other medications being taken, or complicating conditions.

Etiologic Factors and Interventions

1. *Dependency issue.* May involve fear of abandonment, retaliation, or withholding of nurturance if pharmacotherapy is questioned. Pattern of pleasing others in return for real or imagined security emerges in other aspects of life. Interventions include (a) actively sanctioning role of client as informed consumer; (b) teaching assertive ways of coping; (c) encouraging verbalization of dependency needs; and (d) helping client find more stable sources of security.

2. *Need for interpersonal contact.* Interventions include (a) seeking out client for contact at times other than when medication is scheduled to be given; (b) setting limits on medication requests; (c) seeking validation of pattern with client; and (d) helping client find motivation behind the behavior (loneliness, boredom, lack of meaningful relationships) and the appropriate solutions.

3. *Inadequate coping strategies.* Medication is used in place of behavioral means to reduce interpersonal anxiety. *Note:* client may be hoarding medication with the intention of overdosing. Interventions include (a) setting limits on medication use; (b) validating pattern with client; (c) helping client try new ways of reducing anxiety while using medication; followed by (d) trying new methods of anxiety reduction without medication; and (e) observing for indications of suicidal behavior.

4. *Altered thought processes; memory deficit.* Occur frequently in the depressed client whose preoccupation with his own thoughts causes forgetfulness. Interventions include (a) helping client devise reminders (calendars, digital watch alarms, taking medication while watching a favorite daily television show); and (b) supervising self-medication experiences while emphasizing interpersonal avenues to reminders about medication (caution is advised if client wants family members to assume this function—it may be preferable to ask a friend of the client to stand in).

5. *Operative strength.* Forgetfulness may indicate a wish to discover new ways to reduce the symptoms, or a wish to discontinue the medication because it is no longer helpful. Interventions include (a) reevaluating the effectiveness of the medication and eliciting the client's feelings about taking it; and (b) assisting client to develop other ways to reduce symptoms.

6. *Value conflict.* Interventions are discussed under Active Refusal.

Helping the Client Use Medication as a Catalyst for Personal Change □ The proceedings of the Fifth National Conference on Classification of Nursing Diagnoses identified ineffective coping in families and individuals as a diagnostic category (Kim, et al., 1984). The diagnosis is useful in planning interventions with the psychiatric client, as this very general term can be applied to just about any client seeking psychiatric help. Psychotropic medication reduces symptoms and allows health professionals with therapeutic skills to gain the emotional closeness to the client that will help him cope more effectively.

Medication use should always be seen as only one step toward permanent personal change. At times, the dramatic results of taking medication encourage both client and nurse to overvalue its place in treatment, especially since personal change comes only slowly and as a result of hard work.

Psychiatric clients are often unable to adhere to medication regimens after their discharge from the hospital, and interaction with the nurse has been found to be a significant factor in helping them to continue (Battle, et al., 1983). The low compliance rate may be related to client dissatisfaction with medication as a primary provider of the solution to problems. Further investigation, however, may establish that continual interaction with a nurse who helps the client solve the dilemmas of daily living actually enhances the benefits of the medication.

Three nursing diagnoses related to ineffective coping which are frequently associated with psychotropic medication are alteration in thought processes, social isolation, and anxiety.

Alteration in thought processes is related to the psychological defenses with which the client attempts to cope with overwhelming anxiety. Most such defenses alter reality by limiting the input of information. For example, the client practicing denial is slowing the flow of information to himself. His statement, "I don't have problems" can mean "I am not ready to accept my difficulties." The client who hallucinates may be seen as projecting unacceptable urges to something outside himself, thus slowing the recognition of anxiety-provoking aspects of himself. The slowed thinking and responding seen in depression may be viewed as a means of controlling the recognition of overwhelming feeling states. It is essential that the nurse recognize that defenses exist be-

cause the client perceives a danger to himself, and that he will no longer use defenses once the danger has passed. Medication may be helpful in reducing the need for reality-altering defenses, particularly if the manner in which it is given respects the client's coping pattern. Helping the client gain control of his thought processes is an essential key toward achieving self-directed personal change. Two common defenses are presented below with suggested interventions.

1. *Denial.* Expressions of denial about taking medications might be, "I don't need drugs," or "This medication isn't for me." Interventions include (a) presenting facts without challenging the client's defense ("This medication has been prescribed by your doctor" does not challenge whether the client needs it or not); (b) offering the medication in a supportive manner and accepting refusal of it; and (c) providing information in increments (e.g., a progression of information from most important item to least important item would be to state that the pill is medication, that the medication is meant to help, that any uncomfortable feelings associated with it should be reported to the nurse, and that it is desirable for the client to ask any questions he may have about the medication). Further information may be introduced as the client indicates his readiness for this.

2. *Projection.* A client may express projection by saying something like "You're hurting me with that pill." Interventions include (a) reinforcing reality ("I have no need to hurt you and I will not let you hurt anyone else"); and (b) creating an atmosphere of physical and emotional safety by setting limits on behaviors that indicate loss of control, and by making available, on a consistent basis, the service of helpers whose presence is emotionally comforting.

Social isolation is part of the life of many psychiatric clients. Anxiety and social isolation are partners. The client often feels anxious when in the presence of others, and his attempts to cope with his anxiety produce symptoms that give rise to anxiety in others. Constant failure to experience positive interactions with others leads the client into further isolation, and eventually, his life-style supports his dysfunctional relationships. His leisure time becomes empty and remains empty because he lacks the stimulation of other persons' encouragement to try new things. Isolation breeds autistic thoughts and behaviors that further complicate relationships. Psychotropic medications work to reverse symptoms that support isolation. Antipsychotics correct perceptual distortions, antidepressant-antimania drugs correct dysfunctional mood states, and antianxiety agents reduce learned responses to anxiety. The nurse is then able to help the client in his efforts to alter the dysfunctional patterns of interaction and diversional activity which underlie isolation. Interventions include (a) assessing changes in target symptoms when the client is interacting in social situations; (b) validating patterns of dysfunctional behavior with the client; (c) planning interpersonal situations in which the client has an opportunity to try new behaviors while on medication; (d) helping the client apply the new behaviors to periods when he is medication-free; and (e) assisting the client to learn new ways of using his time in creative diversional activity.

Anxiety as a diagnostic term is found in both medical and nursing nomenclature, and is a word frequently used among lay persons. Its widespread use implies that anxiety is a state familiar to us all. Culturally, anxiety is often declared to be a disease process, when in actuality it is the response that prepares us to face the stress of living.

■ Point of Emphasis

The presence of anxiety suggests that some aspect of the client's life is in need of attention. Medication should never be given, however, until there has been an investigation into the source of the anxiety.

The anxiety may be short-lived, as might occur because of a final examination in school, or long-term, as might occur because of bereavement. Regardless of the cause, it may well be that the client will have to endure the discomfort until it is understood and resolved.

Cultural attitudes in our society are intolerant of anxiety; a "quick fix" is encouraged as a means of getting rid of it. The widespread use of alcohol and other drugs, and the praise given to a widow who remains composed throughout the funeral service for her spouse are two examples that demonstrate how our culture handles anxi-

ety. Anxiety over short-term events such as surgery, states of extreme anxiety, and anxiety that no longer seems related to traceable causes are appropriately treated with antianxiety agents. However, whenever these agents are prescribed by nonpsychiatrists, for indefinite periods of time, and in the absence of some other form of interpersonal or behavioral intervention, the nurse should question the appropriateness of the treatment.

The nurse can help the client identify long-term causes of anxiety and develop strategies that may bring about permanent change. This process may begin during treatment with antianxiety medication, and should extend past the time that medication has been discontinued. Interventions include (a) taking a factual, problem-solving approach to identifying sources of anxiety in the client's daily life; (b) encouraging the client to verbalize and being supportive of the client; (c) helping to develop effective ways to handle stress, both when the client is taking medication and after medication is discontinued; and (d) teaching the client to relax without the use of chemicals—as with exercise, diversion, bathing, and conscious control of symptoms.

□ Ethical and Legal Issues in Pharmacotherapy

Pharmacotherapy presents special ethical issues to client and nurse. The capacity to have feelings and to think privately and creatively is one of the attributes that distinguish human from all other forms of life. Psychotropic medications are designed to alter feeling and thinking; consequently, the nurse must approach the issue of pharmacotherapy with caution and an awareness of the ethics surrounding the use of such powerful agents.

To treat clients with psychotropic medication is to control their behavior, to at least some extent. To assume that a person or group can devise standards of optimum behavior for another person implies that behavior can be understood objectively and that the group can act in the best interests of that person. As stated by Fromer, "Acceptable behavior is what society defines it to be, and the designation is often subject to group moods and standards as well as cultural and societal values" (Fromer, 1981). Because psychotropic medications have powerful mind-altering capabilities, they must be treated with caution. Also it must be recognized that helping persons are not immune to disturbances caused by disruptive client behavior. In their zeal to eradicate troubling behavior in clients, helpers may be led to participate in the abuse of psychotropic medication. These abuses have led to suspicion, creating a group of troubled persons whose fear of being imprisoned by medication has left them prisoners of their symptoms. Race, gender, and economic class also may make it more likely that a client will receive medication instead of interpersonal therapies.

ETHICAL NURSING PRINCIPLES IN PHARMACOTHERAPY

1. Use of objective assessment criteria that consider the client as more than the sum of his symptoms helps ensure that medication is given for purposes of treatment and not for punishment or control.
2. The client's rationality should be protected. In the case of psychotropic medication, dose is an important consideration, since too high a dose of even a correct medication can render the client incapable of making rational decisions on his own behalf.
3. Collaboration is essential in pharmacotherapy. Methods that deceive or withhold relevant facts from a client should not be used (Fromer, 1981). An endpoint to treatment with drugs should always be determined and the client should know that the decision to continue medication is always his to make.
4. Medication is an intrusive method (Fromer, 1981). Interpersonal change is nonintrusive and should always be a goal in conjunction with medication.
5. Resistance should always be allowed (Fromer, 1981). Refusal of medication ushers in the process of collaboration.
6. Countertransference reactions, that is nonobjective responses by the nurse, must be worked through in a supervisory relationship since these feelings can become the basis for improper medication use with clients.

Legal issues about psychotropic medication have been numerous, and generally legislation has been enacted to protect the client. Fromer (1981) states that the safest course of action in the interest of protecting the freedom of the client is the assumption that any type of thought is valuable to the person and should be legally protected unless it presents a clear and present danger to others. Such statements do not give much direction to difficult clinical problems such as self-harm and neglect which are dangerous to the client but not necessarily to others. Fromer's principle, however, does remind nurses to be cautious when considering violation of legal rights to individual freedom. The nurse should be aware of legal statutes about the status of psychiatric clients in her care. Involuntary commitment does not necessarily allow involuntary medication of the client. (See the discussion of legal aspects in Chapter 5.) The nurse may be liable to assault and battery charges if she threatens to medicate or actually medicates a client who is refusing medication. In a 1974 ruling regarding the use of organic therapies in California prisons, simple refusal was all that was required to stop a procedure, and treatment could not be performed if the client lacked the mental competence to give consent (Fromer, 1981).

Informed consent is said to occur when the client understands the type of treatment to be given, the risks associated with the treatment, and acceptable alternatives to the treatment; and based upon that information, allows the treatment to proceed. Unless the client has been judged incompetent and has been assigned a guardian, the client alone may consent to treatment. When consent has been given in writing, verbal refusal is all that is necessary to withdraw consent. The nurse should see to it that informed consent occurs before she administers a psychotropic medication, and that she respects refusal as a right of the client. If refusal is approached from the standpoint of ushering in a collaborative process wherein the concerns of the client are addressed and final consent is left to him, medication will remain a safe option. Interpersonal approaches always remain the safest, least-compromising approach to the client's problems.

■ Enrichment Activities

DISCUSSION QUESTIONS

1. Identify an attitude you hold about psychotropic drug therapy. How do you think this at-

titude might affect a client in a positive way? In a negative way?

2. Using Table 15-5 choose the three baseline observations you think are the most important for the nurse to monitor on a regular basis. Discuss your reasons for choosing them.

3. A client refuses to accept his Thorazine tablets. He is taking the drug for the first time. He inspects the pills cautiously and looks suspiciously at you, the nurse. How do you respond? What interventions might you develop with him as part of his care plan? (Use the section Helping the Client to Collaborate in Pharmacotherapy as a guide.)

LEARNING ACTIVITIES

1. Develop a medication card for a client who is being discharged from the hospital and who will be taking medication at home. Choose a medication from the groups presented in this chapter and develop categories of important information for the client to have available. Present the information without the use of technical terms and confusing jargon.

2. Role-play the following situation. Four people will be involved.

   CLIENT: A young woman who is experiencing frightening voices telling her that all the things around her are poisoned.

   NURSE: A caring person who is trying to encourage the young woman to accept an antipsychotic medication.

   CLIENT ALTER-EGO: Whenever the client speaks, you follow the statement with a statement of what you think is really being felt or thought but not said.

   NURSE ALTER-EGO: Whenever the nurse speaks, you follow the statement with a statement about what you think is really being thought or felt but not said.

   Afterwards, discuss your perceptions of what the issues were between the nurse and the client and ways in which the issues could have been addressed.

3. In a classroom case conference, present a client with whom you have worked. Develop the case conference around one or more of the nursing diagnoses described in the chapter. Discuss the relationship of pharmacotherapy to the care of this client and develop interventions that encourage interpersonal change.

4. Develop an outline for a plan to teach a group of community citizens how to be informed consumers of psychotropic medications. Include at least one ethical issue that you would encourage the participants to discuss.

5. Carry out the following simulation: You are employed by a company that produces emergency warning bracelets to be worn by clients taking certain medications. Your assignment is to designate which psychotropic drugs require the wearing of warning bracelets, and to write brief descriptions of emergency situations that can develop while the medications are being taken.

■ Recommended Readings

Boettcher, Elaine G. Preventing violent behavior: An integrated theoretical model for nursing. *Perspectives in psychiatric care,* 21, 2, 1983:54–58. Violent behavior is a source of anxiety for both patients and staff, and drugs are frequently prescribed, along with other measures, to calm the patient. The author presents an assessment tool for identifying unmet needs which may result in acts of aggression and suggests that nurses may find the tool helpful during assessment, thereby helping to determine preventive nursing interventions that will decrease the incidence of violent behavior.

Cordoba, Oscar A. Antipsychotic medications: Clinical use and effectiveness. *Hospital practice,* December 1981:99–104+. The choice of antipsychotic drugs to be used in treating mental illnesses is the prerogative of the physician. However, careful evaluation of presenting symptoms and avoidance of undesirable side effects help guide the physician in his choice. Nurses can benefit from knowing common indications for specific drugs, especially as they provide the continuing assessment and evaluation of therapeutic results and side effects. The use of antipsychotics with such pathological conditions such as Huntington's chorea and Tourette's syndrome is also discussed.

Goldhamer, Paul M. Psychotherapy and pharmacotherapy: The challenge of integration. *American journal of psychiatry,* 28 (April 1983):173–177. A medical article advocating the joint use of psychotherapy and psychopharmacology, which supports the views expressed by the authors in this chapter. A review of medical literature shows validation of the beneficial effects of adjunctive therapies. Several case studies are presented, pointing out transference and countertransference issues.

■ *References*

American Psychiatric Association. *Diagnostic and statistical manual of mental disorders*, 3d ed. Washington, D.C.: A.P.A., 1980.

Battle, Ethel, Halliburton, Audrey, and Wallston, Kenneth. Self-medication among psychiatric patients and adherence after discharge. *Journal of psychosocial nursing and mental health services*, 20, 1983:21–28.

Boettcher, Elaine, and Alderson, Sylvia. Psychotropic medications and the nursing process. *Journal of psychosocial nursing and mental health services*, 20, 1982:12–16.

Conroy, Robert, Smith, Kim, and Felthous, Alan. The value of exercise on a psychiatric hospital unit. *Hospital and community psychiatry*, 33, 1982:641–644.

Durel, Sally, and Munjas, Barbara. Client perception of role in psychotropic drug management. *Issues in mental health nursing*, 4, 1982:65–76.

Fromer, Margot. *Ethical issues in health care*. St. Louis: Mosby Company, 1981.

Gever, Larry. Monitoring lithium to detect toxicity. *Nursing*, 82, 11, 1982:110–112.

Gordon, Marjory. *Nursing diagnosis: Process and application*. New York: McGraw-Hill. 1982.

Hahn, Anne, Barkin, Robert, and Oestreich, Sandy. *Pharmacology in nursing*. St. Louis: Mosby Company, 1982.

Harris, Elizabeth, and Eth, Spencer. Weight gain during neuroleptic treatment. *International journal of nursing studies*, 18, 1981:171–175.

Hemelt, Mary, and Mackert, Mary. *Dynamics of law in nursing and health care*. Reston, VA: Reston Publishing Company, 1982.

Hunn, Susan, Miranda, Cecile, Molyneaux, Vivian, and Warshaw, Catherine. Nursing care of patients of lithium. *Perspectives in psychiatric care*, 28, 1980:214–220.

Jewell, Jacklynn, and Chemij, Marion. Tardive dyskinesia: The involuntary movement disorder that no one really understands. *Canadian nurse*, 79, 1983:20–24.

Kim, Mi Ja, McFarland, Gertrude, and McLane, Audrey. *Classification of nursing diagnoses: Proceedings of the fifth national conference*. St. Louis: Mosby Company, 1984.

Kucera-Bozarth, Kathryn, Beck, Neils, and Lyss, Liny. Compliance with lithium regimens. *Journal of psychosocial nursing and mental health services*, 20, 1982:11–15.

Martin, Edward. *Hazards of medication*. 2d ed. Philadelphia: J.B. Lippincott, 1978.

Peplau, Hildegard. Some reflections of earlier days in psychiatric nursing. *Journal of psychosocial nursing and mental health services*, 20, 1982:17–23.

Pirodsky, Donald. *Primer of clinical psychopharmacology: A practical guide*. Garden City, NY: Medical Examination Publishing Co, 1981.

Turnquist, Arlynne. The issue of informed consent and the use of neuroleptic medications. *International journal of nursing studies*. 20, 1983:181–186.

PART THREE

Lifespan Development and Developmental Crisis

Primary prevention is the focus of this unit. The nurse promotes mental health by assisting individuals and families in meeting the developmental challenges that arise across the life cycle. Through these challenges, individuals develop various coping skills which contribute to their sense of mastery and self-esteem.

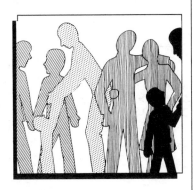

16

Attachment Theory—
Implications for Nursing

Patricia Mayer Ehrhart

Learning Objectives

Upon completion of this chapter, the reader will be able to:

1. Have an understanding of attachment theory at different stages in the life cycle.

2. Describe attachment behaviors in parents and infants, young children, adolescents, adults, and the elderly.

3. Have knowledge of the implications these behaviors have for the nursing of clients in a hospital or institutional setting.

4. Develop sensitivity toward the attachment needs of individuals and families in all age groups and respond to those needs in the clinical setting.

In the past decade, the general population has been exposed to countless media and literary accounts of terrifying hospital experiences. From the fictional *Coma* and *One Flew Over the Cuckoo's Nest* to the numerous nonfiction accounts written by physicians, nurses, and clients, we learn of the negative experiences that might occur in a hospital setting. It is not surprising that even the most stouthearted among us feel enormous anxiety when faced with the need to be admitted to a hospital.

Health providers have the responsibility to study the problems related to hospitalization and then to alleviate, to the greatest possible degree, unnecessary stress and anxiety for the client. One universal problem relative to institutional treatment is that the client is taken from his familiar environment and supportive family to an environment of isolation, unfamiliar machines, uniforms, and strangers. This separation from a spouse, parent, or special other person when the support and comfort derived from the presence of that individual is great, is an issue which should be considered in the nursing plan.

For nearly three decades investigators have been studying attachment theory, or the bonding that develops between persons. These studies have produced significant evidence documenting the negative social and psychological problems that result from the forced disruption of attachment bonds. An understanding of attachment is important for health providers, who must constantly deal with problems arising from such unnatural separation of hospitalized persons from their customary support systems. This chapter explores the theory of attachment as conceptualized by John Bowlby and supported by other theorists. The focus is on theory, types of attachment in various age groups across the life span, and nursing implications.

□ *Attachment Theory*

Bowlby (1975) defines attachment theory as "the propensity of human beings to make strong affectional bonds to specific others" and adds that these behaviors characterize humans from "the cradle to the grave." Numerous studies support the idea that attachment behaviors remain a normal part of human behavior throughout life. This means that just as the infant bonds to the mother, an adult bonds to a special other person. Attachment behaviors are evident in time of fear and

---

TABLE 16-1 Human Attachment Behaviors[a]

Proximal Behaviors

Behaviors that require physical nearness to the object or person for completion of the behavior. This includes physical contact with the object of attachment.

    Touch: A hand placed nonaggressively on a person

    Affection: Warm voice accompanied by hug, kiss, pat

Distal Behaviors

Behaviors that allow the person to maintain a certain distance from the other person yet complete the behavior.

    Smile: The smile must be directed to a specific person rather than being independent of interaction

    Praise: An explicit statement that shows positive recognition of the other person

    Enthusiasm: Clapping hands at what the other has done

    Warmth: Soft voice when interacting

    Positive comments: Directed toward the other person's behavior

    Supportive or encouraging comments: for example "I knew you could do it"

    Eye contact: Direct gaze between the persons

[a] Adapted and reprinted with permission of authors and publisher from Kogan, K.L. and Gordon, B.N., "Interpersonal behavioral constructs: A revised approach to defining dyadic interaction styles. *Psychological Reports*, 1975, 36, 835–846.

---

anxiety as well as times of contentment and joy. Just as the infant or child seeks the parent when fearful, in pain, or anxious, so do the adolescent, the adult, and the elderly seek and receive comfort from a significant other. Table 16-1 describes distal and proximal attachment behaviors which may be observed from infancy to old age.

Essential features of attachment, as outlined by Bowlby, are presented below. An understanding of these features can aid the nurse in providing holistic care to hospitalized clients and their families:

1. In a great majority of human infants, attachment behavior to a preferred figure develops in the first 9 months of life. If bonding does not take place before a child's second birthday, it may never occur. This has lifelong negative implications for the individual.

2. Attachment behavior is directed toward one or a few specific individuals in order of preference (e.g., mother, father, sister).

3. An attachment endures through the life cycle.
4. Persons become emotionally affected when new attachments are formed and when close attachments are disrupted.
5. Attachment has a biological component. Research studies have shown that nearly all species, including the human, demonstrate attachment behaviors and seek protection from the attached figure when in a fearful situation. In most species, for example, some innate behaviors such as clinging (in primates) or imprinting, automatic following of the mother, can be demonstrated which promote attachment behavior.

ATTACHMENT VS. DEPENDENCY

Research has demonstrated that securely attached toddlers exhibit more independence by exploring their environment to a greater extent than do the insecurely attached. Children who are less securely attached to their mothers tend to cling and cry in new situations (Ainsworth and Bell, 1970). Dependency tends to be viewed negatively by society; it is important to keep in mind that the securely attached infant or toddler is better able to develop greater independence and au-

tonomy. This distinction serves in adulthood also. The wife who is totally dependent upon her husband to make her decisions and shelter her in a childlike existence is not exhibiting a healthy level of independence. On the other hand, a wife who retains her individuality and is able to make mature decisions may be as attached to her husband as the woman in the first example but she is not overly dependent upon him.

Table 16-2 distinguishes the psychological aspects that show a person to be dependent on another from the interpersonal and biological aspects that show one person to be attached to another.

AFFECTIONAL PATTERNS IN PRIMATES

Research on attachment behavior has been developing slowly since the 1950s. It appears that attachment behaviors play a significant role in the physiological, psychological, and social development of humans throughout life. Most of the research to date has been done on attachment behaviors observed in primates and human infants.

Harlow (1958), one of the early researchers, theorizes that primates offer a reasonable experimental substitute for the study of man because the primate infant undergoes a long period of development analogous to that of the human child.

TABLE 16-2 Attachment vs. Dependency[a]

Attachment (Interpersonal/Biological)	Dependency (Psychological)
Attachment implies an emotional closeness to a significant other person.	Dependence is not specifically related to being emotionally close to another person.
Attachment is directed to a specific and special person (e.g., a mother and child, a husband and wife).	Dependence is not necessarily directed to a special individual (e.g., an individual may become dependent on a nurse for his care, yet have no emotional attachment to her.)
Attachment implies a close bond to another person, perhaps over the life cycle.	Dependent behavior does not imply an enduring bond. A person can become dependent on a caregiver, a teacher, a boss, for example, without having a warm or lasting relationship.
Attachment is associated with strong emotional feelings that would leave a person in state of distress or despair if unexpectedly separated.	Dependence is not associated with a strong feeling.
Attachment has its roots in ethologically researched behavior.	No biological function is attributed to dependent behavior.

[a] Criteria of Bowlby, (1975).

Studies done since 1958 indicate that a deep and abiding bond exists between infant monkeys and their mothers. It has been consistently observed that when the mother and infant are separated the infant's response is one of protest and despair (Harlow, 1958; Jones and Clark, 1973; Suomi, 1976).

In a study of the pigtailed monkey, the researchers returned the separated infant to an adoptive mother, a childless female in the group. Even though the adoptive female displayed mothering behavior toward the infant, the infant did not demonstrate a return to a normal physiological state (e.g., heart rate and respiration) as predicted. The researchers inferred that the physiological changes seen in the infant were due not to the mother's absence, but to a psychological reaction (Reite, 1978). The separation reaction is similar in man (Reite, 1978; Suomi, 1976) suggesting further that the study of primates enhances understanding of attachment separation among humans.

☐ *Types of Attachment*

PARENT-CHILD ATTACHMENT

Infant Attachment Behavior

Crying, sucking, rooting, and smiling are the earliest behaviors that have been identified (Ainsworth, 1969). Stern (1974) isolated visual contact and the face-to-face (en face) position as the cardinal attachment behaviors in early mother-infant attachment. Moss (1967) emphasized that crying, as well as vocalizing, smiling, and focusing on the mother, were important signals to which the mother should respond.

It is important to understand that the attachment between the infant and either parent is mutual. Mother/father and child have built-in responses and provide feedback to each other. For example, when they look into each others' eyes, a baby will smile and the parent will respond by cooing, laughing, holding, eliciting more smiles from the infant. When the baby cries, the parent will pick him up, comfort him, feed him. The parent is sensitive to the infant's needs and responds to them. Bonding is reciprocal. Erikson's concept of trust vs. mistrust is interwoven into the fabric of parent-child attachment (see Chapter 17). The child trusts that the parent will respond in a predictable fashion, and the parent is sensitive to the child's needs.

Mother-Infant Attachment. The importance of mother-infant attachment (bonding) and its lifelong implications have been extensively reported by researchers. Reite (1978) emphasizes the importance of bonding to maintenance of family and social structure and the child's relationship to them. Disruption of bonding may result in the development of serious pathology, though it is not established with certainty that disrupted infant-mother attachment is a cause of adult social pathology. Among questions yet to be answered are the following: Can an interrupted mother-infant bond correct itself later, for example, when the infant attaches to a new caretaker? Do infants who bonded well with the mother at birth continue to experience effective attachment at 2 or 3 years of age? If a young adult is socially well adjusted is it because of early mother-infant bonding or is it because healthy mutual attachment was operative throughout life? If an infant does not attach early with the mother can he be socialized at a later time? Though the possibility that pathology results from lack of early mother-infant attachment is speculative, a large number of studies, both animal and human, indicate that children and youths who were isolated from parents in early infancy are disturbed (Maccoby, 1980; Klaus and Kennell, 1976).

Father-Infant Attachment. The influx of mothers into the job market has focused attention on the father's role in parenting. Fathers can attach to their infants and parent them very effectively. An important predictor of paternal attachment is participation (or lack of it) in the birth process (Peterson and Mehl, 1978). In the past, fathers were discouraged from participating in the birth process, were refused entry to the delivery room, and had only limited involvement with the neonate during the hospital stay. We now know that the father's involvement should be encouraged, because its absence may have harmful effects as the child grows older. As with the mother, the nurse is in a position to facilitate the bonding process between the father and the infant.

Greenberg and Morris (1974) identified a critical time when attachment should occur between infant and father. This period is identified as the engrossment period, from birth to 3 days, when the father is most receptive to his infant. When the infant is awake and alert during this period, the father responds joyfully and expresses self-esteem. The nurse should be concerned if the father (1) does not talk to the infant, (2) does not gaze into the infant's eyes, (3) fails to touch the infant and hold him close, or (4) does not let the infant hold onto his fingers (Figure. 16-1). Table 16-3 describes attachment behaviors of fathers to their infants and young children.

Two factors that may inhibit a father from bonding may be his familial background (e.g., the way his own father related to him) and his cultural background (e.g., "This is a woman's domain"). Nevertheless, the father's role has been increasingly appreciated in recent years.

> ### ■ Point of Emphasis
>
> *The father's role in the mother/father/child triad has become increasingly significant due to changes in American society. His contribution is irreplaceable and positively affects the entire family (Johnson, 1979).*

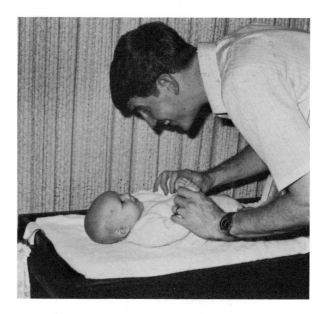

Figure (Photo) 16-1 *Father attachment. The significance of father/infant attachment is becoming more evident in our society. Adaptive father behaviors include talking to the infant, eye contact, touching, and letting the infant hold onto his fingers. (Photo by Chris Ehrhart).*

Attachment often begins for the parents at the time of quickening when the fetal movements are noted by the parents-to-be. Both the parents sense the movements, and often begin to "talk" to the fetus. Some researchers suggest that even this early in its development, the fetus may respond to outside stimuli. The observant nurse may identify cues to the possible future attachment level even during pregnancy. However, the majority of researchers investigating child development stress the importance of immediate attempts to attach from the moment of the infant's birth.

As discussed, attachment formed by the mother and the father to their infant shortly after the birth may have long-lasting effects on the family. The bonding that takes place at this time can be interrupted and altered if the infant is separated from the parent. If the baby is ill and placed in an incubator, the parents are not able to bond effectively during this separation. Studies have indicated that even if the parents and infant are reunited before the family leaves the hospital, changes in the relationship take place. The parent has more difficulty reestablishing the initial affectional bonding (Klaus and Kennell, 1976). Conversely, the mother may be ill (e.g., she may suffer postpartum depression and reject the newborn infant). After recuperation, some mothers have reported difficulty in establishing an affectional tie to the infant for weeks or months. In each of these

circumstances the nurse can facilitate attachment behaviors between the infant and his parents before leaving the hospital and in subsequent home visits.

In the best of circumstances the family unit will arrive home to begin the care of the infant. This is the time that the responsibilities and demands of parenthood call forth patience, cooperation, love, and support between the parents in order to provide the infant with the love and guidance he needs for the next important developmental years.

Parent-Child Attachment Behavior

Maccoby (1980) states that some general behaviors can be expected in children, 2 to 3 years of age, who were securely bonded as infants. These include playing with toys more intensely, interacting without aggressiveness with their peers, exhibiting social leadership, and self-directed behavior.

Those whose parents did not make effective attachments, for example they avoided the child as much as possible or did not respond to the child's sensitivities, demonstrated these behaviors: low frustration level, tantrums, frequent crying, clinging to the mother or anger with her,

TABLE 16-3 Adaptive and Maladaptive Fathering Behaviors[a]

Time/Situation	Adaptive	Maladaptive
Touches child	Freely, uses whole hand, gentle	Infrequent, uses fingertips, rough
Holds child	Holds close to body, relaxed posture	Holds distal from body, unrelaxed
Talks to child	Positive manner, tone; uses appropriate language, speed, content	Uses curt, loud, inappropriate language or content
Facial expression	Makes eye contact, expresses spectrum of emotions	Makes limited eye contact, little change in expression
Listens to child	Active listener, gives feedback	Is inattentive or ignores child
Demonstrates concern for child's needs	Active, involves others, seeks information	Indifferent, asks few questions
Aware of own needs	Expresses feelings about self in relation to child	Gives no expression about self
Responds to child's cues	Responds promptly to verbal, nonverbal cues	Has limited awareness and response
Relaxed with child	Posture, muscle tone relaxed	Posture rigid, tense, fidgets
Disciplines child	Initiates reasonable, appropriate discipline	Does not initiate or uses measures too severe or too lax
Spends time with, visits child	Routinely, utilizes time so that child is involved	Has no routine, no emphasis on child during time spent
Plays with child	Uses appropriate level of play, active, both enjoy	Uses inappropriate play, no obvious enjoyment
Gratification after interaction with child	Father states, appears gratified	Gives no statement or display of gratification
Initiates activity with child	Frequently	Infrequently
Seeks information and asks questions about child	Concerned, asks frequent, appropriate questions	Asks few questions, needs prompting
Responds to teaching	Positive, reinforces instructor, seeks more information	Has low interest
Knowledge of child's habits	Is knowledgeable	Has little knowledge
Participates in physical care	Feeds, bathes, dresses	Allows others to perform tasks
Protects child	Aware of environmental hazards, actively protects	Protective behaviors not exhibited
Reinforces child	Gives verbal/nonverbal responses to child's positive behavior	Does not notice or acknowledge child's behaviors
Teaches child	Initiates teaching	No teaching
Verbally communicates with mother about child	Uses positive, frequent verbal encounter	Gives negative, infrequent communication
Verbally and nonverbally supports mother	Demonstrates support— reassures, touches, guides	Support not obvious
Mother supports father, father responds	Gives positive response	Responds negatively, no response
Speaks of other children	Responds when asked, initiates, shows interest	Shows no interest, no initiation

[a] Johnson, S. H. *High-risk parenting: Nursing assessment and strategies for the family at risk.* J. P. Lippincott, (C) 1979.

ignoring of directions, and aggressiveness toward their peers (see case study below).

As the infant matures, he manifests more frequent attachment behaviors as well as behaviors of longer duration (Moss, 1967). Kogan and Gordon (1975) describe mother-child affective behaviors in 10-year-old children as involving direct praise, hugs, kisses, smiling, enthusiasm, and friendly tone. As described in Table 16-1, attachment behaviors can be both proximal and distal. Proximal behaviors are those that require physical nearness or contact with another person—a touch, a hug, a kiss, a pat. Distal behaviors are those that allow a person to maintain some distance from the other person yet demonstrate attachment behavior (a smile, praise, warm comments, open posture). Over the years, as an individual matures, these behaviors remain essentially the same, though the persons to whom they are directed may be different and one behavior may be more dominant than another. For example, Hollender, et al. (1970) found that the desire of women to be cuddled and held described an attachment behavior of later life. If the attachment experience of infants can be measured and conceptualized, adult functioning can be more sensitively predicted and better understood (Moss, 1967).

Early Childhood. Few data have been collected relative to attachment from toddlerhood to adolescence, and much research needs to be done. Nevertheless, it is established that children from 3 years through preschool begin to comprehend

---

Case Study

In their investigation of pathological failures in attachment, O'Connor and Master (1984) reported on a 2-½-year-old child hospitalized with a presenting problem of severe emotional disturbance and mental retardation.

The child had been delivered normally. Her 1- and 5-minute Apgar scores were 9 and 10, respectively. All of her growth parameters were within the 25th percentile. The mother was schizophrenic and left the maternity hospital, against medical advice, on Day 1. She was discovered 2 days later with the infant, hiding in a broom closet in her home. At 6 days the infant was placed in a foster home where she remained for 14 months. The infant developed normally during this time, that is, she sat at 6 months, crept at 8 months, walked at 11 months, spoke single words at 10 months. She was removed from the home at 14 months after her foster father (to whom she was securely attached) became ill. In her new placement the foster mother found the baby to be difficult to care for and reported that she had the "personality of a schizoid." The pediatrician, who knew that the biological mother was schizophrenic, reinforced this assumption.

After a psychological examination to rule out autism, the child was hospitalized with behaviors of social withdrawal, little language use, inability to play with toys, finger licking, rocking, and vomiting in stressful situations. She was resistant to strangers. There was a decline in physical growth. By 30 months of age, all growth parameters were below the 3rd percentile. On a standardized test, all areas of functioning were below norms for 21 months of age.

The treatment plan included: (1) put one primary nurse in charge of the child's care program to promote sensitivity to her signals and communication; (2) allow the child to participate in the development of separation and reunion rituals with her primary caretaker for example, allow short episodes (several minutes) of separation in which the child could explore, away from the primary nurse; and (3) document the reaction to the separation and the reunion. If the child has attached to the primary nurse the following behaviors would be anticipated: After a brief separation the nurse's presence would reduce stress and the child would continue to explore. At reunion with the nurse, the child would not display anxious resistive behaviors.

Within 1 month, the child's behavior greatly improved. She used language spontaneously, played with toys, no longer appeared depressed, and sought to be near her primary nurse, showing attachment behaviors even after a weekend separation.

One month after hospitalization, the child demonstrated angry anxious behavior after separation from her primary caretaker. The researchers found it significant that even though she had progressed rapidly during the first month in the hospital, her anger, anxiety, and depression were very close to the surface. After 2 months of hospitalization, she was adopted. One year later her development was normal for her age and she was thriving emotionally and physically (O'Connor and Master, 1984). This case study demonstrates the potential pathology that can occur when the infant's attachment is disrupted.

themselves as separate persons from others while children 4 through 12 years are developmentally involved in socialization outside the home and in seeking the influence of others besides their parents. However, even though the child is beginning to explore other attachments in a social setting, the basic attachment is still the parent figure. If the child's psychobiological needs are met by his parents or caregivers through these childhood years, he develops confidently to adolescence.

The Hospitalized Toddler. Hospitalization is one of the first disruptions to attachment that the young child may experience. A toddler may have a very healthy attachment to his parents but experience anxiety, anger, and depression if separated from them during the hospitalization. If the child is placed in this unfamiliar situation where a stranger becomes the caretaker after the parent leaves, the child will usually suffer separation anxiety—he grieves, becomes anxious, has tantrums, becomes angry, or withdraws. Without appropriate nursing interventions, some children may suffer only temporary effects while others experience long-lasting effects.

Branstetter (1969) studied three groups of hospitalized children. In the first group the mother stayed with the toddler throughout the 24 hours in a rooming-in plan. In the second group a mother surrogate stayed with the child during most of his waking hours. (The surrogates were volunteers chosen on the basis of their warm interest in children.) The third group was a mother-absent group, whose parents could not stay with the child. The children in this group were given the usual pediatric care. The study demonstrated that the surrogate-mother group displayed behaviors similar to those of the mother-present group, and the children displayed much less disturbed behavior than the mother-absent group, who displayed behaviors of anger, sadness, and withdrawal.

The following vignette demonstrates a possible hospital situation involving a toddler.

Judy's situation could have developed in another way. Cathy might have remained at her feeling level and engaged in a power struggle or treated the family in a punitive way. She might have opted to ask the mother not to stay at night so that Judy could get used to not having her there. She could have maintained usual staff routine with Judy's nurses changing daily, and would not have sought the surrogate mother. In all likelihood Judy would have progressed from tantrums

---

Vignette

Two-year-old Judy has been admitted to the hospital for evaluation. Each time Judy's mother attempts to leave, Judy screams and becomes inconsolable. Judy's mother would like to stay but feels she is in the way. Judy and her mother have a history of healthy affectional bonding. The hospitalization and the fear of the possible diagnosis cause anxiety in Judy's mother.

The nurse, Cathy, is young. She does not have children. She feels impatient with Judy's behavior (tantrums, refusal to eat, crying) and wonders why her mother can't settle her down. Cathy knows that her own parents would have "put an end to this nonsense" and would have disciplined Judy because Judy is not in pain. Cathy feels that Judy is spoiled, and sees Judy's mother as being overprotective.

Cathy identifies these feelings in herself. She is a good nurse and wants to help this little girl. At a staff conference she shares her frustration with her peers. A staff member suggests that Cathy discuss this problem with the hospital clinical specialist. The clinical specialist shares attachment theory with Cathy and helps her plan nursing care that provides consistently assigned nurses to reassure Judy's mother and make family members welcome and comfortable. The family is involved in Judy's care and a volunteer surrogate mother is available when family cannot be present.

During her hospital stay, Judy becomes her secure and cheerful self again. She is no longer afraid of her nurses and doctors. Her mother is able to leave Judy when necessary with much less anxiety, feeling secure that her daughter is in loving hands.

---

and anger to withdrawal from staff and her parents. She could have had a life-long fear of hospitals and health caregivers. She could have lost trust in her parents, and regaining that trust might take weeks or months. Judy would probably be clinging and insecure whenever her mother left their home. Her parents would have felt cheated by this hospital experience, harboring angry feelings about nurses, physicians, and hospitals for a long time.

Hospitalization in Older Children. Older children who are separated from their parents during hospitalization will usually attach to the nursing staff as parent surrogates. Figure 16-2 depicts the process of establishing an attachment

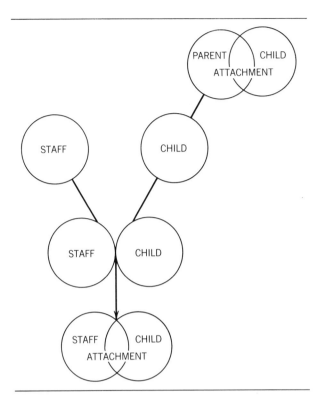

Figure 16-2 *Process of attachment behavior to nursing staff. From Ehrhart, P. Attachment behaviors of hospitalized children to the nursing staff. 1980.*

relationship with caregivers other than the parents.

One study of attachment behavior in psychiatrically hospitalized schoolage children suggests that children from 4 through 12 years of age attach most frequently to members of the nursing staff who approximate the age of their parents. Moreover, these children attach to staff of the same sex, which suggests that they identify with role models as well as parent models. The study also suggests that individual shared time (working, playing, or talking) each day with a primary nurse facilitates the child's sense of well-being (Ehrhart, 1980). The finding has implications about staffing for children who must be hospitalized for a period of several weeks or longer. However, in an acute care general hospital in which the child can be expected to be discharged in a week or two, the parent remains the primary attachment.

ADOLESCENT ATTACHMENT

The nature of attachment changes with adolescence. The parent is no longer of singular impor-

tance, as the teenager moves into wider social circles. During this period, interest shifts from solitary to group activities. The peer attachments made at this time are of paramount importance in the adolescent's psychological, social, and personality development. Ansubel (1954) states that the development and maintenance of peer relationships aid the teenager in accomplishing the tasks of adolescence. He defines these tasks as follows: (1) learning to accept and come to terms with his own body, (2) learning the appropriate sex role, (3) establishing independence from adult domination, (4) achieving adult economic status, and (5) developing a system of values.

The peer group influences the accomplishment of these tasks as the teenager becomes less dependent on parents and gains status in his own right within the peer group. The seeking of new allegiances and values outside the home greatly aids in his emancipation. The peer group also provides the basis for increased heterosexual contacts. Finally, being a successful member of a peer group reduces the teenager's frustration and helps bring stability to this difficult transition period (Ansubel, 1954).

Adolescents progress through several stages of peer attachment. Figure 16-3 depicts these stages from early through late adolescence. In the early stage, peer attachment consists of same-sex cliques (Figure 16-4). In Stage 2 the teen begins to touch base with heterosexual groups. These interactions are of a group nature rather than of paired-off couples. The groups remain in single-sex cliques. Stage 3 represents the beginning of heterosexual relationships while remaining a part of the unisexual transformation into heterosexual groups. At this time the teen is attracted to the opposite sex and in some cases pairs off; however, the attachment to the same sex crowd is still strong and predominent. Stage 4 indicates the transformation into heterosexual groups. Finally, Stage 5 represents the dissolution of the crowd and the formation of couples who are "going steady" or are engaged (Lewis and Rosenblum, 1975).

Although the peer group may be the most important influence on adolescents (e.g., clothes, social activities, type of music), affection for parents, although displayed less frequently at this time, is not altered (Elkind, 1971). The conflict that is often present between teens and parents may stem from their ambivalence. The adolescent has mixed feelings about growing up. Teenagers want to be treated like adults at times, but like

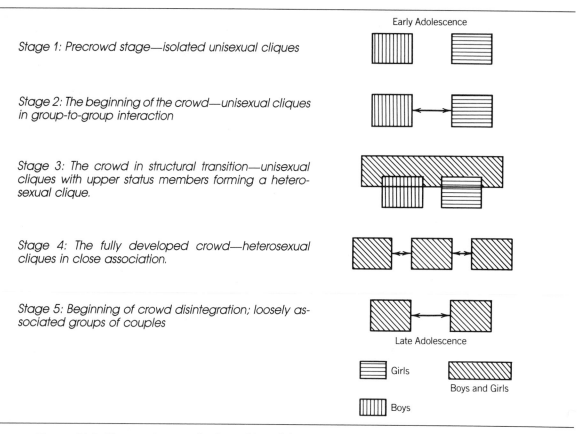

Stage 1: Precrowd stage—isolated unisexual cliques

Stage 2: The beginning of the crowd—unisexual cliques in group-to-group interaction

Stage 3: The crowd in structural transition—unisexual cliques with upper status members forming a heterosexual clique.

Stage 4: The fully developed crowd—heterosexual cliques in close association.

Stage 5: Beginning of crowd disintegration; loosely associated groups of couples

Figure 16-3 Stages of peer attachment in adolescence. From Dunphy, Dexter C. The social structures of urban adolescent peer groups, Sociometry, 1963.

children at other times, on their terms. Parents also have conflicting feelings, wanting their children to be mature and independent but behaving toward them in ways that may promote dependency. Another source of conflict stems from the extreme self-consciousness of the teenager. He looks at his home and family with a more critical eye, "viewing them from the outside" (Elkind, 1971). The adolescent is strongly attached, then, to two groups, family and peers. His attachment to peers helps him to gain independence and meet his developmental tasks while he remains emotionally attached to his parents.

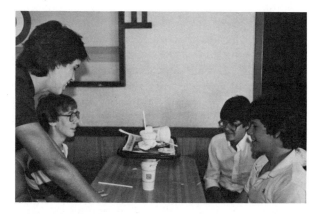

Figure (Photo) 16-4 Adolescent attachment. Peer attachments are of paramount importance in the psychological, social, and personality development of the adolescent. Photo depicts early unisex group (Ansubel, 1954). (Photo by Annette Kutilek).

Nursing Implications

Adolescent attachments should be of concern to the nurse caring for the teen in a psychiatric hospital setting. Bearing in mind the developmental tasks that need to be met, the nurses will set policies that promote peer attachment.

In the acute care setting of a general hospital, the adolescent is dependent and vulnerable, and parent attachment has high priority.

The following vignette demonstrates that attachment can be either inhibited or fostered by the nursing staff:

Vignette

Billy, a 16-year-old quadriplegic, had been in the ICU for 3 weeks following a motorcycle accident. He was alert and responsive but dependent on a respirator. Because he was unable to communicate verbally, his mother developed an effective system of nonverbal communication with Billy. She interpreted his needs to the nursing staff, who worked efficiently to meet his physical needs. It was disconcerting, then, to find that in three consecutive nursing reports, the overriding communication about Billy was the irritation of the staff toward his mother. They reported that she would not leave the room, was demanding and troublesome. The resulting tension transmitted to both client and the mother caused further stress. The patient responded by refusing to try to breathe on his own when taken off the respirator for short periods.

Had the nursing staff understood the reciprocal attachment behaviors and needs of Billy and his mother, several days of distress and setback might have been avoided. A psychiatric nurse assigned to the patient identified the problem and assisted the staff in solving it. The nurse, in a private meeting with the mother, held her hand and gave the mother an opportunity to share her grief. (Nurse: "You must be feeling terrible pain." Mother, beginning to cry: "No one has cared about that before.") The mother's ability to communicate with her son was then included in the plan of care as a valuable aid to the staff whose time was taken up primarily in providing skilled care to Billy. His mother was able to inform the staff of foods her son preferred, and his eating pattern improved. With harmony restored between the mother and the staff, Billy became cooperative again. The mother felt comfortable in leaving the unit for short periods of time as she gained trust in the nursing staff. The staff became caregivers instead of antagonists, creating a milieu in which physical and emotional healing could go on.

ADULT AND ELDERLY ATTACHMENTS

As the adolescent matures into adulthood, his significant attachment develops into deeper and more initimate relationships.

Adults

An adult primary attachment usually denotes an intimate sexual relationship with a significant other. This relationship may or may not culminate in marriage. Loss or separation at this level of attachment will cause great loneliness and distress. Secondary attachments include friends, siblings, and parents who are vital to one's sense of well-being. The loss of these attachments may also cause loneliness and distress. A third level is attachment to a community or an organization. The loss of a special homogeneous group, as occurs when a person moves away from a job, a neighborhood, or a community, can give rise to distress. The degree of distress varies with the level of attachment; for example, a person may have friends but still be lonely if his primary attachment is gone (Parkes, 1982).

The Development and Nature of the Dyadic Bond.
The adult has usually established some effective and strong ties over time. Generally, the greatest of these is with a spouse, followed in strength by ties to children, parents, siblings, and friends. These attachments, made over a long period of time, are deep and rich. It should be noted, however, that the strength of these bonds does not depend on physical proximity of the members. For example, an elderly parent may live hundreds of miles away from a child, but their attachment is enduring in its intensity.

To clarify the quality of a relationship, Troll and Smith (1976) differentiate between the terms *attraction* and *attachment*. They suggest that a long-term relationship proceeds as follows: In the beginning, mutual attraction is high. For example, during courtship a couple disregards each other's faults and exaggerates the desirable qualities (the "love is blind" stage). If the relationship is ended at this point, it is painful, but there is no great void in the lives of the two people. However, if the couple continue to have intimate relations over a long period of time, the novelty and mystery diminish and a more companionable type of love develops. The intense attraction lessens, yet a strong attachment may have formed. At this point, the loss of the loved person will cause much pain and leave a void that may not be filled. Altman and Taylor (1973) describe four levels of interaction in the development of a relationship:

1. Superficial, minimal interaction
2. Friendly interaction: may be acquainted with one component of each other's personality (e.g., coworkers)
3. Warm interaction and knowledge of many facets of each other's personality (e.g., close friends and engaged couples)

4. Stable interaction with intimate knowledge of each other, involving self-disclosure and emotional investment. This level is achieved in only a few relationships. Middle-aged couples who report their marriage "has never been better" have often reached this level of richness and depth.

Reedy, et al. (1981) studied 102 happily married couples (young, middle-aged, and older) in an effort to identify the components of a satisfying love relationship. Their findings suggest that the nature of the love relationship is different at different ages. The younger couples found sexual intimacy and passion very important, while the older couples found tenderness and affection very important. At all ages, however, emotional security (feelings of concern, caring, trust, and comfort) was ranked as most important.

Even though it has long been evident that unwanted separation from an attachment figure causes anxiety, anger, and mourning (Bowlby, 1975), little attention has been given this evidence, especially as it relates to adults. Several important coping mechanisms have been identified that adults use in traumatic or life-threatening situations: (1) keeping stress within manageable limits with denial (often the means of coping with a diagnosis of serious illness); (2) maintaining some measure of hope; (3) believing that one is still valued by a significant other; (4) maintaining valued groups, of which the family is most important; (5) maintaining self-respect (Visotsky, et al., 1961; Hamburg and Adams, 1967; Bowlby, 1975).

Henderson and Bostock (1977) found attachment ideation (thinking about a wife or a girl friend) as the most significant coping mechanism used by survivors of a shipwreck. Other studies indicate the passion with which family members strive to be reunited following a disaster (Bowlby, 1973; Killian, 1952). In the case of adversity, bereavement, or serious illness, it is generally accepted that most people seek and obtain comfort or support from close family members or friends (Henderson and Bostock, 1977, p. 189). Figure 16-5 suggests the comfort level derived from the affectional bond.

Adult Hospitalization. In light of what we have learned about attachment, it is difficult to understand some of the practices seen in a hospital setting. In some critical care units, nurses will invoke an archaic hospital rule that allows 5- or 10-minute visits when in so many instances there is no rationale for doing so. If a patient is comforted and feels more relaxed by the presence of the spouse and the spouse wants to be present, it is irrational to ask that person to keep a lonely vigil in a waiting room. If the patient is dying, the spouse, if present, has an opportunity to share in the death experience. It is a time, however limited, for adjusting to the reality of the eventual loss. Ultimately, this sharing will aid in the grieving process and promote the mental health of the surviving spouse.

■ *Point of Emphasis*

Research findings demonstrate that a patient in an ICU, CCU, or medical surgical area will feel less anxiety, be less susceptible to intense or chronic fear, and will use his call light less if allowed the comfort of the spouse's presence.

The following vignette depicts a situation that may be found in acute care settings:

Vignette

Joe, age 50, was admitted to the hospital because he was experiencing anginal pain. As he was undergoing cardiac catheterization he suffered a massive myocardial infarction. He was moved to the CCU. His condition steadily worsened.

Joe asked his wife to remain with him, and she insisted on doing so. When he awoke from a brief nap, he expressed both verbally and nonverbally his thanks to his wife for staying at his side. He voiced his frustration when nurses asked her to leave, saying "They try to separate us at the most crucial times of our life—when you were giving birth to our kids and now when I may be dying." Joe's wife remained with him throughout the 30 hours that he lived; 30 hours of shared love.

The nurse on the evening shift complained to a physician that Joe's wife was not following the regulation (10 minutes every hour). The physician relayed this message to the wife: "I would like you to stick to the rules. Your constant presence is intimidating the nurse." (The nurse's tasks were to check the monitors and take Joe's vital signs. Even when Joe was awake, she did not touch him, look at him, or address him by name.)

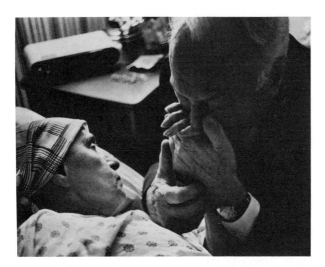

Figure (Photo) 16-5 *Adult attachment. When adult patient is critically or terminally ill, the presence and comfort of a loving spouse can reduce pain, anxiety, and fear. (Photo by Don Doll, S.J.).*

If nurses understood the strength and dynamics of adult attachments, hospitalized individuals and their families could work through pain, grief, and even death with their self-esteem and dignity intact.

The Elderly

Little reliable information is available on attachment behaviors or attachment needs of the elderly. Although research has been done relative to their social and psychological disengagement, results have been conflicting. The attachment of the older person to a significant other is rarely discussed but is often observed by community health nurses, who have an opportunity to see the couple in the home setting. The maturation of a long intimate relationship of partners in the winter of their lives often results in fierce loyalty and total commitment between the partners. They have a long history of sharing events—usually including children and grandchildren. It is a special attachment. In the following section the attachments between older people and their relevance tó life satisfaction are discussed, as is disengagement theory from the standpoint of its relevance to nursing care of the elderly.

Attachment: Significant Others. Studies by Lee (1978) and by Stennett et al. (1972) have demonstrated that elderly married persons have higher morale, a greater sense of well-being, and greater happiness than single, widowed, or divorced elderly. Companionship and the sharing of deep feelings characterize these enduring marriages.

In the United States there is also a steady increase in the number of persons over 65 years of age who marry (Vinick, 1978). Approximately 35,000 couples of whom at least one partner is above 65 marry each year (Papalia and Olds, 1981).

In the absence of a marriage partner or a significant other, attachment satisfaction may be realized through interaction with children and grandchildren. Seelbach and Hansen (1980) found that 8 of 10 elderly persons were content with their family interactions, while institutionalized elderly reported less satisfaction with family relationships, perhaps because they do not see family members often.

Palmore (1975), examined this issue among elderly Japanese and found that they felt well satisfied with their lives because they were integrated into the families of their children and grandchildren. Palmore has proposed that it may be desirable for older persons to live near their children and grandchildren. By being available to help with various household tasks, they feel less isolated at the same time that interaction with family increases.

Attachment to Confidant/Friend. Many elderly have outlived a significant other or do not have a family. For these persons, close friends and confidants provide increased life satisfaction. It is the quality of the friendship that is important. An intimate relationship in which the members can confide in each other is the most valuable in promoting well-being. "A confidant is more important for good mental health and high morale than is high social interaction or role status" (Papalia and Olds, 1981). A study by Miller and Ingham (1976) supports the evidence that having a significant other or a confidant during a period of major adjustment or traumatic life change decreases anxiety and stabilizes mental and physical health. The evidence that significant attachments among elderly people promote high morale and high life satisfaction has important implications for nursing care.

Attachment vs. Disengagement

Some theorists suggest that as a person ages he begins to withdraw from personal attachments and from society in general and that this withdrawal is based on his desires.

> ### ■ *Point of Emphasis*
>
> *Misinterpretation of the disengagement theory has often led to the isolation of terminally ill persons in a hospital setting, isolation of elderly in nursing homes, and isolation of older people in the community.*

Cumming and Henry (1961) proposed that withdrawal on the part of the older person is natural and voluntary and that the withdrawal occurs at three levels: physical, psychological, and social. At the physical level the person decreases his activity in order to conserve energy. Psychological disengagement refers to preoccupation with self, a lack of interest in the world, and a focus on one's own feelings and thoughts. This is accompanied by diminution of mental and emotional energy. Social disengagement is a voluntary reduction in interaction with others that is mutually beneficial.

The theory has been widely defended and attacked; but evidence goes against the theory and indicates that "disengaged older people tend to be more unhappy, lonelier, sicker and die sooner than more active older people" (Palmore, 1975). Support for Palmore's position can be found in his study of elderly Japanese, that relates to disengagement theory in two aspects. First, Japanese elderly are more active and are expected to work to an older age than persons in other industrialized countries. This disputes the idea that people lessen their activity to conserve energy regardless of health, and indicates that the degree of disengagement in an elderly population is determined mainly by the cultural and social structure. Second, the study indicates that the high degree of activity among elderly Japanese is a source of physical and psychological satisfaction to them.

In support of activity as a form of engagement and a degree of life satisfaction, Markides and Martin (1979) found that health and income are factors closely related to life satisfaction—when people are in good health and have sufficient money, they can be more active. These researchers also found that elderly persons who go on outings, such as meetings, trips, and movies, are happier than those who stay home. Neugarten (1978) reports that elderly who are active socially with family and friends and/or who are members of clubs report themselves most content with their lives.

Kalish and Knudtson (1976) identify some of the external forces that may move an elderly person to a state of disengagement. The older person generally has a more difficult time controlling his environment. With more chronic health problems, less financial independence, and diminished status, the older person may become extremely vulnerable. Significant others have often died. Relationships with adult children may not be fully satisfying because of individual schedules, tensions, or physical distance. The personal response and feedback in an elderly person's life may come from the physician, the nurse, or the social worker. These relationships are centered on caregiving rather than emotional support. With the loss of attachment figures and earlier roles, and with diminished activity and emotional support, the elderly person may withdraw and disengage socially and psychologically. Challenges to disengagement theory are important to health providers because some elderly (who need socialization and attachments) are left alone in their home or nursing homes based on the premise that they want isolation and that withdrawal is part of the aging process.

PROBLEMS OF DISRUPTED ATTACHMENT

Disruption of attachment bonds occurs frequently over the life span. These disruptions and separations have been linked to the development of grief, anger, protest, denial, and despair—feelings and behaviors that may on occasion lead to disease, death, or psychopathology. Generalizations based on research cannot yet be made, and the consequence of separation and disrupted attachment is an area in need of investigation. The most significant current research is concerned with the psychological and biological effects of separation in animals and infants.

Prenatal

Mother-infant interaction is present in utero. It is known that the fetus adapts to the circadian rhythms (day-night cycles) of the mother (Reppert and Schwartz, 1983). Stress in the mother during the third trimester of pregnancy is known to have a profound effect on the fetus. The fetus is affected by the "physical, nutritional, hormonal and psychosocial environment of the mother" (Call, 1984).

Infant/Toddler

An attachment disorder can be diagnosed in the infant as early as 1 month of age. When attachment capacities such as sucking rhythms, rooting behavior, gazing and vocal reciprocity with the mother, are absent, and when physical signs, such as low weight gain, poor muscle tone, weak cry, excessive sleep, feeding disturbance (without an organic cause) and apathy are present, this should be considered an attachment failure (Call, 1984).

One of the most difficult disturbances of attachment is the situation of a child who has not been able to develop a stable attachment during the first 2 to 3 years of life. This can happen when a child has been placed in an institution and is moved frequently from one place to another. These children are often unable to make affectional bonds with anyone throughout their lives and are likely at some time to be diagnosed as sociopathic; or, though asocial, may present a superficially social facade (Bowlby, 1975).

The earliest behavioral symptom of disrupted attachment that appears when a child is separated from his mother is protest; this is followed by despair. In the protest phase the child appears acutely distressed. He will cry loudly, strike out, and look anxiously for any sign that his mother is returning. This is followed by the phase of despair when he withdraws and becomes inactive (Bowlby, 1960b). This may occur when an infant or child is separated from parents by hospitalization or institutionalization, or when the parent is separated from the child by illness, wartime service, and so on. A final stage, detachment, may occur in which the child appears to recover and respond to other caregivers, and may reject the parent figure if he or she returns. In most cases, the attachment is rebuilt, though questions arise about the possible influence of detachment in those children who do not reattach.

Infant/Child Abuse/Neglect.

Crying, one of the infant's primary communicative behaviors, signals to the mother that he is hungry, wants to be held, is in distress, and so on. It may be misperceived by the parent as being "bad." Thumbsucking, helplessness, neediness, and dependence can cause parents to project previous bad feelings about themselves onto the infant, which may

elicit punitive, hostile behaviors on the part of the parents or caregivers (Call, 1984).

The alcoholic parent, by reason of his altered mental state, cannot give consistent nurturance to his child. At the one extreme alcoholics may be physically violent when irritated or annoyed, and at the other extreme may be noncommunicative and neglectful. Somewhere in between, the parent may vacillate between needing love from the child and demanding great displays of affection. The child has difficulty making a healthy attachment to this parent. He may be anxiously attached (overdependent, clinging, unable to individuate) and fearful that the parent will leave; he may become ill, or threaten to commit suicide (or actually commit suicide), or will emotionally detach. The anxiously attached child may come into adulthood as an anxious person, smothering his spouse with attention or caregiving and may suffer phobias. At a young age, school phobia may be present; at a later age phobias such as agoraphobia may arise (Bowlby, 1969).

The child who detaches emotionally may proceed through adolescence and adulthood with a borderline disorder of chemical dependency and into adulthood with a personality disorder of chemical dependence; or he may be considered a sociopath. These outcomes are by no means inevitable. Many variables come into play: the developmental period of the child during the loss of attachment experience, the other people in the child's life, the child's constitution and temperament, the child's perception of parental behaviors toward him, and clinical intervention.

Problems in Attachment in Childhood Affecting Adolescence and Adulthood

Bowlby and Parkes (1970) stresses that there is a causal relationship between an individual's experiences with parents and later capacity to make affectional bonds. If the attachment process is anxious, inconsistent, or nonexistent, the child brings this anxiety and loss into adolescence exhibiting clinical symptoms such as depression, aggression, substance abuse, and suicide attempt. If intervention is unsuccessful in adolescence, neurotic symptoms and personality disorders pervade adult interactions. The anger and resentment that underlie the anxiety and loss may be manifested against a weaker person, for example, a spouse or child. Unconscious yearning for love may be expressed in an inappropriate form of care-eliciting behaviors such as "half hearted suicide attempts, conversion symptoms, anorexia nervosa, hypochondria." The individual may present as very needy and clinging to a partner or may "smother" a partner or child with "love." The person may project onto the spouse perceptions from childhood, such as fears of abandonment (Bowlby, 1975). This disturbance in giving or receiving love will be further inflicted on the individual's children, thereby promoting a generational cycle of faulty attachments among family members.

Kagan (1984) points out, however, that an insecure attachment in the first year of life does not always lead to adult pathology, and securely attached infants and children have no guarantee that they will not succumb to stress or disease and need to seek help in the mental health system. For example, cultural and political dynamics change over time, affecting the vulnerability of adolescents and young adults. Indian adolescents in Bombay are anxious because cultural demands are no longer consistent with what they learned when they were closely attached to their mothers. An infant girl who was securely attached to a mother who promoted passivity and dependence toward men would have some confusion in the America of the 1980s (Kagan, 1984). Older children of the 1960s who were securely attached infants displayed behaviors and rebellion totally incongruent with their parents' values. Well-bonded infants and children of the 1970s and 1980s cope with powerful peer pressures to experiment with and use drugs. Adolescents in Japan commit suicide because of the overwhelming pressure to produce high grades in school. Biochemically influenced conditions such as schizophrenia, bipolar illness, and alcoholism disrupt normal attachments in adolescence and adulthood.

Separation and Loss: Grief and Mourning

Disruption of a strong attachment due to death can be healed over time with much consistent support by those who will allow the process of grief, anger, yearning, sadness, and talking about the loved one to take place. Bowlby (1975) noted four main responses that have been recognized in bereaved persons: (1) a numb phase which lasts for hours or weeks and may be interrupted with great distress and/or anger, (2) searching and yearning for the lost person which may last for months or years, (3) disorganization and despair, and (4) reorganization.

Death of Spouse

Widows have reported some sleep disturbance during the first year of bereavement, such as waking up at 3 or 4 A.M. and being unable to return to sleep. They also report other connected losses; loss of "couple" friends, loss of social and/or economic status. Kalin and Carnes (1984) reported on several studies that described the biological correlates of attachment disruption. Several studies suggest an increased mortality due to cardiovascular disease and an impairment of the immune function following conjugal bereavement. Cancer is correlated with death in widowers 6 months after bereavement more frequently than in control groups (Mellstrom, et al., 1982). Severe loss or separation such as the death of a close family member or marital separation was found to be a frequent antecedent to the development of lymphomas and leukemia in children (Mellstrom, et al., 1982; Greene, 1954; Jacobs and Charles, 1980).

The greater the role of the deceased in the life of the bereaved—emotional, social, economic—the greater the distress. A sudden and unexpected loss also causes greater stress during bereavement (Bowlby and Parkes, 1970). The more securely attached the bereaved person was to the one who died, the better is the outcome expected in the course of recovery. If the attachment was anxious or ambivalent the mourning process may be expected to present some disturbed or pathological behaviors. Psychiatric disturbance may also happen to those who had no one to care for and no one to care for them, support them, or listen to them after the loss (Bowlby and Parkes, 1970).

Young Children and Loss

Mahan (1985) presents an interesting example of loss and separation of children in a clinical setting. In the nursery school there was a white guinea pig that the children cared for on a rotating basis. When he died one weekend the children did not know how to respond to the loss or how to express their feelings. A new brown guinea pig replaced the first pig. At first the children thought their old pet had been painted. As Mahan points out, their attachment did not end with death, "death ends a life, but not a relationship." Death to a 3-year-old is not yet a biological fact. Believing that the pet was painted and not actually dead was a protective defense mechanism from the painful reality of the finality of death. Later when the children realized that the new pet was not painted but a new creature their unconscious mourning was expressed by, for example, "losing the lettuce they brought to feed" the new pet. To help the children mourn, the teacher met with them in small groups and helped them appreciate the attributes of both pets. Mahan believes a working through of losses from this secondary world helps prepare them for traumatic loss from their primary world. Working through the loss includes the loving memory of the lost "object" (Mahan, 1985).

Working through the Loss of an Attachment

"The psychodynamic work of mourning is to remember more than it is to say goodbye" (Vaillant, 1985). Vaillant believes that failure to internalize those we have loved or not having loved at all is what causes psychopathology, rather than the loss itself.

That a person loves and remembers the love he has lost is far more important to his mental health than the loss itself. For each love relationship an individual has, the potential for growth and stability increases. In therapy, the therapist can enable a client to increase self-esteem and grow in maturity and awareness by helping him recall lost loves and internalize those relationships. The therapist can help him reach back into his childhood to accomplish this. Vaillant describes the case of two brothers, one of whom had severe character flaws. In their preschool years they lost their father through divorce, alcoholism, and a move to an opposite part of the country. Their strong, overbearing mother remained behind. In adolescence one son rebelled against the mother, performed well in school, crossed the country as well as the barrier of his father's alcoholism, and became friends with him. That brother healed his losses and was able to forge continuing intimate relationships. The other brother was overwhelmed by the mother, sought no reconciliation with the father, left all family members, and ultimately had difficulty in adult relationships. This example supports Vaillant's (1985) statement that "separation/individuation is not inhibited by loss but enabled by loving." In his clinical work Vaillant has found that problems are greater when children live with inconsistent and incompatible parents than when they lose a good parent whose love they can internalize. Adults who internalize the love they had with a deceased attached figure will do their grief work well, will recover in due course, and will retain a comforting sense of the loved one's presence (Bowlby and Parkes, 1970; Vaillant, 1985).

☐ Nursing Process

The purpose in understanding attachment is to translate understanding into action. For example, the nurse can assist the childbearing family to establish attachment bonds and recognize their importance in child development. Nurses can exercise caution to avoid needlessly disrupting important bonds when caring for patients of any age. All nurses need to be aware of the indicators of loss and the pain associated with it.

CLIENT ASSESSMENT ☐ Nurse assessment of attachment behavior is especially important in three respects. First, as the nurse identifies emotional bonds at any point in the life span, she can enhance these in support of the client. Second, if there are no indicators of attachment, she can often facilitate attachment through education, role modeling, or structuring the environment. Finally, she can recognize the process of mourning and loss of significant attachments.

Mother-Infant ☐ Some predictors of the quality of attachment following birth are clues the woman gives during the prenatal period. The nurse in the clinic can assess whether the expectant mother refers to the unborn infant in endearing terms, is gathering together a layette, and whether she envisions herself and her changing body in a positive manner. If the woman has negative reactions to quickening (when the gestation is of approximately 4 months' duration), the nurse should allow ample time at each clinic visit to further assess the expectant mother's feelings and adaptation. The absence of positive responses at this early stage may be a clue to future problems.

The great majority of births occur in a hospital setting, though increasing numbers of women now prefer to give birth at home. The nurse is in a unique position to observe the progress of attachment and encourage it. This is especially true in the case of high-risk infants (premature, handicapped, or born to teenage and single mothers). These infants are particularly at risk of being battered and failing to thrive. The nurse may reduce this risk by facilitating the bonding process.

Observations the nurse should make in her assessment of infant-mother bonding include the following:

1. Does the mother gaze into the infant's eyes and anticipate a response (en face)? The neonate is highly attracted to the shininess and movement of eyes. Eye contact offers great satisfaction to both parent and infant.

2. Does the mother touch the infant? Most new mothers touch the infant from head to toe, first with the fingertips, and then with the entire palm. Skin-to-skin touching and cradling, as depicted in Figure 16-6, is of greater importance than feeding the infant. Nursing the infant, of course, incorporates skin-to-skin touching and closeness, and is ideal for promoting attachment (Klaus and Kennell, 1976).

3. Does the mother talk to the baby? The mother uses a higher pitched voice when talking to her new infant than in normal conversation. The pitch is very important to the neonate's auditory perception (Klaus and Kennell, 1976).

4. Does she hold the baby at other times than when giving direct care?

5. Does she make positive statements about the infant, for example, "My baby is so cuddly"?

6. Is she satisfied with the infant's gender?

Father/Infant □ Fathers often accompany their wives on prenatal visits. At this time the nurse can assess his involvement in the birth process. Does he plan to take prenatal classes with his wife? Does he plan to be present in the delivery room during the birth? Does he "speak" to the unborn infant. After the birth the nurse makes similar assessments for attachment as with the mother (Does he talk to the infant, gaze into his eyes, touch the infant and hold him close, let him hold onto his fingers?).

Parent/Child □ As the child grows, the nurse may suspect a lack of healthy parent/child attachment if the child clings to the parent, whines, is afraid to explore his environment, withdraws, makes minimal eye contact, is not touched and

hugged by the parent, does not engage in reciprocal smiling, or has little or no play interaction with the parent. Table 16-3 presents criteria for assessment of fathering behaviors.

Adolescent Attachments □ Nurse observations of adolescents will take place mainly in general hospital settings, psychiatric units, and in substance abuse programs. If a teenager is hospitalized in a general hospital because of injury or disease, his dependent position will increase his attachment for parents. Nurses in this setting will assess the degree of nurturing the parent provides. If the illness is life-threatening or traumatic, the adolescent may show strong or clinging attachment to the parents; conversely, he may project displaced anger toward them. If the nurse notes either of these behaviors, she can facilitate a desirable outcome of the attached relationships through her interventions.

In a psychiatric milieu or in a substance abuse program, teenagers usually spend several weeks together. The nurse in this setting will have the opportunity to assess relationship development among peers, which is a primary consideration in adolescence. It is these attachments that will help teenagers complete the developmental tasks that prepare them for independence and intimacy.

Adult/Elderly □ Nurse assessments of a threat of disrupted adult attachment will generally take place in a general hospital, psychiatric hospital, nursing home, or community health setting. In a

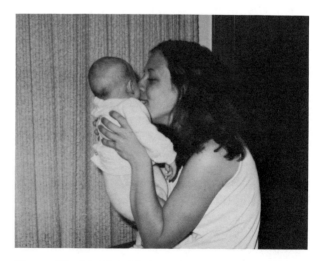

Figure (Photo) 16-6 *Mother-infant attachment. Skin to skin touching and cradling has been found to be of greater importance than feeling. (Photo by David Ehrhart).*

hospital setting, the nurse should assess if the attachment needs of the client to a significant other person are being met. She will judge if there are institutional barriers causing disrupted attachment. The nurse can determine if the client is too timid to have his needs met. Does the client understand client rights to visitation, telephone calls, and so on? Is privacy respected? Is the hospitalized client more content when his significant other is present (e.g., satisfaction is verbalized, anxiety is decreased, demands on the nursing staff are decreased, fear is lessened)? In long-term care, is the person permitted and encouraged to surround himself with familiar objects or mementos such as albums, a favorite chair, or handmade quilt. In all settings the nurse should draw assessments from a carefully conducted interview. Often social isolation, losses and unresolved grief can go undetected unless the nurse does a sensitive and skilled interview.

Humans can survive adversity and loss if they have a primary affectional support network. Widows, for example, cope with the first year of bereavement with less illness or morbidity if they perceive their primary groups as supportive. Persons have been reported to survive traumatic life events, such as being prisoners of war or shipwreck survivors, and experiencing loss of a spouse through death, without risk to physical or mental health if they have a primary group of persons who care specifically for them and their situation (Henderson, 1977; Moddison and Walker, 1967; Glick, et al., 1974; Glosser, 1965).

The above mentioned primary group is a small group of persons consisting of a significant other or close kin and friends who will remain supportive throughout the crisis. A spouse or girl/boyfriend has been found to provide great protection against adversity and difficulties (Brown, et al., 1975).

Often the grieving process is overlooked if a person has lost a spouse due to divorce or death that occurred 6 months or more ago. Yet the grieving process can continue for years depending on the circumstances. If a divorce was sought by one of the partners and not wanted by the other, the hurt, anger, and grief of the injured partner can remain for as long as 5 years. The nurse should also note that anniversaries may precipitate grief and depression in the client who has lost attachment figures.

NURSE SELF-ASSESSMENT □ Each person develops certain beliefs and biases based on familial and social backgrounds as well as on personal experiences. These may color one's view of an unmarried teenage mother, for example, or of a dependent elderly client in a nursing home. The attachment behavior of persons with different cultural backgrounds may seem foreign. The insistence of a Mexican family to have many members of their extended family present in the client's hospital room may be different from the nurse's own family experience. She may recognize important bonds in her life and in so doing, be able to relate to the client's needs in a therapeutic manner. If she is able to identify her biases and her feelings, she will be better able to give sensitive care to the client and family.

ASSESSMENT OF THE ENVIRONMENT □

Infant/Parent □ As stated earlier, to enable the parents and their infant to bond effectively and quickly, the mother should be able to explore her newborn infant with her hands and eyes immediately. These first hours and days have also been identified as the engagement period when the father and infant can bond. This is the time when reciprocal responses (parent to infant, infant to parent gazing and touching) take place. In the past, hospital policies and rules made this difficult if not impossible during the hospital stay. The father was especially deprived of interaction with his infant. However, as attachment theory and research are appreciated, most hospitals have attempted to structure their obstetric units to meet the needs of the family. Birthing rooms are now often part of the hospital milieu where father, siblings, and grandparents can make early contact with the newborn.

Hospitalized Children □ Policy in many children's units has been to allow parents or extended families to stay around the clock with their young children. However, this is not universally true. Many civilian and military hospitals continue to support policy that separates hospitalized children and parents for extended periods. In these cases the nurse should do everything possible to change the restrictive policy and to foster an attachment with a primary nurse.

Adolescents □ In psychiatric hospitals and substance abuse programs adolescents are involved in activities and leisure time with their peers. In a general hospital the nurse will need to assess the adolescent's attachment needs and support the client and family in meeting that need.

Adult/Elderly □ This area is least attended to by researchers and theorists, therefore environmental barriers may be greater. Most hospitals adhere to archaic policies related to visiting privileges and other matters. In a nursing home setting, the nurse has more power to structure the environment to promote attachments. The only barrier may be lack of knowledge. In a general hospital setting, however, the client attachments may be made very difficult by adherence to restrictive policies or routines.

Environmental Factors Influencing Nursing in the Hospital Setting □ With an understanding of attachment theory and its importance to the mental health and social development of human beings, a question may be posed: Can nursing incorporate into the hospital environment the strong affectional bonds that human beings make with significant others? The precepts of holistic health care are often practiced by nurses. Generally, meeting the needs of the client's physical and psychosocial self has been a service that has set nurses apart from most other health care providers. On the surface it may seem a simple matter to implement this aspect of caring in a hospital environment. Yet, as described below, there may be problems that hinder expanded care.

Hospital Administration □ The policies and rules devised by institutions to serve their requirements may at times conflict with certain aspects of holistic care. There is a need to look at a hospital's organizational goals. Etzioni (1961) has defined the human groupings called organizations as being characterized by (1) division of labor, power, and communication responsibilities, deliberately planned to enhance specific goals; (2) the presence of one of more power centers that control the efforts of the organization and direct them toward its goals; (3) substitution of personnel, that is, the power to hire and fire or float personnel to unfamiliar areas.

Changes in an institutional setting depend on the organizational structure. There may be a hidden agenda (e.g., stay within a budget; make a profit), whereas the stated goal is "command few resources." A hospital may have a policy of allowing visitors in the CCU for 5 minutes of every hour. "For the good of the patient" (is the stated goal) while the hidden goal is to remove families

from the area "for the comfort level of the staff" or because "it has always been done that way."

A significant factor that would have a negative influence on implementing attachment is the intense technical background of the physician which ill equips him to understand the psychological and social needs of the client. Another inhibiting factor is the nurse who functions along institutional lines, with little room for more personal elements; for example, the nurse who is passive toward the physician, feels her work space is her private domain, is technically rather than professionally oriented, and has little self-esteem about her own ability to relate or to carry out nursing functions.

The nurse, however, can be an effective change agent. All bureaucracies involve power structures and politics. Nurses who wish to make a difference in their society know that interaction with policy makers is necessary. A committee decides hospital rules and regulations concerning patient care. The nurse can begin by learning who the committee members are, so she can lobby for her concerns. Next, the nurse finds out how committee members are selected, and considers becoming a member of the policy-making body.

Nursing Service □ One excellent definition of nursing service is: to be aware of the client's role within his family and his subcultural group, and of their effect on him and his on them, and to implement care in relation to these influences. A task-oriented definition of nursing service is readily understood, but the psychosocial definition given above is notable because this aspect of service is often overlooked.

Philosophically, nursing service should not have a problem understanding or implementing this concept. Nursing, however, to effect change will have to (1) understand the goals of nursing service and (2) present the service with a plan and objectives that will enhance the service's identity. This offers positive benefits for nursing service as follows:

> *Satisfied personnel.* Caring deeply about other human beings was probably at the core of most nurses' aspirations when they first chose nursing as a career. Greater job satisfaction is possible when the nurse can combine technical skills with the professional capacity to relate to patients and their families.

Cost effectiveness. Cost containment is a significant social issue. Studies indicate that patients with attached persons in close proximity are less frightened and anxious, use their call light less, ask for pain medications less frequently, and free the nurse for other tasks.

Nursing Education □ Zais (1976) defined education as " . . . the process of actualizing human potential." In the past nursing education focused on technical skills. As late as 1976, Fagin reported that consumers perceived the nurse as a technical functional doer. . . . More in evidence today is the nursing school that integrates or teaches psychosocial skills. However, the term psychosocial skills is meaningless unless it is learned as an equal value with technical skills and patient teaching skills. The balanced combination of these values will identify the nurse as professional and enhance her image to consumers and other professionals.

Responsibility to the Consumer of Health Care □ Hospitalized patients and their families find themselves in a dependent and often fearful situation, unaware of their rights or intimidated by the institution or the personnel. It is nursing's responsibility to counsel, inform, and support patients and their families in efforts to gain maximum and humane care for the client. Weisman (1976), who has worked extensively with dying patients, says that "not many patients ask for miracles, but evidence of care and concern."

Problem Identification □ The problem of inadequate or disrupted attachment is significant to nurses practicing in diverse settings and caring for clients of any age. Influencing factors may include (1) significant stressors which delay or impede the bonding process between infant and parents, and (2) separations which disrupt attachment bonds after they have been established. These disruptions may involve chronic illness with prolonged hospitalizations, divorce and geographic or emotional distance from the noncustodial parent, death, or imprisonment.

Inadequate or disrupted attachment in infancy and childhood is believed to influence the capacity to form other attachments throughout life. Theorists studying domestic violence cite attachment as an influence in reducing the likelihood of child abuse (Goldstein, et al., 1985). Both separation anxiety and the process of grief and mourning are relevant to disrupted attachments throughout the life cycle.

NURSING INTERVENTIONS □ With an understanding of the implications that attachment theory has for nursing intervention, the nurse will: (1) teach; (2) structure the environment; and (3) promote attachment of the client to a significant other person. Interventions in the institutional setting occur at all three levels of prevention.

Primary Prevention □ Nurses can assist pregnant women by giving them reading material that explains the importance of bonding and teaches them how to begin attachment even at that stage. If, after the birth of the infant, the parents are hesitant about holding the infant, the nurse can facilitate the bonding by encouragement or support. She can show them how to hold and touch the infant, and how to talk to and look at him.

In the case of a single teenager, the nurse needs to make a referral to a social or home health agency so the attachment process can continue in the home setting.

Secondary Prevention □ As previously discussed, the hospital or institutional setting is an environment that by its very structure, policies, and procedures can foster disruption of attachments. Most age groups across the life span are at risk when placed in these settings. Nursing interventions for these groups are discussed below.

The Toddler. Separation trauma will be decreased if the nursing staff orients the parents to the unit and includes them in any appropriate care. Provision should be made for parents or extended families to stay around the clock with the child, if possible. Consistent staff members should be assigned to care for the child and arrangements made for a surrogate mother or grandmother to offer emotional support if the parents cannot be present.

The Older Child. The same interventions apply to the older child who is in a medical/surgical acute care hospital. In a psychiatric hospital, where children may be hospitalized for several weeks, stress can be alleviated by (1) providing the child with one-to-one time with a primary nurse in order to foster self-esteem and uniqueness; (2) taking into account special needs related to the age and sex of the child; (3) promoting attachment behaviors to the nursing staff by making appropriate assignments that consider the age and sex of the child; and (4) facilitating attachment among peers in order to encourage the child's social development during hospitalization (Ehrhart, 1980).

The Adolescent. As in younger children, the adolescent in a general medical/surgical hospital will be emotionally dependent on his parents during an acute crisis, so the nursing staff can reduce anxiety and stress by including the parents or extended family into the environment to provide emotional support. The adolescent in a psychiatric hospital or substance abuse center, however, has to meet his developmental needs when hospitalized over a period of time. In this setting the nursing staff need to be aware of the importance of peer attachments. This can be accomplished in several ways:

1. Structure ward activities so that adolescents have ample time for interaction with peers.
2. Plan activities so the teen can experience positive dyadic interaction.
3. Divide the adolescent population into small groups to accommodate age and need, in order to maximize the capacity to form peer attachments.
4. Provide a secure milieu so that the adolescent feels free to experiment in forming relationships (Kunes, 1979).

The Adult and Elderly Client. A high risk (but less researched) area for painful disruption of attachment may be found in any intensive care unit or acute care general hospital setting. The nurse is in a unique position to facilitate attachment between hospitalized adults. On a short-term basis she can promote attachment and decrease anxiety and fear by allowing a significant attached person to be present for extended periods or for as long as is desired. She may need to be the patient's advocate in accomplishing this task. It may be necessary to collaborate with the physician as well as other staff members. If policies are barriers she may need to challenge their logic. For the long term, the nurse will be the most effective change agent if she becomes a member of the committee that makes the rules.

There are several interventions that will foster attachment in nursing homes, hospitals, clinics, or in the client's home.

The Therapeutic Relationship with the Elderly Client. First and foremost a therapeutic relationship needs to be established. The one-to-one relationship is the framework by which mutual goals are set, motivational strategies are devised, attachments are fostered, and problem solving begins. This interaction should commence with a warm approach and with respect. Genuine interest in the person must be shown. It can be developed through active listening. Nonverbal communication, such as body positioning, is effective when there is a handicap such as visual or hearing impairment. The nurse should position herself in front of the client at eye level so he can see her face and lip movements. The relationship will be enhanced if it is intimate, involving a degree of self-disclosure on the part of the nurse (Wahl, 1980). The client's self-esteem and sense of control will be increased by allowing him to set the time of the meeting. The length of the session should be limited. Sessions are ended when mutual goals have been met. Because there is emotional bonding in this kind of relationship, ample time must be allowed to prepare the client for any separation so he can adjust appropriately.

Touch. Touch is a very important nonverbal means of communication and should be incorporated into the therapeutic relationship. Burnside (1979) claims that older people soon learn the difference between task-oriented touch and non-task-oriented touch. Elderly are often grossly deprived of the latter form of interaction. The kind and amount of touch an individual appreciates varies from person to person and between cultures. If the touch offered is not acceptable, the client will give clues—either verbally or by turning away. Generally the client will be appreciative of this contact. At first, the nurse can offer a handshake, which is nonthreatening to most people. Burnside recommends a gentle touch on the cheek, shoulder, or the arm as other nonthreatening touches. Holding the client's hand during the interview has been found to be an effective means of contact. If the nurse is giving foot care, a gentle massage is another form of touch that goes beyond task-oriented touch, such as changing dressings or clipping nails, to promote attachment between nurse and client.

Sexuality. The sexuality needs of the older person are often overlooked by health providers as well as family members. Some people, in fact, believe that sexual behavior by older people is distasteful or disgusting. The reality is that human beings remain sensual well into old age or until death. The nurse should be able to address the issue of the client's sexual relationship with his spouse or significant other.

The nurse should remember that sexuality does not refer only to intercourse. The aged person also enjoys being physically close to another individual, being special to one particular person, flirting, being fully human. The sexual self is very much a part of the psychological, social, and spiritual self. Nurses are not always comfortable approaching this issue with a client. They often lack instruction on the sexuality needs of a client and may find it difficult to discuss this topic. It will help the nurse to address the issue if she is comfortable with her own sexuality, has knowledge of physiology, and is aware of different sexual orientations. If she is self-confident about the subject, she can speak to the client in an open and direct manner, which will generally invite open communication. It will help the client feel that his sexuality is not a taboo subject and that it is appropriate to discuss. If the nurse is not comfortable, she should refer the client to another professional.

Residents in nursing homes are at the greatest disadvantage because of the lack of privacy. Nursing home administrators and health providers can help by structuring the environment to allow privacy for clients who wish to be alone with a partner. Arrangements should be made for married couples and those with alternative couple arrangements to room together and maintain some privacy.

Pets. Pets provide another source of attachment to the elderly. The need to love and be loved can be met if the older individual has a pet to care for. Pets provide solace during times of loneliness, depression, and grief. The pet also helps the older person fulfill his need for touching. Some nursing homes now have pets living in the institution for the enjoyment of all the residents. However, this is not as satisfying as having one's own pet.

Tertiary Prevention □
The Confused Elderly. Confused elderly in nursing homes continue to be a population at great risk of isolation and loss of attachment figures. They are often disoriented to time and place and many have severe memory loss.

One group of nursing students fulfilled a nursing course objective by facilitating a group for elderly clients with a diagnosis of confusion, organic brain syndrome, or Alzheimer's disease. The group met twice a week for 8 weeks. Their goals were to (1) promote socialization; (2) increase physical activity; (3) increase sensory stimulation; (4) decrease negative behaviors exhibited by

clients (e.g., calling out in the halls, attempting to leave the facility); and (5) provide respite time for the overworked staff.

Goals and interventions were as follows:

1. *Guide the client through a short series of exercises.* These included range of motion actions such as initiating activities of daily living (e.g., pretending to comb hair or brush teeth) and tossing a beach ball.
2. *Provide sensory stimulation through dancing, singing, and touching.* The music was from the era that most clients enjoyed reminiscing about. The student gave each client a face, neck, and shoulder massage. Elderly in wheelchairs also "danced." The students held the person's hands and guided the chair to the music.
3. *Facilitate reminiscence on selected subjects.* Reminiscence centered on radio shows, seasons of the year, certain flowers, and the like.
4. *Provide a social time with refreshments.*

In order to evaluate their intervention, the students kept a weekly record of positive and negative behaviors for each. Behaviors recorded included *smiles, laughs, sings, other positive signs (claps, winks, dances), talks to others, exercises, disruptive behavior,* and *wants to leave.* Each week the positive behavior increased for each person as negative behavior decreased. By the fourth week every person received a check mark in each positive category. By the fifth week there were no disruptive behaviors and no one asked to leave. The nursing home staff reported that agitated behavior decreased in 50 percent of the clients during the rest of the day. Social behaviors improved generally, with clients talking to each other and looking at each other more frequently. The members became better oriented to time and place. They counted the days between sessions. They knew the sequence of routines and anticipated each one. Some group members became attached to certain students. When one male student was absent because of illness, an elderly lady immediately commented on the absence and refused to dance with the other students that day.

Reminiscence Therapy. An intervention of great benefit to most elderly clients is reminiscence therapy in which the focus is on the person's past life. Reminiscence is viewed by many gerontologists as "an adaptive strategy which compensates for losses and inadequacies in the present" (Ryden, 1981). Successful reminiscing may be a behavioral indication that the aged person is accepting the life that was lived with no regrets for how it was lived or for what might have been done differently (Erikson, 1963). Fostering reminiscence serves to promote interpersonal relationships and thus attachment between older persons. (See also Chapter 13.)

Attachment deprivation is greatest in the nursing home environment where the client may have lost autonomy, life roles, home, and lifelong friends. Here, the surroundings should be arranged to give clients opportunities to interact with each other. Couples should be allowed to enter the nursing home and maintain their privacy, even though one partner may be independent enough to come and go. The community health nurse may encounter many couples who would choose this arrangement if it were possible when one spouse finds it too difficult to care for the other. Because of institutional rules, however, many couples elect to stay at home (even though this puts additional burdens on them) as they do not wish to be separated.

■ *Point of Emphasis*

For a client who has few visitors, the staff, especially nurses, will be the providers of warmth and personal interaction.

EVALUATION □ If attachment in the health care setting has been fostered, the following criteria or outcomes should be met:

1. *The infant.* The parent will touch the infant, hold him close, gaze into his eyes, talk to him, respond to his cries of discomfort.
2. *The securely attached toddler.* The toddler will show a preference for the parent as opposed to others, and he will explore the environment without fear with the parent nearby. He will be distressed if separated from the parent. When the parent returns the toddler will seek contact and will again be able to play or explore. He will also interact without aggression with peers, may tend to be the leader during play, and will be self-directed.
3. *The hospitalized child.* He will become attached to a primary nurse in the absence

of the parent and will be sociable and cooperative with caregivers.

4. *The teenager.* The teenager will have a strong relationship with a peer. He will confide in the peer, and spend recreational time with others in his age group.
5. *The adults.* An intimate or emotionally close relationship will be observed with a significant other person. This may be a spouse, a child, or a friend. In the hospital setting the client will have less fear, sorrow, and anxiety and make fewer demands on the hospital staff if the attached person is present.
6. *The older person.* An older person will interact socially within his milieu, participate in work or hobbies according to his physical and mental ability, and have a spouse, friends, or a confidant with whom he can share information and feelings.

■ *Point of Emphasis*

The anxiety and fear caused when a child or an adult is unwillingly separated from an attached person can be alleviated by knowledgeable, sensitive nursing care.

■ Enrichment Activities

LEARNING ACTIVITIES

Using the concept of attachment, problem-solve each of the following situations. This may be done by discussion or role playing, first in small groups, later for the entire group. Allow class discussion time in your presentation.

1. Betty Jo is an active 2-year-old who was admitted to the hospital for diagnostic testing. It is expected that 1 week will be required to complete the tests, some of which are painful. She is afraid, and screams whenever a stranger approaches her. There are four older children in the ward, none acutely ill. Betty Jo's crib is covered by a net, so she cannot climb out.

   Her mother is anxious about the outcome of the tests and about the intense fear her child is experiencing in these strange surroundings. The mother works during the day and has expressed a desire to stay through the night with Betty Jo. Other family members who have been visiting with Betty Jo are her father and grandmother.

a. Assume the role of the mother. Express your feeling of: (1) worry over the possible diagnosis, (2) the child's fear of being left alone without a family member; and (3) worry about her being "penned in" the crib whenever the family isn't there. Express any other feelings a mother might have in this situation.

b. Assume the role of the charge nurse. Discuss a plan of care with your staff. Consider: (1) different staffing patterns that might be present on a pediatric unit; (2) Betty Jo's age, activity level, fear, and anxiety; and (3) the mother's request to be with her child as much as possible. Discuss the plan of care with the mother and set mutual goals (discuss in your group what these goals will be). Assign your staff and give rationales.

2. Jimmy, who is 14 years old, has recently been admitted to an inpatient psychiatric hospital with a diagnosis of problems of adolescent adjustment. Jimmy is sullen and keeps to himself on the unit. His mother and father have been divorced for 4 years, and he lives with his mother and two younger sisters.

As the team leader of the adolescent unit, formulate a plan of care for Jimmy. When deciding on an activity schedule, consider his psychosocial developmental needs. For his primary staff person, select one of the following members of your staff: (1) Mary, 25 years old, psych. tech.; (2) Mrs. Jones, RN, 60 years old, staff nurse; (3) John, 30 years old, psych. tech.; (4) Judy, RN, 25 years old, charge nurse.

3. Mrs. Kay suffered a myocadial infarction. She is recuperating in the CCU. The staff nurse has asked Mr. Kay to leave the room so "Mrs. Kay can get her rest." Mr. Kay expresses a wish to sit by his wife and hold her hand. The nurse tells him that there are hospital rules that must be followed and she insists that he leave. After he leaves, Mrs. Kay cries and continually asks when he can come back. Mrs. Kay becomes depressed and the psychiatric liaison nurse is called in for a consultation.

While visiting with Mr. Kay, the liaison nurse learns that the couple have been married 28 years. Mr. Kay says, "I know my wife will be more relaxed with me by her side. I know her. I would feel much better too, knowing I was a comfort to her instead of feeling so helpless and useless out here in the waiting room."

Take the role of the psychiatric liaison nurse and consult with the staff nurses. Help them formulate a holistic plan of care, addressing the attachment needs of this family.

4. Mr. Jons, 77 years old, is a resident in a nursing home. His three adult children live in other states. His wife is dead. He keeps several pictures of his grandchildren and their notes to him taped to the wall. Because his family lives far away, Mr. Jons has very few visitors. He had been the president of a small business in town but most of his associates have moved away or died. He is becoming increasingly irritable and aggressive toward the staff.

In light of Mr. Jons's loss of contact with family and old friends, diminished power and control in his life, and separation from home and business, formulate a plan of care addressing the loss of the attachment bonds in his life. Discuss three significant therapies the nursing staff can provide to help Mr. Jons cope with: (a) loss of a confidant; (b) loss of control; (c) adapting to Erikson's final stage of life of integrity vs. despair.

■ *Recommended Readings*

Bowlby, John. The making and breaking of affectional bonds. I. Aetiology and psychopathology in the light of attachment theory. *British journal of psychiatry.* 130, 1977:201–210. The author examines attachment theory as a way of conceptualizing the strong bonds human beings make toward one another. He also deals with the possible consequences when the bond is unwillingly broken. Both healthy and pathological personality development are touched upon, including some common patterns of parenting that contribute to them.

Bowlby, John. The making and breaking of affectional bonds. II. Some principles of psychotherapy. *British journal of psychiatry.* 130, 1977:421–431. Bowlby explores how a clinician can approach the problem of working with a client with disrupted attachment.

Burnside, Irene; Ebersole, Pricilla; and Monea, Helen (eds.). *Psychosocial caring throughout the life span.* NY: McGraw-Hill, 1979. This book interprets concepts, theories, and issues related to healthy developmental aspects of persons across the life span. Part One deals with infancy through adolescence; Part Two looks at the span from young adulthood to old age; and Part Three addresses issues related to the last half of life (A sensitive, caring, and positive final section).

Kagan, Jerome. *The nature of the child.* New York: Basic Books, 1984. In this book about child development, the author challenges many long-held assumptions. He argues that a child's experiences do not necessarily shape his life, that humans have a lifelong capacity to change.

Kandzari, Judith; Howard, Joan; and Roch, Martha. *A developmental approach to assessment.* Boston: Little, Brown & Co., 1981. The focus of this book is on wellness. It gives the nurse direction in promoting and teaching wellness behaviors to family members at all stages of development throughout the life span.

Maccoby, Eleanor. *Social development. Psychosocial growth and the parent-child relationship.* New York: Harcourt Brace Jovanovich, 1980. This book deals with social and personality development of infants and children. It contains a fine section on the development of attachment, including some research studies.

■ References

Ainsworth, Mary D. Object relations, dependency, and attachment: A theoretical review of the infant-mother relationship. *Child development,* 40, 1969:969–1025.

Ainsworth, Mary D., and Bell, Sylvia M. Attachment, exploration and separation: Illustrated by the behavior of one-year-olds in a strange situation. *Child development.* 40, 1970:49–67.

Altman, J., and Taylor, D. *Social Penetration,* Holt, Rinehart and Winston, N.Y., 1973.

Ansubel, David P. *Theory and problems of adolescent development* Ansubel, (David P., ed.) New York: Grune & Stratton, 1954:382–384.

Antonucci, Toni. Attachment: A life-span concept. *Human development,* 19, 1976:135–142.

Ban, Peggy, and Lewis, Michael. Mothers and fathers, girls and boys: Attachment behavior in the one-year-old. *Merrill-Palmer Quarterly,* 1974:195–204.

Bell, Sylvia M. The development of the concept of object is related to infant-mother attachment. *Child development,* 41, 1970:291–311.

Bischof, Norbert. A system approach toward the functional connections of attachment and fear. *Child development,* 46, 1975:801–817.

Bowlby, John. The nature of the child's tie to his mother. *International journal of psychoanalysis,* 39, 1958:350–373.

Bowlby, J., Grief and mourning in infancy and early childhood. *The psychoanalytic study of the child,* 15, 1960a:9–52.

Bowlby, J., Separation anxiety. *International journal of psychoanalysis.* 41, 1960b:89–113.

Bowlby, J., *Attachment loss.* Vol. I, *Attachment.* New York: Basic Books, 1969.

Bowlby, J., *Attachment and loss.* Vol. 2, *Separation.* London: Hogarth Press; New York: Basic Books, 1973.

Bowlby, J., Attachment theory, separation anxiety, and mourning. In *American handbook of psychiatry.* 2d ed. Vol. 6, *New psychiatric frontiers* (Hamburg, David A., and Brodie, Keith H., eds.) New York: Basic Books, 1975:292–309.

Bowlby, J., The making and breaking of affectional bonds. I. Aetiology and psychopathology in the light of attachment theory. *British journal of psychiatry.* 130, 1977:201–210.

Bowlby, J., The making and breaking of affectional bonds. II. Some principles of psychotherapy. *British journal of psychiatry.* 130, 1977:421–431.

Bowlby, J., and Parkes, C. Separation and loss within the family. *The child in his family.* (Anthony E., and Koupernik, C., eds.) New York: John Wiley & Sons, 1970.

Branstetter, Ellemae. The young child's response to hospitalization: Separation anxiety or lack of mother care? *American journal of public health,* 59, 1, 1969:92–97.

Brekenridge, Marian, and Vincent, Lee. *Child development,* 3d ed. Philadelphia: W.B. Saunders Co., 1957.

Brown, G.; Bhrolchain, M.; and Harris, T. Social class and psychiatric disturbance any woman in an urban population. *Sociology,* 9, 1975:225–254.

Burnside, I., Ebersole P., Monea, H., (eds.). *Psychosocial caring throughout the life span,* New York: McGraw-Hill Book Co., 1979.

Butler, R. The life review: An interepretation of reminiscence in the aged. *Psychiatry,* 26, 1963:65–76.

Call, Justin. Child abuse and neglect in infancy: Sources of hostility in the parent-infant dyad and disorders of attachment in infancy. *Child abuse and neglect.* 8, 1984:185–202.

Cohen, Leslie, and Campos, Joseph. Father, mother and strangers as elicitors of attachment behaviors in infancy. *Developmental psychology,* 10, 1, 1974:146–154.

Cohen, Leslie Jordan. The operational definition of human attachment. *Psychological bulletin,* 81, 1974:207–217.

Cumming, E., and Henry, W. *Growing old,* New York: Basic Books, 1961.

Dickens, Charles; Bryson, Rebecca; and Kass, Normal. Companionship therapy: A replication in experimental community psychology. *Journal of consulting and clinical psychology,* 45, 1977:637–646.

Dunphy, Dexter C. The social structure of urban adolescent peer groups, *Sociometry: A Journal of Research in Social Psychology,* 26, 2, (June 1963):230–246.

Ehrhart, Patricia M. Attachment behaviors of hospitalized children to the nursing staff. Master's thesis, University of Nebraska Medical Center, Omaha, 1980.

Elkind, David A. *A sympathetic understanding of the child six to sixteen.* Boston: Allyn and Bacon, 1971.

Erickson, E. *Childhood and Society,* New York: Norton, 1963.

Etzioni, Amitai. *A comparative analysis of complex organizations on power, involvement and their correlates.* New York: The Free Press, 1961.

Fagin, Claire. Can we bring order out of the chaos of nursing education? *American Journal of Nursing,* (Jan. 1976):98–100.

Fleener, Don E., and Cairns, Robert B. Attachment behaviors in human infants: Discriminative vocalization on maternal separation. *Developmental psychology,* 2, 1970:215–223.

Gerwitz, Jacob L. The attachment acquisition process as evidence in the maternal conditioning of cued infant responding. *Human development,* 19, 1976:143–155.

Glick, Ira; Weiss, Robert; and Parker, C. Murray. *The first year of bereavement.* New York: John Wiley & Sons, 1974.

Glosser, W. *Reality therapy: A new approach to psychiatry.* New York: Harper & Row, 1965.

Goldstein, A.; Keller, H.; and Erne, D. *Changing the abusive parent.* Champaign, IL: Research Press, 1985.

Greenburg, M., and Morris, N. Engrossment: The newborn's impact upon the father. *American journal of orthopsychiatry,* 44, 4, (July 1974):520–531.

Greene, W.A. Psychological factors and reticuloendothelial disease. Preliminary observation on a group of males with lymphomas and leukemia. *Psychosomatic medicine,* 16, 1954:220–230.

Hamburg, David A., and Adams, John E. A perspective on coping behavior. *Archives of general psychiatry,* 17, (September 1967):277–284.

Harlow, Harry. The nature of love. *The American psychologist,* 14, 11, 1958:673–685.

Harlow, Harry. Primary affectional patterns in primates. *American journal of orthopsychiatry,* 30, 1960:676–684.

Harlow, Harry, and Harlow, Margaret. Social deprivation in monkeys. *Scientific American,* 207, 1962:136–146.

Harlow, Harry; Harlow, M.; and Suomi, S. From thought to thérapy: Lessons from a primate laboratory. *American scientist,* 59, 1971:538–549.

Heard, D.C. The relevance of attachment theory to child psychiatric practice. *Journal of child psychology and psychiatry and allied discipline,* 22, 1, 1981:89–96.

Henderson, Scott. Care-eliciting behavior in man. *The journal of nervous and mental disease,* 159, 1974:172–181.

Henderson, Scott. The social network, support and neurosis. *British journal of psychiatry,* 131, 1977:185–191.

Henderson, Scott, and Boston, Tudor. Coping behavior after shipwreck. *British journal of psychiatry.* 131, 1977:15–20.

Hollender, Marc H.; Luborsky, Lester; and Harvey, Roberta B. Correlates of the desire to be held in women. *Journal of psychosomatic research,* 14, 1970:387–390.

Jacobs, T., and Charles, E. Life events and the occurrence of cancer in children. *Psychosomatic medicine,* 42, 1980:11–24.

Johnson, Suzanne Hall. *High-risk parenting: Nursing assessment and strategies for the family at risk.* New York: J.B. Lippincott, 1979.

Jones, Byron, and Clark, Dennis. Mother-infant separation in squirrel monkeys living in a group. *Developmental psychobiology,* 6, 3, 1973:259–269.

Jones, Colette. Father to infant attachment: Effects of early contact and characteristics of the infant. *Research in nursing and health,* 4, 1981:193–200.

Kagan, Jerome. *The nature of the child,* New York: Basic Books, 1984.

Kalin, N.H., and Carnes M., Biological correlates of attachment bond disruption in human and non-human primates. *Progress neuropsychopharmacological and biological psychiatry,* 8, 3, 1984:459–469.

Kalish, Richard A., and Knudtson, Frances W. Attachment versus disengagement: A life span conceptualization. *Human development,* 19, 1976:171–181.

Killian, L.M. The significance of multiple-group membership in disaster. *American journal of sociology,* 57, 1952:309–314.

Klaus, Marshall H., and Kennell, John H. *Maternal-infant bonding.* St. Louis: Mosby, Company, 1976.

Kogan, Kate L., and Gordon, Betty N. Interpersonal behavior constructs: A revised approach to defining dyadic interaction styles. *Psychological reports,* 36, 1975:835–846.

Kunes, Mary. Attachment behaviors in hospitalized adolescents. Master's thesis, University of Nebraska Medical Center, Omaha, 1979.

Lee, G. Marriage and morale in late life. *Journal of marriage and the family,* 40, 1, 1978:131–139.

Maccoby, Eleanor E. *Social development, psychological growth and the parent-child relationship.* New York: Harcourt Brace Jovanovich, 1980.

Maccoby, Eleanor E., and Masters, John C. *Attachment and dependency.* In *Carmichael's manual of child psychology* (Mussen, P., ed.). New York: Wiley, 1970.

Maddison, D and Walker W. Factors affecting the outcome of conjugal bereavement. *British J. of Psychiatry,* 113, 1967:1057–1067.

Mahan, Eugene. Some aspects of separation and loss in therapy with disturbed children. *The American journal of psyshoanalysis,* 45, 1 (Spring 1985):35–44.

Markides, K., and Martin, H. A causal model of life satisfaction among the elderly. *Journal of Gerintology,* 34 (1), 1979:86–93.

Mellstrom, D., Nilsson, A., Oden, A., Rudgren, A., and Svanborg, A. Morality among the widowed in Sweden. *Scandinavian journal of social medicine,* 10, 1982:33–41.

Miller, P., and Ingham, J. Friends, confidants and symptoms. *Social psychiatry,* 11, 1976:51–58.

Moss, H.A. Sex, age and state as determinates of mother-infant interaction. *Merrill-Palmer Quarterly,* 13, 1967:19–36.

Neugarten, Bernice L. "Developmental perspectives," *Readings in Gerontology,* (Brown, Mollie, ed.), 2nd ed., St. Louis: Mosby Co., 1978.

O'Connor, M.J., and Master, Ann. Use of the strange situation procedure in the diagnosis of attachment disorders. *Child psychiatry and human development,* 15, 1, (Fall 1984):64–71.

Palmore, Erdman. Sociological aspects of aging. In *Behavior and adaptation in late life* (Busse, E., and Pfeiffer, E. eds.). Boston: Little, Brown & Co., 1969.

Palmore, Erdman. *The honorable elders, a cross-cultural analysis of aging in Japan.* Durham, NC: Duke University Press, 1975.

Papalia, D., and Olds, S. *Human development* 2d ed. New York: McGraw-Hill, 1981:535–565.

Parkes, Colin, M., and Stevenson-Hinde, Joan. *The place of attachment in human behavior.* New York: Basic Books, 1982.

Peddler, J.R. Attachment and new beginning. *International review of psychoanalysis,* 3, 1976:491–497.

Peterson, Gail, and Mehl, Lewis. Some determinants of maternal attachment. *American journal of psychiatry,* 135, 10, 1978:1168–1173.

Pollock, George H. Mourning and adaptation. *International journal of psychoanalysis,* 42, 1961:341–361.

Porter, R., and Laney, M. Attachment theory and the concept of inclusive fitness. *Merrill-Palmer Quarterly,* 26, 1, 1980:35–52.

Reedy, Margaret N.; Birran, James E.; and Schaie, K. Warner. Age and sex differences in satisfying love relationships across the adult life span. *Human development,* 24, 1981:52–66.

Reite, Martin, Seiler, C., and Short, R. Loss of your mother is more than the loss of a mother. *American journal of psychiatry,* 135, 3, 1978:370–371.

Reppert, S., and Schwartz, W., Maternal coordination of the fetal biological clock in utero. *Science,* 220, 1983:969–971.

Ryden, Muriel. Nursing intervention in support of reminiscence. *Journal of gerontological nursing,* 7, 8, (August 1981):461–463.

Schultz, Ned. A cognitive development study of the grandchild-grandparent bond. *Child study journal,* 10, 1, 1980:7–26.

Seelbach, W.C., and Hansen, C.J. Satisfaction with family relations among the elderly. *Family relations,* 29, 1, 1980:91–96.

Singer, Robert D. and Singer, Anne. *Psychological development in children.* Philadelphia: W.B. Saunders Co., 1969.

Stennett, N., Cavter, L., and Montgomery J. Older persons perceptions of their marriage, *Journal of Marriage & the Family* 34, 1972:665–670.

Stern, Daniel N. Mother and infant at play: The dyadic interaction involving facial, vocal, and gaze behaviors. In *The effect of the infant on its caregiver* (Lewis, M., and Rosenblum, L., eds.). New York: John Wiley & Sons, 1974.

Suomi, Stephen, et al. Effects of maternal and peer separation in young monkeys. *Journal of child psychology, and Psychiatry and allied disciplines* 17, 1976:101–112.

Troll, Lilian E., and Smith, Jean. Attachment through the life span: Some questions about dyadic bonds among adults. *Human development,* 19, 1976:156–170.

Vaillant, George, E. Loss as a metaphor for attachment. *The American journal of psychoanalysis,* 45, 1, (Spring 1985):59–67.

Vinick, B. Remarriage in old age. *The family coordinator,* 27, 4, 1978:359–363.

Visotsky, H., Hamburg, D., Goss, M., and Lebovitz, B. Coping behavior under extreme stress. *Archives of general psychiatry,* 5, 1961:27–52.

Wahl, Patricia. Therapeutic relationships with the elderly. *Journal of gerontological nursing,* 6, 5, (May 1980):260–266.

Weinraub, Marsha; Brooks, Jeanne; and Lewis, Michael. The social network: A reconsideration of the concept of attachment. *Human development,* 20, 1977:31–47.

Weisman, Avery D. *On dying and denying: A psychiatric study of terminality.* New York: Human Sciences Press, 1976.

Wise, Susan, and Grossman, Francis. Adolescent mothers and their infants: Psychological factors in early attachment and interaction. *American journal of orthopsychiatry,* 50, 3, 1980:454–468.

Zais, Robert. Curriculum principles and foundations. New York: Harper & Row, 1976.

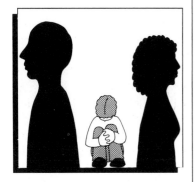

17

Childhood

Stephanie Stockard

Learning Objectives

Upon completion of this chapter, the reader will be able to:

1. Identify factors contributing to the development of mental health in children.

2. Describe the three levels of prevention in relation to child mental health.

3. Explain the role of the family in the development of mental health.

4. Identify stressors affecting a child's mental health.

5. Identify early warning signs of stress in children.

6. Describe the components of a mental health assessment of a child.

7. Explain the role of the child mental health nurse specialist.

8. Identify mental health considerations and nursing implications in care of the hospitalized child.

The mental health of children as a major focus of concern, research, and treatment has evolved only as recently as the past two decades. The National Institute of Mental Health (NIMH) estimates that some 1.4 million children and adolescents could benefit from psychiatric services—a conservative estimate by their own admission. Yet only some 5 to 7 percent of children who are in need of treatment receive it.

The family is the primary system for promoting mental health and preventing mental illness. Within this small system the child receives the basic physical and emotional tools, be they adequate or inadequate, with which he will later interact with the larger system of society. The family is a critical element in the development of a mentally healthy adult. Stressors, both familial and societal, can disrupt the child's healthy self-concept and his ability to learn, grow, and love. Unhealthy parenting, environmental stress, and social pressures may create an emotionally disturbed child who matures into a disturbed adult; as a parent he may foster a similar disturbed development in his own children.

The nurse who has contact with families and children, whether in hospital or community settings, is in a key position to recognize the child's psychosocial needs and intervene to prevent disruption to their being met. She should understand how important it is that the child develop a healthy self-concept, as well as the many problems that may impede its development.

□ *Evolution in the Child*

There is no single moment when a child achieves emotional well-being; it is ongoing through experiences. Positive experiences enhance growth—yet negative experiences may present opportunities to develop problem-solving skills and so advance personal growth.

SELF-ESTEEM

The infant basks in the parent's love. Caring, cuddling, talking, and playing send the message that the infant is worthwhile, important, and protected. The infant feels safe and secure, and trusts his environment; he has a stable base from which to seek opportunities that will later enhance his intellectual skills, foster learning about self and environment, develop physical capabilities, and promote creative expression.

In contrast, the infant whose initial experiences are negative feels uncertain and insecure; he learns that the world is a frightening place, and feels helpless. Later he will fear to take risks to learn, grow, and develop because his early experiences have taught him not to trust the world.

As the child grows, parents allow him greater independence, while still protecting him from experiences beyond his capabilities. Most parents wish to protect the child from emotional hurt as well as physical hurt, but this is often more difficult to do. How can the parent protect the child's self-esteem when he has been emotionally hurt? By listening to him and regarding his feelings as seriously as he does. This will restore the child's sense of well-being so that he can face the world once again. The child feels reassured about his worth, and this increases his self-confidence.

A parent builds the child's self-esteem by praising his actions: "You did well." "Nice work!" "Smart thinking!" "I'm proud of you!" These comments instill a sense of accomplishment in the child. These phrases are in contrast to comments that base acceptability of the child on his behavior as a person: "You're such a good girl when you help me." (And a bad girl when you don't.) "You always do a good job." (You'd better not do a bad job.)

When the child's action must be criticized, the adult should clearly indicate that it is the behavior that is unacceptable—not the child. "I don't like that language." "Toys are not to be broken."

> **■ *Point of Emphasis***
>
> *Convey disapproval of the act. If the child, rather than the behavior, is constantly criticized or belittled, he comes to believe that he is a bad person. Comments such as: "You're so dumb" and "You're a rotten kid" tell a child that he is "bad."*

If the parents consistently display regard for the child, he learns to respect himself. Praising his accomplishments, encouraging and supporting him, and allowing him to do all he can for himself contribute to a positive self-concept and sense of worth. Children also are keenly aware of how parents value themselves, each other, and those outside the family circle, and this too serves as a model for the child.

LOVE

Love has as many definitions as there are people. At the least, it indicates a concern and care for another human being.

■ *Point of Emphasis*

To a child, the parent conveys love in actions rather than in words, because the child's verbal and intellectual skills are not advanced enough that he understands the verbal expression of love.

Bonding-attachment is the first manifestation of parental love. If the pregnancy is welcome, the woman will begin to bond with the fetus. Klaus and Kennell (1982) define a bond as a tie from parent to infant. It is a unique relationship between two people that endures through time. Parental kissing, cuddling, fondling the infant, and gazing at him bespeak the affection felt for him. Attachment is the tie from child to parent (Klaus and Kennell, 1982)—the fetus is literally attached to the mother in pregnancy; at birth it must attach to her for survival.

TEMPERAMENT

Temperament is an early indicator of personality. Thomas and colleagues (1970) have delineated temperament of children as easy, slow to warm, and difficult (Table 17-1). Understanding these types helps adults understand how the psychological or temperamental fit between parent and child at birth influences all their future interactions. For example, a "difficult" child with an "easy" mother may encounter few problems because of the mother's adaptable personality; in contrast, an interaction between a "difficult" child and a "difficult" mother may generate high anxiety.

Medoff-Cooper and Schraeder (1984) studied the development and behavioral styles of very low birth weight infants (VLBW). They found some specific characteristics in both the infants and their parents. First, a large percentage of the babies were at risk for developmental delays, and had a "difficult" behavioral profile. Infants weighing under 1000 grams were at highest risk, with delay in motor skills most apparent.

Second, there were fewer "easy" babies and more "difficult" babies in the VLBW group than in the general infant population. The "difficult" babies were less easily soothed, more withdrawn, and more moody than the other babies.

The home environments of these VLBW infants were less enhancing than others, but this might have been the result of several situations. One possibility was that caregivers found the VLBW's negativity unappealing and provided little stimulation. Another possibility was that the environment made the babies "difficult."

The infant's temperament is not produced in a vacuum. It is one aspect of a child's total personality, and an important early influence on the parent-child relationship.

Family members other than the mother (or other caretaker), school friends, and social setting also play roles. As Chess and Thomas (1982) point out, "blaming the mother" was popular two or three decades back. It is now acknowledged, however, that problems in child development can have other causes.

☐ Prevention of Mental Disorders in the Child

Nowhere is there greater opportunity for prevention of mental disorders than in the field of child development. More so than is the case with adults, early recognition and treatment of problems can prevent chronic disability.

FIRST LEVEL OF PREVENTION

The first level of prevention is being wanted. Responsible sex life, family planning information, and contraception all help give the child a good start—his birth was desired, not accidental. Proper nutrition and medical care of the pregnant woman can prevent some diseases and developmental disabilities in the newborn.

Genetic counseling is becoming increasingly significant. As examples, research now suggests the existence of genetic predisposition in depression and schizophrenia.

Education of parents in child development and parenting skills is essential. The awesome responsibility of parenting is often practiced by persons who have had no instruction in it—nor do they desire the job! Such persons are ill equipped to be effective parents.

TABLE 17-1 The Origin of Personality[a]

Type of Child	Activity Level	Regularity, Rhythmicity	Distractibility	Approach/ Withdrawal	Adaptability	Attention Span	Intensity of Reaction	Threshold of Responsiveness	Quality of Mood
	The proportion of active periods to inactive ones (squirmers vs. sleepers)	Regularity of hunger, excretion, sleep, wakefulness (e.g. short or long naps)	Degree of distractibility from what he is doing (e.g., eating—some ignore, others respond to external stimuli)	Response to a new person or object; initial reaction to any new stimulus (food, people, toys)	The ease with which a child adapts to changes in the environment; ways in which initial reaction is modified	The length of time devoted to an activity and the effect of distraction on the activity (sucking, toys)	Energy of response regardless of its quality or direction (soft cry vs. howl for hunger)	The intensity of stimulation required to evoke a discernible response; various responses to noise, light fabric, response to pain (Sleeps through tornado vs. springs up in bed)	The extent of friendly, pleasant, joyful behavior vs. unpleasant, unfriendly behavior
Easy	Varies	Very regular	Varies	Positive approach	Very adaptable	High or low	Low or mild	High or low	Positive
Slow to warm	Low to moderate	Varies	Varies	Withdrawal	Slowly adaptable	High or low	Mild	High or low	Slightly negative
Difficult	Varies	Irregular	Varies	Withdrawal	Slowly adaptable with difficulty and with much repetition	High or low	Intense	High or low	Negative

[a] Adapted from "The Origin of Personality" by A. Thomas, S. Chess, and H. G. Birch, *Scientific American*, August 1970, W. H. Freeman Co.

SECOND LEVEL OF PREVENTION

At the second level of prevention is early identification and treatment of children with disturbed mental health. Table 17-2 lists warning signs of stress.

Failure to thrive signals early difficulties. During the first year, potential neurophysiological or psychological problems (such as hyperactivity, apathy, or lack of interaction with the mother) may be found. In preschoolers, overactivity, extreme awkwardness, anxiety, inability to separate from the mother, severe isolation, and failure to speak or to reach the usual developmental milestones may suggest emerging problems.

With entrance into school, the child has more or less established his behavioral pattern. It is estimated that 15 to 20 percent of school children have severe learning problems that are first manifested in behavioral problems (Bateman, 1973).

TABLE 17-2 Early Warning Signs of Stress in Childhood

Infancy	Continuous crying followed by withdrawal
	Lack of response to adults and family
	Signs of extreme fear, screaming continuously, or withdrawal
	Extreme anxiety demonstrated in agitation, inability to sleep or play, loss of appetite
	Indifference to caretaking adult
Preschool	Eating disturbances: anorexia, overeating, pica
	Sleep disturbances: wakefulness, frequent nightmares
	Developmental delay: speech delay or disturbance, late motor development, perceptual disturbances
	Physiologic symptoms (no demonstrable disease)
	Chronic constipation
	Small size and weight
	Malnutrition
	Chronic vomiting
	Chronic skin rashes
	Chronic wheezing and rhinorrhea
	Chronic undefined illness that prevent school participation
School age	Signs that are marked or persistent:
	Difficulty separating from mother
	School phobia
	Temper tantrums
	Extreme isolation
	Impulsive, asocial behavior
	Inability to relate to teachers or peers
	Learning problems

Chronic physical disease also has an impact upon both child and family, physically and emotionally. Early-onset diabetes, cancer, and developmental anomalies are examples of conditions in which intervention would be warranted.

Teachers and health personnel in schools, and child mental health and other health professionals are able to identify the child who is likely to experience difficulty. Regular screening of children at critical phases of development—such as age 3 (preschool), 5 or 6 years (first grade), and 8 or 9 (third grade) will measure the child's abilities.

Intervention may occur in the classroom, in various children's groups, in parent groups, or in the community through referral for medical or psychological assessment and intervention. Mental health services are available in inpatient, outpatient, and day-care settings, group homes, residential treatment facilities, or through foster care. If parents are involved, along with the school or other facility, the child stands a better chance of achieving mental health.

THIRD LEVEL OF PREVENTION

The goal of tertiary prevention in severe disorders is to achieve the maximum possible for the individual child, as early discovery and treatment can help the child to maximize his potential. Immediate educational, rehabilitative, social, and psychotherapeutic intervention is needed.

A severely disturbed child may require long-term residential care. If the child remains at home, any problems related to his being there must be resolved, and special schools or day hospitalization programs must be utilized. If the child remains at home, respite care to allow parents occasional relief is essential. A therapeutic milieu and a trained staff, whether in the residential setting or the hospital, are necessities.

☐ The Child Mental Health Nurse Specialist

Traditionally, nurses have worked with children either in the pediatric setting or at the tertiary level of prevention in the psychiatric setting. However, in the last 15 years, the nurse's expanded role allows the nurse interested in child mental health to broaden the services that promote mental health by intervening early.

The services provided by the educationally prepared child mental health nurse specialist may include, but are not limited to the following.

Primary Prevention

1. Educating parent groups about normal growth and development; intervening in common problems of childhood; and establishing support groups for mothers
2. Providing prenatal teaching, programs in nutrition, genetic counseling, family planning
3. Offering family life classes for adolescents
4. Serving as nurse advocates for legislation and funding of programs affecting children

Secondary Prevention

1. Identifying the child likely to experience an emotional disorder through consultation in nursery schools, grade schools, and in the community
2. Intervening in various relationships—one-to-one, group, family—and in a variety of settings—community mental health, private practice, inpatient, day care
3. As a referral source for social, educational, and rehabilitative services
4. As a consultant to other professionals who work with children, such as teachers, child care workers, and other nurses

Tertiary Prevention

1. Developing programs suitable for seriously disturbed children in residential, inpatient, or day-care settings
2. Intervening with disturbed children and their families for the purpose of minimizing the disruptions due to the child's problem, and helping child and family gain the most from rehabilitative programs
3. Participating in and promoting research into the causes of childhood disorders

☐ Mental Health of the Family and the Child

The family has the greatest influence in developing a mentally healthy child; and the child influences the family system. As in any system, each family member (component) affects all the other members (components), and the total family (whole) is greater than the sum of its parts.

The family is a microcosm of society and a vehicle for transmission of values. Styles in family life have undergone a change, however. The traditional family of mother, father, and children remains strong. At the same time, the number of single parent, communal, and foster families has rapidly increased in recent years. Whatever the form, nevertheless, all have the potential to provide the ingredients that contribute to a child's mental health and well-being. To work effectively with a child and his family, the nurse must be aware of the different attitudes and values that family life-styles generate. Obviously, what happens to the child will have an effect on the family—whatever the family's life-style.

THE CHILD IN THE TRADITIONAL FAMILY

The traditional family is idealistically portrayed in the paintings of Norman Rockwell. Though there are many families who manage to meet and overcome the stresses of the modern world and provide an environment that nurtures the child, there are family situations that can give rise to stress in the child.

Marital Discord

Children are far more sensitive to their emotional climate than adults believe. Children are experts at reading nonverbal cues and sensing adult emotions, because it was by these means that they first experienced communication with others. Necessity plays a part, too, since a child learns early that his basic needs are most often met by the parents.

Constant discord in the home evokes fear that these needs will not be met or fears that the parents will abandon him—remember that young children are normally egocentric and see themselves as the center of family life.

A parent who displaces anger toward the spouse onto the child sends a message to the child that he is "no good"—just like the "other" parent. "You're just like your father (or mother)" said disparagingly and repeatedly may not only destroy a child's self-esteem but also prompt behavior that fulfills the prophecy. The displaced parental anger may also be manifested in physical abuse of the child.

The child may identify with the parent of the opposite sex, which can cause confusion about his (her) sexual identification. The child might also adopt defenses used by the parent such as helplessness, hypochondria, or manipulation.

Deprivation of parental affection resulting from parental discord is one of the fundamental causes of psychopathology in children. In contrast, a spouse who is not shown affection by the partner may turn to the child for affection. The child feels overwhelmed by such expectations, or overstimulated by too much affection. The other parent resents the relationship with the child, and a vicious circle ensues.

On the other hand, parents who never openly argue may become role models of inhibition. A young child does not know that anger is a human emotion, can be expressed, and can be resolved without destroying a relationship. If he does not learn to use anger constructively, he will be unable to channel the anger that inevitably arises in family relationships.

Mental Illness in a Parent

Orvaschel and colleagues (1981), studying children of psychiatrically disturbed parents, found that these children had a high rate of psychiatric disorders. An earlier study (Orvaschel, 1979) found that the children of disturbed mothers evidenced differences when compared to children of disturbed fathers or with normal parents. Among these differences were increased tactile sensitivity, greater evidence of clumsy and awkward behavior, and heightened sensitivity to stimulation.

Anthony (1976) found that children of psychotic parents, although appearing imperceptive to the parents' behavior, actually registered, understood, and categorized the event. They recognized the premonitory signs of a psychotic episode. When a parent's psychotic episode was imminent, the children then physically avoided the parent, and denied the event to themselves on a conscious level.

Younger children were more accepting of violent behavior in their parents perhaps because their own aggressive behavior is not yet fully controlled. The early school-age child was frequently frightened by violence because of his own struggle to control aggressive drives.

Anthony (1976) also found that the children of psychotic parents used defensive behavior, including avoidance and distancing through busyness, writing, hobbies, denial of feelings, increased vigilance, hoarding possessions, greater tolerance for the parent, and repeatedly reassuring himself that he was not crazy. These children also experienced many fears, such as illness, "going crazy," loss of memory, dying, or becoming "suddenly stupid."

This research suggests that the child of an emotionally disturbed parent is at risk not only during childhood, but also in adult life.

Substance Abuse

A pregnant woman who uses drugs or alcohol places the fetus at great risk. There may be defective neurological and physical development, as well as structural damage to the fetus.

A child growing up in a family where there is drug or alcohol abuse faces many potential hazards. Money spent to support the habit can cause economic hardships, while the child may be neglected or actually abused because of the parent's physical and emotional condition. Furthermore, legal difficulties due to substance abuse are frequent occurrences. Finally, the children may themselves use drugs or alcohol in their efforts to cope.

A case example illustrates what alcoholism does to the family of an adolescent (see page 324).

The Physically Ill Parent

If the ill parent is coping well with the illness and the family or others can help in those areas where the sick parent cannot function well, then the child will be able to handle the situation. If the sick parent can meet the child's basic needs for care, love, and security, the other parent or family members can provide the physical supportive measures the child needs.

The situation is different, however, if the child has to be the caretaker of the sick parent—the "parent's parent"—or is forced to assume familial responsibilities before he is mature enough to do so.

Although a parent may explain the illness in clear and simple terms, the child may harbor a deep fear that the parent may die or that he himself may contract the disease. Children also frequently believe that their "bad behavior" or angry feelings might have caused the illness. These feelings may be underscored by a distraught relative who tells the child that something he did has caused the illness.

Case History

Cheryl L. was a 15-year-old junior high student who was brought to the family mental health center by her mother. The school counselor had recommended she be brought because of her chronic truancy and resultant failing grades. Cheryl's mother contributed very little to the interview except for nervously smiling and agreeing to Cheryl's statements admitting her truancy and concern about her poor grades. Both Cheryl and Mrs. L. agreed that Cheryl could meet with the nurse therapist on a weekly basis. After several meetings during which Cheryl talked about her two older brothers and an older sister, she confided to the nurse that she had attempted to overdose on an over-the-counter drug for relief of premenstrual tension and that she had told her school counselor about it. This, in fact, was the true reason the counselor had referred her to the mental health center.

The therapist discussed with Cheryl the events leading up to this situation. Cheryl said worry about her grades, about skipping school, and about possible loss of her boyfriend had all contributed to the suicide attempt. She said that her boyfriend had been pressuring her into having sexual relations, and she was frightened because she felt she loved him but didn't want to become pregnant in high school as had her older sister. She had only sketchy information about contraception and feared seeking a contraceptive because her parents "would kill her" if they found out. She was fearful that her refusal to engage in sexual intercourse would make her lose her boyfriend.

In subsequent interviews, Cheryl finally revealed the "family secret." She related that her parents both drank a great deal and would come home around 1 or 2 A.M. nearly every night arguing and fighting. Frequently Cheryl's brothers, both in their 20s, who lived at home and also drank heavily, would join in the rowdyism, often becoming physically aggressive. Unable to sleep because of the noise, Cheryl would lie in bed shaking, with her ears covered. Not uncommonly, one of her parents would come into her room and drag Cheryl in to "referee." Sometimes Cheryl also intervened to protect her mother physically. Of course, no matter whose side she took, she was in trouble.

These fights occurred several times a week, so that Cheryl frequently overslept, was late for school, and often decided to skip school alto-

gether. And, when she did attend class, she often fell asleep. The family situation prompted Cheryl to reveal that she had considered becoming pregnant to get out of the house. Her older sister, to whom she was close, had tried to discourage Cheryl, but this sister lived on the opposite side of town and Cheryl could not spend much time with her.

Cheryl's treatment focused on problem solving in several areas. Living outside the home was not an option, so the nurse emphasized coping skills and supportive measures.

1. Initially, a contract was made between Cheryl and the nurse in which Cheryl promised that she would not attempt suicide again. Rather, when she felt pressure building, she would call the clinic. She did this one time, then contacted friends at school and Alateen members for support.

2. Mrs. L. was willing to come to the health center and meet with Cheryl and the nurse but Mr. L. and the two brothers were not. Mrs. L. confirmed Cheryl's account of the family fights, and expressed concern about Cheryl. Yet she held out little hope that the family situation would change.

3. Cheryl explored ways to avoid becoming physically or verbally involved in family conflicts.

4. Cheryl found an Alateen group in her neighborhood, and this group became her support system.

5. Cheryl arranged for a friend who attended school regularly to call her every morning so she would not oversleep. She made conscious efforts to avoid friends who chronically skipped school.

Cheryl's participation in therapy provided the support she needed and helped her to find alternative behaviors. In a single term she was able to bring her grades up, complete the breakup with her boyfriend, and begin to find friends who helped her stay in school. Her rise in self-esteem and sense of control was gradual, and suffered some setbacks, but Cheryl had the necessary strength to find more constructive ways of handling family problems that she was unable to resolve.

THE CHILD IN A SINGLE PARENT FAMILY

There has been an increase in the number of single parent families in the last decade. Hetherington (1980) estimates that 40 to 50 percent of children born in the 1970s will spend at least some time in a single parent home. On average, these parents remain single for 6 years.

Although death and abandonment contribute to the creation of single parent homes, divorce is by far the most common reason. Also, choice of parenthood by a single person, through either childbearing or adoption, is an alternative family life-style that has gained considerable acceptance by society.

The fact of single parenthood does not automatically create emotional disorders in a child, it does, however, carry greater potential risk simply because the stresses and responsibilities of parenthood are not shared with another adult. Guidubaldi and Perry (1984) found evidence that children of divorce enter school with significantly less social and academic competence than those from intact families, independent of the family's socioeconomic status.

The Child and Divorce

In 1973, over 1 million children lived in families that were involved in divorce action. Recently there has been a rise in the rate of remarriage, with attendant emotional pressure of adjustment to a new family (Jenkins, 1979).

The anxiety-charged atmosphere in a divorcing family has significant effects on the child's emotional well-being. In some families, husbands and wives, although facing dissolution of their marital relationship, may still be able to provide good parenting. Wallerstein and Kelly (1980) found that of the 60 divorcing families they studied, 16 were able to keep their parenting free from marital conflict. However, the emotional energy involved in divorcing makes parenting—another high energy task—very difficult. The children may be highly susceptible to emotional problems.

Jenkins (1979) discussed the following general issues of concern in divorce that have direct impact on a child:

Economic Problems and Child Support.
Economic changes may create many practical problems. Most divorced families experience a decline in their standard of living. Father may be paying child support and perhaps alimony, and maintaining two homes. Mother receiving this payment may be living on less than when the family was intact. Less money may mean relocation, with a resultant loss of friends, support, and recreational outlets and increased risks to personal safety (Hetherington, 1980).

The financial situation may cause the custodial parent (usually the mother) to return to work—another difficult adjustment, particularly for a young child. Child support may be late or nonexistent, thus placing greater strain on the single parent family.

Custody Issues and Court Involvement.
There has been much discussion in recent years about the best means of deciding custody. In most states the yardstick is the best interests of the child. Some researchers, however, believe that not enough criteria have been established upon which to base these decisions (Felner and Farber, 1980). They believe that financial resources, the child's age, and the child's own coping skills are important elements and that further research is needed.

Custody decisions can give rise to violent and bitter quarrels; in desperation the "losing" parent may kidnap the child. This can be especially frightening to a child, who may blame himself for the hostility. Joint custody is one means of maintaining two-parent involvement. The child lives part of the week with one parent and the remainder with the other. Greif (1979) studied 40 white, middle class, divorced fathers. In the families practicing joint custody there was more interaction between father and child, and fathers reported greater comfort in being with the child. Fathers who did not share custody often felt depressed following separation from their children and felt they had lost their parental role.

Emotional Problems and Therapeutic Intervention.
According to Hetherington (1980) feelings of anger, fear, depression, and guilt in children are due not to a single event but to a sequence of events occurring before, during, and after divorce. How a child responds to divorce differs from child to child (Table 17-3).

In their 1979 study, Wallerstein and Kelly found that after the first year following divorce, the preschool child was most vulnerable to stress caused by the divorce, while older children were less affected. Their study also indicated that whether or not the child would once again make normal developmental progress depended heavily

TABLE 17-3 Child's Reaction to Divorce

Temperament of Child	The difficult child may be less adaptable to the changes involved in divorce or the focus of anger by parents.
Cumulative stressors	Changes in housing; care, economic status, relocation, mom returning to work.
Sex differences	Boys were found to have more behavior problems of an aggressive, noncooperative nature, especially with mom. Boys were more likely to be exposed to parental battles and challenge inconsistencies and limits set by mother. Boys were found to receive less support and nurturance than female siblings from mom.
Home conflict	Children exposed to quarrels were often forced to choose sides. Conflict between parents often resulted in manipulation by the child. Single parent children functioned better than those in a conflict-ridden nuclear family.
Father absence	Continued involvement of father with children is helpful, especially with boys.
Support systems	Older children tended to seek support from peers. Low income families utilized more social service systems.

on how well his support system functioned. They also found that after 5 years, over half the children did not consider the divorced family an improvement over the predivorced family. However, in a 10-year follow-up of these families, Wallerstein (1984) found that children who were 2½ to 6 years at the time of the divorce were less burdened with memories of family unhappiness and marital conflict. These children had few conscious memories of the intact family, although most still spoke sorrowfully of their deprivation following the divorce. The children felt close to the custodial mother and appreciated her struggles on their behalf, yet many expressed yearning and concern for fathers who had been and remained troubled following the divorce.

In working with divorcing parents, the nurse needs to be aware of common issues of concern that change during the divorce process (Gardner, 1979). In the predivorce period, parents may wonder if they should stay together for the sake of the children. There is no conclusive evidence that an intact unhappy home is better than a divorced home. Parents should be advised to consider both positive and negative effects of the divorce on the children but this should not be the primary consideration. Another concern at this time is the critical age in the child. Some researchers believe that the preschool period is critical because this is when oedipal conflicts are resolved and sexual identification is accomplished. Others hold that the preadolescent stage is critical because this is the period when oedipal conflicts are again ex-

perienced, as well as the start of heterosexual relationships. There is no conclusive evidence that either time is the critical period. Gardner (1979) states that the earlier the child is deprived of healthy involvement with a parent, the greater the possibility that he will develop psychological symptoms.

Wallerstein's long-term studies seem to suggest that the younger the child at the time of divorce the easier it is for him to cope, provided he has a good support system. Westman (1983) points out that divorce demands a realignment of interpersonal and material relationships, regardless of the child's age. Divorce doesn't erase the past—parents are still parents and the child is still their child. He believes that working through a divorce is a lifelong matter for both parent and child.

At the time of separation parents are concerned about when and how to tell the children. Gardner (1979) advises that a child be given advance notice so he can work through his feelings before the parent departs. A young child, who cannot conceptualize the future, may be told a few days in advance and may not react until the separation has occurred. Parents should also be advised that many times children do not display reaction. This is not because of lack of concern; it is the use of denial.

It is best to be honest with children about the reasons for the separation, and ideally both parents should participate. This lessens the likelihood that one parent will be regarded as the villain, since in most cases both have contributed to the marital breakdown. A parent may be embarrassed to talk with the child about the divorce, and should be helped to overcome this fear. Intimate details of the parents' marital relationship need not be revealed. A simple explanation, such as, "Mommy and Daddy don't love each other anymore and can't live together, but we both still love you," reassures the child that despite parental conflict, he is still loved. Children should be encouraged to express their feelings, and crying should not be discouraged.

It is also helpful for parents to tell the child's teacher about the divorce so that the teacher can be prepared for the child's reactions. The teacher is a consistent figure at a time when home stability falters, and can be a source of comfort to the child.

After the divorce, the child should be allowed to ask questions and discuss the situation, visit the absent parent's new home if possible, and call that parent at will. Children need to review events several times, and may repeat their questions. They may exhibit anger at their own helplessness in changing the parents' decision, and parents may need help in handling their children's expressions of anger.

A child may fear to express anger toward the departed parent or the "at home" parent, feeling that one of them may abandon him. If his anger is repressed unhealthy behaviors may follow. The child should be able to spend time alone with each parent, and siblings should respect each others' time alone.

After a divorce, some unanticipated problems may develop.

Criticism. Parents are often advised not to criticize the former spouse. A child will not trust this situation; if the spouse was such an excellent person, why did the divorce occur? It is more realistic for the parent to be honest about his (her) feelings toward the other parent. Though it is detrimental to the child's welfare to constantly dwell on the parent's shortcomings, it is helpful for the child to learn that no one is "all good" or "all bad." If the divorce was bitter, or unwanted by one of the parties, then of course that parent will find it difficult to follow this advice.

Table 17-4, based on Wallerstein's (1983) research, lists psychological tasks of the child after the divorce. Recognizing these potential problems helps the nurse who works with the child.

Distancing. Children who do not hear from the absent parent, or are frequently disappointed by a parent who forgets about plans to see the child or claims to be too busy should not be reassured that the parent still loves them. As Gardner (1979) points out, such reassurance is confusing because it tells the child love is possible without any direct involvement or communication. Rather than trying to protect the child, who in any case will suspect the parent doesn't care, it is better to reassure the child that he *is* lovable and that he can be loved by other people. When a parent has only minimal involvement in the child's life the child learns that love is not automatic.

The noncustodial parent may, however, be experiencing emotional difficulties that could explain the absence. If the custodial parent is aware of the reason, he (she) can explain it to the child. Wallerstein and Kelly (1980) found that noncustodial fathers who were depressed or felt guilty about the divorce tended to limit their visits to the child. The father's role in the divorce decision and his eagerness to divorce or opposition to it were critical in regard to future visiting. The more control the father had in the decision the more likely he was to visit. If the mother encouraged visiting and the children took pleasure in it, fathers tended to visit more.

■ *Point of Emphasis*

Whether or not a parent visits, the child needs to be reassured of his own self-worth and lovableness.

Hostility. In the postdivorce period, continued hostility between the parents is a common cause of emotional problems in the child. Constant fighting and bickering—which involves parental contact even though negative—furthers the child's hope that the parents might reconsider. Children may often be used as scapegoats for the anger one parent feels toward the other, or may be pressured into choosing sides. The child may be used as a pawn to gain money or concessions, or used as a spy or informer.

■ *Point of Emphasis*

Negative interactions are destructive to the child's emotional well-being. Parents should be supported in efforts to avoid such interactions.

TABLE 17-4 *Psychological Tasks of the Child Following a Divorce*[a]

Task I	Acknowledging the reality of the marital rupture
Features	The child understands family and environmental change in a realistic way.
Obstacles	Child's fantasies and fears of abandonment by the parents or disaster
	Fears of being overwhelmed by painful feelings such as sorrow, anger, and rejection lead to the need for denial
	Use of fantasy to undo reality and reunite parents
	Diminished support from parents and other adults
	Failure to explain the events to children and prepare them for the future
Interventions	Elicit child's fears and fantasies through play, verbalization, or storytelling
	Talk about feelings children are likely to have when their parents divorce and that such feelings are acceptable
	Explain events simply in language appropriate to the child's level of development and prepare the child as much as possible for events that lie ahead
Usual Time Achieved	One year after parent's separation
Task II	Disengagement from parent's conflict and resumption of daily pursuits
Features	Takes pleasure in the school and play activities previously enjoyed
	Psychological distance from the adult developed
	Relative mastery of anxiety and depression surrounding the divorce; child could remove himself from the preoccupation with parental distress
Obstacles	Intense needs of one or both parents for nurturing from the child
	Inability to master anxiety leading to school problems, sexual acting out, or delinquency
Interventions	Recognize need for support and understanding
	Allay fears of rejection and abandonment
	Assist child to verbalize or play out fears and worries
Usual Time Achieved	1 to 1½ years following separation
Task III	Resolving the multiple losses
Features	Child's losses often include one parent, familiar routines, and traditions, the family, home, school, and neighborhood
	Most difficult task because of need to mourn many losses and overcome sense of rejection and powerlessness
Obstacles	Total loss of one parent's presence, or a parent's unreliability makes closure difficult
	Difficulty mastering a sense of being unloveable or unworthy
Interventions	Assist the child in mourning the losses he must encounter through verbalization or play
	Attempt to retain important rituals or traditions or discuss changing them together if they are too painful to reenact without the other parent
	Reassure the child of his self-worth and acceptability
Usual Time Achieved	Many years may be necessary
Task IV	Resolution of anger and self-blame
Features	Children may blame one or both parents for the divorce or blame themselves
	Anger toward parent or parents or self may be intense and long lasting
	Cooling of anger and forgiveness of the parents and/or the self seems to accompany the child's growing emotional maturity
	Child needs to forgive self for wishing for the divorce or for failing to reunite parents

TABLE 17-4 *(continued)*

Obstacles	Undiminished anger alienates the child from the parents
	Anger that correlates with acting out behavior, school problems, and low achievement
Interventions	Encourage expression of anger in appropriate ways such as art, physical activity, drama, play, or storytelling
	Assist the child to forgive himself by dispelling unrealistic beliefs that he was responsible or should have saved the family
Usual Time Achieved	Often, several years
Task V	Acceptance of the permanence of divorce
Features	The living presence of the parents often lends credence to the child's wish that the family be restored
	Acceptance seems more difficult for the younger child and for the child whose parent continued to long for the restoration of the marriage
Obstacles	The child's continued fantasies of reconciliation
	Actual situations where parents might discuss remarriage
Usual Time Achieved	Often lifelong process
Task VI	Achieving realistic hope for his own relationship
Features	Child must resolve issues so that he can have a realistic sense of his capacity to love or be loved
	Child must learn to take a chance on a loving relationship knowing it might fail but hoping it will flourish
	Adolescence provides a time for child to rework the crisis of divorce in conjunction with other tasks, such as who he is, what kind of person he wishes to be
Obstacles	Failure to adequately resolve five previous tasks
Interventions	Assisting in resolution of earlier tasks
	Supporting in efforts to maintain self-esteem and relationships with others
Usual Time Achieved	Lifetime process

ᵃ Based on Wallerstein (1983)

The Nurse's Role

Nurses can assist the single parent family in several ways (Wright and Leahey, 1984).

1. Give the family information on growth and development and the possible effects of the divorce on the child. Custodial fathers especially may lack experience and information about normal developmental stages.

2. Help the parents encourage the child to talk about the divorce and deal with his emotions.

3. Prepare the single parent for predictable stresses, both logistical and emotional. The logistics of day care, babysitters, and transportation may be met through community resources. Predictable emotional stress such as feelings of decreased self-esteem, depression, loneliness, anxiety, and helplessness should be discussed, then handled as they arise.

4. Encourage and assist the parent to mobilize a personal support system to help deal with the long-term affects of the divorce. Norbeck and Sheiner (1982) found that absence of a close friend and lack of people to call on for help contributed to problems of parenting. A woman friend, a male friend, or another mother was the support system for most single custodial mothers.

5. Promote involvement in community groups that focus on providing support for the single parent. Parents Without Partners, Displaced Homemakers, and others are the types of groups that welcome di-

vorced parents. Churches and temples often sponsor such activities.

6. Recognize symptomatic complaints that reflect the stress of the divorce. Often a parent or child reacts to the divorce by exhibiting physical stress that brings him to the health care system.

The Child Whose Parent Has Died

When a parent is facing death, priority is given to his (her) emotional needs; however, the child has great emotional needs, too. If the parent has accepted the fact of death, this should be discussed with the child at his level so that anticipatory mourning and desensitizing may begin (Gardner, 1979). If the dying parent practices denial, this should be respected, as it is difficult to inform the child about the parent's dying in this situation. Nevertheless, the child should be told, in a manner appropriate to his age, that the parent is very ill and may die.

If a child wishes to visit the dying parent and the parent agrees, this may help the child understand what is occurring. If the child does not wish to do so, he should not be forced. In the past, parents and grandparents died at home, and children saw this as a natural part of life. With modern technology, more often death occurs in hospitals, and this has enlarged the mystery of dying. Nowadays, the dying parent may remain at home, if the family so wishes.

If a parent meets an abrupt and unexpected death, as in suicide or a car crash, the child should be given a clear and simple explanation of the event along with reassurance that he was not the cause. Children often fantasize that death of a parent is punishment for their misdeeds or angry thoughts.

There is not complete agreement about the age when a child mourns, but this probably cannot occur until the child develops the capacity to understand the irreversibility of death—usually at age 7 or 8. These children still fantasize about death's reversibility, and may believe the death was due to their bad behavior or wishes. By age 10 or 11, most can conceptualize death and mourn the loss.

The nurse who cares for a dying parent can offer information about the child's probable reactions. She can help the surviving parent to reassure the child that his basic needs of food, shelter, and clothing will be met, and that the child is not ill and has a long life ahead (Gardner, 1979).

The parent should reassure the child that the parent is well and will take care of the child, to allay the child's fears that he may be abandoned.

The parent builds trust by expressing honest beliefs about the other parent's death, avoiding deep philosophical explanations. Whether or not the parent believes in an afterlife, the belief should be acknowledged. A child may attend the entire funeral service, or, if very young, part of it. This helps the child to understand what has happened.

Predictable and normal responses to a parent's death are summarized in Table 17-5. Recognizing the forms that a child's grieving might take and appreciating that mourning this loss is necessary if the child is to establish new family relationships increases the nurse's ability to help the child.

Elizur and Kaffman (1982) believe that bereaved children are extremely vulnerable to emotional problems. In their group of 25 children ages 2 to 10 who had lost their fathers, two-thirds manifested psychological problems and impaired functioning in several areas including family, school, and social. About half were very obviously dis-

TABLE 17-5 Child's Reaction to Death of a Parent

Emotional Responses	Behaviors
Grieving: a gradual release of feelings caused by loss	Clinging to photo or possession of the deceased parent; repeated questions and discussions of the death—to work through fantasies, stories and plays about death
Anger	Rough play Nightmares Demandingness and whining Expression of anger at surviving parent or others Wetting or soiling pants Hitting or biting
Identification with deceased parent	Adopts mannerisms and behavior of dead parent
Feelings of ambivalence existing before the parent's death and continuing	Criticizes substitute parent Idealizes dead parent Overaffectionate and dependent on substitute parent

turbed at 6, 18, and 42 months following the father's death.

Feelings and Behaviors of the Bereaved Child.

Feelings and behaviors that are marked or prolonged may indicate that the child is having difficulty grieving. Like divorce, death is a crisis situation with long-term consequences for the child. But, unlike divorce, the permanence of the parent's absence can eventually be resolved when the child is able to conceptualize death.

A bereaved child may develop a feeling of guilt. He may feel relieved that it was the parent rather then himself who died in an accident, then feel guilty. The child's natural egocentricity also contributes to a sense of guilt because he sees himself (unrealistically) as the cause of various events. The young child believes that thoughts and feelings can cause real situations; thus parental death may be seen as a direct outcome of the child's wishes. In turn, this may give rise to fears that the dead person will return to seek retribution.

The child also may feel anger toward the dead parent for "abandoning" him, then feel guilty because of it. Gardner (1979) recommends that the child be reassured that angry feelings are normal and do not cause harm. Giving the child specific information about the cause of the parent's death can alleviate these feelings.

If the parent committed suicide, there is an even greater likelihood of the child's feeling guilt. The parent who commits suicide probably had been depressed, and may have attributed his depression and ultimate suicide by saying to the children "You're driving me to an early grave," "You're driving me crazy," or "I'm going to end it all." Later the child may feel that it was his fault for not taking enough care of the parent. Often the surviving parent also experiences much guilt and the child senses this. Social responses, religious restrictions on services and burial, and police investigations intensify feelings of shame and guilt.

Some parents use the spirit of the deceased parent to engender guilt and control behavior. Statements such as "This would hurt your mother if she were alive," or "If your father could see you he'd be so ashamed" may control behavior but produce pathological guilt.

Guilt may evoke antisocial behavior, obsessive preoccupation, or proneness to accidents. Antisocial behavior may be the child's way of diminishing his guilt by being caught and punished.

Having more than the usual number of accidents may signal his attempt at self-punishment. His obsessive thoughts of unworthiness, and berating himself for any faults he may have or for misbehaving, may be his way of handling guilt.

Signals that a child is experiencing unusual difficulty mourning a parent's death are summarized in Table 17-6. The child who is unable to mourn, or does so inadequately, may experience emotional difficulty months, even years, later in life.

> ### ■ Point of Emphasis
>
> *The younger the child at the time of a parent's death the greater the possibility that psychological problems will develop. There is evidence that such psychiatric disorders as psychoses, antisocial behavior, alcoholism, and depression, as well as suicide, may have their roots in early parental loss.*

The nurse can help the bereaved child and family by intervening as with divorcing families (pp. 329–330). Group support, as well as family therapy are available for families who have lost a parent. The nurse who assesses the child's understanding of death can help the surviving parent explain the loss to the child.

The Choice Of Single Parenthood

In recent years changes in our society are reflected in the options now available to single persons. Whether male or female, singles can raise children. The single woman who chooses to have a biological child outside marriage, and the unmarried man who adopts a child or raises his biological child alone, are accepted by society.

Perhaps one reason for the changed attitude was the Vietnam War, in which thousands of young American men died (Teplitz, 1979), increasing the female to male ratio. Less restrictive attitudes toward children born out-of-wedlock, the feminist movement, and improved methods of contraception were also factors in the increase in single parenthood.

The single parent and the child may live alone or with friends or relatives who lend support in child care, provide adult relationships, and offer financial assistance. The single adult who wishes to adopt a child can do so provided that adequate care of the child can be assured. A great deal of

TABLE 17-6 Indications of Difficulty in Mourning Loss of Parent

Expected Defenses	Pathological Defenses	Contributing Factors
Denial	Denial continuing after funeral	Usually due to lack of information or discussion of the death
Suppression (conscious) Repression (unconscious)	No expression of feelings about the loss	Social values to "be brave" Need to "protect" the surviving parent Unrealistic guilt about causing the death
Depression	Self-destructive behavior (e.g., suicidal gestures, overeating, oversleeping, substance abuse) Loss of interest in school, friends, activities Apathy Acting-out behaviors (e.g., shoplifting, truancy, running away)	Denial of the loss by significant others Inability to grieve Lack of emotional support and adequate care Child's feeling that if he were not bad, the parent would not have died
Regression	Remains at developmental level at time of death or reverts to earlier level	Overprotection Increased responsibilities Inappropriate expectations for the child's age
Identification	Excessive morbid play Imitation of parent's terminal symptoms	Unresolved guilt No discussion about deceased parent to help child work through fantasies
Idealization	Unrealistic "glorified" ideas about the deceased Child develops unrealistic expectations for self	Idealization of the deceased parent by surviving

research needs to be done to determine differences in outcomes for the child reared in a single parent household.

THE CHILD IN A LESBIAN OR HOMOSEXUAL FAMILY

As acceptance of lesbian and homosexual life-styles increases, gay parents are electing to care for their children and often gain custody following divorce. It is estimated that in the United States 1.5 million lesbian mothers live with their children as a family unit.

A study comparing groups of single lesbian and single heterosexual mothers (Kirkpatrick and colleagues, 1981) indicated that there was little difference in maternal interests or child-rearing practices. It was noted, however, that lesbian mothers, more often than heterosexual mothers, shared living arrangements and child care with a lover. Children in the lesbian family tended to see the lover as a big sister, "aunt," or "second mother," rather than as a substitute father.

Hoeffer (1981) compared the influence of lesbian and heterosexual mothers on their children's sex role behavior (age 6 to 9). She found more similarities than differences, in that the children chose toys and activities based on peer influence, rather than on what the mothers might have chosen.

In his study of 18 gay fathers, Bozett (1981) found they frequently had social difficulties because their life-style was rejected by society at large and their fatherhood was rejected by the gay community. Those who found support for both roles in their social network were most likely to function effectively as fathers.

Though the influence of the lesbian or homosexual parent on the mental health and sex role identity of the child is a recent area of study, and much remains to be learned, it might be reasonable to hypothesize that the parent's self-esteem has a critical bearing on the child's well-being.

THE CHILD IN THE EXTENDED FAMILY

The traditional extended family represents one type of communal living except that the members are generally related by blood or marriage and may or may not live in the same household. Grandparents, aunts, uncles, and cousins still may share a household with a nuclear family unit, although this is not as prevalent as in the past. There are benefits in the extended family living: child care and household duties are shared, and where several generations live together, there may be economic benefits to all.

Multigenerational living gives the child opportunities to understand and experience a wide variety of people and different types of relationships. Conversely, conflicting values of the different generations, illness or incapacity of an older family member, or economic stress caused by the dependency of some members may strain the family system.

COMMUNAL FAMILY LIFE-STYLES

The communal family life-style is characterized by sharing of goals and responsibilities by a group of nonrelated individuals. Children generally are raised by adults for whom this is the assigned task. The amount of time the child spends with the biological parents depends on the philosophy of the particular commune. In some situations, children are raised by nonrelated adults from birth and only visited by their parents. In others, the child is cared for by the biological parents within the framwork of their role in the commune. Nurseries may provide child care by day, and the child may spend the night with his parents.

The child is subject to stress because of difference in values or child-rearing practices among the adults. Some writers are of the opinion that communal child rearing may impair the child's ability to form intimate relationships in later life, because of the lack of an early intimate relationship with one consistent caretaker.

If the values of the communal family conflict with those of society in general, this conflict will be communicated to the child, making his later adjustment to society difficult. He may experience a two-culture conflict, for example, when entering school and learning about the world outside the communal family (Eiduson, 1979). Intolerant attitudes toward the alternative family life-style by surrounding communities may also be stressful.

THE CHILD IN A STEPFAMILY

As a direct consequence of the rising divorce rate, a growing number of families find themselves becoming reformed, blended or stepfamilies. This can also occur through death of a parent and remarriage of the other. What is more often the case, however, is that the "new" family following divorce brings a host of relatives and siblings, a "yours, mine, and ours" situation. A child enters the new family with many fears and questions. Will the new parent take my other parent's place? Will they take all "my" parent's love away from me? Will mom or dad love the new sisters and brothers more than me? Will my stepfather (or stepmother) be mean to me and nice to their kids? What if no one loves me?

The child also faces a real or an imagined loss when the noncustodial parent remarries and establishes a new family. Depending on his age at the time of the remarriage, the child may eagerly accept the new parent, or resent him (her) as an "intruder" who is attempting to replace the "true" parent.

The marital relationship is even more important, if possible, in the reformed family. If the marriage is strong and consistent, agreed-upon discipline is maintained, and each partner trusts the other's sense of caring and fairness for all the children, the transition to the new family system and its development may be relatively smooth. Communication is, obviously, crucial between the parents, and between both parents and children.

Children frequently test their parents' consistency or favoritism toward themselves. They may try to pit the "true" parent against the stepparent to learn if their parent will oppose the stepparent, or because they hope to reunite their biological parents by causing marital discord in the new home. Parents need to understand that the child is seeking reassurance of their love and need to remain united in their approach to the child.

The parents in a stepfamily have two difficult challenges to face at once: adjusting to the new marriage, and learning to parent in the new situation (perhaps for the first time). The influence of ex-spouses and ex-relatives may also create pressures for the new family.

Visher and Visher (1979) list six major areas in which children and stepfamilies often need assistance.

1. *Dealing with loss.* Not only has the child lost a parent through death or divorce, but the child may also have lost friends and school through moving. The close bond forged with the custodial parent after divorce may lessen when the parent remarries—another loss.

2. *Loyalty conflicts.* Children are torn between their parents and often this is played upon by one parent. The child needs to relate to both parents.

3. *Feelings of belonging.* The change in siblings, space and personal belongings is a difficult adjustment. Visiting stepsiblings may disrupt the child's routine during their stay.

4. *Feelings of guilt and anger.* Children frequently feel guilty about the parents' divorce, about the death of a parent, and even about liking the stepparent. Anger may arise at a stepparent who attempts to set limits without first establishing a friendly relationship. The stepparent may also be the target of the child's displaced anger toward the biological parent.

5. *Knowing what is right.* People coming together as a stepfamily have various needs, values, and attitudes. It is unrealistic to expect a child to quickly adjust to new rules, surroundings, and expectations all at once. A stepfamily needs to create its own set of guidelines rather than attempt to force standards held by the former family upon each other. Discussion and negotiation are paramount in establishing the new family guidelines.

6. *Stepsiblings, half siblings, and adult stepchildren.* New relationships take time to develop in the stepfamily. The children should not be pressured to like each other. Parents in a stepfamily need to be told that jealousy among children is to be expected and may be seen in the children's competition for time, attention, and possessions. These are ways to gain the parent's love.

Often stepsiblings get along well with each other, but not with the stepparent. When a child is born into the stepfamily, it often unifies the stepsiblings (Duberman, 1973). However, a stepparent who had had no children may have a child in the new marriage and may feel less affection for the stepchildren.

Many families unrealistically expect deep affection among the siblings and themselves. While this is possible, getting along with each other is more realistic. Stepfamilies need education about changes to be expected in newly formed families.

Nurses who work with children and their families can help families identify the problems and be supportive of the stepfamilies.

THE CHILD IN A FOSTER FAMILY

Moreso today than in past years, children are placed in foster homes. This is because lawmakers and the general public are aware that not all parents are able to provide an environment that is favorable to a child's needs and development. The function of the foster family is to step in and give the child nurturance and protection when the biologic parents are unable to do so.

Foster families generally are reimbursed by the state for the cost of child care. They may be given special training. They may have access to support groups that teach them parenting skills and how to understand the special needs of their foster child, and provide a forum where parental concerns can be shared.

Foster parents vary widely in education, parenting skills, income levels, and motivation for this role. Most enjoy children, desire to provide loving care to the child, and eagerly learn how to best help their child.

A child is usually placed in a foster care home after a court has determined that the home of the biologic parents can no longer provide for him because of parental death, illness, desertion, neglect, or abuse, or because parents and child cannot live together in a normal relationship. A foster family may adopt a child if the biologic parents' rights are terminated or given up voluntarily. A child may live with a foster family on a temporary basis (e.g., during a family crisis) or for many years.

There are several stressors that are unique to the foster care setting and that the nurse needs to understand. First, there is a sense of impermanence that is intrinsic to the relationship and that may prevent both child and foster parents from forming a mutually satisfying attachment. Children who have had several separation experiences from parents, significant others, or previous foster families may view their most recent foster parents warily and avoid becoming attached to them, in efforts to avert a later painful separation. Foster parents need to be helped to understand the difficulties the child may have in forming attachments and must be prepared not to expect unreasonable expressions of affection. Second, though the foster parents know that they want to keep the child and can be trusted to care for him, the child who has had earlier unhappy experiences may not feel the foster adults are to be trusted or believed.

A third stress factor is created by the sense of ambivalence and divided loyalties a child may feel toward both the biologic parents and the foster parents. He may feel guilty because he loves his foster parents, and be confused about whom he really cares about. The situation is worsened should either set of parents attempt to gain the child's affections, particularly when the rights of the biologic parents have been suspended or terminated by the court. Separation from siblings also may be quite traumatic, since siblings tend to "parent" each other if the parents are unable to do so.

Stressors inherent in the foster care system also affect the child. These range from lack of screening and education of foster parents, inappropriate placement, multiple placement with different families, and legal and bureaucratic "red tape." Foster care systems generally are funded by state and federal agencies, and share the problems of many human service agencies—low pay, staff shortages, immense caseloads, and politics. All are detrimental to the child's psychological needs.

☐ *Stressors That Affect Mental Health*

The nurse who works with families in various settings is aware that certain stressors interfere with the child's ability to love, trust, and develop a positive self-image. The effects of poverty, racism, and sexism are summarized in Table 17-7. These social problems frequently form the basis for dysfunctional parenting, child neglect, deprivation, exploitation, abuse, and the rise in numbers of adolescent parents. Multiple separations and institutionalization of children, two more obstacles to a child's emotional growth, are often the results of dysfunctional parenting.

DYSFUNCTIONAL PARENTING

Neglect

How neglect affects a child's mental health depends on the individual child. Neglect is a "disorder of the parent-child relationship characterized by a primary failure of the parents to endow the child with personal value" (Galdstone, 1979). As Guyer (1982) points out, in attempting to define neglect, the community is actually seeking the establishment of "minimal thresholds of acceptable child rearing conduct and standards for the physical environment provided for children." He warns that the possibility of cultural relativity may cause a subjective, class-based preference for certain child-rearing practices.

Because our society includes a variety of cultures and mores, what constitutes neglect is a subjective evaluation. However, deliberate denial of food, shelter, and clothing is evidence of obvious neglect. Neglect of basic human needs, due to either lack of concern or inability to provide, has effects on learning, socialization, intelligence, and physical growth and development. Before the individual can experience the sense of belonging and self-actualization that are essential to mental health, basic physical needs must first be met.

Emotional neglect, although more subjective, is in some ways more traumatic than physical neglect. Who can survive without touching and

TABLE 17-7 Social Stressors Affecting Mental Health

Stressor	Actual or Potential Effect
Poverty: One in five children lives in poverty	Malnutrition, illness, learning problems, low self-esteem, depression, hopelessness, apathy, helplessness, ignorance, isolation, drug and alcohol abuse, psychosis
Racism: View that a person is inferior based upon race	For the victim: low self-esteem, sense of unworthiness, anger, depression For the child who learns to be racist: Displaced anger and hostility, displaced aggression, blames others for his own inadequacies, has problems living harmoniously with others
Sexism: View that a person is inferior based on sex	Low self-esteem, identity confusion, anger, depression, inhibition of expression of natural feelings Women seek psychiatric help more frequently than men, and are often hospitalized for psychiatric illness

being touched, holding and being held, cuddling and being cuddled? Many children, while physically cared for, do not receive the emotional nurturing essential for healthy self-esteem. In infancy, lack of touching and stimulation can cause failure to thrive. In older children, the absence of nurturance and affection can give rise to behaviors designed to elicit the needed affection. Some behaviors are healthy, others are unhealthy. If emotional needs are not met by the parents, many children turn to a relative, a neighbor or teacher, even an older sibling. A child may attempt to get needed attention by misbehaving, indiscriminately seeking affection, or by withdrawing into fantasy. The child who is "starved" for affection expends so much energy in having this need met that there is little left for other pursuits such as learning and social relationships. If a child receives little or no emotional interaction from a parent, including listening, touching, holding, and positive reinforcement, the child perceives himself as unlovable.

Deprivation

Galdstone (1979) defines deprivation as the "parent's valuation of the child as a nonhuman item." Since the child's humanity is denied, he is deprived of human interaction. The deprived child is treated in accordance with the misperception the parent or caretaker has about *what* the child is. The parent treats the child not as a biological being but as a "vehicle for an idea, agency for power, or item to employ in a practice" (Galdstone, 1979). The child may be subjected to rigid discipline or be given total freedom; may be forced to follow special diets or rituals; or may be treated like an animal. He may be physically confined to a closet or a cellar; there may be no safeguards to prevent injuries (e.g., the child will be burned to show him that fire is hot).

The parents of the deprived child are intense and possessive in their attachment to him, yet fail to recognize his human needs. They will oppose any attempt to remove the child from their custody when the inevitable results of deprivation— failure to develop physically and emotionally— occur. After 6 to 9 months, the child is behaving more bizarrely than the neglected child. Self-induced vomiting, incessant thumbsucking, and autistic behavior may develop (Galdstone).

Exploitation

The exploited child is used by the parents to fulfill or defend against unconscious desires that they

have not mastered. The child, although valued as a human being, compensates for parental defects and alleviates the parent's psychic conflict (Galdstone, 1979).

The child appears precociously mature, acting and speaking more like an adult. He may be aware that mom or dad depends too heavily upon him but may see this behavior as natural. The parent experiences extreme anxiety, has difficulty separating when the child begins preschool or is otherwise separated, and may take the child home. The parent is usually unaware that the child's development is being twisted to satisfy his or her own needs.

The child may be sexually exploited until he realizes that this does not happen in other families, and may develop symptoms that require medical attention. Exploitation generally does not receive attention from social agencies, because the affected children are not neglected or abused. Unless some unusual behavior is evident, and an outsider witnesses the parents' behavior, the child will not receive help.

The full impact of this exploitative relationship usually is observable in adolescence. Children whose parents have imposed unusual or rigid moral prohibitions will have difficulty distinguishing and satisfying their own desires. Because they have been severely inhibited, they are unable to care for themselves or relate to others. Other manifestations of exploitation, such as a parent who satisfies aggressive or sexual drives vicariously through the child, may be observed in adolescent antisocial behavior or sexual promiscuity. Psychosomatic complaints or self-destructive activities also appear in pre- or early adolescence because of the skewed relationship.

The nurse who works with the neglected or deprived child must be able to function without the reciprocal recognition response that usually develops in a relationship. The child who is neglected and has had no recognition has not learned how to give it back. A one-to-one, consistent relationship, characterized by a great deal of affection, is essential. The child should not be smothered with love, and may need small doses at first to avoid overstimulation. However, the nurse should be consistently available.

Abuse

Child abuse is a complex problem, caused by environmental and parental stess. In recent years, a great deal of research and literature has focused on child abuse, increasing public awareness of this problem. In 1968 mandatory reporting laws on child abuse were passed in the U.S, and in 1975 the United States Child Abuse Prevention and Treatment Act was passed (Smith and Pagan, 1979). This act prohibits physical or mental injury, sexual abuse, negligence, or maltreatment of a child under 18 years of age by the person responsible for his or her welfare.

In a study of 30 physically abused children (Kinard, 1982) it was found that the younger the child was during the period of abuse, the greater the evidence of emotional problems as measured by standard psychological tests. Ability to master aggression, to separate from the mother, and to develop a positive self-image was impaired. Severe verbal or physical abuse was related to tantrums, hyperactive behavior, aggressiveness, avoidance of peers, and bizarre behavior. The children who remained with the mother after the abuse was reported had greater problems with attachment and separation than did those who were placed in foster homes.

Intervention in cases of child abuse includes psychological counseling for both parent and child, and placing the child in a foster home. Family therapy appears to be the most effective treatment, focusing on improving family relationships.

ADOLESCENT PARENTS

The number of teenagers who become parents has risen dramatically in recent years. Adolescent pregnancy, affecting over 1 million teenage girls per year, is the major health problem of adolescence. These young mothers are at high risk for the development of toxemia. Their babies are more likely to be premature, to have physical anomalies, to be smaller than normal; and their mortality rate is more than twice the normal rate. They constitute the majority of very low birth weight (VLBW) infants, and tend to have a "difficult" temperament.

Both adolescent mothers and fathers most often are unmarried, school dropouts, runaways, and truants, and have histories of drug and alcohol abuse. Many adolescent mothers are victims of physical and sexual abuse or incest.

The high birth rate among adolescents in light of the wide availability of contraceptives reflects the immaturity of these youths as well as a lack of sex education.

Children of adolescent parents are an "at risk" group. As Schwartz (1979) discusses, they often have multiple caretakers, which makes for much greater difficulty in their ability to form trusting relationships. Each caretaker has individual expectations about the child and consequently develops a unique pattern of interaction with the child. The latter, confused and unsure of how to behave, may then misbehave, giving rise to anger and frustration in the parent, who may simply give up and let the child "run wild."

Schwartz (1979) points out that young parents have difficulty setting limits firmly and consistently because they have not achieved control of themselves. The adolescent parent may give up in sheer frustration and set no limits for the child, which creates greater anger in the parent and a great deal of insecurity in the child.

Elster and Panzarene (1983) reported that teenage fathers had few concerns about parenting because of the other problems brought on by the crisis of fatherhood—vocational, economic, and social. Secondly, adolescent parents tend to have inadequate impulse control, and, having the normal positive and negative feelings about their children, may express their negative feeling physically. Lack of understanding and education about a child's needs and behavior at various developmental stages may result in a belief that the bad behavior is deliberate, leading to harsh punishment of an infant who cries continuously because of a gassy stomach, or a toddler who is practicing autonomy by using the word "No!".

The direct relationship of adolescent parenting and emotional problems in children is clearly documented. Poor school performance, truancy, disruptive or withdrawn behavior, and legal difficulties characterize the majority of children raised by child-parents. A British study conducted over a period of 5 years compared the development of single children born to both younger and older mothers (Wadsworth, et al., 1984). The children born to younger mothers scored lower in tests of vocabulary and behavior than the other group. They were also more active and distractable and had less impulse control. These differences were attributed to the social immaturity of the younger mothers. Also, on the average, the children of younger mothers were smaller in stature and had a smaller head circumference.

Schwartz (1979) indicated that many adolescent mothers have histories of assaultive and violent behavior and themselves had single, adolescent parents. Thus a destructive cycle of troubled children and their child-parents has developed.

Aggressive and disruptive children, with a diminished ability to form personal relationships, are difficult to help in the mental health setting.

When the adolescent parent chooses to keep the child, as an ever-increasing number do, ethical issues such as the rights of the child to consistent loving care need to be examined. Individual rights of the parent must be balanced with rights of the child.

The nurse who works with adolescent parents must remember that parent and child are simultaneously going through significant developmental adjustments. Economic, educational, and vocational support and encouragement must be available to these parents, to interrupt the cycle of poor parenting and thus enhance the child's mental health.

MULTIPLE SEPARATIONS AND INSTITUTIONALIZATION

The key problem in multiple separations or institutionalization of children is the lack of a consistent, nurturing caretaker. The establishment of trust in the early years of life is critical, if the child is to develop healthy relationships. Moreover, the stimulation consistently provided by the caretaker is the impetus for the child's neurological and psychological growth. Multiple separations and institutionalization often go together. The institutionalized child usually experiences frequent separations, due to legal or bureaucratic maneuvers or to staff or caretaker changes. Multiple separations occur as well for the child who is sent from relative to relative, or who has only sporadic contact with his parents.

■ *Point of Emphasis*

When a child experiences the hurt, anger, and despair associated with frequent separation, he learns that attachment to others is painful and to be avoided. The price the child pays by avoiding significant relationships is the ability to have his needs for nurturance and love met. He learns to mistrust the world and the people in it.

The child may feel that it is dangerous to love or become attached to anyone because that person will abandon him, as have other significant people; normal dependency and the wish for nurturing and closeness are repressed and denied. As the child grows older and continues to avoid relationships his capacity to understand the feelings of others is also compromised. He may never be able to achieve deep meaningful relationships with others.

The child may also learn that negative behavior draws the attention of adults more readily than positive. Depending on his developmental level, he may believe that the reason people abandon him is because he is bad, worthless, and unlovable. Low self-esteem and shame is engendered. Negative behavior may be the child's unconscious attempt to punish his "bad self" and thus reinforce his sense that he is a "bad" person.

A case example illustrates how multiple separation affects a child (see page 339).

☐ *Assessment Of The Child*

Assessment of the child includes not only physical, emotional, and developmental information about the child, but about the family, the school and the social environment. Assessment focuses on the child's current functioning and is a basis for problem identification, intervention, and evaluation. Sample questions and statements are included to facilitate communication between the nurse and the family. Information may or may not be available in certain areas, and the nurse should ascertain where or from whom additional pertinent information might be obtained in order to develop an accurate assessment. Records of physical examinations, psychological tests, and educational evaluations can be released only with parental permission; they provide important information. Table 17-8 contains a general guide to assessing the child.

When a child is being interviewed it is helpful to have a playroom available. Since a child frequently is unable to place feelings into words, the playroom allows nonverbal expression of feelings through play. This part of the interview should be conducted with the child only. It is important to deal directly with the reason the child has been brought to see the nurse therapist. The child may or may not have a notion about what is happening and be eager or reluctant to share it. The nurse may say "It seems you've had several fights at school and your mother is worried about it. What do you think?"

Sometimes posing the question, "If you had three wishes, what would they be?" may reveal the child's concerns. It is essential to remember that the nurse, as a complete stranger, may elicit little verbal interaction from the child during the initial interview. On a nonverbal level, however,

Case Study

Jimmy, an 11-year-old boy, was brought to the child psychiatric inpatient unit by his grandparents. For the preceding several months, his behavior was marked by fighting, temper tantrums, annoying other children, and forms of aggressive behavior in school and at home. His grandparents finally felt unable to manage the behavior any longer and brought him to the unit. Jimmy had lived in no fewer than eight places. Abandoned by his mother at age 11 months, he was cared for by an aunt until age 3, after which he lived in three foster homes, then with his grandparents, then in a residential home for boys, and finally again with his grandparents. His mother's and father's whereabouts were not known. No one knew who his father was, and his grandparents did not know if his mother (their daughter) was still alive. The grandparents, although admitting they could not handle Jimmy and did not want to care for him, felt it was their moral duty to take responsibility for him. Although they expressed a desire that he "be straightened out," they rarely visited him and refused to participate in conferences with the staff.

Jimmy was a physically attractive child who quickly elicited friendly responses from the staff and could be very friendly and charming to staff and peers. However, whenever a staff member tried to form more than a superficial relationship, Jimmy's level of anxiety rose and he became so negative and aggressive he would often have to be isolated from the other children. The nursing staff felt very angry and frustrated toward both Jimmy and his grandparents—it seemed that their efforts were in vain.

In a care conference, several staff nurses and a student nurse who was working with Jimmy reviewed his history. They could understand how the loss of several significant adults made efforts at positive relationships not only painful for Jimmy but unfamiliar to him. Jimmy's experience had been that people he loved left him, and this must

have happened because he was not a good kid. His negative behavior was both a defense against forming attachment with its possible loss, and a way of unconsciously reinforcing his image of himself as unacceptable.

The staff described their feelings of frustration and became able to see that they had not accepted Jimmy's level of behavior. In their desire to make him "well" they wanted to show him that a positive relationship was possible in a very short time, even after his lifetime of loss. They then reassessed their goals in light of what they might realistically hope to achieve. Their new goals included:

1. Assigning one staff member to spend time each day with Jimmy even when his behavior was negative
2. Giving that person responsibility for meeting Jimmy's needs and requests every day
3. Ignoring negative behavior as much as possible, and acknowledging positive behavior
4. Trying to involve his grandparents by explaining how separation was affecting Jimmy, and explaining to them the meaning of his behavior

Jimmy's grandparents did not wish to have him return to their home; at the same time they would not relinquish custody. They also refused to become involved in his treatment. When Jimmy became aware of this situation and recognized that his grandparents did not want him to return to their home, his aggressive and negative behavior rose dramatically.

Unfortunately, the outcome of Jimmy's treatment was not positive. Although alternative placements were suggested, Jimmy's grandparents decided to bring him home though they were no better able to understand or deal with his behavior.

the child may express feelings in several ways, through mannerisms, playfulness or hesitancy, or guarded behavior.

PSYCHOLOGICAL ASPECTS OF CARE OF THE HOSPITALIZED CHILD

The nurse who cares for the child hospitalized because of physical illness cannot effectively provide

care without understanding certain psychological aspects of child development. These are outlined in Table 17-9. In addition, recognizing the impact of the child's illness on the family is critical to providing interventions that promote growth for both child and family. The pediatric nurse and the psychiatric nurse liaison can collaborate with other members of the health team to ensure that a holistic approach is followed in caring for the child.

TABLE 17-8 Assessment Guide

General Information: Informants—child, parents, and/or significant adult
- Child's name (and nickname)
- Birthdate
- Family name (if different)
- Family tree
  - Who lives in child's home?
  - Has child lived in other homes?
  - Relationship with family members
  - Significant people to child who live outside of the home

Presenting Problem: Informants—child, parents, and/or Significant Adult
- Child's view: Does he feel different or are things different in his life?
- Parent or adult's view: What brings them for help?
- Recent stressors in family
  - Death
  - Divorce/Remarriage
  - Birth of sibling/new stepsiblings
  - Physical or emotional illness of significant person
  - Moving
  - New job/loss of job for parent
  - New school, teacher, or grade for child

Child's Physical, Developmental, and Social History: Informants—Mother and/or Father
- Mother's prenatal, labor, and delivery and postpartum history
  - Pregnancy: planned/unplanned
  - Mother's physical health/complications: pregnancy through birth
  - Emotional stressors during pregnancy (e.g., divorce, death)
  - Family history of alcoholism, substance abuse, depression, psychosis, other mental disorders
- Developmental history: Informants—mother and/or father
  - Child's general temperament (easy, difficult, slow to warm)
  - Response to feeding
  - Sleeping patterns
  - Response to others
  - Attention span
  - Developmental milestones
    - Sat up
    - Turned over
    - Talked
    - Walked
    - Toilet trained: day/night

Social history: Informants—child, parents, or significant adult
- Educational assessment
  - Grade level
  - Relationships with teachers/peers
  - Attitude toward school
  - Formal educational assessment (from school)
- Recreational assessment
  - Favorite activities
  - Likes and dislikes
  - Use of drugs or alcohol (if applicable) how often? with whom? how much?
- Religious/ethnic/cultural assessment
  - Child and/or family's religious beliefs
  - Child and family's attitude toward their race or cultural group
- Economic assessment
  - Family income sources
  - Changes in income
- Child's strengths (talents, personality traits, skills)

Physical assessment (by nurse)
- General appearance (e.g., hair color, eye color)
- Height, weight
- Physical limitations or handicaps
- Bruises, cuts, abrasions (size and location)
- Dental condition
- Psychomotor status
- Recent medical history and physical should be available

Current Psychological and Developmental Status (done by nurse, based on observation and Erikson's tasks)
- Psychological status
  - Child's orientation to person, place, time as appropriate for age
  - Child's verbalization and communication with others
  - Child's nonverbal behavior/parent's nonverbal behavior with child
  - Child and family's communication and nonverbal interaction with each other
- Current developmental task expected for child's age
- Actual developmental level based on observation and history

TABLE 17-9 *Emotional Problems Arising from Hospitalization and Nursing Interventions*

Period	Features	Interventions
Infancy		
Anaclitic depression	At risk: Institutionalized premature or sick infants Withdrawal and apathy Lack of touch and stimulation delays normal neurological and emotional development	Consistent, loving care Tactile, visual, and auditory stimulation Limit overstimulation such as constant bright light and noises from machinery
Disturbance of bonding	Early, prolonged separation interferes with attachment-bonding Impairment of future human relationships	Involve parents in child's care Emphasize touching, holding, and talking Allay parents' fears of hurting a frail, ill child
Toddler		

Separation anxiety	Security threatened by absence of significant adult
	Parent does not "exist" if not visible at this age
	Three phases of anxiety:
	  Protest: screams, cries, clings, has tantrums
	  Despair-preoccupied with mother's return, remains vigilant
	  Detachment appears uninterested in the parent, as defense against painful feelings
		Prepare parents to regard this behavior as normal
		Allow liberal parental visits or overnight visits
		Consistent care by same nurse
		Do not feel inadequate if child cannot be consoled—only the parent can console child
		Reassure parents that detachment will decrease and responsiveness return with resumption of normal activities

Negativism	"No" is assertion of toddler's separateness from parent. Hospitalization limits opportunities to exercise control	Allow choices if any exist; do not offer choices if there are none Do not give long, reasoned explanations Prepare child by giving brief explanation immediately before each step of a procedure Expect dislike of painful procedures and strange environment Give praise and comfort after unpleasant procedures
Support of internal control	Control of behavior not completely internalized New environment tests immature coping skills	Develop familiar routine Bring familiar objects from home Provide consistent care Set limits on behavior in a firm, consistent manner Watch behavioral changes as early indicators of physical changes (e.g., restlessness, whining or excessive quietness)
Preschool and School Age		
Body image	Preschooler begins to see self as separate from parent and learns that his body can help him explore the world Devlops an understanding of sexuality Fears mutilation and body intrusion (blood "leaking out," or "folding up like a balloon")	Observe child's play and drawings Stories about "other children" may represent the child's fears Ask child why he thinks he's here Mention that children his age often fear something might happen to them Tell child simply what to expect and what body part is involved A child with global effects of illness needs help to express feelings of "ugliness" of "differentness" Provide wigs, caps, ribbons for hair loss Help child feel attractive (fix hair, paint fingernails)
Feelings of guilt and punishment	Hospitalization may be seen as punishment for wrongdoing or "bad" thoughts or feelings	Assure child that feelings, thoughts and behaviors have not caused the hospitalization Counsel parents to avoid using threats of injections or leaving the child in the hospital as a way to get him to cooperate

THE FAMILY OF THE HOSPITALIZED CHILD

A child's long-term hospitalization affects the entire family. Parents—the most critical element in the child's life—need to be supportive of the child so they can master the crisis. Nurses need to work with parents and other family members by including them as team members whose interest and cooperation are essential.

The Siblings

The siblings of the hospitalized child are greatly affected and the nurse needs to assist parents in dealing with several situations that may arise.

Jealousy. The parent's natural anxiety about the ill child and absence from the home may create anger and jealousy in other children. Parents should be counseled to accept a sibling's verbal expressions of anger. Providing time alone with the sibling will help the parent understand that child's feelings. However, an exhausted parent may have little time to spend. Caretakers may relieve the burden somewhat, though whether relatives or friends, they cannot entirely substitute for the parent.

Behavior Problems. In an attempt to get parental attention, many children will act out in negative ways. The parents should understand that this usually is a reaction to stress within the family; giving the children more attention will help.

Illness. The sibling may view illness as a means of getting attention; by feigning illness, he may gain his parents' undivided attention. The parents should recognize the child's underlying need for attention and offer it in healthy ways.

The Parents

Parents are perhaps the most critical element of a child's hospitalization. Their understanding and support often makes the difference between a severely traumatic event or a relatively minor crisis.

Nurses must work with parents by educating them and enlisting their cooperation. The nurse is not a parental substitute but a professional caregiver who includes parents as members of the health care team. However, parents differ in their ability and desire to care for the hospitalized child. The nurse should explain to the parents why they are asked to give care, and should offer instruction and assistance with procedures delegated to them. Feelings of inadequacy and anxiety may be interpreted by the nurse as "not caring."

Sometimes a distraught or angry parent may displace feelings of anxiety, guilt, or fear upon the nurse. The nurse should recognize that outbursts of criticism about the child's treatment or persistent questions often represent parental efforts to cope with stress, and should not be personalized. Rather, the nurse should recognize the underlying anxiety and try to relieve it as much as possible. Parents are not always objective about their children. The nurse may expect reasonableness in situations in which a parent finds it too difficult to be reasonable.

The Absent Or Uncooperative Parent. Absent or uncooperative parents often are a cause of anger and blame placing among staff. Why is the parent absent? Why does s(he) not cooperate? Job demands, heavy home responsibilities, inability to obtain child care, or lack of transportation may be the cause. The parent may be frightened and uncertain about how to behave.

☐ The Nurse's Self-Assessment

Before beginning to work with children and their families, the nurse should feel certain that she will not impose her own cultural and moral beliefs about child rearing upon others. The nurse may become aware of rescue feelings, in which she wishes to save the child from "uncaring" parents. Angry feelings, especially about a dying child, may accompany the sense of helplessness and hopelessness. The nurse may then find herself avoiding the child and family or engaging in superficial conversation or giving false reassurance.

■ Enrichment Activities

DISCUSSION QUESTIONS

1. Discuss various parenting styles.
2. Compare parenting beliefs of various social, cultural, and ethnic groups using your own culture as a springboard.
3. Discuss feelings nurses may have about the abusive or neglectful parent.

4. Discuss the impact of poverty, racism, and sexism on the child's self-esteem.

5. Explore the influence of self-esteem on behavior.

6. Discuss the composition of several families and the differences among them.

7. Discuss the influence of the federal government system upon the care and protection of children.

8. Assess the presenting developmental level of a hospitalized child and compare to expected levels for that age.

LEARNING ACTIVITIES

1. Observe a child at each developmental stage at play in a home, child care center, preschool, or school setting.

2. Tape-record and observe a one-hour interaction between a parent and a child. Note how the parent communicates with the child. Count the number of times the parent gives the child positive/negative verbal or nonverbal messages. Count the number of times the child gives the parent positive/ negative verbal or nonverbal feedback.

3. Tape-record a family meal in which two or more children are above three years of age. (1) Who speaks most often? (2) Who interrupts or is interrupted most often? (3) What is the topic of conversation? (4) What is the main style of parent communication with the child? (listening, giving direction, providing information, setting limits, suggesting topics of conversation).

4. Make arrangements to observe a class of a course in family life in a local junior or senior high school.

5. Do a mental health assessment of a child of any age and compare to expected development level. Plan and teach a unit on parenting of a specific age level.

6. Attend a community group meeting of parents who have abused their children.

7. Attend a community group meeting that teaches parenting skills (e.g., Parent, Toughlove).

8. Read and evaluate some books that focus on promoting mental health. Recommended: *About Dying,* S.B. Stein, *My* *Grandpa Died Today,* Joan Fassler, *The Boy with a Problem,* Joan Fassler, *Don't Worry Dear,* Joan Fassler, *I Have Feelings,* Terry Berger, *My Very Special Friend,* Lucille Hein, *That New Baby,* S.B. Stein, *All Alone with Daddy,* Joan Fassler, *One Little Girl,* Joan Fassler, *Grandpa Didn't Wave Back,* Rose Blue, *Making Babies,* S.B. Stein, *Billy and Our New Baby,* Helen S. Arnstein.

■ Recommended Readings

Fagin, C. *Nursing in child psychiatry.* St. Louis: Mosby Company, 1972. The first comprehensive look at the nurse's specialized role in the mental health care of children.

Fagin, C. *Readings in child and adolescent psychiatric nursing.* St. Louis: Mosby Company, 1974. A selection of readings pertinent to nursing in child adolescent psychiatric nursing.

Middleton, A., and Pothier, P. The nurse in child psychiatry: An overview, *The clinical nurse specialist,* Contemporary Nursing Series. New York: American Journal of Nursing Company, 1970; *Nursing outlook,* 18 (May 1970):52–56. Discusses the various roles that are part of the nurse's specialty in psychiatric mental health nursing.

Joint Commission on Child Mental Health. *Crisis in child mental health: Challenge for the 70's.* New York: Harper & Row, 1969. The report of the commission to investigate mental health needs of children in the United States. Although the report was issued some years ago, the problems in identifying children in need and providing care for them have intensified.

Pothier, P. *Mental health counseling with children.* Boston: Little, Brown & Co., 1976. Covers all aspects of mental health counseling with children. Developmental tasks, problems, and interventions are discussed. The nurse's therapeutic relationship with the child is examined. Treatment interventions in groups, individual counseling, and family counseling are all discussed.

Pothier, P. Developmental stages and interventions with children. In *Psychiatric nursing* (Kalkman, Marion and Davis, Anne, eds.). New York: McGraw-Hill, 1974. Discusses developmental tasks and expected behaviors. When there is interference in a child's development, the child may exhibit unhealthy behaviors. Identifying the problems and intervening to resolve them is the focus of the chapter.

Sahler, O.J. *The child and death.* St. Louis: Mosby Company, 1978. Deals with various aspects of death, the child's perception and understanding of death, the dying child, parents of the dying child, and staff reactions to a child's death.

■ *References*

Anthony, E.J. How children cope with a psychotic parent. In *Infant psychiatry: A new synthesis,* (Rexford, E.N., Sander, L.S., and Shapiro, T., eds.). New Haven and London: Yale University Press, 1976.

Bateman, B.D. Educational implications of minimal brain dysfunction. In *Children with learning problems: Readings in a developmental interaction approach.* (Sapir, S.G., and Nitzburg, A.C., eds.). New York: Brunner/Mazel, 1973.

Berlin, I.N. Secondary prevention. *Basic handbook of child psychiatry,* Vol. 4. New York: Basic Books, 1979.

Berlin, I.N. Tertiary prevention. *Basic handbook of child psychiatry,* Vol. 4. New York: Basic Books, 1979.

Berlin, I.N. The role of the school in early identification and prevention. *Basic handbook of child psychiatry,* Vol. 4. New York: Basic Books, 1979.

Berman, S. The psychodynamic aspects of behavior. *Basic handbook of child psychiatry,* Vol. 3. New York: Basic Books, 1979.

Bozett, F.W. Gay fathers: Evolution of gay father identity. *American journal of orthopsychiatry,* 51, 3 1981:552–559.

Chess, S. Development theory revisited. *Canadian journal of psychiatry,* 24, 1979:101–112.

Chess, S., and Thomas, A. Infant bonding: Mystique and reality. *American journal of orthopsychiatry,* 52, 1982:213–222.

Crisis in child mental health: Challenge for the 1970's. Joint Commission on Mental Health in Children, 1969.

Duberman, L. Step-kin relationships. *Journal of marriage and the family,* 35, 1973:283–292.

Eiduson, B.T. Alternative life styles. *Basic handbook in child psychiatry,* Vol. 4. New York: Basic Books, 1979.

Elizur, E., and Kaffman, M. Children's bereavement reactions following the death of the father II. *Journal of the American academy of child psychiatry,* 21, 1982:474–480.

Elster, A.B., and Panzarene, S. Teenage fathers: Stresses during gestation and early parenthood. *Clinical pediatrics,* 22, 1983:700–703.

Felner, F.D., and Farber, S.S. Social policy for child custody: A multidisciplinary framework. *American journal of orthopsychiatry,* 50, 1980:341–347.

Galdstone, R. Disorders of early parenthood: Neglect, deprivation, exploitation and abuse of little children. *Basic handbook of child psychiatry,* Vol. 2. New York: Basic Books, 1979.

Gardner, R.A. Death of a parent. *Basic handbook in child psychiatry,* Vol. 4. New York: Basic Books, 1979.

Gardner, R.A. Divorce. *Basic handbook in child psychiatry,* Vol. 4. New York: Basic Books, 1979.

Gardner, R.A. Marital Problems. *Basic handbook of child psychiatry,* Vol. 4. New York: Basic Books, 1979.

Greif, J.B. Fathers, children and joint custody. In *Annual progress in child psychiatry and child development.* (Chess, S., and Thomas, A., eds.). New York: Brunner/Mazel, 1979.

Guidubaldi, J., and Perry, J.D. Divorce, socioeconomic status, and children's cognitive-social competence at school entry. *American journal of orthopsychiatry,* 54, 1984:459–468.

Guyer, M. Child abuse and neglect statutes: Legal and clinical implications. *American journal of orthopsychiatry,* 52, 1982:73–81.

Hetherington, E.M. Divorce, a child's perspective. In *Annual progress in child psychiatry and child development.* (Chess, S., and Thomas, A., eds.). New York: Brunner/Mazel, 1980.

Hoeffer, B. Children's acquisition of sex role behavior in lesbian-mother families. *American journal of orthopsychiatry,* 51, 3, 1981:536–544.

Jenkins, S. Children of divorce. In *Annual progress in child psychiatry and child development.* (Chess, S., and Thomas, A., eds.). New York: Brunner/Mazel, 1979.

Kinard, E.M. Experiencing child abuse: Effects on emotional adjustment. *American journal of orthopsychiatry,* 52, 1982:82–91.

Kirkpatrick, M.; Smith, C.; and Roy, R. Lesbian mothers and their children: a comparative survey. *American journal of orthopsychiatry,* 51, 3, 1981:545–551.

Klaus, M.H., and Kennell, J.H. *Parent-infant bonding,* 2d ed. St Louis: Mosby Company, 1982.

Kornfein, M.; Weisner, T.S.; and Martin, J.C. Women into mothers: Experimental family lifestyles. In *Women into wives, Sage annual of women's policy studies,* Vol. 2. (Chapman, J.R., and Gates, M.J., eds.). Beverly Hills, Ca: Sage, 1977.

Langmeier, J., and Matejcek, Z. *Psychological deprivation in childhood.* St. Lucia, Australia: Queensland University Press, 1975.

Medoff-Cooper, B., and Schraeder, B.D. Developmental trends and behavioral styles in very low birth weight infants. *Nursing research,* 31, 1984:68–73.

Norbeck, J.S., and Sheiner, M. Sources of social support related to single parent function. *Research in nursing and health,* 5, 1982:3–12.

Orvaschel, H.; Sarnoff, M.; Schulinger, F.; and Rock, D. The children of psychiatrically disturbed parents: Differences as a function of the sex of the sick parent. *Archives of general psychiatry,* 36, 1979:691–695.

Orvaschel, H.; Weissman, M.M.; Padian N.; and Lowe T.L. Assessing psychopathology in children of psychiatrically disturbed parents. *Journal of the American Academy of Child Psychiatry,* 20, 1981:112–122.

Schwartz, B. Adolescent parents. *Basic handbook in child psychiatry,* Vol. 4. New York: Basic Books, 1979.

Smith, S., and Pagan, D. The battered young child. In *Modern perspectives in the psychiatry of infancy.* (Howells, J.G., ed.). New York: Brunner/Mazel, 1979.

Stockard, S. The child's concept of death. Manuscript. August 1975.

Teplitz, Z. Changes in morality and social behavior. *Basic handbook in child psychiatry,* Vol. 4. New York: Basic Books, 1979.

Thomas, A.; Chess, S.; and Birch, H.G. The origin of personality. *Scientific American* (August 1970):106–107.

Visher, J.S., and Visher, E.B. Stepfamilies and stepchildren. *Basic handbook in child psychiatry,* Vol.4. New York: Basic Books, 1979.

Wadsworth, J.; Taylor, B.; Osborn, A.; and Butler, N. Teenage mothering: Child development at five years. *Journal of child psychiatry and psychology,* 25, 1984:305–313.

Wallerstein, J.S. Children of divorce: A preliminary report of a ten year follow-up of young children. *American journal of orthopsychiatry,* 54, 1984:444–458.

Wallerstein, J.S. Children of divorce: Psychological tasks of the child. *American journal of orthopsychiatry,* 53, 1983:230–243.

Wallerstein, J.S., and Kelly, J.B. Divorce and children. *Basic handbook of child psychiatry,* Vol. 4. New York: Basic Books, 1979.

Wallerstein, J.S., and Kelly, J.B. Effects of divorce on visiting father-child relationships. *American journal of psychiatry,* 137, 1980:1534–1539.

Westman, J.C. The impact of divorce on teenagers. *Clinical pediatrics,* 22, 1983:692–697.

Wright, L., and Leahey, M. *Nurses and families: A guide to family assessment and intervention.* Philadelphia: F.A. Davis Co., 1984.

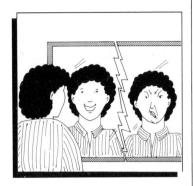

18

Adolescence

Mary Kunes-Connell

Learning Objectives

Upon completion of this chapter, the reader will be able to:

1. Define the concept of adolescence.

2. Describe the physical, emotional, interpersonal, cognitive, and moral development of the adolescent.

3. Identify the role of the nurse in primary prevention with adolescents.

4. Utilize the nursing process in assessing and planning for the needs of the adolescent at the primary level of prevention.

The term adolescence derives from the Latin term meaning "to grow up." However, for the person experiencing adolescence and for those who interact with adolescents, "to grow up" would appear to be an overly simplistic way of explaining the extensive physiological, emotional, and social restructuring that a person must undergo to successfully enter adulthood. The vagueness of this term and its meaning have prompted many persons to develop their own interpretations about this period. These interpretations have created confusion among nurses and other mental health professionals who take an active role in guiding the adolescent through this reconstructive period. Before growth and development and the nurse's role in facilitating it can be discussed the nurse must have a basic and functional definition that provides a framework for understanding adolescence. This definition will be derived from present viewpoints regarding adolescence and weaknesses inherent in these viewpoints.

One definition regards adolescence as a stage or period of development occurring between the **ages** of 12 and 18 (Erikson, 1968). This theorist believes that during this age span certain developmental tasks must be attained. This view of adolescence offers a guideline for placing the adolescent period into a useful perspective. A weakness with this definition, however, is that it is taken literally, and does not account for variation in age and maturity. The definition might foster the notion that no one under the age of 12 is biologically, emotionally, or socially prepared to face the tasks of adolescence. It may also suggest that puberty occurs magically at the age of 12 years. Rapidly advancing technology, changing social mores, advances in education, and higher standards of nutritional and medical care have brought about more rapid biopsychosocial growth in young people. Thus, a person of 9, 10, or 11 years may undergo the physical, cognitive, and emotional changes indicating entrance into adolescence. At the other end of the continuum, it is often believed that an individual 18 or older is legally classified as an adult and should have accomplished the tasks of adolescence. But this may not be true, as increasing numbers of 18- to 22-year-olds remain within the educational system and delay career choices, economic independence, marriage, and starting a family. Thus adolescence may be prolonged, with many tasks not being accomplished by the age of 18 years.

A second weakness in that definition is the idea that a particular task *must* be accomplished—a task that is usually different from, and more advanced than, the tasks of previous stages. It could imply that the tasks of earlier stages are never again reviewed or built upon. A workable definition must therefore be less narrowly defined in terms of age; and greater emphasis must be placed on the natural biological, emotional, cognitive, and social changes that occur between childhood and adulthood and the issues related to these changes.

A definition can be derived that will offer a general, yet comprehensive, understanding of the adolescent period. If she is to understand adolescence, the nurse needs to understand ego development. Successful passage through adolescence culminates in establishing an ego identity capable of relating in the adult world (Erikson, 1968). The concept of ego identity can be best understood by a view of the adolescent as an individual who is in constant interaction with his physical, psychological, and interpersonal environment and who, in order to successfully interact with this environment, needs to acquire a set of guidelines with which to orient himself. The ego or ego identity is, in essence, the set of guidelines by which the adolescent can realistically interpret, analyze, act on, and master this environment (Adams, 1976; Erikson, 1968; Loevinger, 1966).

According to this definition, the ego is basic to understanding human development, as the behaviors exhibited by an individual are the manifestations of his ego's attempt to respond to and solve the problems he experiences. Adolescence then can be defined as the sum total of the ego's response to the physiological, cognitive, and emotional demands placed on the developing person as he attempts to gain a clear sense of self, and to meet the challenge of adulthood. At the start of adolescence there are numerous changes, which are so profound and rapid that the person's ability to cope with them is taxed and his sense of self—

■ *Point of Emphasis*

A definition of adolescence should not be so narrow as to merely focus on a specific age range or a specific list of tasks to be accomplished. Rather, the definition should stress that adolescence is one of dynamic change from which issues evolve that must be confronted for successful entry into adulthood.

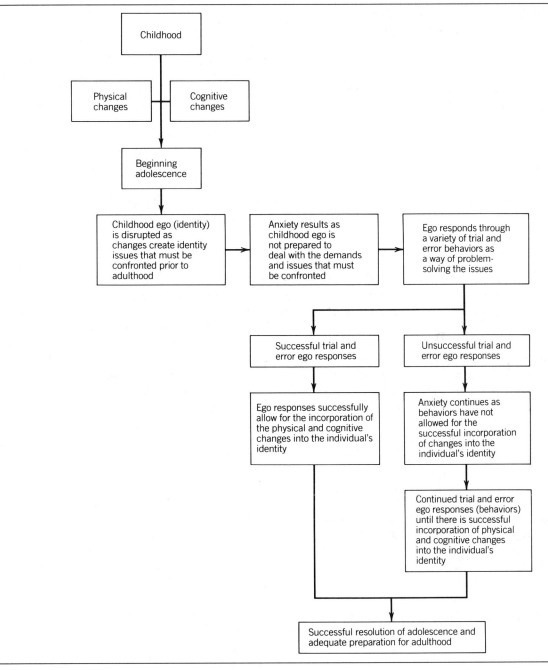

Figure 18-1 Dynamic process of healthy adolescent development.

self-understanding—is diminished. There is inner tension, as the ego is temporarily unable to assimilate the changes and integrate them in stable fashion. The ego responds to these demands by developing a number of behaviors that may appear strange and erratic; they are, nevertheless, a way to enable the person to advance to the next level of development—adulthood. Figure 18-

1 depicts this transition period between childhood and adulthood.

This chapter focuses on three elements: (1) the physical and cognitive changes that occur with adolescence; (2) the identity issues arising from these changes; and (3) the multifaceted role of the nurse in facilitating an adaptive response to these changes.

☐ *Theoretical Viewpoints on Adolescent Development and Identity Issues*

It is not always possible to alter physiological or cognitive development; however, the nurse is capable of facilitating positive responses to those changes provided she has a clear understanding of the changes and the identity issues that the adolescent faces in preparing for adulthood.

PHYSICAL-SEXUAL DEVELOPMENT

Though one's biological identity is determined prior to birth, sex role behaviors associated with biological identity become more firmly established during the adolescent years. Physical development peaks in the early years of adolescence and there are very few overt physical changes during the later adolescent years.

The early years of adolescence are marked by an increase in the release of the growth and gonadotropic hormones. This increase is responsible for the many changes in height and weight, production of the secondary sexual characteristics, and menarche in girls and ejaculation in boys.

The growth spurt occurs approximately 1 to 2 years earlier in girls than in boys. At about the age of 9 the girl begins to experience marked growth in height, peaking at approximately age 12. This growth slows and finally stops at age 15 or 16. These changes in boys do not usually occur until age 11. Peak growth occurs at about age 15, slows, and stops at age 18 or 19. Along with changes in height come changes in body proportions. In both boys and girls the head, the extremities, the hands, and the feet develop faster than the trunk. This gives the adolescent an awkward, lanky appearance.

Another change is the way body fat and muscle mass are distributed. Both boys and girls have a marked weight gain during the early adolescent years. The girl will gain 30 to 40 pounds over a 3- or 4-year period beginning at puberty. Girls gain weight earlier and have proportionately more fat than boys. In girls the fat is distributed primarily in the breasts, abdomen, and thighs. In boys the weight changes are more variable, ranging from 10 to 70 pounds over 2 to 4 years (Hurlock, 1973). Though the boy's weight gain is primarily due to an increase in muscle mass, there is some fat distribution in the abdomen and breasts; in fact the breasts may become a source

of temporary concern for the boy as he fears that he may develop female characteristics.

The secondary sexual characteristics also emerge during early adolescence. In girls the first visible sign of puberty is early breast development. This is followed by the growth of pubic hair. Axillary hair, and possibly facial (upper lip) hair begins to develop. The apocrine glands become active and the characteristic body odor begins to develop. The sebaceous glands also are more active; the facial pores enlarge, giving rise to characteristic "adolescent acne" and "greasy hair." Along with these external changes there are rapid internal changes culminating in menarche: the ovaries and uterus develop; the vaginal mucosa thickens; and a vaginal discharge appears. The girl may be unaware of these events before menarche. Initially the menstrual periods may be irregular, which can cause embarrassment to the teenage girl.

In boys the secondary sexual characteristics are initiated by enlargement of the testes and the scrotum, followed by penile growth. Pubic, axillary, and facial hair begins to appear. The apocrine and the sebaceous glands become increasingly active, and acne usually occurs. More apparent in boys than in girls is the voice change: Initially, the boy's voice becomes high-pitched, and it often cracks; finally the voice is lower and deeper. As in girls, there are coincident internal physical developments. Sperm is released with ejaculation. The boy's feelings and thoughts associated with ejaculation are similar to the girl's feelings and thoughts associated with menarche. The first ejaculation may take the form of a nocturnal emission ("wet dream"). The first ejaculations may not mean that the male is capable of reproduction as sperm may not be fully matured.

Issues Related to Physical-Sexual Changes

The physiological changes of adolescence bring with them issues of self-identity that must be addressed in order for the adolescent to develop a strong sense of self able to meet the challenges of adulthood. The adolescent is confronted with three main issues or tasks: (1) developing a positive body image and a positive attitude toward his emerging sexuality; (2) redefining one's self as independent from parents and siblings; and (3) redefining one's self and his role in relation to society's expectations.

Positive Sexual Body Image. The physical changes of adolescence create a need in the adolescent to alter the sense of physical identity. Body image becomes a source of deep concern, and the adolescent seems to be obsessed with his physical self. This preoccupation often is manifested as frequent complaints or vague pains—complaining that often labels the adolescent as a hypochondriac out to seek attention from others. However, these vague pains are often the consequence of actual organic changes and are completely real for the individual. The adolescent is also plagued with worries over his changing body. While the girl may express anxiety because she is taller and heavier, the boy is just as concerned over his smaller, thinner frame. He feels that he will "never catch up." The girl, on the other hand, fears that her "gigantic" stature will last forever and she may become an "old maid." Each is concerned about complexion and noticeable new body odor. Each constantly compares him/herself with peers. This comparison never seems to yield a positive or satisfactory response and the adolescent becomes vulnerable to mass media promotions about "beautiful people." Adolescents may spend considerable amounts of money and time on skin care and body products, and experiment with fad diets and clothing styles. It is not unusual for the adolescent to spend an inordinate length of time in the bathroom preparing for school or a date, to take two or three baths a day and change clothes just as often.

A more important issue for both sexes is the attitude toward menarche, ejaculation, and masturbation (Godenne, 1979; Hurlock, 1973; Lidz, 1976). Though all are natural aspects of development, their acceptance is often determined by the attitudes conveyed to the adolescent by significant others. No matter the content of instruction by formal sex education classes or by books—it is often overshadowed by the learned affective attitudes. If, for example, the parent or significant adult figure in the girl's life either avoids the topic of menstruation as a normal part of sexuality or sends her negative verbal or nonverbal messages about it, then she will be led to believe that menstruation is "dirty" or "unnatural." This may, in turn, lead to overall negative feelings about her body and her emerging sexuality. Boys often are taught nothing about the normalcy of nocturnal emissions and ejaculation. The unprovoked ejaculations may therefore be seen as foreign to the self and as a regression to the stage of autonomy versus shame when he was unable to control his body processes (Godenne, 1979). Unless he understands the physiology of ejaculation he will find this a period of time fraught with shame over his body.

Masturbation is another source of worry for both sexes. The negative attitudes surrounding masturbation are derived from two sources: (1) myths about the effects on the body, for example, blindness will follow, and (2) the moral codes of the culture, society, and religion. The act of masturbating places the adolescent in a dilemma. On the one hand, there is a need for an outlet to relieve the turbulent sexual feelings, and masturbation is a normal outlet for the release of this tension. On the other hand, this most often used tension reliever provokes guilt and shame because of parental and moral teaching (Godenne, 1979; Lidz, 1976). The need to seek immediate relief outweighs teaching, and guilt is aroused, accompanied by a belief that it is abnormal to have sexual thoughts and to masturbate.

Other emotional implications result from the changing body image. There are rapid mood swings and frequent fantasizing or daydreaming. Adolescents are known for their unpredictable and unprovoked mood changes, which seem to shift from minute to minute, and for being overly sensitive to the remarks of others. These shifts are partly due to the increase in hormone production and its release, and partly due to the adolescent's responding to others' view of his physical self. The adolescent makes quick responses to the verbal and nonverbal communication of others about his physical self. A compliment, either verbal or nonverbal, elicits a positive change in mood while a stare or a giggle may be perceived as an attack on the adolescent and may elicit a negative mood shift. These quick changes, if not understood, may mistakenly be regarded as the result of emotional disturbances.

The constant preoccupation with body and ideal image leads the adolescent to fantasize. Fantasy serves as a common sexual outlet that allows the release of the emerging sexual tensions in introspective hypothetical situations. The fantasizing lets the adolescent enter situations in which the desired self-image is affirmed. Some fantasizing is healthy—it protects the adolescent's inner self (ego) and facilitates the ability to cope with real-life changes that can upset both the physical and the emotional balance (Josselyn, 1971).

The adolescent's interpersonal relationships are an important vehicle by which he shapes the personality. Interpersonal relationships with significant others (both peers and significant adults) serve as a frame of reference by which the adolescent validates the self-image, and often serve to determine certain sex role behaviors. The young adolescent develops a concern about whether this ideal image can be maintained and whether it will be validated by others (Hurlock, 1973; Lidz, 1976; Newman and Newman, 1976). To validate this ideal self-image, the adolescent may develop a "crush" on a person or indulge in hero worship (Josselyn, 1971; Hurlock, 1973). The crush is directed toward an adult outside the family, and it marks one of the first breaks from family ties. The object of the crush may be a person known to the adolescent, such as a teacher or a coach, or it may be someone physically out of reach, such as an actor, or a rock star (Lidz, 1976). The adolescent chooses an idol based on the latter's ability to validate the adolescent's ideal self-image. Though the adolescent may not choose the object on the basis of sexual drives or instincts, the adolescent's behavior toward the idol, if known to the former, may be consciously or unconsciously sexually oriented (Josselyn, 1971). The emergence of an idol crush is of frequent concern to the family: until now the adolescent has tended to idealize the family and rely on the family members to gain an understanding of "male" and "female" and the associated behaviors; now much of the adolescent's conversation and action is imitative of those of the idealized figure. The family may perceive this as a breaking away from them and an abandonment of family values.

Developing a body image, whether positive or negative, requires a great deal of effort on the part of the adolescent. Childhood responses to the environment are no longer adequate, and the youth becomes increasingly introspective and sensitive to the environment. This introspection is necessary as the adolescent struggles to develop an ego strong enough to face the challenge of adulthood. Therefore, these responses, despite their unpredictability, should be accepted and understood as a necessary means to resolve the conflicts generated by a developing body.

Independent Identity. Adolescents must search for an identity independent of their identity within the family. With the acquisition of an adult physique the adolescent senses a need to put away childish thoughts, emotions, and actions and to behave more like an adult. To accomplish this task the adolescent feels a need to break away from or become independent of the family—the first step on the journey to adulthood. A physical breaking away from the family is not feasible now because this would require financial security that is not available to most adolescents. Because physical independence is not possible, the adolescent opts for a symbolic independence by emphasizing peer relationships over familial. Developing and maintaining peer relationships serves a threefold purpose: (1) attainment of an identity independent of that associated with belonging to a particular family group; (2) an outlet for the release of sexual tensions that cannot be expressed within the family; and (3) a vehicle of acceptance for feelings and behaviors that the adolescent thinks the family could not understand.

During the early adolescent years the teenager will break away from the family by gravitating to others of the same sex (Lidz, 1976). One possible explanation for same-sex orientation may be that the adolescent is uncomfortable with physical changes and does not want to risk rejection by the opposite sex. It must be remembered that the girl is now taller and heavier than the boy. Furthermore, other physical characteristics may not be fully developed, causing the adolescent to be ill at ease about his or her appearance in front of members of the opposite sex. Therefore the first step in developing a heterosexual relationship is to develop an accepting relationship with a member of the same sex. These developing relationships, though natural and positive steps on the road to future heterosexual relations, often bring about a fear that liking a member of the same sex is tantamount to being homosexual. This feeling can precipitate premature dating and sexual acting out as a way to ward off the strange sensations.

During the middle years of adolescence, heterosexual relationships emerge as the method by which the teenager continues to move away from the family. Heterosexual peer relationships can serve to release sexual tensions that the adolescent may feel the family cannot understand. These early relationships take place within a mixed group of boys and girls coming together for various activities. This group situation provides some safety from the still-threatening one-to-one relationship and allows the adolescent an opportunity to experiment with more adult behaviors and gain support and response from both sexes. This helps the youth to decide what behaviors are appropriate and should be incorporated into the self. In essence, the adolescent is attempting to establish and validate masculinity or femininity.

As s(he) becomes comfortable with the masculine or feminine identity as accepted by the group, the next step is to develop an opposite-sex relationship apart from the group (Lidz, 1976). With dating comes experimentation with sexual behaviors ranging from kissing and "necking" to sexual intercourse. It must be remembered that the sexual experimentation of the adolescent years may not always equate with a love relationship.

The development of an independent identity is far more complex and involves more than establishing relationships outside the family. However, these relationships are important to independence, because peer relationships provide an arena for developing and testing new sexual roles and behaviors that cannot be tested within the family. The peer group becomes the major source of support and means of validating the emerging sexual feelings. If this group were not available, the adolescent might remain inner-directed in thoughts and feeling and never successfully work through thoughts and feelings and incorporate them into the self. Furthermore, gravitating toward the peer group allows the adolescent to move beyond dependency on the family. This is a necessary step that helps prepare the adolescent to successfully meet the challenges of adulthood.

Sex Role Prescriptions. Sexuality also becomes important as the adolescent attempts to define his place in society. The adolescent must make a choice and feel comfortable with it—to accept the traditional roles that society assigns based on gender identity or to develop his own role regardless of society's expectations.

Sex role behaviors have undergone profound changes in recent years. Throughout history society has consistently reinforced certain behavioral characteristics according to sex. Traditionally, the man has been categorized as assertive, task oriented, and practical; the woman, as submissive, passive, emotional, and relationship oriented. Although this role assignment continues into the present day, it has been weakened by economics and education. No longer are role behaviors prescribed merely on the basis of sex; today the teen can choose from among various roles and behaviors. Dellas and Gaier (1975) define three roles available to women: (1) the traditional and conventional passive/dependent role; (2) the traditional male role of independence and achievement; and (3) a combination of the conventional female role with the less conventional male-oriented role.

The conventional role depicts the woman as a passive person whose basic goal is to develop and nurture a family and maintain a home. At the other extreme is the male-oriented role characterized by a striving for independence and a self-reliant career. Domestic activities are often postponed or sacrificed for the development of the career. The third role attempts to compromise between the conventional and the contemporary—the woman attempts to balance a career and need for independence and achievement with a family and a desire to nurture. She attempts to establish her competence in both the personal and the professional components of her life. She may experiment with a variety of roles during adolescent years and when asked what she will do when she is older, she may give a different reply each time.

Men may also choose from among alternatives. The man has as many choices as the woman, though he may have a more difficult time choosing. Society is generally accepting of the woman who has a career, yet frowns on the man who prefers nursing to a business career.

Though sex role identities and behaviors begin in childhood, it is during adolescence that the individual is faced with making some choices that may permanently affect ego identity. Adolescents must decide whether to finish high school, get married, go to college, find a permanent job, or do whatever it takes to determine the role that is to be adopted.

■ *Point of Emphasis*

Physiological changes occurring in the adolescent force him to confront the following issues: (1) developing a sexual body image that is ego syntonic, (2) establishing an identity apart from the identity associated with the family, and (3) developing sex role behaviors that are ego syntonic.

COGNITIVE DEVELOPMENT

Adolescent cognitive development is not as well understood as physical development because the changes in cognitive structure are not as rapid or as readily apparent as the physical changes. The adolescent is slowly moving away from the realm of the concrete into the realm of the abstract. He now begins to reflect on the unknown. No longer does he have to experience a situation in order to understand how he will respond now or in the future. Rather, he is able to hypothesize about the actions that could be performed, and the various consequences of these particular actions. This phenomenon is known as reality testing a situation (Mosey, 1970). The adolescent is now successfully able to recognize and appreciate that "If I do this . . . then this will happen."

■ Point of Emphasis

Even though a majority of adolescents will develop a level of cognitive abstraction, they will often use a combination of concrete and abstract abilities to problem-solve complex situations.

Changing cognitive patterns force the adolescent to confront further identity issues that must be resolved, or at least begin to be resolved, before meeting the challenges of adulthood. The main issue that faces the adolescent in the cognitive realm centers on his ability to construct a code of moral behavior that is ego syntonic (can be comfortably incorporated into his sense of self) while not coming into conflict with society's code of behavior.

Moral Code Of Behaviors

When the child or adolescent exhibits concrete thought patterns, he seems correspondingly to exhibit a concrete level of moral judgment and behavior. He blindly believes that (1) an act is bad only if he is punished (e.g., stealing is "wrong" only if he gets caught); (2) an act is good as long as it is not punished and, simultaneously, meets his own needs regardless of the needs of others (e.g., stealing is okay if no one finds out, even though he impinged on the rights of others); or (3) an act is right or wrong based solely upon the teachings of significant others (e.g., if a significant other says that stealing is wrong he unquestionably believes that the act is wrong).

Behavior of this stage is often impulsive, and consequences are not thought through. The adolescent does not possess the ability to analyze his behavior based on the internal "rightness" or "wrongness" of the act. Rather, he analyzes all behavior in light of the external controls placed on the behavior. His id (impulsive behavior) is being controlled by a strict superego (conscience) that dictates what is right or wrong behavior. This is because the adolescent is not yet sophisticated

enough for the ego to take over and analyze actions with regard to their effects on others in his environment.

As cognitive patterns mature so do levels of moral judgment. Ideally, adolescence should be a period of development when the ego becomes sufficiently strong to mediate between the young superego and the id. This mediation involves an analysis of the appropriateness of actions based not on the external consequences provoked by the actions, but on the action's effects on the self and others in the environment (Josselyn, 1971). Behaviors on the part of the adolescent and his adult significant others are consistently being critically analyzed by the adolescent. No longer is he content to behave in a particular fashion because the adult or because society says that he should act that way. Most adolescents believe that there needs to be a more valid reason for their actions.

Experimenting with drugs and experiencing sexual intercourse are areas of concern to the adolescent. He struggles between the verbal teachings of family and society about the "wrongness" of drug use and sexual experimentation and their nonverbal messages sanctioning these behaviors. For example, many parents preach the evils of drugs yet sometimes drink to excess. Society, through the mass media (e.g., soap operas), condones the use of drugs and sexual experimentation. Society also conveys messages about a "male" standard vs. a "female" standard (e.g., it is permissible for adolescent males to be sexually active, but not for adolescent females). These double messages make it difficult for the adolescent to develop a set of consistent guidelines that will help him to solve complex problems.

In his attempt to question the family's value system and establish his own independent code, the adolescent may blindly adopt the value system of his peer group. To be accepted by his peers, the adolescent often feels he must conform to their standards of behavior. There may be both positive and negative aspects to this: positive if the peer group's standards of behavior are congruent with expectations to respect the rights of others; negative when their behaviors do not respect the rights of others (e.g., gang behaviors).

It is hoped that ultimately the adolescent will transcend the level of behaving to gain approval or to avoid punishment to a level of respecting the right of others while promoting law and order (Mitchell, 1975b; Muuss, 1976). However, this will occur only when the struggle between peer group influence and parental influence creates enough inner tension that the adolescent must develop a code of behavior that decreases the tension. Most adolescents discover that a suitable compromise is to determine what effect their behavior has on others, which usually comes after a period of experimenting with certain behaviors and responses (Josselyn, 1971; Mitchell, 1975b).

Developing a code of morals is not easy for the adolescent as he must establish a set of behaviors that not only satisfactorily meets his own needs, but also respects the needs of other individuals and of society as a whole. He must realize that the principles he follows may not be suitable for others who live in different situations. Finally, the adolescent must realize that developing moral standards is not a one-time event, but a lifelong process of evaluation and change (Mitchell, 1975b).

□ *Nursing Process in Primary Prevention with Adolescents*

Though the changes that occur during adolescence are normal and to be expected, the adolescent himself often is not aware of this fact. Thus he may develop an undue anxiety that is incapacitating and that affects his ability to effectively deal with these changes. The nurse becomes involved in primary prevention with adolescents to prevent this immobilization before a full-blown emotional disorder arises.

The nursing goals in primary prevention are to promote a sense of well-being in the adolescent and to avoid an emotional disorder by: (1) helping the adolescent and his significant others to understand the normal developmental processes of adolescence; (2) fostering the development of adaptive problem-solving skills; and (3) removing barriers to healthy development (e.g., parental confusion about "what teens want and need," which can lead to over- or undercontrol).

To accomplish these goals the nurse must have a thorough understanding of the anxiety-provoking physical and cognitive changes of adolescence. And she must have a working knowledge of nursing process in relation to the potential needs and problems facing the adolescent.

The potential of the nursing process in primary prevention may be overlooked if the health professional believes that the sole purpose of primary prevention in adolescence is merely to teach *all* aspects of normal growth and development to *all* adolescents regardless of the needs of the particular adolescent population with which she is dealing. This attitude does not allow for focused teaching and consultation (e.g., adolescent girls may require a different teaching focus than adolescent boys).

ASSESSMENT □ If the goal of nursing care is to provide comprehensive yet individualized services, a thorough evaluation must be performed, emphasizing: (1) a thorough physical and psychosocial assessment of the adolescent with a focus on the identification of probable areas of need; (2) a self-assessment on the part of the nurse; and (3) an environmental assessment focusing on the various environments with which the adolescent interacts (e.g., home, school, leisure facilities).

Client Assessment □ The nurse must assess the physical and psychosocial status of even a healthy adolescent in order to determine if there exist potential areas of need that should be addressed. A workable framework to guide the nurse is Maslow's hierarchy of basic human needs. This framework affords the nurse a holistic view of the adolescent. Table 18-1 presents a framework for the nurse's assessment.

It must be remembered that most adolescents are hyperresistive and may fear intrusion into their world. Therefore, the assessment interview should follow accepted principles of communication:

1. Show that you respect the adolescent by introducing yourself and describing the purpose of the interview.
2. Avoid beginning an interview with intrusive or probing questions. Begin by showing interest in the adolescent as an individual discussing hobbies, interests, likes, dislikes.
3. Avoid a patronizing attitude such as "talking down" to the adolescent, or speaking about him (using third person) with his family, when he is present.
4. Avoid biased or leading statements that would compel the adolescent to respond to what he thinks you want to hear. These types of questions also stifle the adolescent's ability to discuss openly his thoughts and feelings. "You haven't been sexually active, have you?" is an example. More appropriate would be "Tell me about . . ." statements.

TABLE 18-1 Nursing Assessment of the Adolescent[a]

Basic Human Need	Interview Questions	Physical Assessment

Oxygenation	1. Questions may focus on allergies:
	  (a) Have you experienced any allergy difficulties?
	  (b) If so, to what are you allergic?
	  (c) What symptoms do you experience due to your allergies?
	  (d) Do these allergies affect your activities of daily living?
	2. Questions may focus on smoking patterns:
	  (a) Do you smoke?
	  (b) If so, how long have you been smoking?
	  (c) How many cigarettes do you smoke per day?
		1. Baseline vital signs: All should be within adult ranges.
		2. Laboratory tests: CBC with special emphasis on HGB, HCT, RBC (due to the nutritional intake of the adolescent, for example, erratic meals, junk food (often the adolescent misses the iron and vitamins needed for development of blood cells, resulting in anemia). Also, the adolescent female experiencing menstruation may develop anemia due to loss of iron and blood.

Fluid and electrolyte balance and nutrition	1. Questions should revolve around normal nutrition patterns:
	  (a) Identify dietary habits through a 24-hour recall. (A 24-hour recall identifies daily eating habits and gives the nurse a picture of the adolescent's daily caloric intake and protein intake.
	  (b) Identify your favorite foods.
	2. Identify patterns of weight loss and weight gain.
	  (a) Have you ever attempted to lose/gain weight?
	  (b) If you have lost/gained weight, how much was lost or gained? How long did it take to lose or gain?
	  (c) What kinds of diets have you tried?
	  (d) Have you taken any medications to facilitate the loss or gain?
	  (e) What other methods besides dieting have you used to lose weight (e.g., vomiting, fasting, over-the-counter diet aids)?
		1. Determine height and weight.
		2. Determine muscular strength and tone (muscular strength and tone may be indicative of protein intake). Adolescents require adequate protein because of muscle growth.
		3. Laboratory tests:
		  (a) Blood chemistry: be aware of levels of Ca^{++} and alkaline phosphatase (alkaline phosphatase may be above normal limits)—important in understanding normal bone development in adolescents
		  (b) CBC (review under oxygenation)
		  (c) Urinalysis (may be of significance if there is reason to believe that protein levels may be abnormal, e.g., excessive tissue breakdown)

Rest and sleep	Tell me about your sleeping habits. 1. Approximately how many hours of sleep do you require per night? 2. Do you take naps? 3. Are there times when you feel tired even when you have not been active.	
Mobility and exercise	1. Describe a day's activities. 2. What types of sports/exercise do you become involved in? 3. How often do you participate in exercise/sports per week? 4. Do you have any handicaps that prevent you from taking part in activities?	1. Check posture for signs of slumping. 2. Bend-over test to indicate spine curvature (scoliosis is common in adolescence and may affect self-esteem).
Sensory awareness	People take drugs or alcohol for a wide variety of reasons—some take drugs because it makes them feel better, others because it relieves stresses that they feel at school/home, others because it gives them a different physical sensation. 1. Have you ever used or do you now use drugs or alcohol?	

TABLE 18-1 (continued)

Basic Human Need	Interview Questions	Physical Assessment
	2. If so, which ones? 3. How often do you use drugs? 4. Are there certain days or times that you feel a strong urge to use drugs? 5. What physical changes do you experience when you use drugs? 6. Do you continue to experience changes after you've "come off" this drug?	

Sexual reproduction	1. Both sexes: It is normal for adolescents to have concerns about their sexuality as they are experiencing sexual changes.
	  (a) What concerns are you experiencing at this time? (Appropriate question either in this category or under self-esteem. This question may also serve to bring out any myths a girl might have, e.g., one can get pregnant by swimming in the same pool as a male).
	  (b) Tell me what you know/understand about the physical sexual changes that you are experiencing at the present time (gives the nurse a clue about the client's sexual knowledge).
	  (c) As the adolescent grows, he often experiments with varying forms of sexual activity. Are you sexually active? In what ways?
	  (d) What resources have you used to learn about sex/sexual functioning?
	2. Females
	  (a) Have you started to menstruate?
	  (b) When did you have your first period?
	  (c) Describe your cycle of periods (e.g., length of time between periods, amount of bleeding, physical sensations associated with your periods).
	  (d) If you have pain or bloating, do you take any medications to alleviate the feelings?
	  (e) If you are sexually active, are you concerned about becoming pregnant? What do you know about contraception (birth control)? Do you use any form of birth control?
	3. Males:
	  (a) Many young males experience the normal occurrence of a "wet dream" (may need to define this). Do you understand what a wet dream is? (Have him describe.) Have you ever experienced a wet dream?
	  (b) What changes do you notice about yourself (physically/emotionally) as you are growing? (Good question to check out awareness of body)
	  (c) How do you see your role/responsibility in sexual relationships?
		1. Physical examination:
		  (a) Breast examination to determine breast development
		  (b) Examine patterns of pubic/axillary/facial hair
		  (c) Examine testicular development
		2. Laboratory values: Gravindex
		3. Assess verbal and nonverbal behaviors that indicate level of comfort of the client when discussing his body, for example, eye contact, body movements, hesitant verbal responses

TABLE 18-1 (continued)

Basic Human Need	Interview Questions	Physical Assessment
Self-esteem	1. Tell me how you would describe your physically? 2. What would you describe as you best physical feature? 3. If there were one feature that you would change, what would it be? 4. Describe your "ideal self"; we often daydream about what we would like to look like or like to do when we get older. What kinds of daydreams do you have about yourself? 5. Finish the following sentences for me: "The best thing about being a teenager is . . . ." "The worst thing about being a teenager is . . . ." 6. What does it mean to you when someone tells you to act "feminine/masculine"? (How would you define femininity/masculinity?)	1. Describe the individual's physical attributes, for example, complexion, makeup, hairstyle, dress, weight (general appearance often affects self-esteem or may be indicative of how a person feels about himself). 2. Identify verbal and nonverbal behavior that indicates esteem levels, for example, eye contact, tone of voice, hesitancy in giving answers, self-derogatory remarks.

Love and belonging	1. Family
	  (a) Who makes up your family? Describe the members of your family.
	  (b) Has your relationship with any members of your family changed since you have become a teenager? In what way has this relationship changed?
	  (c) Describe your relationship with your individual family members
	  (d) How would you define "closeness"? Do you feel close to anyone in your family? If so to whom?
	2. Peers:
	  (a) What is a friend? (or What is important in friendship?)
	  (b) When you describe friendship in this way, tell me about the individuals whom you call your friends.
	  (c) Are most of your friends male or female?
	  (d) Are most of your friends younger or older than you, or the same age?
	  (e) When you get together with your friends, what kinds of things do you do?
	  (f) How do you respond when your friends do something that you consider wrong or that you don't want to do? (Or have him finish the following sentence, "When my friends do something I don't want to do, I. . . .") The above question not only looks at peer pressure, but views the developing moral code.
		If the family is present, identify the communication dynamics between the family members.

ᵃ Note that many aspects of the physical assessment may be performed by or ordered by the physician. However, it is the responsibility of the nurse to have a knowledge of the results in planning care.

5. The adolescent should be helped to feel that the thoughts, feelings, and situations he is experiencing are normal for his age group. Rather than asking "Do you daydream?" it might be better to say "Often, as an adolescent grows up, he naturally daydreams about how he will look or what he will do in the future. Can you tell me about some of your daydreams?"

6. Avoid moralizing. The adolescent will not be open with you if he senses that his every statement will be judged.

7. Above all, listen carefully. Don't interrupt. Don't assume you know what he is about to say and finish the sentence for him. Adolescents often complain that "no one listens."

Self-Assessment □ Adolescents often engender powerful feelings in nurses who must interact with them on a daily basis. These feelings can be positive if they enhance the nurse's ability to intervene or negative if they inhibit effective intervention. Anger, frustration, and rejection are commonly felt.

Frustration and anger often go hand in hand. Nurses experience frustration when they set unrealistically high expectations. This can happen if the nurse has not resolved her expectations of herself. She may want the adolescent to become what she herself could never become. As a result her attitude may convey "I know what's best since I've been through it myself." This attitude is reflected to the adolescent in unrealistic expectations that he rebels against as he tries to establish his independence. The nurse fails to see the adolescent as an individual in his own right with his own set of needs and reactions to these needs; she views him only as an individual who may have experienced what she had earlier experienced and who could benefit by her wisdom. She feels frustrated and angry.

Because adolescents behave impulsively, they will often speak or act in haste. Repeatedly, the adolescent may be unable to express his thoughts and feelings in appropriate fashion. Therefore, rather than sending a clear verbal message, for example, "I'm upset with my parents' decision to ground me," he may verbalize this concern by saying "You (the nurses or doctors) can't help me— I don't want to talk to you." The adolescent can also express his frustrations in other ways (e.g., the "silent treatment" or rebellion). These negative verbal and nonverbal messages are often perceived as rejection by the nurse, and she will tend to avoid, rather than explore, the feelings and thoughts that prompted the negative behavior.

The nurse who desires to increase her ability to work with the adolescent must analyze her own thoughts and feelings about the adolescent experience, through a thorough exploration of her past experience, value system, and the value judgments that may have been attached to the adolescent experience. The nurse should ask herself the following questions:

1. When I think of the term "adolescence," what thoughts, feelings, and attitudes immediately enter my mind? Which of them are positive and would serve to enhance my ability to function effectively with adolescents? Which of them are negative and would serve to inhibit my ability to function effectively with adolescents?

2. Do I identify (or tend to overidentify) with particular aspects of an adolescent's growth and development? Do I relate to any particular aspects of adolescent growth and development? Are there any aspects of my own adolescence that are difficult to relive? If so, why? What did I do to resolve these difficulties? Will these difficult aspects of my adolescence affect my ability to work effectively with adolescents? Are there aspects of my adolescence that will enhance my ability to intervene with the adolescent population?

3. What are my expectations of adolescents? Are my expectations realistic in regard to a particular adolescent's present level of development? What are my beliefs about sexuality, education, drug use, and religion? What value judgments do I make about adolescents? Do I attempt or have I in the past attempted to impose my own value system on someone younger than myself?

4. Are there any particular subject areas that I find uncomfortable to discuss, such as sexuality, drugs, death/suicide?

5. If I were to take a close look at my overall communication skills, I would describe my communication patterns as: patronizing, supportive, confrontive, facilitative, flexible depending upon the situation.

6. Are there any changes in communication patterns that I must make when working with adolescents?
7. Overall, what strengths do I bring with me when working with adolescents?
8. What weaknesses must I strengthen if I am to work effectively with adolescents?

Environmental Assessment □ To gain a comprehensive picture of the adolescent, the nurse must assess the various environments in which he functions on a daily basis. The environments of home, school, and leisure are those the nurse may want to explore with the adolescent and his significant others.

Home

Family Structure

1. "Who makes up the family in this household?" The answer identifies the family situation the nurse is to work with (e.g., nuclear family, extended family, nontraditional family).
2. "Who makes the decisions in the family?" This question could be further delineated by asking "Who makes the rules in the family?" It is important to identify the process of decision making in the home, especially as the adolescent becomes more responsible and capable of making decisions.
3. "On an average day approximately how much time does the family spend together?" "Is there any special time set aside each day for the family to be together?" "What activities do the family do together?" These questions are designed to determine the actual personal contact time that exists among family members.
4. "Does each family member have a place within the house where he can go to enjoy privacy?" This question has importance as an adolescent often seeks solitude.
5. Describe ways in which your family demonstrates their respect or lack of respect for you?
6. Describe ways that your family allows you to take control over situations?
7. Do you think that your parents trust you? How do your parents show their trust or mistrust?

Questions 5 and 6 are designed to evaluate the family "climate," that is their attitudes of respect and caring vs. attitudes of control, punishment, or disinterest. These questions should be addressed to the adolescent as well as to the family members.

Household Organization

1. What are the duties of each family member that keep the household functioning effectively? This question serves a twofold purpose: it assesses the adolescent's perception of adult obligations and it provides clues to determining how much responsibility is given to the adolescent.
2. What are the general rules of the household?
3. Are there different rules for different children? (If so, describe these rules).
4. Are the rules adhered to at all times and in all situations? (If not, when are they not followed?)
5. How does the family discipline the children?
6. Who is the main disciplinarian within the family, or is discipline shared?

School

Structure

1. What type of school does the adolescent attend? (Elementary, junior high, senior high, special education, parochial, or public). This question helps the nurse understand the school's philosophy.
2. How many students attend?
3. What is the disciplinary code of the school? Determine if the adolescent and his significant others perceive that code as fair.

Activities

1. Please describe a typical day spent in school.
2. Can you describe your extracurricular activities?
3. Tell me about your accomplishments in school.
4. Are there any parent organizations related to the school? If so, determine the level of

parental involvement in these organizations.

5. Have you ever had to transfer from one school to another? What was the reason? How did this affect your school work and your friendships?

Leisure

1. Tell me about your leisure activities and where they take place.
2. How do your parents feel about these activities?
3. Can you tell me how much time and money you devote each week to these acitivities?
4. Do you have a job? How many hours do you work per day or per week?

PROBLEM/NEED IDENTIFICATION □ Following the assessment, the focus of primary prevention is not on the identification of existing problems but rather on the identification of areas of potential problems. If these areas of need are dealt with, the nurse may be able to prevent undue stress and resulting emotional difficulties. Even when assessing a healthy adolescent, the nurse will discover that there often is a lack of knowledge or skills to effectively deal with many normal situations.

A major area of need centers on the development of a healthy self-esteem, including a positive body image. Remember that the adolescent is undergoing tremendous physical changes. Furthermore, many of his activities involve food, the "slumber party," the after-the-game pizza. The adolescent may develop the habit of eating a lot of food, especially junk food. Overeating combined with the normal growth process can encourage becoming overweight approaching obesity. Even a minor gain in weight does not fit the scheme of the adolescent's world—he wants to be as attractive as possible to his peers, or he risks being ridiculed. His anxiety about his body image may cause him to follow unsafe fad diets. Some adolescents, especially girls, carry this concern to the extreme, and it may go on to anorexia nervosa, bulimia, or both.

The adolescent also expresses concern, both verbally and nonverbally about his sexuality. If these concerns go unnoticed, he may become unduly preoccupied with his sexual image, and resort to various forms of acting out behavior to establish his sexual identity.

For healthy self-esteem, the adolescent needs to develop effective coping skills to enable him to handle the normal changes going on in his life. It often happens, however, that the multiple physical and emotional changes taking place within a relatively short span of time put demands on the adolescent that he is not yet able to deal with. This temporary ego inability heightens his anxiety and impairs his ability to readily adapt and cope with changes. Life is difficult for him, because he has not yet established a firm set of values on which to base his problem solving. The adolescent facing questions about drugs and premarital sex, among other issues, finds these matters vexing because the value system he had held at an earlier time is now under question. He is unsure whether the teachings of his parents are appropriate to his emerging life-style. And because the value system itself is undergoing change, he has little to guide him.

Another potential problem revolves around the relationships between the adolescent and his significant others, especially his parents. Often, his acting out behavior is due to an inability to communicate his needs on a verbal level. Adults, on the other hand, send inappropriate messages because of their inability to actively listen and reflect on what the adolescent is trying to communicate. Communication between adults and teens may also be hampered because each harbors stereotypes of the other, for example, "teenagers never listen" or "parents never understand." This is a no-win situation for everyone. Table 18-2 summarizes the potential problem areas of adolescence and the goals of primary prevention.

NURSING INTERVENTIONS IN PRIMARY PREVENTION □ To promote the development of a healthy adolescent personality the nurse takes on the role of teacher, consultant, and program planner. As a teacher in the community she focuses on three target groups: (1) adolescents, (2) parents, and (3) significant caregivers in the community. Teaching can take place in a wide variety of nonpsychiatric settings including schools, parent associations, church groups, and physicians' offices. The role of consultant and program planner is closely associated with the teaching aspect of nursing. The nurse consults with parents and professional caregivers and works as program planner in the design of community recreational and school learning experiences that will maximize the adolescent's potential to meet his developmental needs. Community youth groups, PTAs,

TABLE 18-2 Potential Adolescent Problems: Goals and Interventions for Primary Prevention

Assessment Category	Major Areas of Need	Goals of Primary Prevention	Interventions	Evaluation Criteria
Fluids, electrolytes, nutrition Rest, sleep Mobility, exercise	Potential problem of self-esteem: inadequate physical body image related to rapidly changing physical status due to poor nutritional habits	To promote a sense of wellness in the adolescent and to avoid an increase in emotional disorders by increasing the awareness of the adolescent and his significant others regarding the normal developmental changes and the feelings and behaviors accompanying the developmental process of adolescence	Teaching and program planning in the following areas: Growth and development Physical growth and development Emotional growth and development Interpersonal growth and development Cognitive and moral growth and development	Active participation by significant others or adolescents in the program Knowledge base and communication skills before and after the program presentation
Sensory awareness	Potential problem of sensory awareness relate to the use of drugs as a substitute coping mechanism		Coping skills: Values clarification, exercises and discussions in areas of sexuality, drug use, religion, self-destruction Positive problem-solving techniques	
Sexuality, reproduction	Potential problem of self-esteem: inadequate sexual body image related to a lack of sexual knowledge or inadequate sexual knowledge regarding body changes	To promote a sense of wellness in the adolescent and to avoid an increase in emotional disorders by fostering the development of adaptive problem solving skills.		
Self-esteem	Potential problem of self-esteem: ineffective individual coping skills related to a questioning of present value systems thus providing no coherent set of values as a guideline for problem solving	To promote a sense of wellness in the adolescent and to avoid an increase in emotional disorders by removing barriers to healthy development	Communication skills: Active listening techniques Assertiveness techniques Use of "feeling" statements Communication techniques in adolescent-authority conflicts	
Love and belonging	Potential problem of love and belonging disruption of role relationships related to the ineffectual communication patterns between adolescents and adults			

schools, community action groups, and Ys are examples of groups in which such consultations can take place.

Self-Esteem Needs □ Innovation in program planning is the key to success. It is not appropriate, with either the adolescent or his adult significant others, to rely merely on lectures to address the teen's self-esteem needs. Rather, the nurse must plan programs that will elicit feedback and active problem solving by all the participants.

To enhance the teen's body image the nurse first discusses the normal physical and sexual changes of adolescence. She goes on to describe normal psychosocial needs associated with the physical changes. Finally, she explains the normal emotional and behavioral responses of both the adolescents and their caregivers to these changes. Teaching about normal physical and psychosocial growth and development is based on the premise that predictability about one's body and emotions will help the person prepare both physically and psychologically for these changes and thereby avert a potential crisis.

Teaching is best done in small groups. One method involves audiovisual media (movies, books, pamphlets, cassettes) that can be viewed or read by all participants, followed by discussion. Another strategy is to hold "rap sessions" with adolescents and parents or other caregivers. In these informal sessions, there is less structured discussion of concerns. The more formal lecture can be the method for reaching larger groups within a brief period of time.

The development of effective individual coping skills is facilitated by clarifying the teen's value system. This is a sensitive realm, and it cannot be dealt with merely by teaching normal growth and development and normal values. Helping the teen to establish values requires that he have opportunity to express himself and relate his experiences and actions to others so he can elicit feedback from them. He should see that there is more than one response to a situation. Group sessions allow the adolescent to think through plans of action and develop responses that suit his life-style. Role playing is an effective group technique that enables the adolescent to test new patterns of responses in such controversial areas as sexuality, drug use, and religion.

Love and Belonging Needs □ Communication is at the forefront in understanding the adolescent's need for love and belonging. Because communication patterns between the adolescent and his caregivers are undergoing changes, he often believes that no one understands him. He feels inhibited from sharing thoughts and feelings with others. If the caregivers are unaware that his behaviors are normal, they are at a loss as to how to respond to the "silent treatment" or rebellion. Then both sides withdraw from communication, and problem solving is impeded. To prevent such a dead end, the nurse works with the parents, teaching them how to convey the message that they accept the adolescent as he is.

Parenting is not a skill that comes naturally to someone just because he has reached a certain age or become a parent. Parenting is learned. Parenting issues often surface during adolescence when there arise conflicts and questions relating to independence and decision making that are often not encountered during childhood. These issues require parents to learn new ways to communicate. Parents often experience frustration with their teens because they "can't get their child to listen." Parenting skills can be divided into three categories: active-listening skills, general communication techniques, and conflict-resolution skills (Gordon, 1970).

Adolescents complain that their parents "never listen." Listening is an art involving one person restating the other's position in order to (1) validate correct understanding and (2) communicate that the message has been accurately perceived (Gordon, 1970). Active listening establishes a climate of trust, respect, support, interest, and acceptance for the adolescent. If the teen senses an open, nonthreatening atmosphere, he will feel free to express his needs, feelings, and concerns to others.

There are certain general communication skills that can effectively enhance or inhibit interactions with adolescents. Though these skills can be used with anyone of any age, it is especially important to use them with teens. The adolescent's ego is fragile so that a slip of the tongue can be perceived as a "put down." If he feels put down by parents he may refuse to talk with them. A common feeling on the part of the teen is "I can't talk to them, they don't understand me—all they want to do is put me down."

A most important parenting skill involves conflict resolution. Gordon's (1970) three methods for resolving conflicts are presented in Figure 18-2.

Method I (Gordon, 1970) illustrates a type of

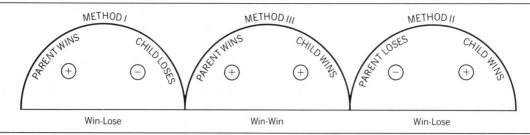

Figure 18-2 *Methods of conflict resolution. Adapted from Thomas Gordon, Methods of conflict resolution, 1979, P.E.T. Parent Effectiveness.*

problem solving whereby the parent chooses the solution to the problem and imposes this solution onto the teen. The situation seems to be "solved"—however, in reality it is nowhere near being solved. The child may submit to the parents and ultimately be unable to make any decision on his own. Even into adulthood he may develop a dependency in relationships—that is, he never develops a sense of autonomy. At the other end of the continuum, the teen may become aggressive in seeking his indepencence and rebel against the decision, perhaps becoming labeled "trouble-maker." Method II puts the locus of control in conflict resolution almost exclusively upon the teen. The parents, often in an attempt to keep the peace, allow the teen to determine the solution. As with Method I, this method does not, in reality, produce a winner. The parents are frustrated with their "vulnerability" and "weakness." The teen does not develop a sense of responsibility for others when solving problems. He often develops the attitude that he must win or have his own way which does not promote a sense of impulse control in conflictual situations.

According to Gordon (1970, p. 237), there does exist a method that can produce a two-sided win. Method III involves a series of steps that, if done in a *mutual* manner, can produce successful resolution to parent-teen conflicts. Gordon outlines the steps as follows:

Step 1: Mutually identify and clarify the conflict/issue

Step 2: Mutually generate a number of possible alternative solutions

Step 3: Discuss the pros and cons of each possible solution

Step 4: Mutually determine the best acceptable solution

Step 5: Mutually determine strategies for implementing solution

Step 6: Mutually evaluate the solution

The nurse also works with the adolescent to promote effective socializing skills. His messages to his parents must not be accusatory or degrading to their attempt to work with him. He must learn to listen carefully to their messages and formulate responses that convey an understanding of them while asserting his own ideas.

To enhance successful communication skills, the nurse needs to arrange settings in which both parents and adolescents can practice as they are being taught. Such arrangements might include: (1) lectures or seminars on parent-adolescent communication followed by role-playing various conflicts; (2) video presentations on themes involving normal parent-adolescent conflicts, followed by discussion; (3) innovative table games that involve active communication by all participants; and (4) support groups that focus on problem solving in communication.

> ■ *Point of Emphasis*
>
> *The role of the nurse in primary prevention emphasizes teaching, consulting, and program planning in the areas of growth and development, coping skills and values clarification, and communication skills between adults and adolescents.*

EVALUATION IN PRIMARY PREVENTION □ Ideally, evaluation is a long-term activity focusing on whether or not families who took part in the programs eventually need to seek formal psychiatric assistance to resolve their problems. Because long-term data gathering may not be feasible, it is often more practical to seek immediate feedback from those who participated in the programs. If the level of knowledge is higher after participation in the program than it was before, and the new skills are being used effectively, then the nurse's efforts may be said to be successful.

■ Enrichment Activities

DISCUSSION QUESTION

In a small group, identify and discuss your value system as it relates to drugs, sexuality, and religion. Following a discussion of your personal values answer the following questions:

1. Do you think that your value system comes into conflict with the value system of today's adolescents?

2. How will your value system enhance/inhibit your ability to work with today's adolescents?

3. In what ways can you prevent your values from interfering with your delivery of care?

LEARNING ACTIVITIES

Form groups of three students:

1. Choose a target group of adolescents, parents, teachers, or other significant caregivers.

2. With this target group identify an area of need that could be dealt with through planning a program of anticipatory guidance.

3. Plan and implement this program.

■ Recommended Readings

Blos, Peter. *Adolescent passages.* New York: International Universities Press, 1979. Blos views adolescence from a psychoanalytic standpoint. He discusses adolescent development as a "second individuation" in which the adolescent relives all earlier stages of development in order to reach adulthood. Blos then discusses the development process in the adolescent who is having a difficult time mastering his environment and its implications for nursing.

Gordon, Thomas. *Parent effectiveness training.* New York: Peter H. Wyden, 1970. An excellent resource for the nurse who may be planning programs for the lay caregiver. Thomas discusses communication techniques that can be used between the caregiver and the child or adolescent. Special emphasis is placed on the technique of active listening in conflict situations.

■ References

Adams, Gerald R. Personal identity formation: A synthesis of cognitive and ego psychology. *Adolescence,* 12, 46, 1976:151–164.

Beard, Margaret T. Interpersonal trust, life events and coping in an ethnic adolescent population. *Journal of psychiatric nursing and mental health services,* 18, 11, 1980:12–21.

Blos, Peter. *Adolescent passages.* New York: International universities press, 1979.

Brook, Charles. Growing Pains. *Nursing mirror,* 151, 1980:19–21.

Critchley, Deane L. Mental status examinations with children and adolescents: A developmental approach. *Nursing clinics of North America,* 14, 3, 1979:429–441

Dellas, Marie, and Eugene L. Gaier. The self and adolescent identity in women: Options and implications. *Adolescence,* 10, 39, 1975:399–407.

Dennis, Lorraine, and Joan Hassol. *Introduction to human development and health issues,* Philadelphia: W.B. Saunders Co., 1983.

Duncan, Jane W. The problem(s) of the adolescent in the family. *Psychiatric annals,* 12, 3, 1982:301–316.

Erikson, Erik H. *Identity: youth and crisis,* New York: Norton, 1968.

Faulkenberry, James R., and Murray, L. Vincent. Adolescent sexual behavior. *Health education,* 10, 1979:5–7.

Finkelstein, Jordan W. The endocrinology of adolescence. *Pediatric clinics of North America,* 27, 1, 1980:53–66.

Fox, Kathleen. Adolescent ambivalence: A therapeutic issue. *Journal of psychiatric nursing and mental health services,* 18, 9,. 1980:29–33.

Godenne, Ghisline D. Sexual development of children and adolescents. *Nursing clinics of North America,* 14, 3, 1979:475–482.

Gordon, Thomas. *Parent effectiveness training.* New York: Peter H. Wyden, 1970.

Hauser, Stuart T. Loevinger's model and measure of ego development: A critical review. *Psychological bulletin,* 83, 5, 1976:928–955.

Hogan, Rosemarie. Sexual problems of adolescence. *Human sexuality: A nursing perspective.* New York: Appleton-Century-Crofts, 1980.

Hubschman, Lynn. Why bother coming out of adolescence? *The journal of current adolescent medicine, 3, 2,* 1981:21+.

Hurlock, Elizabeth B. *Adolescent development* 4th ed. New York: McGraw-Hill, 1973.

Iveson-Iveson, Joan. Not so sweet sixteen. *Nursing mirror,* 151, 1980:18.

Josselyn, Irene M. *Adolescence,* New York: Harper & Rowe, 1971.

Katchadourian, Herant. Adolescent sexuality. *Pediatric clinics of North America,* 27, 1, 1980:17-27.

Langford, Rae W. Teenagers & obesity. *American journal of nursing,* 81, 3, 1981:556–559.

Lerner, Richard M.; Orlos, James B.; and Knapp, John R. Physical attractiveness, physical effectiveness, and self-concept in late adolescents. *Adolescence,* 11, 43, 1976:313–326.

Lidz, Thomas. *The person,* New York: Basic Books, 1976.

Loevinger, Jane. The meaning and measurement of ego development. *American psychologist,* 214, 1966:195–206.

Logan, Richard D. A reconceptualization of Erikson's identity stage. *Adolescence,* 18, 72, 1983:943–946.

Mitchell, J.J. Moral dilemmas of early adolescence. *Adolescence,* 10, 39, 1975a:442–446.

Mitchell, J.J. Moral growth during adolescence. *Adolescence,* 10, 38, 1975b:221–226.

Mitchell, John J. Adolescent intimacy. *Adolescence,* 11, 42, 1976:275–280.

Mosey, Anne C. *Three frames of reference for mental health.* Thorofare, NJ: Charles B. Slack, 1970.

Muuss, Rolf E. Kohlberg's cognitive-developmental approach to adolescent morality. *Adolescence,* 11, 41, 1976:39–57.

———— The implications of social learning theory for an understanding of adolescent development. *Adolescence,* 11, 41, 1976:60–83.

Newman, Philip R., and Newman Barbara M. Early adolescence and its conflict group identity versus alienation. *Adolescence,* 11, 42, 1976:261–273.

Satir, Virginia. *Conjoint family therapy.* Palo Alto, CA: Science and Behavior Books, 1967.

Stanton, Michael. The concept of conflict at adolescence. *Adolescence,* 9, 36, 1974:537–545.

Weller, Leonard, and Luchterhand Elmer. Adolescents' perceptions of their parents. *Adolescence,* 12, 47, 1977:367–379.

Woods, Nancy F., and Mandetta, Anne F. Sexuality throughout the life cycle: Prenatal life through adolescence. *Human sexuality in health and illness,* 2d ed. St. Louis: Mosby Company, 1979.

Woods, Nancy F., and Mandetta, Anne F. Preventive intervention. *Human sexuality in health & illness,* 2d ed. St. Louis: Mosby Company, 1979.

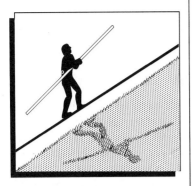

19

Adulthood

Diane M. Dodendorf

Learning Objectives

Upon completion of this chapter, the reader will be able to:

1. Describe the current theories of adult development.

2. Identify the developmental tasks of young and middle adulthood.

3. Define a developmental assessment and its underlying support.

4. Explain the developmental basis of typical adult problems.

In recent years there has been a great increase in research into adult development and in public interest in the findings. While there is much to recommend the study of adult development in itself, the importance of developmental psychology for nursing lies in the applied areas. Applied developmental psychology provides insights to help the nurse understand and care for clients.

Developmental processes continue throughout life; they do not end with adolescence. The study of young and middle adulthood has implications for children and the elderly as well. Children are cared for by adults and are bonded in the most intimate relationships that humans experience. The events and relationships of childhood have an impact in adulthood in a multitude of ways. Early adult experiences have implications for later development in middle and late adulthood. The adult years are a stage of human life that is interrelated to a much larger whole of an individual's life span and a family's history.

Another distinction about adult development is the infinite variety of adult experiences. While there may be maturational events that are nearly universal in adulthood, one's childhood, adolescence, family, personality, educational experiences, and cultural mores make universal solutions or adaptations impossible. For example, while marriage is a nearly universal maturational event, there is almost unlimited variety in the structure and functioning of an individual marriage. This chapter outlines common developmental themes in adulthood, but the reader must remember that variation around the average is greatest in the adult years, in contrast to little variation in the childhood years. (For example, 90 percent of infants take their first steps at approximately the same time.)

The first part of this chapter covers the theoretical and research aspects of adult developmental psychology and provides support for the later section on developmental assessment, nursing intervention, and evaluation. This chapter focuses on mental health problems only as they relate to developmental issues; the emphasis is on normal, maturational processes of adulthood.

■ Point of Emphasis

Developmental theories attempt to define universal themes that adults deal with throughout adult life.

☐ Developmental Theory and Research

DEVELOPMENTAL THEORIES

A number of early theorists from several disciplines considered adult development. The theories of the pioneers described below are not to be considered as separate from each other—each of these men and women contributed to the others' work in the development of their ideas and writings; they are not necessarily contradictory and may even be complementary to each other. One can think of these theorists as viewing different aspects of the same thing, all trying to answer the question "Why?"

Early Theorists

Charlotte Buhler. An early disciple of Sigmund Freud, Charlotte Buhler (1968) was one of the first to study adult development within the complete life cycle. Goal setting was a central theme in Buhler's psychosocial stages. She believed that the period from age 15 to 25 consisted of rudimentary goal selection with experimentation and preparation for meeting those goals. During the next stage (25 to 45 years) the goals were set, specific, and relevant for each individual. The work of meeting the goals is the major activity of this stage. Adults aged 45 to 65 are involved in assessing the goals and their achievement in whole or in part as established in early adulthood. Later adulthood (65 years on) is the culmination of goal setting and achieving in a public sense, with private acknowledgment of failure or success. If a middle-aged person has had physical strength and attractiveness as a goal in life, that person may feel negative about aging when physical strength is diminishing and youthful attractiveness is no longer possible; whereas, if one's goal was to achieve warm and positive family relationships, then it is possible to see that goal richly accomplished in middle and late adulthood. Aging may not seem negative if one can realize those goals to which a great deal of time and attention have been given.

Arnold Van Gennep. Arnold Van Gennep (1960) was an anthropologist whose pioneering idea of "rites of passage" has helped us to understand the course of adult development. Van Gennep studied several cultures and noted the rituals that indicated changes in adult status. These rituals were observed in primitive cultures as well as in industrialized countries.

He noted several consistencies in the observation of rites. First, certain universal events across cultures were recognized: betrothal, marriage, pregnancy, childbirth, initiation (entering adulthood), aging, menopause in women, and death. Second, while the individual was the focus of these rites, the entire community or tribe participated in them. Third, there was order to these rites—they occurred to all persons in predictable fashion.

Each rite encompassed three phases: separation from the group; transition (learning stage); and reincorporation into the group. The first phase involved the isolation of the individual or group of individuals from the group. This detachment was necessary in order for the second phase to be effective, that is, for some new learning to take place. For example, in some cultures the woman in labor was isolated from the community. After delivery, the new mother was restricted by tribal beliefs to certain behavior, diet, and dress. The new learning involved "mothering." The third phase was the return of the individual to the community. The purpose of the separation was to enhance learning but also to allow the community to see the woman in her new situation. The new mother returned to the community as an adult of status, a woman able to bear children, and typically she had greater say in group affairs.

Another, more familiar, example is the honeymoon. The newlyweds are encouraged and expected to take a trip after the wedding, away from family and friends. After this separation, during which the man and the woman have bonded as a couple, the pair returns to be regarded by family, friends, and the community at large as a couple, no longer as two individuals.

If one understands these phases of a rite of passage, one can appreciate them as they occur in day-to-day life. One can come to recognize the less public, more private rituals that people have created to mark developmental milestones. With the industrial revolution and more recently the technological revolution, there are fewer widely accepted rituals, ceremonies to mark transition from one group or social situation to another. This disregard for rituals, or the complete absence of rituals for some events (adoption, divorce, stepparenting), has left a void in many people's lives. Not only do we need to have developmental tasks set and assessed; we need overt markers to let us know where we are and how we are doing.

> ■ **Point of Emphasis**
>
> *No single developmental theory can answer every question related to adult development.*

Erik Erikson. Erik Erikson (1950) was the first to describe a psychosocial theory of adult development that included the entire life span from childhood to old age. His focus was on the emotional/affective aspect of development. He conceived of each of the eight stages as an intense conflict between two opposing poles. At the end of each stage there was either a positive or a negative resolution to the dilemma, the resolution of which influenced the next developmental stage.

Table 19-1 is a visual representation of Erikson's stages of the life span. The resolution of the intense feelings common to each stage comes at the end of the stage. As one positively resolves an earlier stage, the person is positively predisposed to coping successfully with the subsequent stage. Applications of this theory have been made in parent training and in counseling. The therapist attempts to resolve earlier negative resolutions in a positive way, thus facilitating further affective development.

Erikson's model incorporates the internal (psycho) action as described by Freud and introduces the external (social) action from and toward the environment. Erikson emphasizes that the individual is within the social environment, not separated from it. The interaction or conflict of each stage then takes into account the external demands from the environment *and* the internal wants and needs of the individual.

The four psychosocial crises from infancy and childhood (see Chapter 17) have implications about young and middle adulthood. Examples of the trust vs. mistrust resolution are infinite; a trust in oneself and in one's significant others is absolutely critical to a positive self-identity and to the establishment of relationships such as friends, spouse, children, and work colleagues. During toddlerhood the conflict revolves around "autonomy or shame and self-doubt." The confidence in one's self-control and self-expression stems from the resolution of this stage. Erikson also believes that the latter experiences of love and hate have their origins in these first two psychosocial struggles. The positive resolution of the "initiative vs. guilt" conflict is the enjoyment of doing. Healthy assertiveness and the "dare to do" attitude are examples of initiative, while chronic

TABLE 19-1 Stages of the Life Span

Stage	Psychosocial Crises	Radius of Significant Relations	Related Elements of Social Order	Psychosocial Modalities	Psychosexual Stages
1	Trust vs. mistrust	Maternal person	Cosmic order	To get To give in return	Oral-respiratory, sensory-kinesthetic (incorporative modes)
2	Autonomy vs. shame, doubt	Parental persons	"Law and order"	To hold (on) To let (go)	Anal-urethral, muscular (retentive-eliminative)
3	Initiative vs. guilt	Basic family	Ideal prototypes	To make (= going after) To "make like" (= playing)	Infantile-genital, locomotor (intrusive, inclusive)
4	Industry vs. Inferiority	"Neighborhood," school	Technological elements	To make things (= completing) To make things together	"Latency"
5	Identity and repudiation vs. identity diffusion	Peer groups and outgroups; models of leadership	Ideological perspectives	To be oneself (or not to be) To share being oneself	Puberty
6	Intimacy and solidarity vs. isolation	Partners in friendship, sex, competition, cooperation	Patterns of cooperation and competition	To lose and find oneself in another	Genitality
7	Generativity vs. self-absorption	Divided labor and shared household	Currents of education and tradition	To make be To take care of	
8	Integrity vs. despair	"Mankind" "My kind"	Wisdom	To be, through having been To face not being	

Source: "The Worksheet" is reprinted from *Identity and the Life Cycle* by Erik H. Erikson, by permission of W.W. Norton & Company, Inc. Copyright © 1959 by International Universities Press, Inc.

experiences of guilt over one's actions are examples of the negative resolution of this stage. The fourth psychosocial crisis of "industry vs. inferiority" is the foundation for future attitudes toward work and work behavior. One's sense of competence and a satisfaction with a job well done come from a successful resolution of the "doing" and its evaluation, first by others, and then by self.

The last four stages are particular to adulthood. "Identity vs. role diffusion" is the conflict that develops during late adolescence and early adulthood. Preoccupation with one's essential character and one's value orientation leads to periods of depression and elation, all experienced on the way to a clear self-definition. "Intimacy vs. isolation" logically follows the attainment of a

self-identity in Erikson's theory. This unique task requires young adults to form an intimate relationship with someone who is not a family member. An Eriksonian definition of intimacy "includes the ability to experience an open, supportive, tender relationship with another person, without fear of losing one's own identity in the process of growing close." (Newman and Newman, 1984, 384) Intimacy implies the ability to engage in mutual empathy and mutual regulation of needs.

The seventh psychosocial stage (middle adulthood), "generativity vs. stagnation," is a pressured concern for the well-being of future generations. The obligation to care for one's children, grandchildren, or simply the younger generation is a factor in the survival of the species. The skills of the middle-aged adult are refined, and have the power to influence others and to continue long afer one's death. The last stage is "integrity vs. despair." The older adult, after considerable thought (reminiscing), generally comes to accept past decisions as being good and right. The aging individual must pull together all the events, persons, judgments, and outcomes of a lifetime and integrate all of them into a whole that is positive (integrity) or negative (despair). There is more information about this psychosocial stage provided in Chapter 20 on Aging.

Robert Havighurst. Robert Havighurst (1972) organized what we know about adult development into developmental tasks to be accomplished. Others have followed with other schemes of developmental tasks, but Havighurst is considered the conceptual "father" of developmental tasks. He defines a developmental task as "a task which arises at or about a certain period in the life of an individual, the successful achievement of which leads to his happiness and to success with later tasks, while failure leads to unhappiness in the individual, disapproval by the society, and difficulty with later tasks" (p. 2).

Havighurst's specific developmental tasks for each adult stage are listed below:

Early Adulthood	Selecting a mate
	Learning to live with a marriage partner
	Starting a family
	Rearing children
	Managing a home
	Beginning an occupation
	Assuming civic responsibility
	Finding social groups
Middle Adulthood	Achieving adult civic and social responsibility
	Establishing and maintaining an economic standard of living
	Helping teenage children become responsible, happy adults
	Developing adult leisure activities
	Relating to the spouse as a person
	Accepting and adapting to physiological changes
	Adjusting to aging parents
Later Maturity	Adjusting to declining physical strength and health
	Adjusting to retirement and reduced income
	Adjusting to the death of a spouse
	Establishing relationships within one's age group
	Meeting social and civic responsibilities
	Establishing satisfactory physical living arrangements

Newman and Newman (1984) combined the theoretical approach of Erikson with Havighurst's notion of developmental tasks. An outline of this combination of stage-specific developmental tasks with the corresponding psychosocial crises is represented in Table 19-2. These dual concepts of psychosocial crises and developmental tasks are useful in constructing developmental assessments. Once the crises and tasks are defined, one can measure one's progress in mastering those tasks. Developmental assessment tools are based on the crises and tasks defined for each age group.

Family Development. Evelyn Duvall (1977) has been a foremost leader in the area of family development, following the pioneers Waller and Hill (1951). Duvall described the stages a family goes through from courtship to marriage, to first pregnancy, to child rearing, to launching children, to retirement and death. Using the model of developmental tasks from Havighurst, Duvall has listed developmental tasks for the family at each stage. Table 19-3 is an outline of the developmental tasks by stage.

There are other "family forms" that are the result of economic, legal, social, and cultural pressures on families. The single-parent family is typically a single, divorced, or widowed woman with children. This woman is subject to all the stresses of parenting and breadwinning without a partner and with distressed (due to divorce or death) children. There is a growing number of male single-parent households, but their employment and financial problems are usually less difficult. Single parents are plagued with feelings of guilt associated with their areas of weakness—women are concerned about breadwinning and time spent away from children, while men are concerned about nutrition and household management.

Another result of the rising number of divorces and remarriages is the blended or stepfam-

TABLE 19-2 Developmental Tasks/Psychosocial Crises

Life Stage	Developmental Tasks	Psychosocial Crises
Prenatal (conception to birth)		
Infancy (birth to 2 years)	Social attachment Sensorimotor intelligence and primitive causality Object permanence Maturation of sensory and motor functions Emotional development	Trust vs. mistrust
Toddlerhood (2–4)	Elaboration of locomotion Fantasy and play Language development Self-control	Autonomy vs. shame and doubt
Early school age (5–7)	Sex identification Concrete operations Early moral development Group play	Initiative vs. guilt
Middle school age (8–12)	Social cooperation Self-evaluation Skill learning Team play	Industry vs. inferiority
Early adolescence (13–17)	Physical maturation Formal operations Emotional development Membership in the peer group Heterosexual relationships	Group identity vs. alienation
Later adolescence (18–22)	Autonomy from parent Sex role identity Internalized morality Career choice	Individual identity vs. role diffusion
Early adulthood (23–34)	Marriage Childbearing Work Life-style	Intimacy vs. isolation
Middle adulthood (35–60)	Management of the household Child rearing Management of a career	Generativity vs. stagnation
Later adulthood (61–)	Coping with the physical changes of aging Redirection of energy to new roles Acceptance of one's life Developing a point of view about death	Integrity vs. despair

Source: Newman and Newman, *Development Through Life*, 3rd ed., Homewood, Ill, Dorsey Press, 1984 pp. 46 and 384.

TABLE 19-3 *Family Developmental Tasks* [a]

Married Couple Stage
Finding, furnishing, and maintaining their first home
Establishing mutually satisfactory ways of supporting themselves
Allocating responsibilities that each partner is able and willing to assume
Establishing mutually acceptable personal, emotional, and sexual roles
Interacting with in-laws, relatives, and the community
Planning for children
Maintaining couple motivation and morale

Childbearing Stage
Adapting housing arrangements to the young child
Meeting present and future costs of childbearing
Assuming mutual responsibility
Facilitating members' role-learning
Communicating with one another in the family
Planning for future children
Relating to relatives and others
Maintaining motivation and morale
Family rituals and routines

Preschool Stage
Supplying adequate space, facilities, and equipment for the expanding family
Meeting predictable and unexpected costs of family life with small children
Assuming more mature roles with the expanding family
Maintaining mutually satisfying intimate communications in the family
Rearing and planning for children
Relating to relatives
Tapping resources outside the family
Motivating family members

School-age Stage
Providing for children's activity and parents' privacy
Maintaining financial solvency
Furthering socialization of family members
Upgrading communication in the family
Establishing ties with life outside the family
Developing morally and building family morale

Teenage Stage
Providing facilities for widely different needs within the family
Working out ever-changing financial problems
Sharing responsibilities of family living
Keeping the marriage relationship in focus
Bridging the communication gap between the generations
Keeping in touch with relatives
Widening the horizons of teenagers and their parents
Maintaining the ethical and moral stance that is meaningful to them

Launching Young Adults
Rearranging physical facilities and resources
Meeting the expenses of a launching center family
Reallocating responsibilities among grown and growing children
Coming to terms with themselves as husband and wife
Maintaining open systems of communication within the family and between the family and others
Widening the family circle through release of young adult children and recruitment of new members by marriage
Reconciling conflicting loyalties and philosophies of life

Middle Age Parents
Providing for comfortable, healthful well-being
Allocating all resources for present and future needs
Developing patterns of complementarity
Undertaking appropriate social roles
Assuring marital satisfaction
Enlarging the family circle
participating in life outside the home
Affirming life's central values

Aging Family Members
Making satisfying living arrangements as aging progresses
Adjusting to retirement income
Establishing comfortable routines
Safeguarding physical and mental health
Maintaining love, sex, and marital relations
Remaining in touch with other family members
Keeping active and involved
Finding meaning life

[a] Source: Adapted with permission from Evelyn Duvall, *Marriage and Family Development.* New York: Harper and Row, 1977.

---

ily. With the acquisition of a second spouse, there are his children, her children, and their children; more kinship systems; and thus roles and relationships that are painfully created rather than evolving through customs and traditions.

Other forms of family are the dual-career or dual-earner families, the married but childless family, and the "I created my own" family. In the dual-career family, both parents are working outside the home. While there are financial and emotional benefits in this arrangement, the stresses include limitations on time spent with children and with each other. The assignment of household tasks is usually quite different from that of the traditional family; father and children may be expected to take on more responsibilities at home, and some tasks may be delegated to paid domestic and child care help.

Today, more couples choose to remain childless, and these adults consider this arrangement to be just as legitimate and satisfactory as one of a family with children. The deemphasis on child-rearing in our culture and the greater emphasis on women's careers have contributed to this alternative form of family. The same cultural forces have given rise to an increase in the number of people remaining single throughout adulthood. These persons "create" their own families by establishing close, intimate relations with others in the community. Rituals such as Thanksgiving dinner, are continued with one's chosen "grandparents," "parents," "brothers," and "sisters." Communes are another example of "family creation."

DEVELOPMENTAL RESEARCH

The five current researchers described next have worked in the area of adult development. Each of the five acknowledges the prior contributions of the pioneer theorists. Most of these researchers identify themselves clearly as being in one theoretical camp. Their goal is to study the phenomenon, to test hypotheses as they construct a theory, and to produce the data that will support that theory or will negate it.

Daniel Levinson

Daniel Levinson (1978) and his team intensively studied adult male development by means of biographies and interviews with 40 men over several years. Levinson's theoretical orientation is Eriksonian but he puts greater emphasis on the relation between the self and the world. Figure 19-1 illustrates the "eras" across the life span. The developmental process is the periodic constructing of a "life structure," stabilizing it, modifying or drastically changing it. "The concept of life structure—the basic pattern or design of a person's life at a given time—gives us a way of looking at the engagement of the individual in society" (p. 41). The three perspectives of the life structure are: (1) sociocultural—class, religion, ethnicity, family, politics, occupation; (2) self—wishes, conflicts, anxieties, talents, skills, moral values, ideals; and (3) participation in the world—relationships and roles as citizen, husband, father, friend, worker.

The "novice" phase of adulthood includes a transition to adulthood from adolescence, marked by three distinct periods. The transition involves separating from the adolescent world and giving up the dependency on adults. This Early Adult Transition is also the time for initiative in terms of work and career. This is the time of selection and preparation. The stage of Entering the Adult World signals the creation of the first life structure. Numerous choices are made, and this is the heart of the evolving life structure. Age 30 Transition is the second stage and the time when a man reviews his first life structure and evaluates its usefulness to him. Changes or modifications will be made at this point to serve as the continuing life structure for the next stage of early adulthood, Settling Down, which is just as it sounds—a time of building the nest, creating a niche for oneself in society. The other task of this period is to strive for advancement and achievement. Thus, at the same time that there is stability (nest) there is improvement and change (advancement). The nurse may know a client who "settles in" quickly after a second marriage. The divorce and second marriage involved significant change, yet the person will say his goal was to be involved in a stable, secure relationship. The security that comes of working for a particular company may involve numerous changes in both place of residence and professional colleagues, as a person is transferred from one office to another on a planned career path.

During middle adulthood, Levinson proposes for men another transition (Midlife Transition) and three stages that follow. The majority of the men in Levinson's study found this period of time painful. They reviewed their goals of early adulthood and appraised its successes or failures. At this time the adult is initiating another life structure to serve him through middle adulthood. Entering Middle Adulthood is the first stage, and a major task is individuation. A man must develop a much deeper relationship with himself; he comes to realize he is a combination of opposites—"polarities." This deepening self-awareness may result in internal or external changes or both.

Age 50 Transition is similar to the previous transition in that the adult evaluates his second life structure constructed throughout the middle adult years, and makes certain alterations or adjustments in his course. Culmination of Middle Adulthood is the final stage of the middle years and is similar to the Settling Down period of young adulthood. Satisfaction with the previous structures and modifications of these (as well as the ability to make changes and move in other directions) can bring a sense of fulfillment during these years. Long-term marriages can be transformed into new patterns of relating to each other. A career change that seems quite drastic may, in fact, grow out of a long-term slowly developing hobby.

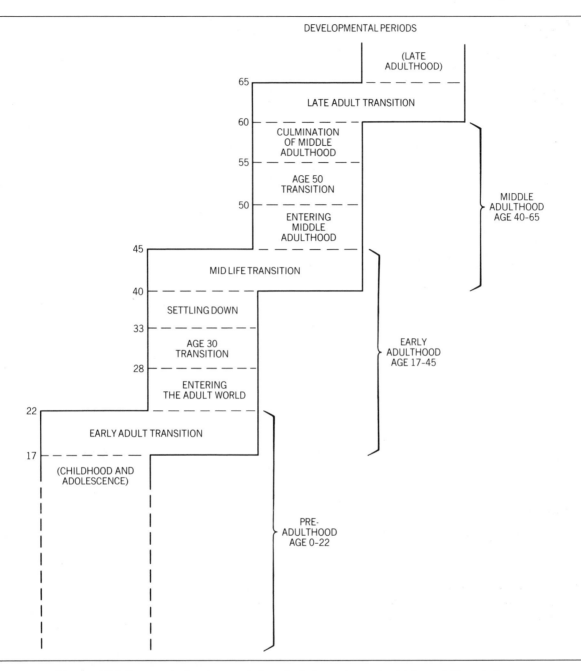

Figure 19-1 *Eras and developmental periods in early and middle adulthood. From Daniel Levinson's* Seasons of a Man's Life, *1978, reprinted by permission of Alfred A. Knopf, publisher.*

Roger Gould

Roger Gould's (1978) theory of adult development comes closer to a "psychotherapeutic" approach. Gould believes that the process of maturing depends on the giving up of irrational and childish notions—"myths"—that a person has relied on to protect him as a child and an adolescent.

There are four major false assumptions that a person must intellectually and emotionally abandon: (1) I will always live with my parents and be their child. (2) Parents will always be available to help when I cannot accomplish a certain task myself. (3) My simplified version of a complicated inner reality is correct. (4) There is no real death or evil in the world.

The first major false assumption is challenged in the first stage, Leaving Our Parents' World, ages 16 to 22. Gould cites various false assumptions as components of this stage that must be challenged and mastered. Each major false assumption has subassumptions, that is, particular myths that underlie the one central illusion of that period.

Irrational childhood fears about not becoming a competent adult dominate Gould's first stage. Young adults are overly sensitive toward older adults, and yet the pressure to become self-reliant may cause young adults to be strident about their decisions. If a young person gives up his obstreperous position he may fear that the parents will see his vulnerability, and he will continue to need their protection.

The second false assumption is dealt with in the I'm Nobody's Baby Now stage, ages 22 to 28. Opening Up To What's Inside is the third stage; it includes ages 28 to 34 and the third myth about one's complicated inner reality. Gould's Midlife Decade, ages 35 to 45, focuses on the final illusion about evil in the world and in oneself. Each of these stages represents a conflict between childhood notions and adult realities. Gould suggests some risk taking in order to clearly discriminate between the two views. The end goal is an integrated view of the world.

TABLE 19-4 Schematic Table of Adaptive Mechanisms[a]

Level I: Psychotic mechanisms (common in psychosis, dreams, childhood)
Denial (of external reality)
Distortion
Delusional projection

Level II: Immature mechanisms (common in severe depression, personality disorders, and adolescence)
Fantasy (schizoid withdrawal, denial through fantasy)
Projection
Hypochondriasis
Passive-aggressive behavior (masochism, turning against the self)
Acting out (compulsive delinquency, perversion)

Level III: Neurotic mechanisms (common in everyone)
Intellectualization (isolation, obsessive behavior, undoing, rationalization)
Repression
Reaction formation
Displacement (conversion, phobias, wit)
Dissociation (neurotic denial)

Level IV: Mature mechanisms (common in "healthy" adults)
Sublimation
Altruism
Suppression
Anticipation
Humor

[a] Source: Copyright 1977 by George E. Vaillant, *Adaptation to Life*, p. 80, reprinted by permission of Little Brown & Company.

George Vaillant

George Vaillant's longitudinal study (1977) of adult males encompasses a period of almost 40 years. In 1939 a group of Harvard undergraduates were selected on the basis of their mental health and were followed until they were in their 60s. The focus of the study was "ego mechanisms of defense"—the intraphyschic defense mechanisms involved in managing environmental demands and instincts and wants.

The uniqueness of Vaillant's work was that it grouped defense mechanisms into a hierarchy of less to more mature (Table 19-4). Vaillant found that those men who were highly adaptable in defense patterns had the most satisfactory external adjustments, that is, better life outcomes. Vaillant also found that certain defense mechanisms were more frequent at certain age periods, and that the defense mechanisms tended to be more mature with more mature ages. For example, the immature mechanisms of fantasy and acting out, which are common in young adulthood, are replaced by altruism, anticipation, and humor.

Bernice Neugarten

The most outspoken proponent of adult development is Bernice Neugarten (1975). Her focus has been on men and women in middle age. Neugarten is best known for her study of perception of time vis-à-vis age. Increasingly, time is viewed as "time left" rather than "time since birth" (Neugarten's "social clock"). The adult assesses his passage through time as being either similar to that of other adults of corresponding age ("on time") or too early or too late ("off time"). Increased self-understanding and a sense of greater body fragility are also part of the personality adaptations; greater tolerance within sex roles is apparent when grandfather can be quite nurturant and grandmother quite assertive.

Lawrence Kohlberg

Following Piaget's work on cognitive development, Kohlberg and colleagues (1983) studied the cognitive aspects of moral development. Kohlberg was interested in the *judgments* about right and wrong rather than in the affective components (guilt) or the behavioral (actual transgressions). He constructed a six-stage theory of moral development, based on responses to hypothetical moral dilemmas.

In the first two stages, Level I, a person conceives of right and wrong depending on the pain or pleasure derived from the act; "If it feels good, it's okay." After successful socialization and a higher level of cognitive development, Stages 3 and 4 of Level II involve a reliance on others for constructs of right and wrong. In Stage 3, it is significant others, such as the family, who influence these judgments. In Stage 4, it is larger social groups, such as a particular religious faith, or the military. Level III, Stages 5 and 6, constitutes the development of an individual conscience based on universal principles that guide one's behavior. In his recent work, Kohlberg has eliminated Stage 6 and created two parts to Stage 5. He has indicated that the moral dilemmas of our time may arise because persons are at different moral stages rather than that they simply disagree over an issue.

Carol Gilligan

Carol Gilligan (1982) has challenged Kohlberg's theory of moral development. In Kohlberg's six stages, women seemed to "get stuck" at Stage 3. Women were concerned with other people rather than moving on to abstract, individualized principles by which to judge whether an action is moral or immoral. Gilligan argues that women have a different mode of experience, "a different voice." For girls and for women, continuing a relationship and being concerned about the impact on others of one's actions is more important than a conflict of ideas. For example, if a woman responded that a particular action was wrong (or right) because of its impact on a significant relationship, she would be considered Stage 3 in Kohlberg's hierarchy. Gilligan analyzes the reasoning as indicating that abstract principles have less relevance for women, real life people more. Gilligan believes that this attitude should be viewed as a strength and not as a weakness. According to Gilligan, different does not mean deficient.

> ■ *Point of Emphasis*
>
> *Assessment tools are the bridges that allow application of abstract theory to individual clients.*

ADULT DEVELOPMENTAL ASSESSMENT □ As in other sections of this text, developmental assessment is discussed from the aspects of client assessment, family and environmental assessments, and self-assessment by the nurse. All of these factors are important to the nurse's ability to identify the mental health needs of adult clients and to promote self-awareness and professional growth.

Client Assessment □ Table 19-5 provides an organizing framework that may be useful in planning a developmental assessment. The theoretical expectations can be identified for the age/stage of the person to be assessed. Appropriate interview questions can be developed that may elicit the person's views and experiences about the theoretical issues. During and following the interview, the subjective and objective data concerning the client's development can be listed opposite the theoretical content for comparison and analysis of the person's unique strengths, weaknesses, needs, and perspectives. The nurse can prepare an assessment tool for young adults and for middle

---

TABLE 19-5 Developmental Psychosocial Assessment Tool Young or Middle Adult

Expected	Compared to	Observed
Developmental Tasks (Newman and Newman's for each stage)		
Psychosocial Crisis (Erikson's developmental stages)		
Thought Processes (cognitive development, moral development, learning, memory, attention, perception)		
Language Development/Changes (communication: verbal, nonverbal, delays, articulation)		
Physical Growth and Development/Changes (milestones, rate, emotional reaction to, body image, growth indicators such as height, weight, and health concerns)		
Emotional Development (moods, temperament, expressiveness, mode of expression, personality factors)		
Interpersonal Relations (significant others, social attachments, supports, resources)		
Common Stresses and Responses to Stress (typical stresses and problems of each age group and usual ways of dealing with stresses and problems)		
Work/Leisure/Play (amount of time, balance of work and play, kind of leisure or play, attitude toward work and play)		

adults by completing the "expected" side, listing the typical tasks, concerns, and issues of the age group, and by formulating key broad questions to introduce each topic. Copies can be made for future use. With the completion of several assessments comes an appreciation for not only commonalities in developmental issues but also the uniqueness and variability of individuals and their experiences. Analysis of strengths and weaknesses in relation to current and future tasks of development permits identification of needs and planning for primary or secondary prevention strategies.

The Young Adult □ Components of assessment have been identified by Colarusso and Nemiroff (1981). These include the person's attitude toward his body and its use, including body image, sexuality and sexual experiences, the desire for children, the dawning sense of one's personal history, with related awareness of time limitation and attitude toward illness and death. Work-related factors include choice of a career, financial decision making, role in a mentoring relationship, and overall aspects of creativity. Components related to interpersonal relationships include one's independence from parents and the ability to relate to them on an adult level, friendship patterns and capacity for personal intimacy, and conceptualizing one's role in society. Leisure or playtime activities and religious attitudes and practices should also be assessed in young adults.

The Middle Adult □ Significant aspects related to physical changes of growing older in the period from ages 40 to 60 include altered body image manifested in declining strength and agility, the menopause/climacteric, and some alteration in sexual functioning and activity levels. Attitude toward time is altered (from time lived to time left) as the person experiences illnesses and the death of aging parents and contemporaries. Work attitudes to be assessed include the position and relative balance of work vs. relationships and play, one's position as a mentor, the sense of creativity, and financial attitudes that affect both present life-style and future retirement. Interpersonal attitudes and relationships focus on intimate relationships, friendships with people of various age groups (both new and of long duration), and with aging parents. Perspectives on the changing role of the middle adult in society are also important to assess (Colarusso and Nemiroff, 1981).

An additional organizational structure for assessment is outlined in Table 19-6. It is organized around an alphabetic mnemonic to promote recall of the categories that influence developmental issues; affect, body, communication/cognition, development, economic, and family/future assessments (Dodendorf, 1981). Some content areas for assessment and suggested key questions are addressed in the following discussion.

Affect □ The major components to be assessed under the category of affect include current feeling states and predominant emotional patterns, personal attitudes and issues related to mood and feelings, and current stressors, coping strategies, and supports.

Emotions and Mood. □ It is helpful to inquire about the presence of feelings of loneliness, guilt, "the blues," or serious depression. If the person experiences any of these, it is important to determine the frequency and degree to which they

---

TABLE 19-6 Developmental Assessment for Adults

Affect:	Moods
	Self-esteem
	Stressors
	Coping
Body:	Physical handicaps
	Chronic illness
	Pain
	Body image
	Sexuality
Communication and Cognition:	Listening
	Clarification
	Assertiveness
	Conflict resolution
	Thought
	Reasoning
	Judgment
	Intelligence
	Memory
Development:	Tasks
	Issues
	Concerns
	Adjustments
	Prior developmental mastery
Economics:	Needs/Resources
	Life-style
Family:	Family of origin—issues and relationships
	Current family—issues and relationships
	Family stressors
	Family as support system

occur. Ask if the person considers himself to be an anxious/nervous person or a moody person, and ask him to describe the responses and circumstances that lead to this conclusion. Inquire whether he is more quick to feel hurt or angry than most people. How does he feel about himself in general (self-esteem)? Many people find it difficult to respond to this question. It may be helpful to ask them to describe themselves as they think others might, to rate how they feel about themselves on a scale of 1 to 5 with 1 being "Don't like myself at all" and 5 being "Like myself a lot." This scale is not a valid measure of self-esteem; however, the self-rating may prompt further discussion into areas of self-dissatisfaction.

Stressors □ Current problems and life changes (even positive occurrences) should be discussed. Adults often experience significant changes such as promotion, transfer, or career change; increase or decrease in number of family members related to births, children leaving or returning home, marriages and in-laws, assisting elderly parents with living arrangements; injuries or illnesses; losses and grief; and common problematic events such as parent-child conflict, marital conflicts, and financial ups and downs.

It is important to keep in mind that the relative degree of stress depends upon the current overall status of the person and his coping, the severity of the stressor, and the number of stressors occurring in a particular period of time (Clements, 1983). Consideration of the multiple changes that occur when a divorced woman with children remarries illustrates the potential stressors even in a planned, happy event. While the couple is working out their new relationship, the children must work out relationships with the new stepparent. Conflicts may occur around concerns of the natural father, former friends, new friends, and family (which includes an additional group of in-laws). If the marriage also involves moving to a new home, neighborhood, town, or state, and a change in jobs, then the stressors are further compounded.

In addition to assessing the number and severity of life stressors or life change, it is necessary to identify the related effects on the person's functioning and personal resources. He may describe feeling exhausted, tense, and irritable with decreased patience and ability to solve problems. Physical symptoms such as sleep problems, headaches, gastrointestinal distress, or increased susceptibility to minor illnesses may be reported.

Coping □ Assessment of coping includes inquiring into both current ways of handling feelings and stressors and how stressors were handled in the past. Does the person believe that his coping skills are adequate for most or all of the situations he has been called upon to deal with, or does he perceive deficits in this area? Less-than-adequate coping skills in the past influence future vulnerability to stress and affect self-control in terms of one's sense of competence or mastery.

Body Image □ Many severely handicapped and disfigured people manage to live highly successful and satisfying lives, while some individuals, with minimal or no deficits, are seriously disabled by their perceived unattractiveness or functional deficits. It has been demonstrated that loss of physical function and chronic illness are often associated with lowered self-esteem (Antonucci and Jackson, 1983). Pain may have a significant effect on body image.

The young adult may have a variety of feelings associated with body image ranging from embarrassment or shame to pride and satisfaction. Many people possess physical attributes they would like to change, such as losing or gaining weight, or changing some parts of their body. What are the person's attitudes and desires toward his body? What, if anything, is being done to bring about desired changes? Is the amount of time spent "working out" or on other bodily activities suggestive of healthy self-care or preoccupation? Is the body image realistic? Anorectic people see themselves as fat when they are excessively thin; and many persons exaggerate the significance of particular features into a belief that they are ugly when in fact they are attractive.

Initially it is valuable to identify any physical deficits that have a potential to influence the individual's self-concept, including body image and self-esteem. These deficits may affect either appearance or function; the most important aspects are not the deficits themselves but the person's attitude and perception of how (or if) they interfere with particular role functions or interpersonal relationships.

Sexuality □ Assessment of sexuality includes sexual role attitudes and practices as well as sexual behavior. The person's view of self as a man or woman needs to be described. Does he or she seem comfortable and satisfied with his or her sex role and sex life? Problems in this area can be stressful for young adults as they develop relationships and experiment with various sexual roles and practices, as well as for middle-aged adults who may experience gradual decline in frequency and intensity of sexual responses along with concern about their attractiveness based on the physical changes of aging. (Further details on assessment of sexuality are found in Chapter 21.)

Communication □ Does the person communicate effectively in order to relate to others in personal and work roles? Listening, responding, assertiveness, and conflict resolution can significantly influence relationships with peers, family members, and co-workers. The person with low self-esteem may lack assertiveness and be ineffective in significant aspects of communication. This ineffectiveness in turn may further lower self-esteem (Fensterheim and Baer, 1975). Questions that ask, for instance, if the person would describe himself as assertive, nonassertive, or overly aggressive and as a good or a poor listener may help to screen for communication problems. If the person describes communication difficulties, it is helpful to explore their nature, what underlying attitudes exist in relationship to them, and what behaviors and interpersonal consequences result.

Cognition □ In adulthood, the person has achieved full development of abstract thought and reasoning processes. Judgment generally continues to improve based on accumulation of life experiences. Intelligence, memory, and learning abilities do not decline in middle age unless organic mental problems are present, such as those secondary to problems of oxygenation, chronic alcoholism, or exposure to toxic substances (e.g., heavy metals). Older adults may require more time to process/learn new information, but learning does occur. The mental status examination includes components that can be used for further assessment in this area (see Chapter 10).

Development □ Assessing developmental status of the adult involves an overall assessment of basic psychosocial factors such as those identified by Erikson, and the age-related stage issues identified as developmental tasks and concerns.

Prior Personality. □ Erikson (1950) identified central issues to be resolved in personality development related to trust, autonomy, initiative, industry, and identity during childhood, adolescence, and adulthood. Some questions that focus on this information are:

1. Has trusting people ever been a problem to you?
2. Have you tended to doubt yourself a lot, to feel ashamed or embarrassed?
3. What do you remember of grade school? Did you do well? Did you make friends?
4. What are some of your most vivid memories of childhood?
5. Would you describe yourself as a leader or a follower in most things?
6. Did you have a hero/heroine or idol that you hoped to emulate when you grew up? Describe the qualities you admired. Have you developed some of those desirable qualities?
7. If you could sum up your high school experience in a few words, what would they be?
8. How many years of education have you had? What would you describe as your attitude and accomplishments in high school and college (if applicable) regarding academic subjects? Social and sports activities? Dating?
9. When did you leave home and why did you leave?
10. Describe the years after you completed your schooling? Describe your feelings on graduation—were you confident of your plans or unsure?

Young Adult □ Young adults strive for intimacy and the establishment of a career. Intimacy is the ability to bond to another in a loving relationship while retaining a sense of personal identity. Inability to form and sustain intimate relationships is associated with loneliness and decreased ability to cope effectively with stress. Components of intimacy have not been consistently defined but generally includes emotions (warmth, caring, closeness), self-disclosure (sharing personal information), and sensitivity to the needs of the other (Chelune and Waring, 1984). Related questions might include:

1. Have you ever had a close and lasting relationship with another person (not a family member)? If so, ask for further description. (How did you feel toward the other

person? How did that relationship differ from other friendships?)

2. Do you currently have a close relationship with someone that permits sharing of intimate thoughts and feelings?

Couple relationships can be further explored to determine aspects that enhance the relationship and meet the needs of the partners. Inquiries might include the level of open communication between the partners, similarity of preferences in friends and leisure activities, shared intellectual or social pursuits, and level of satisfaction with the sexual relationship. What would the couple describe as the strengths and weaknesses of the relationship?

If the person has children, it is helpful to ask for ages and descriptions. (Tell me a little about each of your children.) Ask if parenting is different from what was expected and if so, in what way. Are there particular parental skills or knowledge that he would like to develop or improve on? What other persons are helpful in sharing some of the demands of parenting (e.g., spouse, family, friends)?

Work-related questions are significant to adults, particularly in American culture. "What do you do?" is one of the initial questions asked of new acquaintances. Occupational status and achievement affect identity, self-esteem, and social standing. Most young adults have significant adjustments to make in initiating, maintaining, and changing careers. Inquiries include:

1. Do you have a particular goal for your life right now? What is your dream/hope for your life in 5 years? In 10 years?
2. What is your occupation? Are you considering changing jobs or careers? How do you feel about your work? What differences would you describe from your expectations before starting a career? How much of your time do you devote to work activities in any average week? Are you satisfied with the amount of time you have for leisure? What sort of activities do you pursue for recreation? How often?

Middle Adult ☐ Many of the questions for the young adult also apply to the middle aged. It is also helpful to inquire what changes, if any, have occurred in priorities or values since younger years. A sense of caring for others and leaving

something of value creates a need for accomplishments, in parental pride, in work achievements, or in mentoring relationships. The nurse could ask:

1. What would you say you've accomplished in life?
2. When you look back on your goals as a younger person, how would you say you are doing in relation to them?
3. How has your sense of time changed since you were younger? Has this affected your values or life in any way?
4. What are your feelings about marriage and family? (If not married or has no children, are there any regrets?)
5. Many people begin to feel restless and less content as they enter the 40s or 50s. Would you say this was characteristic of you? Would you describe this as a midlife crisis? How did/do you cope with these feelings?
6. What are the feelings associated with menopause (women) or any perceived changes in sexual capacity (men)? Are they perceived as a problem?
7. What were or are expected to be the best years of life?
8. (If applicable) If your children have left home and thus require less time and attention, has your relationship as a couple changed? Many grow closer, others drift apart.

Economics ☐ Financial realities influence one's sense of self-worth, life-style, and ability to meet comprehensive needs. Rather than inquiring about the amount of money a person earns (which most people consider to be personal information), it is generally acceptable to ask if the person's income is satisfactory to him and if it is adequate to meet his needs. Many people are comfortable in terms of having adequate food, shelter, and security but would prefer a more affluent life-style. Others may not have sufficient income to provide basic family necessities. Economic decision making can be a source of conflict in families. It is often helpful to inquire how the family handles money and if they are satisfied with this arrangement.

Family ☐ In this chapter the focus on family assessment is in relationship to the developmental needs of the individual adult. (Refer to

Chapter 12 for a discussion of the family as an entity in itself.) Questions relating to roles, values, and issues revolving around dependence and independence include:

1. What is a central concern in your family (e.g., togetherness, education, hard work)? How has this influenced your values and view of yourself?

2. What roles do you tend to play in your family (e.g., harmonizer/peacemaker, black sheep/scapegoat, little mother/organizer)?

3. Would you say that you are relatively dependent upon or independent from your original family in the following areas: living arrangements (live separately or in family home); personal decisions (e.g., job, purchases, future choices); financial support; emotional support; socialization (e.g., time spent with members in leisure or recreation activities).

4. Have you established a family of your own yet? Please describe.

5. Are there significant people whom you consider family who were not mentioned because they are not blood relatives?

6. If you are married or part of an intimate relationship, what are significant characteristics that attracted you to that person? Are you still attracted? What adjustments have you had to make?

7. Do you have/expect to have children? What does having children mean to you?

8. Does your family provide you with the degree of closeness and support you need?

9. How do you resolve problems or differences of opinion in your family? Are there any changes you would like to make in your family life?

10. Whom are you most likely to seek out for advice or assistance when you have problems or concerns?

Family members may have differing developmental needs depending upon their stage in life. For instance, the need for increasing independence on the part of the late adolescent or young adult in the launching phase may conflict with the heightened sense of generativity, the need to nurture the development of the younger generation on the part of middle-aged parents. Or the couple who chose to have children later in life may have a sense of being "off-time" as they struggle with the demands of child care while their friends may be experiencing increased freedom as their older children become independent.

Questions that may elicit some of these issues might be:

1. Have you ever experienced a sense of being "out of step" with other people in your age group?

2. What would you say are the pressing concerns of each of the family members in your house?

3. Are any of these needs of other family members particularly difficult to deal with at this stage of your own life? How do you handle these different needs? Are you satisfied with the results?

4. Do you anticipate any future needs or difficulties?

Self-Assessment □ The nurse needs to be aware of her own developmental needs and concerns. Self-awareness may promote greater acceptance of one's own needs and those of others. For instance, an inability to tolerate the intrusive questioning and advice giving of an older co-worker may be easier to accept if the young nurse can acknowledge her own need for autonomy and her feelings of having only recently made progress in working through these issues with her own mother. Once feelings of being told what to do are resolved, then the young person can seek (and selectively use or ignore) advice in an equal relationship.

The nurse's awareness and comfort level about particular developmental issues such as sexuality, intimacy, conflict, and loss will influence the quality of relationships with clients of various age groups and the ability to collect and analyze pertinent developmental information. (Self-awareness is discussed fully in Chapter 4.)

PROBLEM-NEED IDENTIFICATION □ Many nursing diagnoses are applicable in the identification of developmental needs and problems of adult clients. A positive diagnosis, coping—potential for growth—is indicative of the challenges to healthy individuals and families that are posed by the changes, transitions, and adjustments across life-span development. Primary prevention strategies can be planned to further promote the coping capacity of healthy people. Problems may arise in several general areas such as role activity, sexual functioning, self-concept, parenting, and coping. See Table 19-7 for a presentation of some common problems identified under specific nursing diagnoses.

NURSING INTERVENTION □ One of the basic premises of developmental psychology is that development will proceed naturally in a supportive or adequate environment. People do not need to be pushed toward the next phase of development because there is an inherent tendency within each person to learn, to grow, and to develop new skills. The environment enhances these maturational strivings by providing social expectations, opportunities, and challenges for further development. For example, young adults feel a need to try out their independence by making their own decisions, seeking their own living arrangements, and trying out occupational roles. A successful career woman of 35 may experience a sense of longing to have a child before the biological clock runs out. The businessman of 40 may begin to ask himself: "What have I accomplished?" "What has it cost me?" "What potentials or paths have I neglected in order to get where I am?"

Where development is stalled or distorted, there is generally an identifiable barrier to growth and task attainment. Work role efforts may be hampered by past experiences that impede successful resolution of issues such as industry and initiative. A positive identity and efforts to reach intimacy are influenced by body image, social skills and confidence. Experiences with illnesses, disability, disfiguring handicaps, or prejudice can present barriers to self-confidence and interpersonal relationships.

Generally stated, the activities of nurses in relation to adult development should be directed toward understanding developmental issues and tasks, educating and supporting clients according to their developmental needs, and identifying and influencing potential barriers to the attainment of developmental tasks. This chapter focuses on normal adult development and primary and secondary levels of prevention. Tertiary prevention is discussed in the chapters on behavioral and mental disorders.

PRIMARY PREVENTION □ Primary prevention emphasizes recognition and removal of potential hazards to healthy development and promotion of effective stress management and coping. Some types of nursing interventions include communication in a therapeutic relationship, client education and skill development relevant to maturational needs and adjustments, and environmental management of health care settings to eliminate artificial barriers to developmental needs. Crisis theory and intervention (Chapter 22) provide insights and strategies for assisting clients with developmentally related stressors.

Couple Relationships □ Young adults may have difficulty in working through the normal adjustments of living together in intimate relationships. There are issues of sexual values and practices, finances, life-styles, and degrees of closeness vs. privacy to be resolved. Long-standing single friendships must be readjusted in terms of the demands of the couple relationship. A wife may say "He can't stand my best friend so I only meet her for lunches now" or "His weekly night out with the boys drives me up the wall—they act like they're still in college!" Any or all of these issues may create tension and conflict. The nurse may assist by listening, by helping the client to iden-

---

TABLE 19-7 Nursing Diagnoses and Typical Problems in Adult Development

Communication, Impaired	Coping, Family
Marital conflicts	(Potential for growth)
Power conflicts	Healthy family seeking
Life-style conflicts	growth in response to transitions

Self-Concept Alteration	Coping, Ineffective
Unwanted pregnancy	(Family or individual)
Infertility	(Potential or actual)
Sexual difficulties	Unhealthy approaches to
Unhappy singlehood	dealing with stressors in opposite column

Role Alteration	Others Applicable
Separation/divorce	Potential for violence
Competency crisis	Stress
Career dissatisfaction	Social isolation
Adjusting to marriage and/or parenting	Grieving
	Knowledge deficit

Parenting, Alterations in
Parenting stresses
Inadequate knowledge of children's needs

Source: Adapted from Gordon, M. (1982). *Manual of Nursing Diagnosis.*

tify priority issues, and then to formulate strategies for communication and initiation of problem solving between the partners. It may be helpful for the couple to learn and practice active listening and conflict resolution strategies in order to enhance their problem-solving abilities.

Child Rearing □ Having children brings new problems as well as new joys. Parenting involves renegotiation of customary tasks as the demands of infants and growing children place new burdens on the time, energy, and resources of the parents. Values about discipline, scheduling activities, and parenting roles may differ since each parent was raised in a different family setting and now both must build a new family structure together. Various forms of parenting education and support can be helpful, including, for example, such things as recommending informational resources on child development and health and providing direct parent education to individuals, couples, or groups. Nurses also often offer telephone information services to new parents during their initial adaptation to the new baby. These 24-hour call-in lines provide answers and reassurance about immediate concerns. The nurse may refer parents to various community services for parent effectiveness training, talking-with-teens programs, and other services for families with school-age or adolescent children.

Lifestyle and Career Stressors □ Single adults may experience loneliness and a sense of isolation as peers pair off, marry, move into child-centered activities, or leave town. Special efforts may be needed to reexpand one's social circle by pursuing professional, leisure, and special-interest group activities. Career concerns may also be experienced around choice of occupation, job performance, co-worker relationships, competition, and competency. These concerns are shared by married and single adults. Stress is commonly identified in women who wish to combine career interests, marriage, and parenthood—and in the families of these women. Couples who may have been raised in families with traditional sex roles and values attempt, with varying degrees of success, to negotiate new roles and task assignments. The divorce rate attests to the fact that adjusting to marriage is not easy for most couples regardless of life-style or circumstances.

Additional stressors for young adults may include unplanned pregnancies and the decisions related to choosing among alternatives such as abortion, relinquishment for adoption, single parenting, or "forced" marriages. On the other hand, for the couple who want a child and cannot have one, infertility can be equally stressful. Because of the divorce rate, many families have additional complications to resolve such as second marriages and the need to form new blended families which must meet the needs of "his children," "her children," and "their children."

Middle-aged adults may be nearing peak years in career earnings and responsibilities or, on the other hand, may experience layoffs or cutbacks in employment and the spectre of age discrimination in starting over with a new company or a new career. Conflicts with the teenager may occur over issues of binding and letting go as the adolescent strives for identity and independence while the parent may seek to hold on to the more familiar and satisfying parent-child relationship. The parents must strike a balance by not setting the teenager adrift (premature and excessive freedom) and not clinging too tightly (thwarting growth) while acknowledging the normalcy of what can be a stormy phase in family life.

Chronic illnesses may begin to manifest themselves in middle age including cardiopulmonary problems, degenerative conditions, diabetes, and complications of long-standing alcohol abuse. In addition to family, career, and health concerns, the "generation in the middle" may have to assist aging parents with difficulties in managing their everyday lives, terminal illnesses, and/or the pain of being widowed.

The tasks of young and middle adulthood are demanding, since intimacy and generativity are the soul of one's being and encompass the hopes for a lasting contribution in the world. The nurse who works with these adult "activists" has an impact on many others through their family, work, and social networks. Health teaching, counseling, health care, and referral services have significant impact in primary prevention.

Strategies for Intervention □ Primary prevention approaches that may be of particular value pertain to the common adult concerns of communication, parenting, and stress adaptation. Several approaches are discussed briefly here (see Chapter 22 for detailed information relevant to crisis theory and intervention).

Improving Communication □ Depending on the type of communication problem, it may be appropriate to teach skills of active listening, conflict resolution, and/or assertiveness training. Active listening was developed by Thomas Gordon (1970) as a basic communication technique to improve the listening skills of parents and teachers. These strategies are also equally valuable in promoting listening among peers, spouses, and co-workers. The process relies on developing skills in: (1) nonverbal attending behaviors, such as taking the time to sit down and really listen carefully without formulating one's own responses while the other person is talking, and (2) observing the nonverbal aspects of the other's behavior. Additional skills are developed in paraphrasing, sharing nonverbal observations, clarifying, summarizing, and validating both the content and the feeling components of the message. Only if one has truly understood another's view is it possible to engage in valid problem-solving or conflict-resolution activities.

Conflict resolution requires that the people involved agree to meet and discuss the conflict. The discussion should start with a statement of the problem from the "initiator" with the "receiver" listening actively and validating his understanding of the problem as stated. He may ask for further clarification as needed. Next, the receiver presents his view of the problem and the initiator assumes the active listening role. Validation and clarification also follow this step. Completion of the preceding steps ensures that both parties have stated their position and been heard by each other. Now alternative solutions can be explored together. One person can ask for modifications in the other's behavior. Once the parties come to a decision about what steps will be taken, a follow-up discussion can be planned to evaluate the effectiveness of the plan and the level of satisfaction each person experiences with the new approach. This process has been referred to as a "fair fight" (Marriner, 1984, 184). Destructive strategies such as name calling, digging up old wounds, and sidetracking the discussion are ruled out.

Assertiveness training provides information on basic personal rights and helps participants distinguish between nonassertive, assertive, and overly aggressive behavior. Techniques of responsible, assertive communication are taught (e.g., "I messages") and role-modeled. Participants practice until the skills are developed in role play and peer evaluation sessions (Fensterheim and Baer, 1975).

Promoting Parenting Effectiveness □ Client teaching, support groups, and role supplementation may be effective interventions to improve parenting confidence and effectiveness. Teaching strategies for child growth and development include providing printed booklets appropriate to the child's age group, instruction and discussion, and media presentations. The nurse should evaluate the client's ability to understand and apply the content on an individual basis. Many support groups for parents emphasize education in parenting skills to prevent potential problems of neglect or abuse.

Role supplementation is an approach developed by Meleis (1975) that promotes role change adjustment. Role changes in individuals bring about corresponding changes in significant others. For instance, as the woman adopts the role of wife in the marriage relationship, expectations are communicated about the husband role, and vice versa. Role taking and role clarification are components of role supplementation. Strategies that have been found useful include role modeling by family and health professionals; the use of supportive groups, called reference groups, which permit exploration of feelings and experiences associated with the role; and role rehearsal through case study applications (Moorhead, 1985).

Stress Adaptation Support □ Techniques that foster effective coping by building up the health and adaptive capacity of the client include relaxation training, nutrition education, and exercise counseling. Crisis intervention strategies emphasize an active problem-solving approach which focuses on perception, informational needs, support systems, identification of feelings, and generating effective coping strategies. (See Chapters 22 and 23 on crisis and on mind-body relationships.)

SECONDARY PREVENTION □ Early identification and intervention with the groups at risk may minimize dysfunctional adjustments. The nurse in the hospital may identify problems of mother-infant attachment, parents who were abused as children, and adults with disabling, chronic, or disfiguring conditions likely to negatively influence self-esteem and interpersonal relationships. Special programs and follow-up in the community designed to provide active support and continuing assessment may be able to reduce the incidence of neglect, abuse, and depression in these target populations. The on-going assessment of these populations permits early referral into treatment should efforts to prevent abuse or depression, for instance, not be successful.

■ Enrichment Activities

DISCUSSION QUESTIONS

1. Discuss one topic, such as "Watergate," "nuclear disarmament," or "good parent" with a number of adults of both sexes, of different ages and socioeconomic backgrounds. First, identify the political, moral, religious, and personal philosophy or beliefs that influenced the comments of each of the adults. Secondly, identify the cognitive and personality characteristics that distinguish their answers from each other. Are there any similarities due to developmental stage?

2. Discuss the ethical issues involved in nursing assessment and intervention. What responsibilities does the nurse have in these professional activities?

3. Identify some current rituals. What rituals could be revived? What rituals could be created that would facilitate the mastery of adult developmental tasks?

LEARNING ACTIVITIES

1. Do a psychosocial assessment of yourself, being as honest as possible. Ask for feedback from a roommate or a close friend. What do the comparisons indicate? How would you feel if someone else knew this much about you? Does who that someone is make a difference?

2. Do a psychosocial assessment of someone you know well. How much do you know already about that person without consulting him/her? Next, collect the information that you need to complete the assessment. Evaluate the assessment and ask your friend for feedback. How would you feel if this person knew as much about you?

3. What role did personal development play in the lives of the theorists described in this chapter? Study the biographies of Buhler, Erikson, Neugarten, or others to gain an appreciation of the significant persons, events, decisions, and environments that correlate with their theories.

■ Recommended Readings

Goodman, Ellen. *Turning points: How people change through crisis and commitment.* New York: Doubleday, 1979. Newspaper columnist interviews people about personal crises, and their survival and growth. Ms. Goodman has a wonderful writing style, enjoyable to read.

Rubin, Jerry. *Growing (up) at 37.* New York: Warner Books, 1976. An account of adulthood from a former Yippie of the 1960s who is now a stockbroker. Gives a double perspective: young rebel and middle-aged conservative.

Sheehy, Gail. *Passages: Predictable crises for adult life.* New York: E.P. Dutton, 1974. A readable, popular, and less scholarly review of the stages than the Levinson and Gould studies. Sheehy focuses more on women than on men.

Ullman, Liv. *Changing.* New York: Alfred Knopf, 1977. Autobiography of a famous actress who is politically active. Many developmental themes and many well-known names.

■ References

Antonucci, T., and Jackson, J. Physical health and self esteem. *Family and community health,* 6, 2, 1983:1–9.

Buhler, C. The developmental structure of goal setting in group and individual studies. In *The course of human life* (Buhler, C. and Massarik F., eds.). New York: Springer, 1968.

Burnside, I.M.; Ebersole, P.; and Monea, H.E. (eds.). *Psychosocial caring throughout the life span.* New York: McGraw-Hill, 1979.

Chelune, G., and Waring, E. Nature and assessment of intimacy. In *Advances in psychological assessments,* vol. 6 (McReynolds, P., and Chelune, C., eds.). San Francisco: Jossey-Bass, 1984.

Clements, I. Stress adaptation. In *Family Health: A theoretical approach to nursing care* (Clements, I., and Roberts, F., eds.). New York: John Wiley & Sons, 1983.

Colarusso, C.A., and Nemiroff, R.A. *Adult development: A new dimension in psychodynamic theory and practice.* New York: Plenum Press, 1981.

Dodendorf, D.M. *DPAT: Dodendorf psychological assessment tool.* Manuscript, 1981.

Duvall, E. *Marriage and family development,* 5th ed. Philadelphia: J.B. Lippincott, 1977.

Erikson, E. *Childhood and society.* New York: Norton, 1950.

Feldman, H.S., and Lopez, M.A. *Developmental psychology for the health care professions: Part 2. Adulthood and aging.* Boulder: Westview Press, 1982.

Fensterheim, H., and Baer, J. *Don't say yes when you want to say no.* New York: Dell, 1975.

Gilligan, C. *In a different voice.* Cambridge: Harvard University Press, 1982.

Golan, N. *Passing through transitions.* New York: The Free Press, 1981.

Gordon, T. *Parent effectiveness training.* New York: New American Library, 1970.

Gould, R.L. *Transformations: Growth and change in adult life.* New York: Simon & Schuster, 1978.

Havighurst, R. *Human development and education.* New York: Longman, 1972.

Kohlberg, L.; Levine, C.; and Hewer, A. *Moral stages: A current formulation and a response to critics.* New York: Karger, 1983.

Lambert, V., and Lambert, C. *The impact of physical illness.* Englewood Cliffs, NJ: Prentice-Hall, 1979.

Levinson, D. *The seasons of a man's life.* New York: Ballantine Books, 1978.

Longo, D.C., and Williams, R.A. *Clinical practice in psychosocial nursing: Assessment and intervention.* New York: Appleton-Century-Crofts, 1978.

Marriner, A. *Guide to nursing management,* 2d ed. St. Louis, MO: Mosby Company, 1984.

Meleis, A. Role insufficiency and role supplementation. *Nursing research,* 24, 4, 1975:264–271.

Moorhead, S. (1985). Role supplementation. In *Nursing interventions: Treatments for nursing diagnoses.* (Bulechek, G. & McCloskey, J. eds.). Philadelphia: W.B. Saunders, 1985.

Morgan, A.J., and Moreno, J.W. *The practice of mental health nursing.* Philadelphia: J.B. Lippincott, 1973.

Neugarten, B. Adult personality: Toward a psychology of the life cycle. In *The human life cycle* (Sze, W.C., ed.). New York: Jason Aronson, 1975.

Newman, B., and Newman, P. *Development through life,* (3d ed.) Homewood, IL: Dorsey Press, 1984.

Scott, C.S. Young and middle adulthood. In *Medical applications of the behavioral sciences* (Braunstein and Toister, eds.). Chicago: Year Book Medical Pub., 1981.

Snyder, J., and Wilson, M. Elements of a psychological assessment. *American journal of nursing,* 77, 2, 1977:235–239.

Vaillant, G.E. *Adaptation to life.* Boston: Little, Brown & Co., 1977.

Van Gennep, A. *The rites of passage.* Chicago: University of Chicago Press, 1960.

Waller, W., and Hill, R. *The family: A dynamic interpretation.* New York: Holt, Rinehart & Winston, 1951.

Wolman, B.B. (ed.). *Handbook of developmental psychology.* Englewood Cliffs, NJ: Prentice-Hall, 1982.

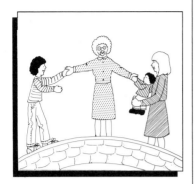

20

Aging

Linda R. Phillips

Learning Objectives

Upon completion of this chapter, the reader will be able to:

1. Describe the impact that selected characteristics of the aging population (e.g., life expectancy, living arrangements, marital status) have on the delivery of nursing and mental health services.

2. Describe the impact that social attitudes and interpersonal expectations have on the incidence and prevalence of mental health problems among the elderly.

3. Identify how the negative views of health professionals toward the elderly have influenced definitions of mental health, diagnosis, and treatment of mental health problems, and the provision of supportive or preventive mental health services.

4. Describe the relationship between intrapersonal changes of aging (e.g., changes in cognition, learning, personality, and sensory-perception) and the mental status of elderly individuals.

5. Identify the general guidelines applicable for assessing the mental health status of elderly clients.

6. Do a nursing assessment of the mental health status of an elderly client that includes consideration of (a) self-presentation, (b) presenting symptoms, (c) historical and cultural influences, (d) behavioral and functional abilities, (e) physical status, (f) environmental influences, and (g) psychosocial status.

7. Plan a program for primary prevention of mental health problems for an elderly client using knowledge of the principles of anticipatory guidance.

8. Plan a program of secondary prevention of mental health problems for an elderly client using selected nursing intervention techniques.

9. Describe the three levels of evaluation appropriate in planning and delivering mental health services to the elderly.

The elderly constitute one of the most visible and challenging minorities served by health professionals in the United States. Although, according to the 1980 census (Statistical Life Bulletin, 1981), individuals over age 65 constitute only about 11.3 percent of the total population, it is difficult for health professionals in any specialty to avoid contact with this group. Despite their relatively small numbers, the elderly use most of the services in acute care facilities, long-term care facilities, public health and home health agencies, and ambulatory care settings. Elderly clients are frequent care recipients in critical care units, psychiatric inpatient units, and community mental health centers. Contact between health professionals and elderly individuals occurs even in settings that seem remote to a geriatric population such as pediatric and maternity units, as the elderly frequently serve as significant others for clients in these areas. Therefore, whether the nurse claims to have primary interest in caring for the elderly or not, virtually every nurse in the United States spends some portion of time in contact with elderly people. Knowledge about the needs and concerns of this group is essential.

Viewed from one perspective, there is nothing unique about growing old. Nothing happens to an individual between the ages of 64 and 66 that is magical. Aging is a universal human experience which begins at the time of conception. It is continual, irreversible, and inevitable. Adding chronological years does not create an automatic risk to either physical or mental health. Aging does not necessarily jeopardize autonomy, personal worth, self-determination, or ego integrity. In truth, the aging process, whether viewed as the slice of time between 20 and 30 years of age or the slice of time between 70 and 80 years of age, is essential for personal growth, personality de-velopment, self-actualization, and the acquisition of coping skills and knowledge. A person at age 80 is no different from a person at age 20. He is first, an individual; second, a person of worth and integrity; third, a person with strengths and weaknesses, joys, and problems; and last, a person who happens to have lived for 80 years.

Viewed from another perspective, however, there are some unique features associated with the later years just as there are unique features associated with being a teenager or a young adult. Some of these are related to the normal physiological and psychological events associated with biological aging, some are related to pathological processes that are more prevalent among elders than among younger individuals, some are related to the social conditions that impact aging in our society, and some are related to the developmental tasks that arise as an individual plans for the end of his life and views the termination of life among those he loves. As a result of these unique features, promoting mental health among elderly clients requires specialized skills and strategies that are similar to but different from the skills required for other age groups.

The purpose of this chapter is to explore some of the factors related to understanding, assessing, and promoting mental health among elderly clients. Consideration will be given to developing background information about aging that relates to our conceptions of mental health. The areas to be explored include: (1) characteristics of the elderly in America; (2) the impact of the community on the aging individual; and (3) intrapersonal changes of aging and their relationship to mental health. Assessment parameters, areas of problems and needs, intervention strategies, and evaluation methods that are appropriate for promoting mental health among an aging population will be given.

☐ *Characteristics of the Aged in America*

DEMOGRAPHIC CHARACTERISTICS

There is an old saying: "A person has essentially two choices; either to grow old or to die young." Every year, more and more individuals take the first option as witnessed by the fact that currently there are 25.5 million individuals over the age of 65 years among the total 226.5 million American citizens (Statistical Life Bulletin, 1981). Life expectancy in the United States has been slowly but steadily increasing over the past years. A male child born in 1980 can expect to live 69.4 years, and a female child born in 1980 can expect to live 77.2 years (Statistical Life Bulletin, 1980). Of the 25.5 million elderly in the United States, 15.2 million are females and 10.3 million are males (Statistical Life Bulletin, 1981).

To this point the elderly have been roughly defined as all individuals over the age of 65 years. To speak of them in this manner is misleading because it implies that all individuals over 65 years of age belong to one homogeneous group and consequently are all quite similar. To compare a 70-year-old with a 90-year-old and assume they are the same is as ridiculous as comparing a 15-year-old with a 35-year-old and assuming they are the same. To deal with this problem the total elderly population is usually divided into rather arbitrary categories for the purpose of discussion, for example, the "young-old" or those between 65 and 79 years of age, and the "old-old" or those who are 80 years old or older.

There are some striking differences between the young-old and the old-old population. The young-old constitute a group that generally requires less in terms of physical, mental, and supportive health care services. On the other hand, old-old individuals tend to have quantitatively more health problems and require more of the health care system. In 1980, old-old women outnumbered old-old men by 2 to 1 while young-old women outnumbered young-old men by 3 to 2 (Statistical Life Bulletin, 1981).

Equally significant to health care delivery and assessment of the elderly as the number of older individuals requiring services are some of the other characteristics of the elderly population. About one-half of the men who survive to 85 years of age are married and about three-quarters of those men are still married to their first wives. About one-half of the women who live to be 70 are married and about three-fifths of those women are still married to their first husbands. Before the last few years, marriage, remarriage, and divorce were rare among the elderly. In 1975, for example, only 1 percent of all brides and 2 percent of all grooms were 65 years of age or older (Glick, 1979).

SOCIAL CHARACTERISTICS

Although the most common living arrangement for individuals over the age of 65 is to be married and to live with a spouse in a single-family house or apartment, that is by no means the only living arrangement represented. About 15 percent of all elderly men live alone with the percentage increasing to 35 percent by age 85, and 43 percent of all elderly women live alone with the percentage remaining fairly stable across the age span. Four percent of the men and 6 percent of the women over the age of 65 live in an institutional setting (including rest homes, long-term care facilities, room-and-board facilities, and mental institutions) (Glick, 1979). Although the chances of being institutionalized increase with increasing age, only 14 percent of the men and 27 percent of the women over 85 reside in institutional settings. Another living arrangement for the elderly is living with someone else such as children, other relatives, or friends. In 1975, 7.4 percent of all elderly men and 22.8 percent of all elderly women lived with someone else. Although there has been a slow but steady decline in the numbers of elderly people who live with kin in the past 50 years, significantly more elderly in all age groups live with their kin than are institutionalized (Mindel, 1979). Alternative living arrangements, such as living with friends of the same or opposite sex, individuals living with paid "live-ins," and group living situations, although not unheard of among the elderly, are fairly uncommon.

So that the wrong impression is not conveyed, more needs to be said about the living alone phenomenon among the elderly. In our society, there has been a myth perpetuated that we used to take much better care of our elderly. In the good old days, Grandma, Granddad, Mom, Dad, and the kids all lived together so that when grandparents were old, they had someone to care for them. Not only does this myth generate guilt among adult children and contribute to strongly judgmental attitudes toward them, but a number of fallacies are associated with it. First, we never took any better care of the elderly in our society than we do right now. Historical researchers have documented that the three-generation family never existed in America on any large scale (Mindel, 1979). With the limited life expectancy of yesteryear, an elder who survived much beyond his own child rearing was quite rare. As a result, the care of large numbers of elderly in American is a new problem. There are no rules that we can rely on to solve the problems, and there are essentially no real role models who can teach us how elderly people should be cared for.

A second fallacy associated with the myth is that just because an elderly person lives alone, he is necessarily isolated from his family or his social supports. As a matter of fact, despite our current geographic mobility, a large number of elderly people who live alone maintain a residence that is in close proximity to children and siblings. Elderly people who relocate to be close to their children are not at all unusual (Glick, 1979), but regardless of where they live, they and their families tend to maintain regular and close contact. Due to the widespread use of the long-distance telephone, even when families live far from an elderly member, the communication among them is probably better than was ever possible before.

The myth's third fallacy is that the situation of most elderly people who live alone represents abandonment by their families. This is simply not the case. Most elderly individuals value their independence, and when they feel they have a choice, prefer to maintain their own residences (Mindel, 1979). Second, if children were truly abandoning their elderly relatives, then as soon as elderly people became disabled they would be institutionalized by their families. This is not true. Several surveys, for example, Shanas (1979) and Brody, et al. (1978) have shown that there are large numbers of elderly living in the community who have severe functional impairments and multiple health problems. Not only are the needs of many of the community-dwelling elderly intense, but the number of ill and frail elderly living in the community is about two times the total number residing in institutions at any time. Finally, if the elderly were truly abandoned by their children, the family would not provide a significant amount of support to the elderly at home. Contrary to this view, aging and the problems that are sometimes associated with aging in our society remain a family affair. The bulk of the home health services provided in this country to the aged and chronically ill comes from family members (Brody, et al., 1978). If an ill elderly person is married and his spouse is well, the spouse is

the major source of help and support. The relatives, however, tend to step in and help as soon as the spouse is unavailable. Although both sons and daughters help with the care of elderly parents, the bulk of the responsibility for care falls to daughters (daughters-in-law) regardless of their employment status and other family responsibilities. The amount of help that a daughter provides increases sharply with the increasing age of the parent (Lang and Brody, 1980), which is particularly important when one considers that as the parent ages, so does the daughter. Many daughters who are in the young-old category themselves are currently providing intense, time-consuming services for their old-old parents, many with the support and concern of their own middle-aged daughters (Brody, 1981).

To summarize, the elderly are a nonhomogeneous minority group whose number is growing. A number of major characteristics of the group have been identified in this discussion, several of which relate to the relationship between the elderly and their major sources of help and support. The aging person is not an island. Aging does not occur separately from other people and other events; it is a social phenomenon. The social nature of aging impacts both the views and expectations that the elderly person has for himself and those that others hold for him.

■ *Point of Emphasis*

The social forces surrounding the aging process are powerful enough to shape and alter (1) the behaviors that elderly people display, (2) the ways their behaviors are viewed by others, and (3) the feelings elderly people have about themselves and others—in short their mental health.

The next topic to be explored, therefore, is the impact that society-at-large has on the elderly person and the ways in which this impact affects the elderly person and his mental health status.

☐ The Impact of the Community on the Aged Person

SOCIAL VIEW OF AGING AS PERSONAL DECLINE

In our society, aging is predominantly viewed as a time of personal decline. Most health professionals and lay persons believe that individuals reach a peak of personal growth and potency during the middle adult years and then experience physiological, psychological, and sociological deterioration during the later aging process, which eventually leads to death. Aging is commonly seen as an endpoint and not as a life goal.

In the past 25 years, researchers and practitioners who deal with aging have in a number of ways supported the position of aging as personal decline. For example, a great deal of time, effort, and money has been devoted to describing the ways in which the elderly are psychologically and physiologically different, thus setting them apart from the rest of us. Much research has concentrated on the liabilities and problems associated with aging, and little has focused on the ways in which elderly people contribute to society and experience personal growth and satisfaction. In many ways, the view of aging as personal decline has been perpetuated by such fields as geriatric medicine, gero-psychiatry, social gerontology, and geriatric nursing—because their emphasis is on the differences and the problems of the elderly and not on the positive attributes and strengths of elderly people. Although the practitioners in these fields would deny having a negative approach to aging, by virtue of their focus, aging is seen as a disease and intervention is seen as the process of correcting defects. In practice, the positive aspects of aging and the growth potentials of aging people are rarely emphasized, even by those working in the fields of aging (Levine and Levine, 1980).

On the one hand, the concept of aging as personal decline is partially truthful and has served some useful purposes. There are physiological and psychological changes that occur with aging that cannot be ignored. Some of these changes affect the ways in which elderly people are able to function, particularly in society as it is currently structured. Despite controversy that rages over the appropriate definition of mental health among the elderly and the difficulty with identifying the causes of mental problems among the elderly, there is evidence that a sizable proportion of this population experiences some form of emotional distress at some time during the aging process. In fact, problems may be more frequent with advancing age in our society. There are estimates that between 12 and 40 percent of all people 65 years or older experience psychological difficulties (Reifler and Eisdorfer, 1980). The incidence of functional mental disorders such as depression and paranoid states seems to be disproportion-

ately high among the elderly (Butler, 1975; Pardes, 1981) and approximately 25 percent of all suicides occur in the over-65 population (Butler and Lewis, 1982). It is estimated that up to 60 percent of the elderly in long-term care settings have some form of emotional distress that interferes with their daily functioning (Burnside, 1978). Because of the work done in geriatric medicine, gero-psychiatry, social gerontology, and geriatric nursing, there is a greater awareness of the ways in which those elderly who experience difficulties can be helped.

On the other hand, the view of aging as personal decline is untrue and has served to insidiously perpetuate stereotypes of all elderly people as incompetent, ineffective, dependent, and in need of protection. As a result, the elderly are pervasively seen as victims of their own biology, trapped by social and economic problems and by inevitable, untreatable, and chronic physical and mental ailments that make them more and more vulnerable with advancing age. (It is interesting that treatment of women and blacks has been similarly justified in the past because they were seen as victims of their own biology.) Although there are physiological and psychological changes and sociological losses associated with the later stages of aging (just as there are with the stages of aging throughout the life span), not every elderly person is affected in the same way or to the same degree. Most elderly people adapt to the changes and cope with the losses with a minimum of interference to their daily lives. As a matter of fact, the majority of elderly people are functioning in the community without the assistance of either health professionals or supportive services. In addition, the relationship between the individual and society is delicate and intimate; figures about the incidence of mental problems among the elderly do not, in any way, consider that relationship. There is no way of knowing, from our current research, the degree to which some elderly people "fail" because they internalize the view of aging as personal decline. There is also no way of knowing if decline could be prevented and if more elderly people would experience success in their later years if society were structured in a way that supported rather than complicated the normal changes of aging. As Levine and Levine (1980) note:

> Clearly we cannot wish away that decline which accompanies aging—some physical and psychological capacities do deteriorate. However, at what rate would they decline if the treatment of old age in our society were different? How could the struc-

ture of our society be changed so that it minimized the consequences of these losses? What gains in capacity with advancing years are masked by the generalized expectations of losses and what losses are imagined where they do not exist?

All of these are questions that we have not begun to address.

SOCIAL BREAKDOWN MODEL

Of all the theories of aging that have been used to explain the behaviors of elderly people, one of the most useful in describing the relationship of society to individual behavior is the Social Breakdown Model proposed by Kuypers and Bengtson (1973). Specifically stressed in this model is the idea that the societal view of aging as personal decline is internalized by the elderly person and leads to the individual experiencing both segregation from society which results in declining function and competency, and declining competency and functioning as a result of self-labeling. A cycle is established in which the elderly person's expectations are positively reinforced by those around him in the form of behaviors directed at "taking over for him" and "protecting him" and by the inevitable losses that are a part of every individual's development at whatever age. A negative pattern is established in which personal gains and autonomous functions become masked by the overwhelming and pervasive negativity surrounding the aging experience.

From this perspective, the behaviors displayed by an individual elderly person can be viewed as a response to strong social forces that ultimately determine the elderly person's view of his own well-being and mental health and other people's view of the elderly person's competency and mental health. Physical and mental failings become sanctioned, supported, self-fulfilling prophecies.

EFFECT OF STEREOTYPES ON HEALTH PROFESSIONALS

Health professionals, of course, have not been immune to stereotypes and negative images of the elderly. These images affect (1) the ways in which elderly people are perceived and assessed by health professionals; (2) the ways in which health services are delivered to the elderly population; (3) the types of health care services that are available to elderly people; and (4) the degree to which the health care system is accessible to the elderly consumer. This impact has been particularly pronounced in the area of mental health services. Until recently, the psychoanalytic tradition of delivering mental health services has predominated in our society along with its assertion that people over the age of 50 are unable to change and therefore are not amenable to treatment (Freud, 1949; Butler, 1975).

The impact of the societal image of aging on the provision of mental health services to the elderly has been evidenced in a number of ways. First, a disproportionate number of emotional and functional difficulties of elderly clients are tagged as being caused by senility or organic brain syndrome thus placing them outside of the realm of treatment. Individuals with these so-called diagnoses are usually dumped out of the health care system and are as a result offered custodial rather than restorative or rehabilitative services. The probabilities of physical illness or treatable mental illnesses are often overlooked as diagnoses after an individual has attained the age of 65. Second, community mental health services and outpatient treatment facilities have been repeatedly found to be wanting in the services they provide to the elderly (Reifles and Eisdorfer, 1980; Burnside, 1978). Only about 2 percent of the patients served by community mental health centers are over the age of 65 (Pardes, 1981). Third, as a whole, the psychiatric community has been unwilling to explore treatment alternatives tailored to the needs of the elderly, insisting that clients in every age group adhere to the same set of treatment rules. For example, many mental health workers have been unwilling to make home visits to the homebound elderly, insisting that this population come into the clinical setting for services.

The societal image of aging has had an impact on the distribution of funding to pay for mental health services and on the focus of the treatment provided. Health care providers have failed to lobby effectively to affect the reimbursement available to the elderly for mental health services. Medicare, for example, severely limits the amount reimbursable for outpatient mental health services (Pardes, 1981). In addition, the focus of reimbursable services for third-party payers in this country is on crisis and disease. To be eligible for reimbursable service, the individual must have a documentable mental illness with a certifiable diagnosis. No monies are provided for either support or prevention. As a result, the mental health services provided to the elderly tend to be episodic and palliative. There is no way of estimating how common depression, paranoid states, or suicide would be among the elderly if time and money were devoted to prevention rather than disease.

The societal image of aging has affected even the distribution of manpower available to provide care for the elderly. The number of professionals providing health care and mental health services to the elderly is sadly disproportionate to either the numbers of elderly people or to the needs of this group. For example, despite estimates that 60 percent of the elderly in long-term care facilities experience mental health problems, the client-to-professional nurse ratio in those settings is quite low, and lower still is the client-to-social worker ratio and the client-to-psychiatrist/psychologist ratio. In comparison to the total number of elderly living in the community and the numbers of health care providers specializing in their care, the ratios are just as dire (Lansley and Robinowitz, 1979). The needs and concerns of the elderly population have been devalued in our society just as those providing care to the elderly have been accorded low prestige, low status, and low salaries among health professionals.

DEFINITIONS OF MENTAL HEALTH AND THE ELDERLY

The view of aging as personal decline has had a tremendous impact on the way mental health has been defined for the elderly population and on the ways in which assessment and diagnosis of mental health problems have been done. With few exceptions, mental health has been considered to be a single concept, measurable by one set of criteria. Definitions of mental health have focused on the "principle of primacy" (Birren and Renner, 1981)—which asserts that the events of early life have greater cognitive and emotional impact on an individual than events occurring during any other slice of time. This principle has been used to rationalize the idea that mental health is mental health regardless of the individual's age and that it can be appropriately defined for all age groups based on observations of the behavior and coping patterns of young adults. There has been a tremendous void in serious studies or observations of matured adults. Studies of the emotional well-being of healthy elders have been almost nonexistent. There has been little success in establishing a definition of mental health in terms of unequivocal observable, behavioral indicators. Although this is true for all age groups, the problem is most acute for the elderly population because few people have a clear picture of what "mentally healthy aging" looks like apart from how they conceive of "mentally healthy middle-aging" among middle-class adults (most particularly among men).

Birren and Renner (1981) state that definitions of mental health have most commonly been based on two concepts: (1) normalcy and (2) lack of distress. Both of these present problems, particularly among the elderly population. Normalcy, for example, reflects a statistical concept that indicates the most frequently expressed feelings or behaviors of the majority of individuals. It does not address the enormous diversity among people or the behaviors and feelings that are outside of the range for the majority but nevertheless belong to the normal distribution. Normalcy also implies conformity (an expectation commonly held for elderly people in the health care system) and reflects little regard for situational or cultural variables that impinge on the individual. Depending on the situation, conformity, itself, may be a reflection of "abnormalcy" more than of "normalcy." In addition, the concept of normalcy carries with it certain value judgments that reflect what the majority of individuals in a given society consider to be "normal" (Birren and Renner, 1981).

The concept of lack of distress in some ways is more useful as a definition of mental health than some others but even it has its limitations. Distress is often situationally determined and justifiably felt. The world as experienced by many elderly people *is* distressing. Society does not make it easy to be distress-free during the later stages of the life span. As the saying goes, "Just because I'm paranoid doesn't mean they're *not* out to get me." For an elderly person, feelings of righteous distress may predominate over the individual's affective tone and there still may be no compromise to the individual's overall positive view of self, acceptance of self, life satisfaction, or success at *being*, each of which, according to Birren and Renner (1981), may be more reflective of mental health among the elderly than the presence or absence of distress. Likewise, the elderly individual may even experience a compromise in the sense of worth and integrity along with the distress, but following multiple and continual assaults from society and little preparation and support for aging, isn't that reaction more "normal" than any other?

To summarize, a large number of individuals

do experience mental health problems in their later years. When aging is set within the context of the social forces surrounding the aging process, however, it becomes clear that mental health problems are probably not an inherent property of aging.

■ *Point of Emphasis*

Mental health problems among the elderly may represent the results of aging within a social context that is less than supportive to the needs of this portion of society.

The elderly, as a group, receive less support for their problems than do individuals in other age groups, they receive fewer services from fewer well-qualified professionals, and they have less access to the mental health care system. The services they do receive tend to be episodic and crisis-focused, and elements of prevention and rehabilitation are frequently absent. In addition, the social images of aging have influenced our definitions of mental health and mental illness among the elderly.

Social images are not the only variables that influence mental health. Certain intrapersonal variables also have an influence on the ways in which individuals feel about themselves and the ways in which they interact with the human and nonhuman environment. The next section of this chapter will explore some of the key intrapersonal variables that impact the mental health status of the aging individual.

☐ *Intrapersonal Changes of the Later Years and Mental Health*

Growth and development is characterized by changes that occur in an individual's behavior, outward appearance, and perceptual abilities. From birth to death, individuals experience physiological and psychological changes that affect communication, interaction, cognition, and mentation. Since these intrapersonal changes are often used to establish normative expectations for how well an individual will be able to function and perform socially, they become indicators of mental health status for all age groups. Unfor-

tunately, because views of the elderly have been complicated by negativity, myths, and stereotypes and because, until recently, the growth and development literature has focused on the young and middle-aged, the intrapersonal changes experienced by the elderly have tended not to be considered as essential to either growth or development. In addition, researchers and practitioners have had a continuing problem in determining which changes of the later years are the normal result of increasing age and which occur as a result of pathological processes that sometimes complicate aging. This section will explore some of the current beliefs about the developmental intrapersonal changes experienced by old adults and the effect of these on mental health. The areas to be considered include: (1) cognition, psychomotor function, and learning, (2) personality, and (3) sensory-perceptual function, since these most directly impact the assessments we make of an elderly person's interpersonal, mental, and emotional competency.

COGNITIVE ABILITIES

Cognitive abilities among the elderly have received a great deal of attention by gerontologists in the past years. Despite the persistence of widespread stereotypes about the developmental changes of aging that make an individual less able to think and learn, many of the research findings contradict previously held beliefs.

INTELLIGENCE

Substantial evidence suggests that intelligence (particularly verbal intelligence) is not affected by aging. Although discrepancies can be found between the test scores of younger and older individuals, there are many variables that affect the performance on intelligence tests that do not have an effect on the individual's actual intelligence. For example, the older person usually has more anxiety in testing situations, less test-taking experience, and less interest in the test material than do younger subjects who have been raised in an environment that has stressed the importance of test taking. Older subjects are more likely to see the complexities in situations than are younger people and therefore have more difficulty making definitive choices about the right answers on a test. In addition, factors commonly not considered in interpreting tests of intelligence are the individual's overall health status at the time of testing and his current life experiences. Poor health and current life stress do affect intelligence test scores and are likely to affect older subjects more frequently than younger ones. Despite these problems, when longitudinal studies (those that test the same individual repeatedly over time and use the person's own scores as the basis for individual comparisons) are conducted, the results demonstrate that people tend to retain their intelligence over their entire life span, and the effects of aging are minimal (Ebersole and Hess, 1981; Butler and Lewis, 1982).

PSYCHOMOTOR FUNCTION

Developmentally, there is a general slowing of psychomotor function with advancing age. Older people require more time to respond physically to a situation, and the speed of response is particularly slowed if the task requires fine movements, fine coordination, or is timed. The speed with which an individual responds is complicated by a couple of factors. For example, elderly individuals usually display generalized muscle weakness that may be the result of disuse atrophy more than of neuromuscular deterioration. Elderly individuals also tend to display more caution and less risk taking with advancing age, and may be slower because of the need to be more sure of a "correct" response. Both of these may affect the speed of reaction but may not necessarily reflect psychomotor deterioration (Forbes and Fitzsimmons, 1981).

LEARNING

Under the umbrella of learning are a number of related concepts that affect the elderly individual's ability to process new information. These include memory, problem-solving abilities, and cognitive styles. While long-term memory is probably not affected by the aging process, there is evidence suggesting that older people do experience some decline in short-term memory. This decline is termed "benign senescent forgetfulness"—a complicated concept since any number of young people are just as forgetful as their older counterparts but discuss their forgetfulness less. It is actually very difficult to determine whether healthy older individuals are more forgetful than they once were or whether they simply concentrate more on their forgetfulness and worry about it more than they did when they were younger. Some authors

have suggested that older people are forgetful because they have quantitatively more information to process, more stress and worry, and more memories to sift through than do the young whose memory stores are relatively empty. Older individuals may be more selective about the information they choose to remember, with the choice being based on the relevance of the information to the individual's need state. Many elderly people find benign senescent forgetfulness to be very anxiety-producing, despite its lack of pathological significance.

Problem-solving abilities probably do not decline with age. In fact, as Forbes and Fitzsimmons (1981) note, the elderly most likely have a decided advantage over the young in problem-solving situations that require a reliance on past experience. Solving new problems that have no relationship to past experiences, however, may be as difficult for the old as it is for the young. Some authors feel that solving new problems may be even more difficult for the old, based on some recent research in the areas of cognitive style. An individual's cognitive style is related to two types of intelligence: crystallized and fluid. Fluid intelligence arises from the nondominant hemisphere of the brain and is usually associated with innovation and creative problem solving. Artistic expression and putting abstract concepts together in new ways are examples of the types of thinking associated with the use of fluid intelligence. Crystallized intelligence arises from the dominant hemisphere of the brain and is associated with rote learning, logical problem solving, and drawing on past experiences in new situations. Examples of the use of crystallized intelligence include application of the scientific method and of nursing process. The use of crystallized intelligence is constantly reinforced in our society through the educational system and emphasis on logical thinking. Conversely, there are few sanctioned opportunities provided for individuals to expand and refine their use of fluid intelligence in our society. As a result, many authors feel that the ability to use fluid intelligence begins to decline during adolescence (Ebersole and Hess, 1981). Crystallized intelligence tends to predominate among the elderly, which means that it may be more difficult for some elderly people to problem-solve and learn if they have no experience to draw on for help. Although the capacity to problem-solve and learn remains undiminished throughout the life span, the ways in which the elderly learn may be quite different from the ways used by the young.

PERSONALITY

Any number of myths are associated with defining the "aged personality." The elderly are believed to be more resistant to change and more rigid, more conservative, more quarrelsome, more hypochondriacal, more passive and dependent, more withdrawn, and more tranquil either than the young or than they once were. None of these is true.

> ### ■ Point of Emphasis
>
> *There actually is no such thing as a personality structure that can be attributed to the elderly any more than there is a single personality structure common to middle-aged people.*

Each elderly individual is a unique composite of personality characteristics formulated over a lifetime of experience. Throughout the years, an individual carries a developing, growing, and unique way of interacting, coping, and using defense mechanisms that he has found to be successful.

There are, however, certain common socialization experiences that most elderly people are exposed to during their lifetime that may have an effect on their observable behavior and may reflect the direction of personality development in later years. For example, from reviewing empirical data, Palmore (1979) suggests that, as a group, the elderly tend to be more politically active, more law abiding, and more altruistic in volunteering their time and money than are younger people. He also observes that the elderly tend to be more dependable and more vigilant and therefore make better and more reliable workers than do young people. Hayer (1976) states that the elderly tend to have more stable value systems, put more emphasis on the value of life, display less pretense, and demonstrate more wisdom and better judgment than the young. In many ways, elderly people tend to be released from the "shoulds" of society and are, as a result, freer to express their personalities honestly and openly. Many elderly are simply more certain about and more willing to express what they believe to be true than the young.

Butler and Lewis have identified some features of the lifelong personality structure that are more adaptive in later years than are some other characteristics. These include a "sense of self-es-

teem, candor, the ability to relate easily with others, independence and self-motivation, and a sense of usefulness" (1982, 204). Defense mechanisms that have been identified as being particularly adaptive in later years include insight, denial, the use of activity, and the use of humor. Defense mechanisms that are seen as maladaptive among younger people which may be quite useful to the aging individual in view of the ways in which our society deals with the elderly include (1) obsessive-compulsive personality traits which may help the individual late in life to fill empty hours and to structure his world in a consistent, comfortable manner; (2) schizoid mechanisms which may help "insulate" the individual from loneliness and isolation; and (3) dependent personality traits which may help the individual accept the help of others if and when he is unable to care for himself. Projection is a particularly maladaptive defense mechanism when carried into the later years.

SENSORY-PERCEPTUAL CHANGES OF AGING

Virtually every sensory ability is affected in some way by the aging process. The major sensory changes of aging are outlined in Table 20-1 as is their effect on perceptual function. Individual assessment, however, is required to determine the degree to which any aging person is impaired by the changes he experiences.

An individual's sensory-perceptual functioning is extremely important to his mental competency and mental status. There is a direct, reciprocal relationship between the degree to which an individual is able to perceive and interpret his environment and the degree to which he is able to interact successfully and competently. In addition, decreased sensory function can produce reversible confusional states among the elderly and can lead to the misdiagnosis of the irreversible confusional states (Wolanin and Phillips, 1981). Many studies have shown the importance of this information to mental health assessments of the elderly. H. Weinberg (1975) and Snyder et al. (1976) demonstrated a relationship between decreased vision and decreased mental competency. As early as 1928, Greenwood showed a relationship between eye patching of the elderly and bizarre behavioral manifestations and "mental symptoms." Hearing loss has been associated with apathy, sleep disturbances, anxiety, insecurity,

TABLE 20-1 Sensory Changes of Aging and Effects on Perceptual Function[a]

Sensory Changes	Effects on Function
Visual Apparatus	
Hypertrophy of corneal cells and flattening of endothelial cells	Light transmission decreases, need for more external light to produce image on retina, distortion of sight (astigmatism)
Decreased opacity of sclera	Image "wash out," more striking color contrasts required
Increased number of "floaters"	Black spots perceived in visual field
Loss of accommodation in the lens	Presbyopia or loss of near vision
Lens becomes thicker and protein pigments accumulate in lens	Alteration in color vision particularly for shades of brown, beige, and blue
"Yellowing of the lens"	Bright reds and yellows are seen best; senile cataracts
Arterial and venous occlusions in blood vessels	Loss of some portions of the visual field (senile macular degeneration)
Size of pupil decreases and diameter narrows (senile miosis)	Decreased light reaching retina, more time required to accommodate for light-to-dark changes
Changes in exterior orbital structures, decrease in tear formation	Chronic irritation of cornea and conjuctiva, dryness and discomfort
Outward deviation of eyeball (exotropia), loss of orbital fat pad, and ptosis	Mechanical changes in field of vision
Obstruction of nasolacrimal ducts	Excessive watering of the eye Distortion of vision
Auditory Apparatus	
Presbycusis	Progressive loss of hearing in the higher frequencies, loss of sound discrimination usually manifested by ability to hear but not to understand (phonemic regression) and inability to separate background noise from other sounds
Tactile and Proprioceptive Apparatus	
Mild to moderate loss of sensation appearing earliest and most evenly in feet, legs, and end of spine	Generalized somesthesia in affected area
Decreased vibratory sense and localization sense, pattern is caudocephaled with face dominant over hand, and thigh dominant over foot	Difficulty perceiving being touched in two spots at the same time
Decreased temperature sense	Difficulty recognizing temperature extremes both for locally applied heat and for cold and ambient temperatures
Decreased pain sensitivity	Requires less pain medication, difficulty responding to dangerous or painful stimuli
Decreased position sense	Some difficulty determining the placement of lower extremities
Olfactory and Gustatory Apparatus	
Decreased number of taste buds and decreased sensitivity of those remaining	Difficulty determining the differences in tastes, need more seasoning to keep food from tasting flat
Decreased olfactory reception	Difficulty determining the differences in odors, need more stimulation to recognize odors

[a] Adapted from Phillips, 1981.

399

and physical complaints (Ramsdell, 1970). Perron (1974) demonstrated a relationship between hearing loss and anger, erratic behavior, and acting-out behavior among the elderly.

Interference with mental function becomes even more severe when a person has multiple sensory impairments. Eisdorfer (1960), Weiss (1965), and O'Neil and Calhoun (1975) demonstrated a relationship between lower scores on mental status tests and overall compromised sensory functioning. Ziskind (1960) documented a relationship among hearing loss, the ability to communicate in the dominant language of the culture, and the appearance of "mental symptoms" among elderly people who had cataracts. When any elderly person has difficulty seeing and hearing and when these sensory losses are complicated by a language problem, the likelihood that the person will display or experience mental symptoms such as delusions, paranoia, illusions is increased manyfold.

Another complicating factor in sensory loss among the elderly and the appearance of mental symptoms is the effect of the environment and the amount and type of sensory input available within the environmental setting. Elderly individuals, like the young, can experience mental effects as a result of sensory underload (deprivation), sensory alteration, monotonous sensory input, and sensory overload. The effects of these states can include delusions, hallucinations, irritability, restlessness, anxiety, panic, emotional lability, and an inability to concentrate or problem-solve (Wolanin and Phillips, 1981). These effects are particularly severe when the elderly person has a sensory loss and suddenly finds himself in an environment that is new or different; an environment in which either the elderly person's usual orienting cues are missing or one in which it is difficult for him to determine the pattern and meaning in the setting.

To summarize, as we age each of us experiences intrapersonal changes which have an influence on our behavior and social interaction. The amount of change experienced by a person, however, is not predictable. In order to determine the unique way that each individual compares to the expected norms and to identify the specific ways in which nursing intervention will be most effective individually, a detailed assessment is necessary. The next section will therefore identify the major areas of consideration in conducting a mental health assessment for an elderly client.

□ *ASSESSMENT*

Mental illness and mental health among the elderly are intimately related to the individual's ability to function successfully in the environment, to communicate effectively and maintain social ties, and to maintain a stable, optimal level of physical health. Among the elderly, the mental health status cannot be separated from the individual's physical well-being or from insidious signs of physical illness that are manifest in the form of "mental symptoms." A complete mental health assessment, therefore, whether for the purpose of promoting a mentally healthy state or for identifying specific mental health problems, must include physical and environmental considerations along with the assessment of the overall presentation of self, historical and cultural influences, behavioral and functional abilities, and psychosocial dimensions.

GENERAL GUIDELINES □ Before considering each area of the mental health assessment in detail, there are several general guidelines for assessing the elderly that should be discussed. One key issue is the need to demonstrate genuine concern, consideration, and respect for the elderly individual. Respect for an elderly client as an important, unique, and worthy human being can be demonstrated in a number of ways.

1. Listen actively and attentively and give undivided attention.
2. Allow sufficient time for interaction—the elderly are generally slower in the speed with which they formulate responses to questions and "tell their stories." This slowness does not reflect indecision, incompetence, decreased intelligence, confusion, or a lack of cooperation. Slowness of response is even more profound when communication with the elderly person is complicated by either a hearing loss or a language problem.
3. Curb the urge to be impatient, to ask someone else who is in the room such as a family member, and to interrupt the elderly person in midsentence or midthought—asking someone else will probably yield misinformation since the answer received will be phrased in another person's perspective and not from the point of view of the elderly person.

4. Communicate clearly and avoid unintelligible slang.

5. Respect the elderly person's right to confidentiality and privacy. Intense and repeated questioning about topics that may be sensitive economically, emotionally, or socially is inappropriate with the elderly.

6. Respect the elderly person's right to control what and how much he reveals about himself; to determine to whom the information will be given; and the timing of self-exposure. Violating the confidence of an elderly person to anyone—health care colleague or not—without the elder's expressed permission is unforgivable. If the information that is being gathered will be shared, the elderly person has a right to know with whom and for what purpose before the interview is conducted.

7. Adhere to strict conventions of social courtesy. Address the elderly person formally, using his full name until instructed to do otherwise; introduce yourself formally, telling the person the purpose of your contact, and be extremely sensitive to conventions of privacy and delicacy.

Closely aligned with the issue of respect is the issue of client advocacy. Along with all of its other meanings, advocacy, when applied to caring for an elderly client and assessing his needs, means that the health care provider believes what the elderly person says and is willing to give him the benefit of the doubt, over and above everyone else. Strange as it seems, it is not at all unusual, in practice, that health care personnel do not take seriously what an elderly person says. Rather, they seek confirmation of the elderly person's story from some younger person such as a family member or a co-worker or they simply act as if the elderly person's word is humorously suspect.

■ **Point of Emphasis**

An advocate for the elderly listens actively and attentively to the words used by the client, seeks clarification and redefinition from the elder for a complete understanding of impressions and experiences, and totally believes that the descriptions offered reflect a true reality even if the facts differ from the descriptions offered by someone younger.

There always seems to be an underlying assumption in interaction with an elderly person that he could not possibly know what he is saying because he is, after all, forgetful, old, or senile.

ASPECTS OF A MENTAL HEALTH ASSESSMENT FOR THE ELDERLY □ The mental health assessment of an elderly person can be roughly divided into several overlapping dimensions: (1) presentation of self; (2) presenting symptoms; (3) historical and cultural influences; (4) behavioral and functional abilities; (5) physical status; (6) environmental influences; and (7) psychosocial status. Although the nurse may choose not to collect all of this information at one sitting or to obtain some parts of the needed information from the client's record, each of these aspects should ultimately be explored, analyzed, and interpreted in developing a total picture of the mental health status of the elderly client.

Assessment of the Presentation of Self □ An assessment of how the elderly person presents himself should include observation of (a) his overall physical appearance; and (b) his dominant affective tone or mood state.

Physical Appearance. The nurse should carefully note the person's appearance during each assessment session. Attention should be given to both the client's physical characteristics and to the manner in which he is dressed and groomed. Unusual physical characteristics are very important to notice because these can have multiple meanings, each of which needs to be explored as the assessment proceeds. For example, the elderly person who presents with a blank facial expression may be displaying a sign of depression, Parkinson's disease, hypothyroidism, or hearing loss, each of which is known to be associated with "mental symptoms" among the elderly. Only further assessment can reveal the significance of each unusual physical characteristic that is noticed. Deterioration in grooming, inattention to dressing, or unusual forms of dressing and grooming can each be associated with multiple causes such as depression, psychosis or confusion, or untreated visual problems. Dressing with multiple layers of clothing is a peculiarity displayed by individuals who are confused just as it is of individuals who are anemic or suffering from problems of thermoregulation (hypothermia). Odors should be noted as well and efforts made to differentiate their possible causes and identify their possible meanings. Body odor due to lack of personal hygiene may be a sign of confusion or it may simply be a sign of a lifelong habit or "cultural imperative." The odor of urine may reflect the inattention to toileting habits sometimes displayed by confused, depressed, or psychotic elderly; or it may reflect incontinence due to an untreated urinary tract infection or due to perineal relaxation that the person finds too embarrassing to mention.

Affective Tone. The client's dominant affective tone can be partially determined from observation. Like younger clients, the elderly often display facial expressions and body postures that reflect their inner conflicts, anxiety, or depression. Simple observation of the elderly to determine affective tone should, however, be done cautiously; ultimately this observation should be confirmed verbally with the client because these indicators tend to be less reliable in the elderly. For example, among the elderly who experience aging changes that affect voice quality, the tone of the voice may be unrelated to affective tone. Tears and weeping, which are common among the old-old who experience age-related changes of the orbital structures, are often completely unrelated to feelings of sadness or depression. Using observation to infer affective tone or mood state among the elderly serves as only a starting point for further assessment and exploration.

Assessment of Presenting Symptoms □ Each elderly person should be given the opportunity to describe his own problems in his own words. Although information gathered from the family or those living with the client may be helpful in completing the picture, the primary source of information needs to be the elderly person. During the assessment of presenting symptoms, the nurse needs to listen closely to the words used. It is not uncommon, because of culture and socialization, for elderly people to concentrate attention on the physical aspects of problems or to somaticize the problems. Although recognizing the importance of looking into somatic symptoms, the nurse needs to be able to elicit information about feelings, and to give permission to the elderly person to discuss the meaning he attaches to the physical symptoms.

Assessment of Historical-Cultural Influences □ In the absence of a historical and cultural perspective, it is very difficult to place the problems described by an elderly person into a context from which inferences can be drawn. For example, if the elderly person complains that he is forgetful, the nurse must obtain the historical view of his particular forgetfulness. He may always have been forgetful, even at age 20, but may now, at age 80, be frightened or disturbed about it. If his family reports that he is argumentative, it is important to trace with the family members the ways in which the elderly person has always handled conflict and disagreement. For some reason, families often expect that when the elderly person has reached age 75 and has moved in with them, he will change his basic personality pattern and become cooperative, compliant, sweet, and pleasant. Many families need help to recognize that the behavior patterns that the elderly person shows are not new; rather, they are firmly established.

Whatever the client's national origin, religion, and native language, it must be assumed that he adheres to certain cultural norms and standards of behavior that are not dictated by his having lived during a different time in history. These cultural differences can affect basic aspects of behavior such as how often the person changes clothes, how often he bathes and washes his clothes, his customary diet, and the timing of his meals. More complex aspects of behavior are also affected by culture, for example, his expectations about the behavior of his family members and the health care providers around him; his decisions about the appropriate uses of money; his attitude toward social courtesy and privacy; and how he treats his personal possessions and his "space."

Collected in the assessment of historical and cultural influences is information about the individual's educational, marital, and work role history. Information about previous and current living arrangements and life-style should also be collected in this portion of the assessment.

Assessment of Functional Abilities □ Maintenance, instrumental, and cognitive behaviors and functions must all be considered in the assessment of an elderly person.

Maintenance Functions. These functions include all those related to personal management and comfort such as the ability to bathe, dress, groom, ambulate, eat, and use the toilet (Lawton and Brody, 1969). The degree of independent function in each area and the amount and type of help required should be noted. When the elderly individual is living in the community, it is also important to note who is available within his social network to provide help when needed.

Instrumental Functions. Instrumental functions are more complex than maintenance functions. They are the tasks required for community living such as the ability to use the telephone, prepare meals, obtain groceries and other personal items, arrange for and use transportation, self-administer medications and other health care remedies, perform housekeeping duties, do laundry, and manage finances (Lawton and Brody, 1969). Again, the nurse should note the extent of independent function in each area, the amount and type of help required, and who is available to provide help.

Cognitive Functions. These functions include all the activities related to orientation, direction following, memory, problem solving, using judgment, and communicating.

Although orientation is the most basic of these functions, in some ways, it is the most difficult to assess because it can be judged only in view of the circumstances of the assessment. For example, although it is probably impossible for an oriented elderly person not to know his own name, it may be quite reasonable for an oriented elderly person to mistake those around him for other people from his family or his past if he has been suddenly relocated or has poor sensory-perceptual abilities. Depending on the circumstances, the likelihood that an oriented elderly person will be aware of the exact date and time, and of his location, may be quite slim. For example, if he has suddenly been relocated or hospitalized and has not had contact with either calendars or newspapers recently, he may know the name of the city he is in but not the name of the exact place. He may also display his orientation by being able to mention the general time of the year or the month but may not be able to state the exact date or time of day. Orientation to purpose is another dimension that should be assessed. For example, a person could not be considered oriented if he was observed trying to use a hair brush for eating his eggs but he may be considered oriented if he was observed using a hairbrush to remove the lint from his clothing (Wolanin and Phillips, 1981).

The normal healthy young adult is able to correctly follow no more than three directions given at the same time. We can expect no more of the elderly person. Direction following is assessed by giving the elderly person two directions to follow, for example, "Please grasp the side rail and hand me a tissue." If he is able to follow these two directions, a third is added. If he is unable to follow these two directions, only one is given. In order to gain the cooperation of the elderly person during this assessment, the nurse should make the directions simple and physically possible for the client. They should also be relevant to his situation and should not be ones that will make him appear foolish. "Please stick out your tongue and pat your stomach" would be an example of an inappropriate test for direction following (Wolanin and Phillips, 1981).

Short-term memory can be tested by asking the individual to describe some relevant and important event that happened to him that day, for example, what he had for breakfast or who his visitors were. Short-term memory can also be assessed by asking the individual to remember some information, such as the names of three objects in the room, or your name and position, at the beginning of the assessment session; then asking him to retrieve the information at the end of the session. Long-term memory can be tested in a number of ways. Among all of the benefits associated with life review (Butler and Lewis, 1982), one of the most important is to test long-term memory. Long-term memory can also be tested by asking the elderly person to relate some historical facts that you know for sure he is aware of, for example, "Name the date that we celebrate as Independence Day."

Problem solving and judgment are related to the ability to (1) identify the purpose and use of objects, and (2) classify objects and events according to their similarities and differences. For example, the individual could be shown a hair brush, a comb, and a piece of soap. He could then be asked the purpose of each, how each is related to the others, and how each is different from the others. The ability to calculate is also related to problem solving and judgment. Tests involving simple addition, subtraction, multiplication, and division assess the ability to calculate. Both problem solving and judgment are involved in household and financial management and can be assessed from those perspectives.

Communication is considered throughout the assessment process, and special notice should be taken, during assessment of functional and behavioral abilities, of the ability to use and recognize words that are presented verbally and in writing. Adequate vision and hearing are, of course, essential for these tasks. If the person has difficulty communicating by one means, such as the verbal, try other means to test his abilities to communicate. Gestures, pantomime, and drawing represent various approaches to assessing ability to receive information, understand it, and respond appropriately.

Assessment of Physical Status □ No mental health assessment for the elderly is complete without giving consideration to physical status.

Physiological Factors. The following is a partial list of physical problems that affect mental status: (1) hypoxia caused by respiratory inadequacy, circulatory inadequacy particularly involving problems with the cardiac pump; perfusion inadequacy particularly involving problems of cerebral edema, and inadequacy of the oxygen-carrying capacity of the blood (as in the various anemias); (2) hypotension and hypertension; (3) hypothermia and hyperthermia; (4) problems of glucose metabolism including both hypoglycemia and hyperglycemia; (5) hypocalcemia and hypercalcemia; (6) malnutrition and undernutrition; (7) dehydration; (8) failure of the renal mechanisms leading to increased levels of nitrogenous wastes in the blood; (9) disturbances of electrolytes, particularly potassium and sodium; (10) asymptomatic infectious processes that are unrecognized due to lack of hyperthermic reaction; (11) traumatic head injuries caused by recent, supposedly benign falls; (12) drug interactions, iatrogenic and self-induced drug abuse; (13) alcohol abuse; and (14) sensory-perceptual deficits.

■ *Point of Emphasis*

Failure of any body system can be the causative agent of mental symptoms among the elderly.

It is essential that this fact not be overlooked and that health care providers not act on the mistaken idea that behavioral changes and mental problems among the elderly are simply a fact of growing old and that they are neither treatable nor preventable.

Sensory-Perceptual Factors. Sensory-perceptual problems are intimately related to the mental health of an elderly client. Visual problems should always be carefully assessed. Even though the client wears corrective lenses, do not assume that there is adequate correction for a visual problem. The date and time of the last eye examination should be ascertained. In addition, the nurse should test visual acuity both for distance and for reading, the ability to distinguish colors, the functional visual field, and sensitivity to light and

brightness, darkness and shadows. The purpose of this assessment is to assess functional vision so that care strategies and environmental manipulations can be planned to enhance the existing visual capacity and increase the likelihood of appropriate interactions.

The sensory problem most intimately related to mental health problems among the elderly is hearing loss—which is known to be related to anxiety, depression, and paranoid states. It is not uncommon for an elderly person seen by health care providers for evaluation and treatment of a mental or physical problem to have a long-standing hearing deficit that has not been recognized, evaluated, or treated. The recognition and treatment of hearing problems among the elderly are complicated by the denial that many elderly people and their families practice as a means of dealing with hearing loss and by the embarrassment they feel about being unable to hear. In our society, hearing loss arouses little sympathy or concern on the part of either family members or health care professionals probably because of its invisibility and the frustration involved in attempting to communicate with a hearing-impaired individual. Each elderly person with even a slight hearing loss, however, deserves the opportunity and encouragement to have his hearing professionally evaluated and to have a comprehensive plan originated that identifies strategies to maximize the best possible functional hearing. These strategies include the use of hearing aids accompanied by appropriate teaching and counseling, lessons in speech reading, lessons in signing, the use of pantomime and alternative visual forms of communication, and the identification and use of the tone, volume, and sound combinations that are best perceived by the individual. During the mental health assessment, the nurse should ascertain the degree to which the person is able to perceive the spoken word, his functional hearing, and the extent of medical attention he has received for a hearing problem. Presbycusis, the hearing problem most common in old age, affects (1) the ability to understand words that can be heard at normal volumes (phonemic regression), (2) the ability to understand certain letter combinations (such as f, th, s, and sh—particularly at the beginning of words), (3) the ability to hear high tones (there is usually more difficulty with female voices than male voices), and (4) the ability to screen background noises from speech. The following is a crude assessment technique for detecting problems with recognition of words and letter combinations often associated with presbycusis: Face the client. Using a normal tone, say each of the words that follow and have the client repeat what he hears: smart, off, with, that, will, cat, room, all, jaw, does (Shore, 1978). The information thus gathered allows communication with the client to be structured so that words that he finds easiest to understand are used most commonly. As a general rule, lowering the pitch, using a normal tone, (shouting does not help), speaking slowly, clearly, and distinctly while facing the client, avoiding those letter combinations and words that are most problematic to the client, and screening out background noises are all strategies that should be used in the assessment and intervention for hearing loss among the elderly (Phillips, 1981).

The person's ability to perceive sensory input via touch should also be assessed since many misperceptions and anxieties arise from misinterpretation of touch input. Ability to perceive hot and cold, pain and pressure, two-point localization, light and deep sensations, and proprioceptive input are also part of the mental health assessment (Phillips, 1981).

Assessment of Environmental Influences □ The client's environment should be assessed for pattern, meaning, variability, consistency, and stability. A history should be taken that reveals the types of environments and inputs that the client is most familiar with, and his current environment should be assessed for its similarity to them. All aspects of the environment should be considered including other persons and their characteristics; the sights, sounds, and odors most commonly encountered; the activity levels, and cyclic influences within the environment. Some research has shown that exacerbation of mental symptoms and bizarre behaviors such as wandering and acting out among the elderly are related to cyclic or unexplained changes in the environmental activity level. Uniform orienting cues, such as message boards, should be identified that can be used to help the person understand the activity going on around him and to predict what is going to happen next. Ways of making the environment work for the advantage of the elderly person should be identified.

Assessment of Psychosocial Status □ The keys to assessing the psychosocial status of an elderly client are (1) establishing a respectful, caring rapport; and (2) developing a method of communication that permits as much information flow as possible, limits the amounts of misunderstanding, and permits expression of a pace comfortable to the older person. Unlike younger clients, many of whom are easily able to discuss their feelings and thoughts frankly, many elderly people have never exposed their intimate ideas to any other person, particularly a person they barely know. Raised in a culture that discouraged self-exposure, that considered medical and nursing practice to be concerned only with fixing physical ills, and that was suspicious of psychiatric techniques, many elderly people are unaware that discussing their thoughts with a health professional is permissible under any circumstances. Because self-exposure is so alien, many elderly people use techniques that limit the amount of information they provide during interviews. One such technique is using socially "nice" expressions to shut off the discussion. Another is somaticizing conflicts, worries, and fears and discussing only the physical problems they are encountering. A third such technique is using symbolic or metaphorical language which to the sensitive listener reveals a great deal but to the unperceptive individual reveals nothing. In metaphorical language, poetic statements (often quoted bits of poetry or biblical phrases) reveal inner feelings but only within the context of the entire poem or passage. Symbolic statements such as "my light will soon go out" to refer to death or "they are trying to poison me" in reference to feelings of rejection from significant others are also a part of this language pattern (Wolanin and Phillips, 1981). As a result, psychosocial assessment of an elderly client requires careful and intense listening, the clarification and reclarification of ideas, enormous patience and sensitivity, and a permissive, accepting attitude on the part of the health professional.

Three interrelated dimensions are usually considered in gathering information for a psychosocial assessment of an elderly person. These include (1) psychological state, (2) developmental satisfaction, and (3) social effectiveness. Each of these areas is considered in the discussion that follows along with some suggested ways of eliciting information. The questions suggested are meant only to be guides in helping you identify some ways of helping the elderly person to discuss his thoughts and feelings. Creativity and sensitivity are required so that assessment questions can be tailored to fit the personalities and styles of both the client and the nurse.

Psychological State. Psychological state can be thought of as being composed of five separate facets: (1) the client's view of self, (2) his thought content, (3) affect and mood, (4) stress management and coping styles, and (5) behavior.

Since it is easy for an elderly person to internalize a view of himself as useless, incompetent, and worthless, helping him to describe his picture of himself yields information that may relate to a number of mental health problems common to aging. The questions and statements presented below may be helpful in determining an overall assessment of the client's view of self.

1. Tell me what it's like for you to be 72 (or whatever his age).
2. Tell me about what aging is like.
3. Tell me about what *your* aging has been like.
4. What is the ideal old person like? Tell me what most old people are like.
5. How are you like the ideal old person? How are you different?
6. If you had to describe yourself in three words, what would they be?
7. How do you feel about growing older?*

A word of caution—the elderly person needs to know that whatever he says in response to these or other questions is all right, that he is not being judged, and that you are willing to accept all of his answers. Old people are noble and courageous as well as petty and fearful. They are nice and kind as well as cruel and hateful—just like the rest of us. Their answers during an interview will reflect many facets of being human, and they need to know that it is all right that they are nothing more and nothing less than human.

Bodily perceptions and image of bodily function are a part of the client's view of self. Therefore, it is essential to include the client's view of his body in the assessment of his view of self. The questions given below may be helpful in eliciting information about the elderly person's bodily perceptions. During the assessment of bodily perceptions, the nurse should be alert to references to sexual function within the overall discussion. Since elderly people are not the asexual creatures they are often thought to be, and may find that discussion of their bodies makes them feel com-

fortable about discussing sex, the nurse should be prepared to handle interview content at this time related to sexual function, sexual expression, and the inhibition or prohibitions associated with sexuality.

1. What is your physical body like?
2. Does your body function differently now than it used to? In what way? How does this affect you?
3. How does your body feel right now? How did it feel when you arose this morning? Can you recall how your body felt when you were 40?
4. What is your greatest problem with your body? How does that make you feel?
5. What do you like best about your body? Least?*

Another aspect of the individual's view of self is his assessment of his own assets or resources and liabilities or weaknesses. These assessments may encompass money, financial security, and housing; knowledge, intelligence, education, and experience; coping strategies; social supports, social networks, and social ties; cultural stability; religious and philosophical beliefs; life view; health, health behaviors, and health orientation (Antonovsky, 1979); and personality characteristics. Presented below are questions and statements that might be helpful in eliciting information about personal resources or assets. Resources should be viewed both in the present and from a historical perspective to provide an overall picture of the positive characteristics the elderly person attributes to himself.

1. Tell me about the periods when you felt most successful. Do you think you were different then, or much as you are now?
2. Tell me about your greatest strengths.
3. Tell me about your happiest times. What about you makes you happy?
4. What was the most important thing you have done in your life? What personal characteristics of yours made it happen?*

Below are questions and statements that might be helpful in eliciting information about personal liabilities or weaknesses. Liabilities are best assessed when the emphasis is on the here and now and the individual is not permitted to ruminate over real or imagined deficits from the

---

* Questions presented in this section are based on Wolanin and Phillips (1981).

past. Since the purpose of this interview is assessment and not therapy or counseling, every effort should be made to help the person consider his liabilities realistically, focusing mostly on the liabilities impacting his life right now (Wolanin and Phillips, 1981).

1. What is your greatest weakness right now?
2. Does anything interfere with the way you live today?
3. If you could change one thing about yourself, what would it be?
4. When you got up this morning, did you think about something you had to face that would be difficult to deal with?
5. How do your personal weaknesses influence your life?*

The thoughts that recur, preoccupy the cognitive domain, and cause anxiety and worry are often related to the needs dominant in the person's life. Because of the negative influences and events experienced by many elderly people, there are certain patterns that constitute common themes for thought content among them. These include loss, rejection, powerlessness and uncertainty, grief, separation, loneliness, hopelessness, helplessness, anxiety, ambivalence and conflict, anger, and vulnerability. These themes are sometimes expressed directly through verbalization and behavior, and at times they are expressed indirectly, such as through symbolic language or in dreams. The exploration of thought content can reveal, in addition to the client's needs and concerns, the presence of delusions, hallucinations, illusions, suicidal thoughts, paranoid ideation, and obsessional thoughts. Some questions and statements that might be helpful in assisting an elderly person to explore his dominant thought content are listed below.

1. Tell me what you think about most of the time.
2. Do you worry? What sorts of worries do you have?
3. Sometimes all of us have thoughts that keep coming back and bothering us, thoughts we just can't seem to get rid of. Do you have any thoughts like that? Tell me about them.
4. Some people think that they have crazy thoughts. Do you have thoughts that you think are really crazy? Could you tell me about them?
5. Do you daydream? What kinds of things do you think about when you daydream?
6. Dreams at night sometimes make us think during the day. Have you had any dreams lately at night that have caused you to think about them the next day?*

Although it is usually necessary to help the elderly person interpret the meanings associated with these thoughts and to identify the feelings that underlie them (techniques more consistent with therapy and counseling than assessment) simply giving the client permission to verbalize these thoughts often provides a great sense of relief.

Some questions and statements that might be helpful in exploring the elderly client's thoughts and feelings about suicide and death are given below.

1. Do you ever think about dying?
2. How do you imagine your death will occur?
3. Have you ever considered taking your own life?
4. Have you ever made a plan to take your own life?
5. Under what circumstances would you think it would be all right to take your own life?*

Geriatric suicide is an important topic to consider separately since elderly individuals, particularly elderly men, are at high risk for suicide, a risk that increases exponentially with increasing age (Miller, 1978; Butler and Lewis, 1982). There are some important facts about geriatric suicide that the nurse should know. First, it is not usually a spontaneous event but, rather, well planned over a long period of time. Suddenly making or changing a will, giving away prized possessions, and purchasing the means for the suicide are signs that can be recognized by sensitive health professional's and significant others. If approached, the elderly person is usually willing to discuss his plan openly and honestly. Second, geriatric suicide is rarely simply attempted or threatened. Rather, those elderly who intend suicide are skillful and methodical in their ability to complete the act, regardless of whether or not they live in an institution. Suicide threats are not used by the elderly to manipulate those around them. An elderly person who indicates a desire and plan to commit suicide has a great likelihood of being wholly serious and of successfully completing the act. Third, suicide among the elderly is commonly provoked by precipitating events that are the "straws that break the camel's back," such as (1) loss of independence (suicide often occurs immediately before or after an institutional placement); (2) loss of status; (3) loss of a spouse (suicide within 1 year after the death of a spouse is not at all uncommon); (4) loss of income; and (5) the compounded multiple losses associated with the aging process. Geriatric suicide is often associated with addiction to drugs or alcohol, acute intoxication, confusion, mental and emotional problems, and multiple physical problems (Miller, 1978). Geriatric suicide can be active (e.g., intentionally taking an overdose or using a pistol) or passive (e.g., refusing to eat or to seek medical attention for an acute illness). Suicide-homicide pacts between elderly spouses or siblings are not uncommon and often occur after one of the duo has been permanently institutionalized.

Affect and mood are best assessed by exploring the topic with the client and verbally confirming any observation-based inferences about posture, body language, facial expressions, or behavior. Below are presented some questions and statements that might be helpful in assessing the client's affect and mood.

1. What is your life like most of the time?
2. Is there one emotion that best describes how you feel most of the time?
3. How do you feel about your life, right now? How do you feel about your life generally?*

The elderly client's affect and mood can range from a neutral position of comfortable and pleasant to elation and euphoria on the one pole and withdrawal and apathy on the other.

Although stress is a part of everyone's life, there is little doubt that excessive stress or multiple stressors that occur in a short period of time can adversely affect physical and mental health. The list below offers some questions and statements that may be helpful in assessing the total amount of stress the individual has experienced in his lifetime and in recent years. In addition, some of the questions deal with how the individual has previously coped with stressful events. This portion of the assessment serves to identify the client's strengths on which crisis intervention and future counseling can be based.

1. Has your life changed in the past 2 years? (Exploration of recent deaths, retirement, divorce, income reversals, moving, physical changes, and so on, is helpful.)
2. Tell me about the deaths that you have known about in your lifetime. (Unresolved grief and the stress associated with it can arise from the deaths of parents, spouse(s), children, confidants, friends, pets, business associates.)
3. Have you been sleeping and eating well?
4. What was the worst thing that ever happened to you? How did you deal with that situation?
5. Was there a time when you experienced a great stress? How did you cope with it?*

Observing the elderly client, discussing his behavior with other individuals who are close to him, and discussing behavior patterns with the elderly person himself are all ways of assessing behavior. There are two points that are particularly important to remember. First, when health care providers (or family members) react negatively toward an elderly person, the cause is most commonly the elder's behavior. Although his attitudes, feelings, or ideas might be considered unusual or troublesome, these are not usually the basis of interpersonal conflict. Rather, conflict usually arises when the behaviors of the elderly person are seen as "inappropriate," "disruptive," or as somehow jeopardizing the health professional's role definition. Examples of behaviors of elderly clients to which health care providers and family members react most negatively are given below. Because helping professionals usually define their roles toward the elderly person as "in his best interest," any behavior of the elderly person that makes him less accessible to being helped or that interferes with the desires of the health professionals to help other clients arouses particularly negative feelings.

Talking too loudly and too much
Interrupting and dominating the conversation
Demanding attention
Wandering
Refusing to eat
Refusing to talk
Being confused or disoriented
Being incontinent

Smearing feces

Being detached and withdrawn

Refusing help

Refusing medications and medical treatments

Actions that are interpreted as suicidal

Second, behavior is best understood within the context of its underlying motivation. Behavior is caused; and dealing effectively with an individual's behavior involves paying attention to the underlying cause. Rarely are intervention strategies effective if attention is directed only at the behavior. For example, a behavior of many elderly people that health professionals find troublesome is what Burnside (1981) calls "overloading." Overloading is demonstrated when an elderly person tries to say too much, too rapidly, in too little time; and when he uses ploys to keep the other person involved in the interaction past the time when the latter wants to terminate it. Fear, anxiety, and loneliness often underlie overloading. Dealing with overloading requires giving attention to the fear and anxiety and not to the behavior itself. The focus of assessing behavior and behavior patterns, then, must be on the reactions that others have to the elderly person's behaviors and on the underlying causes of the behavior as much as on the behavior itself.

Developmental Satisfaction. Accomplishing age-related developmental tasks contributes to the satisfaction the elderly person has with his own life (Kurtz and Wolk, 1975) and undoubtedly enhances his feelings of self-respect and self-worth. Ebersole and Hess (1981) have presented an excellent discussion of the developmental tasks of aging. Using data from Peck (1968), Havinghurst (1972), Ebersole (1976a), and Butler and Lewis (1982), Ebersole and Hess have divided the developmental tasks of the elderly into those that are intrinsic and those that are extrinsic, and then have related each to Maslow's human needs hierarchy (1962). Ebersole and Hess's scheme can serve as the basis for assessment parameters to determine the degree to which an individual elderly person has accomplished or managed the developmental tasks appropriate for his age. It should be emphasized, however, that not all elderly people are the same nor does one elderly person remain the same throughout his later years. As individuals progress through the years from 60 to death, the developmental tasks on which they focus can be expected to change and

evolve, with some tasks taking priority depending on the overall life circumstances, the individual's growth needs and personal style. For example, some developmentally "normal" elderly individuals choose to continue "middle-aged" activities such as maintaining successful work roles late into life and some developmentally "normal" elderly individuals quite late in life choose to reactivate tasks usually associated with young adulthood such as parenting. The activities described by Ebersole and Hess represent the developmental tasks that the majority of elderly individuals focus on with advancing years but they are certainly not the only "normal" tasks available to the aging individual.

Social Effectiveness. The last facet of the psychosocial assessment of an older adult involves gathering data that can be used to determine the elderly individual's social effectiveness. The socially effective elderly person is one who is able to establish, maintain, and use social networks and interpersonal relationships to meet basic human needs. The greatest threats to social effectiveness among the elderly are those related to his ability to establish and to maintain social networks. As people age, so do their significant others. As a result, by attrition alone, the number of individuals available to serve as members of the elder's social network decreases with time. Many elderly individuals have difficulty activating new relationships to replace those that are lost through death, disability, and institutionalization.

Among the elderly, social ties can be thought of as being grouped into three potentially overlapping but often distinct networks: affinal, affectional, and service-giving, each of which focuses on meeting different human needs. Determining the adequacy of one network does not indicate the adequacy of the others.

The affinal network is composed of all those living individuals to whom the elderly person is related either by blood (consanguinal relationship) or by marriage (acquired relationship). On one level, if the individuals in the affinal network serve no other purpose in the elderly person's life such as giving support or sharing confidences, this network is of the least importance for the elderly person's social effectiveness. On another level, in some cultures, the affinal network takes precedence regardless of whether it serves another purpose and its simple existence provides support and feelings of belonging.

The affectional network is composed of all those individuals who provide love, affection, and support to the elderly individual. More and more in our society, the affectional network extends far beyond the affinal, with friends fulfilling more of the individual's need for love and affection and having more importance than family members. The affectional network is defined solely from the perspective of the elderly person and is determined by his estimate of the strength of the bond. It includes his self-defined significant others (regardless of the actual relationship) and his confidants, lifelong friends and companions, neighbors, correspondents, and church affiliates. Determining the overall quality of interactions with these individuals is an important assessment task.

The service-giving network is composed of all those individuals who provide some type of help to the elderly person. The type of help given may range from running errands and providing transportation to supplying actual physical, emotional, or financial care. This network often has formal or informal organization with specific individuals performing certain selected tasks and one individual acting as the service coordinator. Usually self-selected or appointed family members, significant others, friends, neighbors, church affiliates, and community agency personnel form the core of the service-giving network. Many elderly people could not maintain themselves in the community or return to community living following an institutionalization without the existence of such networks.

☐ PROBLEM IDENTIFICATION

Following a complete mental health assessment, problems may be identified or inferred in any of the three major areas discussed. Regardless of where in the health system the elderly client is encountered there are two sets of problems that commonly arise.

NORMAL PROBLEMS ☐ Normal problems arise from the simple process of living and growing old. These problems, which are summarized in Table 20-2, are often related to certain emotional reactions common to the aging population including grief (mourning), guilt, loneliness, depression, anxiety, sense of diminished importance, helplessness, and rage. These reactions are often associated with certain defense mechanisms includ-

---

TABLE 20-2 Common Emotional Problems of Aging[a]

Losses
  Loss of relationships with people
    Loss of significant others and confidants
    Loss of peer group and collegial relationships
  Financial losses
  Loss of possessions
  Awareness of declining health
    Deterioration of own health
      Discomforts and pain
      Confinement and immobility
      Physical changes
      Monotony of daily encounters
      Absence of personal privacy
      Enforced idleness
      Awareness of death
    Deterioration of significant others' health
      Confinement
      Burden of caring for others
Rejection
  Feeling forgotten
  Being forgotten
  Feeling unworthy or unacceptable
Powerlessness
  Powerlessness against others and the world
    Vulnerability; being a spectator
    Unreliability of others
    Unpredictability of others and "the fates"
    Indignities and dependence
    Being exposed to propaganda
      Being "talked into" accepting something that is not wanted
      Having information withheld
      Not receiving accurate information
  Powerlessness against time
    Not knowing the duration of confinement
    Sensing a meaningless existence
    Sensing threats to life and health

[a] Used with permission, Wolanin, M. O., and Phillips, L. R. *Confusion: Prevention and care.* St Louis: The C.V. Mosby Company, 1981.

---

ing denial, projection, fixation, regression, displacement, counterphobia, idealization, rigidity, selective memory, selective sensory perception, and exploitation of age and disability (Butler and Lewis, 1982). The first set of problems are the focus for primary prevention of mental illness among the elderly in that intervention is centered on strengthening existing resources and preventing crisis and disorganization.

MENTAL ILLNESS ☐ The incidence of mental illness increases as individuals age, and the types of mental illnesses that the aging population display are as varied as the types seen among a younger population. There are, however, certain mental illnesses that are more commonly seen as individuals age.

Depression. This is probably the most common mental health problem among the elderly. Depression among the elderly can be bipolar or unipolar, and the symptoms can range from transient "blues" to psychotic withdrawal and suicide. The symptoms of the depressed elderly most frequently take the form of a somatic complaint such as chronic pain, sleep disturbances, and gastrointestinal disturbances; apathy; and indecision. Depression is therefore often overlooked as a primary diagnosis because the individual is seen as a "crock" or hypochondriac or as senile and confused (Butler and Lewis, 1982; Wolanin and Phillips, 1981).

Paranoid Disorders. Although a certain number of individuals with lifelong or chronic classic paranoia do live to be old and are therefore seen by health professionals for treatment (often for the first time), classic paranoia among the elderly is actually quite rare. Classic paranoia is defined as a disorder "marked by an elaborate, well-organized, paranoid system in which the person may consider himself or herself remarkably endowed with superior ability and power" (Butler and Lewis, 1982, 68). Most of the paranoia displayed by the elderly is of short duration and is associated with periods of increased stress or illness. Often, the delusions are discrete, circumscribed, and related to specific fears (Butler and Lewis, 1982).

Organic Disorders. Organic disorders can be thought of as being of the reversible type (the most commonly encountered) and of the irreversible type. Reversible confusions can be related to physiological, social and economic, cultural, psychological, environmental, and sensory-perceptual problems. Reversible confusions are also frequently related to acute alcohol intoxication and iatrogenic drug overdoses. Of the irreversible confusions, the most common type is organic mental disorder of the Alzheimer type. Irreversible confusions among the elderly are also caused by multi-infarct disease and by the chronic effects of drug or alcohol abuse (Wolanin and Phillips, 1981).

Anxiety and Hypochondriasis. Both of these are probably related to the realities of aging with the individual's increasing awareness of his vulnerability as well as to other psychological factors. Hypochondriasis is sometimes used by the elderly as a means of reducing anxiety by avoidance of problems and by reducing isolation and loneliness (Butler and Lewis, 1982).

Secondary prevention is the focus of intervention for the second set of problems identified. The goals of nursing intervention are to reduce symptoms and distress, restore functions, and prevent further disorganization.

☐ *PRIMARY PREVENTION*

Although it is not possible to identify specific preventive measures that would be applicable for every individual elderly client the nurse encounters, there are some general guidelines that can be used in planning interventions and preventing further problems for elderly persons experiencing the normal mental health problems of aging.

> ### ■ *Point of Emphasis*
>
> *The goal of primary prevention is to mobilize the individual's self-healing powers and inner resources for maximum resistance against the normal assaults of living and aging.*

HELP THE CLIENT EXPLORE HIS FEELINGS ☐ Exploring thoughts and feelings requires an empathic listener who first gives permission to the expression by gentle questioning and by displaying interested, unrushed demeanor, and then accepting the individual and his verbal expressions in a nonjudgmental manner. An empathic listener stresses the normalcy of the content and helps the individual recognize his right to have his own feelings. This listening process involves restating ideas, gently probing for clarification, and the use of reflective techniques. The empathic listener is active and verbal and shares a great deal of himself in the interaction process. The nurse must approach the elder as an adult who is a colleague in the healing/helping process and must resist the urge to follow role models who communicate with the elderly in paternalistic platitudes and false reassurances. Only two equal and involved adults can establish the trust and respect required to therapeutically explore and resolve feelings.

HELP THE CLIENT DEAL WITH LOSSES ☐ As we have seen, every individual experiences some losses as he progresses along the life continuum. There are three basic ways of helping individuals deal with losses that are a part of life: planning, replacing, and accepting.

Planning □ Although we have no way of knowing for sure which losses will occur and which will not, based on statistical frequency some losses can be anticipated and planned for. These include the loss of employment through retirement, various role losses, loss of parents through death, and (particularly for women) loss of a spouse. There is, of course, no way to plan completely or to totally anticipate the impact of these losses, but making life changes in middle age often takes the edge off the chaos that can accompany loss. Preretirement planning can help the individual find ways to alleviate to some extent the economic problems and isolation that often accompany retirement. Helping the individual to identify and develop vocational interests and other social outlets may make a measurable difference in the types of problems encountered at retirement. Planning for loss of a spouse is also possible. A merging or blurring of role tasks associated with one or the other sex is not uncommon among couples as they grow older. This blending of responsibilities should be encouraged and supported: men should be encouraged to develop skill and pride in cooking and household management tasks and women should be helped to learn the skills required for financial management and mechanical maintenance. Interestingly enough, for a great many couples who experience marital dissatisfaction during the middle years, this role blurring begins to serve as the basis for new areas of interaction and interest during the later years of their marriage.

Replacing □ Many losses are not literally replaceable, for example, the loss of one's parents or the loss of long-standing, loving relationships between spouses who have shared a good marriage. It is possible, however, to figuratively replace lost companionship, intimacy, and support through deepening the remaining relationships or expanding the social circle and finding new relationships. In the process, although the earlier love object is not actually replaced, new love objects are discovered as is the joy of developing intimacy, perhaps at a new or different level. Similarly, roles can be replaced, for example, work roles can be replaced by volunteer roles or parenting roles can be replaced by grandparenting or volunteer grandparenting roles.

Accepting □ Accepting losses is probably the most difficult of the three options, particularly if the loss was not anticipated and is not accompa-nied by attempts at replacement at some point. Grief and grief reactions are a normal part of living and aging. Elderly people need permission to experience the acute grief reactions that accompany loss and to establish and live through mourning rituals that are a necessary part of eventual acceptance. Providing opportunities for the grieving elderly person to express his feeling of loss and rage and to reflect on and remember the lost love object within his own individual time frame is an important part of facilitating acceptance. Nurses can be particularly influential in this process. Sometimes families, in their concern and love for the elderly person, have unrealistic expectations about the speed with which the loss will be resolved. They shut off communication prematurely and don't allow the reminiscence and rumination necessary for successful grieving. Nurses can help elderly people and their concerned others to appreciate the normalcy in grief reactions, and they can help family members give the elderly person the necessary time to grieve.

HELP THE CLIENT MOBILIZE HIS RESOURCES □ Through discussions and by listening, the nurse can help the client recognize and mobilize his personal resources and sources of strength. Often the elderly resolve some of the issues surrounding their personal values, philosophy, and religion, put to rest past conflicts and anxieties, put the significance of past failures into perspective, and find meaning in their lives. Through techniques such as life review and reminiscing, the elderly person can be helped to recognize and value the ways in which he has been most effective in the past, his personal strengths, and his resources.

Nurses can also be of assistance in helping an elderly individual mobilize his social resources. For example, nurses can help the client recognize the need to expand his social circle whenever losses begin to diminish the number of potential social contacts. Nurses can help him identify individuals in the community who might be potential sources of service or emotional support, and can make referrals to community agencies to supplement existing resources. Since families tend to asume more responsibility for service and emotional support as the elderly person ages, the nurse can help the family members find respite by identifying methods of organizing and coordinating services that will assume part of the burden for total care. Moreover, if specific stress-producing situations are identified during the assessment, such as the lack of proper housing or the presence of financial concerns, the nurse is in an excellent position to help the client identify and mobilize community resources to help.

HELP THE ELDERLY CLIENT AGE SUCCESSFULLY BY PROVIDING HEALTH EDUCATION □ Nurses have primary roles as teachers of the elderly and their families. Knowledge of relevant topics can help them avoid some of the more common problems.

Facts about Aging □ Elderly individuals need factual information about the normal changes associated with aging and what to expect of their aging bodies. The elderly are not immune to the myths about aging, and often live up to the negative expectations because they don't know any other way to behave. For example, many older men and women may discontinue sexual activity around the late middle years simply because they have been conditioned to believe that older people aren't supposed to enjoy sexual activity. Simple factual education can help dispel such myths and the negative behavior that arises as a consequence. Relatedly, many unfounded anxieties and fears can be dispelled by giving factual knowledge.

Wellness □ Elderly people need information about how to remain physically and emotionally healthy with advancing age—diet and exercise, where to go for hearing and vision testing, what to expect of assistive devices, how to seek help in the community for financial and housing problems, how to seek health care, and what to expect of the health care system are all areas of concern. The problems of drug use, alcoholism, drug interactions, and alternatives to drug use are key educational issues. The elderly also need information about some of the more complex problems they face in community living. For example, how to prevent accidents, how to prevent being victimized, and how to avoid becoming a target for crime are essential topics. Assertiveness training is extremely important, particularly in helping elderly women learn to become their own advocates.

Family Living □ Both the elderly and their significant others need to learn how to listen and how to interact openly. Teaching them ways of establishing two-way communication when the elderly person has a hearing or visual problem is a great service that a nurse can perform. When family members have lived apart for many years, it is difficult for them to resume living together as a family, and teaching about these matters is therefore a contribution to the mental health of all the parties involved.

Stress □ The elderly have long been ignored in educational programs that focus on stress reduction and stress management. This is a prime area for both educating the elderly and for promoting their mental health. They can be taught ways of identifying their own optimal stress level and how to reduce the stressors of daily life through such means as meditation and guided imagery, physical activity, planned diversion, and socialization.

HELP THE CLIENT DEVELOP IN THE ROLES OF TEACHER AND ACTIVIST □ Although role loss is common to aging, two roles that may emerge and develop are those of Elder as Teacher and Elder as Activist. Developing these roles helps the person find new ways of contributing to his own welfare and to the welfare of society. The first of them, Elder as Teacher, can be facilitated every time that you, the nurse, have contact with an elder. Each elderly person for whom you care has something important and unique to teach you. Permit this role to evolve as you share yourself with the elderly client and develop in your own role as nurse. The second role, Elder as Activist, can also be facilitated in the health care setting. This role takes root and develops when the power for decision making is shifted from the health care provider to the health care recipient. To enact the role of activist, the elderly client must become the major decision maker in areas that concern his health and welfare. Some elderly individuals naturally assume the role of activist but others must be helped to see that role and be invited to take part.

□ SECONDARY PREVENTION

Intervention in acute mental illness occurs in the hospital, in specialized gero-psychiatric units, general psychiatric units, and general medical-surgical units; in the extended care facility; in all types of ambulatory care settings, including day care; and in the home.

The basic interventions available for secondary prevention include (1) early case finding; (2) monitoring and intervention in health problems that affect mental function; (3) monitoring the use of drugs; (4) individual counseling and support;

■ *Point of Emphasis*

The most effective secondary prevention programs are those in which a multidisciplinary approach is followed and in which the professional nurse serves a primary therapeutic role as well as a coordinating function.

(5) group work; (6) family counseling; and (7) environmental manipulation. These are, of course, variously applied depending on the nature of the problems.

EARLY CASE FINDING □ Early identification and treatment is essential to a favorable prognosis in all mental health problems experienced by the elderly. As demonstrated by Coetzee (1980) in a study of depression, clients had the most favorable response to therapy when community health nurses became actively involved in early case finding, treatment, and coordination of services. This study also suggested that the community health nurse was the health team member most likely to perform the case-finding function well. This is partially because nurses are educated in the use of assessment techniques that identify the psychological and physical origins of disease. Regardless of the setting in which the nurse contacts the elderly person, investigating the relationship between the client's presenting physical symptoms and potential mental health problems is an important facet of the nurse's role in preventing deterioration from undiagnosed mental health problems.

MONITORING AND INTERVENING FOR HEALTH PROBLEMS THAT AFFECT MENTAL FUNCTION □ Mental health can be affected by a multitude of physical problems ranging from poor nutrition and hydration to immobility or poorly controlled diabetes.

■ *Point of Emphasis*

A psychiatric diagnosis does not preclude the possibility that other health problems are producing or exacerbating the mental symptoms, a fact frequently overlooked when the elderly are treated in psychiatric settings.

Among the health team members, nurses are often in the best position to identify potential health problems, to monitor the progress in identified health problems, to assist the client to modify his life-style in favorable ways, and to alert the primary physician to changes in health status that require further study. Careful attention should be given to all aspects of the client's health including sensory-perceptual function, cardiac and respiratory status, nutritional and fluid status, and daily exercise routine. The importance of even simple aspects of health care cannot be overestimated.

MONITORING THE USE OF DRUGS □ In the United States most of the medications prescribed are taken by persons over the age of 65 (Krupka and Verner, 1979; Ebersole and Hess, 1981). Adverse drug reactions; idiosyncratic drug reactions; reactions from drug-drug, drug-alcohol, and drug-food interactions; and unintentional overdoses that result from a failure of metabolic, excretory, and detoxification mechanisms must never be overlooked as the initial or continuing cause of mental symptoms among the elderly. Drug problems result from the misuse of prescription drugs usually arising from misunderstood directions, from misuse of over-the-counter drugs, and from the use of illicit drugs (Raffoul, et al., 1981; Peterson and Thomas, 1975). Interestingly enough, although drug use can produce mental symptoms, drug therapy is the treatment most frequently prescribed for mental health problems among the elderly. Psychotropic agents can cause as many problems as they resolve if they are not properly regulated and monitored. Guidelines that can be used to monitor the use of drugs among the mentally ill elderly are listed below. Laboratory tests should be done to measure cumulative blood levels of drugs and to prevent overdosing. Physical and behavioral symptoms should be monitored, with special attention given to the appearance of the most frequent side effects such as syncope, orthostatic hypotension, tardive dyskinesia, depression, confusion, agitation, dry mouth, constipation, cardiac decompensation, hypothermia, increased ocular pressure, and reduced ocular accommodation (Green, 1978; Bachinsky, 1978; Ebersole and Hess, 1981).

1. The nurse should ascertain the reason for prescribing every drug for an elderly client. This is particularly important when the drug is being given to cause behavior modification and may have been prescribed more for the convenience of the staff or family than the relief of the client.

2. A minimal amount of the least potentially dangerous drug should be used initially. The smallest dose possible should be given when therapy is initiated; if symptoms are not relieved, the dose can be slowly increased. If there is a choice, a minor tranquilizer is preferable to a major tranquilizer, based on the susceptibility of the elderly to develop tardive dyskinesia.

3. The smallest number of drugs possible should be prescribed to deal with a single problem and the smallest number of different drugs overall should be given to one individual.

4. Giving a different drug before the drug that was given initially has reached maximum effectiveness should be discouraged.

5. Side effects and adverse reactions should be continually monitored in assessing the client's status.

INDIVIDUAL COUNSELING AND SUPPORT □

Ebersole and Hess (1981) report that all of the following are effective treatment modes for mental health problems among the elderly: psychoanalysis, psychotherapeutic reminiscence, brief psychotherapy and crisis intervention, somatotherapy, behavioral therapy, reality orientation, resocialization, and remotivation. The type of therapy chosen depends, of course, on the client's problems. Although some of these require specialized training not usually within the repertoire of nurses who have had a general education, there are some guidelines, summarized below, that may help the nurse establish therapeutic relationships with elderly clients.

1. Active, empathic listening, tactful exploration of unresolved conflicts, and the identification and clarification of feelings are helpful in reducing the anxiety that often accompanies acute mental symptoms. Counseling the elderly often requires that the nurse be willing to confront personal feelings about issues such as death, disability, sexuality, separation, and dependency.

2. The nurse must be willing to offer the affection, respect, and protection that the elderly person needs. In many instances, she must be prepared to assume the role of surrogate family member and to provide the love and affection that may be unavailable from other sources.

3. Major goals in counseling and support include acceptance of the aging process, reduction of stress and other symptoms, resolution of conflicts, mastery of the past, identification of the meaning and emotional gratification of past experiences, validation of feelings, and increased self-esteem.

4. Activities that promote the elderly person's competence and attractiveness are most likely to increase self-esteem.

5. Promoting social and personal competence is of utmost importance for persons who have acute mental health problems.

Intervention strategies include those that increase the person's likelihood to succeed such as one-to-one practice sessions in both social interaction and the performance of functional tasks; progressive planned training sessions that begin at the client's level of competence and slowly move toward mastery of more complex tasks; and guided socialization in which the nurse helps one elderly person interact successfully with another. If he is likely to fail at interacting competently in a large group, those techniques should be used on an individual basis before the person is exposed to a larger group (Wolanin and Phillips, 1981).

GROUP WORK □

Four types of groups are available to help cognitively impaired, psychologically disturbed, and depressed elderly individuals: (1) reality orientation (2) remotivation (3) resocialization and (4) reminiscing (Ebersole and Hess, 1981). The structure and size of the group and the group process which whould be of most benefit to the elderly person are determined by the client's level of orientation, social competence, and presenting problem. Before instituting a therapeutic group with the elderly, the student should refer to Chapter 5.

FAMILY COUNSELING □

Most elderly clients have family members and significant others who are intimately involved in their situation and are concerned about their well-being. Nurses play an influential role in facilitating communication between these family members for the purpose of (1) expressing feelings, needs, and concerns, (2) making realistic plans and decisions based on appropriate expectations of all family members, and (3) resolving conflicts that surround the aging and living experience. The focus of family counseling should be individual to the extent that each member (including and especially the elderly person) is given the opportunity and privacy to express his feelings and concerns about the family unit, and group-centered to the extent that interactions are planned during which communication is face-to-face, as open and honest as possible, and involves all concerned individuals. Group-centered interaction is particularly critical when plans and decisions are being made so that the elderly person has as much opportunity as the other family members to express his opinions and preferences.

Mental health problems frequently activate the need to evaluate the current living situation and to decide if it meets the needs of everyone involved. Whether or not the elderly person should live with one of his kin is a decision frequently made at this time. Presented below are questions that the elderly person and his family should carefully consider before finalizing any decision.

1. What does the elderly person currently need in the way of supervision, social input, and personal service? Who is available and willing to help? In what way are the client's needs likely to change in the future?

2. What are the available options for living arrangements? Which alternatives are most acceptable to the client? Which alternatives are most acceptable to the family members? What community resources are available to provide service and support to the family unit?

3. If the elderly person moved in with kin, would he have personal and private space for sleeping? toileting? cooking? socializing? How much room would be available for his personal belongings? What arrangements could be made for the storage or disposition of items for which there is not room? Is this arrangement acceptable to the client?

4. How will responsibilities for the care of the elderly person and his expenses be arranged among the client, members inside the household and other related individuals outside the household? How often will related individuals outside the household visit, offer service, and provide financial support?

5. For what length of time are the involved persons prepared to maintain the new living arrangement? At what point is the living arrangement likely to become unacceptable? Will termination or another arrangement be necessary from the perspective of the client and the other family members?

6. What does each person in the situation expect? How closely matched are these expectations?

After the elderly person and his family have made the decision about living arrangements, the need for nursing intervention and counseling does not stop. At many points during the adjustment period, families need factual information about what to expect, ways to communicate and cope, and what community resources are available to supplement services and provide respite. In addition, having ongoing counseling and support sevices available permits the individuals to explore and share feelings and reconcile differences.

ENVIRONMENTAL MANIPULATION □ By carefully structuring the client's environment, the nurse promotes independence, self-esteem, and a sense of well-being. The key points in environmental manipulation are summarized below.

1. Changes in the environment that facilitate rather than inhibit the elderly client's functioning (also termed creation of the facilitative or prosthetic environment) help to increase both independence and self-esteem. For example, independent toileting is facilitated when (a) clothing is chosen that the elderly person can remove himself, (b) furniture is arranged so that bathrooms are accessible to a wheelchair or a walker, (c) assistive devices are affixed in the bathroom that permit independent transfer, and (d) visual problems are identified and steps taken to help the client distinguish the bathroom door from other doors. Creating a prosthetic environment requires that the person's limitations be identified and the environment be structured to make every activity as easy to do as possible.

2. Sensory stimulation that is pleasant, consistent, and planned with the client increases the sense of well-being and decreases the feeling of isolation. The elderly person needs to have the opportunity to

choose the forms of stimulation that are most desirable to him and needs permission to discontinue activities whenever he so desires.

3. Although sensory deprivation brought about by monotonous input and social isolation increases mental symptoms, the elderly client also needs the opportunity to escape continual stimulation. Simply turning on the television and leaving it on all day or shuttling the elderly person from one activity to another without providing rest periods may exacerbate rather than alleviate the symptoms. Privacy and solitude are necessary, too, and need to be included in the activity schedule.

4. Confusion and anxiety are created when the client is unable to sense any consistency, pattern, or meaning in the activities going on around him. Helping him find meaning in these activities in view of his sensory disturbances, helps him to achieve a sense of control over his environment.

5. To achieve a sense of control over the environment, the client must have the opportunity to touch, manipulate, and explore his surroundings. Providing the client with limited ambulation the opportunity to explore and find meaning in his environment is important.

6. Touching increases well-being, decreases isolation, and promotes trust. Many elderly people are "touch hungry," and the pleasant input provided by hand holding, placing an arm around the shoulder, or giving a gentle massage helps the elderly person "keep in touch" with reality.

To summarize, the professional nurse has an important role in secondary prevention of mental health problems among the elderly whether treatment occurs on an inpatient or an outpatient basis. The nursing role goes beyond simply coordinating the services provided by paraprofessionals. The nurse is a primary therapist. Because of the holistic nature of nursing, the professional nurse brings to the treatment setting the skills and knowledge necessary for comprehensive, wellness-oriented care for both the elderly client and his family. The nurse plays an important role also in the rehabilitation (tertiary prevention) of chronically mentally ill elderly clients.

□ EVALUATION

The Standards of Care established by the American Nurses' Association Gerontological Nursing and Psychiatric Nursing Sections (as adapted for use by the nurses in the client's locale or treatment agency) serve as the overall basis for the evaluation component of the nursing process. Based on these standards, evaluation involves both summative or outcome aspects (evaluation based on the individual goals for care established with the client and his family) and formative or process aspects (evaluation based on the way in which the care is delivered and the response that the client and his family demonstrate to specific nursing therapies).

■ Point of Emphasis

The evaluation of outcomes is possible only to the degree that (1) the care the patient receives is goal directed and based on individualized observation and assessment, (2) the goals are realistically focused on the client's needs and assets, and (3) the goals focus on the behavior that the client will display as a result of the prescribed nursing actions. The evaluation of process is possible only to the degree that (1) the professional nurse has consistent, therapeutic contact with the elderly client and his family during which observations can be made of the response to treatment and (2) the nursing process is applied in strategic manner for each individual client.

The evaluation and reevaluation involved in nursing process go on day-by-day, hour-by-hour. This activity is directed at modifying intervention strategies for goal attainment. It is also a terminal activity in which the nurse can judge the overall effectiveness of the interventions that were prescribed for one client. It is well to remember that goal attainment for many elderly clients is a much slower process than it is for younger clients. The evaluation plan must reflect a larger time frame so that neither the nurse nor the patient gives up on nursing intervention too soon.

■ Enrichment Activities

LEARNING ACTIVITIES

1. Acquaint yourself with your local community with regard to age distribution, health needs,

health care, and mental health resources and the prevailing attitudes toward the elderly.

a. From your local or state vital statistics bureau obtain the most recent data available on age distribution, gender distribution, income distribution, marital status, and living arrangements. From your local health planning office obtain the most recent data available on the health needs and health status of the elderly in your area.

b. Go to the largest shopping center in your area on a weekday morning or to a local bank on the third or fourth of the month. Observe the proportion of those who appear to be elderly (60+) to others in the area. Observe the proportion of those elderly who appear to have physical or mental limitations and the proportion of apparently well elderly. Compile a list (with documenting observations) of the types of possible mental or physical problems observed and a list of your observations that lead you to believe that an elder is well.

c. Identify the local community resources that provide supportive or mental health services to the elderly and their families. Visit one agency and observe the types of services provided, the ages and types of clients served, the prevailing treatment focus of the agency (primary, secondary, tertiary prevention, palliation, and so on) and the prevailing attitudes of the health care providers toward the elderly.

d. During a seminar session compare your observations in each area with those of your classmates. Synthesize your observations by summarizing your findings, identifying met needs and document ongoing needs of the elderly in your community, identifying the prevailing attitudes of community health care providers toward care of the elderly and projecting the greatest need for nursing intervention in your community.

2. Select three well elderly individuals: one who is 65 to 75 years of age, one who is 75 to 85 years of age, and one who is above 85 years of age. All should be living in the community and should be willing to discuss their life situations with you (some may be ones you met during your trip to the shopping mall or the bank). Contract to meet these individuals for 1 hour weekly for at least 4 weeks. During the first week establish rapport by obtaining a personal history up to early adulthood, including information about childhood, education, and family of origin. Explore with them the major decisions they made during this time, who helped them, who didn't, what they consider their major successes, failures, and disappointments. Keep notes on the interview. During the second week focus on middle age. Explore major decisions; major successes, failures, and disappointments; major rewards; effects of physical changes on self-image; changes in self-concept, self-awareness, and life goals; and coping styles, personal resources, and supports. In the third meeting focus on the later years. Explore major decisions and factors that influence his life-style; successes and strengths; weaknesses and fears; rewards and burdens; effects of physical changes on self-image and physical functioning; changes in self-concept, self-awareness, and life goals; and coping styles, personal resources, and supports. During the fourth week summarize with the client and terminate. If you need additional time with any of your clients, contract individually with them. Summarize the major themes discussed by each informant from your interview notes. Attempt to view the aging process through the eyes of your client, as you summarize your findings. Focus on aging as a time of growth and learning. Compare the experiences reported by the three informants. How do they differ, how do they correspond, and how does advancing age influence views of aging? Identify major threats to mental health and well-being in each informant and the areas in which the nurse can offer primary prevention. Identify at least three social changes that would make aging more successful and easier for each informant. Share your observations with your classmates.

3. Select one client over the age of 65 who is in a general hospital for treatment of an acute or a chronic physical illness. Perform a comprehensive mental health assessment and then plan an intervention program with the client, the focus of which is primary prevention. Include consideration of personal resources, strengths, family and social networks, and community resources as you both plan the intervention program. Evaluate the plan of care.

4. Select one client over the age of 65 in whom the *primary* diagnosis is indicative of a mental health problem. Perform a comprehensive

mental health assessment. Explore with him and his family and social support network the role of the social and physical environment in the mental health problem. Discuss whether and how this illness might have been prevented. Plan an intervention program with the client the the focus of which is secondary prevention. Include consideration of personal resources and strengths, family and social networks, and community resources as you both plan the intervention program. Evaluate the plan of care.

■ *References*

Antonovsky, A. *Health, stress, and coping.* San Francisco: Jossey-Bass, 1979.

Bachinsky, M. Geriatric medications: How psychotropic drugs can go astray. *R.N. magazine,* 41, 1978:50.

Birren, J.E., and Renner, V.J. Concepts and criteria of mental health and aging. *American journal of orthopsychiatry,* 51, 1981:242–254.

Brody, E.M. "Women in the middle" and family help to older people. *The gerontologist,* 21, 1981:471–480.

Brody, S.; Poulschock, S.W.; and Masciocci, C.F. The family caring unit: A major consideration in the long-term support system. *The gerontologist.* 18, 1978:556–561.

Burnside, I.M. (ed.). *Working with the elderly: Group processes and techniques.* North Scituate, MA: Duxbury Press, 1978.

————. Mental health and the aged. In *Nursing and the aged.* (Burnside, I.M., ed.). New York: McGraw-Hill, 1981.

Butler, R.N. Psychiatry and the elderly: An overview. *The American journal of psychiatry,* 132, 1975:893–900.

Butler, R.N., and Lewis, M.I. *Aging and mental health: Positive psychosocial and biomedical approaches.* St. Louis: Mosby Company, 1982.

Coetzee, D. Secondary prevention of depressive illness among the elderly. *SA medical journal.* (October 1980):571–574.

Ebersole, P. Developmental tasks in late life. In *Nursing and the aged.* (Burnside, I.M., ed.). New York: McGraw-Hill, 1976a.

Ebersole, P. Reminiscing and group psychotherapy with the aged. In *Nursing and the aged.* (Burnside, I.M., ed.). New York: McGraw-Hill, 1976b:214–230.

Ebersole, P. A theoretical approach to the use of reminiscence. In *Nursing and the aged.* (Burnside, I.M., ed.). New York: McGraw-Hill, 1976c:139–154

Ebersole, P. Establishing reminiscing groups. In *Working with the elderly: Group process and technique.* (Burnside, I.M., ed.). North Scituate, MA: Duxbury Press, 1978:237–254.

Ebersole, P., and Hess, P. *Toward health aging: Human needs and nursing response.,* St. Louis: Mosby Company, 1981.

Eisdorfer, C. Developmental level and sensory impairments in the aged. *Journal of projective techniques,* 24, 1960:129–132.

Forbes, E.J., and Fitzsimmons, V.M. *The older adult: A process for wellness.* St. Louis: Mosby Company, 1981.

Freud, S. *Collected papers,* Vol. 4 (Jones, Ernest, ed.; Riviere, Joan, trans.). London: Hogarth, 1949.

Gelperin, E.A. Rehabilitative psychiatric nursing for chronically ill, elderly patients. *Journal of the American Geriatrics Society,* 21, 1973:566–568.

Glick, P.C. The future marital status and living arrangements of the elderly. *The gerontologist,* 19, 1979:301–308.

Green, B. The politics of psychoactive drug use in old age. *The gerontologist,* 18, 1978:525.

Greenwood, A. Mental disturbances following operation for contracts. *Journal of the American Medical Association,* 91, 1928:1713.

Havinghurst, R.J. *Developmental tasks and education,* New York: David McKay Co., 1972.

Hayer, J. Positive aspects of aging. *Journal of gerontological nursing,* 2, (January/February 1976):19.

Krupa, L., and Verner, A. Hazards of drug use among the elderly. *The gerontologist,* 15, 1979:129.

Kurtz, J., and Wolk, S. Continued growth and life satisfaction. *The gerontologist,* 15, 1975:129.

Kuypers, J.A., and Bengtson, V.L. Competence and social breakdown: A social-psychological view of aging. *Human development,* 2, 1973:37–49.

Lang, A., and Brody, E.M. Patterns of family support to middle-aged, older and very old women. Paper prepared for 33d annual meeting of the Gerontological Society of America, San Diego, CA: November 1980.

Lansley, D.G., and Robinowitz, C.B. Psychiatric manpower: An overview. *Hospital and community psychiatry.* 30, 1979:749–755.

Lawton, M.P., and Brody, E. Assessment of older people: Self-maintaining and instrumental activities of daily living. *The gerontologist,* 9, 1969:179–186.

Levine, J., and Levine, W.C. *Ageism prejudice and discrimination against the elderly.* Belmont, CA: Wadsworth Publishing Co., 1980.

Maslow, A. *Toward a psychology of being.* Princeton: D. Van Nostrand Co., 1962.

Miller, M. Geriatric Suicide: The Ariena Study. *The gerontologist,* 18, 1978:488–495.

Mindel, C.H. Multigenerational family households: Recent trends and implications for the future. *The gerontologist,* 19, 1979:456–463.

Oberleder, M. Managing problem behaviors of elderly patients. *Hospital and community psychiatry,* 27, 1981:325–330.

O'Neil, P.M., and Calhoun, K.S. Sensory deficits and behavioral deterioration in senescence. *Journal of abnormal psychology,* 5, 1975:579–582.

Palmore, E. Advantages of aging. *The gerontologist,* 19, 1979:220.

Pardes, H. The aging: Mental problems. *New York State journal of medicine,* (April 1981):788–804.

Peck, R. Psychological development in the second half of life. In *Middle age and aging.* (Neugarten, B., ed.). Chicago: University of Chicago Press, 1980.

Perron, D. Deprived of sound. *American journal of nursing,* 74, 1974:1057–1059.

Peterson, D.M., and Thomas, C.W. Acute drug reactions among the elderly. *Journal of gerontology,* 30, 1975:552–556.

Phillips, L.R.F. Care of the client with sensoriperceptual problems. In *Confusion: Prevention and care.* (Wolanin, M.O., and Phillips, L.R.F., eds.). St. Louis: Mosby Company, 1981:171–267.

Raffoul, P.R.; Cooper, J.K.; and Love, D.W. Drug misuse in older people. *The gerontologist,* 21, 1981:146–150.

Ramsdell, D.A. The psychology of the hard-of-hearing and deafened adult. In *Hearing and deafness.* (Davis, H., and Silverman, S.R., eds.). New York: Holt, Rinehart & Winston, 1970:453–461.

Reifler, B.V., and Eisdorfer, C. A clinic for the impaired elderly and their families. *American journal of psychiatry,* 137, 1980:1399–1403.

Shanas, E. The family as a social support in old age. *The gerontologist,* 19, 1979:168–174.

Shore, H. Sensory deprivation. Paper presented to Mainstreaming the elderly, conference, University of Kansas, Overland Park, Kansas, 1978.

Snyder, L.H., Pyrek, J., and Smith, K.C. Vision and mental function of the elderly. *The gerontologist,* 16, 1976:491–495.

Statistical Life Bulletin. State variations in longevity. Metropolitan Life Insurance Company (January–March 1980):10–14.

Statistical Life Bulletin. Changes in the age profile of the population. Metropolitan Life Insurance Company (July–September 1981):3–4.

Weinberg, H. On adding insult to injury. *The gerontologist,* 16, 1975:4–10.

Weiss, A.D. Role and importance of sensory function in aging. In *Duke University Council on Gerontology: Proceedings* 1961–1965, (Jeffers, F.D., ed.). Durham, N.C.: Duke University Regional Center on Aging, 1965.

Wolanin, M.O., and Phillips, L.R.F. *Confusion: Prevention and care.* St. Louis: Mosby Company, 1981.

Ziskind, E. Observations of mental symptoms in eye-patched patients: Hypnogogic symptoms in sensory deprivation. *American journal of psychiatry,* 66, 1960:895.

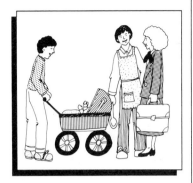

21

Sexuality

Mary Lou Haberman Orchard and Daniel Murphy

Learning Objectives

Upon completion of this chapter, the reader will be able to:

1. Demonstrate an understanding of the complex nature of sexuality and the role of the nurse in promoting sexual well-being.

2. Describe changes in the American concept of sexual "normality" over past decades and identify biological, psychological, and social components of sexuality.

3. Recognize that overtly sexual behaviors may be manifestations of covert nonsexual motives or needs.

4. Distinguish among various forms of sexual expression including parameters of sexual behavior, alternative lifestyles, and the psychosexual dysfunctions.

5. Identify means by which nurses can enhance their self-awareness and effectiveness in assessment and support of client sexual well-being.

6. Apply knowledge of nursing process in assisting clients to cope with a variety of sexually related issues in health and illness.

7. Evaluate the effects of the health care setting and professionals' attitudes on client sexual well-being.

Sexuality is a component of human being-ness that is, by nature, complex. Broadly, it includes concepts of gender identity, gender role, and physiological functioning. In addition, realities of specific sexual behaviors, language, attitudes, beliefs, and values serve to enhance its complexity. Perhaps this is why sexuality and sexual well-being have, for a long time, been an area largely ignored by nurses as an essential, integral part of the process of caring for another human being.

It is only within the last 10 to 15 years that human sexuality has become a generally recognized legitimate area of concern for nurses. Like death, sexuality is an essential part of life. And, like death, integrating the reality of sexuality into professional practice can be anxiety provoking at first, also challenging, and eventually quite satisfying.

The purpose of the first part of this chapter is to provide an overview of information about various components of sexuality. The second part provides avenues for guiding the nurse in developing understanding and skill about sexuality and promoting sexual well-being within the health care delivery system.

□ *Trends in Understanding Human Sexuality*

WHAT IS "NORMAL?"

Contemporary views about sexual normality are affected by a number of factors—scientific discoveries, changing cultural values, personal expectations and limitations, technological improvements, and therapeutic interventions. Normality as a concept is no longer absolutely right or wrong, a static concept to be followed blindly. Individual and cultural attitudes and values must be considered, as well as the Diagnostic and Statistical Manual of Mental Disorders (DSM III) classification.

The past two decades have been characterized by profound changes in ideas about healthy, or normal, sexual behaviors, and those that should be diagnosed as unhealthy. These changes parallel a shift in theoretical views about human sexuality. Earlier psychiatric definitions of abnormality focused on specific genital activities—homosexual acts, masturbation, necrophilia. The most widely accepted classification of maladaptive behavior today is found in the DSM III (1980). In addition to addressing such behaviors as pedophilia, fetishism, and transvestism, this revision also includes gender identity disorders and problems of sexual desire. Adjustment problems created by homosexual orientation are considered, rather than homosexual behavior per se.

SCIENTIFIC DISCOVERIES

Scientific discoveries have paved the way for alterations in our concepts of normality. For example, Freud's dual orgasm theory in women was predominant through the 1950s. Therapists viewed the clitoral orgasm as "immature," and women who could not achieve orgasm through vaginal stimulation were considered to have a psychological disorder. A series of experiments by Masters and Johnson (1966) destroyed the Freudian myth by demonstrating that there was no difference in the physiological orgastic response in women, regardless of the locus of stimulation. They further suggested that the vagina was devoid of sensory nerve endings and concluded that all orgasms are based upon stimulation of the clitoral system. However, contemporary sexologists cannot be complacent about "facts" related to human sexuality. Not only is the trigger for orgasm independent of clitoral stimulation (the locus is between the vagina and the urethra, named the Gräfenberg spot), but the physiological reactions are quite different from those of clitoral orgasms. These researchers have even presented evidence of female ejaculation!

THEORETICAL CHANGES

With the advent of discoveries about physiological sexual functioning, theorists and therapists alike are recognizing the complex roles that the human mind and body play in creating and developing a sense of sexual well-being. That organic impairment (e.g., chemical imbalance or vascular disease) may be causing sexual dysfunction is now as often considered in treatment planning as is intrapsychic conflict. The concept of stress is now often incorporated into the search for understanding impaired sexual well-being. For example, when the realm of the client's biological, psychological, social, and spiritual experience is considered, the theoretician or therapist may see that expectations for certain levels of sexual satisfaction might be unrealistic at the present time and help the client to adapt to or minimize stressors in order to facilitate sexual well-being. Also, the idea that sexual behavior is learned has led to the development of behavioral therapy techniques that are often helpful for persons with simple sexual dysfunction.

Most theoreticians and qualified therapists now use an approach to understanding and promoting healthy sexuality that recognizes and respects the complex interplay of the whole human person, not exclusively his intrapsychic processes, or physiology, or behavior.

CHANGES IN CULTURAL NORMS

Cultural norms have undergone significant shifts over the past 20 years. Oral-genital behaviors are now accepted as positive acts between people, women are expressing the need for sexual equality at all levels of their existence, and religious organizations are openly struggling with changing standards of sexual behaviors—such as homosexuality, abortion, premarital intercourse, contraception, and male superiority. Antiquated laws regulating sexual activities are under review in most states, reflecting changing cultural values. Many penalties for sexual behaviors between consenting adults are being eliminated or reduced in severity. Rape is viewed as an aggressive act, wherein the shame of the crime is placed upon the assailant, rather than upon the victim. Laws protecting the rights of women and children are being enacted.

SEXUALITY AS A LEGITIMATE HEALTH CONCERN

Health professions now consider the sexual behavior or problems of clients as legitimate areas for intervention. Concerns clients have regarding their own sexuality are as much in the province of the nurse as in that of the psychologist. Sexual matters are incorporated into the treatment plan for persons with cardiac problems, diabetes, spinal cord injury, mastectomies, and prostatectomies, to name a few.

Current trends in nursing education place additional pressures upon the nurse, especially in the area of human sexuality.

■ *Point of Emphasis*

Sex is not merely the copulative act of generation, but includes a vast array of human activities and attitudes: physical sexual relations with self and others; self-image; sexual preferences; emotions such as joy, guilt, fear, and expectations; and parenthood roles. Health problems and corrective medications may interact with several facets of sexuality.

To treat the total needs of the client may require in-depth consideration of sexuality. This situation was addressed by S.P. Hirsch, (1977) of the National Institute of Mental Health and the National Cancer Institute: "In hospitals, the norm for staff, clients, and friends is to pretend sexuality doesn't exist." Dr. Hirsch continues, "I suggest that sexuality become an ongoing topic of discussion for the staff of oncology services, particularly those working with children and adolescents. I would suggest self-help groups assist in opening up for discussion and exploration the areas of human sexuality and the cancer patient, just as they did with the issue of death and dying."

A holistic approach often requires that the nurse assume roles that conflict with that of the nurturant, obedient caretaker. This in itself creates problems in many health-care institutions, but involvement in the area of sexuality may introduce additional difficulties for the nurse, with colleagues and clients alike. Clients may regard the concerned nurse as a seductive person, complicating the client-nurse relationship. Despite recent advances in medical education, many physicians are not trained to deal with a client's sexuality, and could perceive the involved nurse as a threat.

Social taboos surrounding nudity, bodily elimination, and privacy still abound, and the hospital setting may provoke embarrassment in clients. For many, the only refuge from this intrusion of modesty is the sterile, clinical approach of the nurse. To introduce discussion of sex into the treatment plan may lead to false assumptions related to seduction, or may reflect incorrectly upon the nurse's own sexual attitudes and desires. Those who are comfortable with their own sexuality, and who can comfortably discuss sexual difficulties with clients, may be viewed with suspicion by those who cannot do the same. In spite of these pitfalls, the client's sexuality is often an integral part of the total health program. Involvement in this area is personally rewarding to the practitioner, for to become competent in dealing with the sexual problems of others, one must first examine, cope with, and accept one's own sexuality. In addition, clients will generally have a more positive outlook on their own recovery.

☐ Components of Sexuality

While some still attempt to discover singular motives for or causes of specific sexual acts, most present-day authorities consider this a simplistic approach in light of contemporary research findings. Sexuality is viewed as an interaction between biological and psychosocial factors. John Money (1965) has described a model of psychosexual development which identifies several important variables.

BIOLOGICAL ASPECTS OF SEX

The typical genetic code for a male is 46, XY, and that for a female is 46, XX. Under certain conditions a child may be born with an extra chromosome, or with one missing. Either of these situations affects maleness or femaleness. Two of the most frequent conditions of chromosomal abnormalities are a 47, XX pattern, identified as Kleinfelter's syndrome, and a 45, X pattern, labeled Turner's syndrome. The Kleinfelter's individual is typically a sterile, relatively passive male with a tendency to have developed breasts and a low sex drive. Turner's syndrome females are also sterile, amenorrheic, and suffer a variety of external and internal physical abnormalities. A more complete description of genetic abnormalities, including hermaphroditism, may be found in Money (1972).

Until the sixth or seventh week of gestation, the gonadal structures of males and females are identical. At this stage of development, the Y-chromosome controls the release of H-Y antigen, which stimulates the development of the gonads into testes (Haseltine, 1981). The testes additionally secrete müllerian inhibiting substance (MIS) which causes the female müllerian duct system to degenerate (Francoer, 1982). In the absence of the actions of H-Y antigen and MIS, the primordial gonads always develop into ovaries, regardless of chromosomal coding. The principal sex organs of males and females develop from the same embryonic tissue. We will return to this fact when discussing the similarities between male and female experiences of orgasm.

In the absence of positive chemical action all human embryos will develop into females, regardless of chromosomal coding. It is possible that these results could occur from surgical or external chemical intervention that prevents the production of H-Y antigen or MIS. Some feminist writers have used these data to raise provocative issues. Sherfey (1972) believes that since only female development is autonomous, male development should be considered as adaptation of female structures. "Thus it seems that nature's basic plan is to make a female and that the addition of a Y-chromosome produces a variation." (Hyde, 1982).

GENDER ROLES

Every stable society has sexual scripts, or roles, that men and women are generally expected to follow. Many of these roles serve a positive function in that they help maintain order by assigning certain tasks by sex. They also aid in psychological adjustment by providing standards against which we may judge masculinity and femininity. When such roles become stereotyped, or solidified so as to restrict growth, they serve a negative function.

> ■ *Point of Emphasis*
> *Social roles exert powerful influences upon sexuality.*

Although all cultures expect a type of sex role and sexual behaviors, there are no generalizable sexual behaviors or roles that hold for all societies. The only consistent finding has been that only males can impregnate and only females can gestate and lactate. Gender expectations vary among cultures. Margaret Mead has provided stark contrasts of gender roles of continuous societies of New Guinea (1935). Arapesh parents are expected to cooperate in child rearing, and share the responsibility of providing a warm, safe, and supportive environment for the children. Distinctions are not made between boys and girls as to assigned tasks, toys, or games. The neighboring Mundugermor are radically different, and physical violence and an atmosphere of suspicion and mistrust of other family members are the rule. Women are violently aggressive, and children are taught that no one is to be trusted, including the parents. The Tchambuli, another New Guinea tribe, present a third contrasting set of roles. The mother is responsible for supporting the family through weaving and fishing for food. Tchambuli men depend entirely on women for their survival, and devote their lives to decorating their bodies, playing music, and coquettishly attempting to win the favor of women. Others (Malinowski, 1929; Ford and Beach, 1951) have documented similar varieties among scores of cultures. Traditional Japanese and Iranian women are considered subservient to men, while Swedish women are independent. Masturbation, oral-genital acts, and intercourse are taught to children in some societies, denied them in others. These educational experiences help shape the concept of what "good" men and women are.

Double standards also exist in abundance. Islam, one of the major religions of the world, generally has a positive view of sex, but primarily for the men. Copulation using any bodily orifice is acceptable, even if both partners are male, yet clitoridectomy is still commonly practiced among certain Islamic sects, for sexual pleasure is restricted to males. Men are allowed to take several wives, but wives are not allowed to talk in the presence of men and are expected to eat in a separate room after the men have finished.

■ *Point of Emphasis*

People experience difficulties when the actual roles and sexual practices of a society conflict with the stereotypes of the culture.

In the United States, many men and women are experiencing challenges to traditional sexual role stereotyping. Social forces such as divorce, economics, and the women's movement have created new opportunities for people to function in varied and alternative roles. For example, as the divorce rate has increased, the number of single parent households has also grown. Whether as fathers or mothers, single parents face problems related to demands on time and energy for wage earning and parenting. For this population, getting needs met for intimacy and physical sexual fulfillment can be particularly difficult. Death of a spouse also creates demands for the survivor to create new modes of getting needs met to maintain sexual well-being.

As the economic and social situation changes, more and more women are entering the work force. This phenomenon creates demands on both men and women to reorder the notion of "acceptable" male and female behavior. Men in traditionally male occupations (e.g., law, medicine, construction, business) are challenged to incorporate women into the unspoken yet powerful normative behaviors related to networking, language, and standard practice. Women in these occupations are challenged to learn what may be new and different normative behaviors (e.g., assertiveness) in order to function effectively in their roles.

As the social atmosphere regarding occupational choice has become more flexible toward gender, men have also entered traditionally female occupations (e.g., nursing and elementary education) in greater numbers. In these occupations, men sometimes face challenges related to expectations of others for stereotypical "male" behaviors and sometimes risk having their personal sexual preference questioned.

The impact of those phenomena on the sexual behaviors of individuals is currently not well described in the literature. However, it might be speculated that as sexual role behaviors change and diversify, some degree of personal conflict may occur within sexual relationships with spouses or significant others. Personal beliefs and values, cultivated since childhood, can be challenged in often unexpected ways as people venture into new modes of occupational and relational functioning. The nurse must be alert to the actual and potential difficulties created by such change and strive to understand the person's situation. The importance of acceptance and communication between partners cannot be overemphasized. Both men and woman may, at various times, experience anxiety, confusion, and self-consciousness about sexuality. Such experiences are part of the human condition, need to be respected as such, and responded to with empathy and support.

PARAMETERS OF SEXUAL BEHAVIOR

The purpose of this section is to either familiarize the reader with various aspects of sexual behavior or to serve as a reminder of them. It is of vital importance that the nurse know what types of behaviors human beings engage in so she can avoid making responses of disgust or shock when clients have questions, concerns, or learning needs about specific sexual behaviors. Ways of increasing comfort about sexual behavior are discussed in the second section.

Sexual Fantasy and Dreams

Sexual fantasy and dreams have been known to be a rich and common source of sexual stimulation (Kinsey, et al., 1948; 1953). There is great similarity in the fantasies of both men and women. However, women are more apt to imagine being forced into sexual activities (in the absence of pain or genuine violence), having sexual relations with a member of the same sex, or performing sexual acts that they would never do in reality. Men have more frequent fantasies about having sex with a stranger, having sex with several people at the same time, or forcing someone into sexual activities (although the victim soon capitulates and becomes a willing partner). Male fantasies tend to focus upon specific sexual acts and themes of power, while female fantasies revolve around romantic, seductive scenes (Hunt, 1974; Sue, 1979).

■ *Point of Emphasis*

Sexual fantasy is a normal, healthy part of people's lives.

Friday (1973; 1980) provides evidence that any dream content, however bizarre, may be normal. It is not uncommon for people to have fantasies involving them in antisocial or anticultural acts (e.g., raping or being raped; becoming a prostitute or strip-tease dancer; homosexual behaviors). Some of Friday's respondents did live out their fantasies, and they found the reality far less pleasurable than the fantasy. Under certain conditions fantasies can be considered maladaptive or potentially pathological: (1) when they become a substitute for, or an escape from, human interactions; (2) when they become obsessive and interfere with social relations and personal growth; or (3) when they become compulsive, leading toward an acting out of antisocial behaviors.

Autoeroticism

Masturbation refers to genital self-stimulation for sexual gratification and is very common in our society. Social attitudes toward self-pleasuring have undergone drastic changes during the past half-decade. In the early 1900s masturbation was considered to be physically and psychologically harmful, leading to acne, senility, physical debilitation, and insanity. Onanism (masturbation) was a classification of mental disorder, and many religions labeled this behavior as sinful.

Present attitudes are considerably more lenient. The extent of masturbation among males has remained relatively constant at 90 to 94 percent (Kinsey, 1948; Hunt, 1974). There has been a gradual and progressive increase in the extent of female masturbation from two-thirds in the Kinsey (1953) and Hunt (1974) surveys to 78 percent (Miller and Lief, 1976) or 82 percent (Hite, 1976). Further evidence of the growing acceptance of masturbation is revealed in the data on married respondents. Almost 75 percent of married men and women masturbate (while married) an average of 24 and 10 times a year respectively (Hunt, 1974; Levin and Levin, 1975).

Today, few physicians, psychologists, or psychiatrists warn about excessive acts of masturbation. The basis for physical or mental pathology has failed to be supported. Some religions, for example, Roman Catholic and Orthodox Judaism, still proscribe self-pleasuring as a sin. For individuals accepting these values, the act would have negative impact. It should be pointed out that some people never masturbate (6 to 10 percent of men, 25 to 35 percent of women), and that many others experience this infrequently during their lives. While in the minority, they should not be considered abnormal or disordered.

■ *Point of Emphasis*

Nurses need to remember that masturbation is a normal activity that accompanies growth and development of body image and self-awareness throughout the lifespan. Masturbation may be triggered by other motives: sexual pleasure and release; completion of unsatisfactory sexual interactions; curiosity; self-exploration to discover bodily responses; reassurance that sexual response is still functional; a temporary substitute for a partner from whom one is separated; boredom; tension release; and as an aid to sleep. The hospital experience frequently exacerbates several of these conditions simultaneously, and nurses should anticipate an increase in such activity among hospitalized patients.

Oral-Genital Behavior

Hunt (1974) has observed that oral-genital stimulation has shown the greatest increase in acceptance of all sexual activities during the past few decades. These behaviors may be the final stage for achieving orgasm or may be preliminary to intercourse. One partner may stimulate the other unilaterally, they may take turns, or they may stimulate each other simultaneously (sometimes called "sixty-nine").

Cunnilingus. Cunnilingus is the use of the mouth and lips to lick or suck on the clitoris, labia, vulva, and introitus. Each woman has her own preferences of types and locations of stimulation. Techniques include: gentle sucking of the clitoris or labia minora; changes in speed or pressure of the flicking tongue; simultaneous stimulation of the vagina with a finger. The variations are endless. Good communication with the partner about personal preferences provides the best guide.

Women who allow themselves to totally accept this activity find it extremely stimulating, and for some this is the only way of achieving orgasm.

Fellatio. Fellatio is stimulation of the penis and the scrotal area with the lips, tongue, or mouth. Methods of stimulation include: nibbling or lightly touching the penile shaft or glans with the tongue; gently sucking on the shaft and glans. Most men do not enjoy actual blowing on the penis. Fellatio is a highly stimulating activity for most males. Bodily cleanliness is essential with either cunnilingus or fellatio. Some women reject fellatio out of fear of the male ejaculating into their mouths. While semen is relatively tasteless, and harmless when swallowed, some view this with revulsion. Men also may find cunnilingus repugnant, viewing the vulva as an organ of bodily elimination. On the other hand, many men and women find the aroma and taste of the genitalia arousing. Men have experienced erection while performing cunnilingus, and some women have had orgasm during fellatio. As in all matters, open discussion about likes and dislikes is important in order to maximize pleasurable experiences.

Penile-Vaginal Intercourse

While sexual intercourse (coitus) is the most common sexual technique employed by couples, great variations in intromission are possible. Within this decade, some states established laws that allowed the male-superior position as the only legal act of intromission. The variations, too numerous to list, are beyond the scope of this text, and clients may have to be informed that any position that is enjoyable and mutually acceptable is normal. Some advantages and disadvantages of the basic positions are described—other variations center around standing, sitting, lying, and kneeling.

Man-on-Top, Face-to-Face. Man-on-top, face-to-face is often referred to as the missionary position. This is the most frequently used style in the United States. Even among experimenting couples, this becomes the standard. It is the best position for those attempting to achieve pregnancy and also leaves the woman's hands free to hold and caress her partner. This position does not work well when the man is extremely heavy or should avoid exertion, when the woman is obese, or in the late stages of pregnancy.

Woman-on-Top, Face-to-Face. This position provides a great deal of clitoral stimulation and allows the woman maximum control over her own stimulation. Thus it is the optimum position for female orgasm during intercourse. It also allows the man to caress her body during coitus. Additionally, it aids the man who wishes to delay orgasm, or if he is tired or should avoid strenuous activities for health reasons.

Rear-Entry. Rear entry is highly stimulating to some who are becoming bored with sex and provides an opportunity for the man to stimulate the breasts and clitoris of the woman during intercourse. Care should be taken during thrusting, for this position allows deep penetration, and men with long penises may cause the woman pain.

Side-by-Side. Used with either front or rear entry, this position is advantageous for gentle, prolonged intercourse. It may be used when either partner is fatigued, when one is obese, or when the woman is in the advanced stages of pregnancy.

Anal Intercourse

Intercourse by inserting the penis into the anal opening is practiced by heterosexuals, by homosexual males, and rarely by lesbians using a penile substitute. While some couples find it highly arousing and obtain great pleasure from it, most Americans have strong negative attitudes about anal sex, viewing that part of the body as unclean or disgusting, or feeling that the act itself is perverted. Some have reservations on religious grounds, as this type of intercourse precludes pregnancy. Some prefer it for the same reason, enjoying sex without the fear of pregnancy. Fewer than 25 percent of Hunt's (1974) sample had attempted it even once, while 43 percent of Levin and Levin's respondents (1975) had done so. The majority of the respondents were under 35 years of age.

Couples trying anal intercourse encounter several problems. The anal sphincter muscles must be conditioned to relax, and first attempts must be slow and gentle to avoid pain. The anus does not contain natural lubricants, so a commercial lubricant must be employed. Frequent indulgences may cause fissures around the anal opening. Finally, some anal bacteria are infectious to the vagina and the male urethra.

Homosexualities

A homosexual is a person who prefers, or exclusively requires, sexual interactions with someone of the same sex. The variety of definitions used by lay people often confuses issues related to homosexuality and lesbianism. Many definitions have been tendered. The majority of Americans view this form of sexual expression with disgust, considering it as abnormal and obscene. They believe it is an illness that can be cured; that homosexuals are a threat to society, particularly to children; and that liberalized thinking fosters an explosive growth in this form of behavior. The data show most of these myths to be untrue.

There are many varieties of homosexual experiences. Situational homosexuals are those who engage in same-sex activities because of long-term separation from opposite-sex members. Examples of this are found in prisons and at isolated military establishments. When members of the other sex are available, these individuals revert to heterosexual life-styles. Latent homosexuals are defined as those who would desire same-sex relations, but who refrain from it. The term is falling out of use because of former meanings in Freudian terminology. Covert homosexuals ("closet homosexuals") are those who actively engage in same-sex relations, but who do so surreptitiously, maintaining an external appearance of heterosexuality. Overt homosexuals make no attempt to disguise their orientation. A further distinction must be made between those who engage in a transitory relationship out of curiosity, or during a period of confusion in sexual identity, and those who make an informed, mature choice.

Kinsey (1948, 1953) found that 37 percent of men and 13 percent of women had had a homosexual experience. The varieties of situations reported led him to propose a scale that reflects the degree in involvement and has proven quite helpful. At one end of the scale (0) are found those who are exclusively heterosexual in desires and behaviors. Kinsey found 63 percent of males and 87 percent females to belong in this category. The scale progresses through several other categories, concluding with class 6, those who are exclusively homosexual in desire and behavior. Kinsey found that 2 to 3 percent of men and 1 percent of women were at this end of the continuum. These data have been given support through the years by Hunt (1974) and several other researchers in the United States and Europe. The extent of exclusive homosexuality has remained remarkably stable

for over 30 years, showing neither increases or decreases.

No single factor has been found that is responsible for the development of same-sex desires. Biological theories, whether endocrinological or hormonal, have not received support. Social factors, such as a domineering mother and an indifferent father, have been noted in a few studies, but in others appear to have no effect. Bell and Weinberg (1978) believe there are many different types of homosexual life-styles, each having its own set of causative factors. They espouse the term "homosexualities" to emphasize that there is no single homosexual personality.

■ *Point of Emphasis*

Homosexuality is considered a psychiatric disorder by the American Psychiatric Association only if it is ego-dystonic, that is, a source of distress for the patient.

Earlier studies had shown that homosexuals experienced more adjustment problems than heterosexuals, but the gay population studied were already in therapy, and they were being compared to heterosexuals out of therapy. When homosexuals not in therapy and heterosexuals not in therapy were compared, no differences were discovered.

While the percentages of exclusive homosexualism are small (2 to 3 percent of men), the numbers in our society are significant—over 2 million men. Nurses should anticipate that some of their clients or their health care colleagues will have this orientation. Clients may have concerns about their sexual adjustments but hesitate to discuss them with the doctor or nurse, fearing disapproval. They may also feel uneasy about the possible visits of their homosexual partner.

The preceding section has provided information about various human sexual behaviors that are usual or normal. The behaviors are among the ways in which human beings promote, maintain, and enhance growth, intimacy, and sexual well-being with each other.

The following section on Psychosexual Disorders describes human behaviors and experiences that are not considered to be usual or normal. With most of the behaviors, there are characteristics of dissatisfaction, absence of a sense of sexual well-being, and, with the paraphilias, dynamics of exploitation and victimization.

The discussion covers behavior patterns for which diagnoses have been formulated. These diagnostic categories are taken from the DSM-III, which includes others not discussed here (see Appendix B).

PSYCHOSEXUAL DISORDERS

Gender Identity Disorders

Transsexualism. Transsexualism connotes the desire for gender identity that is opposite to the person's anatomical sex. Affected individuals often express very painful feelings that they are trapped in the body of the opposite sex. Diagnosis must include at least 2 years of extreme dissatisfaction with the assigned sex and a desire to be free of the offensive sex organs. Most transsexuals have healthy bodies with normal chromosomal makeup and healthy sex organs. Causative factors have not been identified, although most authorities lean toward a social learning explanation. Early treatments through psychotherapy proved unsuccessful in alleviating the mind-body disharmony (Tollison and Adams, 1979). Surgical procedures, coupled with hormone treatments, gained popularity during the 1960s and 1970s. Persons with this condition experience a great deal of distress and need to have warm, respectful, and empathic responses from health care providers.

The majority of individuals presenting for transsexual surgery are men. Male-to-female candidates must typically undergo a year or more of psychotherapy in order to eliminate inappropriate candidates, such as: people with schizophrenia; people undergoing temporary, severe psychological stress; unstable persons who may not be ready to accept the disadvantages of this irreversible surgery. Because homophobia is still rampant in our society, persons with ego-dystonic homosexuality may seek to have the surgery done so that they won't be considered homosexual. In the late stages of psychotherapy, candidates begin to receive hormone treatments, which will be a lifetime need. They are expected increasingly to wear clothing of the adopted sex, and to begin other-sex role behaviors (e.g., to use other-sex bathrooms). Surgery has been more successful for male-to-female transsexuals than the reverse. In the former, testes and penis are removed, an artificial vagina is implanted, and (occasionally)

breast implantation may be done to increase breast size. Female-to-male surgery includes breast removal, (occasionally) a partial or complete hysterectomy, and implantation of a prosthetic penile device.

Physiological sexual responses in transsexuals are impaired, sometimes seriously, but for many this is a small price to pay for being free from their previously detested body. Long-term evaluations have led some experts to question the efficacy of such surgical procedures, and some medical centers, such as Johns Hopkins, have suspended performing them until reliable findings become available.

Transsexuals face many legal and social problems. Few states recognize the person as changed. Nor do the Social Security Administration and most insurance companies. Consider the situation for a hospitalized patient: Is he/she to be placed with a male or a female roommate? Which records have to be maintained by the physician?

Nurses should review their own feelings about caring for such an individual. Through understanding the complexity of the condition, nurses may learn to respond with respect, genuineness, and compassion.

Paraphilia

Paraphilia includes sexual preferences that rely on unusual, atypical experiences or fantasies for sexual gratification. These objects or situations become the focal point of sexual activity. Professionals prefer this term to "sexual deviancies," because some behavior that deviates from the norm may not be a disorder (e.g., celibacy in a cleric). Paraphilia may center around an inappropriate object (child, animal, leather gloves), or a particular act (inflicting, or receiving, pain). Paraphilia is characterized by preoccupation, repetition of the behavior, and by the essential nature of the experience to achieve sexual release. It is more frequent in men than in women.

There is often a thin line between paraphilia and less intensive desires or fantasies. Many men are aroused by filmy lingerie or by the thought of sexual activities with a juvenile, as occurs in the novel *Lolita*. Similarly, women may be aroused by a man's hairy chest, or his firm, tight buttocks. Each of these desires could be magnified to the point of psychological dependence, could become a prerequisite for sexual arousal, and could become a form of paraphilia.

Fetishism. Fetishism is a pathological displacement of sexual interest to an object—the fetish. The fetish is commonly a piece of female attire, such as a brassiere, panties, high-heeled shoes, or gloves, but may be any object, or material, such as items made of fur, rubber, or leather. The person prefers that the fetish be involved in any sexual activity or requires its presence to achieve sexual gratification. Care should be taken in identifying body parts as fetishes. Americans are well known for their intense interest in the female breast—which is considered normal—while sexual desire focused on the foot is frequently identified as fetishism. A man may masturbate, using feminine underwear to enhance satisfaction, or a woman may use a vibrator to reach orgasm, both done in the absence of a desired partner. These are considered only as masturbatory aids; a fetish is the particular underwear, or a particular type or shape of vibrator, that is necessary to reach orgasm.

Some fetishists maintain large collections of objects, such as underwear, and may maintain catalogs listing the owner of the object, and the time and date of collection. Distinction must be made between actual dependence upon certain pieces of apparel for sexual arousal, and the sight of a person wearing sexually provocative garments.

Transvestism. Transvestism is repeated cross-dressing, that is, wearing women's clothes, by a heterosexual male. In the early stages of this behavior one of the primary purposes is to achieve sexual excitement. Sexual release may be achieved through masturbation or heterosexual intercourse. This diagnosis is restricted to men, though individuals may cross-dress for various reasons. Present social customs sanction the wearing of men's clothing by women. Jeans and pantsuits are considered asexual dress; a woman wearing a man's T-shirt, but no brassiere, may be considered a sexually arousing stimulus to men, rather than a transvestite. Male entertainers may cross-dress for professional purposes.

As discussed earlier, transsexuals wear opposite-sex clothing, because they see this as appropriate for their perceived sex. Some male homosexuals go out "in drag" (cross-dress) to attract other men for sexual relations. In these cases, the purpose is other than to exert sexual arousal through the wearing of the clothing per se, hence it is not transvestism.

Zoophilia. Zoophilia is an abnormal sexual fondness for animals and is a rare condition. Bestiality is the legal term for a single, isolated sexual act involving an animal. In the Kinsey (1948, 1953) studies, 8 percent of men and 4 percent of women reported having such contact, but Hunt (1974) found much less. Women reported having body contact more frequently than men, and men more frequently masturbated, using the animal for arousal. While contact between the animal's mouth and the human genitals was equally reported by men and woman, actual coital activity was extremely rare among women (Kinsey). Bestiality is very uncommon today, occurring but once in an individual's lifetime. Some prostitutes engage in "shows" with trained animals, but the women perform these acts for money rather than for sexual gratification.

Pedophilia. Pedophilia is sexual activity of an adult with a prepubertal child. According to DMS III, a minimum difference of 10 years of age between the participants is required for this diagnosis; activity between an adolescent and a much younger child is a special case. Individuals may have become involved in these sexual activities out of curiosity or ignorance, or in the absence of an acceptable partner. Child-adult sexual activities are viewed with horror, outrage, and disgust by most Americans. The harshest punishments are demanded, particularly for homosexual pedophiles. Men convicted of this crime do not fare well in prison either and are frequently raped or beaten by other convicts, who call them "short eyes." These attitudes result from stereotyping the pedophile, and from the effects these activities have upon the young victim. It is commonly believed that pedophiles are lecherous old men, strangers lurking near schools and playgrounds, waiting to lure young girls into their cars. The experience is generally believed to be debilitating to the child; children are believed to be sexually innocent and pure, devoid of sexual feelings, desires, and curiosity. Current research contradicts these beliefs.

Convicted pedophiles are older than most sex offenders. Approximately 5 percent are senile, and from 15 to 20 percent are mentally retarded. The majority, however, demonstrate no significant psychological or organic difficulties. In 85 percent of reported cases, the offender is a family member, a friend of the family, or a neighbor. Given the reluctance of parents to report in order to protect the child from publicity or the inclination to "protect the family name," fewer family-related cases are recorded than actually occur. (Public health nurses are often suprised at the number of adult-child sexual activities that are unreported). Eighty percent of reported incidents occurred in the home of the adult and usually consisted of kissing and genital fondling. Oral-genital contact occurred in 15 percent of the cases, and only 2 percent report actual penile intromission (Gebhard, et al., 1965; Kolodney, et al., 1979).

The sexual episodes usually last for a brief period, prolonged encounters being the great exception rather than the rule. While some children carry emotional scars for years, most do not appear to suffer any long-term trauma unless the activities resulted in violence or pain (Gagnon, 1965). It is considered by many professionals that the trauma experienced usually results from the severe negative reactions of adults, rather than from the sexual interaction itself (Francoer, 1982).

In spite of the general taboo against such behavior, adult-child contacts are very common in our society. One of every four female respondents in the Kinsey survey indicated that sexual contact with an adult had actually occurred or that an adult had attempted to have such contact.

Landis found 30 and 35 percent of college men and women, respectively, had had childhood experiences with adults they labeled as sexually deviant (cited in McCaghy, 1971). When these data are pooled with the number of children reporting incestuous relations, it becomes clear that the nurse must be cognizant that adult-child sexual interactions are a relatively common experience in this country.

Exhibitionism. The confusion between standards of socially acceptable and unacceptable behavior is clearly illustrated by exhibitionism. Legally, men and women may wear sexually provocative clothing (e.g., tight fitting jeans, "see-through" blouses, or low-cut dresses, skimpy bathing suits, open unbuttoned shirts), may undress on stage, or may swim nude at public beaches. On the other hand, if a woman in passing is offended by seeing the penis of an intoxicated man as he urinates in an alley, the man may be arrested as an exhibitionist.

Exhibitionism is almost exclusively a male act, and the majority of victims are women and young girls, usually complete strangers to the man. Sexual satisfaction results from the shock, fear, or disgust reflected by the victim. Ejacula-

---

■ *Point of Emphasis*

Exhibitionism is a repeated and preferred method of obtaining sexual gratification by exposing the genitals to unsuspecting and unwilling victims.

---

tion may occur at the scene, but more typically is achieved through masturbation at some future time, if at all.

Exhibitionists are timid, nonaggressive, and emotionally and sexually inadequate. While a few cases of molestation or sexual attack following the incident have been reported, most exhibitionists have difficulty relating to members of the opposite sex, and many of them experience erectile failure in heterosexual encounters (Gebhard, et al., 1965). Exhibitionism accounts for one-third of sexually related arrests, probably because of the public nature of the act and the timidity of the man. Nurses should be cautious in applying the label of exhibitionist, or "dirty old man" to clients who deliberately or flagrantly expose their genitals. The man may be reassuring himself of his masculinity in spite of his infirmity, may be rebelling against the bureacracy of the institution, or may be trying to regain control of the male-female role in the hospital setting. The best way to cope with this behavior, in the park or in the hospital, is to remain calm and treat it casually (Brecher, 1978). Suggestions are made later in the chapter about utilizing these "cues" from clients as an opening to a dialogue about the client's sexual concerns.

Voyeurism. It is not abnormal to experience a desire to observe other individuals in a nude, or partially nude, condition. Legal avenues for this sexual outlet include male and female beauty contests, strip-shows, movies, and commercial pornography. "Peeping" behavior is not uncommon within the family setting, around college dormitories, or in the hospital. Where such behavior results from aroused curiosity or during particular psychosexual stages of development, there is little reason for concern.

Voyeurism means spying on unsuspecting people, usually strangers, who are in the act of disrobing, are nude, or are engaging in sexual activities. The voyeur prefers this method, or uses it exclusively, to achieve sexual gratification. While looking, he often masturbates and fantasizes about the victim. Rarely does the voyeur desire actual contact with the victim. A man who enters the building where the activities are going on is dangerous, however. He is more likely to commit real crimes such as robbery and rape (Gebhard, et al., 1965).

Voyeurism is exclusively a male crime. Women are not arrested for this activity, nor do men prosecute them as victims. (The spied-upon male is more likely to be arrested for exhibitionism!) Convicted men tend to be shy and socially unskilled, and to have few close friends. Their sexual histories reveal delayed sexual development, and they experienced petting and coitus at a later age than most men (Smith, 1976).

Psychosexual Dysfunctions

A human being's sexual response cycle consists of the following four phases: (1) appetitive, (2) excitement, (3) orgasm, and (4) resolution. When a person experiences a psychosexual dysfunction, inhibition in the cycle most often occurs in one or more of the first three phases. According to the DSM-III, clients will usually report subjective dissatisfaction with desire or pleasure as well as objective performance.

The experience of psychosexual dysfunction may occur after a period of normal functioning, or it may be a lifelong problem. In addition, psychosexual dysfunctions may occur with all sexual partners in all situations (including masturbation), or they may occur only with certain partners in certain situations. Persons may also experience varying degrees or frequency of dysfunction.

The following section briefly describes the psychosexual dysfunctions as identified by the American Psychiatric Association. It is important for the reader to remember that most nurses are expected only to assess sexuality in their day-to-day practice and that treatment of psychosexual dysfunctions should be done only by those properly trained and qualified.

Inhibited Sexual Desire. According to the DSM-III, two diagnostic criteria are used in identifying a client's problem as inhibited sexual desire. The first is that there is a persistent and pervasive inhibition of sexual desire. Determining "persistent" and "pervasive" in context is a matter of considerable psychiatric clinical judgment. The second criterion is that the disturbance is not caused exclusively by organic factors (e.g., physical conditions or medications).

Some partners may report discrepancies in levels or degrees of sexual desire. This is not nec-

essarily indicative of inhibited sexual desire, but may indicate a need to explore other factors such as communication patterns, fatigue levels, and psychosocial stressors.

It is important for the nurse to remember that degrees of sexual desire may be affected by drugs such as sedatives, antiadrenergics, anticholinergics, antiandrogens, antihistamines, and drugs used for weight control (Hyde, 1982). Depression, alcohol abuse, cardiac disorders, cancer, diabetes, and treatments for these illnesses can seriously affect the level and degree of sexual responses of both clients and their partners.

> ■ *Point of Emphasis*
>
> *Sexual desire may be affected by drug use, physical conditions, and psychosocial stress.*

Inhibited Sexual Excitement. Inhibited sexual excitement in men is also referred to as erectile dysfunction. It is the inability to achieve an erection firm enough to accomplish vaginal intromission, or to maintain erection long enough to achieve orgasm. An earlier term, impotence, is no longer employed, for it signified a loss of power, and was associated with an inability to impregnate.

An important distinction must be made between primary erectile dysfunction and secondary erectile dysfunction. Some men have never been able to maintain an erection to orgasm (primary erectile dysfunction). This is a serious condition and always requires a thorough physical examination and sexual therapy. Secondary erectile dysfunction occurs when the man had been able to maintain erections in the past, but can no longer do so. Alcohol ingestion and fatigue are common causes of secondary erectile dysfunction. Fear, anxiety, guilt, or a deteriorating interpersonal relationship may also contribute to its occurrence.

According to the DSM-III, inhibited sexual excitement in women is identified when there is partial or complete failure to attain or maintain the responses of sexual excitement until completion of the sexual act. As with other psychosexual dysfunctions, the diagnosis is made by careful assessment when the disturbance is not caused exclusively by organic factors.

Inhibited Female Orgasm. Inhibited female orgasm, or orgasmic dysfunction, is the inability of a woman to reach orgasm and is the most common female sexual problem reported by sex therapists. Some women have never been able to achieve orgasm, while others are dissatisfied with the frequency of their responses. When orgasmic dysfunction is related exclusively to organic factors (i.e., physical disorders), it is not considered to be inhibited orgasm. Generally psychosocial factors are the basis for the disturbance; such factors may include guilt, lack of knowledge, disintegrating or undeveloped partner relationships, or inadequate communication patterns. The condition can frequently be resolved by learning through self-exploration, or by a partnership characterized by open communication, caring, and safety.

Inhibited Male Orgasm. According to the DSM-III, inhibited male orgasm is diagnosed when there is recurrent and persistent inhibition of male orgasm as manifested by a delay in or absence of ejaculation following an adequate phase of sexual excitement. As with inhibited female orgasm, this diagnosis is assigned when the disturbance is not caused exclusively by organic factors. The problem frequently can be resolved by giving attention to psychosocial factors such as intrapsychic conflict, interpersonal communication, "permission," and specific behavioral changes (Reid, 1983).

Premature Ejaculation. Premature ejaculation is possibly the most commonly reported sexual concern of men, and one of the most difficult to diagnose. Initially, this condition was identified in males who ejaculated before intromission, or within 5 seconds after. More recently, premature ejaculation has been defined as ejaculation within 2 minutes after intromission, or within ten pelvic thrusts. To add confusion, some defined it in terms of partner satisfaction, as when the woman was orgasmic less than 50 percent of the time. Presently the DSM-III accepts the man's subjective appraisal as a basis for diagnosis—that is, whether the man feels he has "reasonable" voluntary control of ejaculation and orgasm during sexual activity.

As with inhibited sexual excitement (erectile dysfunction), a distinction must be made between premature ejaculation that has always been present in the man's experience (primary premature ejaculation) and disturbance that has oc-

curred following a period of normal functioning (secondary premature ejaculation). It is also important to remember that those with this disturbance are not deficient in sperm production.

Treatment of premature ejaculation is most successful when the "squeeze technique" is taught to the man and his partner (Reid, 1983).

Functional Dyspareunia. Recurrent and persistent genital pain associated with coitus, but not caused exclusively by a physical disorder, lack of lubrication, or functional vaginismus, is diagnosed as functional dyspareunia.

This disorder is considered a physiologic manifestation of emotional conflict (Reid, 1983) and treatment should consider psychodynamic issues. Behavioral approaches are often recommended, but should not be exclusively employed (Reid, 1983).

Functional Vaginismus. Vaginismus is involuntary muscular contractions and spasms around any object at the vaginal entrance. These spasms close the vaginal opening so tightly that intercourse is impossible or extremely painful. This condition may be brought about by fear of pain, pregnancy, or discovery, or by previous painful experiences such as sexual assault or a careless pelvic examination.

Like functional dyspareunia, the condition often has serious emotional associations that need to be understood through psychodynamic exploration (Reid, 1983). Behavorial approaches with desensitization techniques are also utilized, but should not be the sole approach in treatment (Reid, 1983).

☐ *Sexuality and the Health Care Delivery System*

To promote and support the sexual well-being of clients, the nurse needs to consider and be aware of issues in the health care system that influence sexual well-being, the impact of health disruptions on sexuality, and nursing process in promoting sexual well-being. The next section of this chapter addresses these matters.

In any health care delivery system issues of privacy, power, separation, and desexualization potentially threaten sexual well-being. In hospitals, clinics, nursing homes, doctors' offices, and the community, nurses are in a position to minimize the effects of these issues and to maximize sexual well-being through the use of nursing process.

PRIVACY

The Privacy Problem

Webster has defined privacy as "the quality or state of being apart from company or observation; the freedom from unauthorized intrusion." Privacy is often suspended when a person enters a health care delivery system. Consider the invasion of physical and psychic territory that occurs when, in the course of examination or treatment, clients not only experience close physical proximity and contact from one or more strangers, but also attention toward, touch of, and exposure of private body parts. Children, adolescents, and the elderly may be particularly vulnerable to such invasion due to psychosexual development factors and cultural mores. For many people, touch, exposure, and attention toward any body part (not exclusively the genitals or breasts) may be uncomfortable.

In many settings, there is still professional insensitivity to a client's sense of modesty. Unfortunately, it is not uncommon for examinations and procedures to occur with undrawn curtains in hospitals and for baths and treatments to be given behind open doors in nursing homes. Nurses working in the community sometimes forget that although the elderly person lives with a son or daughter, there may be strong familial taboos against children touching parents' genitals when giving personal care such as a bath. This type of insensitivity to modesty can interfere with the teaching of home care of the ill person.

Persons institutionalized in hospitals or in nursing homes find themselves accessible to health care providers and auxiliary personnel (cleaning people, dietitians, and others) 24 hours a day and often have little control over who enters their space and when entry occurs.

Institutionalized persons also suffer from lack of privacy when alone with their sexual partners. Rarely is privacy with one's partner considered to be a client's right once he has entered a hospital or nursing home.

Client Responses to Diminished Privacy

Responses to diminished privacy vary from person to person. Some people may feel humiliation,

shame, or embarrassment. Others may become frustrated and angry about being exposed and about the lack of sensitivity on the part of health care providers. Feeling helpless to protect or regain their privacy, some clients may become depressed. Lack of privacy may be particularly difficult for those people who are institutionalized over a long period of time.

What Nurses Can Do

Nurses can take the following actions to prevent or minimize the traumatic effects of privacy invasion:

1. Evaluate "privacy policies" in the work setting; if they are not present, or are inadequate, create and institute them.
2. With the client's permission, post "Do Not Disturb" signs that are to be respected by all personnel.
3. Incorporate "alone time" into the individual's care plan.
4. Always close doors, pull drapes, and use covers when giving any treatment or performing any procedure that requires giving attention to the client's body or discussing personal topics (includes diagnosis, treatment plans, discharge plans, and so on).
5. Be sensitive to a person's cultural, familial, religious, and personal values about modesty.
6. Be an advocate for the client in respect to privacy: alert others (physicians, students, auxiliary personnel) to the issue of privacy and demand respect for the issue.
7. Support and provide uninterrupted time alone for clients and their partners. If this is not possible in the client's room, provide a special quiet and private place.
8. Assure confidentiality regarding sexuality at all times.

Nursing Response to Client's Masturbation

A situation that can be embarrassing to both the nurse and the client arises when the nurse enters the client's room and finds the client masturbating. Sensitive handling of this situation can help increase the client's sense of sexual well-being. The most appropriate response to such a situation is: "Excuse me, Mr. (Ms., Mrs.) T. Here, let me give you some privacy." Inform the client that you will be back in a short period of time, for example, 15 to 20 minutes. Close the door and post the "Do Not Disturb" sign. If the client later apologizes or seems to be behaving or relating differently to you, there is fertile ground for discussion of the meaning of masturbation to the client and affirmation of the normality of the behavior.

POWER

The Power Problem

The need for health care and entry into the health care system diminishes the client's power. Webster defines power as "possession of control, authority, or influence over others." Power is diminished in the health care system for several reasons: (1) The client who is ill in an institution or bedridden in any setting is dependent on strangers to meet needs for nutrition, mobility, eliminations, safety, and so on. (2) Frequently power is diminished when clients become dependent on others for information about bodily functions or disease.

Another subtle yet pervasive factor in diminution of client power lies in the attitudes and expectations of health professionals that clients conform to institutional rules, follow treatment plans, and maintain an attitude of gratitude toward the health care provider.

Client Responses to Diminished Power

In addition to reacting to elements that are inherent in the health care delivery system, clients may have conscious or unconscious responses to actual or perceived loss of power. These responses may manifest themselves in sexual behavior. For example, the man who makes sexually provocative remarks or openly masturbates may be perceiving his illness as a loss of control and thus a threat to his self-image. His ability to embarrass others may be the only means he thinks he has to control an otherwise uncontrollable situation. Likewise, the woman who acts in a sexually provocative way to male health care providers may be using a usually successful behavior to control a frightening situation.

Professional expectations that clients conform to rules may affect masculine or feminine control habits and thus threaten sexual self-image. For example, the male or female executive who is usu-

ally the one giving the orders may find it difficult to be in a subordinate position to other people. Since most nurses are women, some men may have difficulty handling a relationship where the control and dominance seems to be reversed; thus, conflicts may arise about control and dominance in relation to sex roles. Cultural factors, including traditional sex roles, may play an important part in this problem.

Finally, some clients may find it particularly difficult to be cared for by other people and, in coping with their discomfort, may be solicitously concerned about the sexuality of the nurse, for example, by asking questions about her marital status or social life.

What Nurses Can Do

There are several actions that nurses can take to improve the client's sense of power and reduce the need for maladaptive behaviors.

1. Acknowledge the presence of the power issue to self, others, and the client.
2. Find out what is most troublesome to the client and provide concrete means for the client to resume some control. For example, give the client the power to make decisions about the scheduling of procedures, personal hygiene, or who may visit and when.
3. Whenever possible, permit the client to walk instead of riding in a wheelchair, sit up instead of lie down, and ask questions instead of merely listen to descriptions of plans. By involving clients in their health care and encouraging and allowing them to function as independently as possible, the nurse can reduce threats to control.

SEPARATION AND LOSS

Separation from significant others and one's usual daily experiences may have distressing effects on the client's sexual well-being and/or relationships. It is important to recognize the variety of losses clients experience when institutionalized.

The Loss of Touching

For many people the need for comfort from touching is augmented by illness. Institutionalization interrupts one's usual way of having the need for touching met. The touch of strangers is sanctioned in our society when one is occupying a sick role. However, the touch of health care providers may, whether consciously or unconsciously, be interpreted by the client as carrying a different meaning; that is, a sexual connotation may be ascribed to touch. Some people may not be able to allow themselves to be comforted by the touch of the health care provider and therefore translate touching into something sexual. There is nothing inherently bad about this type of meaning assignment. The important point is that nurses recognize it and not be unconsciously seductive.

Interruption of Partnership Communication Modes

Another loss that occurs when clients are institutionalized is that the usual roads of partnership communication and bond maintenance are interrupted. For people who have very close relationships, the effects of separation may be as deleterious for the well partner as for the sick one. It is important for the nurse to keep in mind that worries about the welfare of the partner may be a hindrance to the client's focusing his energy on healing. Men or women may seek to relate with the health care provider in ways that mimic the partner relationship in the area of sexuality. One may see this with delusional or confused people. In such a case, it is very important that the nurse provide reality orientation and empathic responses to the client so as not to cause any embarrassment or shame when the period of confusion or delusion passes.

Loss of Sex-Role Activities

With illness and/or hospitalization, clients may lose the usual ways they had of carrying out their sex roles. For example, one may find the man who, unable to be the sexual aggressor and provider for the family, expresses his frustration about this through sexual behavior. Careful examination of the meaning of the current illness and institutionalization to the client may help to clarify the issue and decrease anxiety.

Loss of Familiar Tactile Experiences

A fourth subtle but influential loss is the loss of customary tactile experiences. Being institutionalized, the client does not feel the crispness of the autumn wind, smell the blooms of spring, or feel the intensity of the summer sun. Institutional clothing has the same texture as does the bedding.

Gone from one's daily experiences are the variety of textures of bedding, street clothes, pajamas, and so on. The impact of this loss can be seen as a loss of a reality-orienting part of daily life, and may numb the ability to feel. The outcome of such a loss may be a heightened need to feel something other than hospital bedding and clothing. Thus, pats on the bottom, breast caresses, or touches of the nurse's face may not be overtly sexual gestures at all, but rather an attempt by the person to touch something different, to assure himself that there are other tactile sensations than those associated with institution life.

Client Responses to Separation Experiences

Feelings related to separation losses may go unspoken. Clients may be concerned about their work, family, recreational, or religious obligations. Loss of ability to fulfill commitments may threaten the client's sex-role activities and thus sexual self-image. Clients may feel guilty and sorrowful about not meeting their partner's sexual needs or they may worry about their partner seeking sexual release or alliance with others during the period of institutionalization. Some clients may be concerned that their partner is less able to cope with the illness-imposed separation because the couple's usual sexual intimacies are lacking.

What Nurses Can Do

Nurses can take action to minimize the effects of separation on sexual well-being in the following ways:

1. Facilitate a pass home, if possible.
2. Encourage partner visits and provide privacy either in the client's room or in another area.
3. Be sensitive to feelings that may be unexpressed regarding the impact of separation on the client's sense of sexual well-being.
4. Allow wearing of personal clothing and provide for alternative tactile experiences.

DESEXUALIZATION

The Desexualization Problem

Insensitivity to or denial of the complexity and reality of human sexuality results in desexualization of clients and health care professionals.

Desexualizing Attitudes and Beliefs. Some attitudes and beliefs that have a desexualizing effect are:

1. Sick people are not sexual.
2. Sexuality is present only in the bedroom and not at all times of our lives.
3. Sexuality means only genitally oriented behavior.
4. Dealing with sexuality is not within the scope of the health care professional's repertoire and should not be.
5. Sexuality is too personal an issue for health care professionals to discuss with clients, particularly when they are ill or injured.

The effect of these attitudes and beliefs is that an entire system of human functioning and need goes unacknowledged. By ignoring or distorting sexuality, clients are denied an opportunity to learn and grow in this area of human-beingness. The belief that sexuality is not present at all times of a person's life can create an atmosphere where sexual concerns are effectively negated. This occurs particularly with children, the elderly, the ill, the physically disabled, and those with other than heterosexual orientation. Unvalidated assumptions about gender, age, marital status, appearance, occupation, behavioral idiosyncracies, emotional status, mental ability, physical status, ethnicity, and religion can also lead to desexualization.

Desexualizing Behaviors

In any setting, ignoring cues about sexual concerns, making jokes about sexuality, making demeaning comments about sexual issues, and avoiding a sexuality assessment can lead to client desexualization. Other desexualizing behaviors include: expecting clients to wear uniform clothing that permits easy access to and exposure of the body; failing to attend to the client's needs for personal grooming to enhance the sense of attractiveness; removing personal belongings that may have special significance (e.g., clothing, jewelry, photographs); being insensitive to such physiological factors as menstruation and morning erection; and failing to acknowledge the client's independence despite the sick role.

Client Responses to Desexualization

Clients may react to a desexualized climate through sexual acting out in order to gain reassurance about their attractiveness, ability to function sexually, and affirmation of their sexual being. Nurses may also see depression as a response to a desexualized climate.

What Nurses Can Do

Nurses can take action to reduce system-induced effects of desexualization. These include:

1. Assert to others every person's right to receive sexual health care.
2. Permit and encourage wearing of client's own clothing whenever possible.
3. Conscientiously attend to needs for personal grooming.
4. Allow and encourage the presence of personal belongings that are meaningful to the client's sense of sexual attractiveness.
5. Learn the facts of physiological sexuality and keep these in mind when providing daily care.
6. Be sensitive to psychological and sociological influences on sexual behavior and use this information in planning and providing care for clients.
7. Become aware of one's own assumptions about sexuality in certain groups of people (such as, children, the aged, working women, divorced or widowed women or men, homosexuals, other ethnic groups, religious groups others).

Nurses can also reduce the effects of desexualization by being prepared to deal openly with difficult situations that frequently arise in the course of daily work with clients. These include client-to-client attraction in the psychiatric setting, client-nurse attraction in any setting, and nurse-client attraction in any setting.

Client-Client Attraction in the Psychiatric Setting. It is not unusual for psychiatrically hospitalized clients to form opposite-sex or same-sex liaisons while in the hospital. Finding clients in bed together or embracing in a closet can be a disruptive event. In order to maximize the therapeutic potential of such behavior, the psychiatric team must establish clear rules about such behavior and communicate them to clients upon admission.

> ### ■ Point of Emphasis
>
> *Ignoring or punishing sexual behavior has the effect of denying a person's sexuality. Therefore, it is important to use sexually related incidents or relationships as a catalyst for discussion and examination.*

Examining the positive or negative effects of the relationship with both of the involved clients can help them to realize how this behavior is a self-affirming or harmful thing for each of them. Such liaisons are not always negative, and for some clients, the ability to form a close and, perhaps, sexual relationship with someone else may be a mark of progress. Kietner and Grof (1981) provide an excellent discussion of this issue.

Client-Nurse Attraction in Any Setting. It is also not unusual for clients to develop feelings of warmth and sexual attraction toward their health care providers. The basis for this may be a transference phenomenon and in some cases indicative of maladaptive relationship formation, nevertheless the feelings are real and not to be dealt with lightly. The man who "falls in love" with his nurse or the woman who "falls in love" with her doctor may be motivated by needs to express gratitude for the care received. It is also possible that such experiences are generated by feelings of genuine respect and attraction.

There are a variety of ways to deal with the situation. General principles include:

1. Acknowledge to the client that you understand the feelings.
2. Provide clear verbal and nonverbal limits to your involvement by explaining your professional role.
3. Avoid rejection of client either verbally or nonverbally.
4. Talk the situation over with a trusted colleague or supervisor. It is important to request consultation with someone knowledgeable and caring in order to sort through your own feelings about the situation, and thus be more objective in giving care.

5. If the situation is too difficult to handle or interferes with your ability to provide quality nursing care, request that your care of the client decrease in frequency.

Nurse-Client Attraction in Any Setting. A less common but not unusual experience occurs when nurses find themselves physically and emotionally attracted to clients. Again, the motivation for such attraction may be complex, but the feelings are real and must be dealt with. Once aware of such feelings, the nurse should discuss them with a trusted colleague or mental health consultant. The effect of acting on one's feelings of sexual attraction to clients could be detrimental to the client and interfere with the therapeutic relationship.

> ### ■ Point of Emphasis
>
> *Issues of privacy, power, separation, and desexualization have tremendous impact on clients' sexual well-being in all settings.*

FACTORS INFLUENCING THE IMPACT OF HEALTH DISRUPTION ON SEXUAL WELL-BEING

A person's sexual well-being can be adversely affected by health disruptions and treatments. Sexuality can be affected by both the nature of the health disruption and treatment and the meaning that the client and/or partner attaches to the health disruption. The purpose of this section is to examine the various ways that sexual well-being is affected by health disruption and treatments.

The Nature of the Health Disruption Can Affect Sexuality

Four types of health disruption and treatment are considered: the type of illness (acute vs. chronic), health disruption as an insult to a major organismic system, surgical intervention, and drug therapy.

Acute vs. Chronic Illness. When an illness is acute, that is, self-limited in time, the deleterious effects on sexuality may not be as profound as when the illness is chronic. In acute illness, the sick role is more easily accepted by both the ill and the well because an end to it is in sight. There is usually no need for radical alteration in self-image or role activities.

Often, maladaption in the realm of sexuality occurs with chronic illness related to physical, emotional, and life-style changes that affect self-image and self-esteem. A large element in the threat to sexual self-image during chronic illness in our society is the acceptance of or coping with the expectations of the sick role. Another characteristic of chronic illness that may impact on sexual well-being is the cyclical "Some days I feel good, other days I don't" experience. The nurse can use this aspect of chronic illness by counseling clients to take advantage of their good days to fulfill sexual activity.

System Insults, Surgery, and Drugs. Another way of looking at health disruptions in order to assess and understand their impact on sexual well-being is to be aware of any insult to the neurological, cardiovascular, hormonal, or phychic system of the person. All of these systems have a role in satisfactory sexual functioning, and an alteration in any one can impact on sexual well-being. Surgical interventions (e.g., ostomy, mastectomy, hysterectomy, prostatectomy) and drugs (Table 21-1) can also influence sexual well-being. (See Recommended Readings and References.)

TABLE 21-1 *Effect of Drugs on Sexual Function*[a]

Drugs That May Enhance Sexual Function
Steroid hormones (hormone replacement)
    Androgens
    Estrogens
Clomiphene citrate (increased libido and potency)
Levodopa (Increased potency)
Bromocriptine (Increased potency)

Drugs That May Adversely Affect Sexual Function
Antihypertensives (impotence or delayed ejaculation in men, decreased desire in women)
    Guanethidine
    Methyldopa
    Clonidine
    Reserpine
    Phenoxybenzamine
    Spironolacotone

Antipsychotics (impotence or inhibited ejaculation in men, decreased responsiveness in women)
    Thioridazine
    Chlorpromazine
    Prochlorperazine
    Trifluoperazine
    Triflupromazine
    Perphenazine
    Fluphenazine

Antineoplastics (sterility or impotence in men)
    Alkylating agents
    Antimetabolites
    Alkaloids
    Antitumor antibiotics
    Nitrosoureas
    Steroid hormones

Monoamine oxidase inhibitors (impotence or inhibited ejaculation in men, difficulty in achieving orgasm in women)
    Pargyline
    Tranylcypromine
    Phenelzine

Sedatives–Hypnotics–Opiates (impotence or inhibited ejaculation in men, decreased libido in women)
    Morphine
    Methadone
    Barbiturates
    Chlordiazepoxide
    Diazepam
    Lithium carbonate

Tricyclic antidepressants (impotence or inhibited ejaculation in men, delayed orgasm in women)
    Imipramine
    Desipramine
    Amitriptyline
    Protriptyline

Steroids (decreased libido in males and females)
    Cyproterone acetate

Miscellaneous (impotence in men, decreased libido in women)
    Disulfiram
    Disopyramide
    Clofibrate
    Fenfluamine

Social Drugs That May Alter Sexual Function
    Alcohol (impotence in males with prolonged use)
Sedatives–Hypnotics–Opiates (impotence or inhibited ejaculation in males, decreased libido in women)
    Barbiturates
    Methaqualone
    Benzodiazepines

Stimulants (dose-dependent responses)
    Amphetamines
    Cocaine
    Caffeine

Hallucinogens (disinhibition and heightened responses in both sexes; decreased sexual activity)
    Marijuana (disinhibition and reportedly enhanced responsiveness)
    Amyl nitrate (enhanced sexual pleasure)

[a] Source: Stohs, S. J. Drugs and sexual function *U.S. pharmacist*, 3, 10, 1978:51–68.

The Meaning of Health Disruption to Client and/or Partner

Threat to Gender Identity. If a woman has always believed that her femininity and sense of womanhood were dependent on her breasts, a mastectomy could profoundly affect her sense of sexual attractiveness and worthiness. If a man had always thought that the uterus is what defined his partner as a woman, then a hysterectomy can affect his perception of her. Obviously, those people who believe that the ability to achieve erection is what "makes a man a man" will be deeply affected by illnesses, treatments, and injuries that inhibit the erectile response.

Alteration in Sex Role Functioning. If a man or woman is no longer able to fulfill the previous sex-role obligations because of chronic illness or incapacitating injury, then the value placed on these activities is threatened as is the sexual self-image and sexual self-esteem. The man who no longer is able to support his family financially may be seen as less of a man by his partner, and their sexual relationship may suffer.

Alteration in Quality of Sexual Response. Some men or women who had been functioning with great sexual satisfaction before illness may find their adequacy of response affected by the illness or treatment. This can be very distressing to both the individual and the partner unless they are able to redefine the meaning of the diminished response and develop other ways of relating satisfactorily to each other.

Alteration in Relationship Dynamics. Relationship dynamics are affected by any change. Illness, injury, or treatment-imposed alterations in sexual well-being are likely sources of stress. If, because of illness, clients must alter their usual activities (in particular taking on more responsibility than they had before), the potential for the build-up of resentment and anger is great, and can be sexually destructive unless sensitive intervention occurs early. One way nurses can help prevent this type of deterioration is to provide anticipatory guidance regarding the feelings and situations which may arise in the course of role-change that occurs during illness.

Threat to Reproductive Capacity. For many people, threats to reproductive capacity are particularly distressing, and for those who value biological parenting, anything that interferes with fertility can affect sexual well-being. It is not uncommon that depression follows a hysterectomy—an understandable emotion in women of childbearing age. Less well understood is that women past that age become depressed after hysterectomy; perhaps this is because even though they can no longer bear children, the presence of the uterus represented the hope they once had that they could bear children. For people who see sexuality as a means primarily for reproduction, anything which removes or reduces that capacity can have a profound effect on the pleasure associated with sexual intercourse.

Alteration in Modes of Tension Release. Masturbation and sexual activities with others may be seen as a form of tension release. An impairment or a treatment that interferes with one's usual way of relating sexually to oneself or others can therefore increase tension, and unless the person learns other ways to release tension, he may do this in sexually inappropriate ways. In assessing the client's sexual health, the nurse should ascertain whether tension release was a benefit of the client's sexuality. If so, and the illness, injury, or treatment is interfering with adequate sexual functioning, the nurse can teach the client other ways of achieving relaxation.

Alteration in Ways of Maintaining Intimacy. For many partnerships, sexuality is a key to maintaining intimacy and closeness and an affirmation of the relationship. Both verbal and nonverbal communication are important components of sexual relations. When the customary communication is impaired, partners may experience frustration, depression, and anger. Grief over this loss must be worked through before new ways of relating are accepted and established. The role of the nurse in effecting this process is fourfold: to assess the impact of impairment on the relationship, to provide information about how the impairment or treatment affects sexuality; to offer sustained support during the grieving and relearning process; and to evaluate the progress of relearning and of the partnership.

Alteration in Recreation. Clients who have valued their sexuality for recreational purposes also experience loss when previous levels of sexual functioning are impaired. It is important for the nurse to accept this meaning so she can understand the grieving that occurs. For some clients, sexually maladaptive behavior may be related to their inability to fulfill their need for recreation.

Developmental Task Achievement. The client's developmental stage also bears on the impact of illness, injury, or treatment. Developmental issues arising in childhood, adolescence, middle age, and old age may increase a person's vulnerability to stress due to health impairment; then too, a partnership's healthy psychosexual development becomes especially vulnerable during the critical periods of attachment, commitment, pregnancy, lactation, and departure of children. For example, the teenaged woman with an ileostomy due to ulcerative colitis may worry about her sexual attractiveness; the elderly stroke victim may be distressed that he is no longer able to caress his wife in customary ways; the person terminally ill may have special needs for expression of sexuality.

The Client's Gender

Disruption to health may affect men and women differently because of their different anatomical structures. It appears that men have disruptions of sexual functioning more frequently than women. This may be because their central nervous system plays a greater role in coordinating sexual functioning. Little research has been done on the effects of health impairment on women, a lack that may be due to the fact that male sexual functioning is more readily observed, men are more likely to report dysfunctions, and most researchers in sexuality have been men. Women's sexual responses do not seem to be affected as early or as severely with the onset of chronic disease or aging.

It is also to be noted that the sexual organs of women are largely internal. Thus, there is greater potential for misconceptions and fantasies to arise about sexuality and health impairment in women.

Other Threats to Sexual Well-Being

Sexual well-being may be threatened also by psychological reaction to health disruption and treatment (Table 21-2). There are also specific health disruptions that often have a predictable and generalized direct effect on sexual functioning,

---

TABLE 21-2 Psychological Reactions to Health Disruption and/or Treatment that may Interfere with Sexual Well-Being

Reaction		Examples of Causes of Reaction
Fear	*Of*	the unknown
		sex-role failure
		loneliness
		inability to be able to give/receive sexual satisfaction
		hurting partner or being hurt during sexual activities
		asking for information
		rejection by partner
		ability to find or keep sexual partner
Grief and its components (anger, depression)	*Loss of*	ability to fulfill sex-role responsibiities
		body part
		previous level of functioning (mobility, sexual response)
		previous sexual self-image
		former ways of giving/receiving sexual pleasure
		energy available for sexual activity
		hope for dream fulfillment (biological parenthood)
		privacy/power (in health care delivery system)
Embarrassment/shame	*About*	losses
		appearance
		odors, appliances, prostheses
		lack of information regarding sexuality/sexual functioning (vocabulary, positions for sexual activity)
Role conflict	*When*	partners must reverse sex-role responsibilities
		partner must be caregiver *and* lover
Invalidism	*When*	partner or client assumes health disruption or treatment means sexual activity is harmful or impossible

among them diabetes, spinal cord injury, and multiple sclerosis. Any impairment that interferes with respiration (e.g., emphysema, heart disease, obesity) may affect sexual functioning. Mental and emotional disturbances may interfere with satisfactory and appropriate sexual behavior.

Other experiences related to illness, injury, or treatment may also directly or indirectly interfere with sexual well-being (Table 21-3).

■ *Point of Emphasis*

Although treatments may decrease the client's sense of sexual well-being, pain relief, corrective surgery, and mental health care may have the positive outcome of enhancing sexual well-being.

TABLE 21-3 Illness/Treatment Experiences that may Directly or Indirectly Interfere with Sexual Well-Being

System	Experience
Integumentary	Dry skin
	Itching
	Scars
	Wounds/drainage
	Alopecia
	Rashes
Sensory	Vision impairment
	Hearing impairment
	Odors
	Tactility impairment (e.g., secondary to stroke, feeding tubes)
	Pain
	Temperature impairment (ability to differentiate hot/cold)
Neuromuscular	Weakness
	Immobility
	Intrinsic (spinal cord injury, multiple sclerosis, stroke)
	Extrinsic (casts, IVs)
	Balance disturbance (amputations, spinal cord injury, multiple sclerosis, other)
Gastrointestinal	Nausea
	Diarrhea
	Constipation
	Vomiting
	Anorexia
Genitourinary	Burning
	Itching
	Odors
	Catheters
	Lack of vaginal lubrication
Cardiovascular	Fatigue
	Palpitations
	Hypoxia
Limbic (emotions)	Anxiety
	Depression
	Grief
	Fear
	Apathy

□ *Nursing Process in Promoting Sexual Well-Being*

SELF-ASSESSMENT □ In general, nurses have the most frequent contact with clients in all settings, and through their interpersonal relationships with clients, their contact is on a more intimate level than that of most other health professionals. To be able to provide quality care to clients, they need to feel comfortable and confident about their abilities, and to be fully aware of their own attitudes about sexuality.

Personal comfort level is made up of several elements: being self-aware, possessing accurate information, having effective communication skills, acknowledging and accepting personal and professional limitations, and accepting the rights of clients to sexual health care. A high personal comfort level can be developed, and it is up to the nurse to take the initiative toward its achievement.

■ *Point of Emphasis*

The nurse's personal comfort level about sexuality is the most important factor in therapeutic intervention with clients.

Self-Awareness □ Becoming self-aware is an ongoing process. The nurse who does not accept her own attitudes and beliefs about sexuality may attempt—consciously or unconsciously—to influence clients with different frames of reference. Moreover, such an attitude can block communication about and effective intervention in matters related to the client's sexuality. Table 21-4 lists some questions that will encourage self-awareness in the nurse.

Accurate Information □ Many persons who communicate with clients about their sexual concerns report that the absence of accurate infor-

---

TABLE 21-4 Questions to Help Encourage the Nurse's Self-Awareness

How do I feel about myself as a woman (man)?

What characteristics of my body, personality, and social roles do I associate with my sexuality?

What are my attitudes, feelings, and beliefs about:

Male and female roles	Menopause
Menstruation	Venereal disease
Masturbation/self-pleasure	Pregnancy
Same-sex sexual activity	Sexuality in children
Same-sex sexual attraction	Sexuality in the elderly
Orgasm	Sexuality in handicapped persons
Ejaculation	Sexuality in mentally retarded
Erections	Nudity (my own and others')
Lubrication	My genitals
Breasts/nipples	The genitals of others
Oral-genital activity	Frequency of intercourse
Anal intercourse	Positions for intercourse
Bisexuality	Multiple sex partners
Nonmarital sex	Abortion
Contraception	Sexuality of nurses

How did I come by these attitudes, feelings, and beliefs?

What sights, sounds, smells, fantasies, interpersonal experiences arouse me sexually? What are "turn-offs" for me sexually?

Do I accept myself as a sexual human being?

Do I accept nurses as sexual human beings?

How comfortable am I discussing sexuality issues? What do I tell myself in order to inhibit myself from discussing or thinking about my own or others' sexuality?

Am I willing to learn accurate information and increase my self-acceptance and my acceptance of others' sexuality?

How do I feel about answering these questions?

---

mation along with the presence of misinformation is a frequent cause of client dissatisfaction with sexual functioning. Unlike respiration, digestion, elimination, and cognition, sexual functioning is not always taught in schools, so many people must gather the pertinent information for themselves. For centuries, information about sexuality was passed on verbally from generation to generation, colored by the teller's personal views. Nurses can offer clients an important and needed service by giving them reliable information about sexuality. Listed below are some specific steps the nurse can take:

1. Attend workshops and seminars, and enroll in courses dealing with human sexuality.

2. Read widely about sexuality. Do not ignore the literature on the history of sexuality in religion or art or information about cultural aspects of sexuality.

3. Get a solid background in the physiology of sexual functioning and the effects of ill-

ness, disability, drugs, and treatments on sexuality.

4. Learn informal terms related to body parts, sexual behaviors, and sexual orientation.

5. Consult with persons who have expertise in the area of sexuality.

6. Pay close attention to the client's description of his sexual experience.

7. Consider using a guide such as the one shown in Table 21-5.

CLIENT ASSESSMENT ☐ The nurse's sense of comfort and confidence about providing sexual health care are enhanced with her use of well-developed and sensitive communication skills (see Table 21-6). Role-playing, tape recording, and videotaping are effective in fostering good communication. Communication will be enhanced if (1) the nurse feels comfortable about employing the client's terms and (2) the nurse seeks clarification from the client when she does not understand a term or phrase he has used.

TABLE 21-5 Hanson's Concepts of Sexuality and Sexual Health Care Essential to Nursing Practice[a]

All people are sexual.

The physiological component of sexuality is greater than the reproductive system, and, in fact, permeates the entire body.

The sexual self evolves as an integral component of total physiological, psychological, and sociological development; indeed, sexual differentiation/development begins at conception and continues until death.

A person's state of health/illness will affect that individual's sexuality biologically, psychologically, or sociologically.

The physical sexual response cycle affects each body system and therefore has potential to affect symptoms of some illnesses.

Therapeutic modalities, including hospitalization, may affect the sexuality of the patient and his family. Such effect may be perceived as either positive or negative.

Conception, pregnancy, pubescence, and menopause are physiological and psychological events that affect aspects of sexuality, particularly sexual identity, sexual role behavior, and sexual expression.

An individual or family unit, although sexually independent, is very much affected by the sexual milieu of the community and society.

The nursing process is the means through which the nurse provides sexual health care.

[a] Source: Hanson, E. Sexuality curriculum and the nurse. In *Sex education for the health professional.* (Rosenzweig, N., and Pearsall, F. P., eds.). New York: Grune & Stratton, 1978:188–192. Used by permission of E. Ingvarda Hanson, R.N., M.S.N. and Grune & Stratton, Inc.

TABLE 21-6 Interviewing to Obtain Sexual Information—Some Dos and Don'ts[a]

Do	Don't
Obtain information about all need areas	Focus only on sexuality
Provide privacy	Obtain information when others are present or take copious notes
Strive for an unhurried atmosphere	Check your watch, tap your foot
Maintain an attitude that is frank, open, warm, objective, empathetic	Project discomfort, become defensive
Use nondirective techniques when possible	Ask many direct questions
Have a prepared introduction to state purpose of interview	Be vague about the purpose of the interview
Use appropriate vocabulary	Use street terms
"Check out" words to ensure patient understands	Assume the patient understands what you're saying
Adjust the order of questions according to client's needs	Follow a rigid form
Give the client time to think and answer questions	Answer questions for the client
Recognize signs of anxiety	Focus on getting information without recognizing patient feeling
Give permission not to do something	Have preset expectations of the patient's sexual activity
Listen in an interested but matter-of-fact way	Overreact or underreact
Identify your attitudes, values, beliefs, and feelings	Project your concerns or problems on to the patient
Identify significant others	Assume that no one else is involved in the patient's/client's sexual concerns
Identify philosophical religious beliefs of patient/client	Inflict your moral judgments on the patient
Acknowledge when you don't have an answer to a question	Pretend you know when you don't

[a] Hogan, Rosemarie. *Human Sexuality: A Nursing Perspective.* Appleton-Century-Crofts, New York, 1980. 246. By permission.

TABLE 21-7 Who Can Assess and Intervene in Sexual Functioning?[a]

	Professional Competence Required	Levels of Assessment	Levels of Therapeutic Intervention
Level 1	Professional nurse	Health history: Screen for sexual functions and dysfunctions	Limited education —Limited information about sexual feelings, behaviors, and myths —Refer to levels 2 or 3 if necessary
Level 2	Professional nurse with postgraduate training in sex education and counseling	Sexual history	Sex education and counseling —Specific information about sex and sexuality —Concise suggestions about sexual fears and adaptations to illness and anticipatory guidance —Refer to level 3 if necessary
Level 3	Professional nurse, physician, psychologist, social worker—all qualified as trained sex therapists	Sexual problem history	Sex therapy —Individual or group therapy —Couple therapy —Refer to level 4 if necessary
Level 4	Psychiatric nurse clinician with an MSN, physician, psychologist, social worker—all with subordinate specialty in sex therapy	Psychiatric and psychosexual history	Eclectic approach —Intensive individual psychotherapy, sex therapy, and marital therapy
	[There is linear relationship between the depth of a patient's sexual problems and the kind of professional competence that is needed to assess and treat them.]		

[a] Watts, R. J. Dimensions of sexual health. *American journal of nursing*, 79, 9, 1979:1570. Used with permission.

Nurses who are not comfortable communicating about sexuality should recognize this fact and request that another member of the team handle this component of care; in the same way, clients who are uncomfortable about discussing sexuality should in no way be punished by avoiding them or judging them. The nurse's role is to leave the door open to communication by telling the client that a qualified person is available if the client wishes to discuss sexuality (see Table 21-7).

Nonverbal Communication □ Sensitivity to certain aspects of nonverbal communication can enhance the client's sense of sexual well-being as well as facilitate discussion about sexuality. The setting for the discussion of sexual concerns should be a quiet, private place that is free from distraction and interruption. Such a setting can be created by closing doors and speaking quietly; if this is not possible, then seek out a space that provides more privacy.

The nurse's posture and gestures should convey openness and receptiveness—an accepting attitude. Clothing should not be revealing or skirts very short. It is important to be conscious of one's facial expressions when discussing sexuality because clients are often acutely aware of the nurse's response as reflected in her facial expression. A look of shock or disgust can instantly foreclose further discussion. Any touching of the client must be done with discrimination so that it will not be misinterpreted.

Listening for Cues □ Because each client experiences sexuality individually and because the client may be reluctant to speak directly, the nurse listens for cues about his sexual concerns (see Table 21-8). Listening for cues not only gives her information about his concerns, but it also provides information about the terms the client uses and understands.

Verbal Communication □ Clients may not be able to discuss sexuality openly because of embarrassment, fear of appearing ignorant, feelings about sexuality as an unacceptable topic for discussion, or anxiety sensed because the nurse herself feels anxiety about the topic. The nurse needs to remember that the client's and/or partner's response to actual or perceived threats of dimin-

TABLE 21-8 Cues Clients and/or Partners Give that May Indicate Concerns about Sexuality

Nonverbal	
Cues in Interview	Blushing, breaking eye contact, tearfulness, clenched fists, wringing hands
Others	Reaching/touching nurse's breast, buttocks, other body parts
	Openly masturbating
	Deliberate exposure of genitals
	Putting nurse's hand on genitals
	Seductive sounds or smells (e.g., perfume or pleasurable moaning when touched)
Verbal	
Direct	Sex jokes
	Bragging about sexual activities
	Asking about the nurse's sex life
	Comments about nurse's body build, size of breasts, buttocks, and so on
	Offering gifts in return for "sexual favors"
	Requesting caresses in genital area
Indirect Concerns about Self/ Partner	I don't feel the same about my partner
	My partner doesn't feel the same about me
	I've lost my manhood
	I've lost my power
	I can't perform like I used to
	I can't get hard like I used to
	I'm not horny any more
	I have difficulty with my nature
	My desire has changed
	I don't feel desirable
	His/her desire has changed
	I don't get wet
	My ability to be a woman (man) has changed (is gone)
	My partner isn't the man (woman) he (she) used to be
	I'm not the man (woman) I used to be
	What will my partner (spouse, lover, boyfriend, girlfriend) think/do now?
	My personal love life is . . .
	My wife (husband) doesn't understand me
Indirect Concerns about Relationship	We're not as close
	Our relationship is changed (different)
	My personal life is changed (different)
	The magic has worn off
	The spark's not there
	We don't click anymore
Questions	Will I still be able to get hard?
	What will happen to my relationship?
	What will this drug, surgery, do to my relationship (personal life, ability to perform)?

ished sexual well-being will be determined by that individual's unique experiences, personal values, religious beliefs, sexual self-concept, and accuracy of information about sexual functioning.

Guidelines for Information Gathering □ Information gathering about sexuality is developed in the format of the sexual history and should be a part of any nursing assessment. Woods (1979, 1984)* has described a useful three-question form for obtaining information and using it to enhance sexual well-being. It is called "A Brief Sexual History."

---

* From Woods, Nancy Fugate: Human sexuality in health and illness, ed. 2, 1979, ed. 3, 1984, The C.V. Mosby Co., St. Louis.

The history includes only three questions. The first addresses the person's sexual roles.

Has anything (illness, pregnancy) interfered with your being a (wife, mother, father, husband)?

This question may be revised to specifically address life events, health problems, or hospitalization as the situation requires.

The second question deals with the way the person views himself or herself as a sexual being.

Has anything (for example, heart attack) changed the way you feel about yourself as a (man, woman)?

The third item addresses sexual function directly.

Has anything (for example, surgery, disease) changed your ability to function sexually?

Woods reported that "many clients proceed to state their concerns about masculinity, feminity, and sexual functioning without further prompting."

Another way to gather information about sexuality is to include questions about sexual functioning during the review of systems in the health history. The most appropriate place for sexuality questions is after the review of the reproductive system in women and after the review of the genitourinary system in men.

An important principle in information gathering about sexuality is to proceed from less sensitive issues to more sensitive issues. For example, when taking a sexual history in a woman, begin with issues of menstruation, proceed to questions about intercourse, and then ask questions about masturbation. If taking a more detailed history, one would include questions about childhood sexual education and experiences, details of current sexual activity, and current relationship dynamics.

Universality, Review, and Unloading the Question □

Verbal communication about sexuality can be facilitated through the use of three approaches: statements of universality, review statements, and a technique of unloading the question. Statements of universality assume that human beings have common experiences, yet allow for the uniqueness of each individual within an experience. An example of a statement of universality is: "Many people wonder if they will be able to have erections after prostate surgery. Have you wondered that about yourself?" Review statements assume that the client already possesses some information; the purpose of a review

statement is to bring that information to the client's awareness. If the client is not aware of the information, then it is being presented in a nonthreatening way. Example: "As you know, the cervix sits atop the vagina and expands when the baby is ready to be born." The technique of unloading the question is used in order to gain as well as give information about variation in sexual behaviors. An example of unloading the question is: "Some women have orgasms in dreams, some when masturbating, some during intercourse and other sexual activities, and some women report not having orgasms at all. In general, when do you have an orgasm?"

PLANNING AND INTERVENTION □

Knowing when and how to intervene is a problem faced by many nurses. Planning interventions will depend on the personal comfort level of the nurse and the unique patient needs.

Levels of Intervention □

Annon (1976) has described four levels of intervention in sexual counseling: (1) permission giving—simply letting the client know both verbally and nonverbally that sexuality is an acceptable topic of concern; (2) limited information—limited by the nurse's own information and skill in sexual counseling; (3) specific suggestions—should be given only if one is knowledgeable in the area; and (4) intensive therapy—should be practiced only by someone trained and certified to be a sex therapist.

Principles of Teaching about Sexuality □

When teaching about sexuality it is useful to have the client's partner present. This ensures that both people receive the same information, and gives them an opportunity to discuss it and return with questions or requests for clarification.

If the teaching involves sexuality and surgery, it should be done both before and after the surgery. Similarly, it should be done before the start of certain drug therapies (e.g., antihypertensives) and after the therapy has begun. A person who is to have a certain type of surgery (for example, prostatectomy) or is to have a certain drug regimen (for example, antihypertensives) may have heard that the treatment will affect erectile ability. Often, unfounded beliefs become self-fulfilling prophecies, so the nurse should ascertain what the client believes will happen to his sex life as a result of the treatment. Such fears can affect the client's compliance with the medication regimen. The nurse conveys accurate information without giving false assurance. Periodic evaluation of sexual functioning is indicated so that the nurse can intervene before dysfunctions become ingrained.

Accept Limitations and Refer □ Nurses should know who are qualified, reputable professionals in the area of sexuality in their institution and community. The client's permission should be sought before referral to another person is made. An alternative is to give the referral information directly to the client and encourage him to follow up. Nurses in all settings must accept the right of clients to receive health care in the area of sexuality regardless of age, gender, socioeconomic status, or sexual orientation.

EVALUATION □ The nurse should be aware that evaluation of both self and client is an ongoing process, and she should take responsibility for its initiation and maintenance. First, she must know herself. Second, she should seek out and be open to receiving new information. Third, she must evaluate the effectiveness of interventions regardless of the level on which they take place. The following are criterion measures: (1) client will verbally express increased satisfaction with inter- and/or intrapersonal experience; or (2) nonverbal sexual acting out will diminish (i.e., in the institutionalized client).

■ Enrichment Activities

The following are some ways in which self-awareness about sexuality can be enhanced. They can be used in classroom discussions or in informal settings.

1. Recall how information about sexuality was learned. What were your sources of information? Friends? Older siblings? Parents? Books? Movies? School? Church? Did you actively seek information or did you hear or read it and not discuss it with anyone?

2. Identify attitudes and beliefs about sexuality in your early environment: family, school, community, church. What were the acceptable sex roles for men and women? Was sexuality a secret? What words were used for masturbation, intercourse, petting, pregnancy, venereal disease, erections, menstruation, ejaculation? What were the attitudes toward people who

were unmarried and pregnant? What were the attitudes toward sexuality of divorced or widowed people?

3. Examine your own feelings about being a man or a woman. Use the "Table of Questions to Stimulate Awareness" (Table 21-6) by yourself, or with a trusted other. Small group discussions may also be useful.

4. Pay attention to your feelings that are generated by discussion about aspects of sexuality and use this awareness to stimulate introspection.

5. Practice discussing sexuality topics with friends and colleagues.

6. Identify what actions and traits you associate with sexuality, for example, voice pitch, facial hair, gestures, touching, clothing, and hairstyles.

■ Recommended Readings

Hogan, R.M. *Human sexuality: A nursing perspective.* New York: Appleton-Century-Crofts, 1980. A thorough presentation of the biopsychosocial aspects of sexuality and the role of the nurse in guiding the client to attainment or maintenance of sexual health. Addresses sexual problems throughout the life cycle. Particularly comprehensive information on health deviations and sexuality with an informative chapter on sexuality and the mentally retarded and mentally ill individual.

Lion, E.M. *Human sexuality in nursing process.* New York: Wiley, 1982. A well-documented book which systematically integrates information about the biopsychosocial aspects of human sexuality with values clarification exercises for the student in order to enhance self-awareness. Nursing process in relation to a variety of sexuality problems is illustrated with case examples.

Mims, F.H., and Swenson, M. *Sexuality: A nursing perspective.* New York: McGraw-Hill, 1980. An important book for conceptualizing and implementing nursing education and nursing practice in relation to sexual health care. Clearly presents a way to bridge the gap between research/theory and nursing practice. Excellent chapters on the legal aspects of traditional and nontraditional life-styles, sexuality and dying, and advanced intervention and research from a nursing perspective. Useful learning activities for the student at the end of each chapter.

Woods, N.F. *Human sexuality in health and illness,* 3rd ed. New York: McGraw-Hill, 1984. A useful text that addresses the role of the nurse in providing sexual health care from a holistic perspective. The chapters on preventive intervention, restorative intervention, adaptation to hospitalization and illness, sexuality and chronic illness, and sexual adaptation to changed body image provide a good foundation for further study and for practice. The questions for review which follow many chapters are particularly thought provoking and stimulating.

■ *References*

American Psychiatric Association. *Diagnostic and statistical manual*, 3d ed. Washington, D.C.: APA, 1980.

Anderson, M.L. Talking about sex—With less anxiety. *Journal of psychosocial nursing*, 18, 6, 1980:10–15.

Annon, J. The PLISSIT model. A proposed conceptual scheme for the behavioral treatment of sexual problems. *Journal of sex education and therapy*, 2, 1976:1–15.

Bell, A.P., and Weinberg, M.S. *Homosexualities: A study of the diversity among men and women*. New York: Simon & Schuster, 1978.

Brecher, E.M. *Treatment programs for sex offenders*. National Institute of Law Enforcement and Criminal Justice, U.S. Department of Justice, Washington, D.C., 1978.

Bullard, D.G., and Knight, S.E. (eds.). *Sexuality and physical disability: Personal perspectives*. St. Louis: Mosby Company, 1981.

Crewe, N.M. Sexually inappropriate behavior. In *Behavior problems and the disabled: Assessment and management*. (Bishop, D.S. ed.), 120–141. Baltimore: Williams & Wilkens.

Francoeur, R. *Becoming a sexual person*. New York: Wiley & Sons, 1982.

Friday, N. *My secret garden*. New York: Pocket Books, 1973.

Friday, N. *Men in love*. New York: Delacorte, 1980.

Ford, C. and Beach, F. *Patterns of sexual behavior*. New York: Harper & Row, 1951.

Frontiers of radiation therapy and oncology, 14, 1–33. New York: Karger, 1980.

Gagnon, J.H. Sexuality and sexual learning in the child. *Psychiatry*, 28, 1965:212–228.

Gebhard, P.; Gagnon, J.H.; Pomeroy, W.B.; and Christenson, C.V. *Sex offenders: An analysis of types*. New York: Harper & Row, 1965.

Green, R. (ed.). *Human sexuality: A health practitioner's text*, 2d ed. Baltimore: The Williams & Wilkins Co., 1979.

Hanson, E.I. Effects of grief, associated with chronic illness and disability, on sexuality. In *Grief responses to long-term illness and disability*. (Werner-Beland, J.A. ed.). Reston, VA: Reston Publishing Company, 1980.

Hanson, E.I. Sexuality curriculum and the nurse. In *Sex education for the health professional: A curriculum guide*. (Rosenzweig, N., and Pearsall, F.O., eds.). New York: Grune & Stratton, 1978:188–192.

Haseltine, F.P., and Ohno, S. Mechanisms of gonadal differentiation. *Science*, 211, 1981:1272.

Hirsch, S.P. Proceedings of the American Cancer Society, 2d National Conference on Human Values and Cancer. Chicago, 1977.

Hite, S. *The Hite report*. New York: Macmillan, 1976.

Hogan, R.M. *Human sexuality: A nursing perspective*. New York: Appleton-Century-Crofts, 1980:144, 246.

Hunt, M. *Sexual behavior in the 1970s*. Chicago: Playboy Press, 1974.

Hyde, J.S. *Understanding human sexuality*, 2d ed. New York: McGraw-Hill, 1982.

Katchadourian, H.A., and Lunde, D.T. *Fundamentals of human sexuality*, 3d ed. Chicago: Holt, Rinehart & Winston, 1980.

Kietner, G., and Grof, P. Sexual and emotional intimacy between psychiatric inpatients: Formulating a policy. *Hospital and community psychiatry*, 32, 3, 1981:188–193.

Kinsey, A.C.; Pomeroy, W.B.; and Martin, C.E. *Sexual behavior in the human male*. Philadelphia: W.B. Saunders, 1948.

Kinsey, A.C.; Pomeroy, W.B.; Martin, C.E.; and Gebhard, P.H. *Sexual behavior in the human female*. Philadelphia: W.B. Saunders, 1953.

Kline-Graber, G., and Graber, B. *Woman's orgasm: A guide to sexual satisfaction*. Indianapolis: Bobbs-Merrill, 1975.

Kolodny, R.C.; Masters, W.H.; Johnson, V.E.; and Biss, M.A. *Textbook of human sexuality for nurses*. Boston: Little, Brown & Co., 1979.

Kroah, J. How to deal with patients who act out sexually. *Nursing '73*, 3, 12, 1973:38–39.

Levin, R.J., and Levin, A. Sexual pleasure: The surprising preferences of 100,000 women. *Redbook*, September 1975.

Lion, E.M. *Human sexuality in nursing process*. New York: Wiley, 1982.

McCaghy, C.H. Child molesting. *Sexual behavior*, 1, 1971:16.

Malinowski, B. *The sexual life of savages in north-western Melanesia*. New York: Eugenics, 1929.

Masters, W.H., and Johnson, V.E. *Human sexual response*. Boston: Little, Brown & Co., 1966.

Masters, W.H., and Johnson, V.E. *Human sexual inadequacy*. Boston: Little, Brown & Co., 1970.

Masters, W.H.; Johnson, V.E.; and Kolodny, R.C. *Human sexuality*. New York: Little, Brown & Co., 1982.

Mead, M. *Sex and temperament in three primitive societies*. New York: Morrow, 1935.

Medical aspects of human sexuality. New York: Hospital Publications, Inc.

Miller, W.R., and Lief, H.I. Masturbatory attitudes, knowledge, and experience: Data from the Sex Knowledge and Attitude Test (SKAT). *Archives of sexual behavior.* 5, 1976:447–467.

Mims, F.H., and Swenson, M. *Sexuality: A nursing perspective.* New York: McGraw-Hill, 1980.

Money, J. (ed.). *Sex research: New developments.* New York: Holt, Rinehart & Winston, 1965.

Money, J., and Ehrhardt, A.A. *Man and woman, boy and girl.* Baltimore: Johns Hopkins Press, 1972.

Mooney, T.O.; Cole, T.M.; and Children, R.A. *Sexual options for paraplegics and quadriplegics.* Boston: Little, Brown & Co., 1975.

McRae, I., and Henderson, G. Sexuality and irreversible health limitations. *Nursing clinics of North America,* 10, 3, 1975:587–597.

Pettyjohn, R.D. Health care of the gay individual. *Nursing forum,* 18, 4, 1979:367–393.

Reid, W.H. *Treatment of the DSM-III psychiatric disorders.* New York: Brunner/Mazel, 1983.

Robinault, I.P. *Sex, society, and the disabled: A developmental inquiry into roles, reactions, and responsibilities.* New York: Harper & Row, 1978.

Rohme, M.W. The public health nurse as sexual counselor for spinal cord injured men. *Sexuality and disability,* 2, 1, 1979:8–15.

Sadock, B.J.; Kaplan, H.I.; and Freedman, A.M. (eds.). *The sexual experience.* Baltimore: Williams & Wilkins, 1976.

Sadock, B.J., and Sadock, V.A. Techniques of coitus. In *The sexual experience.* (Sadock, B.J., et al. eds.). Baltimore: Williams & Wilkins, 1976.

Sedgwick, R. Myths in human sexuality: A social-psychological perspective. *Nursing clinics of North America,* 10, 3, 1975:539–550.

Sherfey, M.J. *Nature and evolution of female sexuality.* New York: Random House, 1972.

Siemens, S., and Brandzel, R.C. *Sexuality: Nursing assessment and intervention.* Philadelphia: J.B. Lippincott, 1982.

Silbert, D.T. Human sexuality growth groups. *Journal of psychiatric nursing and mental health services,* 19, 2, 1981:31–34.

Smith, J., and Bullough, B. Sexuality and the severely disabled person. *American journal of nursing,* 75, 1975:2194–2197.

Smith, R.S. Voyeurism: A review of the literature. *Archives of sexual behavior,* 5, 1976:585–608.

Stephens, G.J. Mind-body continuum in human sexuality. *American journal of nursing,* 70, 1970:1468–1471.

Stephens, G.J. Creative contraries: A theory of sexuality. *American journal of nursing,* 78, 1978:70–75.

Stohs, S.J. Drugs and sexual function. *U.S. pharmacist,* 3, 10, 1978:51–68.

Sue, D. Erotic fantasies of college students during coitus. *Journal of sex research,* 15, 1979:299–305.

Thomas, S.P. Bisexuality: A sexual orientation of great diversity. *Journal of psychiatric nursing,* 18, 4, 1980:19–27.

Tollison, C.D., and Adams, H.E. *Sexual disorders: Treatment, theory, research.* New York: Gardner Press, 1979.

Wasow, M. Sexuality and the institutionalized mentally ill. *Sexuality and disability,* 3, 1, 1980:3–16.

Watts, R.J. Dimensions of sexual health. *American journal of nursing,* 79, 9, 1979:1570.

Weideger, P. *Menstruation and menopause: The physiology and psychology, the myth and reality.* New York: Alfred Knopf, 1976.

Weinberg, J.S. *Sexuality: Human needs and nursing practice.* Philadelphia: W.B. Saunders Co., 1982.

Whitley, M.P. Seduction and the hospitalized person. *Journal of nursing education,* 17, 6, 1978:34–39.

Woods, N.F. *Human sexuality in health and illness,* 2d ed. St. Louis: Mosby, 1979:79–80; 3rd ed., 1984.

Yeaworth, R.C., and Friedeman, J.S. Sexuality in later life. *Nursing clinics of North America,* 10, 3, 1975:565–573.

PART FOUR

Nursing Process and Life Events

Primary prevention remains the focus as situational events or stressors are introduced and crisis theory is addressed. Concepts of stress, coping, loss, and mental retardation are addressed as challenges that interact to influence health and well-being. These concepts are equally applicable in general hospital, community, and psychiatric settings.

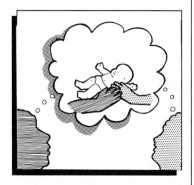

22

Crisis

Susan I. Cullen

Learning Objectives

Upon completion of this chapter, the reader will be able to:

1. Define a crisis event.

2. Discuss the historical development of crisis theory.

3. Identify the difference between a developmental crisis and a situational crisis.

4. Identify the difference between generic and individual crisis therapy.

5. Discuss ways of implementing primary, secondary, and tertiary prevention.

6. Use nursing process to assist a client experiencing a crisis.

During the past two decades the terms "crisis theory" and "crisis intervention" have become increasingly popular with those in health care fields. Although crisis theory has not been without its critics, it has become accepted as a short-term, intensive treatment approach in selected situations.

Nurses are involved in a variety of settings and have a unique opportunity to identify and intervene with clients who are experiencing crises. After developing an understanding of the levels of crisis prevention, the characteristics and definition of a crisis event, and nursing process as it applies to the crisis situation, the nurse can use her skills to promote the client's ability to deal with the crisis event.

□ *Crisis: Historical Perspective*

The works of Freud and other early analytic theorists are influential in the development of crisis theory. These works provide a theoretical basis for understanding the individual's development and response to his environment. They propose that all behavior has a cause and that the individual's earlier life experiences have a profound influence on his later development. The individual who fails to maintain a healthy life-style is one who is unable to learn from experience and develop appropriate behavior. Instead, this person clings to past experience and fails to integrate the past and the present.

Erik Erikson (1963) also believes that the past influences the present and describes this concept in terms of developmental phases. According to Erikson, the ego develops through a series of phases in an orderly, sequential manner. While progressing through the developmental process, each stage presents a crisis for the individual. The crisis is related to changes in the physiological and social events the person is experiencing. Erikson points out that successful completion of one stage is dependent on successful completion of previous stages. If a stage is not managed appropriately, the individual develops attitudes and beliefs that may cause emotional distress. If the process is accomplished effectively, an individual will emerge from each stage with an increase in his sense of judgment, sense of inner unity, and capacity to function. Early in each stage, the capacity to cope with the changes is immature. The individual must develop new approaches to problem solving and use these to supplement the old, familiar methods of coping, which begin to fail. During this time of upheaval or "crisis," the individual is most vulnerable, as well as most open to change.

Erich Lindemann (1979) is recognized as one of the founders of crisis theory. Much of Lindemann's work has focused on the grief response and how it is related to crisis intervention. In 1944, he conducted studies of the survivors of the Coconut Grove (Boston) Nightclub fire, in which more than 100 people died. Based on this work, he identified the normal grief response as having five characteristics: somatic distress and sensorium alterations, preoccupation with the image of the deceased, feelings of guilt, hostile reactions, and loss of usual patterns of conduct. These five characteristics, and a sixth which is thought to be more significant of a pathological response, are described with examples in Table 22-1.

Lindemann identifies the normal grief response as acute, having an identifiable onset. Also, it is seen as time limited and occurring through an identifiable sequence of stages. This is similar to other crisis events and responses.

The theorist most widely known in the development of crisis theory and crisis intervention is Gerald Caplan. Basing his ideas on theories put forth by others, he stresses the growth potential for the client during a crisis state. Caplan (1961) postulates that during the upheaval that occurs in the crisis period, the individual is open to change because of increased vulnerability. With a client who is overwhelmed by a crisis, the value of this approach becomes obvious.

Another important feature of Caplan's theory is emotional homeostasis. Individuals are continually confronted with problems and the resulting stresses, yet the threats are generally short-lived, and emotional balance is maintained. This is achieved through the use of habitual problem-solving methods. For example, when a child becomes ill, the mother takes the child to the doctor, receives a prescription for medication, and reassures both herself and the child that everything will be all right. Although there continues to be stress, a state of crisis has not developed, as both are comfortable with the problem-solving methods that have been used. Crisis occurs only when the habitual problem-solving methods fail and homeostasis is disturbed. The result is disequilibrium, or state of crisis. In the example, if the mother was not able to get the child to the doctor, or if the medication had been ineffective, a crisis state might have occcurred.

■ *Points of Emphasis*

Caplan stresses that "crisis" refers to the individual's emotional response to an event rather than the event itself. According to this view, crisis is an individual matter.

The nurse must recognize the degree of emotional response if she is to identify the importance of an event to the client, even though she may not consider the event as particularly stressful. The client's response must not be seen as silly or one of overreaction, but must be viewed from the perspective of the client himself.

Caplan's theory is the foundation upon which other theorists have built an expanded crisis theory, which includes the social group in which the client lives and according to which a crisis event is not only an individual matter but also includes those involved in the person's social system.

A crisis event may affect the individual client,

TABLE 22-1 Grief Response	
Characteristics	**Client Behavior and Feeling Response**
Somatic distress and sensorium alteration	Complaints of diminishing or lack of strength Deep, sighing respirations Shortness of breath Lack of appetite (may report not feeling hungry or that food does not taste good) Complaints of tightness in throat or difficulty swallowing Complaints of feeling nauseous Complaints of tightness in chest Describes feeling a slight sense of unreality in relation to present life events Describes feeling distanced from others emotionally
Preoccupation with image of the deceased	Image of lost individual remains vivid May mistake others for the deceased May be oblivious to surroundings Describes feeling he may be going insane
Feelings of guilt	Engages in much soul searching for evidence of not doing "enough" and being negligent or somehow responsible for the loss Participates in much wishful thinking about what might have been, for example, "I wish I had done. . . . before he died." Feels upset about negative feelings he had or has toward the deceased Self-accusation focused on an exaggeration of minor omissions toward the deceased
Hostile reaction	Feelings of loss of warmth toward others Irritability and anger toward others Feelings of not wanting to be bothered by others
Loss of usual patterns of conduct	Describes feelings of restlessness Inability to maintain an organized pattern of activity Daily routines may be maintained but are no longer automatic—Simple work activity may require much effort Describes no longer enjoying activities done in the past that were shared with the deceased
Appearance of traits or beliefs of the deceased	Borders on a pathological response to grief Begins to pursue hobbies not previously enjoyed because they were hobbies of the deceased Begins to dress or alter appearance so as to appear more like the deceased Begins to change beliefs or values to parallel the beliefs and values that were held by the deceased May develop behavior traits (e.g., a particular way of standing or talking) similar to those of the deceased

his family, and his social system. The determination of whether or not a crisis exists lies in the balance between the perceived threat of the event and the resources available to the individual for coping with it.

☐ *Definition of Crisis*

Stress is present during a crisis but does not in itself constitute a crisis event. It is important for the nurse to differentiate between stress as a part of daily living and stress as part of a crisis event. Stress may be felt as the tension that results from situations occurring in the normal course of living. It may result from both positive and negative situations: your car stalls on the highway, you spill coffee on your clothes after you've dressed for dinner, you start a vacation, or a friend comes to visit. Stress produces a crisis only when the usual coping mechanisms fail.

> **■ *Point of Emphasis***
>
> *A crisis is a temporary state in which the individual perceives a threat to himself, his self-concept, or his life goals. A loss or a need to change causes the individual to undergo a transition. The usual problem-solving methods are not enough to relieve the tension and reestablish homeostasis.*

Caplan states that a crisis typically evolves in four phases that are distinct but may overlap.

PHASES OF A CRISIS

Phase One

A traumatic event occurs causing increased tension. The first response is to use familiar problem-solving methods to reduce the perceived discomfort. The individual's effort is to solve the problem and restore a sense of emotional equilibrium. For example, a nursing student receives a failing grade on an examination. She may approach another student in hopes of hearing that the latter also did poorly, so that she may feel that it was not her personal failure, but rather a defective test.

Phase Two

If the usual problem-solving methods fail, the stress level increases. At this point, the crisis has not yet occurred, but the individual feels upset and ineffectual. Functioning begins to be disorganized. She makes more trial-and-error attempts to solve the problem. Continuing the example, the student learns that the other student had, in fact, received a high mark. She then may approach the teacher, saying she was not well the day of the test and would like an opportunity to retake it or to take another test. If the teacher refuses the request, she may ask another student to petition for a new test or for a better curve on the test grades.

Phase Three

The continued failure to resolve the problem causes a further increase in tension for the individual. At this time, emergency measures are used. The coping mechanisms may be one of the following: to redefine the problem so as to make it accord with past experience (the student may say to herself that this test contained "a lot of math" and she never was "good at math" anyway, but knows she does well in other areas); to define certain aspects of it as unsolvable and unimportant (the student may decide that this course is inconsequential and she doesn't care whether she passes); or to resign herself to the problem by giving up a goal as unattainable (the student may feel unhappy about not passing the test and realize that there will be no way for her to change the situation immediately, but she will need to work harder in the future). If these emergency measures do, in fact, solve the problem, then the emotional equilibrium is restored and the tension reduced.

Phase Four

If the problem is not resolved through the phase-three efforts, the tension level will continue to rise. Caplan calls this the "breaking point." The result is extreme personality disorganization. The client will describe feelings of helplessness and cognitive confusion, for example, the inability to define problems, evaluate reality, or formulate possible problem-solving approaches. In the example, the student may begin to state that she feels overwhelmed by schoolwork and not able to separate her failure in one test from her work in other courses, and begins to believe she is failing at everything she does. She could also describe feeling tired all the time, and may sleep most of the day rather than attend classes.

TABLE 22-2 Phases of a Crisis

Phase	Behavioral Manifestations and Feelings
One: Initial impact of traumatic event	Describes feeling anxious, helpless, hopeless, or panicky
	May complain of gastric distress, feeling of shortness of breath, weakness, or fatigue
	Reports difficulty in problem solving, feeling unable to think or having a "rush" of thoughts
	May give up efforts to change or indulge in frenzied activity trying to do more than is possible
	Attempts to use the habitual or usual coping mechanisms
Two: Disorganization with attack or retreat	May describe feeling increasingly tense and helpless
	Uses more unusual coping mechanisms in a trial-and-error attempt to resolve crisis or may become more rigid in thinking and unresponsive to attempts by others to help
	Defense mechanisms of repression, denial, rationalization or projection may be used
	May withdraw or become overactive
	Self-esteem is threatened
	Behavior and problem solving become increasingly disorganized
Three: Emergency state with resolution or defeat	Tension and anxiety continue to rise
	Self-esteem continues to be threatened
	Recurrence of complaints of physical illness such as feeling weak, being tired, gastric distress
	May rationalize and redefine the problem or "give up," becoming overwhelmed and depressed
	Begins to use emergency methods of coping, again, in a trial-and-error manner
	Crisis may be resolved at this time and emotional equilibrium restored—Tension will be reduced as a result
	If crisis unresolved, tension continues to increase
Four: breaking point	Major personality disorganization occurs
	Describes feeling helpless and hopeless
	Begins to have cognitive confusion: begins to feel unable to define the problem, and thoughts are completely disorganized
	May begin to evidence disorientation to time, place, person
	May totally withdraw from others
	May become depressed
	Crying frequently for long periods
	Self-image and self-esteem very low
	Can become psychotic

In severe states of crisis, there may be perceptual confusion in the temporal or spatial sense as well. A client may not be able to remember what day it is, where he lives, or where he is. His intellectual capacity appears to be at a standstill. The crisis has evolved. Table 22-2 summarizes this process and some of the reactions that occur.

CHARACTERISTICS OF A CRISIS

A crisis can be further described by certain typical features:

1. A crisis is generally self-limiting. It will be resolved in some way within a period of a few weeks (approximately 6 weeks). The

resolution may mean that the client is coping at a higher level of functioning, at the precrisis level of functioning, or at a lower level of functioning. The crisis itself, however, will be resolved.

2. The outcome of the crisis period is primarily affected by the actions of the individual (persistence in seeking resolution and use of support offered) and the support available from others. Although antecedent factors such as the client's personality, past experience, and the nature of the problem will affect the outcome, they are not the most important factors.

3. During the crisis period the client actively desires to be helped by others. Two things happen. First, the client will generally increase the number and intensity of his signals to others to indicate he is in distress. This is an attempt to engage assistance. Second, he will be more responsive to feedback. This helps explain why a crisis is an opportunity for growth as well as a time of increased susceptibility to illness.

☐ *Types of Crises*

Although the phases and characteristics of a crisis event are present in all crises, the crisis event may be classified in two ways: as a developmental or expected, internally generated crisis; or as a situational, externally generated crisis.

DEVELOPMENTAL OR MATURATIONAL CRISIS

A developmental or maturational crisis is one that is expected and internally generated. Understanding the psychological, physical, and social aspects of personality development is essential for understanding the developmental crisis. Erik Erikson's theory of personality development is well recognized and accepted as a basis for developmental crisis theory.

Erikson (1963) states that development occurs when an individual is confronted by growth problems from the point of birth until death. A progression through a sequence of phases takes place in a healthy manner, with the completion of one phase setting the stage for the next phase. Failure to master the problems or crises that occur in each stage brings about a higher risk of illness in the

next stage. This is most easily understood if compared to a structure made up of a child's building blocks. If each block is in place and solidly supports the block on top of it, the structure won't fall. If blocks are missing, the structure is unsteady and likely to fall. Erikson describes the eight stages or "building blocks" of the developmental process in terms of specific life tasks to be accomplished by the individual. Although ages at which each stage typically evolves are identified, they may vary from person to person yet remain within normal limits. Table 22-3 describes the eight developmental stages.

SITUATIONAL CRISIS

Situational crises are externally generated. The individual is unable to cope with external events which may be either anticipated (death of an elderly relative, marriage) or unanticipated (illness, loss of a job, an unexpected death).

Anticipated Situational Crisis

The anticipated situational crisis requires that the individual make role changes and adjustments in the way he relates to others. These changes are similar to those occurring during the developmental stages. Unlike the developmental crisis, though, not everyone experiences all of them. As with the developmental crisis, an inability to make the expected role changes gives rise to a crisis.

When individuals are expected to change in the way they relate to the family or to society, there is stress, and there may be a crisis during the adjustment period. In order for the person to make role changes, three factors must be present:

1. The person must be able to envision himself in the new role. He will be able to do this if he has had effective role models and appropriate education to prepare him for the change. For example, parenting classes for future parents help them define and meet their new responsibilities. This experience can both educate them and help them see themselves as parents.

2. Interpersonal resources must be available. The person needs the ability to communicate with others in order to define and clarify expectations about the new role. Good communication skills will enable the individual to request assistance and support

TABLE 22-3 Developmental or Maturational Stages

Stage	Infancy: First 15 to 18 months of life
Task	Trust vs. mistrust
Description	Infant develops either a basic feeling of trust or an attitude of mistrust. If needs met regularly—fed when hungry, changed when wet, given affection readily, and not left for long periods of time—child's confidence in others grows. Trust in self also begins—begins to take chances. If environment seen as hostile—needs carelessly or infrequently met—child begins to doubt the dependability of others.
Correlation to psychoanalytic theory	Oral phase—sucking, chewing, and biting viewed as pleasurable. Libido and aggressive drives poorly differentiated and "love" expressed through symbolic devouring of others through the mouth, as with food. Trust develops as the destroyed object reappears as happens with food.
Failure to achieve task	Lack of trust. Person will withdraw and feel estranged from others.
Goal of nurse	To reestablish the basic state of trust through providing consistency and dependability in her contacts with the client.
Stage	Early Childhood: 15 to 18 months up to 3 years old
Task	Autonomy vs. shame
Description	Begins to learn to regulate own behavior. Attempts to increase self-control and not lose confidence in own ability while striving to keep parental affection and esteem. Developmental focus is to gain bowel and bladder control. Needs firm, sensitive, and realistic expectations by parents. If expectations too rigid, child will not exert self-control. Soiling himself in presence of peers and others produces shame. Successful completion of task produces a sense of autonomy.
Correlation to psychoanalytic theory	Anal phase—highly interested in excretory process. Child frequently seen to present the feces to the parent as a gift or uses it to play or paint with. Mud, lipstick, or crayons often used as substitutes to represent the feces.
Failure to achieve task	Person feels and expresses shame and doubt about himself. Can be manifested behavior that is either compulsive in self-restraint and compliance or evidenced by willful and defiant behavior. More simply, the client can focus on feelings about being dirty or soiled, focus on bowel functions—moving too much or too little—and express inability to recognize his own accomplishments.
Goal of nurse	To assist individual to develop more ways to be reassured of self-worth and decrease compulsiveness of his behavior.
Stage	Late childhood: 3 to 5 years old
Task	Initiative vs. guilt
Description	Child begins to explore the environment more completely. Parallel play (playing alongside other children) begins. Rules of society and family begin to have an impact. Child begins to develop goals and have a sense of purpose. Limits about what is acceptable are starting to be recognized. Takes initiative and expresses resentment toward anyone who thwarts his needs. Resentment can be expressed through wishes to "get rid of the other person." Guilt feelings develop in response to these wishes. Guilt feelings must be balanced by feelings of worth for healthy development. Occurs as the child is reassured by others he is important and others need not be eliminated for him to retain importance.
Correlation to psychoanalytic theory	Oedipal period—Freud describes phenomenon of the "death wish" when child wishes the same-sex parent dead so that the parent of opposite sex is entirely available just to him. Guilt feelings produced by wish cause child to fear punishment.
Failure to achieve task	May result in an overly developed conscience. The conscience becomes rigid and automatic, limiting the client's judgment and ability to pursue fulfillment of his own wishes.
Goal of nurse	To help the client begin to challenge his excessive guilt feelings while recognizing the societal limits. Discovering the feared "out of control" behavior does not occur as one loosens control is a major concern for this person.
Stage	School age: 6 to 12 years old
Task	Industry vs. inferiority
Description	Child enters school and spends increasing amounts of time away from home and family. Identification rather than competition with the parent of the same sex begins. Works to incorporate the same-sex parent's image. Adult tasks in the form of school responsibilities and helping at home become important. In healthy development, child begins to recognize his abilities and accomplishments of mastering tasks and relating with others. Needs to have this recognized by parents and others as well. Strong family relationships emerge providing a sturdy emotional base for turmoil of adolescence.

(continued)

TABLE 22-3 *(continued)*

Correlation to psychoanalytic theory	Latency period—Provides the time for alliance with own sex. Children are somewhat disdainful of members of the opposite sex.
Failure to achieve task	If child receives mostly negative responses to his accomplishments, he may feel that he "will never be any good at anything" and lack motivation to continue trying. In the adult becomes expressed through severe criticism of one's abilities; the person seems always to "take the easy way." The client will withdraw from risks and others.
Goal of nurse	Help the client to recognize his achievements by challenging the harsh self-criticism from a realistic perspective. Recognition of his abilities will need to start with external praise, and gradually the child will be able to reinforce his own sense of worth.
Stage	Adolescence: 12 to 20 yers old
Task	Identity vs. role diffusion
Description	Maturing of the endocrine system and development of adult primary and secondary sex characteristics are accompanied by psychological and social developments. Awakening of sexual drives and the control demanded by society cause conflict and tension. Sex drives controlled by: sublimation (use of athletics, work, school, and social activities), masturbation, sex play with friends, erotic dreams. If behaviors are not approached with compassion and understanding, the anxiety and guilt can be overwhelming. Another major issue is the definition of an identity as emerging adult. Begins to be expected to make long-term commitments to both a career and relationships. Concept of love expressed initially through friendships, intense sharing, or a feeling of oneness. Love then takes on a sexual aspect and definition of what is desirable in a long-term partner becomes important.
Failure to achieve task	Begins to feel powerless and alienated from others. Confusion about identity is prevalent. Adult may behave primarily in an antisocial manner as a way to keep a perception of uniqueness. Also expressed through persistent conflicts about personal beliefs (e.g., conservative vs. liberal values), career choices, and relationship issues.
Goal of nurse	To assist the client in identifying a clearer image of himself in relation to others. In addition, learning to compromise between conflicting belief's and learning to delay gratification are important for the client.
Stage	Young adulthood: 18 or 20 to 25 years old
Task	Intimacy vs. isolation
Description	Two conflicting desires present—wanting to begin building a secure future and wanting to extend the irresponsibility of youth. Can appear as a time of wastefullness and aimless activity yet in reality provides a time for consolidating the various aspects of one's personality and social roles. Result can then be an integrated adult identity. Integrated identity allows for establishment of true intimacy with others. Begins to separate from the nuclear family and expand relationships to include others at a level demanding commitment. Can be a time of birth of first child and the resulting changes in responsibilities and roles.
Failure to achieve task	Adult will feel fragmented and isolated. There will be an inability to achieve intimacy with others. Adult is unable to "settle down" long enough to meet goals in work or in personal relationships. Frequently described by others as "jumping in and out" of things. Relationships are kept on a superficial level.
Goal of nurse	To help the client establish increased integration of his personal identity. Help him to sort out his ideas of who he is, what he wants to be, and what he thinks others want him to be. This will enable him to identify more clearly a reasonable place for himself within the social structure.
Stage	Adulthood: 25 to 65 years old
Task	Generativity vs. stagnation
Description	Person evaluates his productivity and on that basis postulates what he can look forward to accomplishing. During this period one begins to develop more platonic relationships and expand one's focus to value intellectual and physical skills in nonwork-related activities as well as work activities. If not, stagnation and boredom may develop. Early part of period, often time of marriage and birth of children, may continue to work on task of previous period. Career establishment may still be of concern. "Mid-life crisis" time is years of middle to early 40s. Important as time when person begins to evaluate goals in terms of actual achievements. Also recognition of physical deterioration or loss of youth becomes more evident. Person may have feeling of pressure that "time is running out." Apparent that productive life span is limited, one's children are growing and less in need of care, and one's own parents may be in (or moving toward) a time of

TABLE 22-3 (continued)

	needing additional care. May define marriage as too costly for his own development or see marriage to a younger partner as a way to extend his own youth. If successful completion of this period, individual is able to incorporate the realities of life and define realistic goals. Depression and lowered self-image give way to new sense of purpose. Unsuccessful coping leaves individual in a struggle looking for youth and youth's goals.
	Middle age: 42 to 65 years old. Brings about the ability to relax and accept one's spouse as a help and support rather than a source of a problem. Competitiveness decreases as he feels more positive about the contributions he has made. Personal values and ideas begin to take precedence with less effort spent on trying to please others at a cost to the self. Focus on material achievements and social status is reduced with increased enjoyment of daily life. Approaching death is accepted as part of the life cycle causing less fear of dying and greater appreciation of life. Accomplishments likely to be viewed as having been successfully achieved, even if not what hoped for as a youth.
Failure to achieve task	Individual has low self-esteem and depression is more or less constant. May be viewed by others as foolish and immature as he attempts to retain a youth that is no longer present or appropriate.
Goal of nurse	To help the client accept the current physical status and evaluate his life achievements more realistically. Important to help him to begin planning for major role changes.
Stage	Old age: 65 years old to death
Task	Integrity vs. despair
Description	Acceptance of one's life as unique and having had value is needed. Redefinition of continued contributions allows for relinquishment of leadership to the younger person. Losses may happen, causing stress: physical strength and stamina are less; illness more frequent; senses diminish (vision, hearing, taste, touch). Loss of physical ability may cause person finally to lose his home and necessitate moving into a supervised living setting (nursing home). Loss of job through retirement and possible resulting changes in economic status. Losses in relationships due to death of family and friends. Will need to "let go" of the people he is losing and "expand" relationships to include new people so he does not become isolated. All these losses cause increased dependence on others with less sense of independence remaining for individual. Being able to accept help and support of others is central to adjustment. Also being able to accept the realities of limitations and adjust realistically is important.
Failure to achieve task	The person who is not able to evaluate and integrate his life experiences into his personal image feels despairing. He looks to the past as all-important rather than seeing the future as having promise. Life may seem to short, and may be filled with regrets. A sense of failure in relation to one's life goals will persist.
Goal of nurse	To help the client establish and maintain a sense of identity and self-worth based on his current functioning. While some isolation and withdrawal seem inevitable, a gradual disengagement from society seems a worthwhile goal so that these feelings can be limited. The amount of involvement should be satisfying without being overwhelming.

from others when he needs it. Healthy interpersonal resources will also allow for flexibility about goals so that goals can be adjusted as his roles change. For example, the birth of a child may shift the focus away from emphasis on a person's career or marital relationship to parenting and providing for the child. Drawing upon his own resources and receiving support from others permits the individual to achieve a balance between these roles rather than to sacrifice one for the other.

3. Others must accept the individual's new role. To assume a new role successfully, others in the person's social system must recognize the necessity of change and adjust their relationships with him. General systems theory states that a change in a person or within a system necessitates change in all other parts of the system. If the new role is not accepted by others in the social system, they may sabotage the person's efforts to change his role. In response, he may experience confusion about the role and his ability to assume it. This confusion is the result of another's nonacceptance rather than lack of actual ability to effect the role change. For example, as the young adult attempts to assume a more adult role and separate from the family by

assuming greater independence, the parents may either attempt to remain in authority or may move toward support and toward suggestions which can be accepted or rejected by their child. If the parents are unable to accept the separation and increased independence of their child, they will attempt to keep the child in a dependent position. Messages that their child makes poor choices about friends and work are examples of ways in which the parents retain control.

Typical role changes that may result in an anticipated situational crisis are presented in Table 22-4.

Unanticipated Situational Crises

The unanticipated situational crises are unexpected, chance events. The individual does not consider them a possibility and is therefore unprepared for their occurrence.

1. *Failure to achieve.* A demotion, loss of economic security, or academic failure are common unexpected and unwanted events. Failure to achieve identified goals can bring about self-recrimination and overwhelming feelings of guilt, anger, frustration, shame. The result may be a poor self-image with a tendency to withdraw from or be aggressive toward other people.

2. *Death of a significant person through circumstances unrelated to old age.* Death is an expected part of the life cycle, and grieving is part of the life experience. Grieving occurs in response to loss of something or someone of value. However, if the loss is unanticipated, this premature separation (a person dying "before his time") can complicate the grieving process because of the anger and guilt felt by the survivor. These feelings can be intensified by the perception that "life has not been fair."

3. *Illness or hospitalization.* Illness requires role changes, from an independent to a dependent position, or toward decreased capability. The self-image must be adjusted to include the "recent" physical limitations. Making these changes includes a grieving process in which the client will mourn the losses. The nurse must recognize that admission to the hospital for even a minor illness can precipitate a crisis for the client. If the illness causes long-term or permanent limitations, the crisis will be even more intense.

4. *Victim crisis.* Another type of unexpected situational crisis is a victim crisis. These crises result from aggression by another person or by some factor in the environment. The aggressive act may be physical or emotional. Examples of victim crisis include family abuse (spouse, child, elderly), rape, murder, assault, war, theft, and natural disasters. The victim crises of family abuse and rape are particularly traumatic. It may be difficult for the nurse to identify whether the victim maintains silence out of feelings of shame and guilt, or because he feels responsible for the event. Society frequently reinforces such feelings. An example is the message often conveyed about a rape victim, such as these: her dress was too seductive; she should not have been out alone; she not only "asked for it, but probably enjoyed it."

In all victim crises, the nurse needs to pay special attention to the degree of anger and guilt experienced by the person. Medical care is obviously essential.

☐ *Crisis Intervention*

Although crisis therapy is not the same as short-term therapy, it is similar in its emphasis on resolving immediate problems, rather than on restructuring the individual's personality.

> **■ *Point of Emphasis***
>
> *It is important to note that crisis therapy differs from traditional psychotherapy in its assumption that the client's health and social adjustment were normal before the crisis event. In contrast, the assumption of traditional psychotherapy is that an existing psychopathology caused the person to seek therapy. Emotional crises are normal events in the life of a well-adjusted individual rather than a signal drawing attention to an underlying illness.*

The nurse who responds quickly and actively to a client experiencing a crisis can help him to reach several objectives: the immediate problem is effectively resolved; coping mechanisms are restored to either the precrisis level of function or to an improved level of function; and maladaptive behavior does not develop.

Crisis therapy may be divided into two categories—the generic and the individual.

TABLE 22-4 Role Changes in Anticipated Situational Crisis

Role	Description
Beginning nursery school or kindergarten	Stressful, as it is the first time the expectation is clear that the child will be away from mother and family for periods of time. May be stressful for parent as well as child.
Beginning independent living	Occurs because the child has left home for school, work, or marriage. Importance of this change is the development of an image separate from the family.
Marriage	The beginning of a shared intimate relationship. May include legal sanction or be at symbolic level. Important change is the forming of a primary family, with increased responsibilities and intimacy with another.
Birth of a child	Beginning of parental responsibilities may be planned or unexpected event. Major role changes occur. If child is born with a disability, identity as a parent may be further impaired due to feelings of anger, fear, and guilt.
Loss of spouse, child, or parent	Loss of others may be through physical separation, emotional distancing, death. As child moves on to form his own primary family, parents may feel lost and unsure about what their purpose is and lack the means to meet their needs with others. Can apply as well to the child's reaction of losing the parent or an adult losing the spouse. Person may move away, changing allegiance (as in divorce), or die.
Career changes	Promotions or job changes are usually pursued but cause conflict and stress due to increased responsibility. Assuming more responsibility can affect both the work setting and personal relationships. The extent of the crisis depends on the demands (e.g., need to relocate) that accompany the career change. An unanticipated, unwelcome change occurs with the loss of a job or demotion.
Economic changes	An increase in income, although positive, can cause much stress. Conflicts arise between wanting to balance spending money with wanting to save. Need also arises to evaluate how the financial change affects personal relationships. A reverse in fortunes causes similar stresses, and roles and individual identity must be renegotiated.

GENERIC THERAPY

The generic approach is based on the belief that there are certain psychological tasks and problem-solving behaviors that must be achieved in order to resolve a crisis. For example, Lindemann's study of bereavement identifies psychological responses and tasks he believes to be universally exhibited whenever a person experiences a loss. These responses and tasks form a behavioral pattern that will be readily apparent in the client in crisis. The use of denial, for example, is a typical, expected behavior.

Personal psychodynamics and features, for example, age and sex, are not of great concern in planning the interventions. Rather, specific interventions are effective for all clients experiencing a particular type of crisis such as the crisis of bereavement. The crisis event is the element common to all. In the individual's crisis experience, the focus is on his ability to resolve each phase of the crisis.

TABLE 22-5 Levels of Prevention

Level	Goal	Examples
Primary	Prevent the crisis and maintain emotional homeostasis	Premarital counseling for engaged couples Prenatal classes for expectant parents Support groups in school for children facing developmental tasks Vocational counseling Community education classes on subjects of assertiveness, stress management, development of leisure skills, and relaxation techniques Pre-retirement support groups Support groups or individual counseling for families with a terminally ill member Presurgery counseling to plan for adjustment in body-image changes Community disaster planning
Secondary	Early identification of a crisis to prevent development of maladaptive behavior	Support groups for people experiencing loss of spouse Support groups for parents who have lost a child Counseling for patient having significant body image changes due to surgery (e.g., mastectomy, amputation) or an accident Support groups for victims of abuse Support groups for victims of rape Individual, group, or family counseling for a person experiencing a crisis
Tertiary	To prevent further decompensation of coping skills and reduce long-term disabling effects	Group therapy for chronically ill persons Support groups for the physically disabled Alcoholics Anonymous for the alcoholic Narcotics Anonymous for drug abusers Remotivation groups for the aged Counseling for the individual having a delayed grief response Resocialization groups for chronic psychiatric patients

Benefits of the generic approach include the following:

1. It can be practiced by health professionals in several disciplines as well as by non-professionals, since an ability to assess individual psychodynamics is not necessary. Interventions are based on anticipated patterns of behavior.
2. It can be easily taught, as it specifies appropriate interventions for situational and maturational events that are common to the lives of most people.
3. It provides a theoretical basis for devel-

opment of preventive (primary, secondary, and tertiary) mental health programs.

INDIVIDUAL THERAPY

The individual approach differs from the generic one in that it focuses on the psychological tasks and problem-solving activities that each client must complete in order to resolve his unique crisis experience. There are no predetermined tasks or expected behaviors. Intervention is designed to resolve the particular situation that precipitated the crisis. It is important that this approach be carried out by mental health professionals, as it involves understanding of the client's biopsychosocial processes.

The individual approach should be employed in the following situations:

1. Clients who are experiencing a crisis that includes elements of both a situational and a maturational crisis.
2. Clients who respond to a crisis by having suicidal and/or homicidal feelings.
3. Clients who have not responded to treatment in which the generic approach has been used.
4. Clients experiencing a crisis for which there is not a generic theory already established.

Although different, the generic and individual approaches are compatible, and elements of each may be used in planning interventions.

LEVELS OF PREVENTION

Theories of crisis and crisis intervention stress that a crisis event is an opportunity for growth as well as a threat to health. Prevention is important in dealing with both the precrisis events and actual crisis intervention. The nurse can be involved with the client on all three levels of prevention as summarized in Table 22-5.

Primary prevention is self-explanatory. It is accomplished through direct education of a population at risk, as well as through consultation with service-oriented professions that deal with such a population, for example, schools, police departments, or medical-surgical treatment settings. The goal is to help the client learn coping skills that can be used in working through the developmental stage of a crisis, experiencing only moderate distress—in short, anticipatory guidance. Helping people by providing education and planning for expected developmental stages or probable situational crises events (parenthood, marriage) may forestall later crises.

Secondary prevention identifies a crisis event early, the aim of intervention being to prevent the development of maladaptive behaviors. Its purpose is twofold: (1) to shorten the period of disequilibrium, and (2) to promote a return to a healthy state of functioning. This is the time when crisis therapy is practiced.

Tertiary prevention occurs after the acute phase has resolved. Its purpose is to mitigate any long-term disability due to the crisis, by helping clients develop new ways of coping.

SELECTION OF CLIENTS

Initially the nurse must decide which clients will benefit more from crisis intervention than from traditional forms of psychotherapy. There are two criteria that will help the nurse make this determination: (1) The problem must be of short duration, to help ensure that active, short-term intervention will prove effective. This is especially true if intervention is begun early in the crisis. (2) The client must be motivated toward treatment. Because of the time limitations inherent in crisis intervention, there is not sufficient time to work with a client who is resistant to treatment. Both client and those in his support system should desire that treatment be given.

Once the decision is made about the form of treatment, the nurse will want either to refer the person to a more appropriate treatment setting, or begin to implement the intervention.

□ Nursing Process

As discussed earlier in this chapter, the nurse can be effective in helping the client to both prevent and resolve crises, applying the nursing process in various crisis situations. A case example (p. 469) illustrates crisis theory and the nursing process.

ASSESSMENT □

Self-Assessment □ Positive involvement with the client in crisis requires that the nurse be aware of her own feelings about the crisis. If she does not understand her own feelings, her own views and biases may interfere with her ability to intervene. This could send a clear message to the client that his distress is out of proportion to the crisis experience. The client then would not only feel unhappy about the crisis itself, but unhappy as well about his feelings.

The nurse needs to have a clear understanding of the client's unique needs so that her own attitudes will not interfere with her ability to deal with the client. Negative or overly protective judgments about the crisis, the client's response to it, or the client himself, are not helpful.

Client Assessment □ Aguilera and Messick (1982) define three factors that determine the existence of a crisis: (1) perception of the event; (2) situational supports; and (3) coping mechanisms that affect an individual's ability to maintain equilibrium and resolve his problems. The client should be assessed for strengths and weaknesses using the following guidelines:

1. *Determine the precipitating event*. The client may be aware of feeling stressed but may not be able to recall the cause. The nurse needs to identify the event that caused the trauma. If the event and the resulting feelings occurred nearly simultaneously, the crisis event can probably be easily identified. If symptoms of the crisis appear after the event itself, however, both nurse and client may identify the precipitating event only after comparing the appearance of symptoms with the occurrence of recent events in his life.

2. *Determine the extent of disruption that has occurred as a result of the crisis event*. The nurse needs to explore the client's ability to meet basic needs (e.g., food and hygiene). With the increased anxiety, the client may become immobilized and unable to provide for his basic needs. To evaluate the situation, ask direct questions, such as "When did you last eat? Are you able to sleep? How much time are you spending with others? Where do you spend most of your day? Are you able to concentrate on your work?"

3. *Determine the client's perception of the event*. The subjective meaning of a crisis event determines which coping mechanisms will be used. As each of us perceives and processes information in a unique way, the nurse needs to know whether the client's perception of the event appears realistic, or is distorted so as to cause the client not to recognize the relationship between the crisis event and the resulting stress, or to make the event seem more threatening than it is.

Ask the client to define the event in terms of his goals and identity, and his relationships with others. For example, "What effect do you think this will have on your life-style? What effect do you think this will have on your goal of obtaining a job? What do you think your friends will think about this? What do you think your family feels about this?"

4. *Determine presence or absence of situational support*. Most theorists agree that positive reinforcement from the environment is essential to maintain self-esteem. During a crisis period, supports may act as a positive factor to reinforce the client's confidence and self-esteem. On the other hand, criticism or absence of support threatens self-esteem. Family or friends may withhold sup-

port. The client may fear rejection and isolate himself. Ask questions such as, "Have you told your wife? How did she respond? Have you talked with anybody about this? Whom do you usually turn to when you're upset?"

5. *Determine the client's coping mechanisms*. Stress is a daily experience in a person's life. Learned patterns of response to stress help a person maintain a sense of equilibrium, and this occurs largely without conscious effort. These defense mechanisms are healthy, and give the person greater confidence about his ability to cope with various situations.

In a crisis, the defense mechanisms fail. In an effort to reestablish equilibrium, the individual consciously focuses on the problem and increases his efforts to resolve it. One result may be that the defenses become pathological, for example, the existence of the crisis may be denied, or the client may persist in dealing with the crisis inappropriately even though a positive outcome is not achieved. To assess the coping mechanisms, the nurse can ask, "What have you done so far? How do you usually react to frustration, anger, or fear? What else have you thought about doing? Does talking about your feelings help? Are you sleeping or eating more?"

6. *Determine the extent of emotional disruption*. A careful evaluation of the person's feeling state is necessary. Does the individual feel hopeless and helpless to change the situation? Does he harbor suicidal or homicidal feelings? Ask specific questions: "Are you feeling sad? How much trouble are you having with feelings of wanting to hurt yourself? Are you feeling you want to hurt someone else? Do you have a plan to hurt yourself or someone else? Do you feel things can ever change?"

The assessment phase provides baseline data from which to make a nursing diagnosis and establish treatment goals and interventions. Remember that family, friends, and significant others must be involved as much as possible. Assessment gives information about the client's strengths and areas of need and the availability and strengths of his support system.

This is the time when the nurse-client relationship begins to be established. In view of the time limitations of crisis intervention, it is essential that the nurse convey warmth, empathy, and a genuine desire to help.

PROBLEM IDENTIFICATION AND INTERVENTION □
Through nursing diagnosis, the nurse can readily

communicate to others the nature of the problem and approaches to its resolution. General guidelines that help the nurse establish the diagnosis are given below:

1. *Focus on the problem.* The nursing plan needs to be based on concrete, identifiable issues related only to the present crisis. There is a temptation to go on to long-term issues, but this is not appropriate.

2. *Always be aware of the client's ability to function independently.* Dependency on others is generally an issue of concern in planning nursing care. Some clients feel angry and upset about needing to become more dependent, and have difficulty allowing others to help; others may become more dependent than is necessary or helpful during the crisis period. By clearly identifying the problems, the nurse can develop a care plan that reinforces the client's strengths while effectively meeting his dependency needs.

3. *Problems stemming from external events, such as the loss of a loved one, may aggravate the crisis for the client.*

The plan of intervention aims toward fostering growth in the client. The nurse needs to decide how much she should do for the client, and how much he can do for himself. Reinforcing the client's strengths and actively mobilizing his support system are integral to intervention. Client and nurse together should identify ways in which he can care for himself. This helps overcome feelings of helplessness and worthlessness.

The nurse must not become so engrossed in the plan of care that she ignores the client's expression of his thoughts and feelings. By actively listening to what the client has to say and by responding to him, she encourages him to express his feelings freely. Negative feelings should be acknowledged, as well as positive ones.

An example will demonstrate. A man who lost his wife related feelings of anger and resentment toward her for "dying on him." He felt extremely guilty about this anger. The nurse helped him to understand that his anger was caused by his loneliness and hurt at having lost his life's mate. She explained that this anger at the deceased is a natural grief reaction, and she encouraged him to further express his feelings.

Guidelines that can help the nurse to develop appropriate interventions are given below.

1. *Focus on the problem areas of the client's life.* Maintain the focus on the problem at hand and resist the temptation to look at others. For example, "Can you tell me how that relates to what is happening for you right now? I know this is important to you, yet I'm not sure how it is affecting your feelings about this current problem. I think we are getting away from what we were talking about. Can we move back to the problem we were discussing a few moments ago?"

2. *Utilize the client's strengths.* When implementing care, the nurse should ask herself: "Is this something that he can do himself?" "Doing for" the client should steadily decrease as intervention progresses. As an example, a client may need to have much assistance with physical care following surgery. As his physical state improves, he is encouraged to take over the care as it is safe for him to do so. The client's desire to resume independent functioning is a strength that needs to be recognized and reinforced.

3. *Involve the support system.* Recognize that because a support system consists of individuals, each member will respond to the client's problem in a unique way, which may not always be useful to the client. An example will demonstrate. In a rape case, significant others frequently express their support of the victim. What may happen, however, is that they become overwhelmed by their own feelings of guilt and anger about the rape, and begin to withdraw or even to blame the victim.

To help the client, the nurse must accept and incorporate cultural and life-style differences, without allowing her own value system to interfere with effective treatment. The nurse must take care not to impose a personal judgment about the "insensitivity" of family and friends or exhibit anger toward them. Instead, by providing opportunities for them to express and work through their feelings, she will keep the support system involved in a positive way.

4. *Keep the plan realistic and time-limited.* Structuring the interventions can help reduce the client's sense of being overwhelmed or hopeless. Set a time for meetings, decide the number of sessions to be held, and clarify expectations about what is to be accomplished. Also convey to the client that by evaluating the situation on a continuing basis, different approaches can be taken, should a particular approach fail.

5. *Be aware of the need for anticipatory planning.* As the crisis resolves, the client will frequently "drop from sight." Follow-up needs to be planned, to help reinforce the changes in the client. This reinforcement then becomes a preventive measure against future crisis events.

In addition to the general interventions de-

TABLE 22-6 Intervention Guidelines

Crisis Event	Intervention
Maturational crisis	Increasing the individual's awareness of the underlying conflict, which is usually related to a developmental task.
	Patterns of behavior must be identified and explored with the individual.
	Greater emphasis on the past than in other types of crisis therapy.
	Intervention must be directed to the developmental issue as well as the manifest problem, which is usually evidenced through acting out or ``role challenging'' behavior (e.g., using drugs, sexual promiscuity).
Situational crisis	
Role changes	Frequently involve a threat to the self-image.
	Special need for helping others in the client's family or support system to recognize and accept the change in the client's role.
Inability to become a parent (infertility)	Discuss threats to self-esteem; will commonly see self as defective or view the infertility as punishment for being ``bad'' or unworthy.
	Discuss how infertility may affect sexuality and relationship with partner.
	Promote involvement in support groups for infertile couples in order to increase the emotional and informational support available to them.
	Often, clients are reluctant to discuss the problem because of feelings of shame or feelings that others do not appreciate the importance of the situation to them.
Divorce	Allowing for expression of guilt generated as a result of feelings of failure or feelings of relief that marriage is ended. Self-image threatened; may see himself as a ``bad'' person
	Assisting client to locate and engage resources for legal protection of rights.
	Assisting client to problem-solve about ways to meet needs with spouse absent.
	Recognizing the intensification of earlier feelings of anger and pain during the divorce.
	Identifying the multiple losses perceived by the client, for example, financial, role changes (spouse to single), and social as social network frequently changes.
Victim of abuse	Engaging social supports for the protection of the victim (e.g., child welfare, shelter, or foster-home settings).
	Providing for medical treatment of the victim since physical trauma is frequently present.
	Self-esteem threatened, victim often feels much guilt and responsibility for the sexual or physical assault against self.
	Denial is a defense mechanism for both the victim and family.
Victim of rape	Providing for medical treatment and support during the examination.
	Planning for follow-up medical treatment in case of pregnancy, infection, or venereal disease.
	Engaging social supports (e.g., legal aid,), helping victim to plan a way to tell members of support system.
	Providing support and education for the family and friends of the victim.

TABLE 22-6 (continued)

Crisis Event	Intervention
Victim of disaster	Evaluating for homicidal and/or suicidal feelings because of the intense anger and guilt victim commonly feels.
	Providing for medical treatment for any injuries sustained.
	Providing for meeting of basic needs if necessary (i.e., food, shelter, clothing).
	Recognizing that crisis response may be delayed and prolonged due to magnitude of trauma. Frequently there are multiple losses—loss of family members, loss of belongings, and personal injury.

scribed above, there are more specific interventions that may be useful in individual situations. See Table 22-6.

EVALUATION □ Evaluation is the appraisal of the client's response to the nursing interventions. Establishing clear expectations aids the evaluation process.

Anticipatory planning is a part of the evaluation process, offering a means of reinforcing coping mechanisms. This type of planning also helps the client see that a similar approach may be useful should other crises threaten. The client should play an active part in the evaluation phase, just as in other stages of crisis therapy.

Successful resolution of the crisis event is indicated as follows:

1. The client is able to verbalize an understanding of the crisis event and his response to it. He views the experience in a realistic manner.

2. The client can identify coping mechanisms that were helpful to him and can understand how to use them if faced with another crisis.

3. The client may still express regret or sadness that the crisis event occurred, but will no longer have feelings of rage, despair, or bitterness.

4. The client does not describe intense anxiety in relation to the crisis event. Instead, the stresses he feels are only those of normal living and can be managed with his intact coping mechanisms.

Case Study

The case example describes a nurse working in the medical-surgical setting with a client who is experiencing an unanticipated situational crisis. Although the interventions are specific to this case, the nurse will be able to use this discussion as a basis for dealing with clients in a variety of settings experiencing a variety of crisis events.

Mrs. Martin, 36 years old, was seen in consultation at a general hospital. She had been admitted to the hospital for surgery after a breast mass had been noted. The nursing staff and her physician were concerned because she was very agitated, and related to the staff in an angry and demanding way. She was constantly using her call light, and when the nurse would arrive at her room, she would express anger that the nurse was slow in responding or that the nurse had not

done what she wanted. Mrs. Martin expressed fears of being "full of cancer" and would state that she knew this was why she wasn't getting good care in the hospital. The nurses were angry and frustrated, as they felt they were giving Mrs. Martin good care.

Assessment, Problem Identification and Intervention

The first visit with Mrs. Martin was spent in obtaining both information from the chart and from the client herself. It became clear that her behavior was unusual and began with her admission to the hospital. Mrs. Martin described her anxiety

(continued)

when the mass was first discovered, but had become increasingly upset when she was admitted to the hospital. Based on information that indicated her behavior had changed radically with the failure of her coping mechanisms as a result of her hospitalization, the nurse decided that Mrs. Martin was experiencing a crisis and would benefit from crisis therapy.

During the initial visit, the nurse encouraged Mrs. Martin to talk about her feelings and thoughts regarding the lump and the impending surgery. Mrs. Martin described her feeling of terror, she "knew" that the lump indicated that she was going to die from cancer. (Nsg. Dx.: Ineffective coping due to anxiety resulting from inadequate information.) In addition, Mrs. Martin expressed fears about her husband's reaction to the discovery of the lump. She stated, "Even if I don't die, I probably will have to have my breast removed. He won't want to live with half a woman." (Nsg. Dx.: Ineffective personal coping as a result of a threat to the body image.) Although she and her husband had had a supportive and close relationship with each other in the past, Mrs. Martin began to distance herself from him by criticizing his efforts to reassure her. She let him know his frequent visits were unnecessary and that he should keep himself busy with his job. (Nsg. Dx.: Disruption of family communication patterns as a result of anxiety and withdrawing behavior.)

Mrs. Martin indicated a desire to work with the nurse. They agreed to meet on a regular basis while Mrs. Martin was in the hospital, with one follow-up visit after her discharge. The focus of their meetings was clarified by identifying goals based on the nursing diagnosis. The goals also were based on what Mrs. Martin specified she wanted to change. For example, she was aware of, and felt bad about, the distancing behavior with her husband. She stated, "I really want him to be here. I don't understand why I get so angry when he comes." They discussed how her lashing out at others might be a way of expressing her anger and fear about the breast mass.

The nurse returned later in the day to meet with Mrs. Martin and her husband. She encouraged both Mr. and Mrs. Martin to talk about what it would mean to them if they learned that the lump was malignant and a mastectomy was required. In the discussion, Mr. Martin was able to remain supportive to his wife, while recognizing both the threat the lump posed to her and her fear that he might want to leave her.

With only minimal support, Mrs. Martin was able to verbalize the feelings and beliefs that motivated her ineffective coping behavior. It became clear that one of her strengths was her ability to express feelings when given the opportunity and encouragement to do so. The nurse was then able to explore them with her, gaining a more realistic perception of the possible outcomes of the surgery. In addition, Mrs. Martin began to talk with the nursing staff about her fears and concerns, rather than lashing out and distancing herself from them.

During the hospitalization, the mass was found to be malignant and a mastectomy was performed. Mrs. Martin expressed many angry and confused feelings about the outcome. She voiced, "Why me? What have I ever done?" She felt the cancer was a punishment that was "uncalled for." (Nsg. Dx.: Ineffective coping as a result of anxiety in response to threatened self-esteem.) Viewing the occurrence of a crisis event as punishment, or feeling consumed with guilt, are common reactions among clients experiencing a crisis.

The nurse worked actively to help Mrs. Martin define the problem as an illness rather than as something she had willfully brought on herself. This was done by exploring ways in which she believed she had caused the illness (e.g., "I never did eat right. . . . I should have had more check-ups") and by reality testing these beliefs with her. The nurse frequently encouraged her to express her anger and guilt feelings, conveying a message that these feelings are a normal response to loss.

As Mrs. Martin was able to problem-solve more effectively and begin to plan for her own care, she began to make changes in her daily schedule to allow time for adequate rest to facilitate her recovery. She also was able to talk about her negative feelings rather than acting them out in an inappropriate manner. She joined a group of mastectomy clients who helped her adjust to the life-style changes and body image changes that occur after a breast removal.

Evaluation

Mrs. Martin was able to resolve the crisis and to begin functioning in a manner that allowed her to plan for her care and receive support from her husband. She also verbalized a realistic perception of the event, recognizing that some feelings and events occur even though she could not find reasons or causes for them. Part of the evaluation process was to help Mrs. Martin identify which coping mechanisms were most useful to her, so that she might use them in the event of a future crisis.

☐ *Alternative Crisis Intervention Services*

The structure in which crisis therapy is done can vary. As each of these forms of treatment is discussed, the nurse is reminded that the interventions already covered are applicable to each of these settings.

INDIVIDUAL COUNSELING

As the term states, this service is directed to one person and engages his available support system. The actual treatment may be based on either generic or individual theory. The case example was of individual counseling.

CRISIS GROUPS

A group therapy structure is employed. The group may be ongoing, with clients contracting for a period of time; this results in a constant change in the group population. Another style is for the population to remain constant, with the group as a whole contracting for a period of time. The group format usually employed is generic crisis counseling. Members are selected because they all are experiencing a common crisis (e.g., rape victim groups, mastectomy groups, retirement planning groups, and premarital groups).

FAMILY CRISIS COUNSELING

The focus is on the entire family when the crisis event is seen to be shared by all members. The death of a family member, the birth of a child, and a natural disaster are typical events that may involve the family.

TELEPHONE CRISIS LINES

The use of "hot lines" at crisis centers has become an increasingly popular means of crisis intervention. The ability to provide immediate intervention is believed to be effective. This is not the treatment of choice for the entire crisis period, but is effective at the start of crisis work. Referrals for follow-up treatment are an important service offered, as is the initial intervention.

Regardless of the form of crisis therapy used by the nurse, it is important for her to keep in mind that the client is experiencing a transition and is susceptible to change. During the crisis the nurse can have a significant impact on the client's coping abilities in the current crisis and in future difficult periods. This treatment requires quick and decisive action by the nurse, hence creativity and flexibility in approach are necessary.

■ Enrichment Activities

DISCUSSION QUESTIONS

1. Explore your definition of crisis, talking about the factors that cause a crisis.

2. Discuss the differences/similarities of the developmental and situational crises.

3. Discuss how crisis intervention compares to the nursing process and how it is effective as a means of treatment.

4. Discuss the grief response in relation to crisis theory.

5. Discuss the crisis sequence, identifying important client behavior in each sequence.

LEARNING ACTIVITIES

1. Identify common crisis events according to the developmental stage of your client. Develop a plan with the client based on primary or secondary prevention, according to his present need.

2. Identify a recent crisis event that you have experienced. What coping mechanisms did you use?

3. Develop a plan of primary prevention appropriate to the community in which you live. Attempt to include nontraditional health-care providers.

4. Identify primary, secondary, and tertiary programs presently operating in your community.

5. Role-play a crisis call and evaluate the responses identifying the problem, interventions, and the rationale for the intervention.

■ Recommended Readings

Aguilera, D., and Messick, J. *Crisis intervention: Theory and methodology.* St. Louis: Mosby Company, 1982. Good basic text, easily read, that covers a variety of crisis events and applies crisis interventions in an understandable way. In addition, compares crisis therapy with other forms of treatment.

Burgess, A., and Baldwin, B. *Crisis intervention theory and practice: A clinical handbook.* Englewood Cliffs, NJ: Prentice-Hall, 1981. Includes a typology of crisis as well as treatment strategies for each. Is easy to read and understand. Good handbook for anyone in the mental health field, as well as the client himself.

Golan, N. *Passing through transitions: A guide for the practitioners.* New York: Free Press, 1981. Gives a complete discussion of the developmental transitions that occur throughout the life span. In addition, covers some common situational crises that occur during these developmental stages. Offers therapeutic strategies. Includes case examples to integrate theory.

Johnson, E., and Williamson, J. *Growing old: The social problems of aging.* New York: Holt, Rinehart, & Winston, 1980. Discusses the adjustments and tasks faced by the elderly client. Explores the support system and the environmental factors influencing individual coping. Losses occurring during this life period are discussed. Good book for increasing the understanding by the nurse of the problems and resources of the elderly population.

■ *References*

Aguilera, D., and Messick, J. *Crisis intervention: Theory and methodology.* 4th ed. St. Louis: Mosby Company, 1982.

Bassuk, E., and Apsler, R. Are there sex biases in rape counseling? *American journal of psychiatry,* 140, 1983:305–308.

Bassuk, E., and Gerson, S. Chronic crisis patients: A discrete clinical group. *American journal of psychiatry,* 137, 1980:1513–1517.

Bassuk, E.; Menden, S.; and Apsler, R. Geriatric emergencies: Psychiatric or medical? *American journal of psychiatry,* 140, 1983:539–542.

Braulin, J.; Rook, J.; and Sills, G. Families in crisis: The impact of trauma. *Critical care quarterly,* 5, 1982:38–46.

Caplan, G. *An approach to community mental health.* New York: Grune & Stratton, 1961.

———. *Principles of Preventive Psychiatry.* New York, Basic Books, 1965.

Colton, P.; Drake, R.; Whitaker, A.; and Potter, J. Dealing with suicide on a psychiatric inpatient unit. *Hospital and community psychiatry,* 34, 1983:55–59.

Dixon, S., and Sands, R. Identity and the experience of crisis. *Social casework,* 64, 1983:223–230.

Erikson, E. *Childhood and society.* New York: Norton, 1963.

Faria, G. Toward a clarification of role loss. *Social casework,* 64, 1983:26–32.

Ferraro, K., and Johnson, J. How women experience battering: The process of victimization. *Social problems,* 30, 1983:325–339.

Golan, N. Using situational crisis to ease transitions in the life cycle. *American journal of orthopsychiatry,* 50, 1980:542–550.

Hagen, D. The relationship between job loss and physical and mental illness. *Hospital and community psychiatry,* 34, 1983:438–441.

Hart, C. Psychiatric mental health nursing consultation: A two model system in a general hospital. *Issues in mental health nursing,* 4, 1982:127–147.

Hatton, C., and Valente, S. Bereavement group for parents who suffered a suicidal loss of a child. *Suicide and life threatening behavior,* 11, 1981:141–156.

Hension, J. Strategies for suicide intervention by telephone. *Suicide and life threatening behavior,* 12, 1982:176–184.

Lindemann, E. *Beyond grief: Studies in crisis intervention.* New York: Jason Aronson, 1979.

McEvoy, Q.; Brookings, J.; and Brown, C. Responses to battered women: Problems and strategies. *Social casework,* 64, 1983:92–96.

Moynihan, B., and Duncan, J. The role of the nurse in the care of the sexual assault victims. *Nursing clinics of North America,* 16, 1981:95–100.

Philips, I. Opportunities for prevention in the practice of psychiatry. *American journal of psychiatry,* 140, 1983:389–395.

Ressler, R. K.; Burgess, A.; and Douglas, J. Rape and rape-murder: One offender and twelve victims. *The American journal of psychiatry,* 140, 1983:36–40.

Sheehy, G. *Passages: Predictable crises of adult life.* New York: E.P. Dutton, 1976.

Terr, L. Time sense following psychic trauma: A clinical study of ten adults and twenty children. *American journal of orthopsychiatry,* 53, 1983:244–261.

Thurnher, M. Turning points and developmental change: Subjective and objective assessments. *American journal of orthopsychiatry,* 53, 1983:52–60.

Weick, A. A growth-task model of human development. *Social casework.* 64, 1983:134–137.

Zusman, J. Psychiatric and mental health services in disaster relief. *Topics in emergency medicine,* 4, 1983:57–65.

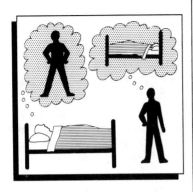

23

Mind-Body Relationships

Geraldine Renschler Newton

Learning Objectives

Upon completion of this chapter, the reader will be able to:

1. Discuss major theoretical concepts related to mind-body relationships.

2. Identify assessment factors related to the client's physical condition, psychosocial status and belief systems.

3. Identify assessment factors in the client's environment, including family dynamics, cultural factors, and conditions at home, work, and in the hospital setting.

4. Describe characteristics of the nurse that might interfere with nursing care and discuss appropriate interventions.

5. Analyze assessment data and formulate nursing diagnoses.

6. Discuss interventions at the primary, secondary, and tertiary levels.

7. Discuss self-regulation techniques.

8. Discuss evaluation of interventions at all levels of prevention.

Although there has been an awareness of mind-body relationships over the centuries, the greatest advances in understanding have occurred in the twentieth century. The broad and complex field of psychosomatic medicine is changing and growing rapidly since the mid-1970s after two decades of struggle for survival. As many as 50 percent of clients are being treated for illnesses with mixed physiologic and emotional components. Nurses have access to this population in all settings and age groups and therefore need to understand the psychosocial dimensions of health and illness, develop skills in applying the nursing process with this group, and become familiar with strategies that can be used to modify the effects of stress in themselves and others.

Various terms have been used to describe mind-body interactions. *Psychosomatic* was first used in 1818 by Johann Christian Heinroth, a German psychiatrist. Later the term *somato-psychic* was introduced to describe the physical illnesses that contributed to psychological disturbances. *Psychophysiologic* appeared in the first and second editions of the *Diagnostic and Statistical Manual of Mental Disorders*. It was used to classify conditions with physical symptoms caused by emotional factors and involving a single organ system, usually under control of the autonomic nervous system. Specifically included were psychiatric disorders with somatic symptoms, physical disorders with reactive psychological disturbances such as depression or anxiety accompanying a chronic illness, and the classic psychophysiologic disorders as discussed in the section on specificity theory. The most recent classification (DSM-III, 1980) is *psychologic factors affecting physical condition*. It includes all of the criteria applied to "psychophysiologic" as well as any physical condition in which psychological factors are significant in either initiation or exacerbation. In the present chapter, the term *psychosomatic* is used in the interest of tradition and brevity, with the understanding that it includes the broad definition given in DSM-III.

The purpose of this chapter is to provide a broad overview of mind-body relationships so that the student will be equipped to apply its general concepts to specific situations. The major focus is on the psychological factors contributing to health and illness within a holistic framework. Other aspects of the topic such as coping with acute and chronic illness, loss, and anxiety are discussed in detail in other chapters.

☐ *Theory*

Ancient philosophers and physicians such as Socrates, Hippocrates, and Galen discussed mind-body relationships in their writings. Scientific thought did not become significant in medicine until the end of the nineteenth century. By that time psychiatry existed as a discrete entity but was alienated from the practice of medicine. The scientific foundations of psychosomatic medicine were laid in the early twentieth century with the contributions of Freud, Pavlov, and Cannon. Freud developed a scientific approach to personality and introduced the phenomenon of the unconscious. Pavlov discovered the conditioned reflex. Cannon identified the fight-or-flight reaction and the concept of homeostasis. The psychosomatic movement, which began in Germany and Austria in the 1920s and in the United States in the 1930s, proceeded along two paths, one psychiatric and mainly psychoanalytic, the other psychophysiologic.

SPECIFICITY THEORY

The 1930s were the setting for specificity theorists Flanders Dunbar and Franz Alexander. Dunbar identified specific personality profiles associated with specific illnesses: for example, Type A behavior associated with coronary heart disease as identified by Friedman and Rosenman (1974). The person is characterized by a sense of time urgency or "hurry sickness," an obsession with numbers, ceaseless striving for achievement, and aggressiveness and hostility expressed in a tendency to compete with and challenge other people. Alexander proposed that specific unresolved, unconscious conflicts were the cause of specific somatic disorders. For example, the person with essential hypertension was identified as having a conflict between expressing hostility and losing the affection of others. A lack of assertiveness is the defense developed to control the hostile impulses. Resentment increases when the person cannot reach his goals because of his passive attitude; then greater control of aggressive feelings is needed. This vicious circle results in chronic tension and eventually in illness. Similar dynamics were proposed for other classic psychosomatic disorders, namely, bronchial asthma, ulcerative colitis, thyrotoxicosis, rheumatoid arthritis, neurodermatitis, and duodenal peptic ulcer.

Alexander also included inherited or early acquired constitutional vulnerability and a precipitating life situation as necessary to the manifestation of disease. Although significant progress was made by these studies, they did not investigate the intervening psychophysiologic mechanisms, and psychotherapy was not always sufficient to alter the course of illness. Consequently, by 1955 the concept had lost its appeal and over the next two decades the whole field of psychosomatic medicine lacked credibility.

GENERALITY THEORIES

The generality theories propose that many factors contribute to illness. Specific attention is given to the individual's susceptibility to illness, physiologic mechanisms, and conscious variables such as conscious emotions, thought processes, and social and environmental conditions. These theories were formulated during the period from 1940 to 1960 which was also characterized by an emphasis on research in neuroanatomy, neurophysiology, and neuroendocrinology.

Stress theory was one of the major developments of the period. The term *stress* was first used in its current meaning in the 1940s, although Cannon had used it earlier in describing his studies of the fight-or-flight response. From Hans Selye's extensive research (1956) with laboratory animals came the definition of physiologic stress as the "nonspecific response of the body to any demand made upon it" or "the wear and tear exerted upon the body" (1965) and the General Adaptation Syndrome (GAS) and its relationship to morbidity and mortality.

The GAS consists of three phases of physiologic adaptation: alarm, resistance, and exhaustion. The organism responds to a stimulus through the alarm and resistance stages and, depending on the force and duration of the stressor and the resources of the organism, tissue damage may or may not occur. The body's tendency to return to a steady state or balance in known as *homeostasis*. If this does not occur, exhaustion, characterized by illness and finally death, ensues. *Stressors* may be pleasant or unpleasant, internal or external, physiologic or psychosocial (Selye, 1974). The degree of adaptation required by an event can be measured by the Social Readjustment Rating Scale (SRRS). Stressors identified as "life change events" by Holmes and Rahe (1967)

are shown in Table 23-1. Each value point assigned to a life event item is called a life change unit (LCU) and is intended as a measure of adjustment. The higher the LCU score the greater the life crisis (Table 23-2) and the more likely a person is to become ill.

Stress is always present in all organisms and varies in response to stressors; in the broadest sense, it is a constant interaction between individual and environment (Garbin, 1979). The organism's response to its environment, known as adaptation, coping, or self-regulation, varies with each individual and is affected by perceptions, conditioning, and genetic predisposition. Two types of coping have been described: direct action, in which the person prepares to meet a threatening situation, and palliation, which is an attempt to control emotions and physiologic factors so that general function is improved (Lazarus, 1977). The word stress has many meanings. It has been described as an external force or pressure, an internal response, a variable that can or cannot be measured, and a state of the human organism. Selye (1980) has proposed the use of the term *distress* to describe experiences that are unpleasant or disease-producing and *eustress* to describe those that are pleasant or curative. Other authors (Hinkle, 1977; Mason, 1975) have suggested that the word stress has been useful in the past; but with recent knowledge of mind, body, and environment, it is possible and preferable to refer to the interaction of specific variables rather than to the concept of stress.

Other major theorists have expressed other viewpoints. Harold Wolff saw psychosomatic disorders as adaptive biologic responses to symbolic threats and studied the mediating mechanisms between symbolic stimuli and physiologic changes. Reusch interpreted psychosomatic illness as communication at a preverbal level, that is, by means of the autonomic nervous system. Grinker applied a theory of regression in which parts of the organism regress to an earlier stage of development (Wittkower, 1977). Janis (1969), in his work with surgical patients, developed the "work of worrying" concept which emphasizes the use of information and anticipatory fear as constructive elements in preventing emotional and physical complications. Engel (1968) is known for his identification of the "giving up—given up" complex in which the individual feels helpless and hopeless after a significant loss and is thus more susceptible to illness.

TABLE 23-1 Social Readjustment Rating Scale[a]

Number	Life Event Item	Mean Value
1.	Death of spouse	100
2.	Divorce	73
3.	Marital separation from mate	65
4.	Detention in jail or other institution	63
5.	Death of a close family member	63
6.	Major personal injury or illness	53
7.	Marriage	50
8.	Being fired from work	47
9.	Marital reconciliation with mate	45
10.	Retirement from work	45
11.	Major change in health or behavior of a family member	44
12.	Pregnancy	40
13.	Sexual difficulties	39
14.	Gaining a new family member (e.g., through birth, adoption, oldster moving in)	39
15.	Major business readjustment (e.g., merger, reorganization, bankruptcy)	39
16.	Major change in financial state (e.g., a lot worse off or a lot better off than usual)	38
17.	Death of close friend	37
18.	Changing to different line of work	36
19.	Major change in number of arguments with spouse (e.g., either a lot more or a lot less than usual regarding child-rearing, personal habits, etc.)	35
20.	Taking on mortgage greater than $10,000 (e.g., purchasing a home, business)	31
21.	Foreclosure on mortgage or loan	30
22.	Major change in responsibilities at work (e.g., promotion, demotion, lateral transfer)	29
23.	Son or daughter leaving home (e.g., marriage, attending college)	29
24.	In-law troubles	29
25.	Outstanding personal achievement	28
26.	Wife beginning or ceasing work outside the home	26
27.	Beginning or ceasing formal schooling	26
28.	Major change in living conditions (e.g., building new home, remodeling, deterioration of home or neighborhood)	25
29.	Revision of personal habits (dress, manners, associations, etc.)	24
30.	Trouble with boss	23
31.	Major change in working hours or conditions	20
32.	Change in residence	20
33.	Changing to new school	20
34.	Major change in usual type and/or amount of recreation	19
35.	Major change in church activities (e.g., a lot more or a lot less than usual)	19
36.	Major change in social activities (e.g., clubs, dancing, movies, visiting)	18
37.	Taking on mortgage or loan less than $10,000 (e.g., purchasing a car, TV, freezer)	17
38.	Major change in sleeping habits (a lot more or a lot less food intake, or very different meal hours or surroundings)	16
39.	Major change in number of family get-togethers (e.g., a lot more or a lot less than usual)	15
40.	Major change in eating habits (a lot more or a lot less food intake, or very different meal hours or surroundings)	15
41.	Vacation	13
42.	Christmas	12
43.	Minor violation of law (e.g., traffic tickets, jaywalking, disturbing the peace)	11

[a] Williams, C.C., and Holmes, T.H. Life change, human adaptation, and onset of illness. In Longo, D.C., and Williams, R.A., *Clinical Practice in Psychosocial Nursing: Assessment and Intervention.* New York: Appleton-Century-Crofts, 1978, p. 72. Printed with permission.

TABLE 23-2 Life Crisis Categories and Life Change Unit (LCU) Scores[a]

Category of Life Crisis	LCU Score
No life crisis	0–149
Mild life crisis	150–199
Moderate life crisis	200–299
Major life crisis	300 or more

[a] The LCU score includes those life event items experienced during a 1-year period. Williams, C.C., and Holmes, T.H. Life change, human adaptation, and onset of illness. In Longo, D.C., and Williams, R.A., *Clinical Practice in Psychosocial Nursing: Assessment and Intervention*, 1978, New York: Appleton-Century-Crofts, p. 76. Printed with permission.

HOLISTIC THEORY

The holistic view is a logical expansion of generality theories. It emphasizes the social and cultural environment in addition to biological and psychological factors. For example, family functioning, working conditions, urbanization, poverty, crowding, migration, and life-styles are being studied in relationship to health. Religion and spirituality are other factors in the holistic approach. Slater (1981) suggests that religion has the potential for healing and for influencing a cultural shift away from materialism, aggressiveness, and competitiveness which are known to affect health. Spirituality, defined as a person's basic assumptions about life and what makes it worthwhile, will contribute to illness in the presence of conflicting values, beliefs, or goals (Tubesing, 1980). Lipowski (1977) describes the holistic view as affirming the uniqueness, complexity, and the general systems view of human beings as well as the doctrine of the multicausality of all disease. It demands an interdisciplinary approach.

■ **Point of Emphasis**

Holistic theory proposes the multicausality of all disease, that is, social, cultural, biological, psychological, and spiritual determinants.

Current theories, practice, and research are based on two assumptions (Lipowski, 1977), the first being that symbolic activity (i.e., conscious and unconscious perceptions, thoughts, memories, imagery, and fantasies) affects all levels of functioning, including the cellular level via the nervous system. It is believed that stress increases an organism's vulnerability to certain diseases by producing an immunosuppressive effect (Rogers, et al., 1979). Also, social and biological functions, through the nervous system, affect symbolic activity. For example, the presence of pain will influence a client's thoughts and fantasies. These assumptions are represented in Reiser's Bio-psycho-social field model (Figure 23-1), which illustrates the relationships of various functions according to the holistic view. An example of this assumption as applied to cancer appears in Figure 23-2. The second assumption is that each individual has specific patterns of cognitive, emotional, behavioral, and physiologic reactions to specific stimuli. These factors influence which life situations and changes are most likely to result in a particular illness. Some of the responses are genetic and some are learned, and many can be modified with treatment or self-regulation.

PSYCHOLOGICAL FACTORS AFFECTING PHYSICAL CONDITION

It follows that if the holistic view is accepted there will be no "psychosomatic disorders." Rather, the focus will be on the major chronic diseases and the associated psychological factors occurring in

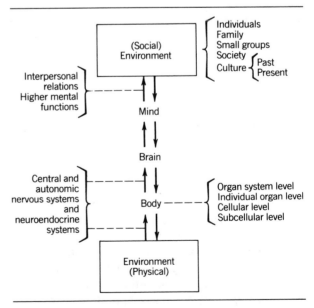

Figure 23-1 *The biopsychosocial field (From: "Theoretical Concepts in Psychosomatic Medicine" by Morton F. Reiser in American Handbook of Psychiatry, Second Edition, Volume 4, edited by Silvano Arieti and Morton F. Reiser. Copyright (c)1975 by Basic Books. By permission of Basic Books, Inc., Publishers, New York.)*

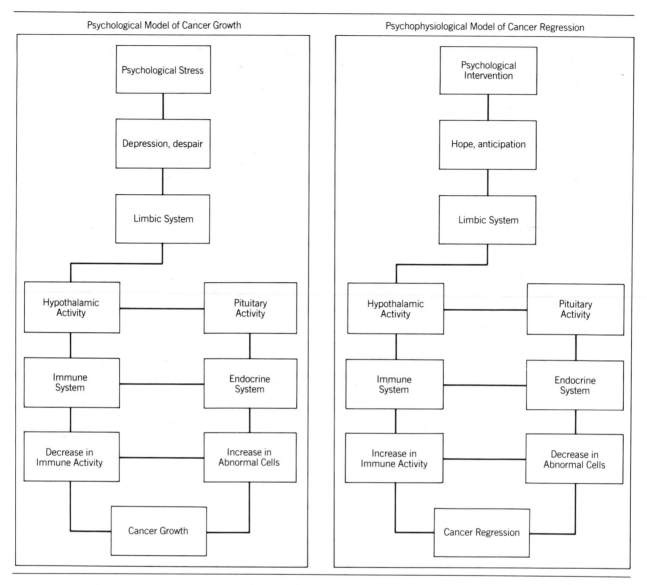

Psychological Model of Cancer Growth   Psychophysiological Model of Cancer Regression

Figure 23-2 *Psychophysiological model of cancer growth and regression. Reprinted with permission from Archterberg, J., Simonton, O.C., and Matthews-Simonton, S., Stress, Psychological Factors and Cancer. Fort Worth, Texas: New Medicine, 1976:6–7.*

the development, course, and outcome of all disease. This supports the development of a psychosomatic approach to the explanation of illness (Weiss, 1977) and to the reduction of disability and premature death. Psychological factors associated with selected conditions are listed in Table 23-3. Although certain psychosocial factors have frequently been associated with certain physical conditions, the relationships have not been established as fact and no general theory of etiology and pathogenesis has been accepted. The complexity of illness and of the human organism demands continued investigation.

Most research in psychological factors affecting physical condition was done before or during the 1950s; retrospective and case study approaches were used. In a prospective study begun in 1946, Thomas and Duszynski (1974) found that medical students who later committed suicide, were psychologically disturbed, or developed malignant tumors reported less closeness to parents in early life and more pathological content (as demonstrated in the Rorschach test) than the control group. The personality configuration consisted of denial and repression, self-containment, rigidity, and a strong commitment to social

TABLE 23-3 *Psychological Factors in Selected Conditions*

Condition	Factor
Hayfever	Feels helpless, overwhelmed
Bronchial asthma	Feels helpless and "shut out"; maternal narcissism and domination; object loss and threat of loss
Emphysema	After disease has developed, normal emotional expression is beyond maximum physiological capacity
Tuberculosis	Occurs in setting of high life change; prognosis better with higher coping ability; susceptible when sensitive, anxious, emotionally labile; strong dependency and affectional needs
Coronary artery disease	Significant loss, multiple life changes, overwork, job dissatisfaction, upward mobility, outwardly controlled, loneliness
Myocardial infarction	Occurs after sustained activity followed by sudden let-down
Essential hypertension	Feels threatened and has to be ready for "anything"; inability to handle aggressive and hostile impulses; object loss
Stroke	Feels lack of control of life and environment and failure to meet own expectations; usually a period of sustained and relatively severe emotional disturbance often intensified before onset
Migraine headache	Occurs after sustained period of high activity followed by sudden let-down; rigid, perfectionistic, ambitious
Lower back pain	Feels need to run away but must stay
Tension headache	Occurs during periods of increased psychological tension
Rheumatoid arthritis	Object loss; self-sacrificing, overconscientious, unable to show hostility; extremely dependent on maternal figure; shyness and social inadequacy in juveniles, life change units during year prior to onset more than twice those of controls
Duodenal ulcer	Object loss; feeling of being deprived; once present, any stimulus that increases secretion (anger, anxiety, euphoria) may produce pain or bleeding
Ulcerative colitis	Feels injured and degraded and would like to get rid of responsible agent; would like situation to be finished; sustained feelings of rage, resentment, and anger might produce condition; object loss; obsessive-compulsive personality
Obesity	Conditioning in the mother-child relationship; no specific personality profile; overeating when upset; difficulty identifying hunger and satiety (strong need for external control); overeating due to fear of hunger; associates bigness with strength, power, and sexual potency (males) and fertility, "giving," and evidence that spouse can provide for her (females)
Anorexia nervosa	Precipitated by traumatic events (separation, bodily changes of puberty, sexual experiences and failures); being in control of one's body and one's life is basic issue
Hyperthyroidism	Inability to handle aggressive and hostile impulses; psychosexual insecurity; overcompensating self-sufficiency, ambition, striving for independence

(continued)

TABLE 23-3 (continued)

Condition	Factor
Diabetes mellitus	Onset with or soon after emotional disturbance associated with significant persons or situations; passive, dependent
Addison's disease	Depression, apathy, negativism, irritability, suspiciousness, agitation
Cushing's syndrome	Depression with anxiety or retardation
Cancer	Early experiences of depletion and loss reawakened by later losses and depression; loss of significant relationship several months to 2 years prior to diagnosis; pre-neoplastic feelings of hopelessness, helplessness, and despair; chronic underlying feelings of emptiness, resentment; selfless and undemanding, easy to please and unaggressive; pattern of self-sacrifice, patience, self-effacement, self-containment, inhibition, rigidity, repression, regression
Leukemia	Loss of a significant person (children and adults)
Epilepsy	Seizures precipitated by emotional stress (especially temporal lobe epilepsy)
Multiple sclerosis	Psychic disturbances contribute to problems in differential diagnosis; may be expression of cortical disintegration and reintegration at lower level in response to psychogenic or organic trauma; loss
Dysmenorrhea	Attitudes of hopelessness, self-abnegation, self-sacrifice; repressed fear, guilt, conflicts
Amenorrhea	Response to stressful experiences (physical danger, object loss)
Fertility problems	Stress may induce spasms of smooth muscle
Obstetric complications	Higher anxiety levels and use of fewer repressive defenses
Menopause	Fears (sexuality, aging)
Impotence (male)	Conflicts due to fears, anxiety, anger, or inexperience
Pruritus (generalized)	Guilt, anger, boredom, irritation
Chronic urticaria	Excessively compliant or demanding and vindictive; anger in response to loss
Atopic dermatitis (neurodermatitis)	Response to loss of love; submissive, helpless, and docile, or ambitious and provocative; decreased self-confidence affects work and social life
Allergies	Life change and stress precede onset of episodes
Pain	May be a nonverbal message to important individuals or a communication for help; develops in certain periods and settings (e.g., with real or fantasized loss); exacerbated by anxiety or depression; diversion of attention can modify response; tolerance influenced by psychological state; somatic preoccupations and reactive depression associated with chronic and psychogenic pain; pain complaints related to cultural and extroversive factors and degree of extroversion and neuroticism

norms. Schwab and Traven (1979) found that in a 3-year period the risk of developing psychosomatic symptoms and conditions was significantly higher in persons of lower socioeconomic status, suggesting that environmental conditions may be a contributing factor. Another group (Bartrop, et al., 1977) found that T-cell lymphocytic function was significantly depressed after bereavement, indicating that grief might be a triggering factor for latent disease. The effect of hypnosis on the immune system was described in another study (Hall, 1982). Lymphocyte counts were significantly increased on two measures at 1 hour and 1 week after hypnosis of 20 well subjects in a laboratory setting. Split-brain research (Sperry, 1976) reinforces the holistic view of psychosomatic medicine. The right side of the brain has been identified as a center of subjective consciousness which may very likely be a higher force in the brain than that which directs physiologic activities. Perception, imagery, emotion, cognition, values, and insight are functions of the right brain. In the past, these phenomena of the mind had not been identified with the physical brain and skepticism about their validity was always present. Also, because the right side of the brain is activated in meditative states, many of the self-regulation activities such as hypnosis, meditation, and biofeedback are supported by these research findings. The trend in research is to focus on conscious emotions and cognitive processes and their relationship to physiological processes.

☐ Nursing Process

ASSESSMENT ☐

The Client ☐ When providing nursing care in the hospital or the community for a client in whom psychological factors are affecting his physical condition, a physiological assessment is of primary importance. The assessment should include a healthy history, examination of the basic systems, and information on the client's health behaviors (Simmons, 1980), such as nutrition, sleep and rest, physical activity, personal hygiene, substance misuse, therapeutic regimen, noncompliance, and difficulties with technical procedures related to the condition. Information from the medical examination, treatment plan, and other therapists (physical, speech, occupational, respi-

ratory) will be part of the data base.

A thorough psychosocial assessment (as presented in Chapter 10) is equally important. This will include the patient's affect and behavior, perception of the problem, peer and family relationships, significant life events, coping patterns, support systems, leisure activities, cultural background, and values. If a psychiatric diagnosis such as depression or anxiety has been established, that should be assessed for level of severity. More specific for a psychosomatic condition would be an assessment of the level of stress. For example, the Holmes-Rahe Social Readjustment Rating Scale (Table 23-1 and 2) will help determine if the client is experiencing a life crisis and to what degree. Levels of anxiety and depression (discussed in other chapters) are indicators of stress. Other factors are evidence of long-term dissatisfaction or conflict, balance or imbalance in life-style, and flexibility. For example, the "workaholic," lacking in play and exercise, is often susceptible to illness. Use of defense mechanisms can promote optimal physical and psychosocial functioning. For example, clients experiencing cardiac and respiratory distress need the mechanisms of suppression, withdrawal, and repression to conserve oxygen. Even those mechanisms that do not appear to be constructive should not be confronted except in a long-term psychotherapeutic relationship. Further, coping abilities can be assessed in terms of cognitive and affective responses, the cognitive usually being more effective. Similarly, long-term coping mechanisms are usually more effective than short-term ones (Table 23-4).

■ Point of Emphasis

The most effective coping methods are those that involve thought rather than emotional processes and those that extend over a period of time rather than those that are limited to an immediate reaction.

Another area of assessment is that of belief systems. Influenced by culture and religion, people have certain beliefs about themselves, health and illness, the health care system, and the effectiveness of various prescribed treatments. Behavior is determined by the subjective perceptions of the client rather than by the objective environment. An assessment of belief systems includes client readiness to act in the interest of his health,

TABLE 23-4 Coping Methods[a]

Short-Term Methods	Long-Term Methods
I use alcoholic beverages.	I talk it out with others (friend, relative, or professional).
I daydream.	
I try to see the humorous aspects of the situation.	I try to find out more about the situation.
I don't worry about it. Everything will probably work out fine.	I believe in a supernatural power who cares about me.
I sleep more.	I work it off by physical exercise.
I use food and food substitutes (smoking, chewing gum, eating more).	I take some definite action on the basis of my present understanding.
I get prepared to expect the worst.	I draw on my past experiences.
I curse.	I make several alternate plans for handling the situation.
I use drugs.	
I become involved in other activities to keep my mind off the problem.	
I cry.	

[a] Copyright © 1977, American Journal of Nursing Company. Reprinted from *Nursing Research*, March–April, Vol. 26, No. 2.

his perception of his susceptibility to the physical condition and of its severity, and the perceived benefits and costs of preventive action or treatment (Mikhail, 1981).

The effect of placebos is evidence of the power of beliefs. Although the placebo is commonly defined as the inactive substance used in control studies of drugs, the effect is also the result of the doctor-patient relationship, life-style changes, and the client's determination to get well (Cousins, 1981). One study found the placebo to be 55 percent as effective as the medication with which it was compared regardless of the power of the medication (Evans, 1974) (e.g., whether it was aspirin or morphine). It is also necessary to distinguish wish from belief (Werner-Beland, 1980). For example, a client may wish to be well but may believe that the family would be better off without him. This may help to explain the discrepancy between what clients say about recovery and their apparently contradictory behavior. Beliefs can affect behavior, but may also affect the organism physiologically at the cellular level (Simonton, et al., 1980). To add to the complexity of belief systems, there is evidence that they are altered only with extreme difficulty (Rokeach, 1968), usually only under conditions very threatening to a person's physical or mental well-being.

A characteristic identified recently in some clients is alexithymia. They "have a marked difficulty in expressing feelings in words, and . . . do not have fantasies appropriate to or expressive of

feelings, their thought content being dominated by the details of the events in their external environment" (Nemiah, 1977:199). The will to live or "predilection to death" (Hutschnecker, 1977; Weisman and Hackett, 1961) also has been identified as a factor in the likelihood of recovery from serious illness. Feelings and attitudes about illness are other areas for assessment and are discussed in Chapters 25 and 26. Psychological factors may be associated with specific conditions although it is often unknown whether they are contributing to, concomitant of, or a response to illness.

Environment □ One of the most important factors in a person's environment is the family, which may include others who have a strong emotional relationship to the individual. The social groups with which a person is identified, including the family, may be the most powerful influence toward normal development and more rapid recovery from illness. Therefore, an assessment of family dynamics is necessary. Guidelines for a general assessment are found in Chapter 12. In their studies of families a member of which has a psychosomatic illness in which at least one child had diabetes, asthma, or anorexia nervosa, Minuchin, et al. (1978:33) identified five characteristics of family functioning that are significant when clustered (i.e., one alone is not significant). Although some of these characteristics are found in normal families, they are not clustered; also,

2. Overprotectiveness. Members overly concerned for each other; hypersensitive to tension and conflict; children's personal and social development inhibited; children feel great responsibility for protecting the family and sick child may use symptoms in response to tension and conflict, thus reinforcing the illness.

3. Rigidity. Members must maintain the status quo; change and growth very difficult; very vulnerable to outside events such as changes in occupation or death of relatives.

4. Low Tolerance for Conflict. Strong religious or ethical code used as rationale for avoiding conflict; problems and conflicts remain unresolved.

5. Child's Involvement in Parental Conflict. Result of parents' inability to resolve conflicts between them: (a) triangulation—child is forced to take side of one parent or the other; (b) parent-child coalition—child has established an alliance with one parent against the other; (c) detouring—parents have coalition but suppress conflicts and unite in protecting or blaming the sick child.

Meissner (1977) has identified other family dynamics. Relationships with the mother are significant in many illnesses, and are characterized by dependency, ambivalence, the threat of loss of the relationship, and maternal projections in which the mother believes her ideas and impulses are those of the child. The influence of the mother on the child is greater than that of the father with regard to attitudes about health and bodily functioning. Increased tension in the marriage may contribute to exacerbations of illness in any family member. It is suggested that a relatively infantile personality organization is often present in the form of inadequacy as well as hyperadequacy, and this is seen in family interactions, for

Beyond the family interactions, the nurse must assess other areas of influence. The community health nurse might be a good resource at this point. What conditions exist in the client's home with regard to finances, personal space, noise, temperature, sanitation, light, safety, lifestyle, and the neighborhood? Similarly, working conditions could be a source of distress, for example, relationships with peers, supervisors, or subordinates; overwork, too much responsibility, or no opportunity to use one's potential; no participation in planning; "burn out," depression, and safety. Cultural factors must also be considered. Persons of certain races or other minority status often are disadvantaged socially and economically, and frequently traditions, religious practices, and value systems interfere with optimum physical and mental health. Urbanization, migration, and rapidly changing life-styles are also significant factors. If the client is hospitalized the treatment setting is also significant and needs to be assessed for disturbances related to noise, light, temperature, and relationships with members of the health care team.

Nurse □ During the assessment of the client and the environment there is a need for awareness of the effect of such information on the nurse and the planning and implementing of interventions. What are her thoughts, feelings, values, and behaviors? In many cases the client has a severe illness or overwhelming socioeconomic problems, and may be noncompliant. Nurses' working conditions may also be a source of stress. Studies have reported the presence of stress in nurses in ICU (Weiner and Caldwell, 1981), oncology (McElroy, 1982), and most recently in hospice nursing (Barstow, 1980; Moser and Krikorian, 1982). Moser and Krikorian also measured the satisfaction of hospice nurses. Whatever the nurse's responses to the client are—positive, negative, or indifferent—self-awareness will help her to see whether

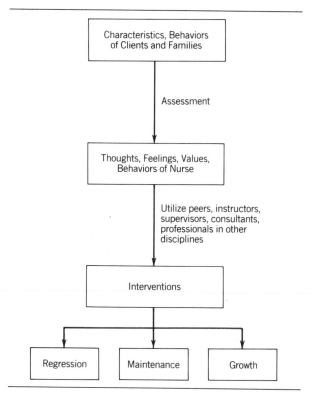

Figure 23-3. *Nurse's response to clients and families.*

nursing care is being blocked or enhanced (Figure 23-3). For example, the degree of frustration and helplessness that the nurse experiences may be an indication of the client's level of depression. Resistance toward authority (the nurse) may be one of the psychological factors accompanying the illness and can then be seen as a symptom or problem worthy of planned intervention rather than a response of anger or withdrawal. Many clients are anxious and/or depressed, and often their lives are in danger. The nurse may feel anxious and overly responsible toward clients who have a life-threatening illness. It is also possible that the nurse might identify with a client because of age, sex, or illness. Illnesses and responses to illness are very complex and require the problem-solving experience of others, such as peers, instructors, supervisors, consultants, as well as professionals in other disciplines. Even though the nurse may identify significant destructive psychodynamic factors, it must be remembered that the client is not aware of them. Therefore the nurse must be supportive rather than confrontational and should refrain from offering explanations of unconscious psychodynamic processes. Similarly, such a thought as "it's all in the person's head" is

obviously a gross misunderstanding and oversimplification of the problem.

■ Point of Emphasis

Psychodynamic factors that might influence illness are usually unconscious and explored only in a long-term psychotherapeutic relationship. The role of the nurse is primarily to offer support rather than to confront or explain psychodynamic processes.

Because of the complexity of illness and the accompanying feelings of helplessness and frustration, there is sometimes a tendency to blame someone. Even though people can take responsibility for their health and illness, many factors remain outside the control of the individual and family; or the adjustment required may be beyond their available resources (e.g., education, finances, and social support). Specific vulnerabilities for individuals cannot yet be predicted. To know that certain conditions (e.g., heart disease, cancer, arthritis, and respiratory diseases such as bronchitis) are known as "afflictions of civilization" (Pelletier, 1977) and are associated with the culture of industrialized countries, will give the nurse less tendency to blame and more appreciation for the complexity of disease and its treatments.

The nurse may also become aware of a discrepancy between what the client has been taught and the behavior she observes, and needs to keep in mind that change is difficult and slow and in some cases may not proceed in the expected direction due to fears, hopelessness, or helplessness. The nurse may have feelings of failure or guilt when the client is not compliant. Perhaps she can relate to the client therapeutically but finds that the family arouses feelings of anger or frustration. Again, the family may be feeling helpless and reacting to loss, and needs to become part of the nursing care plan.

In the face of such obstacles, what can the nurse do to remain an effective, mentally healthy caregiver? It is beneficial to utilize the expertise of other nurses and members of other disciplines for problem solving and as a professional support system within the treatment setting. Staff support groups have been instituted in many settings, for example, oncology (Baider and Porath, 1981; Epting, 1981), ICU (Weiner and Caldwell,

1981), and general units (Scully, 1981). Seeking more information about a particular illness and various approaches to treatment through reading or in-service education might be helpful. Because part of nursing is caring, the nurse is often affected by lack of progress, exacerbations, and deaths of clients and needs to allow for personal grieving in these situations. Similarly, she needs to guard against emotional overinvolvement in work. Practicing some of the self-regulation techniques such as relaxation, meditation, and exercise on a regular basis is highly recommended (Hartl, 1979; Donovan, 1981). The intensity of work should be balanced with vacations, leisure activities, and support systems outside the work setting.

PROBLEM IDENTIFICATION ☐ Identification of unmet needs of the client and nursing diagnoses flow from the subjective and objective data gathered from the assessments. The nurse formulates short- and long-term objectives and determines priorities.

From physiologic data, deficits in functioning of the basic systems can be identified including problems related to pain and health behaviors. For example, if a client in pain has a reduced appetite the problems are identified as Comfort, Alteration in: Pain; and Alteration in Nutrition: Nutritional Deficit. If a client reports sleeping difficulties and boredom and is observed to be smoking heavily and remaining in night clothes most of the day, as a depressed person might, the appropriate problems would be Sleep Pattern Disturbance, Diversional Activity Deficit, Coping Ineffective (Individual); and Health Management Deficit: Personal Hygiene. For the client with hypertension who wonders if it is really necessary to take so many pills the problem would be Noncompliance, Potential: Medication.

As a result of the psychosocial assessment, other problems will emerge. The recently diagnosed diabetic client who fears she may have to change jobs because of her diagnosis and also has difficulty concentrating will have the problems of Anticipatory Anxiety (Moderate) and Anxiety, Moderate. The problem of Independence-Dependence Conflict, Unresolved could be applied to a situation in which the husband prefers not to have the wife work outside the home when she desires to do so, or in the area of psychosocial development, (e.g., an adolescent wanting to participate in activities that do not meet with the parents' approval). The socioeconomic disadvantaged sin-

gle parent may have the problems of Self-Esteem Disturbance; Social Isolation; Home Maintenance Management, Impaired; Sexual Dysfunction; and Parenting, Potential Alteration in. The upwardly mobile middle management person with workaholic characteristics, unaware of and unable to express emotions appropriately may have the problems of Health Management Deficit: Overwork; and Coping, Ineffective (Individual). Analysis of data related to stress such as life change events or long-term dissatisfaction might result in Translocation Syndrome; or Coping, Ineffective (Individual). Symptoms of anxiety or depression, when they are associated with chronic illness, might be identified as Anxiety, Mild or Moderate; or Depression, Reactive (Situational). When coping mechanisms and beliefs are assessed the problems of Coping, Ineffective (Individual); and Spiritual Distress might be identified.

Problems related to environment will focus on family dysfunction, deficits in the home, work or treatment settings, and on cultural impediments. Family dynamics often focus on the issue of authority which would be the basis of an Independence-Dependence Conflict, Unresolved problem. Data related to the home such as sanitation and safety would result in a problem of Home Maintenance Management, Impaired (Mild, Moderate, Severe, Potential, Chronic). Work-related conditions which contribute to anxiety, fear, or anger would be Coping, Ineffective (Individual). Fears of known and unknown events which a client experienced in the hospital would be problems of Anticipatory Anxiety (Mild, Moderate, Severe); or Anxiety (Mild, Moderate, Severe) depending on the situation and the observed behavior. Cultural data that might interfere with the client's health are usually related to conflicts in values or beliefs and would be a problem of Spiritual Distress.

INTERVENTIONS AND RATIONALE ☐ As in other professions the relationship between the client and the professional is basic to all interventions. Unless the nurse can convey the attributes of competence, caring, and hope, interventions will be in jeopardy. Effective interventions also require collaboration with other disciplines. The complexities of illness demand the expertise of the entire health care team. Although interventions are presented for the primary, secondary, and tertiary levels of prevention (Table 23-5), many techniques used at the tertiary level can be practiced for primary prevention, and many interventions at the primary level can be practiced at the sec-

TABLE 23-5 *Nursing Interventions for Psychological Factors Affecting Physical Condition*

Level of Prevention and Setting

Primary prevention: hospital, clinic, home, school, community organization

Intervention	Rationale
Promote good prenatal care	Health of mother has effect on health of fetus
Education of parents in child development and effective parenting techniques	Neuroendocrine responses established in early years
Teach appropriate self-regulation techniques to well people at all ages	Tension is a factor in most illnesses and relaxation techniques are beneficial
Educate people about effective coping mechanisms	Coping ability can affect health and illness
Teach effective communication skills, including appropriate expression of emotions	Impaired communication is a factor in many illnesses
Educate about emotionally healthy family relationships	Many illnesses related to dysfunctional families
Teach people to recognize stressors	Some stressors can be controlled by client
Educate people about a balanced life-style	Some illnesses related to excesses in work-related activities

Secondary prevention: hospital, clinic, home, school, industry, screening program

Intervention	Rationale
Recognize physiologic and psychosocial signs and symptoms of illness and refer for medical diagnosis and treatment	Prognosis usually better with early treatment
Utilize crisis intervention skills with client and family	Clients and families often anxious during diagnostic and early treatment phase of illness
Support constructive coping mechanisms and beliefs	Constructive coping and beliefs sometimes affect the course of illness
Monitor environmental stressors in the treatment setting	Stressors often more easily controlled by nurse than client in treatment setting

Tertiary prevention: long-term outpatient in clinic, home, work setting; periodic hospitalization for evaluation and treatment; stress management units, holistic health centers

Intervention	Rationale
Monitor prescribed medical and psychosocial regimen and implement nursing care measures	Accountability of a professional nurse
Refer to community health nurse, social service, health department, county extension service, community mental health center, clergy, and self-help groups for deficits in health behaviors and in home and work settings	Multidisciplinary effort necessary in treatment of long-term illness
Practice therapeutic communication and problem-solving skills with client and family	Discouragement and fatigue often present in clients and families
Develop knowledge of self-regulation techniques	Better able to support client in therapeutic efforts

ondary and tertiary levels. For example, relaxation is effective as a treatment as well as for prevention of illness, and education appropriate at the primary level can be introduced and reinforced during diagnostic and treatment phases.

Primary Prevention □ Interventions at the primary level are concerned with prevention of illness and can be implemented in settings where well people will be affected by the health care system (e.g., hospitals for newborns and mothers, well-child clinics and doctors' offices, homes, schools, community organizations, and legislative bodies). Nurses and other health care professionals are present in these settings officially or as members of the community and can give direct service or act as resource persons. The main emphasis is the promotion of physical and mental health in individuals and families, including a stress reduction approach to living. This could be accomplished through education and reinforcement of strengths. Perhaps more could be done through legislation similar to that in European countries which have legislated mandatory well-child care and protection of children from spanking.

Secondary Prevention □ Secondary prevention focuses on early diagnosis and treatment and occurs in locations where diagnostic procedures are available or screening programs are provided. These can take place in hospitals, clinics and doctors' offices, homes, schools, and industry. Screening and testing are often offered in shopping centers, at health fairs, and through self-assessment questionnaires found in the media. An alert nurse can be a case-finder in any setting. This is also time for utilizing crisis intervention skills to clarify the client's perception of the problem, provide realistic information, and assist the client in identifying alternatives. Also, the course of an illness might be altered if constructive coping mechanisms and beliefs are supported at this time.

Tertiary Prevention □ Interventions at the tertiary level emphasize rehabilitation and prevention of complications, and clients are often seen as long-term outpatients in clinics and doctors' offices, in their homes, or places of employment. Periodically they may be hospitalized for evaluation or treatment and they may be referred to stress management units, holistic health centers, pain centers, psychotherapists, support groups, or self-help groups in order to gain additional coping

skills and support. Nursing interventions are those related to chronic illness with an emphasis on direct service, maintenance of family functioning, and the coordination of multidisciplinary efforts. The nurse must be familiar with the self-regulation techniques in current use so she can be supportive of the client. Most of these techniques are taught by specialists such as psychiatrists, psychologists, physical therapists, and nutritionists or by assistants under their supervision. Some nurses who have the appropriate skills, preparation, and access to consultation (e.g., psychiatric clinical nurse specialists) are providing direct service (Brallier, 1980), but the role of most nurses is to facilitate the referral process and provide support of the client during treatment.

Self-Regulation □ By definition, the client has a great responsibility for the success of these treatments. Participation rather than just being the object of treatment is required and many involve skills learned with practice. Most of these therapeutic modalities are in their infancy, and research is needed to determine which are most effective for each individual. They are used in addition to the prescribed medical regimen and in collaboration with the health team in order to insure the client's safety. For example, relaxation and meditation might require alterations of dosages of insulin, anticonvulsant and antihypertensive medication.

Biofeedback □ Biofeedback is the process of learning voluntary control over involuntary body functions. The word describes a feedback of physiological information, usually by means of an instrument which provides the client with such information as body temperature, heart rate, blood pressure, muscle tension, or brain waves. Biofeedback has been used as successfully as or more so than conventional treatments in more than 50 major medical and psychological problems (Brown, 1977). A partial list of conditions for which muscle biofeedback (electromyogram or EMG) has been practiced includes anxiety, phobias, tension and migraine headache, insomnia, alcoholism, drug abuse, asthma, essential hypertension, duodenal ulcer, colitis, muscle spasms with pain, nerve-muscle injuries (stroke, paralysis), cerebral palsy, and dystonia. Cardiovascular biofeedback is used to control atrial and auriculoventricular arrhythmias, premature ventricular contractions, essential hypertension, and migraine headaches. Skin temperature biofeedback is used in Raynaud's syndrome and migraine headaches, and as a relaxation procedure. Gastrointestinal biofeedback has been tried in functional diarrhea, fecal incontinence, esophageal spasm, and gastric acid secretion. Brain wave biofeedback (electroencephalogram or EEG) has been used in neuroses, psychoses, behavior problems, pain, insomnia, and epilepsy. Biofeedback is a promising treatment approach because of its relative success, simplicity, low cost, and safety for the client (Ray, et al., 1979).

Relaxation □ There is a variation of relaxation technique that does not involve audio or visual feedback. Jacobson's progressive relaxation (1974) was introduced early in this century and consists of systematically contracting and relaxing muscle groups in order to develop an awareness of relaxation. He demonstrated that relaxation of voluntary muscles can generalize to smooth muscles of the gastrointestinal and cardiovascular systems thereby producing excellent clinical results in many types of illness. An awareness of muscle relaxation usually precedes or is an integral part of other forms of deep relaxation.

Hypnosis □ Although hypnosis is probably the oldest form of treatment, it remains one of the most controversial. Therapy under hypnosis consists of short sessions during which the hypnotherapist assists the client in reaching a trance state for a specific purpose. During this altered state of consciousness between wakefulness and sleep, the client is more receptive to suggestion than in the waking state. It has been used successfully in the treatment of pain (Zahourek, 1982), cancer (Newton, 1982; Margolis, 1982), bronchial asthma, cardiac arrhythmias, peptic ulcer, migraine and tension headaches, obesity, and many other conditions (Peterfy, 1977). Some advantages of hypnotherapy are short duration of treatment, usual immediate and recognizable results, decrease in use of drugs, and the relatively short period of time needed to train hypnotherapists.

Autogenic Training □ Having its roots in hypnosis and often referred to as "autohypnosis," autogenic training is practiced in a relaxed position and a state of "passive concentration"; that is, an absence of effort or concern about relaxation. This passive attitude is essential to all methods of meditation. In this state the individual repeats messages of relaxation such as "My arms and legs are heavy. My arms and legs are warm. My heart beat is calm and regular. It breathes me. My abdomen is warm. My forehead is cool." This method has been applied to a number of diseases and conditions (Shealy, 1978).

Meditation □ Meditation had its origin in the Eastern religions. Benson's "relaxation response" (1975) is based on the principles of transcendental meditation. The instructions incorporate four essential elements: (1) a quiet environment; (2) a repetitive mental device such as the word "one"; (3) a passive attitude, which is perhaps the most important; and (4) a comfortable position. This is practiced for 20 minutes once or twice daily. LeShan's (1975) variation of this method consists of counting each breath up to the fourth one and then beginning again.

Visual Imagery □ Visual imagery may be added to meditation for the purpose of changing habits, setting goals (Gawain, 1978), or altering the course of an illness, as the Simontons have done with cancer patients (1980). While in a meditative state, the client visualizes the cancer as consisting of very weak, confused cells; the treatment and white blood cells destroy the cancer cells; the cancer shrinks; dead cells leave the body; and the individual is again energetic and healthy. This is done three times a day.

Yoga □ The word yoga means "to unite" and its purpose is to develop harmonious functioning of the personality through increasing self-control and decreasing the impact of environmental influences. Self-control at cortical, autonomic, and peripheral levels can be acquired by the use of prescribed exercises involving posture, breathing, bodily movement, and concentration. Studies show it is effective for patients with psychoneurosis and asthma (Vahia and Doongaji, 1977). Formulated 2500 years ago, it is the foundation of biofeedback—which is more widely accepted, studied, and used in this country.

Exercise and Stretching □ Physical exercise on a regular basis can reduce the effects of stress and promote healing, specifically an increase of arousal, improvement of self-esteem and body image, relief of anxiety and reactive depression, and maximization of intellectual and psychomotor development (Shephard, 1983). The aerobics programs outlined by Cooper (1977) have been effective in cardiovascular conditions, diabetes, peptic ulcers, lung diseases, obesity, back pain, arthritis, glaucoma, and depression. Aerobic exercise increases the amount of oxygen in the body and includes running, walking, swimming, cycling, tennis, skiing, rope skipping, dancing, and others. In their treatment program for cancer patients the Simontons (1980) recommend 1 hour of exercise three times a week. Stretching also has a relaxing effect on the mind and body (Anderson, 1980) as muscle tension is reduced and coordination and circulation are improved.

Massage, Acupressure, and Reflexology □ Massage is a passive form of exercise well known to most nurses in the form of a backrub. Increased circulation, more rapid elimination of waste (lactic acid), and relief of tension are some of the physiological effects. One study (Longworth, 1982) measured the effects of slow stroke back massage, a slow, rhythmical, gentle, light stroking done in one direction with the hands in continuous contact with the skin. It was found that a relaxing effect resulted if the massage was done for 6 minutes and that this was due to habituation to the tactile sensations rather than the manipulation of the muscles. It was recommended that this type of massage be used to induce relaxation and sleep instead of the vigorous massage that is more traditionally given. A psychological effect of massage is acceptance as conveyed through touch, which encourages people to be more aware of their bodies (Downing, 1972). Acupressure, the application of pressure to certain points of the body, has been used mainly for pain relief. Reflexology proposes a relationship between various organs and nerve endings in the soles of the feet and palms of the hands. Massage of these areas produces relaxation, increased circulation, and pain relief.

Therapeutic Touch □ This technique (Krieger, 1981) is derived from the ancient art of laying on of hands and is based on the concept of human beings as energy fields which interact with other energy fields in their environment. In illness the flow of energy is blocked and in treatment the interaction between the energy fields of the practitioner and the patient allows the energy to resume its flow. This is accomplished as the practitioner enters a meditative state and then concentrates on the client and the intent to heal. Therapeutic touch is a misnomer since it is most effective when the hands are 2 or 3 inches from the body. The process lasts about 20 minutes during which the patient experiences profound relaxation, heat in the affected area, and peripheral flushing throughout the body. This safe intervention is being used increasingly by nurses who, after learning the skill, have been able to help clients experience relaxation, relief of acute and chronic pain, reduced fever, and increase in blood circulation to a wounded area. The most experienced practitioners have been able to influence blood pressure, thyroid, and diabetic disorders. Studies have documented that therapeutic touch significantly affects hemoglobin levels, brain waves, and state of anxiety, and brings about a generalized relaxation response.

Psychotherapy □ Psychotherapy, for individuals and in groups, has been used in addition to routine medical regimens to alter the anxiety and depression often associated with illness. In a review of controlled studies, Conte and Karasu (1981) found that eight of 13 studies whose research designs were acceptable showed greater physiologic improvement for clients receiving psychotherapy than for clients receiving medical treatment alone. There are times when psychotropic drugs are indicated to facilitate the healing process, specifically minor tranquilizers and antidepressants (Solow, 1977). It is recommended that pharmacotherapy be accompanied and in some cases replaced by psychotherapy. Some psychotherapeutic principles are utilized in more informal group approaches such as self-help groups of bronchial asthma, anorexia nervosa, obesity, and many other conditions (Newton, 1982). Effective ways of living are learned in parenting, assertiveness training and widows' groups.

Nutrition □ Research continues to provide new information in the field of nutrition. In recent years the optimum diet not only includes foods from the basic four food groups, but also encourages the use of reduced amounts of preservatives, sugar, salt, red meat, and fewer processed foods. Increased amounts of whole grains, fresh fruits and vegetables, poultry and fish are recommended. Caloric intake should not exceed the physical need (Cheraskin et al., 1975). Dietary guidelines for Americans proposed by the Department of Agriculture and the Department of Health and Human Services (1980) are: eat a variety of foods; maintain proper weight; reduce intake of total fat, saturated (hydrogenated) fat, and cholesterol; eat food with adequate starch and fiber; avoid too much sugar; avoid too much sodium; drink alcohol in moderation if at all. The use of vitamin and mineral supplements is still controversial, and studies continue on associations with some of the major chronic physical and mental illnesses (Kirschmann, 1979).

Laughter □ Humor has long been known to be a tension reliever and coping mechanism (Robinson, 1978) but laughter is only recently becoming an identifiable intervention. Norman Cousins' (1981) experience with ankylosing spondylitis (a serious collagen disease) is probably the most widely publicized account. Having knowledge of Selye's work on stress and the relationships between negative emotions and negative chemical changes in the body, he reasoned that perhaps positive emotions such as love, hope, faith, laughter, confidence, and the will to live might produce positive chemical changes. He watched old "Candid Camera" and Marx Brothers films and discovered that 10 minutes of genuine belly laughter produced 2 hours of pain-free sleep as well as a noticeable drop in the sedimentation rate.

Play □ Defined by Simonton (1983) as "any activity (or lack of) with no socially redeeming value," play is recommended for cancer patients and well people alike for 1 hour a day. It is valuable in reducing stress on a short-term basis and is also a step toward the formation of a healthier life-style.

Music □ This modality has been found to be particularly helpful for people who have extreme pain. Studies have shown (Bonny and Savary, 1973) that there are certain wavelengths in sound that are exactly the same as the wavelengths in muscles. Music therapy helps to relax the muscles and reduce the pain. Another technique is to use music of different tempi which will be a distraction, diverting the person's attention from the pain, and thus bringing some relief.

EVALUATION □ Evaluation of interventions includes the subjective and objective responses of the client and family, the nurse, and other dis-

---

Case Study

Mrs. F., a 40-year-old homemaker, was hospitalized to undergo a mastectomy. Her nurse found her to be pleasant, quiet, and cooperative. Her attitude toward the loss of a breast was one of resignation. Inquiries about her family revealed that she was married, had two teenage children, and a 2-year-old boy. She had been working as a secretary before the youngest child was born. She expressed some fears related to radiation and chemotherapy. These were relieved somewhat by information she was given about the procedures; she then expressed some concern about child care which would be needed while she traveled daily from her nearby town for radiation treatments. The nurse reflected Mrs. F.'s feelings of frustration related to caring for a 2-year-old and hiring babysitters, and then explored the matter with Mrs. F. The nurse, noting that Mrs. F.'s teenage daughter had not visited, learned from Mrs. F. that her daughter had run away from home, probably would not finish high school, and was not on good terms with her father. The nurse encouraged Mrs. F. to verbalize her feelings of loss and helplessness in the situation and asked about sources of support among family members, friends, and her church.

Soon after beginning radiation therapy Mrs. F. was interviewed by a psychiatric clinical nurse specialist in the unit. She confided that she was worried about finances; was tired but couldn't sleep; her husband had a drinking problem; she hadn't cried since her condition was diagnosed though previously she was able to; and her sister had been very persistent in trying to persuade her to try a questionable and unproven cancer treatment. Assessing the lack of support within the family and Mrs. F.'s possible depression, the nurse specialist made plans to see Mrs. F. on a regular basis during her treatment. Her sleep improved and during a discussion of her losses and feelings of hopelessness, she cried. At one point she missed some treatments; a phone call revealed that she was not sure the treatments were worth the effort. The nurse specialist empathized with Mrs. F. and encouraged her to continue treatments and counseling sessions. During the next few weeks after Mrs. F. returned for treatment, the nurse specialist was able to assist in identifying some of Mrs. F.'s personal strengths and supports in the community, to suggest some assertive measures to follow toward her sister, to explore some goals for relaxation, work, recreation, and exercise; and to inform her of a self-help group in the community for post-mastectomy patients and another for spouses of people with drinking problems. Mrs. F. was able to express her feelings of sadness and inadequacy about her daughter, and became more confident in her ability to cope with her numerous problems and to complete the prescribed treatment.

ciplines at all levels of prevention. At the primary level the nurse evaluates teaching, documenting evidence of learning. At the secondary level the effectiveness of referrals needs to be evaluated for appropriate follow-through. Another concern is the adjustment of the client and family to diagnosis and early treatment. At the tertiary level short-term and long-term expected outcomes of identified problems must be evaluated.

Prognosis depends on many factors. The literature suggests that clients with high psychosocial coping ability have a higher probability of recovering (Backus and Dudley, 1977) and the dimensions of support, cohesion, and affiliation generally have a positive effect (Moos, 1977). Holmes and Masuda (1974) have identified specific attitudes toward life among stress-resistant persons, namely an openness to change, a feeling of involvement in what they are doing, and a sense of control over their lives. Because behavioral treatments are not refined, it is difficult to make predictions, and more research is needed. Illness, specifically chronic illness, is very complex. Progress is slow because the health professional is working with clients who have well-established patterns of living and beliefs which are extremely difficult to change. (See case study on page 490.)

■ *Enrichment Activities*

DISCUSSION QUESTIONS

1. Discuss various theorists and their contributions related to stress theory.

2. Describe a holistic view of illness.

3. Differentiate between "psychosomatic disorders" and a "psychosomatic approach" to the explanation of illness.

4. Describe family dynamics that predispose people to illness. If these are also present in normal families, how are the members protected?

5. What self-assessment and self-care measures for the nurse can one use to enhance nursing care?

6. What are the characteristics of interventions at the primary, secondary, and tertiary levels?

7. Discuss personal and professional experiences related to the use of self-regulation techniques.

LEARNING ACTIVITIES

1. In a small group, describe a client from your nursing experience. Each group member identifies feelings, motives, values, and reactions experienced in the care of that client. Discuss the importance of this awareness and identify resources if assistance is indicated.

2. Describe hypothetical interventions for any client with a chronic illness at the primary, secondary, and tertiary levels. How would these interventions be evaluated?

3. Experience the "relaxation response" by using Benson's method as described or with the assistance of a structured relaxation exercise on audio tape borrowed from a library, stress management unit, or counseling center.

4. Choose five self-regulation activities. Describe how each would be used at the primary, secondary, and tertiary levels.

■ *Recommended Readings*

Bahnson, C.B. Stress and cancer: The state of the art. Parts 1 and 2. *Psychosomatics*, 21, 1980:975–981 and 22, 1981:207–220. A comprehensive review of the literature, a case report, and a review of research relating to possible intervening psychophysiologic processes (neurologic, endocrine, and immunologic) are presented by an authority in the field.

Benson, H. *The relaxation response.* New York: Avon, 1975. A description of a method to induce the relaxation response as well as its rationale and a report of research on hypertensive clients are included.

Krieger, D. *Foundations for holistic nursing practices: The renaissance nurse.* Philadelphia: J.B. Lippincott, 1981. Ancient and modern holistic health practices are reviewed and a contemporary holistic approach to nursing is proposed incorporating Rogers' conceptual model of unitary man. Clinical papers supporting this approach are included.

Lipkowski, Z.J. Psychosomatic medicine in the seventies: An overview. *The American journal of psychiatry,* 134, 1977:233–244. The history of psychosomatic theory, the current holistic view with underlying assumptions, and trends in research are discussed in detail.

Pelletier, K.R. *Mind as healer, mind as slayer.* New York: Dell, 1977. A review of stress theory, major diseases associated with stress, and methods for controlling stress are included.

■ *References*

Achterberg, J., Simonton, O.C., and Matthews-Simonton, S. *Stress, psychological factors, and cancer.* Fort Worth, TX: New Medicine, 1976.

Anderson, B. *Stretching.* Bolinas, CA: Shelter Publications, 1980.

Backus, F.I., and Dudley, D. Observations of psychological factors and their relationship to organic disease. In *Psychosomatic medicine: Current trends and clinical applications* (Lipowski, Z.J., Lipsitt, D.R., and Whybrow, P.C., eds.). New York: Oxford University, 1977.

Bahnson, C.B. Stress and cancer: The state of the art. Parts 1 and 2. *Psychosomatics,* 21, 1980:975–981 and 22, 1981:207–220.

Baider, L., and Porath, S. Uncovering fear: Group experience of nurses in a cancer ward. *International journal of nursing studies,* 18, 1981:47–52.

Barstow, J. Stress variance in hospice nursing. *Nursing outlook,* 28, 1980:751–754.

Bartrop, R.W., Lazarus, L., Luckhurst, E., Kiloh, L.G., and Penny, R. Depressed lymphocyte function after bereavement. *The lancet,* 1, April 16, 1977:834–836.

Benson, H. *The relaxation response.* New York: Avon, 1975.

Bonny, H., and Savary, L. *Music and your mind: Listening with a new consciousness.* New York: Harper & Row, 1973.

Brallier, L.W. Holistic health practice: Expanding the role of the psychiatric-mental health nurse. In *Community mental health nursing: An ecological perspective* (Lancaster, J.). St. Louis: Mosby, 1980.

Brown, B.B. *Stress and the art of biofeedback.* New York: Bantam, 1977.

Bruch, H. Anorexia nervosa. In *Psychosomatic medicine: Its clinical applications.* (Wittkower, E.D., and Warnes, H., eds.). New York: Harper & Row, 1977.

Caldwell, T., and Weiner, M.F. Stresses and coping in ICU nursing. I. A review. *General hospital psychiatry,* 3, 1981:119–127.

Cheraskin, E., Ringsdorf, W.M., and Brecher, A. *Psychodietetics.* New York: Bantam, 1976.

Conte, H.R., and Karasu, T.B. Psychotherapy for medically ill patients: Review and critique of controlled studies. *Psychosomatics,* 22, 1981:285–315.

Cooper, K.H. *The aerobics way.* New York: Bantam, 1977.

Cousins, Norman. *Anatomy of an illness as perceived by the patient: Reflections on healing and regeneration.* New York: Bantam, 1981.

Diagnostic and statistical manual of mental disorders. 3d ed. Washington, D.C.: American Psychiatric Association, 1980.

Donovan, M.I. Study of the impact of relaxation with

guided imagery on stress among cancer nurses. *Cancer nursing,* 4, 1981:121–126.

Downing, G. *The massage book.* New York: Random House and Berkeley, CA: The Bookworks, 1972.

Engel, G. A life setting conducive to illness: The giving up-given up complex. *Annals of internal medicine,* 69, 1968:293–300.

Epting, S.P. Coping with stress through peer support. *Topics in clinical nursing,* 2, 1981:47–59.

Evans, F.J. The placebo response in pain reduction. *Advances in neurology,* 4, 1974:284–296.

Freedman, A.M., Kaplan, H.I., and Sadock, B.J. *Modern synopsis of comprehensive textbook of psychiatry.* Baltimore: Williams & Wilkins, 1976.

Friedman, M., and Rosenman, R.H. *Type A behavior and your heart.* Greenwich, CT: Fawcett, 1974.

Garbin, M. Stress research in clinical settings. *Topics in clinical nursing,* 1, 1979:87–95.

Gawain, Shakti, *Creative visualization.* New York: Bantam, 1978.

Hall, H.R. Hypnosis and the immune system: A review with implications for cancer and the psychology of healing. *American journal of clinical hypnosis,* 25, 1982:92–103.

Hartl, D.E. Stress management and the nurse. *Advances in nursing science,* 1, 1979:91–100.

Hinkle, L.E. The concept of "stress" in the biological and social sciences. In *Psychosomatic medicine: Current trends and clinical applications* (Lipowski, Z.J., Lipsitt, D.R., and Whybrow, P.C., eds.). New York: Oxford University, 1977.

Holmes, T.H., and Masuda, M. Life change and illness susceptibility. In *Stressful life events: Their nature and effects* (Dohrenwend, B.S., and Dohrenwend, B.P., eds.). New York: Wiley, 1974.

Holmes, T.H., and Rahe, R.H. The social readjustment rating scale. *Journal of psychosomatic research,* 11, 1967:213–218.

Hutschnecker, A.A. *The will to live.* rev. ed. New York: Prentice-Hall (Cornerstone Library), 1977.

Jacobson, E. *Progressive relaxation.* Chicago: University of Chicago, 1974.

Janis, I.L. *Stress and frustration.* New York: Harcourt Brace Jovanovich, 1969.

Karasu, T.B., and Steinmuller, R.I. *Psychotherapeutics in medicine.* New York: Grune & Stratton, 1978.

Kirschmann, J.D. *Nutrition almanac.* rev. ed., New York: McGraw-Hill, 1979.

Krieger, D. *Foundations for holistic health nursing practices: The renaissance nurse.* Philadelphia: J.B. Lippincott, 1981.

Kutash, I.L., and Schlesinger, L.B., *Handbook on stress and anxiety: Contemporary knowledge, theory, and treatment.* San Francisco: Jossey-Bass, 1980.

Lazarus, R.S. Psychological stress and coping in adaptation and illness. In *Psychosomatic medicine: Current trends and clinical applications* (Lipowski, Z.J., Lipsitt, D.R., and Whybrow, P.C., eds.). New York: Oxford University, 1977.

LeShan, L. *How to meditate.* New York: Bantam, 1975.

Lipowski, Z.J. Psychosomatic medicine in the seventies: An overview. *The American journal of psychiatry*, 134, 1977:233–244.

Longworth, J.C.D. Psychophysiological effects of slow stroke back massage in normotensive females. *Advances in nursing science*, 4, 1982:44–61.

Looney, J.G., Spitzer, R.L., and Lipp, M.R. Classifying psychosomatic disorders in DSM-III. *Psychosomatics*, 22, 1981:6–8.

Margolis, C.G. Hypnotic imagery with cancer patients. *American journal of clinical hypnosis*, 25, 1982:128–134.

Mason, J.W. A historical view of the stress field. Parts 1 and 2. *Journal of human stress*, 1, 1975:6–12, 22–36.

McDonald, R.L. The role of emotional factors in obstetric complications: A review. *Psychosomatic medicine*, 30, 1968:222–234.

McElroy, A.M. Burnout—A review of the literature with application to cancer nursing. *Cancer nursing*, 5, 1982:211–217.

Meissner, W.W. Family process and psychosomatic disease. In *Psychosomatic medicine: Current trends and clinical applications.* (Lipowski, Z.J., Lipsitt, D.R., and Whybrow, P.C., eds.). New York: Oxford University, 1977.

Melzack, R. Psychologic aspects of pain. *Research publication of Association for Research in Nervous and Mental Disease.* New York: Raven, 1980.

Mikhail, Blanche. The health belief model: A review and critical evaluation of the model, research, and practice. *Advances in nursing science*, 4, 1981:65–82.

Minuchin, S., Rosman, B.L., and Baker, L. *Psychosomatic families.* Cambridge, MA: Harvard University, 1978.

Moos, R.H. Determinants of physiological responses to symbolic stimuli: The role of the social environment. In *Psychosomatic medicine: Current trends and clinical applications.* (Lipowski, Z.J., Lipsitt, D.R., and Whybrow, P.C., eds.). New York: Oxford University, 1977.

Moser, D.H., and Krikorian, D.A. Satisfaction and stress incidents reported by hospice nurses: A pilot study. *Nursing leadership*, 5, 1982:9–17.

Nemiah, J.C. Alexithymia: Theoretical considerations. *Psychotherapy and psychosomatics*, 28, 1977:199–206.

Newton, B.W. The use of hypnosis in the treatment of cancer patients. *American journal of clinical hypnosis*, 25, 1982:104–113.

Newton, G.R. Self-help groups: Can they help? *Journal of psychosocial nursing and mental health services*, 22, 1984:27–31.

Pelletier, K.R. *Mind as healer, mind as slayer.* New York: Dell, 1977.

Peterfy, G. Hypnosis. In *Psychosomatic medicine: Its clinical applications* (Wittkower, E.D., and Warnes, H., eds.). New York: Harper & Row, 1977.

Poser, C.M. Trauma, stress, and multiple sclerosis. *Bulletin of the American Academy of Psychiatry and the Law*, 7, 1979:209–218.

Ray, W.J., Raczynski, J.M., Rogers, T., and Kimball, W.H. *Evaluation of clinical biofeedback.* New York: Plenum Press, 1979.

Reading, A., and Wise, T.A. (eds.). Symposium on psychiatry in internal medicine. *Medical clinics of North America*, 61, 4,1977.

Reiser, M.F. Changing theoretical concepts in psychosomatic medicine. In *American Handbook of Psychiatry.* 2d ed. Vol. 4. New York: Basic Books, 1975.

Robinson, V.M. Humor in nursing. In *Behavioral concepts and nursing intervention* (Carlson, C.E., and Blackwell, B., eds.). Philadelphia: J.B. Lippincott, 1978.

Rogers, M.P., Dubey, D., and Reich, P. The influence of the psyche and the brain on immunity and disease susceptibility: A critical review. *Psychosomatic medicine*, 41, 1979:147–164.

Rokeach, M. *Beliefs, attitudes, and values.* San Francisco: Josey-Bass, 1968.

Schaefer, C.E., Millman, H.L., and Levine, G.F. *Therapies for psychosomatic disorders in children.* San Francisco: Jossey-Bass, 1979.

Schwab, J.J., and Traven, N.D. Factors related to the incidence of psychosomatic illness. *Psychosomatics*, 20, 1979:307–311, 315.

Scully, R. Staff support groups: Helping nurses to help themselves. *Journal of nursing administration*, 11, 1981:48–51.

Selye, H. *The stress of life.* New York: McGraw-Hill, 1956.

Selye, H. The stress syndrome. *American journal of nursing*, 65, 1965:97–99.

Selye, H. *Stress without distress.* Philadelphia: J.B. Lippincott, 1974.

Selye, H. The stress concept today. In *Handbook on stress and anxiety: Contemporary knowledge, theory, and treatment* (Kutash, I.L., Schlesinger, L.B., et al.). San Francisco: Jossey-Bass, 1980.

Shealy, C.N. *90 days to self-health.* New York: Bantam, 1978.

Shephard, R.J. Physical activity and the healthy mind. *Canadian Medical Association journal*, 128, 1983:525–530.

Simmons, D.A. *A classification scheme for client prob-*

lems in community health nursing, DHHS Publication No. HRA 80-16. Hyattsville, MD: U.S. Department of Health and Human Services, 1980.

Simonton, O.C., Matthews-Simonton, S., and Creighton, J. *Getting well again*. New York: Bantam, 1980.

Simonton, S.M. In address to Nebraska Hospice Association, Lincoln, Nebraska, April 6, 1983.

Slater, G.R. Disease as a value statement. *Journal of religion and health*, 20, 1981:100–107.

Smith, M.J.T., and Selye, H. Reducing the negative effects of stress. *American journal of nursing*, 79, 1979:1953–1964.

Solow, C. Psychotropic drugs in somatic disorders. In *Psychosomatic medicine: Current trends and clinical applications* (Lipowksi, Z.J., Lipsitt, D.R., and Whybrow, P.C., eds.). New York: Oxford University, 1977.

Sperry, R.W. Changing concepts of consciousness and free will. *Perspectives in biology and medicine*, 20, 1976:9–19.

Sternbach, R.A. Psychophysiology of pain. In *Psychosomatic medicine: Current trends and clinical applications* (Lipowksi, Z.J., Lipsitt, D.R., and Whybrow, P.C., eds.). New York: Oxford University, 1977.

Strain, G.W. The obese patient. In *Psychological interventions in medical practice* (Strain, J.J.). New York: Appleton-Century-Crofts, 1978.

Sutterly, D.C. Stress and health: A survey of self-regulation modalities. *Topics in clinical nursing*, 1, 1979:1–21.

Teitelbaum, H.A. Neurological disorders. In *Psychosomatic medicine: Its clinical applications* (Wittkower, E.D., and Warnes, H., eds.). New York: Harper & Row, 1977.

Thomas, C.B., and Duszynski, K.R. Closeness to parents and the family constellation in a prospective study of five disease states: Suicide, mental illness, malignant tumor, hypertension, and coronary heart disease. *Hopkins medical journal*, 134, 1974:251–270.

Tubesing, D.A. Stress, spiritual outlook and health. *Specialized pastoral care journal*, Lutheran Council in the USA, 3, 1980:17–23.

U.S. Department of Agriculture, Department of Health and Human Services. *Nutrition and your health: Dietary guidelines for Americans*. Home and Garden Bulletin No. 232. February 1980.

Vahia, N.S., and Doongaji, D.R. Yoga. In *Psychosomatic medicine: Its clinical applications* (Wittkower, E.D., and Warnes, H., eds.). New York: Harper & Row, 1977.

Weiner, M.F., and Caldwell, T. Stresses and coping in ICU nursing. II. Nurse support groups on intensive care units. *General hospital psychiatry*, 3, 1981:129–134.

Weisman, A.D., and Hackett, T.P. Predilection to death: Death and dying as a psychiatric problem. *Psychosomatic medicine*, 23, 1961:232–256.

Weiss, J.H. The current state of the concept of psychosomatic disorder. In *Psychosomatic medicine: Current trends and clinical applications* (Lipowski, Z.J., Lipsitt, D.R., and Whybrow, P.C., eds.). New York: Oxford University, 1977.

Werner-Beland, J. *Grief responses to long-term illness and disability*. Reston, VA: Reston, 1980.

Williams, C.C., and Holmes, T.H. Life change, human adaptation, and onset of illness. In *Clinical practice in psychosocial nursing: Assessment and intervention* (Longo, D., and Williams, R.A., eds.). New York: Appleton-Century-Crofts, 1978.

Wise, T.N. Pain: The most common psychosomatic problem. *Medical clinics of North America*, 91, 1977:771–780.

Wittkower, E.D. Historical perspective of contemporary psychosomatic medicine. In *Psychosomatic medicine: Current trends and clinical applications* (Lipowski, Z.J., Lipsitt, D.R., and Whybrow, P.C., eds.). New York: Oxford University, 1977.

Zahourek, R.P. Hypnosis in nursing practice—Emphasis on the "problem patient" who has pain. Parts 1 and 2. *Journal of psychiatric nursing and mental health services*, 20, 3, 1982:13–17 and 4, 21–24.

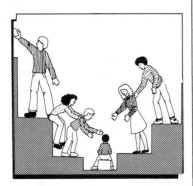

24
Mental Retardation

Rosemarie Hartley and
Cordelia Robinson

Learning Objectives

Upon completion of this chapter, the reader will be able to:

1. Obtain a life-span perspective of the challenges and problems encountered by those with mental retardation.

2. Understand the philosophy that is the foundation of current social policy concerning programs for the mentally retarded.

3. Be aware of major legislative efforts aimed at protecting the civil rights of mentally retarded persons.

4. Recognize environmental constraints and professional biases that impede functional adaptation of mentally retarded persons.

5. Assist clients in acquiring adaptive skills necessary for successful living.

6. Understand the collaborative nature of services needed to maintain optimal functioning of the mentally retarded person in the community.

☐ *Definition and Diagnosis*

The most widely accepted definition of mental retardation is: "significantly subaverage general intellectual functioning existing concurrently with deficits in adaptive behavior, and manifested during the developmental period" (Grossman, 1973, 11). This definition has been adapted by Heber (1959, 1961) and Grossman (1973, 1977) for the American Association of Mental Deficiency (AAMD). Over time several medical and legal definitions of retardation have been in use and have had different emphases (Brison, 1967; Robinson and Robinson, 1976). A commonality among them was their focus on the limitations of the retarded person in meeting the demands of daily living without assistance. With the advent of intelligence testing, professionals often relied heavily or solely on tests that were designed only to measure academic performance and to predict school success. The AAMD definition, on the other hand, requires that in order for a person to be diagnosed as retarded, he must be deficient in both *intellectual performance* and *adaptive behavior*. Definitions of adaptive behavior generally encompass the degree of ability to perform without help the tasks of daily living and those of social competence. In each of these areas, chronological age, social class, and cultural environment are considered in determining behavioral standards.

Unlike earlier definitions, the AAMD definition is only a description of the person's current level of functioning. The definition does not include prognosis because it is difficult to base a prognosis on results of currently available measures.

While the definition adopted considers measurable terms (individual intelligence tests and tests of adaptive behavior), the authors of the AAMD diagnostic manual caution against making a diagnosis strictly on the basis of standardized instruments. Other information about intellectual and adaptive functions and the suitability of the test for a given person must be considered. For example, a number of persons who are diagnosed as retarded have other disabilities as well (physical or sensory disabilities or emotional disturbance). The AAMD definition ". . . avoids specific differentiation of mental retardation from other childhood disorders such as childhood schizophrenia or brain damage" (Robinson and Robinson, 1976, 33).

Because of the nature of the definition, frequently the professional who confirms a diagnosis of mental retardation is a psychologist. In making such a diagnosis, the clinician must consider the appropriateness of a formal instrument such as an intelligence test for a particular person. For example, there are no standardized instruments available that can be used to diagnose mental retardation in infants and toddlers with significant motor disabilities. Standard IQ tests make the assumption that those who are tested have all shared in similar environmental experiences. For those children who have significant motor impairments, this assumption would not apply.

The AAMD definition is also limited in that it identifies retardation as a defect or deficit within the person and thus assumes that the condition can exist even if it is unrecognized or undiagnosed. Mercer (1973) sees a danger in this pathological or clinical model because it may not recognize that different social systems make different demands. Thus, a person may be assigned a status of retardation in one social system (e.g., school) and might not be assigned that status in another social system (e.g., neighborhood). Mercer's view has been labeled the *Social System Perspective* and has had its greatest impact in approaches to persons who, in the clinical or pathological model perspective, are mildly retarded. Her data documenting the disproportionately large number of minority group children in special education classes for mildly retarded children has had in the past 15 years a considerable effect on school policy and on the entire field of retardation.

The AAMD definition, the most commonly accepted in the United States and Canada (Robinson and Robinson, 1976), has changed in its relatively brief history of 20 years, most significantly in the designation of the upper IQ limit considered to be within the range of retardation. In the 1959 definition, persons whose measured intelligence was below one standard deviation from the mean or within the borderline range of 70 to 84 were considered retarded if their adaptive behavior was also considered deficient. Inclusion of persons in this borderline category of intelligence results in a projection of approximately 16 percent of the population as retarded. The changes in the definition adopted in 1973 included the addition of the word *significant* to the phrase *subaverage functioning*. *Significant* is defined as two or more standard deviations from average, and based upon this cutoff score of 69, approximately 3 percent of the population would be retarded.

This change in cutoff score produced a dramatic change in the incidence of retardation based upon the statistical AAMD definition. The practical implications are that many people who test in that range may function reasonably well and with sufficient independence and thus should not be stigmatized by being labeled retarded. On the other hand, being included in the classification of mental retardation may make people eligible for some supportive services that they otherwise might not receive.

CLASSIFICATION SYSTEMS

One of the most common misconceptions about retardation as a diagnostic entity is that persons who carry the label or diagnosis "retarded" are a homogeneous group of persons. This misconception has plagued both behavioral research efforts and clinical intervention programs addressing all issues concerning retardation. Robinson and Robinson (1976) summarized the characteristic lack of homogeneity both in behavior and in causal influences in the following paragraph:

> Retarded children constitute a very heterogeneous group both in their behavior and in the causes of their deficiency. Some children are happy and carefree in their own homes, whereas others are difficult to manage and are impossible to maintain at home. Some have relatively minor handicaps which show up primarily in school achievement, and others are so grossly defective that even in adolescence they have not yet learned to sit, to talk, or to play. Some have maladies which are attributable mainly to the genes they inherited from their parents; others have been injured or diseased; still others suffer mainly the effects of cold or indifferent environments which fail to meet their psychological needs (Robinson and Robinson, 33).

There are numerous approaches that may be taken to classification; however, as Robinson and Robinson (1976, 33) have pointed out, there are three prevalent viewpoints: "severity of the handicaps, etiology of the symptoms, and the symptom constellation or syndrome."

Severity of Handicaps

The current widely accepted nomenclature with respect to severity of symptoms was proposed in 1954 by a subcommittee of the World Health Organization and includes the levels of mild, moderate, and severe subnormality. These terms were proposed to replace the previously widely accepted terms: moron, imbecile, and idiot. As part of the AAMD diagnostic and classification manual (Grossman, 1973), a classification system based upon four IQ levels was proposed and has received general acceptance in the field of retardation in the United States and Canada. This system is presented in Table 24-1.

Each level in this system encompasses one standard deviation on an individually administered intelligence test. As previously noted, a diagnosis based upon IQ alone is inappropriate; there must also be impairment in adaptive behavior to warrant a diagnosis of retardation. The importance of this insistence upon both criteria may be seen in Mercer's 1973 survey data. Mercer (1970, 1973) looked at several approaches to identifying cases of retardation. One comparison involved looking at individuals who met only the IQ criterion versus those who met the adaptive behavior criterion as well. Of 150 persons who met the below-70 IQ criterion, only 45 percent also "failed" the adaptive behavior measure. Also significant was the finding that all the Anglos in the sample met both criteria, while 60 percent of Mexican-American persons and 91 percent of black persons who had IQs below 70 had adaptive behavior scores above the retarded level. From these findings, it is clear that ethnicity or racial differ-

TABLE 24-1 IQ Ranges for Degrees of Severity of Retardation[a]

Descriptive Term	Range in SD Value	Corresponding IQ Range for Tests with SD	
		15	16
Mild retardation	−3.00 to −2.01	55–69	52–67
Moderate retardation	−4.00 to −3.01	40–54	36–51
Severe retardation	−5.00 to −4.01	25–39	20–35
Profound retardation	Below −5.00	Under 25	Under 20

[a] Reprinted with permission from *The Mentally Retarded Child*, Robinson, N. and Robinson, H., New York: McGraw-Hill, Inc., p. 34, 1976.

ence places one at greater risk for a diagnosis of retardation in our culture. This greater risk becomes an indictment of our diagnostic care systems when one considers the fact that there are no data to indicate greater rates of retardation in different racial and ethnic groups, once conditions such as poverty, lack of adequate medical care, and malnutrition are taken into account.

■ Point of Emphasis

Health professionals must recognize that the conditions associated with poverty are associated with and, some argue, cause retardation, particularly in those cases where no specific etiology is identified.

Classification According to Etiology

In classification systems based upon etiology, the primary distinction is made between cases where there is confirmed or presumed pathology as the cause of the retardation, such as disease, trauma, chromosomal disorders, and metabolic disorders, and those cases presumed to be due to psychosocial disadvantage (Grossman, 1977; Robinson and Robinson, 1976). While this approach tries to distinguish between causes such as *exogenous* versus *endogenous* or *mental deficiency* versus *mental retardation*, the reality is that such factors interact in their effects upon development (Anastasi, 1958; Sameroff and Chandler, 1975; Ramey and Finkelstein, 1981).

Classification According to Symptom Constellation

All three prevalent systems for classification of clinical syndromes—AAMD (Grossman, 1977), American Psychiatric Association (DSM-III, 1980), and World Health Organization (1968)—are very similar. It should be noted, however, that the cause of a particular symptom frequently cannot be identified, or a given symptom may have a number of causes. In relatively few conditions have specific treatments been identified (e.g., diet management in phenylketonuria). Prevention of conception is an option to those known to be at risk for genetically transmitted diseases. Prognosis based upon etiology (when it is known) is, in most conditions, uncertain.

☐ Prevalence

The generally accepted prevalence rate of retardation is 3 percent, which approximates the percentage of the population presumed to have an IQ below 70 based upon the normal distribution. Also based upon a normal distribution, most of the individuals with IQs below 70 fall in the IQ range of 50 to 70.

While these estimated figures treat the total population as homogeneous, there are a number of environmental factors that affect the actual prevalence of mental retardation. These are standards and practices in the home, community, age, racial and ethnic background, geographic region, and sex. A good deal of this variability in prevalence figures in subpopulations occurs within the IQ levels of mild retardation.

A number of literature reviews have substantially implicated the conditions of poverty as direct or indirect causes of mental retardation (Hurley, 1969; Haywood, 1970; Robinson and Robinson, 1976; Sameroff and Chandler, 1975). Any successful intervention efforts, be they primary, secondary, or tertiary prevention, must address the conditions of poverty as well as the specific conditions of retardation.

In summary, mental retardation is a complex entity from the perspectives of diagnosis, epidemiology, and, as we will see, treatment. In an effort to illustrate the complexities of retardation, we will take the approach of major life stages in discussing nursing diagnosis and intervention. Those stages will be birth through the preschool years, primary school years, adolescence, and adulthood. Initially, the effects of a mentally retarded child upon parents, individually, and in a family context will be discussed. Since this textbook addresses the field of psychiatric mental health nursing, greater emphasis will be given to those life stages and consequently those individuals most likely to be receiving psychiatric services.

☐ Social Role Valorization

Before the implications of mental retardation in these major life stages are considered, it is essential that the reader recognize that regardless of life stage of the individual and family, particular etiology, or severity of retardation, all persons who carry the diagnosis of retardation have the same basic health and nurturance, physical, nu-

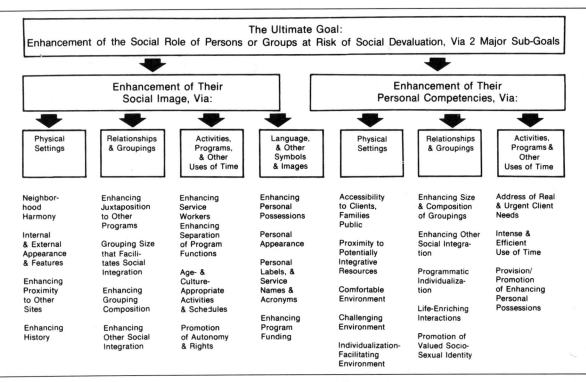

Figure 24-1 Hierarchical structure of social role valorization (formerly known as the principle of normalization). From Social Role Valorization: A Proposed New Term for the Principle of Normalization, Mental Retardation, 21 (6), 1983.

tritional, and emotional needs as any human being. The concept of normalization, or social role valorization, is appropriate in this context (Wolfensberger, 1983). This concept has probably had the single greatest impact upon services for persons who are retarded of any concept or movement in recent history. Wolfensberger (1972; 1980a&b; 1983), the primary interpreter of this concept in the United States and Canada, outlined the major goal of normalization by arguing for use of the term *social role valorization*. In his words ". . . the most explicit and highest goal of normalization must be the creation, support, and defense of [valued social roles] for people who are at risk of social devaluation" (1983, 234). This ultimate goal is accomplished, he contends, by two principles or subgoals: "(a) enhancement of people's 'social image' or perceived value in the eyes of others, and (b) enhancement of their competencies (236). This hierarchical goal structure is presented in Figure 24-1.

These basic human services to support enhancement of social image and competencies should be made accessible to persons who are retarded without the need for segregating them from the rest of society. The nursing interventions

recommended in this chapter are designed to build upon the fundamentals that form this basic level of care.

☐ The Family

CONCEPTUAL FRAMEWORK FOR WORKING WITH THE FAMILY

In addition to use of the concept of social role valorization as a framework for the design of human service systems, a conceptual model is a useful tool to assess and design intervention methods with the family of a person who is mentally retarded. For such a model we suggest the one proposed by Hymovich (1979) for assessing the chronically ill child and family. The key elements in the conceptual model include considering the total family unit at its present stage in the family life cycle as well as the developmental and care needs of each member. The aim is to increase the coping abilities of all family members in their individual and collective mastery of developmental tasks. The family members' functioning is presumed to be affected by such variables as their perceptions, resources, and coping abilities.

Table 24-2 examines resources as one of the areas of concern for evaluation and intervention. Resources include those that are internal, external, personal, or human (such as health, ability to give and receive emotional support), and physical resources (such as income, housing, and physical help from friends and family members).

IMPACT OF A RETARDED CHILD UPON THE FAMILY

The impact of a retarded child upon the family has been extensively studied and reported upon, perhaps as a result of the growing number of early intervention efforts. With public policy changes emphasizing deinstitutionalization, emphasis on community support systems, and the early intervention efforts encouraged by federal law, the relationship of the retarded child and adult to his or her family is receiving increasing attention.

Wolfensberger (1967) noted that the early literature on retardation said little about parents and their response to their child's diagnosis of retardation. He noted that these writings were not empirical and were redundant, and noted further that the parent populations on which they were based were not representative.

The primary issues addressed in the literature of the 1950s and 1960s and still cited today include: (1) the parents' initial reaction to the diagnosis, (2) the continuity or stability in the reaction to the child, (3) the impact of the child on the family unit, (4) parental coping mechanisms, and (5) parent-professional relationships.

In regard to the impact of the diagnosis, Solnit and Stark (1961) and Olshansky (1962) set the tone of the next couple of decades by characterizing the typical parental reaction as one of grief and chronic sorrow. While such frameworks are probably helpful in sensitizing professionals to parents' feelings, the work that has been done in this area has several problems: selection bias among subjects; collection of much of the information sometime after the reported events occurred; absence of individual baselines or contexts within which to interpret the data; the subjective nature of many of the responses; and the lack of stability of many of the measures in categorizing subjects' responses consistently. A prevalent bias is that of the individual investigators' attitudes regarding their own anticipated reaction to the birth of a handicapped child. Few people are neutral in their feelings toward such an event. Such feelings were likely to have influenced the type

of information that was thought to be important in such studies. In addition, many of the words used to describe parental reactions to the diagnosis and circumstances of raising a handicapped child tend to predispose professionals to a negative attitude. Terms such as overprotection, denial, and chronic sorrow, while used initially as conceptual descriptors of stages of reaction, have in subsequent work been used as factual explanations of parental behavior that invariably are seen in a negative frame of reference. It is difficult, especially where mental retardation is involved, to find descriptions of parental reactions that permit a well-adjusted acceptance of the realities of having a handicapped child in a family. The impact is frequently portrayed in negative terms or in unrealistically positive terms.

The difficulty of interpreting parental behavior using the various frameworks that have been proposed was described by Barsch:

> If the parent is militantly aggressive in seeking to obtain therapeutic services for his child, he may be accused of not realistically accepting his child's limitations. If he does not concern himself with efforts to improve or obtain services, he may be accused of apathetic rejection of his child. If he questions too much, he has a "reaction formation" and may be oversolicitous. If he questions too little, he is branded as disinterested and insensitive (1968, 8).

It should also be recognized that much of this literature antedates the recent changes in circumstances of programs for handicapped children. The choices for typical families with moderately to severely handicapped children prior to the 1970s were to institutionalize them or keep them at home with the possible prospect of not having any public schooling. The changes brought about by more recent legislation and the demonstration projects upon which that legislation was founded have been extensive. These changes may limit the generalizability of findings from earlier work to the present.

Despite the warnings regarding possible interpretations or generalizations in this early literature, that work is still an essential reference point for the professional. The consistency found in reports across cultures and across individual circumstances must be given careful consideration. While that consistency could be related to the manner in which the information was collected, it cannot be totally dismissed; the overall issues examined and advances made in this area

TABLE 24.2 Areas of Assessment and Intervention for the Impact Variable: Resources in the Hymovich Model[a]

	Impact variable: Resources Family developmental tasks			
Meet basic physical needs	Assist with individual tasks	Meet needs for emotional support	Adapt organization and management	Function in community
Home structure, location, outdoor play area, sleeping arrangements, adaptations for ill child Health care where, for whom, for what, prevention crisis how paid for, obtain needed equipment, medications etc. for child general health of each family member Finances income: sources stability who contributes who supported insurance, major expenses, cost of illness Clothing appropriate for: weather individual needs Food basic four special diets	Appropriate for: developmental needs, extent of child's disability (specific resources will depend upon developmental needs of each member) What parents do with each child (i.e., recreation, hobbies) Development prior to illness Past experiences Support systems Preexisting family functioning communication patterns decision making feelings of closeness Family values and goals	Individual family member's: temperament, personality, cognitive level, self-concept Relationship between family members Development prior to illness Past experiences Support systems Preexisting family functioning communication patterns, decision making, feelings of closeness Family values and goals	Household membership number, age, sex, relationship Role of each member Role flexibility Availability of external supports	Organizations belong to, i.e.: PTA, church/synagogue, volunteer, parent groups, children's groups, other Specific resources necessitated by child's condition Resources used, i.e., medical, recreational, educational, vocational, transportation, other Day care/babysitting arrangements Attitudes of community

[a] Reprinted with permission from Assessment of the Chronically Ill Child and Family. In D. Hymovich, and M. Barnard (Eds.), *Family Health Care: General Perspectives,* 1979.

of study are critical background for the individual practitioner.

Individual Characteristics of Parents

Wright, et al. (1984) drew conclusions regarding the interpretability and limitations of the literature similar to those pointed out by Wolfensberger (1967) almost 20 years earlier. They then go on to suggest that our models for looking at and interpreting these influences need to take into account the interactions between different parental characteristics, child characteristics, and support systems. This is consistent with Hymovich's model for areas of assessment of family functioning. Some of the most frequently cited factors that need to be considered include coping styles, previous family functioning patterns, resource availability, parents' perceptions regarding the child's problems, and consensus among family members. Such factors are proposed as possible predictors or mediators of the outcomes experienced by the retarded person. Outcomes in this context include both developmental and behavioral functioning of the retarded family member and integration into the family. Implicit within the various proposed models for looking at the impact of a handicapped child upon the family is the assumption that different families and individuals within these families all have unique characteristics. Generalizations that the impact and responses to intervention will be the same for all are inappropriate. The models proposed by Hymovich (1979), Rosenberg (1977), and Wright (1984) offer promise regarding ways to conceptualize the potential family and intervention characteristics.

■ *Point of Emphasis*

Just as individuals who are diagnosed as retarded do not constitute a homogeneous group of individuals, parents and families are not all alike in their reactions.

Parent-Professional Interaction

A clinical example of the tenuous interactions among parent, family, child, and support systems can be illustrated by the following.

In the course of working in a collaborative project whose goals included facilitating needed services to families, the authors were associated with a low-income family whose newest member suffered severe asphyxia at birth, leaving her legally deaf, blind, with severe cerebral palsy, and mentally retarded.

Until the birth of this child, the mother—the pivotal force in the family—had been very successful in organizing family routines and solving family problems. Suddenly, all of the plans for integrating the new family member were no longer usable. The adolescent daughter's imagined interactions with her new sister dissolved in the reality of witnessing the infant's frequent seizures and her inability to follow or smile at her sister's beckoning eyes. Soon after the infant's birth, the adolescent's grades dropped, she became distant and difficult to handle at home, and ultimately took refuge in the home of an uninvolved relative who could devote attention to her needs.

The complexity of care required for the infant in and out of the hospital necessitated the involvement of numerous physicians; specially trained home health care nurses; nurse consultants; physical, occupational, and respiratory therapists; infant educators; respite services; and multiple social services. Portable oxygen tanks, suctioning equipment, continuous feeding apparatus, monitors, orthopedic aids, multiple medications, and complex special treatments became the focus around which family life evolved. Considerable maternal and family stress was expressed in trying to communicate with and understand the therapeutic goals of all the persons who provided services.

The mother's loss of control, which for so long had been sufficient to sustain her family, was expressed in her anger and frustration at the collective system which all too often could not "get its act together" and sometimes was guilty of serious errors of omission or commission.

The professionals were often caught in the web of absolving themselves of blame by projecting it onto others in the system. The mother was labeled incompetent, too ready to relinquish responsibility for care, and a troublemaker by those to whom she turned for help. Her sensitive perception of these categorizations fueled a cyclical process of parent-professional frustration and inertia.

While it was impossible to predict all of the specific crises endured by this family as a result of the infant's fragile medical status, it may have been possible to better anticipate and prepare for the overall impact on the family of the infant and the professional caregivers.

■ *Point of Emphasis*

Frequent parent/interdisciplinary communication focused upon early problem identification, mutual goal setting, clear role delineation, and individual/agency accountability is vital to effecting positive adaptation of family members to entry of a multiply handicapped infant into the family unit. Neglect in the identification of personal biases on the part of the professional can result in emotional injury to the family and others.

Parents and other family members of children who are retarded can be expected to interact with professionals in many disciplines over the course of the retarded individual's care from childhood to adulthood and beyond. Certain behaviors on the part of both family and professionals can facilitate the development of constructive relationships. Specific attitudes and assistance that can be expected by parents from professionals include:

1. Acceptance of the parents as contributing partners in the management of their child's care.
2. Clarification of parent and professional roles and responsibilities as they pertain to the child's care.
3. Knowledge on the part of professionals of the resources available for the child and the family.
4. Information about treatment options that are available, and an explanation of the reasons for the professional's preference for a given option.
5. Opportunity for the parent to participate in setting priorities for care.
6. Opportunity for the parent to ask questions of the professionals in an unhurried and nondefensive atmosphere.
7. Anticipation of issues about the child's care before they become acute problems, and provision of anticipatory guidance as a means of problem prevention.
8. Access to experts who are informed about new developments in techniques of caring for the child.

9. Access to an atmosphere that places the child's needs over issues of professional territories.
10. Maintenance of support and help throughout the child's development.
11. Support and direction that allow the parent personal growth and increasing independence.
12. Professional concern about the child's position within the family, even by those whose areas might be highly specialized.

Parents' responsibilities in their ongoing interactions with professionals, which should be fostered by nurses early in the intervention process, include:

1. Keeping accurate records. During the course of the child's development, he will probably see many different professionals. Since parents are the major source for continuity in a child's care, it is very important that they keep thorough records.
2. Asking questions that are focused toward understanding the rationale for and specifics of any treatment.
3. Reviewing all treatment directions with the professionals to ensure that they will be carried out correctly.
4. Expressing feelings when professionals have done things well, not just when they don't do things well.
5. Telling professionals when a given recommendation is unrealistic for the family situation and jointly working on problem solving that will make it feasible.
6. Being realistic about other family members' needs for respite from day-to-day demands of the care of the handicapped child.
7. Becoming an informed consumer of the services both the child and the family may need.
8. Seeking support through offering support to other parents.

□ *Life Span Issues*

INFANCY AND PRESCHOOL PERIOD

In the past two decades, disciplines concerned with the habilitation and education of mentally retarded children have undergone considerable change. Perhaps the area of greatest change in thinking and consequently in therapeutic approaches is that of management of the period of infancy which, in present context, is defined as the first 2 years of life. A major impetus for this change has been the changing view about the infant. In brief, the infant is no longer seen as a passive and totally dependent organism but instead, as an active learner whose interest in and responses to his caretakers serve to shape their behavior in the same manner as his caretakers' responses shape his behavior, that is, through reciprocal interactions (Bell, 1968; Yarrow, 1979).

Rationale for Intervention with Infants

Initially, the rationale for an emphasis on intervention during a child's first years was largely intuitive. Infancy was recognized as a period during which the child undergoes relatively rapid change, physiologically and behaviorally (Bloom, 1964). The assumption that early experience has a profound and disproportionate impact on development, relative to its time span, long a tradition in the psychoanalytic frame of reference, received new support from the developmental work of the 1960s about the issues of critical and sensitive periods for development of specific structures and behaviors. Developmental psychologists and educators such as Hunt (1961), Bloom (1964), and Clarke and Clarke (1976) analyzed and synthesized findings about early experience and its impact on development. These seminal works served as the rationale and impetus for the program titled Head Start—in the context of which professionals found they could successfully advocate early intervention for children with disabling conditions.

Throughout the 1970s infant programs proliferated, with considerable assistance from federal funding for Maternal Child Health Services and Special Education Programs (then Bureau of Education of the Handicapped) through its Handicapped Children Early Education Program, and from organizations such as the Association for Retarded Citizens and United Cerebral Palsy. With this growth of programs came demands from professionals, especially academicians, for evidence of the scientific validity of these intervention efforts (Denhoff, 1981). At the same time, funding sources demanded greater accountability about program effectiveness and efficiency (Swan, 1981; Zigler and Balla, 1982).

As the results of Head Start program failed to meet the initial high expectations held for it (Horowitz and Paden, 1973), intervention programs for handicapped infants were challenged. The distinction between socially disadvantaged (culturally different) populations and biologically impaired populations of children and their needs and appropriate expectations for intervention efforts was frequently forgotten or obscured. Simeonsson, et al. (1982) reviewed studies published since 1975 in which results of early intervention with biologically impaired infants and young children were reported. They included only interventions "that are exclusively experiential in nature" (p. 636). This included traditional therapies such as occupational, physical, and speech therapy as well as less traditional modes such as vestibular stimulation. They did not include evaluations of pharmacological or dietary interventions in their review. On each of the dimensions by which they analyzed programs, they found incomplete data in many studies, an unfortunate but accurate description regarding the state of the art of early intervention with biologically impaired infants. Where populations were reported, they were small and heterogeneous with respect to subject variables of (1) degree of involvement (severity), (2) diagnostic category, and (3) age. Some studies that involved diagnostically homogeneous populations (e.g., Down syndrome) did not specify diagnostic criteria. These researchers conclude that while 48 percent represents an underestimate of effectiveness. 93 percent represents an overestimate of effectiveness, and offer four explanations (1982, 639) that reflect the methodological and conceptual limitations of the work they have reviewed. These explanations include the conclusion that the handicapped children made progress but statistical significance was not obtained given limited sample sizes. An alternative explanation is that the children made progress but it occurred in domains not measured by the dependent variables. For example, a child's behavior or style of response may have improved but was not documented. Furthermore, maintenance of a certain level of development, or prevention of regression, may also be reflective of success but not recorded.

Nursing Interventions

There are several intervention features that are necessary to the design of an appropriate program. First is the articulation of an underlying program model. Critical elements of such a model include: (1) the identification of the total child whose development is "integrated across behavioral domains" (Sroufe, 1979), (2) acceptance of parents' unique role vis-à-vis their children, and (3) following from that unique role, acceptance of parents as team members of equal status. The other categories of features are procedural and include: (1) statements of specific child and program objectives, (2) use of child and programmatic assessment data to plan and evaluate program effectiveness and efficiency, (3) matching of evaluation methods to objectives, (4) clear delineation of staff roles and responsibilities, and (5) flexibility in program procedures to meet individual child and family needs.

Given these guidelines for an infant intervention program, the nurse's role as an intervention team member will vary with the individual setting. Particularly helpful, however, can be the perspectives of holistic health promotion goals which are integral to the nursing role. If there is to be any teaching of the parent in special care procedures for daily care routines and health promotion, the nurse is well qualified to do this teaching. Also, assisting parents to obtain information and to understand their child's diagnosis and/or symptoms is an important role of nursing in caring for the child. It is at this point in the life cycle of child and family that assisting the primary care physician with the necessary anticipatory guidance for promoting health and facilitating routines is an essential role for nursing.

■ Point of Emphasis

The best guidelines for implementing nursing interventions come from the materials used to promote the well-being of any infant.

ELEMENTARY SCHOOL YEARS

Assessment for School Placement

When a child approaches his fifth birthday, school placement becomes a major concern to his parents. The legal imperative of the least restrictive environment (LRE) that is embodied in the Right to Education for All Handicapped Children Act of 1975 (P.L. 94-142), requires that children ages 5 to 21 be placed in educational environments most facilitating to their developmental needs, yet with the least restrictions upon their interactions and

activities with peers. Newer legislation, the Education for the Handicapped Act Amendments (1983) provides for this intervention from day of birth under a preschool incentive program (Weicker, 1984). Achieving balance between needs and rights has not been an easy task.

A standard intelligence test such as the Wechsler Intelligence Scales for Children-Revised (WISC-R) is most often used to determine the IQ of school aged children. This type of test is not appropriate for all children who are retarded because its norms were established on a population without significant physical or sensory disabilities. Since many of the children who are thought to have problems in mental functioning also have one or more sensory and/or physical impairments, valid and reliable appraisal of their cognitive abilities is often not possible. Ideally, before an educational label is applied to a child, multiple assessment measures should be administered by a team of qualified professionals to identify physical strengths and deficits, cognitive processing abilities, level of emotional maturity, language and communication skills, self-care and social competencies. In fact, however, many school systems still rely heavily or solely on IQ scores. This practice no doubt channels many children into inappropriate educational settings that fail to promote optimal cognitive and social potential.

School Placement and Services

Depending upon the outcome of the assessment procedure, a child will be categorized by the school system as (1) educable, that is, capable of learning academic concepts; (2) trainable, incapable of processing academic information but able to learn basic self-help skills; or (3) severely retarded with the anticipation of some level of custodial care necessary throughout the life span. As a child develops and experiences different life situations in facilitating environments, his abilities may change; therefore periodic and systematic reassessments are essential in order to match educational services to those capabilities. The concept of the Individual Educational Plan (IEP) is based upon the premise of changing status and is legally mandated under P.L. 94-142. Under that law, an interdisciplinary review of a child's school placement must occur no less often than once a year. The educational objectives developed upon a child's entry into a special education program are to be updated to include facilitation of cognitive processing, social competencies, self-help skills, health, and mobility insofar as these variables affect the child's ability to learn.

Services including speech therapy, physical therapy, occupational therapy, behavior management, or psychotherapy may be required to meet these objectives. Funding for these services must be awarded under federal law at no additional expense to parents. Parents are to be active collaborators in the planning and evaluative process, and their signatures on the IEP are necessary to indicate their acceptance. If they are dissatisfied with the plan, they may, under rights of due process, request a special hearing to secure a different placement or additional services. Advocates of the parents' choice may attend the hearing, and additional assessments, obtained through parents' efforts, may be presented for consideration (Jones, 1979). It is not uncommon for groups of parents to band together in class action suits for the purpose of persuading a school system to provide needed services. Ongoing difficulties arise because both sides often interpret funding under the law in different ways, in part because legislators did not clearly define the terms they used in writing the law such as "free" and "appropriate education," nor did they systematically consider the costs associated with implementation until after the law's enactment (Weicker, 1984).

Each state has its own rules for implementation of P.L. 94-142; and several states have expanded the law to include services that begin from the day of diagnosis (which could be the day of birth). Many states have explicitly included nursing among the professions to be represented on interdisciplinary teams that plan, implement, and evaluate services for handicapped children in educational settings.

□ Nursing Process

Interdisciplinary nursing roles include case finding and participating in periodic assessments of the student's level of adaptation and the quality of his educational environment. Coordination of services, parent advocacy, and in-service education for staff are also relevant nursing activities. Identification of areas in which behavior management techniques should be employed to increase self-help skills, health maintenance, and social skills, as well as assisting with their implementation and monitoring, can be incorporated into the nurse's role in educational settings.

ASSESSMENT □

Health Care Maintenance Assessment □ Health care maintenance assessments include all functional areas (i.e., nutrition, elimination, mobility, safety, rest and exercise, communication, and self-esteem). The diversity of need in this population can be illustrated by a review of factors associated with nutrition and fluid assessment.

Because of associated dysfunctions, nutritional deviations involving more or less than body requirements are recurring nursing diagnoses in children who have developmental disabilities. For example, craniofacial deviations observed in children with Down and other syndromes encourage mouth breathing, which is associated with xerostomia (dry mouth) and frequent oral and upper respiratory infections that diminish taste and appetite. Gingival overgrowth is a common side effect of long-term phenytoin therapy. Children who have cerebral palsy are susceptible to stimulation of retained primitive reflexes that make the feeding process difficult, long, and sometimes dangerous. It is not surprising that even the most patient caretakers are tempted to offer those children only foods that are relatively textureless. Not only does such an approach contribute to nutritional and oral motor impairment; it impedes social and cognitive development as well.

Oral-motor physical development and concomitant skills, including the ability to close the lips, to bite, to rotary chew, to locate and move food to the back of the mouth, and to swallow solids and liquids need to be assessed in determining the type of diet appropriate for a specific child. This can best be accomplished through consultation with an occupational therapist.

The child's taste preferences (strong or spicy foods may be preferred because they are more easily located in the mouth), temperature preference (cold or hot is often preferred over lukewarm), and color preferences should be noted.

Caloric needs assessment must take into account physical characteristics and coexisting dysfunction. Because of genetic factors, children with Down and some other syndromes have smaller body stature, increased body fat, and decreased muscle mass. Their metabolic processes are slower and less efficient than those of other children, therefore they usually will require fewer total calories than other children their age. (There are special growth curves available to assess the growth of children with Down syndrome.) Many of these children have cardiac involvement, which limits the amount of energy that is available to expend on the task of eating and in these cases, adequate caloric intake may be seriously restricted. The child who has spastic cerebral palsy has significant impairment of voluntary movements, therefore, caloric needs may be less than for the child who is affected with athetoid cerebral palsy, which is characterized by persistent involuntary movements that increase caloric expenditure.

Allergies or idiosyncratic reactions to certain foods and medical restrictions (such as salt restriction in children with cardiac involvement) need to be identified and considered in meal planning. Vitamin and mineral supplementation and exposure to the sun are important areas to assess if a child is receiving anticonvulsant therapy. Some anticonvulsant drugs are associated with alterations in calcium, vitamins B_{12} and D, and folic acid metabolism (American Dietetic Association, 1981; Simeonsson, 1981).

Because children with craniofacial deviations are mouth breathers and vulnerable to multiple upper respiratory infections, fluid intake needs to be balanced against fluid loss. These children's communication skills and affective responses are often limited, thus recognition of thirst, increasing temperature, or other signs of illness may not be noted by parents or school personnel until serious signs of dehydration appear. If the child is taking anticonvulsant or psychotropic drugs, dehydration can elevate blood levels of these drugs and quickly throw him into toxicity. Lack of bowel movements resulting from inadequate fluid and bulk intake may go unnoticed for days, leaving the child listless and inattentive. Systematic documentation of fluid intake and output can prevent these problems.

Specific data on pica ingestion in children are unavailable. However, Danford and Huber (1982) found that one-quarter of a sample of 991 institutionalized mentally retarded adults had acquired the behavior of consuming nonfood substances such as dirt and garbage. Only one-sixth of the pica ingestors had previously been identified. It would appear to be a good idea for nurses to assess for this problem in school-aged populations.

NURSING INTERVENTIONS □ After a nurse has collected and documented nutritional data in the child's health record, there are several ways to intervene to improve nutrition and fluid intake, as well as the child's developmental status.

Meal planning is best done in collaboration with a nutritionist who is knowledgeable about the needs of handicapped children. In school and in the home, those who prepare the child's meals should be instructed to serve foods so they are separate and attractively arranged on the plate. Food textures need to be preserved to allow the child to identify and move foods about in the mouth; therefore, coarse grinding is usually better than pureeing. When there are energy limits placed on eating, or mechanical feeding problems, foods with high nutrient density should be used to compensate for diminished total intake (Public Health Currents, 1978). Feeding devices that facilitate self-help and coordinated eating movements will need to be purchased or improvised. These include placemats that prevent plates and bowls from moving about, scoopback plates, and specially adapted spoons and cups (Figure 24-2). Consultation with occupational therapists who specialize in this area is advisable. Times for fluid and nutrition breaks may need to be worked into a child's regular school activity schedule. Oral hygiene, to include brushing, flossing, and gum stimulation after every meal, is especially important if the child is taking anticonvulsants.

Parents, school aides, and others involved in feeding the child with special needs will require training in how to position him for feeding, how to avoid stimulation of primitive reflexes, how to develop a reciprocal caretaker-child cueing system, and how to facilitate the child's self-help skills. The assistance of a behavior management specialist may be enlisted to extinguish undesirable behaviors and to ensure that facilitating approaches are consistently being used by caretakers in every feeding situation.

Even the more severely handicapped child often has sufficient perceptual capabilities and memory capacity to be able to recognize consistent approaches used during recurring interactive sequences such as the feeding process. From these experiences he will form expectations which he will communicate through verbal or nonverbal responses to his caretakers. For example, during feeding, a well-balanced reciprocity between the care provider and a multiply handicapped child with severe mental retardation is facilitated by the care provider's consistent timing and sequencing of behaviors that alert the young client that it is mealtime. Structured positioning; use of clear touch cues with accompanying verbal labels; and consistent arrangement of cups, bowls, and plates, will provide the child with a mealtime "script."

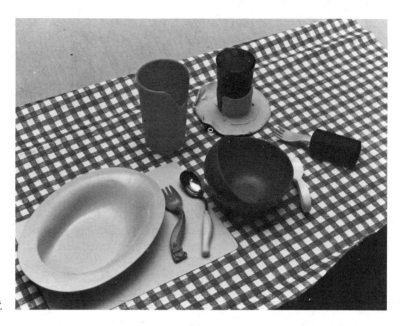

Figure 24-2. Adaptive feeding equipment.

Offering foods of different textures, temperatures, and colors separately will establish an environment that facilitates discrimination of stimuli to which the child can meaningfully respond. Careful observation of postures, facial changes, eye points, or vocalizations that give evidence of preference, readiness for more, displeasure, or need for change in stimuli or rest will allow the care provider to correctly respond to the child's cues. The child will come to realize that he too has some control and autonomy in the situation, and thus he will be less likely to fall into behaviorly inappropriate or disruptive patterns. (See Figure 24-3.)

> **■ Point of Emphasis**
>
> The primary caretaker's understanding of health maintenance and developmental issues is crucial to any nursing goal attainment. This understanding cannot be achieved unless the caretakers are included in every step of the development of specific service programs and the reasons for therapeutic interventions are explained to them.

EVALUATION □ Evaluation of nutritional adequacy may need to be based on kilocalorie by height rather than kilocalorie by weight ratios. The former method is used for children who have chromosomal aberrations and do not follow standard growth curve norms. Measurement of skin-fold thickness may be especially useful. Integrity of gum tissue, dentition, and bone strength need to be evaluated regularly in children who are taking anticonvulsant drugs. Intake and output records are necessary to document achievement of fluid requirement goals.

SAFETY ISSUES □

Potentials for Injury □ The Rehabilitation Act of 1973 mandated that any building constructed or remodeled with the use of federal funds must be barrier free for handicapped persons. While many public building administrations have readily complied, there are more that have not (Weicker, 1984). A simple architectural omission can make life very difficult for a child who has motor, vision, or hearing impairments. Frequent tours of buildings and grounds in which services are provided to children will allow a nurse to identify real or potential barriers and initiate action for their modification.

Systematic monitoring is crucial when it concerns young clients who are taking one or more prescribed drugs. Once written permission to administer drugs in a school or day-care setting is obtained from the legal guardian, the person dispensing the medications should document the name and dosage of each drug, dates and times of administration, whether the child retained or vomited the drug(s), and observed behaviors thought to be related to desired effects or side effects. Behavioral observations in the classroom may be conducted by the nurse whenever a

Position Erica on bean-bag in kitchen to keep you company as you prepare meal. The surround may begin to signify eating time. Picking up cues-verbal/touch sides. Tell her you are going to put her in chair. Show her bib, "Here's your bib. I'm going to put your bib on," with touch cue to chest. Guide her to feel bib. Look for anticipation.	**PRELIMINARY CUES** Helping Mom 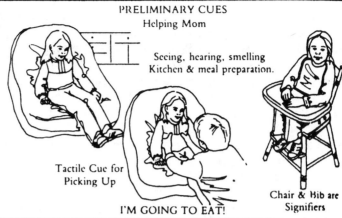 Seeing, hearing, smelling Kitchen & meal preparation. Tactile Cue for Picking Up **I'M GOING TO EAT!** Chair & Bib are Signifiers
Guide her in eat sign & drink sign approximations. Show her spoon or glass each time you change & move slowly toward mouth to see if she visually recognizes. Touch to mouth as cue. Use manual techniques to help lip closure, fade as feasible. Introduce textures gradually. Use food mill. Place bits of food on lateral teeth—touch cue to open & chew.	**FEEDING PROGRAM** Guided EAT sign 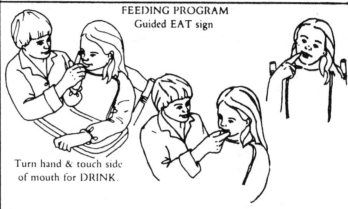 Turn hand & touch side of mouth for DRINK. EQUIPMENT: Cup cut-out, plastic-tipped spoon.
Cognition: Object Schemes. Guide Erica in holding spoon & glass a bit in feeding so that she acquires haptic meaning. We do not expect her to feed herself yet. Cognition: Causality. Pause & ask if she wants more, holding spoon or glass in front, also touching to her mouth. Accept any signal behavior she uses such as move head, vocalize.	**OTHER LEARNING OPPORTUNITIES** So that's what it is! Tying the feeling & action of spoon & cup to experience at mouth. Guide a bit. Ask "More" Guiding hands in more sign.
Cue Erica to hold damp washcloth to wipe her face, then wipe face & hands. Tell her "All done," guiding hands in approximation of finish sign. Cue with hands to each side of trunk when you pick her up. We expect all cues will also be verbal and that strong intonation will accompany cues.	**FINISHING** 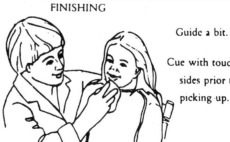 Touch washcloth to face as cue. All done! Guide a bit. Cue with touch to sides prior to picking up.

Figure 24-3. *Situational script for a multihandicapped child.*
Source: A process teaching approach applied to mealtimes: Derived from the individual educational plans of two multihandicapped children by N.M. Fieber. Omaha: Meyer Children's Rehabilitation Institute, 1981 (unpublished).

teacher suspects drug noncompliance, ineffectiveness, or overdose. Close communication between nurse, physicians, teachers, and caretakers will ensure that desired drug effects are maintained. All those who interact with the child need to be alerted to increases or decreases in drug dose, or to the addition of new medications, so that physical and behavioral changes can be monitored.

Blood levels should be assessed at regular intervals in all children receiving anticonvulsants, since metabolic processes vary greatly among children. While the therapeutic goal is to maintain a child in a seizure-free state, the educational goal is to keep him alert enough to be able to learn. If medication leaves a child in a state short of stupor, nothing developmentally is gained by the therapy. Because of its potential interferences with cognitive processing, drug therapy needs to be taken into account when intelligence testing is planned or interpreted.

If several drugs related to different problems are prescribed for the same child, undesirable drug-drug interactions are a potential problem, especially if more than one physician is involved. Over-the-counter drugs may also adversely interact with prescribed medication. The alcohol in cough syrups or antihistamines that are used to relieve common upper respiratory infections can have an additive effect to the depressive action of anticonvulsants.

In settings where multihandicapped children are present, it is necessary to design a comprehensive emergency system including explicit procedures to follow in case of aspiration or asphyxia. Individual medical summary cards that are readily accessible to personnel will facilitate prompt notification of the primary physician and quick transmission of pertinent information to a hospital emergency staff. Portable oxygen and resuscitation equipment should be maintained in a place known to all personnel along with posted emergency phone numbers. Everyone working with multiply handicapped children needs to be trained in CPR.

Development of Self-Concept and School Environment □ As a child acquires the ability to perceive reactions of others toward him, his sense of self will be developed accordingly. Unusual physical appearance, lack of agility, sensory handicaps, communication limitations, seizure disorders, or the motor effects of cerebral palsy all contribute to negative reactions in peers who, according to Erikson (1963), are at the developmental level where conformity and achievement become increasingly important. Concrete categorizing allows school-aged children to make conceptual sense of their world, but mentally and physically impaired children may fare badly in the process if they come to view themselves as lacking in some area of physical, cognitive, or social functioning.

The argument has been posed that mainstreaming of school-aged handicapped children into regular classroom or school activity settings with peers who are not handicapped encourages social isolation because peers will negatively label them and exaggerate perceived differences. However, the school-aged child of average intelligence, according to Piagetian theory (Elkind, 1974), is able to alter his focus from a single characteristic of an object or person and take into account "the whole." The concept of mainstreaming proposes that frequent exposure to and interaction with children who are somewhat different should facilitate incorporation of broad concepts of peer characteristics rather than narrowly defined labels. With time and exposure, classmates will be identified as individuals with certain traits or needs: "Mark is a boy in our class who needs special help with his reading," rather than as specimens reflecting a singular stereotype: "Mark's that retarded kid in the class." In fact, Brightman (1977) noted that school-aged children who used stereotypic labels had based those perceptions on encounters with single individuals.

Diagnostic labels are a necessity in a system that requires proof of need for services requested. Outcomes such as development of a negative self-concept, peer rejection, biased teacher expectations, and difficult adult adjustment have been thought to be negative outcomes of labeling; however, research findings in this area are ambiguous. Faber (1980) suggests that a child often takes on behaviors expected of him under an assigned label, which leads to a desocializing rather than a socializing process. One finding is clear—those who acquire labels don't like them (MacMillan, et al., 1974).

The more able an individual is to discriminate, categorize, and compare differences between himself and others, the more he is going to be disturbed by the ambiguities encountered in interpersonal relationships. In this sense, mildly and some moderately impaired children are more at risk for disturbances in self-esteem than are the more severely affected children whose deficits are so clear that they elicit protective compassion from their peers.

ASSESSMENT ☐ Young persons with mild or moderate mental retardation have been reported to exhibit extreme sensitivity to the reactions of others toward them and to their own consistent failures in meeting others' expectations for social behavior. These self-perceptions are likely to lead to withdrawal from further social interactions in order to maintain self-protection at a time when interpersonal risk taking can facilitate the development of the social skills necessary for later independent living. Inability to use sophisticated defense mechanisms, which are common to persons of average intelligence in maintaining psychological equilibrium, leads instead to the use of more primitive defense mechanisms such as denial. For instance, mildly impaired individuals often do not classify themselves as retarded and therefore tend to set their expectations too high and fail to evaluate their efforts realistically.

By using open, caring communication with young clients and close observation for subtle behavioral changes, nurses in community health, residential, and school settings can help to identify indicators of negative self-concept. Collaboration with teachers and parents and others is necessary to piece together events that precipitate a problem. For example, changes in adult expectations for a child, or changes in family life events, even if these are thought by others to be positive, may negatively affect the child who possesses simple or few coping mechanisms.

INTERVENTION ☐ In order to decrease the misconceptions frequently expressed by school-aged peers, some communities are conducting sensitivity activities. The "Kids on the Block" are an example of these efforts. The "Kids" are a set of lifesize puppets who represent different types of developmentally disabled children. Each puppet comes with a script so that during skits presented to children, common questions and fears are candidly aired. Following these presentations, children in the audience are allowed to question the puppets. The school nurse or teaching staff summarize feelings and facilitate problem solving about peer relationships.

The Special Olympics initiated by the Joseph P. Kennedy Jr. Foundation provides year-round programs for individuals of all ability levels 8

years of age and older, while the Play to Grow Program is available for families with retarded children of any age. Participation in programs worldwide has enhanced the self-concept of hundreds of thousands of persons who experienced the thrill of competition in sports at local, regional, national, and international levels.

■ Point of Emphasis

Prevention of dysfunction in the development of self-concept through systematic case finding, primary prevention efforts, and implementation of early intervention programs should be a primary goal of those who work in the field of mental retardation.

Social Interactions and Sexuality During Adolescence ☐ The adolescent of normal intelligence is highly aware of similarities and differences between himself and his peers. He strives to minimize or eliminate the differences in order to belong to and be accepted by his peer group, and seeks frequent interaction with peers in order to validate and refine his social skills and his emerging beliefs and values. Mildly and many moderately retarded adolescents are keenly aware of the differences among themselves and their age mates. Characteristically bland facial expressions and poorly coordinated body movements along with expressive language limitations impede their abilities to adequately express their perceptions and feelings. Often physical impairments and orthopedic devices restrict the texture of cloth and style of clothing that can be worn, thereby detracting from overall appearance. Association between these young people and their neighborhood peers which, prior to the adolescent stage, was acceptable, may suddenly become prohibited with the onset of pubescence. These restrictions often stem from biases in the general population about the ability of mentally retarded persons to behave in a sexually appropriate manner. All of these factors impinge upon the adolescent's opportunities to engage in social encounters that are necessary not only for gathering information about acceptable modes of behavior but for developing positive coping strategies for dealing with rejection.

Effective social interaction requires an awareness of self and a complex set of cognitive skills.

The abilities to perceive, attend to, and discriminate among physical/behavioral characteristics modeled by others, to store them with related information in memory, to appropriately generalize them to other situations or recombine them in novel ways all are cognitive processes most people take for granted. Yet planning one's discourse with others often involves not only these concrete operational cognitive skills, but also the ability to hypothesize about how any number of different actions might be perceived and responded to by others. This type of hypothetical deductive reasoning is a formal operational skill that emerges during adolescence within the context of frequent and diverse social interactions (Elkind, 1974).

While persons who are more than mildly mentally retarded do not achieve that level of social sophistication, many can, with enough structured interaction, learn the social scripts that are accepted in our society. One area that is frequently overlooked in the preparation of adolescents with special needs for adult roles is that of sexuality.

Sexuality Issues

In today's society every adolescent is bombarded with stimuli colored by sexual themes. Most can share the concerns and feelings prompted by this exposure with close friends and can experiment with casual heterosexual role behaviors without fear of adult interference. These avenues are rarely open to the adolescent who is labeled as mentally retarded.

According to Heshusius (1982), sexual development and sexual drives are similar in all persons, regardless of intellectual level, even though rates of development vary more in the mentally retarded population. Yet social attitudes about acceptable expressions of sexuality may often depend upon the perceived intelligence level of the person expressing the behaviors. For instance, while it is socially acceptable for a young man of average intelligence to reach out and hug his female friend, a similar but clumsy attempt by a mentally retarded adolescent may be construed as an assault. The feedback that accompanies such a perception is so incongruent with the intent of the act that it totally disarms the adolescent and leaves him confused and defenseless.

There is little evidence that either instruction about sexual functions in humans or structured preparation for heterosexual relationships occurs in institutions or community residence settings. Caretakers often deny that residents are capable of true warmth and affection and many places restrict heterosexual interaction even among adults to little more than hand holding. Role modeling by nonprofessional staff often does not incorporate appropriate and sensitive behaviors associated with heterosexual social relationships, and taboos placed on the use of outward signs of affection by residents convey the message that such behavior is wrong.

Masturbation, which is discreetly carried out by most youth in private, is seen by ever-present residence or hospital staff who view such activity as appalling when it is performed by a boy or girl who lacks the cognitive ability to discriminate the environmental cues in which such behavior is safe or acceptable. Outrage and negative sanctions are often swift and harsh, yet rarely is concrete information offered to the individual as to when and where self-stimulation can be carried out without offending others.

Female Sexuality □ Menarche can be a distressing experience for severely mentally and physically impaired females and their families. Contractures and restricted mobility associated with cerebral palsy or seizure disorders (the latter may be exacerbated during menses) can transform a normal developmental event into a major crisis. For the severely mentally retarded female not only is the monthly period not understood, its occurrence along with associated hygienic care (which often must be assumed by the caretaker) is likely to be perceived as a frightening invasion of her body. A survey conducted in one outpatient clinic revealed that some parents rated the problem serious enough to consider hysterectomy as a way of eliminating the periods (Chamberlain, et al., 1984).

Frequency of sexual intercourse among girls with mild retardation in the aforementioned survey approximated that of the normal population. However, most of those who remained sexually active had been victims of sexual assault. Fully one-fourth of that sample had been raped or were victims of longstanding incest. Although concern is most often expressed about the defenselessness of the severely retarded, most of these victims were only mildly impaired.

For the girl who has difficulty understanding and following sequential instructions or cause-effect relationships, conventional methods of contraception pose special problems. For example, use of the IUD requires client cooperation for insertion and is associated with side effects that require prompt identification and reporting (i.e., expulsion, which is especially high in the nullipara, infection, and ectopic pregnancy). Oral contraception requires adherence to a strict schedule and often must involve an adult who is available to administer the pill at the same time every day. However, for many young adults who manage their self-care, behavior management programs can be successfully implemented to achieve compliance if no medical contraindications such as cardiac problems exist. Progesterone acetate (Depo Provera) has been used effectively to prevent pregnancy and is viewed as a satisfactory method by parents (Evans, 1983; Chamberlain, 1984). The American Academy of Pediatrics Committee on Drugs has condoned the drug's use in those instances where risks of pregnancy are significant and the young girl does not understand the consequences of sexual intercourse.

The issue of permanent sterilization is yet unresolved. While states have rescinded inhumane laws that require sterilization prior to deinstitutionalization, statutes about voluntary consent of mentally retarded persons vary widely. The national conscience has been raised to protect the right of consent of persons who are retarded, yet there are those who believe that to deny access because a person is unable to give voluntary consent is also a violation of the right to be protected from the potential harm of a pregnancy (Passer, et al., 1984).

ASSESSMENT OF SEXUALITY NEEDS □ Experiences and cognitive levels within this group of adolescents vary widely, therefore, data should be sensitively gathered about each individual's understanding of human sexuality. The following questions are examples of those to be included in initial assessment: Can the adolescent identify him or herself as male or female? What labels are applied to sexual body parts and what is understood about their functions? How does he or she respond to and describe illustrations depicting sexual embrace or masturbation? What is known about the process of pregnancy and birth? Specially designed charts and manuals as well as anatomically correct dolls are available thorough several national organizations for this purpose (Krajicek, 1982). During an assessment of sexuality, indicators of possible sexual abuse need to be meticulously explored.

For those individuals who have experienced feelings of attraction or affection for another person of the same or opposite sex, there is often a need to express and validate these feelings with someone who can give assurance that they are normal and socially acceptable. Exploration of these issues individually or in groups will allow the nurse to identify misconceptions that arise from disregard of these issues by caretaking adults or from the ambiguous cues gathered by residents from the environment.

NURSING INTERVENTIONS □ There are many creative approaches to assist adolescents and young adults to be socially accepted and to interact successfully with others of the same or opposite sex. Faber (1980) has shown that carefully applied makeup, an attractive hairstyle and functional yet stylish clothing resulted in a decrease in the number of persons being labeled as mentally retarded. Seminars in simple hairstyling and cosmetic use can be arranged in residence facilities, schools, or recreational centers where staff should be encouraged to assist in helping each girl achieve the best possible appearance. Plastic facial surgery may bring dramatic changes that open new doors to social acceptance. For example, correcting of tongue protrusion can improve health status and verbal articulation as well as physical appearance.

Behavior management programs in cooperation with psychologists can be designed to assist young women who are mildly or perhaps moderately retarded to deal effectively with feminine hygiene, contraception, and other self-care behaviors. Victims of sexual abuse may require extensive psychotherapy to repair self-concept and prevent the self-fulfilling prophecy of a sexually "bad" person.

Discussions that center around topics identified by the group and conducted in a language that group members understand should take place in all settings serving mentally retarded adolescents. Physiology, self-care, relationships, and feelings associated with sexual arousal and their acceptable outlets are all areas in which information is needed for responsible decision making. Take-apart models or modeling clay can be used to illustrate body parts or contours during step-by-step exploration of body function. Use of puppets, role play, and pantomime afford nonthreatening ways to express feelings and practice social role behaviors. Planned events such as parties and picnics can provide opportunities to observe and practice heterosexual social skills.

Faber (1980) emphasizes that intervention objectives should deal not only with dispelling misconceptions and reinforcing positive attitudes toward sexuality, but also with identifying and clarifying rights. Instructional units for parents and group-home or day-care staff can help dispel their fears and provide them with alternative models of behavior that uphold and protect the right of persons to express their sexuality.

■ Point of Emphasis

Recognizing the basic need for sexual expression and identifying ways to provide supportive environments and opportunities for responsible and caring heterosexual relationships should be among the primary goals of those who interact with mentally retarded individuals.

□ Transitions to Adult Living

In response to the normalization concept, during the 1970s advocates of the mentally retarded concentrated on emptying the institutions and returning those citizens to functional life in the community. Between 1970 and 1977 there was a 67 percent decrease in the number of persons residing in settings for the mentally retarded (Bruininks, et al., 1980). In spite of this rapid change there has been a continuing debate about whether it is appropriate for those with severe mental impairment to live in community settings. The issues involve continuity in the delivery of follow-up services, social values, and funding.

Deinstitutionalization Efforts

As of June 1981 there remained 283 public residential facilities in the U.S. for the mentally retarded. Most residents were women whose average age was 30; they were severely retarded (Scheerenberger, 1982). A surprising finding of that study was the considerable number of young people with moderate and mild mental disabilities (average age 20 years), who were included in new admissions and readmissions. The data clearly points to a gap in services needed to assist these citizens and their families with community adaptation once school supports cease. Of the reporting institutions, only 39 percent indicated all of their programming needs were met. The most severe deficits were found in occupational and physical therapies. Locked wards were reported

still in use for 12,000 residents because of inadequate staffing, safety concerns, and aggressive acts of clients. Only half of the residents experienced contact with parents at least once a year (Scheerenberger, 1982). Obviously the full intent of the social policy established in the 1970s has yet to be realized.

In an attempt to address the problems of lack of support for the young adult, Congress in 1983 introduced the Education for Handicapped Act Amendment, which broadened the original act to include post-secondary programming for all persons with disabilities. The focus of the extension is to provide supports needed during transition from secondary schools to employment or independent living situations and to facilitate parents' participation in the child's educational and social adaptations (Weicker, 1984).

There are three interrelated goals associated with deinstitutionalization that require funding, policy, and administrative mechanisms:

1. Preventing new admissions through funding to develop community-based alternatives.
2. Establishing habilation and treatment programs to prepare institutionalized citizens for a successful return to community life.
3. Establishing and maintaining a responsive community environment (Bruininks, et al., 1980).

Efforts directed toward those goals have been less than effective and have often resulted in polarization and disillusionment among those involved with the movement (Landesman-Dwyer, 1981). The reasons for these poor results include the absence of uniform legislative guidelines needed to successfully plan, coordinate, administer, and evaluate the transition processes and the community programming associated with deinstitutionalization. Evaluation research is difficult to sort out because of the lack of categorical definitions about characteristics of residential placements, lack of uniform measures for assessing the mental and social competencies of clients before or after placement, and inconsistencies among ongoing supportive and follow-up services.

Residence Models. There are several community residence options for the habilitated institutionalized client just entering the community, or for the young adult who is ready for an alternative living situation apart from his family. Both types of clients are often initially placed in a structured intermediate care facility and moved later to more independent settings. Intermediate care is funded under Title XIX of the Social Security Act of 1971, which provides rehabilitation, education, and training to enhance capacity for self-care or employment (Congressional Record 44720, December 4, 1971).

Community living arrangements range from foster-care situations, in which the resident receives 24-hour supervision in a family setting, to independent apartments, often shared with a normal advocate or peer. Those living in apartments are visited periodically by social service professionals. Hostels or group homes headed by a live-in houseparent provide learning about basic self-help and social skills, and there are residential villages that facilitate sharing of communal work. However, there are far too many boarding houses operated by untrained personnel that offer little beyond bed and board (Bruininks, et al., 1980). With such a wide range of alternatives, it is easy to see why evaluation research is difficult to design or interpret.

Factors thought to be linked to program success are type and size of residence, size of staff, social and cognitive skills of the residents, location and availability of community supports, family involvement, and peer supports—yet few of these have been shown to have any systematic relationship to outcome; in part, this is because of the measurement problems mentioned above. Neither reduced numbers of residents, increased staff, nor large amounts of funding dollars guarantee program success. If the members of a small group home are not motivated toward interaction, their social environment is no more enriched than if they are left to their own resources in a larger setting. Conversely, caring, meaningful interaction can occur in larger, well-managed settings. It is the attitudes, skills, and day-to-day modeling of staff members that have been positively related to acquisition of social skills in clients, rather than higher staff-to-client ratios (Landesman-Dwyer, (1981).

Preparing for and Assessing Transition into the Community

Whether a client is being prepared to leave an institutional setting or to move from a more to less structured community residence, a comprehensive assessment needs to be conducted in order to plan a useful transition training program. Important factors to consider include the client's diagnostic category, measured IQ, physical and mental health status, developmental level, social and communication skills, physical limitations, self-care ability, temperament characteristics, and previous positive and negative social experiences. His future placement, and the functional requirements that will be necessary for meaningful living there must be carefully considered.

For example, investigators presented a shopping list with eight items to members of a group home (mean IQ = 58) and asked them to shop for the items at a local store. Later the subjects were asked why they purchased particular brands of items. While price was an often-cited reason, subjects could not differentiate more from less in their reasoning. The attractiveness of the picture on a can or other similarly inappropriate reasons were offered by many. These subjects never had had firsthand experience of shopping before and therefore had no knowledge of how to discriminate when making choices (Williams and Ewing, 1981).

One thing to keep in mind when planning real-life experiences for mentally retarded persons is that their generalizing ability may be very limited. A behavior learned in one situation cannot be expected to be transferred to another situation unless most of the cues in both situations are the same. For example, comparative shopping skills learned at the grocery store may not be applied when the client is in a clothing store unless the skill has been learned and reinforced in that setting as well.

Although no single competence can be identified that is prerequisite to "making it" in the community, Landesman-Dwyer (1981) noted that the most consistently reported reason for reinstitutionalization was client tendencies toward antisocial aggressive behavior. A poorly prepared person released into a new and strange community setting may exhibit fear, frustration, and anxiety; but because of his limited behavioral repertoire, his responses often are interpreted as being aggressive. As previously noted, institutional settings are not conducive to learning social skills. Nonprofessional caretaking staff members with limited skills in behavior management and poor modeling behaviors may give conflicting and inconsistent messages to the residents about appropriate behaviors. Coercion, punishment, and bribery encourage learned helplessness, characterized by passivity and submission.

Transition shock is a term coined by Coffman and Harrison (1980) to describe the effects of inconsistencies in the perceived meanings of communication and events between former institutional residents and persons who reside in the community. For instance, signals that may have been relied upon in the institutional setting for permission to act are suddenly missing in the community, while on the other hand subtle social cues that most of us take for granted go unnoticed by those who have had no exposure to them. Values that were adaptive in the institution are, without notice, condemned in the community. For instance, institutional life often encourages residents to hoard food or clothing to assure that they have enough for themselves, yet this behavior in the community will quickly be labeled as selfish and deviant.

If the meanings of many events and cues change, the client can be expected to become increasingly unsure of himself, to refuse to make decisions, or to risk encountering any more new situations. He may become withdrawn or suspicious and break down in emotional outbursts or fighting. Sleep disturbances, gastrointestinal upsets, and accidents are characteristic symptoms of transition shock. Sadness, loneliness, or feelings of worthlessness may be expressed in anger and reflect early signs of depression. These transition effects may be evident soon after the environmental change or after several weeks. It may take weeks or months before full adaptation occurs (Coffman and Harrison, 1980).

Follow-up studies indicate that even those who are functioning well regress in acquired skills and become withdrawn during the initial phase of relocation into the community. Grieving for lost peer relationships is common. In some cases involving the profoundly retarded, the relocation has ended in death (Landesman-Dwyer, 1981). These data document the need for adequate preparation for transition and consistent support and follow-up. Nurses functioning in community settings are often called upon to coordinate and provide some of these services.

Role Performance Requirements of Early Adulthood

Employment. The Rehabilitation Act Amendment of 1984 was designed to improve vocational rehabilitation services through mandated state programs. Under this legislation federally funded demonstration projects are to be set up to provide entry of mentally retarded youth into the workforce. In many communities, socialization activity centers have been established to foster skills to ease the person's entry into a work setting after the formal educational program is terminated. Opportunities to work for pay are provided in sheltered workshops where behavior management techniques usually are successfully employed to teach workers how to assemble salable products (Weicker, 1984).

Through the cooperation of three community agencies, including the Maine State Commission of the Arts and Humanities, a sheltered workshop for mentally retarded adults—the Spindleworks—was established in Brunswick, Maine in 1977. This workshop at first made spun products and tapestries of good quality, and later expanded to include basketry, woodcut prints, and clown makeup (Faber, 1980).

Problems that employers must solve in hiring the handicapped concern issues of environmental safety, fair allocation of benefits, and acceptance by other employees—all obstacles that can be overcome, as evidenced by the McDonald's project. McDonald's funded a 2-year project that demonstrated the employability of adults who were moderately or mildly retarded, and whose capabilities were carefully matched to their duties. Attrition was low through both years of the program. The workers were accepted by other employees and they gained financially (Brickey and Campbell, 1981).

Leisure Time. The ability to develop leisure-time activities and a social network of friends and relatives may be critical to the adolescent or young adult's survival in the community and to his perception of himself as a capable and confident human being. However, leisure time programs do not fare very well. There are problems with providing transportation to facilities which are not always barrier free, and suitable friends and companions are difficult to find.

Salzberg and Lanford (1981) described a project that involved pairing residents in community or institutional settings with normal adult volunteers. Partners were matched according to interests, experiences, and preference for leisure-time activities. The physical limitations and skill levels of the clients were also considered. At least once a week each pair of subjects mutually agreed upon an activity, such as attending a movie or the theater, or eating out. Skills, including how to purchase a theater ticket, how to locate a theater seat, and how to applaud were learned for the first time. How to order a meal and how to behave appropriately in a restaurant were learned in actual settings. This approach greatly facilitated the clients' later recall and application of those social skills in addition to providing them with friendship and enjoyable leisure-time experience.

NURSING INTERVENTION □ Whether a nurse is part of an institutional or community residence staff, or functioning as a community mental health nurse, she can provide valuable support and guidance to the client undergoing environmental transition, as described below:

1. Leading support groups. Support groups facilitate expression of fears and anxieties and allow the client to see and hear that similar fears are shared by others. Group settings allow the shy client to pace his own involvement without feeling intimidated. Peer relationships that ease the transition and result in lasting friendship are often positive outcomes of such groups.

2. Structuring role play. Simulations of common social interactions can be first played out within safe supportive environments. Videotaping can augment learning by providing the client with concrete evidence for self-evaluation.

3. Role modeling. Conscious and consistent implementation of the rules of social respect and social conduct, as during nurse interaction with each client and with staff, is a powerful method for teaching social roles.

4. Behavioral analysis. Nurses who interact with mentally retarded persons should be well trained in behavior management theory and its application. Many self-help and social skills can be successfully learned if they are broken down into sequential steps, and consistently monitored and reinforced by all those involved with the client. Conversely, undesirable behaviors can be eliminated and replaced with suitable alternatives without the use of demeaning punishment.

5. Coordinator/advocate. The roles of coordinator and advocate are extremely important during the transition period. The nurse who has established a warm trusting relationship with her clients is the person in whom the clients will confide their fears, frustrations, and needs. Knowledge of community resources and the ability to work collaboratively with other professionals in planning for change will give the nurse a pivotal role in establishing a network of supports for clients.

6. Family support and consultation. Landesman-Dwyer, et al. (1978) noted that when group home residents maintained close contact with their parents, they tended to be socially isolated in their new residential settings. This suggests that the nurse needs to work with families who may have trouble letting go or who need help in forming new relationships with their children. Parents may object to a more independent living situation for the child out of fear that he will not be able to cope with transition. Landesman-Dwyer (1981) reported that among a group of 50 families, 66 percent initially disapproved of their children's community placement; within a year's time only 8 percent still disapproved. Here again, the community health nurse can prevent maladaptive behavior by identifying and explaining these issues to family members before the change is made.

7. Consultation. Providing consultation services to the staff members of residential and community facilities about client needs, modification of staff attitudes and behavior, establishment of measurable and useful goals, and therapeutic intervention to solve day-to-day problems is one of the services offered by masters-prepared nurses (Flagg, 1982).

Ongoing Community Living

Marriage and Parenthood. As late as 1972, one-fourth of the states prohibited mentally retarded persons to marry. This was a carry-over from the Mental Deficiency Act of 1913 which prohibited all such persons to marry (Evans, 1983). At present, women with lower cognitive functioning have a better chance of marrying than do men because they fit comfortably into the traditional homemaking role and are often protected by a male provider (Schulman, 1980). The marriage rate of those who are mildly mentally retarded is only slightly below the national rate (Ingalls, 1978).

Because of the value-laden expectations of our society about parenting, persons with cognitive deficits who become parents are subjected to close scrutiny. They often lose custody of their children because of documented neglect. Data on the frequency of child abuse or neglect are difficult to interpret because of poor study designs and biases. Many times it is the inability of the parent to adequately explain what happened in a given situation rather than his negligence that precipitates a legal action. The review by Schilling, et al. (1982) suggests that up to half of abusing mothers are of borderline intelligence or below, though caution is needed in interpreting these findings because of the lack of uniformity in defining levels of impairment.

When adolescents and young adults are exposed to the responsibilities of child care as demonstrated in hospitals, day-care, or boarding school settings, they frequently recognize their limitations and choose not to have children. Young couples preparing to marry need to have the opportunity to experience parenting behaviors in a caring structured setting.

Self-Perceptions. Literature reporting the feelings of mentally retarded persons who have been living in the community is sparse. One self-evaluation survey conducted by Judge (1983) revealed that many felt a need to conform to social standards and often hid from public view. Those who had normal siblings were aware of the latter's cognitive superiority and of the fact that people disliked and feared them.

Koegel and Edgerton (1982) state that mentally retarded blacks can integrate into cultural and familial networks more easily than whites, nevertheless, their group of blacks were aware of their limitations in language and common knowledge (such as knowing how to spell their children's names). They shied away from everyday interactions with others lest their inappropriate responses betray them. Vacillation between such thoughts as "I'm not dumb, just slow" to the despair of "Why did this happen to me?" reflected their painful perceptions of reality.

There is a tendency by most people to talk to anyone who is labeled as mentally retarded as though that person had the understanding of a 4-year-old, or to talk about him to the parent or caretaker while he is physically present—as though he isn't there at all! The hurt and rejection that the person feels can be measured by his re-

luctance to be part of the mainstream of community life.

Criminal Justice. There is no conclusive relationship between general intelligence and delinquency or criminal behavior, yet the percentage of arrests and convictions of mentally retarded persons is higher than in the general population (Menolascino and McCann, 1983). A number of factors come into play. Often, these persons become involved in criminal activities at the instigation of others, while not understanding the implications thereof, and they frequently are the only ones who remain long enough to get caught. They do not understand their legal rights. They will often confess to a crime just because—for once—someone is interested and willing to listen to them or because they are susceptible to intimidation under cross-examination (Evans, 1983). The public defenders who most often represent mentally retarded persons have little awareness of their clients' mental limitations and therefore do not present realistic explanations for their behavior.

According to Evans (1983), the mentally retarded person, once in jail, is more likely than others to complete his sentence without parole since he often does not qualify for early release. In addition, specific programs to assist mentally retarded persons in preparing for release are rarely viewed as cost effective. It is ironic that a jail sentence for this person, caught in the commission of an illegal act, may be more humane than the alternative of institutionalization until he is deemed fit to stand trial. As Evans (1983) pointed out, the institutionalized individual may be isolated from society for a longer time than if he had served the specific sentence for the crime. In fact, many of these persons end up serving a life sentence for minor offenses that result in little or no incarceration when committed by the normal person.

Social Conscience. The increasing social awareness of citizens who happen to be mentally retarded is reflected in such efforts as the People First organization, which was founded to influence the views of policymakers on issues concerning the intellectually handicapped. Noteworthy publications include the *Milwaukee Citizen*, a newspaper by and for the mentally retarded, and the *Polling Magazine*, as well as publications by individuals. The National Association for Retarded Citizens produces and distributes materials and training packages for parents and others who deliver services to mentally retarded persons.

The Aging Process

If there is little available literature about the feelings of mentally retarded persons, there is less still on the aging process. We do know that persons with Down syndrome seem to age more rapidly than others and are more susceptible to Alzheimer's disease. Features associated with Alzheimer's disease have been found at autopsy of those as young as 40 years, though clinical manifestations are often not identified because of professional or caretaker failure to differentiate symptoms from the expected behavior under the stereotype of Down syndrome (Psychiatric Aspects of Mental Retardation Newsletter, 1982, Down's syndrome).

Richards (1976) summarizes factors associated with increased risk of dying at an earlier age, including complications of congenital heart disease, seizure disorders, and cerebral palsy. Impairment in swallowing, coughing (resulting in aspiration pneumonia), and in general hygiene, along with the other factors, increase mortality in this group whether residing in the community or in institutional settings.

Edgerton and associates (1967) conducted a study of formerly institutionalized citizens 6 years after discharge, about a decade later (Edgerton and Bercovici, 1976), and finally, after 20 years of community living (Edgerton, et al., 1984). The studies included the subjects' ability to maintain a living (which was the criterion originally used to effect their institutional discharge), their available supports and benefactors, marital status, use of leisure time, and feelings of being stigmatized by institutionalization. Based upon the data collected at discharge, the researchers first made predictions about the subjects' status 6 years later. Their accuracy was less than 50 percent, and even when they did predict in the right direction, it was for the wrong reasons. No one factor, even employment, guaranteed success or failure, but combinations of factors seemed to operate together. Most subjects were at least as well off 12 years later as at 6 years after discharge. They valued leisure time and friendships, viewed their low-paying jobs as instrumental rather than as self-defining, and seemed little bothered by their former institutional stigma. Edgerton was struck

by the changing social systems and corresponding values to which he attributed the inaccuracy of his predictions. The rigid work ethic of earlier years had given way to the realization that not everyone could have a job, and financial assistance had become an acceptable alternative.

Fifteen subjects of the original sample of 48, with an average age of 56 years and average IQ of 61.7, comprised the 20-year sample. Only four persons' life situations were worse than they had been a decade earlier; for three people, life had improved; the health of 10 had declined. For some, the aging process offered an explanation of limitations, as though of recent occurrence; most, however, maintained their resilience and zest for life and expressed a belief that desired outcomes were effected through their own actions. This attitude may have been due in part to a nonresponsive social agency system since not one of them had received help from agencies funded to assist mentally retarded citizens (Edgerton, et al., 1984).

☐ Mental Illness in the Mentally Retarded

As we have discussed, the cerebral deficits associated with significant mental retardation limit problem-solving abilities to concrete situations. Often, visual cues given by others in social interactions are not perceived, or are misinterpreted. Receptive language problems, related to both hearing loss and limited cognitive processing, contribute further to confusion about the meaning of social messages, while expressive language limitations frequently lead to the person's inability to accurately convey his own feelings, actions, or intents. Multiple physical handicaps such as cerebral palsy or seizure disorders limit or distort self-expression and contribute to a general lack of self-esteem. All of these factors place the person at greater than average risk of mental illness (Eaton and Menolascino, 1982).

ENVIRONMENTAL FACTORS CONTRIBUTING TO MENTAL ILLNESS

Unrealistic family expectations and related experiences early in the life of the child who has an intellectual deficit may pave the way for later mental health problems. If the child is physically active and suffers mild cognitive impairment, family members and others expect him to achieve normal levels of cognitive, psychomotor, and social competence. There may be negative sanctions such as withdrawal of attention or even of love and affection when those expectations are unfulfilled. Increasing developmental demands and awareness of peers' perceptions of him as slow or different serve to reinforce the child's already negative self-image. Repeatedly falling short of the mark precipitates frustration, anxiety, and fear of failure, which are often manifested in withdrawal or aggression. Because the child physically appears normal and his superficial functioning is adequate, there may be significant delay in the initiation of appropriate therapeutic and educational services. Continued ambivalence, scapegoating, or rejection by others can exacerbate the problem until it reaches critical proportions. The results are often seen in the chronically sullen and defiant youth or adolescent who becomes unmanageable in the classroom and in the community. Available data suggest that many mildly mentally retarded individuals who are admitted to institutions or correctional centers or who turn to drugs or alcohol have had such life experiences (Reid, 1980; Menolascino and Strider, 1981).

At the other end of the spectrum are parents who, when told about their child's mental handicap, react by protecting him from all sources of frustration. This approach severely limits opportunities to encounter life challenges which are necessary in developing effective coping skills. When this situation persists, the child's self-concept remains undeveloped and he becomes solely dependent upon the environment rather than on his own inner resources to guide his behavior.

Serious family disruption is often brought about by unresolved grief over the birth of a child perceived as defective, or by the family's inability to develop effective supports and coping strategies to deal with the stressors associated with caring for the child. The inconsistencies in family members' behavior and in their expectations for one another that result from such upheaval are fruitful grounds for mental pathology in the child and family members as well.

Childhood phobias, which have a greater incidence in mentally retarded children than in the general population, are seen more often in youngsters who experience multiple negative life situations such as separations, frightening natural events, injuries, or threatening experiences involving animals or water. These may be more difficult to identify because the child's retreat or resistance tends to be global and generalized rather than specifically directed (Psychiatric Aspects of Mental Retardation, 1982, Phobic Behavior).

For the young child who is unfortunate enough to have been placed in inadequate institutional surroundings, the risk of interpersonal detachment is great. Multiple caretakers who convey little warmth or caring provide conflicting messages to and expectations of the child. The results of such patterns of interactions are seen in the child's indiscriminate approach to strangers as he attempts to find human affection, and in his general underachievement. If he is later discharged into the community without a comprehensive mechanism of support, adequate adjustment is not likely to occur. Eaton and Menolascino (1982) noted that personality disorders were overrepresented as compared with the general population, and that most of their clients with that diagnosis had mild or borderline retardation and a history of prior institutionalization.

Developmental factors such as the onset of puberty can also precipitate problems. In the mentally retarded population, the timing of changes in hormone levels and/or accelerated growth are often out of synchrony with expected cognitive changes. The resulting disequilibrium may manifest itself in overreaction to even minimal stress.

While the effects of labeling are unclear as to a causal relationship between mental retardation and mental health disturbances, a positive association has been identified between depression and lack of adequate social supports (Reiss and Benson, 1985). Indeed, the myth of the "prince charming" personality (always cheerful and easygoing) believed to characterize persons having Down syndrome, has been dispelled by the diagnosis of severe depression in persons with this syndrome (Sovner and Hurley, 1983). Further, depression may increase in this group if the improvement in educational management, which has significantly raised the measured IQ levels of many with Down syndrome, is not accompanied by an equal effort in addressing mental health needs.

RECOGNITION OF MANIFESTATIONS OF MENTAL ILLNESS

Menolascino and Strider (1981) caution against the tendency toward simplistic diagnoses that place blame for all observed deviations under one category. The individual with impaired cerebral functioning may exhibit behaviors that directly reflect either organic impairment, or the emotional trauma that stems from an inability to cope with environmental demands, or both. The concept of "dual diagnosis" implies a full range of possible combinations of mental disorders and degrees of mental deficiency. It places the burden of proof upon the practitioners, who must provide behavioral descriptions to support their diagnoses.

Descriptions of mental illness in those who are mentally retarded have, until very recently, been based upon observations of persons who were housed in institutions for the mentally retarded. When the negative characteristics of many of those environments are considered, it is easy to recognize the limited validity of such studies. Punitive, judgmental, and highly restrictive attitudes and behaviors of administration and staff, lack of developmentally stimulating activities, untoward effects of medications, and rare opportunities for social, recreational, or sexual expression which prevailed in those settings not long ago would increase the risk of "deviant" behavior in anyone, regardless of intellectual capacity.

More recent data based on subjects living in the community suggest that the types of mental illnesses diagnosed in people who are mentally retarded approximate those found in the general population (Sovner and Hurley, 1983; Eaton and Menolascino, 1982). However, because many of the behaviors that would lead to a diagnosis of mental illness in persons who are not mentally retarded are often erroneously considered as characteristic of those who are, there is a tendency to miss or delay the diagnosis in clients who can least afford it. Well-trained professional staff who carefully assess and document the changes in day-to-day behavior patterns of their clients within structured living, work, educational, or leisure-time settings can assist in the early identification and intervention process. Diagnosis of mental illness in institutionalized individuals is often impeded because of poor documentation of behavioral deterioration over time (Eaton and Menolascino, 1982), and because of misinterpretations of behavior as a result of professional bias and stereotyping (Reiss and Szyszko, 1983).

Since diminished ability to attend to stimuli, memory deficits, hyper- or hypo-activity levels and impulsivity are common characteristics of significant mental retardation or are side effects of prescribed medications, they are not always useful indicators of mental health problems in this population. In clients whose biologic mental impairment already manifests itself in behavioral or motor patterns that in others would be considered signs of mental illness, the professional must look more closely at changes in levels of those behaviors, as well as changes in the client's general mood, intensity of reaction, interpersonal interaction, and vegetative functioning such as weight fluctuations and sleeping patterns (Eaton and Menolascino, 1982).

The need for careful assessment is particularly important in the severely mentally retarded child or adult who routinely exhibits primitive or self-stimulating behaviors such as rocking, hand waving, rumination, or skin picking. At first glance it would seem reasonable to assume these are always deviant behaviors. Yet a person with severe cognitive and sensory motor deficits may have few opportunities to interact with objects or persons to obtain a sense of their properties and stimulus effects upon him. The only alternative stimuli that may be open to him are manifested at this infantile level (Eaton and Menolascino, 1982). This is not to say mental illness does not occur in the severely mentally retarded person. It does, and requires early diagnosis. Diminished eye contact or other changes in interaction style with caretakers may be early indicators of mental illness in this group.

Indicators of specific disorders in those with mental retardation can approximate those seen in the general population. However, some characteristic manifestations are qualitatively different as a function of the limitations on cognitive capabilities of the clients. For instance, manic euphoria will probably not be as infectious as it is in others. Concrete thinking limits the range of flight of ideas and renders them far less clever than when they are generated by a person of normal intelligence. Distractibility and poor judgment are not useful indicators for making a diagnosis of mania because these are commonly exhibited in mentally retarded persons who are not suffering from mental illness (PAMR Newsletter, 1982, Diagnosing Mania), although onset of tantrums and destructiveness may be useful clues (Sovner and Hurley, 1983).

A measured IQ of at least 45 is reported to be necessary to provide a valid self-report of disturbance in mental health (PAMR Newsletter, 1983, Schizophrenia). However, diagnosis of paranoid schizophrenia has been made based upon nonverbal gestures and drawings of perceived attackers in those with lesser capacity. Bizarre rituals and interpersonal distancing are also behaviors associated with schizophrenia in the mentally retarded (Monfils and Menolascino, 1983).

Psychoneurotic disorders which are a common diagnosis in persons categorized as functioning in the high moderate or mild ranges of retardation have been linked to long-term frustration resulting from trying to live up to unyielding demands of others. An impoverished, simple repertoire of defenses leaves the individual open to acts of impulsive behavior, mood swings, and regression as the only means of expressing his distress.

Diagnosis and treatment approaches that are useful in the general population are often useful for the mentally retarded as well. When verbal skills are limited, other ways of eliciting self-expression must be used, for example, Rorschach techniques, drama, and doll play.

Crucial to the treatment approaches designed for the person who is mentally ill are the realignment efforts directed toward family, residence personnel, and others who interact closely with the client. This, for example, will often include planning alterations in value systems and the teaching of a positive means to facilitate social adaptive responses.

Behavior management approaches work well across diagnostic areas because goals for desired behavioral outcomes can be clearly specified. There is a wide range of methods to effect desired change, all of which can be specifically monitored, documented, evaluated, and modified to achieve and maintain the goal state. Psychopharmacologic agents are also useful, especially when there is need to rapidly control socially offensive behavior which might otherwise result in a more restrictive living situation. However, because of the slower metabolic rates of many in this population, the risk of toxicity is increased.

Unless habilitation efforts are emphasized through maximizing vocational and recreational potential as well as strengthening family coping and interaction skills, therapy will have no lasting effect. Active collaboration with community resources such as day-care programs, respite services, and home health care agencies is vital in carrying out long-term follow-up.

■ Enrichment Activities

DISCUSSION QUESTIONS

1. There are both positive and negative outcomes of labeling children in order to get them educational services. What are these outcomes?

How well do the benefits versus the costs of labeling balance each other out in the short term and the long term?

2. What direction do you believe social policy should take regarding the needs of those with intellectual handicaps? Have we gone too far or not far enough?

LEARNING ACTIVITIES

1. Visit your local school district to see what kinds of activities are implemented to facilitate peer acceptance of disabilities. If "Kids on the Block" or some similar activity is available, arrange to observe the presentation, including the question-and-answer session between puppets and students. (For information, write "Kids on the Block," The Washington Building, Suite 510, Washington, D.C. 20005.)

2. Investigate the programs and supports available in your community that facilitate sequential structured transitions to independent living. What steps must be taken to secure this kind of assistance? Are alternative living situations adequate to meet the needs of residents in the community?

3. Look into specific community-based programs that focus upon the friendship and sexuality needs and/or social policy activism for persons who are mentally retarded. How successful are they in meeting their goals? What problems do they encounter?

4. Participate in or observe an infant stimulation session for a client who is at risk for significant sensory, motor, or cognitive delay. These programs are mandated to be provided by your school system by P.L. 94-142.

5. Participate in or observe a behavior management program that is designed to teach a self-help skill to a child who is mentally disabled. This should be available through your school system or local mental health center.

6. Design a teaching plan for a young adult about to enter a semi-independent living situation.

■ Recommended Readings

BY PERSONS LABELED AS MENTALLY RETARDED AND BY THEIR ADVOCATES

Williams, Paul, and Shoultz, Bonnie. *We can speak for ourselves.* Indiana University Press, 1982.

Hunt, Neigle. *The world of Neigle Hunt.* Out of print, but worth finding. 1967.

Perske, R. *Hope for the families.* Nashville, TN: Abingdon Press, 1981.

Perske, R., Clifton, A., McLean, B., Stein, J. *Mealtimes for the severely and profoundly handicapped persons.* Baltimore: University Park Press, 1977.

Perske, R. *New life in the neighborhood.* Nashville, TN: Abingdon Press, 1981.

Roberts, Nancy. *David.* Richmond, VA: John Knox Press. 1968.

INTERVENTION AND TEACHING AIDS

Fisher, Krajicek, and Borthick. *Sex education for the developmentally disabled: A guide for parents, teachers and professionals.* Baltimore: University Park Press, 1974.

Talarico, Ron (ed.). *Taxonomy of behavioral objectives for habilitation of mentally handicapped persons.* Portland, OR: Portland Habilitation Center, 1982.

■ References

American Psychiatric Association Committee on Nomenclature and Statistics. *Diagnostic and statistical manual of mental disorders* (3rd ed.). Washington, DC: American Psychiatric Association, 1980.

American Dietetic Association. Infant and child nutrition: Concerns regarding the developmentally disabled. *Journal of the american dietetic association,* 78, 1981:443–452.

Anastasi, A. Heredity, environment, and the question "how?" *Psychological review,* 65, 1958:197–208.

Barsch, R.H. *The parent of the handicapped child: The study of child rearing practices.* Springfield, IL: Charles C. Thomas, 1968.

Bell, R.Q. A reinterpretation of the direction of effects in studies of socialization. *Psychological review,* 75, 1968:81–95.

Bloom, B.S. *Stability and change in human characteristics.* New York: John Wiley & Sons, 1964.

Brickey, M., and Campbell, K. Fast food employment of moderately and mildly mentally retarded adults: The McDonald's project. *Mental retardation,* 19, 3, 1981:113–119.

Brightman, A. But their brain is broken: Young children's conceptions of retardation. In *Promise and performance,* ACT's guide to T.V. programming for children. Children with special needs (Harmonay, M., ed.). Cambridge, MA: Ballinger, 1977.

Brison, D. Definition, diagnosis and classification. In *Mental retardation: Appraisal, education, and rehabilitation* (Baumeister, A., ed.). Chicago: Aldine-Atherton, Inc., 1967.

Bruininks, R., Thurlow, M.L., Thurman, S.K., and Fior-

elli, J. (1980). Deinstitutionalization & community services. In *Mental retardation and developmental disabilities* (Wortis, J., ed.). New York: Brunner/Mazel.

Chamberlain, A., Rauh, J., Passer, A., McGrath, M., and Burket, R. Issues in fertility control for mentally retarded female adolescents: 1. Sexual activity, sexual abuse, and contraception. *Pediatrics,* 73, 4, 1984:445–450.

Clark, A., and Clarke, A. *Early experience: Myth and evidence.* New York: The Free Press, 1976.

Coffman, T., and Harrison, M. Transition shock and adjustments of mentally retarded persons. *Mental retardation,* 18, 1, 1980:3–7.

Danford, D., and Huber, A. Pica among retarded adults. *American journal of mental deficiency.* 87, 2, 1982:141–146.

Denhoff, E. Current status of infant stimulation or enrichment programs for children with developmental disabilities. *Pediatrics,* 67, 1, 1982:32–37.

Dingman, H.F., and Tarjan, G. Mental retardation and the normal distribution curve. *American journal of mental deficiency,* 64, 1960:991–994.

Eaton, L., and Menolascino, F. Psychiatric disorders in mental retardation: Types, problems and challenges. *American journal of psychiatry,* 139, 10, 1982:1297–1303.

Edgerton, R.B. The cload of competence: Stigma in the lives of the mentally retarded. Berkley: University of California Press, 1967.

Edgerton, R.B., and Bercovici, S.M. The cloak of competence: Years later. *American journal of mental deficiency,* 80, 5, 1976:485–497.

Edgerton, R.B., Bollinger, M., and Herr, B. The cloak of competence: After two decades. *American journal of mental deficiency,* 88, 4, 1984:345–351.

Elkind, D. *Children and adolescents.* 2d ed. New York: Oxford University Press, 1974.

Erikson, E. *Childhood and society.* 2d ed. New York: Norton, 1963.

Evans, D. *The lives of mentally retarded people.* Boulder, CO: Westview Press, 1983.

Faber, M.A. *Social context of helping: A review of the literature on alternative care for the physically and mentally handicapped.* U.S. Department of Health & Human Services, Public Health Service, Alcohol, Drug Abuse & Mental Health Administration, 1980.

Flagg, J.M. Consultation in community residences for the chronically mentally ill. *Journal of psychiatric nursing and mental health services,* 20, 12, December 1982:30–34.

Grossman, H. (ed.). *Manual on terminology and classification in mental retardation.* Washington, D.C.: American Association on Mental Deficiency, 1973.

———. *Manual on terminology and classification in mental retardation.* Washington, D.C.: American Association on Mental Deficiency, 1977.

Haywood, H.C. (ed.). *Socio-cultural aspects of mental retardation.* New York: Appleton-Century-Crofts, 1970.

Heber, R.F. A manual on terminology and classification in mental retardation. *American journal of mental deficiency,* 64, monogr. 1959.

Heber, R.F. A manual on terminology and classification in mental retardation. *American Journal of Mental Deficiency,* 1959, 64, Monogr. Suppl (Rev. ed.), 1961.

Heshusius, L. Sexuality, intimacy and persons we label mentally retarded: What they think—what we think. *Mental retardation,* 20, 4, 1982:164–169.

Horowitz, F., and Paden, L. The effectiveness of environmental intervention programs. In *Review of child development research: Child development and social policy.* Vol. 3. (Caldwell, B., and Riccuiti, H.). Chicago: University of Chicago Press, 1973.

Hunt, J. McV. *Intelligence and experience.* New York: Ronald Press, 1961.

Hurley, R. *Poverty and mental retardation: A causal relationship.* New York: Vintage Books, 1969.

Hymovich, D. Assessment of the chronically ill child and family. In *Family health care: General perspectives.* Vol. 1. (Hymovich, D., and Barnard, M., eds.). New York: McGraw Hill, 1979:280–293.

Ingalls, R.R. *Mental retardation.* New York: John Wiley & Sons, 1978.

Jones, E. PL 94-142 and the role of school nurses in caring for handicapped children. *Journal of school health,* March 1979:147–156.

Judge, C. Self awareness of mentally retarded persons. *Psychiatric aspects of mental retardation newsletter,* 2, 1, 1983: 42–43.

Koegel, P., and Edgerton, R. Labeling and the perception of handicap among black mildly mentally retarded adults. *American journal of mental deficiency,* 87, 3, 1982:266–276.

Krajicek, M.J. Developmental disability and human sexuality. *Nursing clinics of north america,* 17, 3, 1982:371–386.

Landesman-Dwyer, S. Living in the community. *American journal of mental deficiency,* 86, 3, 1981:223–234.

Landesman-Dwyer, S., Stein, J.G., and Sackett, G.P. A behavioral and ecological study of group homes. In *Observing behavior, Volume I: Theory and applications in mental retardation* (Sachett, G.P., ed.). Baltimore: University Park Press, 1978.

MacMillan, D., Jones, R.L., and Aloia, G.F. Mentally retarded label: A theoretical analysis and review of research. *American journal of mental deficiency,* 79, 1974:241–261.

Menolascino, F., and McCann, B. *Mental health and mental retardation.* Baltimore: University Park Press, 1983.

Menolascino, F., and Strider, F. Advances in the pre-

vention and treatment of mental retardation. In *American handbook of psychiatry.* 2d ed. (Arieti, S., ed.). New York: Basic Books, 1981.

Mercer, J.R. Sociological perspectives on mild mental retardation. In *Socio-cultural aspects of mental retardation.* (Haywood, H.C., ed.). New York: Appleton-Century-Crofts, 1970.

———. *Labelling the mentally retarded.* Berkeley: University of California Press, 1973.

Monfils, M.J., and Menolascino, F.J. Mental illness in the mentally retarded: Challenges for social work. *Social work in health care,* 9, 1, 1983:71–85.

Public Health Currents. Nutrition of children with handicapping conditions, 18, 1, 1978:1–6.

Olshansky, S. Chronic sorrow: A response to having a mentally defective child. *Social casework,* 43, 1962:191–194.

Passer, A., Rauh, J., Chamberlain, A., McGrath, M., and Burket, R. Issues in fertility control for mentally retarded female adolescents: 11 parental attitudes toward sterilization. *Pediatrics,* 73, 4, 1984:451–454.

Psychiatric aspects of mental retardation newsletter. Diagnosing mania in the mentally retarded. *PAMR Newsletter,* 1, 3, 1982:9–10.

Psychiatric aspects of mental retardation newsletter. Down's syndrome: A psychiatric perspective. *PAMR Newsletter,* 1, 9, 1982:31–34.

Psychiatric aspects of mental retardation newsletter. Phobic behavior and mentally retarded persons. *PAMR Newsletter,* 1, 11, 1982:41–44.

Psychiatric aspects of mental retardation newsletter. Schizophrenia *PAMR Newsletter* 2, 7, 1983:25–28.

Ramey, C., and Finkelstein, N. Psychosocial mental retardation: A biological and social coalescence. In *Psychosocial influences in retarded performance* Vol. 1. (Begam, M., Haywood, H.C., and Garber, H., eds.). Baltimore: University Park Press, 1981.

Reid, A.H. Psychiatric disorders in mentally handicapped children: A clinical and follow-up study. *Journal of mental deficiency research,* 24, 1980:278–298.

Reiss, S., and Benson, B. Psychosocial correlates of depression in mentally retarded adults: 1. Minimal social support and stigmatization. *American journal of mental deficiency,* 89, 4, 1985:331–337.

Reiss, S., and Szyszko, J. Diagnostic overshadowing and professional experience with mentally retarded persons. *American journal of mental deficiency,* 87, 4, 1983:396–402.

Richards, B.W. Health and longevity. In *Mental retardation and developmental disabilities.* Vol. 8. (Wortis, J., ed.). New York: Brunner/Mazel, 1976.

Robinson, C., and Robinson, J.H. Sensorimotor functions and cognitive development. In *Systematic instruction of the moderately and severely handicapped* (Snell, M.E., ed.). Columbus, OH: Charles E. Merrill Publishing Co., 1983.

Robinson, N., and Robinson, H. *The mentally retarded child.* 2d ed. New York: McGraw-Hill, 1976.

Rosenberg, S. *Family performance prediction study I.* (U.S. OE grant project, number OEG-0-74-7449) 1977.

Sameroff, A., and Chandler, M. Reproductive risk and the continuum of caretaking casualty. In *Review of child development research.* Vol. 4. (Horowitz, F., ed.). Chicago: University of Chicago Press, 1975.

Salzberg, C., and Lanford, C. Community integration of mentally retarded adults through leisure activity. *Mental retardation,* 19, 3, 1981:227–131.

Scheerenberger, R.C. Public residential services, 1981: Status and trends. *Mental retardation,* 20, 5, 1982:210–215.

Schilling, R., Schinke, S., Blythe, B., and Barth, R. Child maltreatment and mentally retarded parents: Is there a relationship? *Mental retardation,* 20, 5, 1982:201–209.

Schulman, E. *Focus on the retarded adult programs and services.* St. Louis: Mosby Company, 1980.

Simeonsson, R. Medication effects in handicapped preschool children. *Topics in early childhood special education,* July, 1981: 61–75.

Simeonsson, R., Cooper, D., and Scheiner, A. A review and analysis of the effectiveness of early intervention programs. *Pediatrics,* 69, 1982:635–641.

Solnit, A., and Stark, M. Mourning and the birth of a defective child. *Journal for the psychoanalytic study of the child,* 16, 1961:523–537.

Sovner, R., and Hurley, A. Do the mentally retarded suffer from affective illness? *Arch gen. psychiatry,* 40, 1983:61–67.

Sroufe, A. Socioemotional development. In *Handbook of infant development* (Osofsky, J., ed.). New York: John Wiley & Sons, 1979:462–516.

Swan, W. Efficacy studies in early child special education: An overview. *Journal of the division for early childhood,* 4, 1981:1–4.

Weicker, L. Defining liberty for handicapped Americans. *American psychologist,* 39, 5, 1984:518–523.

Williams, R., and Ewing, S. Consumer roulette: The shopping patterns of mentally retarded persons. *Mental retardation,* 19, 4, 1981:145–149.

Wolfensberger, W. Counseling the parents of the retarded. In *Mental retardation: Appraisal, education, and rehabilitation* (Baumeister, A.A., ed.). Chicago: Aldine-Atherton, Inc., 1967:329–400.

———. *The principle of normalization in human services.* Toronto: National Institute on Mental Retardation, 1972.

———. The definition of normalization: Update, problems, disagreements, and misunderstandings. In *Normalization, social integration, and community services* (Flynn, R.J., and Nitsch, K.E., eds.). Baltimore: University Park Press, 1980a:71–115.

———. Research, empiricism, and the principle of normalization. In *Normalization, social integration, and community services* (Flynn, R.J., and Nitsch, K.E., eds.). Baltimore: University Park Press, 1980b:117–129.

———. Social role valorization: A proposed new term for the principle of normalization. *Mental retardation,* 21, 6, 1983:234–239.

World Health Organization. *International classification of diseases.* 8th rev. New York: WHO, 1968.

Wright, J., Granger, R., and Sameroff, A. Parental acceptance and developmental handicaps. In *Severely handicapped young children and their families* (Blacker, J. ed.). Orlando: Academic Press, 1984.

Yarrow, L. Historical perspectives and future directions in infant development. In *Handbook of infant development* (Osofsky, J., ed.). New York: John Wiley & Sons, 1979.

Zigler, E., and Balla, D. Selecting outcome variables in evaluations of early childhood special education programs. *Topics in early childhood special education,* 1, 1982:11–22.

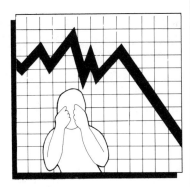

25

Coping with Acute and Chronic Illness

Barbara Geach

Learning Objectives

Upon completion of this chapter, the reader will be able to:

1. Understand the many real or threatened losses entailed in illness.

2. List the adaptive tasks posed by illness.

3. Recognize the coping behavior appropriate to acute and chronic illness.

4. Identify personal and situational characteristics that influence coping.

5. Identify intervention strategies that facilitate family and individual coping.

Before I got sick, I never gave my body too much thought. I took it for granted that it did what I wanted it to. That's all changed now.

Statements like this from clients reveal the serious consequences of physical illness, not just for the biophysical but also for the psychosocial aspect of a person's life. If we pull that statement apart a little, what do we find?

☐ The speaker is a person who has enjoyed good health until recently.

☐ The speaker did not think about his physical status, but just assumed that he'd be able to count on his body to work predictably and satisfactorily.

☐ With the advent of physical illness, both the satisfactory functioning and the predictability have ceased to be certain.

☐ This change *in itself* presents a challenge or threat with which the speaker has to cope—independent of the challenge or threat posed by the illness.

■ *Point of Emphasis*

Among the roles the nurse may assume with physically ill clients is the psychosocial role. This will consist, first, in helping the client to cope with the changes associated with illness. Second, the nurse can act as a facilitator in the adjustment of the client's family to the client's illness. And third, the nurse can act as a liaison between the client and the other professionals responsible for his care and increase these colleagues' awareness of the coping tasks that his illness creates for him.

☐ Basic Terms

In the quotation with which this chapter began, it was unclear whether the client was speaking of an acute illness or a chronic illness. For the purpose of this discussion, acute illness:

☐ Is sudden in onset
☐ Is relatively short in duration
☐ Requires a relatively brief period of treatment
☐ Responds fully to the treatment
☐ Leaves little or no residual effects, and these not disabling ones (A person has an

abdominal scar after an appendectomy, for instance, but this residual effect has no influence on his subsequent functioning.)

Such acute illness has what Strauss and Glaser (1975) have called an expected trajectory, in which the person has acute symptoms, presents himself for treatment, responds to the treatment, recuperates, and gets fully well.

Chronic illness, on the other hand, may have had an initially sudden onset, but generally it

☐ Appears gradually
☐ Lasts a long time (often for the duration of the client's life)
☐ Requires a long period of treatment (which usually only controls or palliates the effect of the illness)
☐ Often requires some special training or remedial efforts on the part of the client, his family, or both, in collaboration with health professionals (A person who has had a stroke, for instance, may never stop taking anticoagulant medication and may need physical therapy to restore functioning and to help other muscles take over the work of the paralyzed ones.)

Of course, a chronically ill person may have occasional exacerbations during which he is acutely ill. These exacerbations may be caused by fluctuations characteristic of the illness; by intercurrent complications to which the illness predisposes the client; or by responses to treatment or to treatment side-effects. But even when the client's chronic illness is flaring up in an acute exacerbation, his situation differs from that of a client with possibly very similar symptoms, but no history of chronic illness. The client, his family, and health professionals all operate differently when the underlying problem is chronic from how they do when it is acute. This is partly because acute illness is appraised quite differently by all concerned.

Both acute and chronic illness call on the client's and family's ability to cope. The specific coping strategies employed, however, are not all the same in acute illness as they are in chronic illness. Coping strategies that are effective and appropriate in an initial emergency may significantly impair the client's and family's functioning if they are continued beyond the acute period of illness or exacerbation.

It is important to know whether a client is suffering from acute or chronic physical illness because, for one thing, this will give information about whether he is still responding to the shock, fear, and pain of acute illness, or is describing a state of affairs that has been going on for some years, since chronic illness was first diagnosed. Or, to put it another way, it is important to know whether the client's statement reflects the disequilibrium characteristic of crisis, or reflects the new pattern of equilibrium which has become established since chronic physical illness was first recognized. This distinction is important both for prevention and for intervention.

For another thing, the sick role for acutely ill clients is markedly different from the sick role for chronically ill clients. Craig and Edwards (1983) explain the difference as follows:

> . . . The acutely ill person relinquishes his normal duties for a temporary period and adopts a new role (sick) for the duration of his illness. For the chronically ill, exemption from normal role obligations is partial, rather than complete; the individual generally gives up his pre-illness role to adopt a less demanding one and/or the sick role on a permanent, but not dominant basis.
>
> The acutely ill person is permitted to accept help and display dependent behaviours as it is understood that this will be for a temporary period only. In chronic illness, the degree of dependence allowed is smaller as prolonged dependent behaviour could pose a major threat to the role performance of the remaining family members. . . .

☐ *Theoretical Concepts*

ILLNESS AS LOSS

It might be asked why illness is such a challenge to client coping. One answer might be that illness presents the client with a variety of real or threatened losses.

Loss is a universal experience. We have all been weaned, left home as little children to start school, and grown out of pastimes and activities. Granted, each developmental loss of this kind is compensated for; new and interesting foods become available once a child can give up the breast or bottle, for instance. Moreover, as Erikson (1968) has pointed out, school is an arena for developing mastery; new competencies make up for the loss of old ones that have been outgrown and set aside. Nevertheless, the old pleasures are lost, even as the new ones take their place.

Illness is a different kind of loss from these, because only rather introspective clients with the appropriate view of themselves and the world they live in can see themselves as gaining in competence or mastering new experience as a result of illness. Unlike new developmental loss, which can be absorbed because the person has previous experience with it, the situational loss of the first serious illness is one for which few adults in the United States are prepared. In fact, Siegler and Osmond (1979) have pointed out that the development of antibiotics and other medications has so greatly shortened the course of many illnesses that many adults have never witnessed serious illness in themselves or other family members. When serious illness has arisen, say in a grandparent, treatment has taken place in medical facilities rather than at home, and death practically always occurs there. Thus, many adults have little idea of the demands that illness may place upon them, let alone of the ways in which they can act to help themselves and make the best possible use of health professionals and health care facilities. The specific losses entailed in illness, as listed in Table 25-1, are expanded upon here.

1. Loss of accustomed bodily functioning. The sick person confronts the partial or complete, temporary or permanent loss of his sense of being able to rely on his body to function efficiently and painlessly, as and when he needs it to.

2. Loss or reduction of contact with family and friends. If the illness requires that the client receive treatment as an inpatient, he is literally taken out of circulation and sees the significant others in his life only when they come to see him. If the illness is severe enough, these visits may be very brief because staff intervene to prevent him from being taxed. Even if the client is able to be at home, there may be so much limitation on his normal activities that he does not have the frequency or type of family and

---

TABLE 25-1 *Losses Encountered in Illness*

Loss of accustomed bodily functioning

Loss or reduction of contact with family and friends

Loss of, or curtailed involvement in, work or study

Loss of accustomed self-image

social contacts that he has previously enjoyed.

3. Loss of, or curtailed involvement in work
or study. Especially if employment demands stamina, strength, and physical coordination, it may have to be suspended or
greatly reduced. This of course leads to a
slowing down of pursuit of career goals and
may even mean these have to be changed.
Earnings are also generally lost or reduced, unless the client is very fortunate.

4. Loss of accustomed self-image. For any
client, the above changes in functioning
lead to changes in his view of himself, at
least to some extent. If he has had a particular role in his family and social circle
and a productive position in his work, the
client has had ongoing experiences which
combine to build and continually reaffirm
a mental picture of himself. Drastic alterations in any of these spheres cause this
process to be discontinued. A new image
will of course ultimately be built, but even
if it is positive and comfortable, the loss of
the old image has to be mourned.

Self-image is not merely dependent on exter-
nals like family, friends, and work; it also relies
on a sense of the predictability of one's own feeling
states. Exposure to painful emotions, such as
rage, guilt, anxiety, and helplessness, is very common during physical illness, and may induce a
feeling of estrangement from the person one
thought one knew best—oneself. Such thoughts
as "This isn't like me" or "I can't believe I'm behaving this way" can indicate that a person's
image of himself is being damaged by the changes
in his feelings, as much as by the other changes
that illness has brought in its train.

■ *Point of Emphasis*

*A person who has fallen ill rarely has to deal with
only one loss at a time. In fact, as Peretz (1970)
has pointed out, one loss usually brings or threatens other losses, as can be seen very clearly in
the following vignette.*

Close analysis of the following vignette reveals
that Mr. Bowes had sustained losses in every
sphere outlined in the previous paragraphs.

Vignette

Alan Bowes sustained a complex fracture of his
right elbow in a fall. He was not in great pain
and the orthopedist was optimistic that full function would be returned to him. So the nurse was
surprised to find that he was intensely depressed
and contemplating suicide. Closer examination
explained his reaction. Alan was right-handed.
He worked as an independently employed ac-
countant. The accident took place late in January—in other words, at the beginning of the busi-
est time of the year. Thus he stood to lose the
bulk of the work on which his family income depended, because the elbow would not be
healed until after April 15th. Additionally, his wife
and children lived a long distance from the medical center and could not come to see him except on weekends. He had become an independent CPA precisely so as to be able to work in
an office at home and see more of them, and
had left a large firm with generous side pay provisions for that reason. He now felt he had lost too
much to be able to tolerate living any longer. He
felt completely helpless and hopeless.

ADAPTIVE TASKS POSED BY ILLNESS

Moos and Tsu (1977) have identified seven major
adaptive tasks which must be mastered by clients
who are ill, if they are to weather the crisis. These
adaptive tasks are listed in Table 25-2.

Pain and Discomfort

The first set of tasks, "involves dealing with the
discomfort, incapacitation, and other symptoms of
the illness or injury itself." Many acutely ill

TABLE 25-2 Major Sets of Adaptive Tasks[a]

Illness-related
  Dealing with pain and incapacitation
  Dealing with the hospital environment and special
    treatment procedures
  Developing adequate relationships with professional
    staff
General
  Preserving a reasonable emotional balance
  Preserving a satisfactory self-image
  Preserving relationships with family and friends
  Preparing for an uncertain future

[a] Source: Moos, R.H., and Tsu, V.D. *Coping with physical illness.*
New York: Plenum Press, 1977.

clients have pain; in fact, it accounts for about 60 percent of first contacts with physicians, according to Suchman (1972). Pain work is important for all clients and has cognitive and affective, as well as physical components (Geach, 1983). Clients must learn to discriminate among various pains and determine which of them is a warning that must be dealt with, and which of them is self-limiting or an inescapable part of illness. If the client decides to seek help, he has the task of explaining his symptoms to others so that they understand them. Quayhagen (1977) even states that pain has to be legitimated, which suggests that communicating one's pain in such a way that this can happen is a large part of the work. Finally, clients must manage their emotional and physical responses to pain, partly so as not to exacerbate their problems and partly so as not to anger and alienate staff or distress their families.

Even if a client is not in physical pain, incapacitation can pose a significant emotional hurdle. Boredom and frustration can be extreme. If the client *can* move but has been told he must rest, these feelings may be so intense that he is incapable of doing so. (See adjacent vignette.)

Hospital and Treatment

The second adaptive task listed by Moos and Tsu (1977) consists in managing "the stresses of special treatment procedures and of various aspects of the hospital or institutional environment itself." Many clients learn how to do this magnificently, while others have a very difficult time. In today's high-technology hospital, clients' capacity to master this adaptive task is severely tested. They are weakened physically by their illness and may have little understanding of what the tests and treatments to which they are required to submit mean. They come to know that certain antibiotics give their saliva an unfamiliar taste, or that other drugs change the color of their urine, affect their digestion, make them drowsy, or alter their vision. Machines hiss, click, and buzz around them even if they are not themselves attached to one. (If they are, especially on a long-term basis, they are vulnerable to changes in body image on an even greater scale than are most clients, as Abram (1977) has shown.) A disembodied voice over an intercom is often the first response to ringing the bell for help. Visitors may create embarrassment by audibly asking questions about staff's activities which clients cannot answer, or by breaking hospital rules.

Vignette

Charlie Davidson, a 57-year-old sheep farmer, had always been up all hours at lambing-time, because the ewes might need help to deliver, and the lambs of ewes that died had to be brought in to be hand-reared. Now he had had a severe myocardial infarction and had been told by his doctor not to work outside in the cold, or he would overtax his damaged heart. Charlie complied for one winter, fretting that his adult sons were not doing as much as he would for the sheep. He sat by the fire and from time to time would ask his wife if there wasn't some little thing she wanted done for her. The following winter, however, he was unable to continue in this way. Even though working outside brought on angina, he could no longer endure the tedium of inactivity. He even denied that the chest pain he experienced had anything to do with his heart, and referred to it as "indigestion."

The client may well experience his first hospitalization for acute illness as if he were an alien experiencing culture shock, so utterly unfamiliar are many of the sights, sounds, and interactions that take place. "Old hands" who have had repeated admissions are often more helpful than staff can be, because they remember the questions they had themselves. The client who has repeated admissions to hospital for tests or treatment is clearly not in the same position as the novice who has been brought in acutely ill for the first time. On the other hand, precisely because the environment is not strange and the events he can expect are known to him, he may be quite depressed and anxious. Familiarity only helps provide confidence if the well-known lessens symptoms. Often, a treatment or test is itself profoundly unpleasant and offers no hope of relief of the condition or its sequelae, but merely lengthens life. Chronically ill clients come to realize this and to view repeated admissions with dread.

Staff Relationships

The third adaptive task "consists of developing and maintaining adequate relationships with medical and other care-giving staff." A thoughtful sociological analysis of patients' work has noted that of all groups of workers, clients are the group whose efforts are both essential and completely taken for granted. Not only do clients' efforts as co-workers seldom get recognition—they are also hardly ever taken into account in planning care, as Fagerhaugh and Strauss (1977) see it. In fact, when it comes to pain, the client's attempts to secure recognition and be a part of planning have at times been observed to create friction or outright hostility between him and staff, according to their study.

Clients tend to be afraid to provoke hostility in any way. During a study being conducted to develop ways to incorporate measures of client satisfaction with care into overall evaluation of quality of care, it was found that many clients were reluctant to offer any negative comments about the nursing personnel (Nehring and Geach, 1973). One respondent, after stating that she had stayed awake all night to watch her intravenous infusion, gave uniformly high ratings to every aspect of nursing care that she had received. She saw no grounds in her sleepless night to complain; perhaps she simply saw watching her intravenous infusion as part of her job, or was reluctant to tell the interviewer her true feelings because of fear of retaliation.

Moos and Tsu (1977) have commented that dealing with staff "can require all the interpersonal skill that [clients] can muster," especially when one considers the variety of questions clients might ask themselves concerning how (if at all) to voice negative feelings about their doctor or their treatment; how to ask for help or medications; how to respond to the staff's behavior toward the clients and to one another; or how to ensure respect for their wishes about how they will be treated if they are dying. Having asked themselves, these clients might try out the solutions they have formulated; but sometimes, their

best efforts at communicating are misunderstood or ignored, as the previous vignette reveals.

If a proper pain history of this client had been taken when she was admitted, much of this difficulty would have been prevented. Fagerhaugh and Strauss (1977) have pointed out that it is essential when admitting a client who is, or may soon be, in a good deal of pain to find out what the previous experience with pain has been. Very few clients have absolutely *no* pain history, though they may have experienced pain rather infrequently. For the nurse, it is important to know what the client did about pain that he experienced. Copp (1974) has pointed out that clients have extremely varied ways of coping with pain intellectually and emotionally. One should also find out, however, what concrete strategies clients have used.

■ *Point of Emphasis*

The concrete strategy the nurse might select to manage pain ought to be similar to the client's, unless the client's approach is likely to cause damage or to endanger him.

Even acutely ill clients who were previously in good health may be aware that in the rare times when they have had discomfort in the past, a particular analgesic, for instance, was unsatisfactory. Thus it ought to be a part of the nursing history to find out just what the pain history has been. It is also useful to remember that the manner in which the pain or discomfort of the present condition is handled is building one more chapter in the client's pain history. If the client is handling the situation well, this may simply be because he has had previous good experience of successfully mastering pain. A nursing goal with any client in pain should be that the client learns more about how to work with pain. This will happen only if his experience is taken seriously, and every effort is made to build in some recognition of his part in the work of dealing with pain. If his experience is disconfirmed (Dangott, Thornton, and Page, 1978) and if decisions are made with other considerations than his experience in mind, however, his pain history will have a shadow of failure and frustration cast over it which will probably affect future episodes of illness negatively.

One example of a consideration other than the client's experience that may affect pain manage-

---

Vignette

Elizabeth Finch had a long history of rheumatoid arthritis, and a long established routine for taking her medication. Yet when she was admitted for tests for a problem unrelated to her chronic illness, she was neither allowed to keep her own medication and deal with the timing and dosage herself, nor even consulted about when she had been finding it most helpful to take what medication. As a result she became quite angry and depressed. The response of staff was to request a psychiatric liaison nurse consultation, as a result of which the misunderstandings were largely resolved and an appropriate regimen was devised. (Example adapted from Mooney, 1982.)

ment is the thought that narcotic analgesia may be addicting. Beaver (1980) has pointed out that "A patient's need for adequate pain control should not be equated with psychic dependence or narcotic addiction." Nevertheless, even dying clients are sometimes undermedicated because staff have this concern, leading both to underprescription by physicians and under-administration by nurses. As McCaffery (1979) has pointed out, pain is what the client says it is and exists when he says it does. Thus it should be what the client says, rather than what nurses or physicians believe is adequate, that determines the pain-control regimen.

Dealing with Unknown Staff.

A different concern in the management of relationships arises from the difficulty some clients have in distinguishing among staff. The hospitalized client may see as many as 30 or more different personnel in a day, and if he is very unsophisticated, he may confide his concerns to staff not directly responsible for the problem at hand, and then wonder why nothing happens. Some clients, on the other hand, believe that nobody but their physicians can deal with any problem or complaint, and wait with long lists for rounds to be made, only to be somewhat hurt that many of their concerns are brushed aside. Clients may often need orientation to the advocacy and liaison aspects of nursing, so

that they make more appropriate use of the time they spend with every staff member. Similarly, nurses need to be sensitive to the fact that many clients see only a blur of white-uniformed figures and have very little idea who among them is responsible for what, at least for a time—and that distinguishing among professionals is a process that can be hastened by adequate communication from nurses. This is particularly necessary if the client is demented, confused, or delirious.

■ Point of Emphasis

However ill the client is, staff should always introduce themselves at least briefly as they start care—even if this takes the form only of saying "I'm Miss Brown and I'm a nurse and that's why I'm shining this light in your eye" while actually carrying out the task. The client may be unable to respond, but may nevertheless appreciate the effort made, and it may help with the subsequent relationship between him and the staff.

Emotional Balance

The fourth adaptive task, according to Moos and Tsu (1977), involves "maintaining a reasonable emotional balance by managing upsetting feelings aroused by illness." Anger, guilt, depression, and fear are among the common responses to illness. Lazarus (1977) has discussed the interaction between a person's deliberate management of his emotional reactions and their "appraisal of the personal and social requirements of the situation" that has evoked these reactions. This may lead the person to do anticipatory work of some kind so as to increase his mastery of the situation—which is only possible, of course, if the person knows or can guess what may happen.

Lazarus calls anticipatory work a form of coping, in that it is an effort to deal with problems that may generate uncomfortable emotions before they arise. The example he gives is of the person who studies for a test; to the extent that this anticipatory work is effective, it permits a benign appraisal of the threat posed by the test, and thus helps the person to regulate emotions.

The person who confronts acute illness may have little or no time in which to engage in such anticipatory work, so this way of regulating emotion may not be open to him. Once the client is beyond the crisis of acute illness, however, he may be helped to do anticipatory work for tests and

---

Vignette

George Harris developed an intestinal obstruction when he was in his 80s and was admitted for surgery at 2 A.M., in great pain, and with much bustle and haste going on all around him. It had been requested that a nasogastric tube be passed before he was taken to the OR. Mr. Harris had already been shaved, and an IV had been inserted, with little discussion from staff, whose one concern was to get help to this critically ill client as soon as possible. When the nurse approached with the NG tube, she told him what she was going to do with it, but did not identify herself as a nurse. The client looked at her firmly and said "Oh, no, you damned well *won't* do that." When Mr. Harris improved, he explained that he did not see why he should submit to a total stranger "shoving something in my nose," and had had only a very hazy grasp of what was happening during the previous preparations. "I was sick as a dog, but I wasn't deaf. Why didn't they say who they were and why they were doing things?"

treatments, as well as to increase his independence in self-care. Nurses often provide explanations before tests and treatments are given. A solid body of nursing research (Johnson, 1973; Johnson et al., 1973, 1975, 1978) indicates that when clients know what is going to happen to them, they are less distressed by procedures than they are when they do not know, or when the information they have been given is irrelevant.

On the other hand, research in psychology (Miller, 1980, 1981) suggests that some clients may typically blunt their situations and do best when they are permitted to ignore most of the available information about what is happening to them. Clients who typically monitor their situations have to be told everything. The following vignettes present examples of blunting and monitoring behavior.

It appears, however, that monitors pay dearly for their knowledge. Miller (1980, 1981) found that they may put up with the immediate impact of a procedure with lower anxiety than the blunters might show at that moment, but their anxiety beforehand and their depression afterward tend to be far more severe than these affects are in blunters. The conclusions that might be drawn are that information-giving should be restricted to those clients it can reasonably be expected to help—clients who are monitors—and that these clients *also* need some special supportive intervention before and after the procedure.

Lazarus points out that the person may seek to affect his emotions directly, for example by drinking or taking anxiolytic medications, rather than indirectly by doing anticipatory work. He adds that much remains unknown about which situations and personal characteristics lead people to select which way of regulating their emotions, based on their cognitive appraisal of themselves and of the problem they confront.

■ Point of Emphasis

The nurse may see many different behaviors in response to apparently rather similar illness situations. The point to remember is that, if Lazarus is correct, much behavior that one sees represents an effort to regulate unpleasant affect.

Vignettes

When Miss Bennett approached to explain the intravenous pyelogram to William Smith, a 37-year-old executive, prior to having him sign the consent form, she noticed that he was not paying attention. He tapped his fingers and his eyes strayed repeatedly to the crossword puzzle which he had been completing when Miss Bennett came in. Finally he said "My doctor's told me everything, I'll sign the paper" and did so. This was quite frustrating to Miss Bennett, who had been told by the physician that Mr. Smith had in fact only been told he had to have "a special kidney test." Yet it was clear that Mr. Smith did not want to know more. Mr. Smith was a blunter.

On the other hand, Joseph Green was something of a trial to staff on the floor, because he invariably questioned what the medications he was given were. This seemed odd because he had few changes of prescription during his hospital stay. After he had received a careful description of the procedures involved in conducting a GI series from his physician, he nevertheless asked his primary nurse to tell him all about it. In the x-ray department, too, he wanted the technicians to explain every step before he would cooperate. Mr. Green was a monitor.

In another article, Lazarus (1974) makes the point that human beings are constantly appraising what he calls their "adaptive commerce" with the environment. The appraisal is cognitive and directed at understanding the significance of what is going on in the environment for the person's well-being. Lazarus believes not only that such appraisals "underlie the ebb and flow of emotional states" but also that cognitive appraisals and self-regulatory processes "are key mediators of the person's reactions to stressful transactions, and hence shape the somatic outcome." Illness, he believes, is "an expression of repeated or persistent forms of adaptive commerce with an environment of some kind," that is, is dependent on *both* environmental changes *and* a particular personality, and also on their interaction.

Not everyone agrees with this definition of illness; even Lazarus admits that there is disagreement about the relationship between stress and illness. Nevertheless, his insight that persons, whether sick or well, are continually appraising their situation and regulating their behavior, so as to deal with it without being overwhelmed by painful emotions, is one that can be very useful for nursing.

As a result of the cognitive appraisal, meaning is attributed to the illness experience. Li-

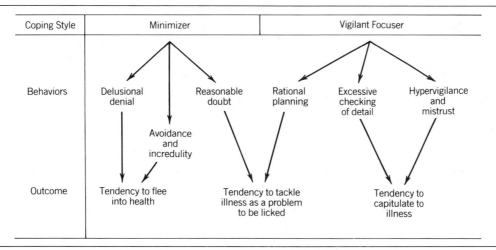

Figure 25-1 *Coping styles, behaviors and outcomes. Based on ideas from Lipowski, Z.J. Physical illness, the individual and the coping process. PSYCHIATRY IN MEDICINE, 1, 1970:91–102.*

powski (1970) has stated that illness may have the following meanings for the sufferer: he may see it as a challenge, as an enemy, as a punishment, as weakness, as a relief from other burdens, as a strategy in his interpersonal battles, as irreparable loss or damage, or as a value, in that it enables him to release higher spiritual or creative energies. Lipowski identifies two major cognitive coping styles, the minimizing and the vigilant focusing styles.

Both of these styles actually can represent a range of behavior from the delusional denial to reasonable doubt of the minimizer, or from the hypervigilance to the rational planning of the vigilant focuser. Lipowski states that persons behaviorally either tackle illness, capitulate to it, or avoid it by fleeing into healthy activity. These behavioral styles fit with cognitive styles: for example, a strong minimizer is more likely to exhibit avoidance and a vigilant focuser is more likely to tackle illness.

■ Point of Emphasis

The meaning of the illness or injury, as articulated on the basis of cognitive appraisal, leads to entirely different feeling-states, and the task faced by each client in managing and regulating his emotions is also entirely different. This suggests that the question of the meaning of the client's illness is crucial in evaluating his coping.

With thoughts such as these in mind, one finds it less puzzling that soldiers wounded in battle often experience little pain from injury that would certainly cause discomfort, at least, if it were inflicted as part of elective surgery. To the soldier, the illness following the wound is his ticket home for at least temporary relief from combat; to the surgical patient, the illness may be disruptive to his way of life, finances, and relationships with others.

It has been noted many times that if the full meaning of an illness is too traumatic to be absorbed, even repeated explanations do not sink in. Burns (1982) states, for example, that the diagnosis of cancer is often denied by both clients themselves and their families. Even if the central fact of illness is not denied, many details go unheard, and staff have to be ready to reiterate information over and over again. On a short-term basis, such denial is probably adaptive. In terms of Lazarus's ideas, it permits the client to regulate the enormously painful emotions that full awareness of the situation might evoke. In the initial few hours, days, or weeks after the bad news, the client usually comes gradually to acknowledge the problem and then may become depressed or angry. On the other hand, he may mobilize his existing resources to address his difficulties rather quickly, in a shortcut from the euphoria associated with still being alive to problem solving, which leaves out the task of working through painful feelings (Beglinger, 1983). Sooner or later, these will have to be addressed, particularly if there are permanent sequelae with which the client will have to live for the rest of his life.

■ **Point of Emphasis**

The most important things for the nurse to recognize about denial in the early period following diagnosis of a serious illness which, if appraised realistically, means serious loss, are that denial is normal and that it is largely unconscious.

In other words, the client is not deliberately blinding himself; emotionally, he simply cannot permit himself to see what may be obvious to all around him. It is sometimes frustrating to know that a person cannot begin to work on ways to use his remaining abilities until he faces what he has lost, and to see that this has not yet happened. The continued truthful, but supportive interaction with helping professionals will usually change this situation over time; meanwhile, it is important to wait out the initial period of denial.

Similarly, a period of depression is normal, though staff may be taken by surprise when a client who had previously been cheerful and cooperative becomes withdrawn, lethargic, and tearful. Yet, if one bears in mind that any serious illness brings loss with it, some mourning of the loss will be expected. This may not appear directly, but may be reflected in expressions of guilt and self-denigration, as may be seen in the following vignette:

Vignette

Jane Kiley, a 26-year-old medical student, sustained crushing injuries to her right lower leg and ankle in a motor-bicycle accident. Because of her career aspirations, the injured leg was not amputated, although this was seriously considered; instead, a long series of repeated skingrafts and other attempts to bring about healing was undertaken. Jane did not respond sadly when first told all the facts, including the poor long-term prognosis for her leg. After approximately 6 weeks, however, she had a sleepless night (rare for her), and was then quite weepy and withdrawn for several days. Since she had been rather cheerful and intelligently cooperative, in spite of pain, some staff were quite surprised by her changed feeling-state. Jane herself was as upset by her plummeting spirits as by the injury's slow healing, and expressed contempt with herself "for losing my fighting spirit."

Much support may be needed for clients who are trying to manage a type of intensity or affect quite foreign to their experience. Jane had been a very successful student and had competently met many challenges. She was not accustomed to becoming depressed in the face of difficulties, being typically a vigilant focuser with a tackling style. She needed help to realize that her sadness was a normal response to the actual loss of certain hopes—for example, that she would finish medical school when her contemporaries did—and the threat that she might lose her leg. She was not so much "giving way to depression" as doing some unfinished grieving over matters that called for grief.

Self-Image

The fifth adaptive task, according to Moos and Tsu (1977), is to preserve a satisfactory self-image, including a sense of competence and mastery. Particularly if the illness or its treatment has permanently changed the client's appearance, he may suffer substantial loss of self-esteem. Krumm (1982), in a review on the adaptation of adult cancer clients, notes that both ostomy and postmastectomy clients take some months to adapt to their changed body image. Hansen (1983) and Savage (1981) both address the necessity of helping this process by encouraging a focus on the whole body as desirable and thus not diminished by removal of a single part, thus promoting a positive sexual identity. Clients who are attached to dialysis machines may come to feel as if they were themselves at least partly machines (Abram, 1977). Mooney (1982) has noted that clients with chronic rheumatoid arthritis often vocalize fear that other family members can "catch" the disease from them, and if a family member does contract it, they may experience guilt.

Examples such as the above indicate that to some degree a person who is ill is at least temporarily suffering from a spoiled identity (Goffman, 1963). Too often, as Mooney (1982) has pointed out, perfectly responsible individuals are stripped of their ability to take responsibility, as in the matter of taking medication for their chronic condition, managing their own care, and so forth. This "sociological sheep-shearing" contributes to their spoiled identity. Where there are social judgments common in the community about the client's condition—for example, in regard to AIDS patients—the spoiling is even more complete, for the client is liable to hear remarks from both professionals and nonprofessionals that increase the damage to his self-esteem.

Another source of damage is the necessity to rely, wholly or partly, on the help of others. Some clients see this as intolerable weakness and infantile dependence. Their bodies may not be disfigured, but the loss of physical autonomy is to them as serious a blow as facial scarring might be to a movie star. Alterations in endurance, strength, power of concentration, and so on can similarly constitute assaults on self-esteem. To the same extent that a person's identity is so bound up with his work that he *is* what he *does*, any loss of ability to work must be experienced as an enormous threat to his self-image. Such a person may express tremendous anger at the slow, palliative, or at best slowly rehabilitative quality of his treatment and may demand more drastic intervention, preferring to risk death than to endure a curtailed existence.

Problems with and for the Family

The sixth adaptive task, preserving relationships with family and friends, can be extremely difficult. Burns (1982) reports that the withdrawal of others from the cancer client can be as devastating as the illness itself. When a family has good solid bonds, these may be preserved by the threat of illness; when the bonds are weak, however, they may be made even weaker as the family confronts the loss or impairment of the sick family member. Intimacy permits the best and most appropriate kinds of support to be provided; but it also creates special vulnerabilities. (A woman's view of herself after mastectomy may be heavily colored by her belief that she is now less attractive to her husband, for example.)

A study (Dhooper, 1983) of 40 families in the first 3 months after the fathers had heart attacks noted that families' anxiety was particularly high in the first month following the heart attack, but there was little reactive illness then. Instead, reactive illness would affect family members during the first month after the client came home to recuperate (usually after about 1 month). However, by 3 months after the heart attack, reactive illness had diminished and anxiety over the client's health had become recognized as something to live with.

During this sort of acute crisis, as at other times, families concentrate their energies on the maintenance of emotional health of the family members, management of finances, household management, and dealing with children and their needs. Fewer than 10 percent of wives required anxiolytic medication in Dhooper's (1983) study,

but a number of them began or resumed smoking and/or overeating. These wives tended to seek both information about their husbands' condition and reassurance from physicians. Some of them prayed. How much they reached out to nonfamily members for help or comfort depended on the extent of their social networks before the heart attack. Children were largely encouraged to continue with their usual activities, but wives might suspend all but absolutely essential household tasks for the first month after the heart attack. By 3 months after the attack, household management was back almost to normal, although there might be modifications to accommodate the needs of the convalescent fathers.

Finances were the least of these families' worries for the first month. Financial strain was, of course, dependent on whether the husband received sick pay, had health insurance and savings, and the like, but the strain did not come to the forefront until after the husband came home. Then, if he had no prospect of returning to work, strain became severe, because obtaining disability monies is a very slow process. Three months after the heart attack, a third of the families were still experiencing financial strain. By that time, any savings had long been used up, and reductions in expenditures had been instituted as far as possible; so if no income was forthcoming and disability payment had not yet materialized, families were severely stressed.

When the subjects were asked about the effects of the husband's illness on family life, about 60 percent felt it was better during the first month after the illness, while 20 percent felt it was worse, and 20 percent felt it was unchanged. By the third month, only 40 percent felt family life was better, while 40 percent felt it was unchanged, and 20 percent felt it was worse. (The data reported did not indicate whether the last of these groups was the same as the 20 percent who felt family life had become worse in the first month, so it is hard to evaluate these figures.)

Dhooper (1983) comments that these families had received little social service intervention and therefore may not have had the support they needed to weather the crisis. (On the other hand, clients with end-stage renal disease in Jamaica did comparatively well at coping with financial and psychosocial problems, despite the dearth of structured social services in Jamaica, as in other developing nations. This raises the provocative possibility that a society that has never known much structured social service both can and does evolve its own creative solutions to the problems of individual members. In turn, one cannot help wondering whether the well-meaning provision of social services in some way weakens or destroys this ability.)

One thing is clear from Dhooper's study: the whole family is affected by illness, and therefore the whole family needs to be considered. This is as true for families of clients with chronic illness as it is for families with an acutely ill member; as Mitchell (1983) has pointed out, the individual has the chronic illness, but families must cope with it. This is not simply a matter of weathering a passing storm. Following acute illness, the concerns are its effects on mental health, finances, and household management. In chronic illness, however, the sick client has lost function in one or more of these four areas: movement, sensing, energy production, or cerebral integration. Family or significant others may have to supplement these fundamental areas to make up for the individual's loss. Moreover, they must learn to live in a state of vigilance to guard against potential crises, because they are in a key position to help to prevent them.

To the extent that the client is aware of all this and capable of interacting so as to affect it, he has a very difficult task. Attending to the needs of friends and family, to the extent that is physically possible, may place the client in an emotional quandary. Not only may the family and friends withdraw from the client; the client may withdraw from them, perhaps feeling that his fear and anger at his illness are too burdensome for them to bear. Both client and family need support, therefore, as they endeavor to maintain communication.

The Future

The seventh task that Moos and Tsu (1977) list is that of "preparing for an uncertain future." This sounds almost impossible, for how can one prepare for what one knows nothing about? And indeed, some clients and families are overwhelmed by this seeming impossibility. It is at times helpful to reflect that the future is *always* uncertain, and that what illness and its sequelae do is to lend shape to what is actually a total unknown for anybody, whether sick or well. Since illness may change the family life-style, for instance, it is essential for family members to collaborate in building the new life-style in such a way that harmonious life together is still possible.

Hall and Weaver (1974) have identified six coping processes which must be used so as to grow into, rather than be crushed by, the uncertain future: cognitive mastery (i.e., achieving a full understanding of the situation and its practical implications); gaining access to community resources; maintaining control over family behavior so that it helps to achieve the client's and family's purposes; formation of coalitions within and outside the family in the service of support and growth; communication; and last, but not least, the choice to grow. Miller (1983) speaks of the powerlessness of illness which the client and his family must combat. Strauss and Glaser (1975) state that chronically ill clients must manage and prevent medical crises, carry out the prescribed treatment regimen, control their symptoms, cope with social isolation, adjust to changes in the course of their disease, and seek financial resources to meet the costs associated with treatment.

THE SICKNESS CAREER

If all of the issues mentioned in the previous paragraph really are systematically addressed by the client, the future must become a good deal less uncertain, in that it is full of tasks that will become as familiar a part of his new life-style as his preillness round of activities was.

In a sense, when he presents himself for treatment, the client has embarked on a decision-making sequence—which Twaddle (1979) calls the sickness career. If the client has started out well, there comes a point when not only has the change in physical status occurred, but also the client decides that it is a change from normal, and, moreover, that it is a significant change. The latter decision depends on the extent to which symptoms interfere with the client's normal activities or characteristics; on the clarity of the symptoms; and on the "tolerance threshold and impression management" of the symptomatic person. Twaddle points out that most people have some symptoms most of the time; but symptoms have to be defined as sickness-related before the client begins to exhibit illness behavior. Other factors affecting these decisions therefore obviously include the familiarity and seriousness of the symptoms (the latter being partly a matter of their frequency and duration). If the symptoms are known to relate, potentially, to diagnoses of illness of uncertain prognosis and with possibly incapacitating consequences, they are likely to be used as the basis for assuming a sick identity. This is partic-

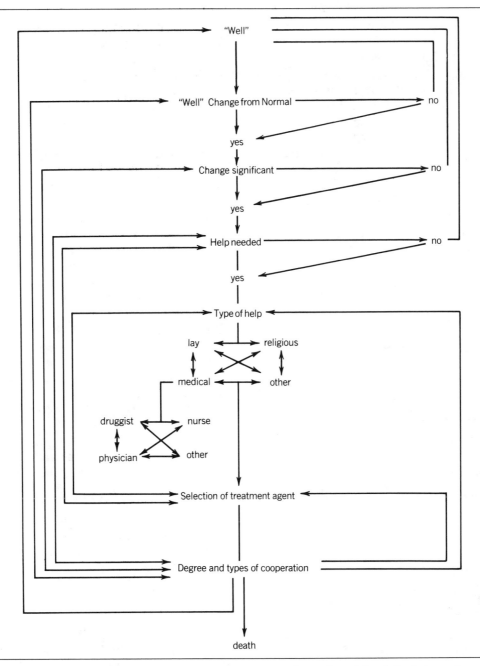

Figure 25-2 *Decision steps in the sickness career. From: Twaddle, A.C. Sickness behavior and the sick role. Cambridge, MA: Schenkman, 1979.*

ularly likely to occur if others are urging the client to get some problem taken care of, or if other crises in his life make withdrawing into a sick identity an attractive or at least a preferable choice.

Twaddle (1979) points out that most people begin by attempting self-care measures and decide that help is needed only if these are ineffec-

tive. Then the next decision comes: what help in particular is needed? The decision to see a professional depends on how much it costs, on the degree of correspondence between lay and professional cultures, and on the number of people consulted. He adds: "In the absence of authoritative laymen, long delays [may result] before a physician [is] seen" in cultures in which the correspondence between lay and professional cultures is low. After the treatment agent has been selected, there is yet another decision as to how much and what sort of cooperation to offer this person.

The chronically ill client has already traversed much of this stepwise career, and spends the rest of his life evaluating his health each day and determining whether he would fare better by seeing a physician or by sitting on his symptoms and enduring them, since the physician may be able to do little. The recovered acutely ill person has traversed the pathway once. If he has made reasonable decisions and the outcome is tolerable, he will have learned a great deal in the process about how to proceed with these decision-making steps in any future episode of acute illness. It is a goal of nursing practice so to handle the client's care during acute illness episodes that such learning is possible.

☐ Nursing Process

ASSESSMENT ☐

Client Coping ☐ In evaluating coping, one might use the seven questions suggested by Weisman (1979):

1. What problems if any, do you see this illness creating?
2. How do you plan to deal with them?
3. When faced with a problem you must do something about, what happens? What do you do?
4. How does it usually work out?
5. To whom do you turn when you need help?
6. What has happened in the past when you asked for help?
7. What kinds of problems usually tend to get you down or upset?

On the basis of the answers to these questions, one should be able to develop a profile of the client's coping. For instance, one should be able to identify what defenses he tends to use and is currently using; whether his basic stance is as active agent or passive victim in his own life; whether he is fundamentally optimistic or pessimistic; the level of his intelligence, motivation, and willingness to learn; the presence of other personal strengths; the extent and supportiveness of his social network; the importance of religion in his life; and the extent to which the illness dam-

ages or threatens to damage his self-esteem, body image, or both. Furthermore, skillful interviewing will also have elicited practical consequences of the illness for the client and his family, and the extent to which he trusts the health care team.

If one comes away thinking: "The client doesn't know what he's in for yet (or has denied the full meaning of his situation), but he's a fighter and always has been; he has a good family life; he's obviously experienced in living and seems willing to learn more; his education is a real blessing; he thinks the world of his doctor; he looks on the bright side; he's dealt with devastating problems in the past and has come through strengthened; and he's found religion helpful"— one has a profile of a client who has coped well and will probably continue to do so. But if, in addition to denial, the answers reflect a fundamentally passive involvement with life; scanty social support; a pessimistic and mistrustful attitude; difficulty in sustaining interest in health teaching or retaining information; limited strengths in other areas; and no particular relationship to a transcendent being, the chances are that both past and future coping have not been and will not be impressive. Most clients, naturally enough, fall between these two extremes as they confront illness.

Note that the questions are addressed to laying bare the client's strengths (if any) rather than his weaknesses. This is necessary because the client's strengths are the aspect that will help him and with which staff should attempt to forge an alliance. Naturally, his weaknesses will come to light as well, but most of the health care team's energy should be directed at circumventing these and building on the strengths.

Using a simple sequence of questions such as that suggested by Weisman will show what the client's "generalized resistance resources" are and have been. This phrase was coined by Antonovsky (1979), who believes that illness consists in large-scale breakdown in a person's resistance due to removal or reduction of enough generalized resistance resources. Talents, friends, family, and religious faith are as important to resistance as immune systems, in his view. Most important of all is an attribute he calls "coherence," defined as "a global orientation that expresses the extent to which one has a pervasive, enduring though dynamic feeling of confidence that one's internal and external environment are predictable and there is a high probability that things will work out as well as can reasonably be expected."

In the case of the aforementioned hypothetical client who was coping well, Antonovsky would state that despite the illness, many of the client's generalized resistance resources are intact and, moreover, he appears to be well-endowed with coherence. The client hypothetically assessed as coping poorly can, in Antonovsky's terms, be seen as lacking in many generalized resistance resources, and particularly in coherence.

As stated earlier, the coping behaviors appropriate to acute illness are not appropriate in chronic illness. Thus the acutely ill person is expected to give up working and become dependent on others, even for the most basic tasks; it is tolerable for him to deny at least some features of his illness and to express negative emotions freely. This is allowed, so to speak, because it is temporary. Chronically ill persons, on the other hand, are expected to undertake regular tasks unless they are completely incapacitated; are expected to appraise their illness realistically; and are supposed to master themselves sufficiently for their negative feelings to be kept under wraps.

Burns (1982) has put this point even more strongly in her discussion of the social role expectations of the dying person. From various sources, she has compiled a list of behaviors which sound almost impossible for any ill person, much less one who is dying and perhaps in great pain, to exhibit. Essentially, the dying person has been expected to die quietly and gracefully, without withdrawing socially or becoming demanding, neither hastening his death nor insisting that impossible cures be tried to prevent it, and, so far as possible, without upsetting the staff. Burns states that "most people would probably become angry and deny that these are socially expected role behaviors. Observing and listening on the average hospital unit, however, may be sufficient to verify the validity of the list."

To a lesser extent, the same stoic independence and care not to upset the caretaker is probably expected of those with chronic illness. A moment's reflection on conversations one has overheard about chronically ill patients being "crocks," "whiners," "kvetschers," and "doesn't respond—basically isn't doing what he's told" reveals the similarity of attitudes toward them to attitudes toward the dying. Needless to say, failure to meet unrealistic expectations such as these is not necessarily a mark of poor coping. The chronically ill frequently have to be more vocal than staff likes, for instance, because they are alert to changes in their own bodies that others cannot perceive until they have deteriorated markedly. A "chronic complainer" may simply be somebody who knows that unless he keeps up a steady barrage, his life may be endangered.

Family Coping □ Weisman's (1979) seven questions could be as effective in assessing family coping as they are in assessing individual coping—what one is seeking is information about family members' ability, collectively and as a family unit, to meet their coping tasks.

Beglinger (1983), in an article addressing the client and his family as a unity, has identified ten coping tasks for critically ill clients and their families:

- ☐ Maintenance of a sense of future
- ☐ Keeping pain at a tolerable level
- ☐ Maintenance of a sense of control
- ☐ Development of a sense of trust in caregivers
- ☐ Maintenance of intimate relationships with loved ones
- ☐ Maintenance of a sense of identity separate from the critical care unit
- ☐ Confrontation of the meaning of loss of self
- ☐ Confrontation of the meaning of loss of a loved one
- ☐ Maintenance of outside obligations without guilt
- ☐ Integration of the meaning of losses

Some of these tasks perhaps apply more to the client than to the family, and vice versa. For example, it is chiefly the family's concern to maintain outside obligations without guilt; but even here, the sick family member, unless he is unconscious, may have a role to play in giving or refusing permission, and thus enhancing or minimizing the guilt the family feels for attending to anyone or anything but him. Comparison of Beglinger's list of coping tasks with Weisman's (1979) seven questions shows how much overlap there is in the assessment questions for families and for individuals.

In addition to confronting Beglinger's tasks, chronically ill clients and their families have to:

- ☐ Integrate treatment into daily living
- ☐ Learn to recognize the signs of disease progression or exacerbation
- ☐ Identify vulnerable periods and adjust lifestyle and treatment regimen accordingly

□ Learn what to expect and when to seek help

□ Learn to recognize and plan for the terminal period of the illness (Mitchell, 1983)

For these families, accordingly, the assessment needs to focus on how they organize their daily lives around the ongoing need to monitor and maintain the sick member. Additionally, the need to have the information they possess about the client's illness and its treatment should be carefully assessed, for without adequate information, they cannot learn what Mitchell (1983) suggests they should.

Often, once the client is home after the initial episode of a chronic illness, and the family confronts the full burden of its responsibility, family members may feel they were not told what they needed to know. They may even say so to the community health nurse. Sometimes, indeed, the health teaching done while in hospital has been too hurried or in other ways inadequate. But the nurse should not be too ready to assume that the family's denial of teaching is accurate.

We have all been in the position of believing we understood something we were told about the difficulties we faced, and yet feeling taken by surprise and overwhelmed when we were actually facing them. It is natural at such times to experience anger and to want to blame somebody for the helplessness and incompetence we feel. "They never told me what it would be like!" The only rational response is: "They really couldn't, beyond a certain point; only *you* could know what it would be like for you," and then to help family members recall and assimilate the information they were given in terms of their own situation. The presence of this sort of anger and perceived incompetence is among the aspects of family functioning that need to be assessed, for intervention will have to be geared to respond to it.

Self-Coping □ It is extremely stressful to care for physically ill clients, especially if they are coping poorly. This is true, even if the nurse is coping well with both her own feelings and responsibilities—it is even more true if she is not. Some indicators of poor coping in oneself are:

1. Emotional numbness
2. Withdrawal from clients
3. Proneness to excessive anxiety, anger, or other unpleasant conditions

4. Forgetting important tasks
5. Forgetting to record care or medications as given

Having recognized that she is having difficulty coping, the nurse should then ask herself whether one of the following issues is at the root of the trouble:

1. She really does not have the knowledge or skill to perform adequately in carrying out physical care.
2. She has the knowledge and skill, but is depressed and angry that the client is deteriorating despite her best efforts.
3. She is aware that the client and family have emotional needs, but is unable to meet them.
4. She is aware that her own emotional responses are colored by past experiences or by stereotypes which interfere with appropriate functioning.

The nurse could come to one or more of these conclusions based on her deeper assessment of such responses in herself as anger, withdrawal, or not performing well. Once she has specified the problem, however, she can seek help to deal with it, as will be discussed in the section on intervention.

PROBLEM IDENTIFICATION □ On the basis of the theory presented thus far, and the assessment approaches that have been suggested, coping problems that can be identified for clients may be listed as follows:

1. Crisis response to acute illness (i.e., a period of acute emotional and cognitive disequilibrium in which the client's normal coping repertoire is not adequate; this is reflected in disorganized behavior and thinking)
2. Denial of acute severity of the illness and its consequences
3. Depression in face of the illness and its accompanying losses:
   a. Loss of accustomed bodily functioning
   b. Loss or reduction of contact with family and friends
   c. Loss of, or curtailed involvement in, work or study
   d. Loss of accustomed self-image

4. Failure to meet adaptive tasks posed by illness:

   a. Dealing with discomfort, incapacitation, and other symptoms of illness

   b. Dealing with the stresses of treatment and the hospital environment

   c. Developing and maintaining relationships with caregivers

   d. Managing upsetting feelings aroused by illness

   e. Preserving a satisfactory self-image

   f. Preserving relationships with family and friends

   g. Preparing for an uncertain future

For families, any of the above problems may be identified, either as experienced by them together with the client or as problems they experience, while he does not, or not to the same degree. For the nurse, problems in coping may be:

1. Difficulty in managing the task demands of the situation

2. Difficulty in handling own feelings and behavior about sickness and death

3. Difficulty in handling clients' feelings and behavior

4. Difficulty in handling client family's feelings and behavior

5. Difficulty in handling co-workers' responses to all of the above and/or to herself

INTERVENTIONS □ In terms of their actual physical illness, both acutely and chronically ill clients have clearly progressed beyond the level of primary prevention; if this had been attempted and had been successful, the individual might not have become sick in the first place. In terms of *coping* with physical illness, however, the primary prevention that is available includes:

1. First aid and CPR classes provided by the American Red Cross and similar community organizations;

2. Emergency medical services with well-publicized phone numbers and points of access;

3. Information available in public places concerning the Heimlich maneuver, antidotes to poisons, cancer warning signs, and so on; and

4. Hot lines provided by support groups for various kinds of client populations, such as the American Cancer Society's services for cancer clients and their families.

By providing information that helps the client or those around him know what to do in an emergency, all of these sources help to facilitate primary prevention in the sense that they may enhance coping and thus prevent the acute illness situation from being made worse because clients do not know what to do. Knowledge does not always lead to better coping, but without knowledge, few clients or families can possibly cope.

Secondary prevention, in terms of coping, consists of such measures as the following:

1. Prompt treatment response when clients seek help

2. Adequate health teaching in hospital

3. Adequate monitoring of self-care once home (e.g., via home visits)

4. Crisis intervention if indicated

5. Assistance with anticipatory grieving if indicated

In these ways early detection and treatment of poor coping can be implemented in order to help the client to master the illness situation. From this perspective, then, intervention directed at client and family coping is very largely a matter of secondary prevention.

Tertiary prevention in the care of chronically sick people is directed at reducing the impairment or disability resulting from their illness. In terms of coping, care should be in the service of preventing any further loss of coping ability. Attendance at support group meetings and visits from community health nurses clearly have this end in view.

Strategies for the Acutely Ill □ Intervention strategies should parallel and be geared to fostering the individual and family coping tasks listed by Beglinger (1983). For example, to maintain a sense of future in critically ill clients, she suggests that the family's and client's understanding of what the physician has told them should be ascertained. If it is realistic and accurate, hope should be fostered, Beglinger believes, even if the prognosis is grim; the decision to hope against hope may simply be a willed decision and, given the uncertainties of treatment, is reasonable. After all, dramatic changes for the better can and do occur.

In speaking of pain control, Beglinger points out that uncontrolled pain can create depression, particularly if the client feels his complaints are being disregarded. She states that the nurse should "act in collaboration with the patient to control his pain [and] openly identify pain relief as a mutual goal of [the nurse] and the patient." She also states that nurses "should familiarize themselves not only with pharmacological but also with non-pharmacological approaches to pain management," including relaxation and guided imagery techniques.

The Intensive Care Experience ☐ Commenting that "the intensive care unit is a setup for powerlessness," Beglinger states that whenever an opportunity can possibly be offered to afford the client some control over what happens to him, this should be done. Powerlessness, she says, is the perception that one's actions will have no effect on the outcome one desires, and every effort should be made, even with the most incapacitated client, to include him at least in nonurgent decisions.

The acutely ill client in a critical care unit is in a position that is very unfamiliar to him, Beglinger reminds us. Both he and his family are likely to put up with the dependency of his position only if they perceive staff as competent. This is particularly true if machines are relied on for aspects of life-support, making the client overwhelmingly aware of the extent to which his life depends on the vigilance of staff as they monitor and use the machines. At all times, staff need to explain at least briefly what they are doing and why. Beglinger suggests that each client in the critical care unit should be assigned one primary caregiver who can be accountable to the family for information and support. Welch (1981) reviews and confirms research showing that this sort of suggestion is applicable to clients with the diagnosis of cancer (often a long-term condition) as well as to acutely ill clients, adding that family stress can be greatly reduced if family members see the client receiving excellent, personalized care that keeps him as comfortable as possible: "The better we practice our oncology nursing skills, the more effective we are at meeting family needs."

Especially if the critical care unit is small, crowded, and busy, it can be very difficult for nurses to help to maintain intimate relationships; the brevity of visits might seem to counteract any such effort. Yet Beglinger suggests that, if family members wish to and are competent, they should be involved in aspects of care. (Care that could be carried out during a very short period include giving the client permitted quantities of fluid, or washing his face and hands.) Beglinger states that whenever possible, the visits should be private. Sometimes, too, family members may need encouragement to discuss topics unrelated to illness while visiting, for they may feel as though mention of how the children are doing at school or what is blooming in the garden was somehow not appropriate. Not only are such topics appropriate, they are essential reminders of the life the client has with his family—and, if all goes well, will continue to have. If the client's condition is sufficiently stable, it might even be valuable for him to see his children—perhaps by being wheeled to an area where they will not have to see other clients *in extremis*. Such brief visits could be useful for them as well as for the client.

Such trips away from the critical care unit may help to impress on the client the important idea that he has a whole identity independent of the unit. Surrounded by "an array of advanced technology," as Beglinger puts it, the client can easily feel as though his universe has contracted to the size of his bed and (if he is on one) life-support system. If he is likely to recover, he will spend short periods, gradually getting longer, being weaned from this apparatus, and it will help the client as well as his family if some of these weaning times coincide with their visits and gradually are permitted to take place away from the machines, say in a dayroom or solarium.

Every client should have a place for a few personal possessions that can be kept in sight, even if this amounts only to a bulletin board big enough for a couple of photographs or a child's drawing and a small shelf with a small bud vase from home, or perhaps a statue or crucifix. Such constant visual reminders of his preillness self can do much to mitigate the depersonalizing effects of acute illness in a critical care unit.

Denial and Coping ☐ Beglinger believes that the client may need help from staff to carry out anticipatory grieving over loss of self (after all, even if he recovers, life after a critical, life-threatening condition can seldom be experienced as unchanged, and the client has a preillness self whose loss he needs to mourn). In relation to cardiac clients, it has been thought for some time that clients with the best prognoses are the ones who tend to deny any fear that they might die (Browne and Hackett, 1967; Hackett, Cassem, and Wishnie, 1968). More recently, however, Thomas and co-workers (1983) did not find the clients they interviewed in a CCU tended to deny their difficulties, and, furthermore, anxiety and denial were not significant predictors of arrhythmias or changes in heart rate during and after the interview. They did not ask the same sorts of questions as the previous researchers had, but concluded, anyway, that since clients in CCUs do have a variety of concerns both about themselves and about their lives and families, they could be encouraged to talk about these without necessarily affecting their prognosis for the worse. It appears that for cardiac clients at least, this is still a matter for debate; but if the sensitive nurse follows the leads the client gives her, she should be able to encourage those for whom it would be helpful to confront and discuss their loss.

Family Coping □ Beglinger's next two tasks are specific to the family, which, she says may need to do anticipatory grieving as much as the client does (or even more so, if he has been a powerful and emotionally impact-laden figure for them). Here the nurse can be of most use by helping the family identify its concerns, express feelings, and make realistic plans. In the first few days of critical illness, the family may experience such disorganization that planning seems impossible. But most families have friends or other family members to turn to, and a gentle question about this may make them realize that however helpless they may feel, they do in fact have resources. Once aware of these, they will not usually take long to use the resources they have.

To do so, however, they may need to be encouraged to continue to maintain their outside obligations without feeling that they have somehow failed or abandoned the client. Of course, as Beglinger points out, if they maintain a bedside vigil for many hours a day and simultaneously try to meet their outside obligations, they will become drained. They may cope better if at least one member is present at all times, and if this seems to be the case, it should be allowed. But the emotional wear and tear may be great, and if the client's condition appears to be stable, they should be encouraged to leave in such a way that they feel able to do so. At the same time, Beglinger cautions that they should not be told that nothing will happen while they are gone; nobody can predict a sudden

reversal. They can, however, be given an honest best guess that so far as the staff can tell, no grievous change is likely. The primary caregiver can help to alleviate anxiety about departure by taking phone numbers and promising a phone call at regular intervals, regardless of how the client is doing, during the family's absence. Such promises must, of course, be kept!

In order to integrate the meaning of losses, the last coping task mentioned by Beglinger, the client and his family may need help to proceed from a "honeymoon" experience engendered by the sheer relief and gratitude that a severe physical crisis has been weathered, to a more realistic appraisal of his situation. The client may be almost euphoric at first, but undoubtedly has some anger and depression about his illness which he will have to integrate if the full meaning of the losses it entails is to become an appropriate part of his plans. Again, a full, and fully communicated, sensitivity to his feelings and those of his family may help the nurse to assist them all in accomplishing this task.

Strategies for the Chronically Ill □ Chronically ill clients may already have mastered many of these tasks before the nurse encounters them, unless she does so when the illness is first diagnosed or during some setback. If she encounters the client at a different point, however—say, during practice in the community—she should recognize that she is dealing with clients who are trying to have some sort of life with their families in spite of the limitations imposed by illness. Thus she should help the family plan days of work and recreation that are compatible with treatment but not so dominated by it that the client becomes his illness. He is, first and foremost, a person, who happens to have a chronic illness. A client whose hands are crippled with arthritis may feel that she cannot go to an alumnae banquet because she cannot use ordinary silverware, yet if encouraged to carry a small kit with implements she can manage, may realize that not only this but other social events are possible. Adult children or friends could be enlisted to scout out places of entertainment, education, or religious worship in which a wheelchair is not a hopeless inconvenience. If clients are daunted at the prospect of managing 10 different containers, they could be encouraged to use compartmentalized containers holding just the medications needed for the period of a trip and to carry a small flask of water. The task of helping chronically ill clients integrate treatment into a life that preserves some semblance of normality for as long as possible is a challenge, but one that calls on the utmost tact and creativity—and thus can be a real joy for the nurse.

In all of this, however, the client must still monitor himself and needs to know the very first signs of difficulty that unless appropriately handled presage graver problems. Faintness and a feeling of unreality, for example, may be the first sign that hypoglycemia is setting in for diabetic clients. It is common to allow newly diagnosed diabetics to experience hypoglycemia while still in hospital so that they know what it feels like. They are advised to carry some source of glucose wherever they go. But an active previously healthy person can still be taken by surprise when an episode occurs for the first time outside the hospital. Diabetics should be encouraged to recognize that repeated hypoglycemic episodes may mean they need to be reevaluated, even if they know very well how to stave them off and do so successfully. Similarly, viral infections that cause vomiting may lead diabetics not to eat and therefore not to take their insulin; they require instruction to recognize that this is not the appropriate response. Mitchell (1983) suggests that the nurse make herself available in person or at least by phone to help with situations such as these, so that times of special vulnerability do not blossom into periods of crisis. For chronically ill clients, crises are best prevented, because frequent repetition of crisis is too demoralizing and physically devastating to be permitted.

For some clients, it is very hard to distinguish between symptoms and signs that are just part of their condition, and those that indicate a need for professional help. At times this may be because of a deficit of information. At others, it is not ignorance so much as financial problems, family difficulties, or other problems that prevent the client from paying proper attention. Families with one parent, other sick members, a history of problems of other kinds with which the family has not coped well, distant members, or members with whom the client has turbulent relationships, are all particularly vulnerable. Moreover, a previously solid unit may become vulnerable to the point of chaos during the maturational crises of either the client himself or other family members (Mitchell, 1983).

If it can be arranged, a consistent relationship with one caregiver, who comes to know the family over a period of years and therefore can help them see trouble coming and prepare for it, should be provided. This ideal may not be very easy to realize. A fair second-best must be in the quality of documentation, which should not merely satisfy bureaucratic requirements, but also give any professional who takes over a realistic profile which can be useful in maintaining continuous, intelligent care that is genuinely sensitive to needs.

Coping with Terminal Illness ☐ With the best of care by the family in collaboration with the health care team, the long battle with ill health must some day be lost. At this stage, if not long before, many clients who subscribe to some faith or another may find it of great comfort, for, as Sevensky (1981) has stated, "that there is a lesson to be learned [from sickness] has sustained many who are faced with what appear to us—the onlooker—to be absurd and empty experiences." Family members may be reluctant to seek spiritual help, regarding this as a capitulation to an enemy—death—which they are determined to fight at all costs. Yet this reluctance may deprive the client of what he most needs, a peaceful death; so the nurse, mindful that helping the client to achieve this is one of her roles, should try tactfully to overcome their resistance. The following vignette may illustrate the value of doing so:

Vignette

Louise Maher's long struggle with cancer was clearly coming to an end, but only her daughter, Betsy, who had discussed the situation fully with a nurse, could grasp this fact. The rest of the family made it clear that all possible efforts were to be made to keep Louise alive; staff tried to do so, even resuscitating her twice despite the injuries that caused (because Louise's metastases-riddled bones were so brittle). The family were bitter with Betsy's request that her mother's clear wish that this cease be respected. Finally, the nurse, knowing the family's Catholic background, suggested that a priest be summoned to see Louise. Betsy bravely did so, over the family's objections, before her mother had slipped into her final coma. At last the family began to be able to deal with the inevitable and to grieve appropriately, and Louise died peacefully one or two days later. Only the total clarity of information that Betsy had had all along from the nurse enabled her to provide the needed strength for her family and to take this last necessary step when it was most needed.

In the meantime, especially when the terminally ill client is dying at home, the nurse can help the family most by herself undertaking and teaching them to undertake comfort measures for the client—and by helping them both to grieve and to plan. All of this will be possible only if, by her interested attitude and concrete availability, the nurse has secured the family's trust.

At times, chronically ill clients have wanted to die at home, but are unable to do so when the time comes. Family members who have had a hemorrhaging or otherwise critically ill client taken to the hospital, only to die there, may be overwhelmed with guilt, may blame themselves for not recognizing that this really was the end, and feel that they failed. Hospital nurses who may have no relationship to the family may be in a poor position to help, but should feel both the freedom and the responsibility to refer the family to the community health nurse who *has* known them, and/or to self-help groups in the area. Some chronically ill clients have been involved in such groups with or without their families all through their illness, and both clients and families have often been found to benefit (Selan and Schuenke, 1982; Winkes, 1983; Wilson, 1982; Dunlop, 1982). Indeed, some of the authors cited describe nurse-led or co-led groups developed specially to help families dealing with various health problems, and bereaved survivors frequently continue to come to such groups because only there can they be sure of hearing from people who truly know what they have endured.

Enhancing the Nurse's Own Coping □ Interventions undertaken by the nurse to improve her own coping are contingent upon her having completed an accurate assessment of self-coping. Based on her assessment, she might try whichever of the following suggestions appears to fit the problem she has identified:

1. She can seek, through her own library research or class attendance, to improve her knowledge and skills.
2. She can discuss her feelings of failure and despair with other nurses; some agencies facilitate this through staff meetings and workshops for the purpose. Some cities have nursing support groups; former instructors can also sometimes be a resource.
3. She can provide frequent small supportive gestures of concern to the client or family, rather than expecting herself to conduct full-scale therapeutic meetings in the heat of a busy day. Also, she could request assistance from members of other disciplines so that the client's and family's emotional needs are addressed by others, if she lacks the time to do so.
4. She can seek counseling or therapy for herself to help her to resolve past conflicts and review the rational basis for the feelings she has toward clients.

In the situation of critical care, many nurses cope by focusing on becoming the best technicians they can be and tending as swiftly as possible to the physical needs that are so pressing. At times this can mean that the emotional needs of not even the client, let alone his family, are addressed. To some degree, this is the result of the nurses' need to cope with the stress of their own situation. It is as if they were saying to themselves: "The only way I can stand the pain and death I am witnessing is to fight both, using all the strategies available to me in the critical care setting." Experienced critical care nurses have frequently said that this way of coping is particularly useful to them in their first year of work in critical care. Unfortunately, the pressure is so great that many nurses do not stay longer than a year, if they stay that long. Clients and families often do not object to the nurse's concentration on physical needs, reasoning that it is necessary to save life. Nevertheless, they would doubtless have no complaint if some attention were paid to their emotional needs.

One reason why emotional support may not be attempted is that the model learned in nursing school involves relatively lengthy periods of sitting with clients and families, listening and talking. So if the pressure of work does not permit a 45-minute session, nurses may feel they can do nothing. This perception is, however, both unrealistic and excessive. The correct use of client's and family's names; a smile on arrival of family members; a brief summary of progress ("He's having a tough time, but he's hanging on"); and willingness to touch both the client and his family in the form of a quick hand-squeeze or an arm around the shoulders—all of this can provide support in a very short time. Moreover, providing such little touches can help the nurse, as well as the family, to cope a little better than either would without them.

With chronically ill clients, the lengthy listening session is physically feasible, but may be very draining, since there may be little the nurse can do but listen to what may seem an endless, repetitive recitation of aches and pains. Many nurses are doers and find it intolerable to hear about suffering that they cannot alleviate by some action of their own. Some cope by curtailing periods spent with the client; others become angry, though they may not express this feeling openly. Such anger arises from the knowledge that one is not omnipotent; one cannot cure the chronically sick client. As soon as this is realized, the unreality of one's expectations both of the client and of oneself becomes obvious. The nurse is then in a position to cope more appropriately than by withdrawing or becoming impatient.

Another issue that can impair the nurse's coping is her personal set of associations to particular diagnoses, age groups, or socioeconomic or ethnic populations. If a near relative went through the same illness as the client, for example, the nurse-client relationship can be heavily colored and even distorted by the nurse's unresolved feelings of guilt, anger, and so on, which were originally evoked by the relative. Also, prejudices and stereotypes about elderly clients versus young ones, poor and ill-educated clients versus rich and well-educated ones, or "typical" Jewish, Irish, Hispanic, or whatever clients, may all create expectations in the nurse that may be quite inaccurate.

Thus, self-awareness is crucial if the nurse is to cope, that is, if she is to help clients to cope while managing her own responses. In more general terms, those nurses cope best who tend to their own physical, emotional, and spiritual needs. Sheer fatigue, inadequate exercise and fresh air, neglected intake of iron and vitamins, or insufficient attention to her own needs for affection, recreation, and spiritual comfort can all diminish coping ability. Thus, appropriate intervention to maintain or restore her own coping largely consists in ensuring that she is fit on all levels to deal with the heavy demands that the care of the sick place upon her.

■ Enrichment Activities

DISCUSSION QUESTIONS

1. Consider the fact (Alleyne, Vassall-Hurd, and Morgan, 1982) that clients with end-stage renal disease in Jamaica did comparatively well at coping with financial and psychosocial problems, despite a dearth of structured social services. In your discussion, attempt to deal with the following questions:
   a. What implications does this have for provisions of social services—does such provision, for instance, actually *impair* people's own capacity to cope?
   b. How can nursing and other health care be delivered in such a way that people are stimulated to use the resources of family, church, clubs, and so on in the community (as do the Jamaicans), rather than relying on public welfare and health care delivery systems?

2. Antonovsky (1979) regards the origins of health and resistance to breakdown as lying in a person's "generalized resistance resources." The most important of these is "coherence."
   a. How would you evaluate the presence/absence of "coherence" in a client?
   b. Do you agree that this variable in some way mediates between other resistance resources and health? Why or why not?

LEARNING ACTIVITIES

1. The next time you have a cold, "flu," or other minor illness, evaluate your coping using Weisman's seven questions. Notice how it feels to think about these questions when you are under the weather. Think about phrasing that might make it easier.

2. List aspects of your situation that reduce the likelihood that this illness will throw you and your family into crisis (good resistance, adequate premises for your care, adequate response from concerned family members, health insurance, sick pay, other).

3. When you have recovered, make a conscious effort to incorporate what you have learned about illness into your planning, interventions, and, particularly, interactions with clients.

■ Recommended Readings

Beglinger, J.E. Coping tasks in critical care. *Dimensions of critical care nursing*, 2, 1983:80–89. A very well-done presentation of the coping tasks of clients and families facing critical illness.

Craig, H.M., and Edwards, J.E. Adaptation in chronic illness: An eclectic model for nurses. *Journal of advanced nursing*, 8, 1983:397–404. Builds on the theory of Lazarus to develop a model for understanding and helping chronically ill clients and their families to adapt.

Lipowski, X.J. Physical illness and the coping process. *Psychiatry in medicine*, 1, 1970:91–102. Sets forth author's ideas about different coping styles. Despite its age, this article is still a classic resource.

Mitchell, P.H. Crisis management for families living with chronic illness. *Washington State journal of nursing*, 54, 1983:2–8. An exploration of coping tasks faced by the chronically ill and their families.

Moos, R.H., and Tsu, V.D. *Coping with physical illness*. New York: Plenum Medical Book Co., 1977. Examines the plight of clients, families, and helping professionals as they confront the crisis of physical illness in various forms, including cancer and kidney failure requiring dialysis. Some chapters have interesting references; all are clearly and interestingly written.

■ *References*

Abram, H.S. Survival by machine: The psychological aspects of home dialysis. In *Coping with physical illness* (Moos, R., and Tsu, V.D., eds.). New York: Plenum Press, 1977.

Alleyne, A.L., Vassall-Hurd, S.A., and Morgan, A.G. End-stage renal disease in Jamaica; How patients cope in a developing society. *Health and social work*, 7, 1982:130–133.

Antonovsky, A. *Health, stress, and coping*. San Francisco: Jossey-Bass, Inc., 1979.

Beaver, W.T. Management of cancer pain with parenteral medication. *Journal of the American Medical Association*, 244, 1980:2653–2657.

Beglinger, J.E. Coping tasks in critical care. *Dimensions of critical care nursing*, 2, 1983:80–89.

Browne, I.W., and Hackett, T.P. Emotional reactions to the threat of impending death. *Irish journal of medical sciences*, 496, 1967:177–181.

Burns, N. *Nursing and cancer*. Philadelphia: W.B. Saunders, 1982.

Copp, L.A. The spectrum of suffering. *American journal of nursing*, 74, 1974:491–495.

Craig, H.M., and Edwards, J.E. Adaptation in chronic illness: An eclectic model for nurses. *Journal of advanced nursing*, 8, 1983:397–404.

Dangott, L., Thornton, B.L., and Page, P. Communication and pain. *Journal of communication*, 28, 1978:30–35.

Dhooper, S.S. Family coping with the crisis of heart attack. *Social work in health care*, 9, 1983:15–31.

Dunlop, J.G. Critical problems facing young adults with cancer. *Oncology nursing forum*, 9, 1982:33–38.

Erikson, E.H. *Identity: Youth and crisis*. New York: Norton, 1968.

Fagerhaugh, S.Y., and Strauss, A. *The politics of pain management: Patient-staff interaction*. Menlo Park: Addison-Wesley, 1977.

Geach, B. Pain memory imagery, experience with pain, orienting information, and distress in response to pain: An experimental study. Doctoral dissertation, University of Pennsylvania School of Nursing, 1983.

Goffman, E. *Stigma: Notes on the management of spoiled identity*. Englewood Cliffs, NJ: Prentice-Hall, 1963.

Hackett, T.P., Cassem, W.H., and Wishnie, H. Psychological hazards of the coronary care unit. *New England journal of medicine*, 279, 1968:1365–1369.

Hall, J.I., and Weaver, B.R. Crisis: A conceptual approach to family nursing. In *Nursing of families in crisis* (Hall, J.E., and Weaver, B.R., eds.). Philadelphia: J.B. Lippincott, 1974:3–9.

Hansen, J.L. Assessing the mastectomy patient's need for special coping strategies. *Journal of practical nursing*, 33, 1983:24–27.

Johnson, J.E. Effects of accurate expectations about sensations on the sensory and distress components of pain. *Journal of personality and social psychology*, 27, 1973:261–275.

Johnson, J.E., Fuller, S.S., Endress, M.P., and Rice, V.H. Altering patients' responses to surgery: An extension and replication. *Research in nursing and health*, 1, 1978:111–121.

Johnson, J.E., Kirchhoff, K.T., and Endress, M.P. Altering children's distress behavior during orthopedic cast removal. *Nursing research*, 24, 1975:404–410.

Johnson, J.E., Morrissey, J.F., and Leventhal, H. Psychological preparation for an endoscopic examination. *Gastrointestinal endoscopy*, 19, 1973:180–182.

Johnson, J.E., Rice, V.H., Fuller, S.S., and Endress, M.P. Sensory information, instruction in a coping strategy, and recovery from surgery. *Research in nursing and health*, 1, 1978:4–17.

Krumm, S. Psychosocial adaptation of the adult with cancer. *Nursing clinics of North America*, 17, 1982:229–237.

Lazarus, R.S. Psychological stress and coping in adaptation and illness. *International journal of psychiatry in medicine*, 5, 1974:321–333.

Lazarus, R.S. Cognitive and coping processes in emotion. In *Stress and coping: An anthology* (Mondt, A., and Lazarus, R.S., eds.). New York: Columbia University Press, 1977:145–157.

Lipowski, Z.J. Physical illness, the individual, and the coping processes. *Psychiatry in medicine*, 1, 1970:91–102.

McCaffery, M. *Nursing management of the patient with pain.* 2d ed. Philadelphia: J.B. Lippincott, 1979.

Miller, J.F. *Coping with chronic illness: Overcoming powerlessness.* Philadelphia: F.A. Davis, 1983.

Miller, S. When is a little information a dangerous thing? Coping with stressful events by monitoring versus blunting. In *Coping and health: Proceedings of a NATO conference* (Levine, S., and Ursin, H., eds.). New York: Plenum, 1980.

Miller, S. Predictability and human stress: Toward a clarification of evidence and theory. *Advances in experimental social psychology*, 14, 1981:204–256.

Mitchell, P.H. Crisis management for families living with chronic illness. *Washington State journal of nursing*, 54, 1983:2–8.

Mooney, N.E. Coping with chronic pain in rheumatoid arthritis: Patient behaviors and nursing interventions. *Orthopedic nursing*, 1, 1982:21–25.

Moos, R.H., and Tsu, V.D. *Coping with physical illness.* New York: Plenum, 1977.

Nehring, V., and Geach, B. Patient's satisfaction with their care: Why they don't complain. *Nursing outlook*, 21, 1973:317–321.

Peretz, D. Development, object relationships, and loss. In *Loss and grief: Psychological management in medical practice* (Schoenberg, B., Carr, A.C., Peretz, D., and Kutscher, A.H., eds.). New York: Columbia University Press, 1970.

Quayhagen, Sr. M. An interactional model for the study of pain. *Communicating nursing research*, 9, 1977:309–318.

Savage, J.S. Effect of crisis on female sexual identity. *Issues in health care of women*, 3, 1981:151–160.

Selan, B.H., and Schuenke, S. The late life care program: Helping families cope. *Health and social work*, 7, 1982:192–197.

Sevensky, R.L. Religion and illness: An outline of their relationship. *Southern medical journal*, 74, 1981:745–749.

Siegler, M., and Osmond, H. *Patienthood.* New York: Macmillan, 1979.

Strauss, A., Fagerhaugh, S.Y., Suczek, B., and Wiener, C. Patients' work in the technologized hospital. *Nursing outlook*, 29, 1981:404–412.

Strauss, A., and Glaser, B. *Chronic illness and the quality of life.* St. Louis: Mosby, 1975.

Suchman, E.A. Stages of illness and medical care. In *Patients, physicians, and illness* (Jaco, E.G. ed.). New York: The Free Press, 1972.

Thomas, S.A., Sappington, E., Gross, H.E., Noctor, M., Friedman, E., and Lynch, J. Denial in coronary care patients—An objective reassessment. *Heart and lung*, 12, 1983:74–80.

Twaddle, A.C. *Sickness behavior and the sick role.* Cambridge, MA: Schenckman, 1979.

Weisman, A.D. *Coping with cancer.* New York: McGraw-Hill, 1979.

Welch, D. Planning nursing interventions for family members of adult cancer patients. *Cancer nursing*, 4, 1981:365–370.

Wilson, L. How to develop a support group for families of open heart surgery patients. *Dimensions of critical care nursing*, 1, 1982:108–116.

Winkes, A. The promotion of adaptation to end stage renal disease. *Nephrology nurse*, 5, January–February 1983:17–19.

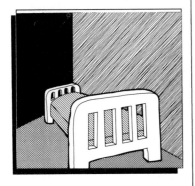

26

Loss: Grief, Death, and Dying

Barbara Gross Braverman

Learning Objectives

Upon completion of this chapter, the reader will be able to:

1. Have an understanding of loss and the grief process.
2. Describe symptoms of normal and dysfunctional grief.
3. Recognize coping behaviors in persons having to deal with death and dying.
4. Develop sensitivity to age and cultural differences in coping with loss, grief, and death.
5. Understand the implications of grief and coping behaviors for nursing care.

Most deaths occur in hospitals. Most often, terminally ill people are treated in hospitals and die there without returning home. However, it wasn't always this way. In times past, death, like birth and illness, all occurred within the confines of the family home.

With the move away from home care, death has become more distant. Dying has become something we not only feel uncomfortable with, but something of which we are afraid. Death has also taken on an element of unreality, with large-scale violence and fatalities becoming part of our daily diet. In the 1940s entire cities—Hiroshima and Nagasaki—were wiped out; in the 1960s and early 1970s we watched televised scenes of the Vietnam War as we ate our evening meal. Today we read about violence and death routinely in newspapers and see them portrayed in children's cartoons and evening television entertainment. We maintain alienation from the realness of death by denying and even avoiding the mention of it. We say, "he passed away" or "departed" when we mean he died, and we say "laid to rest" when referring to the burial. Even sympathy cards rarely make direct references to death, using instead words like "loss" and "sorrow" (Woods and Delisle, 1977).

The denial of death as a natural phenomenon has spread into the health care arena. Since nurses and physicians are taught to care for, maintain, and restore health, death is viewed as a failing of all that is taught. Even the way in which nurses talk about death reflects denial and avoidance, using "it" instead of the word "death" or "dying" (Mood and Lick, 1979).

When denial and avoidance is the approach to death, nurses do both themselves and their clients a disservice. To assist clients through loss, grief, dying, and death, the nurse must recognize, accept, and apply basic principles. This chapter explores concepts of grief, death, and dying with emphasis on coping behaviors and nursing implications.

☐ *Theoretical Perspectives*

NATURAL DEATH

Death as the endpoint in the life cycle can be an active or a passive process. When death occurs passively as a result of a disease process, it is referred to as natural death. The term *natural* emphasizes the inevitability of such a death. Since we expect the death, there may be a less complicated grief reaction. When an elderly ill person dies, we may be saddened or grieved, but we are rarely surprised. Death is the part of the life cycle that accompanies old age and therefore does not come as a shock.

SUDDEN DEATH

Sudden death occurs without prior warning to the person and/or others. It may result from an accident, an environmental cause such as flood or earthquake, or a criminal act. It can also result from an undiagnosed or unrecognized disease process. Since there is no warning and therefore no preparation time, survivors may have a more prolonged or complicated period of grief and mourning.

BENEMORTASIA

Benemortasia is the term used to describe a disease process that is permitted to take its natural course while only palliative, rather than curative, treatment is provided. An elderly comatose client with terminal cancer whose pneumonia is left untreated is an example of benemortasia. The decision to treat or not to treat such an illness is made frequently in hospitals (Young, 1978).

EUTHANASIA

The withdrawal of a therapeutic regimen so that the person may die is referred to as euthanasia. With our ever-increasing technological sophistication, it has become possible to extend life by treating of once-fatal diseases (Young, 1978). Many people believe, however, that in many instances technological know-how is not reason enough to prolong life. The decision to withdraw lifesaving treatment is never an easy one. It is made even more difficult when it involves patients too young or too ill to participate in that decision. The Living Will was developed to aid in the decision making by expressing, through a written document, the wishes of the person involved (Fig 26-1).

MERCY KILLING

Mercy killing differs from euthanasia in that it describes an action taken purposefully to end another's life. Most often it involves people who suffer from a terminal or chronically debilitating ill-

My Living Will
To My Family, My Physician, My Lawyer
and All Others Whom It May Concern

Death is as much a reality as birth, growth, maturity and old age—it is the one certainty of life. If the time comes when I can no longer take part in decisions for my own future, let this statement stand as an expression of my wishes and directions, while I am still of sound mind.

If at such a time the situation should arise in which there is no reasonable expectation of my recovery from extreme physical or mental disability, I direct that I be allowed to die and not be kept alive by medications, artificial means or "heroic measures". I do, however, ask that medication be mercifully administered to me to alleviate suffering even though this may shorten my remaining life.

This statement is made after careful consideration and is in accordance with my strong convictions and beliefs. I want the wishes and directions here expressed carried out to the extent permitted by law. Insofar as they are not legally enforceable, I hope that those to whom this Will is addressed will regard themselves as morally bound by these provisions.

(Optional specific provisions to be made in this space — see other side)

DURABLE POWER OF ATTORNEY (optional)

I hereby designate _____ to serve as my attorney-in-fact for the purpose of making medical treatment decisions. This power of attorney shall remain effective in the event that I become incompetent or otherwise unable to make such decisions for myself.

Optional Notarization: Signed_____

"Sworn and subscribed to   Date _____

before me this _____ day   Witness _____

of _____, 19_____."
                                       _____
                                                        Address
_____   Witness _____
        Notary Public
           (seal)   _____
                                                        Address

Copies of this request have been given to _____

_____   _____

(Optional)   My Living Will is registered with Concern for Dying (No. _____)

Distributed by Concern for Dying, 250 West 57th Street, New York, NY 10107 (212) 246-6962

Figure 26-1 *Living will. Reprinted with permission of CONCERN FOR DYING, 250 West 57th Street, New York, N.Y.*

ness. Although this act may be committed for reasons of mercy and perhaps with the sick person's consent, it is clearly illegal. The moral difference between euthanasia and mercy killing remains controversial.

SUICIDE

Suicide is the taking of one's own life. It may be an active or a passive act. A person may purposefully take an overdose of lethal medication or use another method to actively end his life. The diabetic person who withholds his necessary insulin may be committing suicide passively. Suicide often leaves in its wake feelings of intense anger, helplessness, and guilt in the survivors.

Although suicide may happen abruptly without obvious warnings, very often the person has given both verbal and behavioral clues to his intent. The hospitalized client in pain may state, "I just don't want to hurt anymore." He may say, "I feel like something bad may happen," or he may even bluntly state, "I want to die."

The person may manifest acute behavioral changes. The client who has been markedly depressed may now appear happy or even euphoric. Someone contemplating suicide may begin to put his life in order, pay debts, write a will, or give away cherished possessions. In this way, he may be letting others know of his decision to end his life.

There are several situations in which suicidal thoughts or attempts are most likely to occur. Most often these situations involve significant loss or a series of losses. It may be loss of a significant other or may be any loss that occurs suddenly or without warning. Or the situation may involve a damaging loss of self-image or self-esteem. Chapter 33 discusses suicide and nursing implications in further detail.

☐ *The Dying Person*

In her work with dying people, Kubler-Ross (1969) observed and documented a general pattern of coping with anticipated death. This pattern, often referred to as *coping stages*, begins with denial and continues through the stage of acceptance.

COPING STAGES

Denial

Denial, either partial or complete, is practiced by almost all dying people. It may be employed not only immediately following the receipt of the news, but also to some degree throughout the remaining stages. Denial serves as a protective barrier, temporarily shielding the person from the painful knowledge and allowing him to mobilize other coping methods. Denial may be evident through the person's unwillingness to discuss the illness, in noncompliance with treatment, or in a variety of other ways, such as continuing to plan for an active future. The person's need for denial should not be challenged. Very often, the person's use of denial will fluctuate as a natural part of the coping process; that is, the client may appear to be using denial one moment and then may acknowledge reality the next. Most often denial fades as the process continues and the person moves on to alternative methods of coping.

Anger

Gradually denial gives way to feelings of rage and *anger* as the client demands to know, "Why me?" Although these feelings are in response to his own perceived loss of control, they are often directed outward toward whomever he has contact with. The anger may be displaced onto family, friends, physicians, and, frequently, nurses. When nurses don't understand the anger as a normal response, they may react in ways that intensify the anger. They may spend less time with the client, avoid him entirely, or respond with anger of their own.

Bargaining

The next stage, *bargaining*, is also a necessary but usually temporary approach to coping. The bargain is a wishful attempt to postpone the inevitable. The client believes that if he is "good," he will be rewarded by experiencing recovery or remission. Most such bargains are made with God, and may involve promises to lead a good life, to mend faulty relationships, or to dedicate his life to God. Since generally the promise is kept secret, nurses may be only subtly aware of the existence of the bargain, noting, for example, the client's increased contact with clergy.

Depression

When anger and rage have subsided and "bargaining" is no longer effective, the client may experience a sense of profound loss. This may encompass a variety of losses, such as loss of career, loss of intact body image, and loss of future plans and dreams. The client is experiencing a reactive *depression*, that is, a depression precipitated by the cumulative losses. The client may also experience depression in anticipation of great impending losses, the loss of all love objects, which includes all that has ever been meaningful to him. By expressing his feelings of sorrow now, he may find acceptance of dying an easier process.

TABLE 26-1 Needs of the Dying Person	
Physiological	**Emotional**
To have basic needs fulfilled (e.g., thirst, temperature)	To be treated with respect and dignity
To be provided with sensory stimuli; not to be isolated	To maintain as much decision-making power as possible
To be as pain-free but alert as possible	To maintain a sense of control

the notion of his own impending, inevitable death. Tables 26-1 and 26-2 define some physical and emotional needs of the dying person and the stages of dying.

> **■ Point of Emphasis**
>
> *The dying person copes with anticipated death by use of mechanisms such as denial and anger. Nurses should recognize such reactions as normal.*

Acceptance

Since feelings of anger and sorrow have already been expressed, the final stage is characterized by a sense of peaceful *acceptance*. The client may wish to be left alone now, or spend time quietly with family members and friends. There may be little verbal communication as he may be weak or sleeping a good deal of the time. Although hope generally persists through all stages, the person may now be clearly expecting death. Rather than "giving up," the client has finally come to accept

☐ The Grieving Person

Grief may be defined as a characteristic response to the loss of a valued object, be it person, body part, possession, job status, or ideal (Engel, 1961). It fulfills the criteria of a syndrome, having a relatively predictable course and symptoms. As shown in Table 26-3, these symptoms can be both physical and psychological. There may be fatigue, shortness of breath, and anorexia. There may also be feelings of guilt, sadness and tearfulness, or

TABLE 26-2 Stages of Coping		
Stage	**Behaviors or Symptoms**	**Nursing Actions**
Denial	Unwilling to acknowledge presence of symptoms Refusing tests and/or other procedures Refusing to discuss illness-related matters Continuation of normal activities even when contraindicated	Acceptance and support of the client's denial as a necessary coping method Support of the client's continued activities, unless harmful
Anger	Angry, hostile verbal behavior toward nursing staff and others Angry, hostile nonverbal behavior Increased demands on staff	Understanding of the client's anger as a necessary coping method—don't take it personally Return control to the client whenever possible (e.g., allow the client to decide some issues concerning his care)
Bargaining	Subtle references to promises made, "If I . . . then I may have more time" Wanting to spend more time with clergy or spiritual leaders	Support of the client's spiritual needs, (e.g., arrange for time and privacy with clergy)
Depression	Presence of depressive symptoms (e.g., changes in appetite or sleep, somber mood, crying)	Providing a supportive environment in which the client may ventilate feelings of sadness or grief
Acceptance	May appear void of all feelings Less involved with family, friends, or others May desire to be left alone	Allowing the client quiet time alone or with family Sitting supportively with the client if he desires

TABLE 26-3 Symptoms of Acute Grief

Physical	Psychological
Anorexia	Anger and hostility
Dizziness and lightheadedness	Changes in normal behavior and activity
Fatigue and exhaustion	Disorganization of thoughts and actions
Nausea and vomiting	Guilt and self-blame
Shortness of breath or choking	Preoccupation with the deceased
	Tearfulness and sadness

changes in behavior and anger, all of which are normal responses to acute grief (Lindemann, 1944).

GRIEF WORK

Grief work is Lindemann's phrase for the required readjustment to a loss—which involves three major processes. The first, emancipation from the deceased, requires loosening the attachment bonds. In this process, the survivor must stop depending on the deceased for fulfillment of his needs, which may include emotional, financial, and day-to-day social needs. If the survivor had been depending on the deceased to balance his checkbook, to drive him to and from work, and to go to concerts and movies with him, he must adjust to the absence in all those areas. It is during this first process that one comes to realize how essential the lost relationship has been.

Next, the survivor begins to readjust to his environment. If he has taken a leave from work, he now returns. He may also begin to return to his other life responsibilities such as his family or community roles. Even with this outward return to normal functioning, he still remains inwardly mourning.

Finally the survivor will begin to form new attachments and relationships. Initially he may feel most comfortable with people who have also experienced a recent loss. Later he becomes open to forming relationships with a more diverse group of people.

These three processes in successful or uncomplicated grief reactions can be looked at in detail as a more or less predictable sequence of steps. Although the time involved in completing each sequence differs from one person to another, there should be evidence of progress from one step to the next.

Anticipatory Grief

Anticipatory grief may follow the receipt of news about a terminal or fatal illness. In this step, the mourner may go through all the phases of grief that usually follow loss or death, using this as a mechanism of defense against the inevitable or probable death. This grief work can be done so effectively however, that emancipation and separation from the dying person is complete long before death occurs.

Vignette

The nursing staff observed that the daughter of Ms. Smith, a 56-year-old mother of three, had visited her mother only once in the last week. It seemed odd since the daughter had been in the hospital daily since her mother had been hospitalized, and had been tearful over the diagnosis of terminal metastatic cancer. In discussing the situation, the nurses noted that other family members were calling and visiting less frequently, and that they had become less involved with issues dealing with her care. They wondered whether the family's change in behavior occurred in anticipation of Ms. Smith's impending death.

Disbelief, Shock

When a death occurs, the survivor initially experiences *disbelief and shock*. He is unable to think about the death, or even acknowledge to himself or others that it has occurred. Unable to accept the reality, he may feel numb and devoid of all feeling. This first step, occurring after news of the death, can last just a few minutes or days.

Awareness

As time passes, the shock and numbness begin to fade and there is a sense that something has been lost or is missing. This beginning *sense of awareness* is often described as a hollow, empty feeling in the chest or stomach. There may be anger at those who had been involved in the client's care, often the nurse or other health professionals. There may also be acute behavioral changes—the survivor may appear quite unlike his normal self. Feelings of guilt and self-reproach for what he did or did not do for the deceased may be evident in impulsive and sometimes self-destructive acts. He may cry or scream or behave in a childlike manner, requiring others to do for him.

Restitution

Mourning signifies the beginning of *restitution*. The funeral rituals which confirm the reality of the death help bring on the painful but necessary work of mourning. It is a time of great sadness for all who share the loss, although the sadness may not be experienced by all to the same degree. The group experience of the funeral provides emotional support for the survivors most affected as well as spiritual support that is inherent in the rites.

Resolve

Once the funeral rites have been completed, the survivor must now *resolve* the loss and the pain associated with it. As a result, there is an increased awareness of his own bodily sensations and physical symptoms. Frequently, these symptoms are similar to those that were experienced by the deceased during his terminal illness. If the death occurred due to myocardial infarction, the survivor may experience chest pain. This symptom similarity is usually beyond his awareness and lasts for only a brief time. This stage is also characterized by a growing preoccupation with thoughts of the deceased. Initially these thoughts focus on what significance the loss has for him personally, and later becomes more focused on the person who died.

Vignette

A 24-year-old woman came to the emergency room of her local hospital complaining of chest pain. She described the pain as "sharp shooting pain in the chest, radiating down the left arm." In talking with the nurse the woman revealed that earlier that month she had attended the funeral of a close uncle who had died suddenly of myocardial infarction. The physical examination was benign and the client was diagnosed as having atypical chest pain.

Idealization

Idealization, a process by which all negative feelings are buried and only positive ones are allowed, occurs toward the deceased. The survivor may recall the charitable work the deceased did, but block from memory his stubbornness or other less desirable traits. Through this process, the survi-vor may adopt admired qualities, mannerisms, or ideals that the deceased is thought to have possessed, while denying that the less admired traits existed. Feelings of guilt and responsibility for the death contribute to the initiation of this process.

Completion

The final step is *completion*. As mourning progresses normally, preoccupation with thoughts of the deceased lessens. The mourner is now ready to admit the negative as well as the positive qualities of the deceased and interest is resumed in the outside world and others in it. This process may take a year or more to complete. *Successful mourning* can be said to have occurred when the survivor possesses the ability to recall with comfort and realism both the pleasant and the disappointing aspects of the lost relationship (Engel, 1964).

Factors that Influence the Attainment of Successful Mourning. The more dependent the survivor has been on the deceased person for emotional, financial, or other support, the more difficult it is to resolve the loss. It may be particularly difficult for the survivor of an elderly couple who had relied on each other for safety and security. This is especially true in older people who have few other family supports and have learned to depend only on each other.

In the life process, it is anticipated that the elderly will die before the children. When this natural order is disturbed, mourning may be harder to resolve. The death of a child from a terminal illness or fatal accident is usually more difficult to accept than is the death of an elderly parent or grandparent. It also follows that the closer or more important the relationship between the survivor and the deceased, the greater the impact of the loss (e.g., a parent versus a business associate). Often, the relationship is ambivalent, involving both positive and negative feelings toward the deceased, and the loss may be harder to resolve. There may exist, for example, feelings of sadness over the death and at the same time, feelings of relief over the ending of a difficult relationship—which may lead to guilt in the survivor, who may think that having such feelings makes him a "bad" person.

People who have had few significant relationships will feel the loss of one significant relationship very deeply, as in the example of the elderly couple who primarily have each other. Each sub-

TABLE 26-4 Factors that Influence the Outcome of Mourning

Dependence on the deceased
Age and relationship to the deceased
Number and nature of other relationships
Number and nature of previous losses
Well-being of the mourner
Prior coping skills

sequent loss then adds to the work of mourning. This difficulty is multiplied when the losses occur close in time. A woman whose husband dies and who then loses her house as a result of subsequent financial problems must deal with a double loss.

The survivor's overall health and his previous level of functioning also influence the successful outcome of mourning as do physical and psychological factors, and earlier coping mechanisms. How the mourner has coped with stressful life situations in general will profoundly affect his handling of this particular loss (Table 26-4).

DYSFUNCTIONAL GRIEVING

When grieving does not follow the normal course, it is said to be dysfunctional. Unresolved or delayed grief, and absence of grief are examples of dysfunctional grieving. Other terms that describe dysfunctional grieving include *morbid, pathological,* or *complicated* grief reactions.

Absence of Grief

Absence of grief is seen most often in persons described as independent and self-sufficient and who regard shedding tears as a sign of weakness (Parkes, 1972). These persons have difficulty expressing the full range of emotions, are often isolated, and are fearful of intimacy. Although they do not consciously grieve, they may experience mild to severe physical symptoms such as chest pain, headaches, and insomnia.

Delayed Grief Reaction

An individual who has not experienced grief immediately after the loss (absence of grief) may grieve weeks, months, or even years later. One type of delayed reaction is often referred to as an anniversary reaction, because it is associated with the anniversary of the death. It may be the initial

expression of grief, and it may mark the one-year anniversary, or an anniversary many years later. Sometimes it is a birthday or a family holiday such as Thanksgiving that occasions the grieving.

Grief may be precipitated with the occurrence of another loss, even though the more recent loss is not highly significant—for example, the death of an acquaintance. There is a similarity in feeling generated by loss of any kind.

Another form of delayed reaction is seen in the person who grieves upon reaching the age at which his friend or relative died—the deceased's age has assumed a magical significance.

Grief can be aroused when a friend of a grieving person experiences a similar loss. The more similar these two losses are, the more likely it is that identification will occur, and grief will be precipitated.

Vignette

Mr. Jones, age 54, complained that he suddenly felt sad and had no energy. He could not identify any precipitant but did mention that he was apprehensive because his fifty-fifth birthday was approaching. Mr. Jones also remarked that his father had died suddenly at age 55, and went on to say that he felt he wouldn't live past his own fifty-fifth year.

Euphoria

This inappropriate mood is associated with a definite, emphatic refusal to believe that death has actually happened; along with this, there is a clear sense of the deceased person's continued presence. Another version of this dysfunctional reaction is acknowledgment of death coupled with the claim that it is greatly to the advantage of the survivor. This euphoric mood is quite superficial and can be shattered very easily.

Clinical Depression

Clinical depression gives rise to disturbances in sleep patterns, appetite, level of energy, and sexual interest. There may also be impairment in the ability to think, although the idea of suicide may be entertained. (The treatment of depression and nursing implications are discussed in detail in Chapter 33.)

☐ Cultural Considerations

Culture may be regarded as a regulating system unique to its society. It is within this system that behavior is shaped. Each society instills values, morals, and attitudes in its members during the years of their physical and emotional development. Responses and reactions to life events are acquired through this cultural conditioning.

Culture also serves as the framework within which individuals formulate responses and attitudes toward death and dying. Culture shapes beliefs about the causes of death and the rituals associated with the body, the funeral, and the burial, including practices such as organ transplantation, autopsy, and cremation. Culture influences grief responses and bereavement roles of the survivors. Although the experience of grief is universal, it is cultural factors that determine its expression (Ross, 1981).

DEATH AND DYING AMONG NATIVE AMERICANS

Among American Indians, death is regarded as a normal part of the life cycle. Although it may be believed that the death was caused by the breaking of a taboo, death itself is not feared. During illness, the person is surrounded by family, as it is thought that the spirit of the dying person cannot leave the body unless the family is present. Somes tribes fear to touch the body of a dead person.

Autopsy is strongly opposed because the body must be buried intact and whole. Attitudes toward disposition of the body vary, some tribes practicing burial below ground, others practicing cremation. Grief is expressed outwardly, often through shedding tears, for a prescribed length of time. Afterward the memory of the death is suppressed and rarely discussed. Children are intimately involved in this process, taking part in caring for the dying person, attending the funeral ceremonies, and participating in the mourning practices.

DEATH AND DYING IN THE JEWISH TRADITION

In the Jewish tradition, visitation of the sick is recognized as an important religious obligation. Among Orthodox or traditional Jews, the family stays with the dying person so that his soul will not depart while he is alone. The body must then not be left unattended. The body may not be handled in any way on the Sabbath except by a non-Jew and with the consent of the next of kin (Berkowitz, 1967). Burial may not be delayed. Autopsy, prohibited among the Orthodox, is permitted by more liberal Jews. Plain coffins and simplicity in burial services are emphasized.

Mourning involves five stages that extend over a period of 1 year. The first stage, shiva, is the first 7 days following the burial and includes a prescribed set of mourning customs. The aim of these customs is an acknowledgment of the reality of death, directly and realistically. One of these customs, kriyah, involves a tearing or rending of clothing, as both a visual sign of internal pain and a means of expressing the pain in a culturally approved, controlled manner. The five mourning stages or grief work cycle symbolize first a "going down" or identification with the dead person and then a gradual "coming up" from the depths of sorrow (Moss, 1979).

☐ Grief, Death, and Dying through the Life Cycle

CHILDREN'S GRIEF

Children view death in a markedly different way from adults. A child's perception and understanding of the concept of death depends on his developmental age. (See Table 26-5.)

In the child less than 5 years of age, death is seen as a departure or separation which may be gradual, temporary, and/or reversible. This reversibility is most evident in the child who asks when his deceased family member will be coming home. At this age, a child's thinking is self-centered. When someone dies the child cannot understand that a change has occurred in that per-

TABLE 26-5 Children's Ideas about Death		
Developmental Age	Symbolic Conception	Characteristics
Under age 5	Death as separation	Gradual, temporary
Ages 5–9 years	Personification of death	Seen as resulting from wrong acts; person or object outside of oneself
9 years and above	Death as a natural process	Universal and inevitable

son's body; rather, he is aware of the changes in his own feelings and activities due to the death. For this child, the most painful thing about death is the separation itself, and so a death may initially seem the same as when parents go on vacation. The time period between death and burial may represent for the child a transitory stage between life and death in which the deceased is neither dead nor alive, just simply "not there."

Between ages 5 and 9 years, death becomes personified, that is, death is seen as a person or an object. Dying and death are regarded as bad things that may result from doing things that are "wrong." Often, children visualize death as a skeleton or a ghost and superstitiously fear that talking about death will make it come true. Although this child may accept the definiteness of death, he sees it primarily as a force outside of himself, rather than an internal process.

At about age 9 or 10, the child develops a more adult concept of death, which is now perceived as a process that occurs within himself. Its universality and inevitability also begin to be recognized.

Because developmental age plays such an important part in a child's grieving process, grieving may be severe and traumatic, having a less predictable outcome. In any case, the outcome will be strongly influenced by the manner in which parents and others react to the child's grieving.

■ Point of Emphasis

The developmental age of the child strongly influences his perceptions of death. Nurses must recognize these age-related differences in their interactions with children.

Mourning Behavior

Cultural patterns of grieving legislate a code of mourning behavior for children. In American soci-ety, many of these strongly held beliefs inhibit the normal grieving process. The following are a few of the practices that may inhibit normal grief: (1) excluding children from conversations about death or dying people, (2) excluding children from funeral rites and ceremonies, (3) restricting the expression of grief in instances when children are included, (4) denying the importance of the grieving process in children (Schultz, 1980).

Children should be permitted to grieve. Those who are not permitted may grow up to become adults unable to grieve or express emotions appropriately. They should be included in funeral rites, as their fantasies about death and burial may be far more traumatic than the reality; however, children who strongly refuse to attend should never be forced to go. The ceremonies should be clearly explained before and after the funeral. Euphemisms about death should be avoided, keeping in mind the developmental age of the child. A child who is told his dead aunt or uncle "went to sleep" as an explanation for death may expect the relative to wake up, or may fear going to sleep himself.

Most importantly, a child should be given adequate mourning time. He may not appear to be grieving in the same way an adult might. Instead he may show other symptoms such as poor concentration or behavioral problems in school. This occurs most often with children who are prohibited from grieving or those that are expected to resume their normal activities prematurely. Factors that influence how well a child copes with death are: (1) his chronological age, (2) his developmental age, (3) family support, and (4) the information given about death.

FAMILIES OF DYING CHILDREN

The loss of a child may be one of the most difficult losses to resolve. Since childhood death is less common in American society today, it may be greeted with extreme shock and disbelief when it does occur.

The death of a fetus or a newborn may elicit a severe grief response. Death occurring in utero or shortly after birth may seem unreal to the parents, who have had little or no interaction with the infant. The existence as well as the death of the infant needs to be confirmed. This can be accomplished by: (1) allowing the parents to see, touch, hold, or rock the infant; (2) encouraging them to take photographs of the infant or to keep the infant's identification bracelet; (3) allowing the parents to name the infant, and; (4) having the parents make the arrangements for the funeral and burial.

Pathological grief reactions can ensue if the parents are prevented by hospital staff or others from confirming, both emotionally and intellectually, the death of their infant. It is normal, however, for parents to wonder what their role and responsibility were in the death, especially if it occurred during pregnancy. Parents may ask: Why did our baby die? Did we cause our baby's death? Will it happen again if we attempt another pregnancy?

The risk of a pathologic grief reaction occurring increases when another pregnancy is conceived within 5 months or less of the first infant's death. This may be because 5 months is a less than adequate time for the mourning process to have been worked through. If the parents have not reached appropriate acceptance and resolution, they may regard a subsequent child as a substitute or replacement for the lost baby. As a result, the loss may never be fully resolved and the surviving child may find himself burdened with overwhelming parental expectations.

In general, reactions to a child's death may be related to his age and the cause and suddenness of the death. If a child has a terminal illness, families may have experienced some anticipatory grief. When death is unexpected, as in an accident or an act of violence, grief may take the form of a long period of shock and denial along with strong feelings of anger and guilt. Since parents generally regard themselves as protectors of children, in such cases they may perceive themselves as failing in their protective role. Bereaved parents may even blame each other, sometimes to the point of separating or divorcing.

Siblings may experience the same intense emotions as their parents. They may worry about their role and responsibility in the death. If the sibling is young, normal sibling rivalry or arguing may be feared to have been magically responsible for the brother or sister's death. It is essential, therefore, to include siblings in conversations, interactions, and funeral preparations for their dead sibling.

THE ELDERLY

Loss is a common occurrence among the elderly. The most profound loss may be the loss of a spouse, and there may be few opportunities in this population to find a substitute. Death of friends and relatives, too, comes relentlessly and frequently. These cumulative losses present a special problem. When loss is frequent, there may be little time to finish the required grief work before the next loss occurs. As a result, resolution of each loss may be accomplished to only a limited degree.

One might think that because losses accumulate with age, an elderly person may cope better. Generally, however, the reverse is true. As losses accrue with age, each remaining relationship becomes more strongly valued and harder to part with (Goodstein, 1984).

Along with the loss associated with death, there are other losses common in this population. For the older person who moves to a nursing home, there is a loss of familiar surroundings or family home. There may be loss of body integrity marked by physical deterioration, loss of hearing, or loss of sight. There may be loss of independence due to deterioration in mobility or in mental functioning. For many, this loss may be the hardest to resolve.

Grief symptoms most often take physical forms. There may be chronic pain or anxiety. There may also be mental changes that resemble senile dementia. These somatic equivalents tend to replace the more obvious signs of emotional grief; consequently, grief may go unrecognized and, therefore, untreated. Other subtle signs of grief are a tendency toward self-isolation, hostility, and anger toward family and friends (Dimond, 1981).

Adjustment to loss or bereavement depends upon several factors, including the person's support systems, coping skills, and the significance of the loss. Support systems vary. They may offer emotional aid, material or financial assistance, general information, social contacts, group affiliation, or any combination of these. In assessing a support network, it is important to determine the type of service it provides as well as whether the service meets the particular needs of that individual. Equally important is whether the individual perceives the support as helpful. Without a positive perception, a support system is rarely useful.

TABLE 26-6 Defense Mechanisms

Designation	Description
Compensation	Conscious or usually unconscious mechanism by which a person attempts to make up for a deficiency, real or imagined
Denial	Unconscious blocking of reality from awareness
Displacement	Unconscious transfer of an unacceptable idea or object to an acceptable one
Identification	Unconscious association of oneself with another
Introjection	Unconscious incorporation of another into oneself
Isolation	The separation of an idea from the normally attached feeling
Projection	Unconscious attribution of unacceptable ideas, thoughts, and feelings to another person or group
Rationalization	Unconscious mechanism by which an irrational thought or feeling is made to appear reasonable
Reaction Formation	Development of a socially acceptable interest that is the exact opposite of some unconscious wish or impulse
Regression	Unconscious mechanism by which the person undergoes a return to developmentally earlier patterns of adaptation
Repression	Unconscious removal of unacceptable ideas or feelings from conscious awareness
Sublimation	Unconscious channeling of instinctual drives into socially acceptable behaviors
Suppression	Conscious act of preventing the expression of an unacceptable impulse or feeling
Undoing	Unconscious mechanism by which the person symbolically acts out the reverse of some unacceptable behavior

The person's coping style can be assessed through behavioral clues. Is he surrounding himself with friends, or keeping busy with hobbies? Does he seem to be using denial, isolation, or other defense mechanisms to keep the loss at a distance? Defense mechanisms often constitute healthy coping behavior and should not be discouraged unless they interfere with everyday activities or functions. (See Table 26-6.) Information about how the individual has dealt with loss or stressful situations in the past can be used to help predict how well he will cope with the recent loss. Skills learned in past stressful situations can also be called upon as reinforcement.

How well an elderly person adapts to loss is also influenced by the impact of that loss on his life-style. Does the loss threaten his financial security or future financial state? Will it mean selling a home or moving in with family members? The more drastic the life-style change, the more stressful the loss is to cope with.

☐ *Physiological Changes Associated with Loss and Bereavement*

It has been widely accepted that there is a relationship between the occurrence of stressful life events and the subsequent development of illness. Holmes and Rahe (1967) and others have demonstrated that the likelihood of disease onset increases following periods of intense stress or life change. Both physiological and psychological stress influence the development of disease processes.

A mechanism for the development of disease may be that stress can effect an increase in the number of circulating corticosteroids, which leads to suppression of the immune system and hence

■ *Point of Emphasis*

Although loss occurs frequently to the elderly, the impact of each loss may be cumulative, making resolution more difficult to accomplish.

to increased susceptibility to disease. Studies have demonstrated that measurable immunosuppressive changes occur during prolonged exposure to a type of life stress such as significant loss (Locke, 1982).

Not only do stress and loss effect morbidity, they also affect the mortality rate. There is an increased risk of death among the bereaved, which is greater for male than for female survivors and which appears to be particularly high among those who lose the spouse (Rees, 1967). The reasons for the increased risk have not been clearly established, but one hypothesis is that death may result from the adverse physiological changes that accompany grief (e.g., immunosuppression). Another psychologically oriented hypothesis is that persons who sustain significant loss may begin to disregard their own health needs, resulting in the development of serious illness or exacerbation of chronic illness. It is established that loss and the response to it affect both psychological and physical well-being.

■ **Point of Emphasis**

Stress and loss influence the immune system and the subsequent development of disease. Loss influences mortality rate as well as morbidity.

INTERVENTION □ The goal of nursing care in grief reactions is to support and facilitate the process of grieving or grief work and to identify the presence of dysfunctional grieving when it occurs.

PRIMARY PREVENTION □

The Family □ When the nurse individually or with another health professional must tell the family the news of a death it is best communicated in a private setting and generally to the family as a group. The news of the death should be clear, concise, and factual. Family members may need to hear specifics of the measures that were taken in efforts to prevent death, and may need to have simple facts repeated.

The family may request to see and sometimes to touch the deceased. This helps affirm the reality of the death and should not be denied. Respect and tolerance for cultural or religious practices should always be given. Mourning, like all other customs and rites, is generally a culturally determined process.

The outward expression of grief, in crying or weeping, should be permitted. There is a tendency for nurses to want to "do something" for the mourners such as arranging for sedatives or other medication to be given. As a general rule, sedation is rarely indicated in normal grief and may even be detrimental to the grief process, by delaying or suppressing necessary expressions of emotion. The most valuable intervention in normal grief may be simply to sit quietly with those grieving, express sympathy, and listen.

Nursing Research Findings □ Research involving the grieving spouses of chronically ill clients revealed that the spouses had a number of common primary needs, many of which could be facilitated by nursing intervention. The eight primary needs are: (1) to be with the dying client, (2) to be helpful to the dying client, (3) to be assured of the comfort of the dying client, (4) to be informed of the client's condition, (5) to be informed of impending death, (6) to ventilate emotions, (7) to receive the comfort and support of family members, and (8) to receive acceptance, comfort, and support of health professionals.

Dracup (1978), using those research results, found that staff personnel lacked consistency in their approach to the grieving spouse. Staff members found it most helpful to use a standardized nursing care plan which they devised. Guided by theory and research, nurses can assess the grief process and plan interventions that are helpful and consistent.

The Client □ Crisis theory and intervention was developed from theories of human behavior, including those of Freud, Hartmann, and Erikson. Lindemann and Caplan are credited with making major strides toward the development of crisis theory. (Chapter 22 discusses crisis theory and crisis intervention in detail.)

Crisis intervention is effective with both individuals and families experiencing loss. The characteristics of this method of intervention, which make it particularly appropriate to loss situations, include: (1) a focus on the here-and-now (i.e., the recent loss), (2) the active and direct therapist's role, (3) the primary task of providing support while assisting the client in mobilizing usual, adaptive coping behaviors or in learning new adaptive coping behaviors.

When death or loss of any kind occurs suddenly or without warning, the client may be unable to use his usual coping methods. When the loss is severe, the usual coping methods may no longer work, and a crisis may result. Crisis intervention in loss situations focuses on providing support while helping the client make appropriate use of previously effective coping skills, or helping him learn new coping skills.

■ Point of Emphasis

Crisis intervention is a therapeutic technique effective with clients who are experiencing a death or other kind of sudden loss.

SECONDARY PREVENTION □

Client Intervention □ Most terminally ill clients die in hospitals. An alternative to terminal care in the hospital is available through the hospice movement. Derived from a medieval word for shelter for travelers on difficult journeys, the hospice is designed to relieve the physical as well as the emotional suffering of the terminally ill.

Although the concept of hospice is an old one, the first modern form of hospice care was originated at St. Christopher's Hospice in Syndenham, England in 1967. Seven years later, Hospice Incorporated of New Haven, Connecticut, became the first American hospice. By 1982, it was esti-

mated that there were between 500 and 750 hospice providers in the United States (Buckingham, et al., 1982).

Although the vast majority of hospice clients suffer from an advanced form of cancer, hospice care is available to all persons with a terminal illness. Between 15 and 20 percent of the clients residing at St. Christopher's Hospice have a disease other than cancer, generally a motor neuron disease (Saunders, 1981).

The common usage of the word hospice implies a philosophy of care, rather than a clearly defined program. As a result, this type of approach can be facilitated in many ways, including: (1) wholly volunteer programs, (2) home services, (3) free-standing facilities, (4) in-hospital palliative care units, (5) continued care subacute facilities, and (6) combinations of the above (Thomas, 1983).

Two very different types of hospice programs are offered in the U.S. (Buckingham, et al., 1982). In only a small minority of the states are there statutes specifically guiding the establishment and management of hospices. Where no specific statute exists, the hospice may be licensed under other types of care institutions such as home health agencies or skilled nursing facilities. The category depends upon the types of services offered as well as the organizational structure (Table 26-7).

The overall goal of hospice care is to keep the terminally ill person as pain-free, comfortable, and alert as possible during the final phase of his life. Hospice care emphasizes four major areas: (1) pain and symptom control, (2) client control over his life, (3) client and family considered as a single unit of care, and (4) interdisciplinary team planning for each client and family (Kubler-Ross, 1969).

Family Intervention □ In most hospice programs, control of pain and other symptoms without artificial extension of life is the major tenet. The focus of care is palliative rather than curative as death is the inevitable outcome. The care given to a family unit does not end when the sick member dies but continues for the remaining members through the period of bereavement. This care includes *education*—that is, learning about the member's illness, symptoms, and basic care requirements. In this way the family unit can remain as involved as desired and even provide some of the basic care. They may become skilled at bathing, changing dressings, and in some cases administering medication.

TABLE 26-7 Hospice Facilities in the United States		
	Type 1	**Type 2**
Type of operation	Independent program	Institutionally based program
Location	Services provided to the home	Inpatient program
Staff	Heavily volunteer, with a variety of professional staff	Fewer volunteers and types of professional staff
Types of services	Wide variety of social and psychological services in addition to nursing/medical care	More nursing and medical services, fewer social and psychological services

Respite care, which is periodic relief from daily care, may be given by hospice providers to those families who maintain the terminally ill person at home. Respite care can be given for a few hours or for a few days and can be accomplished by sending a health provider to the home or enabling the client to be admitted to the hospice as an inpatient for a specified length of time.

Emotional support is made available to the family unit throughout the length of the illness and usually continues for about a year following the member's death. Support may be expressed by telephone calls, cards or letters, or home visits.

Nurses are an integral part of the hospice team, which is also comprised of social workers, pharmacists, physicians, clergy, and volunteers. In a many-faceted role, the nurse provides direct care to clients, serves as consultant and teacher to the family, acts as client advocate, and functions as the liaison to the physician and others. In many instances, nurses are the professionals who coordinate the programs.

■ **Point of Emphasis**

Hospice, an approach to care of the terminally ill, emphasizes pain and symptom control as well as providing services for the client and the entire family unit.

Nursing Staff Intervention ☐ Hospice nursing may be quite different from other types of nursing. Whereas policy takes precedent in most nursing settings, client and family beliefs and decisions regarding care are given priority in this setting. Table 26-8 describes the requirements for hospice nursing. Thomas (1983) has discussed the rewards of hospice nursing. These are: (1) greater than

usual autonomy, with more opportunity to practice independently, (2) being a member of a team that shares information and cooperatively plans interventions, and (3) personal growth that is a result of intervention with both the client and the family.

Working with only terminally ill clients is at best stressful, and it can be both physically and emotionally draining. Much of the stress is an inevitable aspect of hospice nursing. To cite only a few of the stressors, there are feelings of helplessness about the inevitability of death, a lack of cooperation by physicians in alleviating the client's discomfort, sadness about the loss of every client, a heavy workload, including 24-hour call, and feelings of guilt about the failure to provide adequate care (Thomas, 1983).

TABLE 26-8 Requirements for Hospice Nursing[a]

A thorough knowledge of anatomy and physiology, and considerable familiarity with the pathophysiology of a number of diseases

Great skill in physical examination and in various nursing procedures such as catheterization, colostomy, and traction care

Considerable knowledge of pharmacology, particularly analgesics, narcotics, antiemetics, tranquilizers, cancer chemotherapy, antibiotics, hormone therapy, steroids, and cardiotonics

Skill in using psychological principles, in both one-to-one and group situations

Great sensitivity in human relationships

Knowledge of measures to comfort the dying in the last hours, and personal characteristics such as stamina, emotional stability, flexibility, cooperativeness, and a basic joie de vivre—a philosophy or faith

[a] Reprinted with permission from the *American Journal of Nursing, Geriatric Nursing*, January–February 1983.

TERTIARY PREVENTION □

Client/Family Intervention □ When the client and the family are not able to resolve the loss in a healthy adaptive manner, referral for psychiatric consultation or treatment is the appropriate next step. A client or family should be considered for psychiatric referral in the following circumstances: (1) The expression of grief is absent, although there may be mild to severe physical symptoms. (2) Depression is extended or severe, interfering with daily functioning (e.g., ability to work, maintain family roles, or attend to personal hygiene). (3) There appears to be any degree of risk of suicide in the depressed client or family members. (Refer to Chapter 33 for clues about suicide potential.)

In general, a client or the family should be referred for psychiatric evaluation or treatment whenever the grief appears to be abnormal in its severity, expression, or duration.

SELF-ASSESSMENT □ Inherent in the practice of nursing care is the knowledge that nurses must deal repeatedly with loss, grief, death, and dying. How a nurse copes with loss has significant impact on how well she can assist her clients to cope. The nurse is seen as the health professional most often designated to assist others to cope more effectively with death and dying. This is so because she has direct and extended involvement with the client and family and because of her perceived role as helper (Freihofer, 1976). Nurses who work in settings where death regularly occurs need to have support systems and resources available to them, and if their institutions do not provide those resources, the nurses themselves must. For example, nurses need educational workshops and programs, professional suport groups, and informal settings that encourage discussion and mutual consultation.

Self Assessment Questions □ To deal effectively with loss, nurses first must become aware of their own reactions and responses, and be willing to examine their own coping methods. The nurse might find it helpful to ask herself questions such as: Am I avoiding contact with clients who are critically or terminally ill? Am I less likely to spend time with or engage these clients in conversation? When the subject of death comes up when I'm with a client, do I offer reassurance, suggest he shouldn't worry, or change the subject? Do I find myself feeling angry with clients, staff, or family, seemingly without reason? Am I unable to discuss my feelings of sadness or grief with my colleagues or family?

■ Enrichment Activities

DISCUSSION QUESTIONS

1. In what ways do nurses and other health professionals inhibit the expression of normal grief in clients and client families?

   In what ways do they promote the expression of normal grief?

   What changes could you make in your clinical setting to facilitate the normal grief process for clients and families?

2. A client tells you he is concerned about his 3½-year-old child. Recently a neighbor died with whom the child had often visited. The child continues to want to visit the neighbor's house, expecting to see him. What information can you give the client to help alleviate the situation?

3. You are the primary nurse for a client recently diagnosed as having metastatic cancer of the colon. Initially the client was pleasant and cooperative but now he has become increasingly uncooperative and demanding. He rings often for what seem to be unnecessary reasons and becomes angry if you are unable to respond immediately.

   What is your explanation for the client's behavior change?

   What kinds of interventions would be helpful for the client and for you?

LEARNING ACTIVITIES

1. Discover the alternatives for terminal care available in your community. Visit a hospice, noting the types of services it offers clients and families.

2. Attend a meeting of a local support group for the bereaved such as:
   > The Compassionate Friends, Inc.
   > National Headquarters
   > P.O. Box 1347
   > Oak Brook, IL 60521

3. Visit a Ronald McDonald House which provides temporary lodging for families whose children are receiving treatment for serious illnesses.

4. Watch the videotape or read a transcript of the program NOVA entitled: "To live until you die: the work of Elizabeth Kubler-Ross."
   WGBH Distribution
   125 Western Avenue
   Boston, MA 02134

5. Explore with classmates, friends, or clergy different cultural customs and attitudes toward loss, grief, and death.

■ Recommended Readings

Kubler-Ross, E. *On death and dying.* New York: MacMillan 1969 Kubler-Ross's first book on her experience with dying people. It is filled with philosophical questions and viewpoints as well as clinical examples that illustrate the psychology of dying. It includes an extensive bibliography on works associated with death and dying up to the 1960s. This book is a classic for anyone interested in reading further on the topic.

Gonda, T.A., and Ruark, J.D. *Dying dignified: The health professional's guide to care.* Reading, MA: Addison-Wesley, 1984. A multidisciplinary approach to care of the dying person that begins with four case studies of people with terminal illnesses. Particularly interesting chapters include principal psychosocial and environmental influences on care of the dying, dealing with roles of health professionals in this context and some basic information about death, including a section on the monetary costs of dying.

■ References

Aguilera, D.C., and Messick, J.M. *Crisis intervention: Theory and methodology.* St. Louis: Mosby and Company, 1974.

Bartrop, R.W., Luckhurst, E., Lazarus, L., et al., Depressed lymphocyte function after bereavement. *The lancet,* April 16, 1977:834–836.

Bender, D.L. (Ed.). *Problems of death: Opposing viewpoints series.* Vol. 8, Anoka, MN: Greenhaven Press, 1974.

Berkowitz, P., and Berkowitz, N.S. The Jewish patient in the hospital. *American journal of nursing,* 67, 11 (November 1967):2335–2337.

Blum, J.D., and Robbins, P.A. Regulation: Current news holds key to hospice licensure. *Hospitals,* 56, 23 (December 1982):91–94.

Bowlby, J. Processes of mourning. *The international journal of psychoanalysis,* 42, 1961:317–339.

Buckingham, R.W., and Lupv, D. A comparative study of hospice services in the U.S. *American journal of public health,* 72, 5 (May 1982):455–463.

Bugen, L.A. Human grief: A model for prediction and intervention. *American journal of orthopsychiatry,* 47, 2 (April 1977):196–206.

Burgess, A.W., and Baldwin, B.A. *Crisis intervention: Theory and practice.* Englewood Cliffs, NJ: Prentice-Hall, 1981.

Campbell, T., and Chang, B. Health care of the Chinese in America. *Nursing outlook,* 21, 4 (April 1973):245–249.

Clayton, P.J. The effect of living alone on bereavement symptoms. *American journal of psychiatry,* 132, 2 (February 1975):133–137.

Clayton, P.J., Halikas, J.A., and Maurice, W.L. The depression of widowhood. *British journal of psychiatry,* 120, 1972:71–77.

Dealing with death and dying. Nursing 76 Skillbook. Jenkintown, PA: Intermed Communications.

Dimond, M. Bereavement and the elderly: A critical review with implications for nursing practice and research. *Journal for advanced nursing,* November 6, 6, 1981:461–470.

Dracup, K.A., and Breu, C.S. Using nursing research findings to meet the needs of grieving spouses. *Nursing research,* 27, 4 (July-August 1978):212–216.

Dupee, R.M. Hospice: Compassionate, comprehensive approach to terminal care. *Postgraduate medicine,* 72 (September 1982).

Engel, G.L. Is grief a disease? *Psychosomatic medicine,* 23, 1, 1961:18–22.

——Grief and grieving. *American journal of nursing,* 64, 9, September 1964:93–98.

Freihofer, P., and Felton, G. Nursing behaviors in bereavement: An exploratory study. *Nursing research,* 25, 5 (September-October 1976):332–337.

Furman, E. Studies in childhood bereavement. *Canadian journal of psychiatry,* 28 (June 1983):241–247.

Garfield, C.A. (ed.). *Psychosocial care of the dying patient.* New York: McGraw-Hill, 1978.

Geltman, R.L. et al. Symptom management in hospice care. *American journal of nursing,* 83, 1 (January 1983):78–85.

Gerber, I. et al. *Perspectives on bereavement.* New York: Arno Press, 1979.

Glaser, B.G., and Strauss, A.L. *Time for dying.* Chicago: Aldine-Atherton, Inc., 1968.

Gonda, T.A., and Ruark, J.E. *Dying dignified: The health professional's guide to care.* Reading, MA: Addison-Wesley, 1984.

Goodstein, R.K. Grief reactions in the elderly. Carrier Foundation Letter No. 99, June 1984:1–5.

Holmes, T.H., and Rahe, R.H. The social readjustment rating scale. *Journal of psychosomatic research,* 11, 1967:148–153.

Kubler-Ross, E. *On death and dying.* New York: MacMillan, 1969.

——*Death: The final stage of growth*. Englewood Cliffs, NJ: Prentice-Hall, 1975.

——*On children and death*. New York: MacMillan, 1983.

Lifton, R.J., and Olson, E. *Living and dying*. New York: Praeger Publishers, 1974.

Lindemann, E. Symptomatology and management of acute grief. *American journal of psychiatry*, 101, 1944:141–148.

Locke, S.E. Stress, adaptation and immunity: Studies in humans. *General hospital psychiatry*, 4, 1982:49–58.

Mood, D.W., and Lick, C.F. Attitudes of nursing personnel toward death and dying: Linguistic indicators of denial. *Research in nursing and health*, 2, 1979:95–99.

Moss, S. The grief work cycle in bereavement. In *Perspectives on bereavement* (Gerber et al.). New York: Arno Press, 1979.

Parkes, C.M. *Bereavement: Studies of grief in adult life*. New York: International University press, 1972.

Primeaux, M.H. American Indian health care practices. *Nursing clinics of North America*, 12, 1 (March 1977):55–65.

Rees, W.D., and Lutkins, S.G. Mortality of bereavement. *British medical journal*, (October 1967):13–16.

Ross, H.M. Societal/cultural views regarding death and dying. *Topics in clinical nursing*, (October 1981):1–16.

Saunders, D.C. The hospice: Its meaning to patients and their physicians. London's St. Christopher's Hospice. *Hospital practice* (June 16, 1981):93–96.

Schultz, C. Grieving children. *Journal of emergency nursing* (January/February 1980):30–36.

Stern, K., Williams, G.M., and Prados, M. Grief reactions in later life. *American journal of psychiatry*, 108, 1951:289–294.

Thomas, V.M. Hospice nursing: Reaping the rewards, dealing with the stress. *Geriatric nursing* (January/February 1983):22–27.

Woods, A., and Delisle, R. Departed, deceased, but never dead. *Psychology today*, 11, 1977:152.

Young, E. Reflections on life and death. In *Psychosocial care of the dying patient*. Garfield, CA: McGraw-Hill, 1978.

Zisook, S., and DeVaul, R.A. Grief, unresolved grief and depression. *Psychosomatics*, 24, 3 (March 1983):247–256.

PART FIVE

Nursing Process and Dysfunctional Life-Styles

All levels of prevention are significant as problems commonly encountered in the hospital and community are addressed: substance abuse; child, spouse, and elder abuse; and personality disorders. The nurse needs particular skills of observation and self-awareness to identify these problems, to refer families appropriately, and to avoid nontherapeutic or punitive approaches.

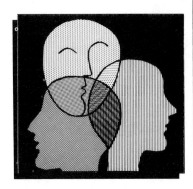

27

Personality Disorders

Stephanie Stockard and Susan Cullen

Learning Objectives

Upon completion of this chapter, the reader will be able to:

1. Distinguish between personality traits and personality disorder.

2. List the factors that influence development of personality disorders and their prevention.

3. Discuss theoretical viewpoints about the development of various personality disorders.

4. Describe preventive measures for the development of personality disorders.

5. Assess behaviors that result in coping deficits due to various personality traits in specific clients.

6. Identify nursing problems arising from specific behaviors and interventions which are pertinent for a client exhibiting specific coping problems.

7. Describe ways to evaluate effective nursing intervention through behavioral changes in a client who exhibits behaviors resulting in a coping deficit.

A personality disorder, by which is meant a life pattern of inflexible and limited behaviors, is a systematic way of relating to others and to society in general that causes problems for the client. The client may experience internal distress or family, social, or work difficulties.

The client with a personality disorder will be encountered in a variety of health care settings. Usually, the personality disorder is not the reason the client requests care. When a physical illness is the focus of care, the client's limited ability to cope with the related stress or anxiety may become evident in dramatic or eccentric behavior. If he is seen in a mental health setting, it may be because of difficulties with the law or domestic problems. Substance abuse, depression, or suicide attempts may be the symptoms of ineffective coping due to the personality disorder. Although a client may not recognize or seek treatment for the personality disorder specifically, the resulting impairment may affect both his physical and his mental capabilities.

□ *General Theory*

Four groups of personality disorders are described in the Diagnostic and Statistical Manual of the American Psychiatric Associate (DSM III) (Table 27-1). Clients with antisocial, histrionic, narcissistic, schizoid and schizotypal, and passive-aggressive personality disorders are described in this chapter in detail, with nursing interventions. Borderline personality disorder, a major personality disorder, is discussed in Chapter 31 since it is often apparent early in adolescence.

The mentally healthy person has the ability to relate to others and understand their needs, shows awareness of self, demonstrates purpose and persistence in pursuing tasks, and accepts limitations realistically. He also is able to perceive reality and cope with stresses in a way that is growth-producing, as well as derive pleasure and enjoyment from life.

The development of personality disorders indicates that the individual's emotional development has been arrested or deviated so that he has difficulty coping with the events of everyday life. It is uncertain what specific factor causes this situation, but it is believed that several factors are involved, including temperament at birth, environment, manner in which the individual perceives and interacts with the environment, and (possibly) genetic/biochemical factors. These fac-

TABLE 27-1 *Personality Disorders*
Behavior: dramatic, emotional, or erratic
Antisocial (also referred to as sociopathic or psychopathic)
Borderline (see Chapter 31)
Histrionic (formerly hysterical personality)
Narcissistic
Behavior: odd, eccentric
Paranoid
Schizoid
Schizotypal
Behavior: anxious, fearful
Avoidant
Dependent
Compulsive
Passive-aggressive
Atypical, mixed, or other personality disorder

tors affect everyone's personality development but some individuals react in a manner that leads to the development of unhealthy life adjustment patterns.

The interaction of personality and environment results in failure to establish constructive adjustment to society, or difficulty in delaying gratification of needs or impulses to act. Studies suggest that factors such as loss or absence of parents, deficient parenting, and critical experiences of the early years may be strong factors in the development of personality disorders.

Primary prevention of personality disorders would appear to begin before birth with effective and responsible parent training. With the extremely high number of adolescent mothers in society today, it is of critical importance to a child's personality development that efforts be made to provide consistent, loving care and parenting education. Sex education and family life classes help prevent the birth of children to parents who are unwilling and/or unable to nurture a developing person.

Since personality development begins in childhood and continues through adulthood, secondary prevention may take place at any point when the child or adolescent begins to exhibit signs of arrested or deviated emotional development. At this time unhealthy patterns can be interrupted if the child or teen receives the needed support through individual, group, or family therapy. In later adolescence and adulthood, personality patterns become relatively fixed. If these become problematic, tertiary prevention is instituted and psychotherapy can be beneficial.

☐ *Behavior: Dramatic, Emotional, Erratic*

ANTISOCIAL PERSONALITY DISORDER

The outstanding behavior of antisocial personality disorder is persistent disregard for the feelings and rights of others. The individual appears to be concerned only for his own needs, without a sense of empathy or sympathy, and lacking either guilt or remorse for transgressions of social or moral codes. He also tends since childhood to have a history of behavior problems, such as lying, stealing, fighting, truancy. In adolescence, there is frequently drinking, drug abuse, and sexually acting-out behavior. A record of poor job performance and lack of close interpersonal relationships are indicators of the antisocial personality disorder in adult life.

According to the DSM III, prevalence of this disorder in the U.S. is higher in men (3 percent) than women (1 percent), although these figures may be influenced by the fact that women are often diagnosed as having other disorders (e.g., hysteria), and many antisocial clients enter treatment through the court system, with which more men than women have contact.

In the past, the individual was considered morally "sick" or "insane" or to be "psychopathically inferior." At a later time, such a person was referred to as a psychopath, or a sociopath. The nurse may hear the terms "psychopath" and "sociopath" used interchangeably to describe antisocial personality disorder.

Cleckley's Theory

There are a number of theoretical viewpoints regarding antisocial personality disorder, the most comprehensive presentation being Cleckley's book, *The Mask of Sanity*. He discusses important factors classically attributed to the antisocial personality, such as apparent lack of anxiety and lack of feeling; a lack of successful methods of treatment is notable also.

Cleckley views antisocial personality disorder as a disorder whose severity, until recent decades, was not recognized and believes this may be due to the convincing "mask of sanity" that the person is able to maintain. There is no loss of reasoning processes as seen in other disorders, no unusual facial or verbal expression, and no tone of voice or inappropriate feeling state that might be evident.

Cleckley postulates that the person differs from the integrated, healthy personality in that he is unaware of, and lacks the ability to become aware of, the meaning of important emotional and interpersonal experiences.

> ■ *Point of Emphasis*
>
> *The antisocial person seems unable to integrate the basic human emotions (e.g., love, fear, hate, caring, friendship).*

The person who does not experience the human emotions that affect most people is able to understand only a superficial level of feelings and motivations of others. This would account for the outstanding indications of antisocial personality disorder: persistent violation of the rights of others, lack of significant attachments, and an apparent disregard for the negative consequences of misbehavior.

It often seems that the antisocial individual flaunts this behavior; however, when caught in a transgression of the law or firmly limited in a social situation, he is dismayed and angry, and feels that the resulting punishment is undeserved and unfair.

Valliant's Theory

Valliant (1975) postulates that anxiety does exist but that it is invisible to family, friends, and therapists for two reasons. First, when the person with antisocial personality disorder begins to experience anxiety, the therapist responds like the client's parents—by not allowing the client to bear anxious feelings. Like the parent who "covers up" for antisocial offspring—posting bail, paying bad debts, and so on—the therapist often fails to acknowledge the feeling of anxiety in the person and fails to expect him to manage it. Secondly, Valliant believes that the antisocial individual transfers his anxiety to the staff or therapist and makes them apprehensive about the client. The staff then believes that the client is unreachable and incurable.

Valliant also argues that the apparent "lack of motivation for change" considered a hallmark of the antisocial individual is, in reality, based on a fear that if he demonstrated his competence, he might be overwhelmed with forbidden thoughts and feelings rooted in childhood. Valliant believes that, contrary to the classic idea that there is no feeling, the antisocial individual "feels too much" and attempts to keep those frightening feelings out of consciousness. Only in long-term treatment where therapy cannot be avoided the real feelings become apparent.

Valliant takes issue with the idea that the antisocial individual cannot experience depression and acknowledge that others matter to him. Instead, he suggests this "incapacity" is a defensive maneuver to avoid terrifying anxiety about close relationships. Because studies indicate that most antisocial individuals were as children "neglected in some way" (e.g., physical or emotional neglect or abuse), it appears that the depression this individual feels is like that of a bereaved child who experiences intense and persistent anger. In both the bereaved child and the child who later appears antisocial, Valliant believes the anger masks the pain of the need for the lost object (parental presence or love and affection). The substance abuse seen in many of these clients may be a way of "blotting out" feeling.

A study of 524 antisocial clients with matched controls (Weiss, et al., 1983) supports Valliant's contention of the presence of anxiety. Further, Weiss challenges the stereotype of a normal mental status in this individual and notes signs of depression, anxiety, irritability, agitation, suicidal thoughts, and difficulties in intellectual functioning.

Moral Development Theory

Link, et al. (1977), studying moral judgment and conduct, demonstrated that a breakdown in any of the six stages of moral development can lead to antisocial personality disorder. The stages are: (1) orientation to one's own primary needs and fear of punishment, (2) unconditioned satisfaction of personal desires, (3) beginning of spontaneous desire to have others think well of one by adherence to social norms, (4) acceptance of authority, (5) acceptance of legal principles, (6) development of conscience.

The authors point out that a breakdown in moral development underlies the glaring discrepancies between knowledge and conduct. In other words, although the antisocial individual apparently knows and can state the "right" or "moral" way of behaving, his conduct does not exemplify these standards. The development of each stage is strongly influenced by the person's early environment and role modeling.

Genetic and Environmental Influences

The genetic and environmental factors in development of antisocial personality disorder are closely intertwined. Studies suggest that a factor may be inherited from the biological father. If the child is separated, even in early life, from an antisocial father and adopted by a father without these traits, the child may develop antisocial personality disorder.

Also, research suggests a possible linkage between biochemical factors such as serotonin and norepinephrine levels seen in aggressive behavior (which frequently characterizes this client). Serotonin is believed to decrease aggressive drives, while norepinephrine sustains them. In the antisocial individual there may be an imbalance of these chemicals—perhaps due to constitutional inheritance or created by factors in the environment that influence the chemical levels.

Stringer and Josef (1983) suggest that some adult antipersonality disorders may be a variant of childhood attention deficit disorder (which may have organic causes). Unfortunately, the small number of subjects and lack of controls makes it impossible to generalize the findings.

Mednick (cited by Locke, 1981) suggests that a defect in the autonomic nervous system prevented the early learning of a "fear response" when the client was a child. Lacking this response, the child's behavior was not modified by fear of punishment or withdrawal of love.

Characteristics and Behaviors

The characteristics, behaviors, and possible etiological factors of antisocial personality disorder are presented in Table 27-2.

Treatment

Successful treatment of antisocial personality disorder has proved futile and frustrating for even skilled therapists because of the individual's reluctance to seek help or to feel assistance is needed. The client's inability to maintain relationships also affects therapeutic alliance.

Further research into biochemical factors promises some hope. For now, treatment is limited to interactional or behavior modification methods. Clear expectations and authority are essential in the relationship. Valliant (1975) suggests the following measures:

TABLE 27-2 Antisocial Personality Disorder

Predisposing Factors	*Adult Behaviors and Characteristics after Age 18*
Environmental	Deceitfulness, lying, "conning"
Unwanted and/or illegitimate child	Egocentricity, narcissism
Parents had unhappy childhood	Selfishness, ingratitude, unreliability
Maternal deprivation	Cynicism, sadism
Desertion, separation, or divorce of parents	Inability to delay gratification
Violence or abuse by parents or others	Inability to see others' acts from their viewpoint
Unreasonable, fantasized parental wishes which the child fails to achieve, resulting in negative attitudes by parents	Severe alienation, detachment, affectionless
	Inability to form meaningful personal attachments
Lack of consistent discipline and warmth	Lack of goals
Institutionalization, foster care, chaotic home life	Recklessness
Characteristics and Behaviors before Age 15	Inability to maintain steady employment
Emotional immaturity/lag in emotional development	Inability to function as responsible parent evidenced by neglect and/or abuse
Domination by primitive drives/impulses	Inability to follow social and legal norms
Frequent temper tantrums and senseless rage	Inability to maintain personal relationships (frequent divorce, separation, desertion, promiscuity)
Stealing	
Persistent lying and deceit	Frequent physical fights or assaults including spouse or child abuse
Uncontrollable behavior	Financial irresponsibility toward debts or family members
Quarrelsome, defiant	
Truancy and school suspension or expulsion	Purposeless travel and/or lack of fixed place of residence
Substance abuse (alcohol and other drugs)	
Frequent casual sexual relationships	Consistent violation of the rights of others
Violations of rules and social codes	

---

1. Self-destructive behavior must be dealt with in a controlled environment where the client is unable to refuse treatment.

2. The client's anxiety should be allowed to increase; the therapist should recognize and control personal anxiety.

3. The mental history given by the client should be viewed cautiously—these clients tend to idealize and fantasize their past.

4. Each destructive defense (e.g., drug use) must be confronted and a substitute for the behavior found. Often 24-hour self-help groups such as Alcoholics Anonymous, church, or drug programs are helpful. Treatment centers specializing in antisocial personality disorder may offer a behavior modification approach. Use of tough confrontation by peers with similar problems (similar to the AA format) has been tried with limited success.

5. Interpreting unconscious feelings or motives is usually nonproductive. Confrontation appears to work best over time in a relationship the client cannot avoid.

In the inpatient setting great skill is needed to maintain a therapeutic milieu for all the clients. This client's frequent use of violent, impulsive, or argumentative ways of expressing anger causes distancing between himself, fellow clients, and staff. Johansen (1983) points out that requirements for control of this client often cause other clients' treatment needs to be overlooked. More timid clients may be victims of overall rules aimed at one or two manipulative clients, and not receive needed support and validation. All clients end up being treated the same in an attempt to avoid "special treatment."

The nurse needs to develop skill in intervening with manipulative, seductive, and/or aggressive behavior, which will be discussed in subsequent sections.

HISTRIONIC PERSONALITY DISORDER

The term "histrionic" is descriptive of a person who is generally overly dramatic, colorful, intensely reactive, expressive, and excitable. Traditionally, this diagnosis was applied only to women, but it is now recognized that behaviors characteristic of the histrionic personality disorder may also appear in men. The DSM III also describes a feature of this person as often "creative and imaginative" as opposed to intellectual achievement and analytic thinking. Although the former characteristics are traditionally "feminine" and the latter "masculine," these characteristics can in fact be ascribed to either sex.

The histrionic person displays a melodramatic seeking of attention and intense response to stimuli, craves excitement, and will create it if none is available. In a group he will seek to focus attention on himself, acting as "the star" or "life of the party" in every situation. Ways of eliciting attention may include dramatic speeches or exaggerated tales of exciting adventures, sexually provocative or bizarre dress, or creation of angry "scenes." Romantic fantasies may be convincingly related or acted out. Many times, on a superficial level, this person may seem very charming, lively and appealing—in fact, he livens up a gathering.

However, there is difficulty in closer interpersonal relationships. He may form a friendship quickly, but once involved, may display demanding, self-centered, and egotistical behavior. He often seems unable to have more than one good friend at a time, and tries to monopolize that person, feeling hurt or rejected if the friend attempts to spend time with others. This possessiveness may lead to manipulative suicidal gestures or threats. The person has strong feelings of dependency or helplessness. The behavior often seems inconsistent, swinging from charm to rage, and may be perceived by others as shallow and lacking genuineness.

Easily influenced by others, the person is quick to adopt "advice" from those in authority that will magically solve any problems. When the advice doesn't work, he tends to blame others, rather than taking responsibility. Frequently, "poor health" or headaches are ways of dealing with stress—which may lead to abuse of alcohol or drugs. Evidence also shows a familial tendency, suggesting a learned pattern of behavior.

The theoretical background of histrionic personality disorder is rooted in Freud's view of hysteria as misplaced sexual drives. However, this all-inclusive diagnosis of hysteria has been broken down into three types for greater clarification: somatization and conversion disorders (see Chapter 32) and hysterical personality disorder (Chodoff 1974).

Kolb (1982) points out that besides the sexual aspects of the client's life, there is an underlying sense of dependency and helplessness. Although the client often exhibits a need for attention through seductiveness, sexual conquest, and exhibitionism, dependency is evident in the desire for a parent-child relationship with other adults. Lack of maternal nurturance due to absence, illness, or maternal egocentricity appears to be a possible factor. A woman with this disorder is likely to have experienced close attachment to her mother and seductive treatment by her father as a child. When the client reached puberty, however, the father was often found to ignore, deny, or condemn evidence of her developing sexuality. As a result the client experienced fear and insecurity about her sexual drives.

The stormy, intense relationships generated by these individuals, their possessiveness, and oversensitivity to rejection provides the vehicle for frequent depression. It is at these times—a loss, breakup of a love affair, or a failure in career—that suicidal gestures or attempts may be made, or abuse of drugs or alcohol may be evident.

The nurse caring for this client will find it helpful to review interventions for a wide variety of behaviors especially seductiveness, manipulation, helpless/dependent, and narcissistic behaviors. She also needs to be alert to expressions of suicidal thoughts, plans, or gestures when the client is rejected by others.

NARCISSISTIC PERSONALITY DISORDER

The term "narcissism" means love of one's idealized self. Based on the DSM-III criteria, the person with a narcissistic personality disorder displays several characteristic behaviors (as described in Table 27-3) causing significant impairment in social or occupational functioning.

The client generally seeks treatment due to a threatened loss of a significant person or to depression accompanying failure of grandiose plans. There is also a risk of substance abuse as the narcissistic individual may have unrealistic belief that he can "control" drug use and not be affected, like ordinary people. Drugs or alcohol may also be abused when the person feels let down by others or when alternatives to grandiose plans and expectations have been exhausted.

Interventions for manipulative, passive-aggressive, or dependent behavior, useful in dealing with the narcissistic client, are discussed in

---

TABLE 27-3 Narcissistic Personality Disorder

Unquestioned and grandiose belief in his greatness or uniqueness with an inflated view of personal achievements or talents. Often is gifted and has won distinctions in some areas, but exaggerates abilities and accomplishments.

Expansive fantasies of power, success, intellectual or artistic brilliance, beauty or love. Capacities and personal limits are often overestimated

If criticized, defeated, or ignored by others, reacts with either total indifference, rage, and/or self-contempt or humiliation. These feelings may precipitate a depression, psychotic episode, or attempts at self-destruction.

Requires constant admiration and attention. Often charming and generous, expects return in the form of admiration or gratitude for favors. Has a great capacity to turn what others might view as flaws into virtues. Others are expected to love him unconditionally.

In interpersonal relationships, at least two of these four behaviors are present:

Expectation of special favors or assistance without any need to reciprocate or earn these favors. Reacts with surprise or anger when people fail to do what is wanted.

Disregard for the rights or personal integrity of others. Often exploits others to further his own goals and plans.

In relationships with others, either overidealizes or devalues the other party.

Inability to have empathy for others or understand how they could be critical or have expectations of him.

---

later sections.

Vignette

Mr. James, a 36-year-old father of one child, initiated treatment following a threat by his wife to divorce him. Following a few sessions, Mr. James and his wife were seen in marital therapy.

Mr. James expressed anger about what he considered to be a lack of appreciation for him on the part of his wife. He listed many ways in which he felt slighted by her. Further, he stated, he had done his wife a favor by "marrying her when he was a big football star and she was just a waitress." When Mrs. James pointed out that by working she had helped him get through school, he was unable to give her any recognition for this and stated that that was what she "should have done." Throughout their marriage there were a number of corresponding incidents. Mr. James pointed out that he could have "written his own ticket in the big leagues" if he had wanted to and hadn't had the responsibility of his marriage.

Mrs. James described living with her husband as similar to having an infant who constantly took and gave nothing in return. She felt the "breaking point" for her occurred when she thought he was competing with their 8-month-old child for attention. She stated he began spending more time with his friends and said all she cared about was "the kid."

☐ *Behavior: Odd, Eccentric*

SCHIZOID AND SCHIZOTYPAL PERSONALITY DISORDERS

Schizoid and schizotypal personality disorders are similar in the lack of ability to form social relationships, but there are distinct differences between them.

In schizoid personality disorder, the person demonstrates emotional aloofness and seems to lack warm or tender feelings for others. He appears to be indifferent to either praise or criticism, or to the feelings of others. Friendships are limited to only one or two persons including family members. The person is a "loner" who is withdrawn and seclusive, and who seems cold and dull in affect.

Usually other-sex relationships are lacking. The person may passively get married because it seems to be "the thing to do." Job functioning is often impaired due to lack of ability to relate to others, although if in a job that requires social isolation such as working only with numbers or abstract ideas, the person may be highly successful.

In schizotypal personality disorder, there are oddities of thought, perception, speech, or behavior that are not severe enough to be considered schizophrenic. The DSM III lists eight such oddities, four of which must be present to meet the criteria for schizotypal personality disorder. These include magical thinking, ideas of reference, social isolation, and recurring illusions or a sense of depersonalization. In communication with others, there may be oddities of speech, inappropriate rapport, suspicious or paranoid ideation, social anxiety, or a hypersensitivity to real or perceived criticism.

Baron, et al. (1983) found that siblings whose parents both had schizotypal disorder were at significantly greater risk for schizophrenia and schizotypal personality disorder than siblings with one normal parent. Siblings with one normal parent and one schizotypal parent were at greater risk than siblings with two normal parents. It would appear there may be genetic, as well as environmental, factors that contribute to the development of this disorder. (See vignette, Tom R.)

Individuals with these types of disorders rarely come to the attention of health care personnel unless their behaviors have caused them legal difficulty or their way of living has caused lack of attention to physical needs. Ability to intervene in withdrawal or helpless/dependent behavior will help this client function more effectively.

PARANOID PERSONALITY DISORDER

The individual with paranoid personality disorder is most often seen in a community or work setting. The person is suspicious and distrustful at all times, expecting harm and trickery. To protect himself, he is hyperalert to the environment, takes unnecessary precautions, and may be very guarded or secretive. He may be pathologically jealous, see hidden meanings and motives in others' behavior, and may selectively see only those "facts" that conform to his beliefs.

Hypersensitivity may be displayed in a "chip on the shoulder" attitude, exaggeration of difficulties, counterattacking at the slightest indication of threat, and general tenseness and inability to relax. The client appears cold and unemotional, humorless, and proud of appearing rational and unemotional. Tender, sentimental feelings are not apparent.

The person, who usually is a man, often seeks treatment only when some very important relationship is threatened. For example, a man who is pathologically jealous may see his wife's social friendliness with others as flirting or disloyalty. Any time spent with other men on a harmless basis is seen as evidence of infidelity. Eventually, the wife may refuse to continue the marriage unless the husband seeks help.

Underlying the paranoid behavior are deep feelings of insecurity and low self-esteem. It would seem that as a child, he experienced the world as particularly hostile and concluded he must always be on guard. He expects harm from others. This leads to loneliness and a sense of isolation. He is unable to trust others enough to reach out and is disdainful of "soft" feelings. The need to be in control and self-sufficient causes this person to seem egocentric and exaggerate his im-

---

Vignette

Tom R. was referred for treatment after being picked up by the police following complaints about loitering at an apartment complex. Tom lived alone in a rooming house near the apartments. He worked as a custodian for a large company and apparently had no family or close friends. His work record showed he did a good job; never had any trouble other than his relationship with co-workers, who described him as unfriendly and suspicious. They stated that Tom "acted odd" in that he would not eat with the others and seemed to actively avoid them. When Tom had been invited to join them on several occasions he responded in a surly manner, stating he didn't like people gawking at him when he ate. When in the hospital, Tom described his solitary life as being best for him as he was a "strong person and didn't need other people." Further, he felt "people just want to take advantage of you if you let them." Tom also expressed the idea that he knew they made fun of him and were "just jealous" although he could not document this with factual information.

His symptoms were not debilitating enough to warrant long hospitalization and he felt no need to change, so he was released. The neighbors did not press charges against Tom because he promised not to loiter at the apartment building anymore.

Tom did not return for treatment following his discharge. He did not see any need to change his behavior or thought patterns and said that being around people made him uncomfortable, thus demonstrating the anxiety precipitated by the closeness of the therapeutic relationship. As expressed in the theoretical presentation, these individuals are frequently found on the fringes of society leading solitary lives—for example among street people.

portance. He is usually rigid and unwilling to compromise.

Kendler and Gruenberg (1982) hypothesized a genetic factor in the etiology of paranoid personality disorder. Studying adults who had been adopted as children from parents with paranoid personality disorder into families without the disorder, the researchers found a higher than expected incidence of paranoid personality disorder. The absence of nongenetic family influences did not eliminate the disorder. Genetic predisposition may influence its development.

Paranoid personality disorder should be distinguished from schizophrenia paranoid type, paranoid disorder, and paranoia (see Chapter 34). In paranoid personality disorder, there are no delusions.

□ *Behavior: Anxious, Fearful*

PASSIVE-AGGRESSIVE PERSONALITY DISORDER

Passive-aggressive personality disorder most often will be seen in the work or social setting as a long-term pattern of behavior. The individuals display procrastination, dawdling, stubbornness, deliberate inefficiency, chronic lateness, and frequent "forgetfulness." For these behaviors to be considered part of a disorder of personality, they must exert a strong negative influence on the person's performance in job and social adaptation. The person may be passed over for promotions or have poor personal relations due to this behavior. It must also be readily apparent that the individual is capable of better performance in these areas. If seeking therapy, he often presents with symptoms of depression.

Underlying this disorder is that the individual feels angry or aggressive but is unable to express these feelings in a direct and appropriate manner. Instead, in almost every area of functioning he uses methods that express the anger indirectly. For example, a worker receives what he considers an unfair job evaluation. Rather than tell the supervisor the evaluation seems unfair or write a dissenting note, the worker signs the evaluation and proceeds to tell his colleagues about the unfairness of the evaluation and injustice of the supervisor. In the social setting, a man may be angry at his fiancée and "forget" her birthday or an important date.

Types

Perry and Flannery (1982) have categorized four types of passive-aggressive clients, all of whom may present similar behaviors but all of whom arrived at that point from various causes:

Anxiety Inhibited. He wants to change but his extreme anxiety inhibits learning. He is usually grossly nonassertive and fits the description for a passive-aggressive personality disorder.

Environmentally Inhibited. He is deficient in social skills and assertiveness, but generally wishes to change. However, this client may be "punished" for attempts to be assertive by a significant person whom he feels unable to leave (spouse, boss). Although he may become more assertive with others, he may be unable to separate from this important person and may continue to accept abuse.

Resentful Vindictive. This client lacks social skills and resents the need to change. He asks, "Why should I change?" and feels that everyone else should change. He tries to thwart the therapist's efforts to help him change by forgetting, procrastinating, displaying "yes-but" behavior, and using other passive-aggressive means.

Existential Choice. He seeks change in his nonassertiveness and may improve in many areas of life. However, leaving the significant person (spouse, boss, or parent) with whom he has the most trouble may not be an option within his values. For instance, a woman may improve her assertiveness in other areas of life and deal more effectively with a demanding elderly parent in the home rather than place the latter in a nursing home. This client recognizes the negative relationship to the important person and consciously chooses to sacrifice herself to meet a valued ideal—caring for her parent.

There is no recent evidence that the disorder occurs at any greater rate in either sex, although the traditional view that women should be "nice" and not "aggressive" may make it more difficult for them to express anger and hostility in a direct manner.

Individuals experiencing this maladaptive pattern of behavior frequently appear to be overly dependent and lacking in self-confidence. Rather than risk disapproval by voicing feelings of anger, or even disagreement, the person harbors the anger and resentment and "gets back" at people by indirect means. The behaviors are difficult to deal with because they are covert in nature. For example, if a person retreats into wounded silence, a spouse or colleague may have no idea of the cause and thus be unable to remedy it. The person's communication skills are severely limited, as his entire repertoire of communicating negative or positive thoughts and feelings consists of nonverbal indirect means. Skill in dealing with passive-aggressive, manipulative, and helpless behaviors is useful with this client.

Vignette

Maggie Martin initially came for treatment because she had been referred by her company's employee assistance program. Included in her admission interview was a long list of job-related counseling slips furnished by her supervisor. When asked what she thought was the reason for her presence at the clinic, she states "I just can't seem to get along with my supervisor. He just doesn't seem to care or understand how hard my job is to do." She explained her problems as being caused "in reality" by the supervisor. While relating her story, Maggie would frequently punctuate sentences with a sigh of exasperation.

It became apparent that Maggie experienced difficulty not only in her job situation, but in her personal life as well. She identified problems in remembering appointments and things others asked her to do such as obtaining her husband's medicine when she was shopping. Maggie expressed confusion at others' response to her behavior stating, "They act like I do it on purpose and I try so hard."

Maggie's treatment involved individual sessions with a nurse therapist in conjunction with participation in an assertiveness training group. Within the group setting it was possible to recognize Maggie's inability to deal with anger directly. When Maggie received feedback from the group about her behavior, she would initially become silent and sullen, later launching an attack upon another member in the group. Maggie had much difficulty recognizing the connection of her feelings and this behavior, just as she had difficulty recognizing how her failure to perform reasonably and to fulfill the job functions were an expression of her anger toward her supervisor.

It might be said that she fulfilled the expression, "Don't get mad, get even." This type of behavior appears typical in the passive-aggressive personality.

Other anxious-fearful behaviors, including compulsive, avoidant, and dependent personality disorders are defined in Table 27-4.

☐ Disorders of Impulse Control

Disorders of impulse control are distinct from personality disorders. They are presented in summary form because they are often observed in the community setting, and usually are not seen in a therapeutic setting unless legal complications require the affected person to seek counseling. According to the DSM III, these disorders have several features in common:

1. There is a failure to resist an impulse to act in a way that is harmful to self or others. The individual may or may not consciously resist the drive or premeditate the act.
2. The individual experiences increasing tension before performing the act.
3. After the act is committed, the individual experiences a sense of release or gratification. The act is in keeping with what the individual wanted to do at that moment, but may or may not be followed by remorse or guilt.

Some types of disorders of impulse control are described in Table 27-5.

☐ Nursing Care of Clients with Personality Disorders

The client with a personality disorder usually does not seek treatment unless the coping deficits created by the behaviors severely impair his ability to function. More often, the nurse will encounter the behaviors that characterize these disorders in the general hospital, outpatient, or community settings. Therefore, it is more useful to assess the client behaviors and examine ways to intervene therapeutically in any situation in which the nurse finds these behaviors problematic.

LIMIT SETTING

Limit setting, which will be discussed in Chapter 30 in regard to children, is equally important

---

TABLE 27-4 *Behavior: Anxious, Fearful*

Compulsive Personality Disorder

Characteristics	Stiff and cold, "stuffed shirt" Trouble expressing tenderness Stingy with material possessions Serious and conventional Perfectionistic Preoccupied with small details Resists authority but insists others conform to his beliefs Exaggerated sense of duty
Causes	Most likely learned behavior Defense against hostile impulses and unconscious aggression
Results	Generates resentment in others by insisting on own way Perfectionism results in narrow focus on trivialities causing poor use of time and low productivity Physical illness: ulcers, hypertension, hives, or myocardial infarction
Examples	Workaholic whose pursuit of perfection destroys relationships and ability to enjoy leisure Religious or political groups who believe theirs is the "right way" to believe

Avoidant Personality Disorder

Characteristics	Fearful of humiliation and rejection Low self-esteem Feels inferior Needs unconditional approval Few friends
Causes	Possibly continually devalued and criticized in childhood Painful relationships with adults Often emotionally or physically abused Lack of warmth and acceptance in family
Results	Fear causes withdrawal from others May have difficulty in job when contact with others required May often become involved in destructive relationships because feels he is not worthy of better treatment
Examples	Abused spouse "Loner" Painfully shy adult

Dependent Personality Disorder

Characteristics	Fears making demands Belittles self Allows others to make his decisions Fears abandonment Clinging behavior
Causes	Devaluation in childhood Physical or emotional abuse in childhood Unresolved loss of significant person in early life
Results	Toleration of humiliating or abusive relationships Feels no control over life Feels like a victim May cause resentment in others due to clinging behavior
Examples	Abused spouse "Clinging vine" Insecure, constantly seeking reassurance Overly apologetic (fears offending anyone)

---

within adult relationships. There are two types of limits: to give direction, and to restrain or restrict. Both are important in establishing and maintaining a therapeutic nurse-client relationship.

Many people perceive a limit as a "punishment" or a severe way of dealing with a person. Some nurses set limits only when they are angry and have been pushed beyond their emotional endurance. When this occurs limits *are* likely to be punitive and diminish the sense of mutual respect that is essential in the therapeutic relationship.

Self-awareness is critical. When the nurse becomes aware of feeling that her own rights are being violated (for example, being verbally abused) it is then limits should be set. The nurse should not tolerate the abuse for several days and then "blow up" in an angry tirade.

The nurse may also recognize that the client is losing control of his behavior, or is acting in a self-defeating or destructive manner. He may also be behaving toward others in a destructive manner. At this time the nurse needs to intervene and set a limit to prevent harm to the client or another person. Limits that are firm and fair, and that are carried out consistently assist clients who have difficulty controlling their behavior to develop responsibility for their own actions. When the client is physically assaultive, limits may be more complex but the principles remain the same (see Chapter 11).

An effective limit: (1) Clearly defines what is expected. (2) Does not decrease self-esteem of nurse or client. (3) Strengthens inner control of client. (4) Recognizes underlying feelings ("I know

TABLE 27-5 Disorders of Impulse Control

Disorder	Predisposing Factors	Characteristics
Pyromania	No information. Onset usually in childhood	Recurring failure to resist impulse to set fires Increasing tension before setting the fire, with release or sense of pleasure after setting fire No obvious motivation such as monetary gain (arson), political or social protests, or terrorism
Intermittent explosive disorder	Alcohol, drugs or past conditions of brain trauma such as encephalitis, head trauma, infantile seizures	Several separate instances of loss of control resulting in assault or property destruction Reactions greatly out of proportion to any precipitating psychological stress Lack of aggressive behavior or impulsiveness between episodes Not due to any other mental disorder (e.g., schizophrenia, dissociative disorder)
Isolated explosive disorder	Alcohol, drugs, or past conditions of brain trauma such as encephalitis, head trauma, infantile seizures	Similar to intermittent, but only a single episode with no previous signs of aggression or impulsivity
Pathological gambling	Parental loss before 15 years Inappropriate parental discipline Exposure to gambling as an adolescent Lack of emphasis in family on fiscal responsibilities High family value on material items	Arrest for forgery, fraud, embezzlement, or other financial crimes while attempting to secure gambling money Failure to clear debts or other financial responsibilities Family disruption due to gambling Illegal borrowing of money Unable to account for lost or won money if this is claimed Absenteeism at work to pursue gambling Need to have another person relieve desperate financial situation (spouse, relatives)
Kleptomania	None known	Recurring failure to resist impulse to steal items not useful or of obvious monetary value Increased tension before the act with relief or pleasure afterward No collaborative stealing or preplanning

you're upset your wife couldn't visit, but I don't like being called names. Let's talk about your feelings"). (5) Is carried out consistently. (6) Offers (when possible) alternatives to the unacceptable behavior ("Mr. Jones, you haven't wanted a bath for two days and will need one today. Would you like to take it at 9 or after lunch?").

The ability to set limits is useful in working with the client because his manner of relating to others often disrupts personal and/or work environment. Disruptive relating is repeated in the way the client relates to the nurse.

MANIPULATIVE BEHAVIOR

ASSESSMENT □ Manipulative behavior may be defined as any purposeful behavior that the individual directs toward meeting certain needs. This broad definition allows a view of manipulation as either a positive or a negative act.

Everyone uses manipulation to some extent in daily life to meet needs. For example, the nurse performs nursing care diligently so that the client recovers to meet her professional needs. This may also meet personal needs in that the client may thank the nurse or others, may compliment the nurse on the care, increasing her self-esteem. On a more conscious level, an employee may plan the right setting and the approach that will be most conducive to receiving a salary increase. Certainly, this behavior succeeds in having needs met but is neither negative nor destructive.

Client Assessment □ Manipulative behavior becomes a problem when it is negative. Richardson (1981) defines three areas in which manipulative behavior may be evidenced. The client (1) undermines the nurse-client relationship, (2) disrupts the entire staff, (3) appears to be working against his own medical recovery or emotional well-being. The client who uses manipulation frequently pits staff members against each other, or other clients against staff by making derogatory remarks about others, giving advice to others that contradicts the plan of care, or choosing "favorite" staff members with whom he will cooperate or communicate.

Manipulative behavior is often seen in the medical or community setting as well as in the psychiatric setting. Bursten (1972) distinguishes between manipulation in which the manipulator is motivated primarily on the basis of situations in which he finds himself and a manipulative personality. Anticipation of danger or discomfort often results in situational manipulation in order to gratify a desire or extricate himself from unpleasantness. In contrast, the person with a manipulative personality is seen as employing manipulative behavior in order to deceptively influence another person. This behavior appears more deliberate and the individual experiences a feeling of exhilaration when the deception is successful.

> **■ Point of Emphasis**
>
> *In assessing the behavior, it is important to distinguish between the behavior as a reaction to a crisis of illness and loss of control (situational) or as a lifetime pattern of behavior.*

The key point in assessing manipulative behavior is that it is generally self-defeating (McMorrow, 1981). The person who utilizes manipulative behavior in its extreme form, such as the person with antisocial personality disorder, eventually encounters difficulties in personal, social, and job-related areas. Legal difficulties may arise from consistent violation of rules.

Flattery and charm may increase the nurse's sense of self-esteem but she should question the purpose of the behavior, if excessive, and monitor her behavior toward the client. She may also feel physically attracted to a seductive, charming client. If these methods fail the client may become hostile or verbally abusive, causing confusion and frustration in the nurse.

Table 27-6 delineates some typical manipulative behaviors prominent in persons with personality disorders. These are ineffective coping behaviors because they are used by the client consistently as a way of meeting needs.

McMorrow (1981) points out that the manipulative client, lacking basic self-esteem and trust in himself, does not trust others. Thus, the manipulator tries to guard a fragile self by controlling others. Establishing trust is essential for a therapeutic relationship.

Self-Assessment □ The manipulative client will elicit many responses, the most prominent feeling being intense anger and frustration. The nurse may feel she has been "had" by the client and that the care and concern shown has been met with ingratitude. Certain client behaviors may bring out other strong feelings. A display of helplessness may bring out the altruistic feelings most nurses possess. These warm feelings, however, quickly give way to frustration when a client appears to refuse to help himself though he is able.

Family and Environment □ The family of the manipulative client may or may not be supportive. If the behavior is brought on by the crisis of illness and hospitalization or the prospect of long-term or only partial recovery, the family may be able to weather the difficult, demanding behavior.

TABLE 27-6 Personality Disorders and Ineffective Coping Behaviors

Antisocial personality disorder	Threats/Intimidation
	Flattery/Charm
	Violation of rules
	Verbal abuse
	Deceitfulness
	Demandingness
	Seductiveness
Histrionic personality disorder	Dramatic threats (e.g., suicide)
	Superficial charm/Flattery
	Helplessness/Dependency
	Possessivenes
	Demandingness
	Somaticization
	Seductiveness
Passive-aggressive personality disorder	Procrastination
	Back biting/Derogating others
	Resistance to changes
	Silence/Pouting
Schizoid and schizotypal personality disorder	Refusal to speak
	Withdrawal
Narcissistic personality disorder	Grandiose demands
	Pouting/Withdrawal when demands not met
	Physical intimidation
	Verbal abuse
	Charm/Flattery
Paranoid personality disorder	Secretiveness
	Withdrawal/Silence
Compulsive personality disorder	Excessive demands or questions
Dependent/Avoidant personality disorder	Withdrawal
	Helplessness
	Silence

The nurse must be alert to cues from the family that their resources for dealing with the client are becoming depleted (e.g., shortened or fewer visits, anger at the client, or undue blaming or criticism of the staff). In these situations, the nurse or the psychiatric liaison nurse can intervene with the family to teach them how to handle manipulative behavior.

In situations in which the manipulative behavior tends to be a way of life for the client, there often will be a noticeable lack of support because of the person's difficulties in relationships. Most often, the last person to "give up" on the client is a parent or spouse. That person may have been supportive all through the client's financial, social, and personal disasters because of his love for the client or because of his own needs that in some way were met by this loyalty. The nurse can help

to teach the significant person to set limits that protect his own physical and mental health and to recognize that the client is unlikely to change. (See vignette, Mr. George.)

The environment created by the person with manipulative behavior is filled with tension and hostility. When he derogates staff or other clients, the atmosphere becomes one of distrust. The staff will wish to get rid of the client in any way possible, by transfer, discharge, or (only half-jokingly) "homicide." These clients are usually assigned to the float or agency personnel because the staff is "sick" of them. Nursing staff will often avoid the client as much as possible and try to ignore his requests, even legitimate ones. Some nurses attempt to meet every demand with sweetness and concern, all the time feeling a growing anger and hostility. An angry divided staff that refuses to care for the client is a good clue that manipulative behavior is taking place.

PROBLEM IDENTIFICATION □ Manipulative behavior is a result of ineffective individual coping. This ineffective coping may be related to a variety of factors, but most often the nurse will see the behavior as a reaction to a situational crisis such as illness or a family or personal crisis. In these situations, manipulative behavior appears as the individual attempts, but fails, to cope successfully with problems. In the *Classification of Nursing Diagnoses* (1982) ineffective individual coping is characterized by two critical factors: (1) Client's verbalization of inability to cope or inability to ask for help; (2) inability to problem-solve. Manipulative behavior is a nonverbal way of asking

Vignette

Mr. George was a 46-year-old seaman hospitalized because he required surgery for treatment of a bowel disorder. He was always very pleasant toward the staff except when he did not receive a requested pass, or his food was not to his liking. At those times he became verbally abusive and intimidating. Mrs. George, his third wife, visited him daily. Her cultural background was different from his, and she spoke little English. When her husband was able to, he walked with her on the hospital grounds. The staff discovered that he was physically abusing Mrs. George while on these walks. Mrs. George refused to discuss the situation with the staff; she continued to visit Mr. George. The staff decided the only intervention possible at the time was to restrict Mr. George to the ward until his discharge.

for help and is self-defeating as a way of constructively solving problems.

In situations where manipulative behavior is precipitated by stress, such as hospitalization or long-term illness, the nurse will be able to identify other problems related to manipulative behavior, such as an inability to meet role expectations, an inability to meet basic needs, or an alteration in the client's social participation.

In the client whose manipulative behavior is more ingrained as a personality disorder, such as antisocial personality disorder, the nurse will be more likely to identify additional ways in which the manipulative behavior is an ineffective coping mechanism. These include verbal manipulation (lying, exaggeration, flattery), destructive behavior toward self or others (suicide gestures, intimidation of staff or other clients) and inappropriate use of defense mechanisms (e.g., denial, regression).

In crisis or prolonged stress situations, most clients are utilizing manipulative behavior to relieve feelings of anxiety and to meet emotional needs, such as those of self-esteem, control, and acceptance from others.

■ Point of Emphasis

In the individual whose manipulative behavior is a prominent personality trait, anxiety or meeting emotional needs does not appear to be the etiological factor prompting such behavior. This person's self-esteem needs are met, not by the outcomes of the manipulative behavior (which may be quite negative) but by the act itself of deceiving, or controlling someone else by the behavior.

The less experienced nurse may be unable to distinguish between the different causes of manipulative behavior, but will easily recognize the behaviors and the problems created. Because manipulative behavior is so self-defeating to the client's physical and/or emotional well-being, the nurse must learn to intervene effectively.

INTERVENTION □ Customary ways in which nurses intervene with manipulative clients do not always prove effective or serve to enhance the client's ability to problem-solve more constructively. Ignoring, avoiding, threatening, refusing care, becoming angry, and trying to transfer or discharge the client are frequent but generally ineffective measures which nurses use in attempting to cope with manipulative behavior. Then, both client and nurse have a problem of ineffective coping!

■ Point of Emphasis

Intervention in manipulative behavior requires self-awareness on the nurse's part and an ability to act, rather than react to the client's controlling maneuvers.

The nurse must also feel capable (if not comfortable) in setting firm limits and following through with expectations (Table 27-7).

EVALUATION □ Richardson (1981) identified outcomes of successful intervention in manipulative behavior. The client can be expected to:

1. Establish trust with the nurse
2. Develop greater awareness of behavior
3. Demonstrate more mature interpersonal behavior
4. Achieve greater self-control
5. Demonstrate an increase in compliance with a specified routine or regimen
6. Experience consistency in the environment
7. Improve problem-solving skills

In addition, the client's ability to work or live in greater harmony with others can be expected. However, for the client who utilizes manipulative behaviors as a life pattern, these changes will appear very gradually.

SEDUCTIVE BEHAVIOR

ASSESSMENT □ Seductive behavior can occur on a covert or an overt level and may be utilized by the client and/or the nurse. Although generally viewed as a maladaptive, manipulative way of behaving it also can be a nondestructive way of meeting needs. Generally, seductive behavior is seen as an expression of sexuality but more broadly defined it is a behavior used in an attempt to gain another's attention and/or receive something desired from that person.

Each of us has used seductive behavior. A child presents a sweet smile and "look of innocence" in an attempt to "seduce" the parent into

TABLE 27-7 *Intervening in Manipulative Behavior*

Intervention	Rationale	Evaluation
Clearly state expectations, rules, and so on to the client	The client must know and understand what is expected in order to follow through	Client follows through expectations or can tell you what is expected
If uncertain of what the client is saying or trying to do, clarify with him N: "You keep getting out of bed and you're on bedrest. Do you know what this means?" c: "Yes, it means I have to stay in bed." c: "Is there some reason you aren't staying in bed?"	The nurse may make hasty judgments about a client's "manipulative behavior" when there may be a valid reason for the behavior	The client can explain what he perceives to the nurse
State clearly why a behavior is unacceptable N: "You are asking other clients for cigarettes. This violates a rule of the group." c: "So what, if they're stupid enough to give it to me." N: "The point is, this behavior takes advantage of people who are afraid to say no to you." c: "I never thought of it like that."	The client may be unaware of what behaviors are causing difficulty	The client is able to relate what is not acceptable; is aware of why a behavior is unacceptable; may or may not agree
Set limits when necessary (see section on limit setting) c: "C'mon—why wouldn't you go out with me? Do you have a boyfriend? Have you ever had sex with a *real* man? I could show you a great time." N: "I don't feel I need to discuss my personal relationships with you. Let's discuss something else." c: "No—what's wrong? Don't you think I'm man enough for you?" N: "If you want to discuss how *you* feel about yourself, I'm willing to do that." c: "Don't you think I'm macho?" N: "I'm interested in what you think about that."	The manipulative client often violates the rights of others—limits need to be set by the nurse to define what will be expected, tolerated, and not tolerated in regard to self and others	The client follows the limits that are set
Suggest constructive alternatives or give choices to a behavior	Allows the client to feel more in control	Client chooses more constructive alternative
Assist the client to express feelings constructively N: "It's frustrating not to be able to get out of bed." c: "Yeah, makes me mad! I get so jumpy!"	Manipulative behavior is a self-defeating way of expressing feelings, often of fear or low self-esteem	Client verbally expresses feelings in appropriate manner
Remain accepting of the client—avoid *acting* in a judgmental way c: "A lot of people are afraid of me—I'm pretty mean." N: "It sounds like you feel good about that." c: "Yeah, I could bust out of here anytime, you nurses couldn't stop me." N: "Are you feeling pretty 'penned up' today?"	The client's behavior invites rejection and avoidance—keep in mind the behavior is motivated by strong needs that are not met	The nurse does not avoid the client or "desert" the client emotionally

TABLE 27-7 (*continued*)

Intervention	Rationale	Evaluation
Recognize reasonable requests and permit them when possible	Not every interaction is an attempt to manipulate—realistic and reasonable care needs to be extended to every client	Reasonable needs are met
Listen carefully to the client and pay attention to what is being said **c:** "The food here is lousy. We got better food at Memorial Hospital." **n:** "You sound really disgusted with the food." **c:** "It's not just the food, it's this whole place. I'm so sick of shrinks and nurses and groups, I could scream." **n:** "You're pretty discouraged about being in the hospital again."	Nurses tend to dismiss the manipulative client as unreasonable, but opportunities to understand feelings and deal more effectively with the client can develop by careful attention to the client	Nurse gains greater understanding of feelings motivating behaviors
Refocus when necessary to topic at hand	Client may try to distract attention from a topic that is uncomfortable or anxiety producing	Client follows routine or specified rules
Give positive feedback when appropriate **n:** "Jim, you did a good job of drawing out Sue and Jerry who are so quiet. They said they really enjoyed the shopping trip."	Manipulative client's behavior may not be reinforced when they are doing what is expected, but everyone needs to be given positive feedback about their behavior	The client uses feedback to continue constructive behavior
Involve all disciplines in the care of the client and be certain the approach is understood and carried out *consistently*	Consistency in approach from all those involved in the client's care reduces opportunities to play one staff member against another; it also makes the environment more predictable for the client	The care plan is understood, written down, and carried out consistently

taking him to the zoo. The adolescent girl flirts with a boy in an attempt to "seduce" him into asking her out. The physically attractive client is charming in an attempt to "seduce" the nurse into giving him better care. This behavior is not necessarily problematic when it is part of a larger framework of behavior patterns.

Client Assessment □ Seductive behavior becomes a problem when it occurs in a negative form or becomes the client's primary means of seeking involvement with others. Seductive behavior then becomes an expression of the anxiety experienced in relation to unmet needs.

Nurses encounter seductive behavior from clients in all settings of practice. Whether in a psychiatric hospital or a medical surgical unit, most nurses can recall having had a client ask them out for a date, being told they had "nice legs," or asked personal questions about their so-

cial life. As with manipulative behavior, it is important to assess if this behavior is occurring as a reaction to a crisis event of if it is a lifetime pattern.

Seductive behavior can occur in many forms. As a reaction to a crisis it can symbolize the anxiety and fear of loss of ability to love or be loved. The client whose self-concept is disrupted by illness, such as a myocardial infarction, prostate surgery, burns, mastectomy, or other injury affecting body image may display seductive behaviors in an attempt to reassure himself he is still a desirable person. As a lifetime pattern of functioning the behavior occurs more deliberately and has been unsuccessful in meeting the long-standing needs. The client's self-esteem remains impaired (Table 27-8).

Self-Assessment □ Many nurses find it difficult to deal with matters related to sexuality. The

TABLE 27-8 Examples of Seductive Behavior

Flirting	Client will give the nurse compliments of a physical nature, for example, "You know, you really have great legs." "You are the cutest nurse I've ever seen." Using nonverbal behavior, for example, winking, making kissing movements with mouth
Use of humor	Joking involving sexual issues Direct—Client laughs and says, "Boy, I bet I could get it up if you'd jump in bed with me." Indirect—"Say, did you hear the one about the nursing student and the intern?"
Flattery	Client praises the nurse and is charming, for example, "John, I feel so safe when you are the nurse moving me. You are so strong." "You are the nicest nurse here. I always feel better when you are on."
Sexually threatening behavior	Client will make threats of a sexual nature, such as, "There's not much staff on at night. A lot could happen before anyone knew what you and I were doing." "I'll get out of here sometime and then I'll give you what you've been asking for."
Socially unacceptable behavior	Exposing self, for example, revealing the breast or genitalia while nurse or other client around; wearing tight and/or revealing clothing; keeping pornographic material around; kissing and fondling other clients and/or visitors in inappropriate setting; masturbating in inappropriate areas; discussing sexual exploits in inappropriate settings
Exploiting others	Approaching other clients sexually who are more vulnerable; encouraging sexual acting out behavior between other clients

seductive client evokes a variety of responses. Some of these are anger, fear, frustration, feeling demeaned and/or taken advantage of, or feeling attractive, desirable, and affectionate toward the client. The nurse's response is affected by many variables including the client's physical appearance, age, the seductive behavior used, the client's identified problems, and the nurse's own comfort with sexuality. The importance of self-awareness should be readily apparent to the nurse.

The client, man or woman, with seductive behavior can initially prove exciting and attractive to the nurse. Flattery and flirting behavior may fill a need for the nurse to be desirable and attractive to others. In response to this, the nurse may then begin to feel guilty about these personal responses and become angry with the client. An attempt to avoid or withdraw from the client is a frequently chosen *ineffective* response.

Fear is another response to seductive behavior when it is more sexually threatening. Asking yourself "What am I afraid this client can actually do to me?" can be helpful in identifying where limits can and need to be set. Giving the patient very open, honest feedback can also help to relieve some of the nurse's anxiety. This of course needs to be done in a nonpunitive way. For example, if

a client remarks about "having you alone" the nurse could reply "It makes me uncomfortable when you make remarks about overpowering me. I wonder what you are wanting from me that you feel a need to try to frighten me."

Feelings of anger and revulsion occur often with physically aggressive seductive behavior. When a client pinches, grabs the nurse, and exposes himself, nurses frequently become either withdrawn or punitive toward the client. With a physically attractive, younger patient the response often is to set harsh limits indicating "you should be ashamed of yourself." With older clients, the behavior is frequently ignored because they are viewed as "not sexual." Whatever the client's age, it is important to recognize how personal attitudes about sex determine one's response. Consistently seductive behavior expresses an underlying need and should not be taken at face value.

As with the manipulative behavior, the nurse's feelings about the seductive client should not be ignored, but instead recognized as valuable cues to assessing the client's needs and behavior.

Family and Environment □ The family of the client who behaves seductively may or may not be supportive of him. With long-standing patterns of seductive behavior, there frequently will be anger if, for example, family members see the client as a "sex fiend," superficial and unable to have a meaningful relationship. There will be little understanding of the anxiety the client feels about being acceptable on any level other than a sexual one.

If the behavior is a crisis response, the family may feel hurt, confused, or disgusted. The nurse can help by explaining the underlying anxiety and how to respond by setting limits. In addition, the nurse must be aware of any family behavior that indicates their own stress and need to withdraw from the client, such as fewer visits, expressing anger at staff ("That doctor's making you this way") and expressing anger at the client ("What's wrong with you? This is important and you're grabbing at me!") The support system is necessary to help the family remain engaged and weather the crisis.

In situations where the behavior is long-standing, those involved with the client have conflicting motives. On the one hand, the seductiveness of the client meets some need of their own, yet on the other hand it has caused frustration and anger. The nurse can be most helpful by supporting the family in identifying their own needs and expectations and the means to be involved with the client in the least destructive manner. This may be done through encouragement of family members to talk with the client about how they are feeling.

■ Point of Emphasis

Long-standing patterns of behavior will not change quickly or easily. Family members themselves may not desire a radical change in the client's behavior because of their own needs.

PROBLEM IDENTIFICATION ☐ Seductive behavior may be a result of several interrelated problems, the most obvious of which is ineffective individual coping—generally encountered in response to a crisis situation. The behavior is a response in an attempt to cope when the usual methods have failed and there remains an increase in stress. As identified in the *Classification of Nursing Diagnosis* (1982) ineffective individual coping includes both the inability to problem-solve and to cope or ask for help. The reason for

the ineffective coping, however, may be body image disturbance (arising from injury or illness) or a disturbance in self-concept. The client exhibiting seductive behavior is having difficulty in these areas and, because of his unique personality and life situations, is unable to cope effectively.

In situational crises, the seductive behavior is utilized as an attempt to reduce anxiety and improve self-esteem. The need to feel in control of the situation, reassurance of acceptance by others, and reassurance of the client's ability to offer something worthwhile to others are prime motivators for the behavior.

The client in whom seductive behavior is a lifetime pattern, such as the hysterical personality disorder, demonstrates other ways in which the seductive behavior is an ineffective coping mechanism (see Table 27-6). This client may be filling some of the same needs as the client in crisis but generally experiences more gratification from the behavior.

INTERVENTION ☐ The nurse's response to the client's behavior is very important. Becoming angry, punitive, avoiding, ignoring, or moving the client to someone else's care are common *ineffective* intervention techniques. In contrast, the nurse who can recognize personal responses and explore the meaning of the client's behavior can provide the limits and feedback allowing for client growth (Table 27-9).

EVALUATION ☐ If the client can understand and increase his control of the seductive behavior, he develops greater self-esteem. Since his behavior generally distances other people and causes greater anxiety, he may become even more seductive in an effort to cope. Greater control of the behavior is evidenced by an increased awareness of and ability to intervene in his own behavior, improved problem-solving ability, increased self-esteem, and the development of more mature and satisfying relationships with others. Both nurse and client will experience a decrease in tension as the behaviors are changed to more constructive coping mechanisms.

NARCISSISTIC BEHAVIOR

ASSESSMENT ☐ Incorporation of self-identity is part of the process of growth and development. Most individuals can identify some disparity between their actual self and the idealized self. The idealized self generally is expressed in terms of

TABLE 27-9 Intervening in Seductive Behavior

Intervention	Rationale	Evaluation
Clearly state limits and the rules within the setting **N:** "John, you must wear a robe while walking in the hallway. Underwear is not considered acceptable attire." **C:** "What!? this covers me more than those bikinis women wear." **N:** "The issue isn't about bikinis, we are discussing that underwear is not permitted in the hallway."	The client must know the expectations in order to be able to meet them—may be confused as to what behavior is not acceptable and causing problems	Client follows through with expectations, such as not wearing underwear in the hallway
Clearly state why behavior is not acceptable **N:** "John, you are putting your arm around Mary and kissing her. That is not acceptable in the day hall area as this is the common area for all the clients and physical contact between the two of you breaks a Unit Rule." **C:** "Mary likes me to do that. I don't think it's any of your business." **N:** "Mary is feeling confused right now and not able to decide for herself. She will do it because you tell her to, not necessarily because she wants you to. Would you want someone else to decide your behavior for you?" **C:** "No, I guess I just thought she liked me."	The client may feel confused why he is unable to do something here which is not a problem elsewhere	Client will verbally be able to identify what is acceptable or not acceptable behavior and the reasons why
Set limits when necessary **C:** "I bet when you're not here you're really a hot ticket." **N:** "Discussing what I do when I'm not here is not how I can be helpful to you. Is there something else you would like to talk about?" **C:** "I'd rather talk about you." **N:** "As I said, that's not an area you and I need to talk about. I am interested in how you are feeling right now."	The client will test limits and at times take advantage of others—limits need to be set so that the client knows what the expectations are	The client will follow the limits set
Set clear expectations for the nurse-client relationship Client pinches nurse. **N:** Mr. Jones, it makes me angry when you pinch me. I don't want you to do that." **C:** "I saw that young guy pinch the nurse. She didn't get mad." **N:** "We are not talking about the other client. We are talking about what just happened. Can you tell me how you were feeling before you pinched me?"	The client will sometimes relate in a sexually aggressive way due to confusion about their relationship with staff—defining the limits can help the client feel more sense of control	Client will comply with the limits and expectations of the relationship
Maintain an accepting, nonjudgmental approach (Client is masturbating while sitting in day hall) **N:** "Mary, would you come with me?' Take patient to quiet, private area. **N:** "Mary, masturbating is a way people express their sexuality and I know that's true for you. The problem is when you do it in public it infringes on other peoples rights." **C:** "I just get so nervous and it helps me."	The behavior of the client stimulates strong feelings in both the nurse and other clients, resulting in rejection and increased anxiety and need for the client to use negative behavior—accepting the behavior as motivated by an underlying, unfulfilled need is important	The client can feel acceptable by the nurse and by others in the environment

TABLE 27-9 (*continued*)

Intervention	Rationale	Evaluation

Assist the client to express feelings appropriately
    c: "I've had so many guys you couldn't count them all."
    n: "I'm wondering why you need to impress me with your sexuality and desirability. Are you afraid you're still not attractive?"
    c: "Aw, what do you know? You're probably a virgin."
    n: "Can you talk about your feelings a little more? You sound both angry and yet scared too."
    c: "You bet I'm scared, who wants a woman with only one boob?"
	Sexualizing conversation frequently is used to mask anxiety about one's acceptance; client may brag as a means to cover fear	Client will express feelings more appropriately

goals and does not cause intolerable anxiety for the individual but in fact can encourage greater growth. For example: an individual may desire to become a nurse. She then goes to school to obtain a degree in nursing, with the eventual result of securing a desired job and functioning in a desired manner. For this person, environmental constraints and personal limitations can be faced and adjusted to, whereas the narcissistic individual may see any barrier as an intolerable threat to self-esteem. For the normal person, the desire to achieve the idealized version of himself is present but not all-consuming as it is with the narcissistic person.

Client Assessment □ The narcissistic individual may be encountered in the medical-surgical as well as the psychiatric setting. The basic motivation in treatment of this person is the presence of depression or psychotic symptoms in response to a severe disappointment in career or personal life. The client may express these feelings through either physical complaints, such as aches and pains, or psychological complaints, such as expression of a low self-concept, feelings of worthlessness, or intense rage at others.

It is important to distinguish between symptoms that occur primarily in response to a crisis situation as opposed to a lifetime pattern of functioning. Clients with the narcissistic personality disorder will consistently exhibit a preoccupation with themselves and their image and importance. In contrast, time-limited symptoms will correlate with an identified, specific threat. The interference with personal, social and/or job-related re-

lationships will be limited and more resolvable. Some typical feelings and behaviors of the narcissistic individual are presented in Table 27-10.

Self-Assessment □ The narcissistic client can provoke feelings such as helplessness, anger, and frustration. Although appearing grandiose and self-important, the client has an underlying need for constant attention, reassurance, and recognition—presenting a challenge to the nurse's understanding.

The need for self-importance can cause the client to elevate the nurse to idealized heights, which may meet the nurse's needs for importance. But since this is an unrealistic perception on the

TABLE 27-10 Narcissistic Behaviors

Interests focused on the self

Inability to feel empathy for others

Inability to defer gratification

Inability to tolerate frustration

Demanding behavior

Feelings of boredom and emptiness

Uncertainty about identity

Lability of mood

Shifting values

Feelings of differentness from others may be expressed in terms of alienation or specialness (haughty)

Intense anger and rage at others

Acceptable behavior chosen as means of gaining attention rather than being based on internalized values

part of the client, the nurse will not be able to live up to the expectations set for her. This results in the client becoming angry and verbalizing feelings of disappointment and disapproval of the nurse. It is difficult not to become threatened and defensive in response to this behavior. A common response by the nurse is anger.

Another form grandiosity can take is the client's expectation that he deserves more attention than any other client with whom the nurse is working. When demands are met, rather than expressing gratitude or even temporary satisfaction, the client will demand even more time and attention. Setting limits on this behavior may be viewed by the client as rejection, increasing the nurse's feelings of frustration. The nurse may then actually reject the client by withdrawing or becoming harsh and unkind in the treatment approach.

Awareness of feelings and personal needs as separate from the professional relationship are important in dealing with this client. The client's intense need for a sense of importance can be overwhelming and evoke many negative responses from the nurse.

Family and Environment □ The self-satisfying demands of this client tend to deplete his support resources, distancing others from him. Family members and friends will frequently describe a feeling of constantly giving without receiving any genuine affection or interest in return. The client's lack of empathy or understanding of others tends to isolate him.

The nurse must evaluate the resources still available to the client, including family, friends, and work relationships. How distant do significant others feel from the client? What behaviors do they find most distressing? Assist the supportive individuals to establish limits in their relationship with the client, permitting them to encourage the client's healthy behaviors without unrealistic expectations for drastic change.

PROBLEM IDENTIFICATION □ Narcissistic behavior is a result of ineffective individual coping which, as with other behaviors, may result from a variety of factors. As a response to a crisis, it may be precipitated by either physical illness or a personal stress due to a change in the individual's relationships. Usual coping mechanisms have failed and the narcissistic behavior is an ineffective attempt to regain stability.

Narcissistic behavior is primarily related to disturbance in self-concept. The individual finds it difficult to relate to others because his view of self is so distorted. His behavior becomes narrowed toward rebuilding and maintaining his idealized view of self. This is evidenced in problems such as alterations in role relationships (unable to meet demands as a spouse or parent), alterations in communication patterns (uses flattery or threats with others), manipulative behavior (uses others for own need gratification), and impaired value-belief patterns (changes values according to environmental influences). Although this behavior can be present in both situational crisis responses or as a lifetime pattern of functioning, the same types of interventions are used.

INTERVENTION □ Working with narcissistic behavior commonly elicits negative responses from staff. Ignoring or becoming angry and punitive in treatment will reinforce the need for the client to defend against others in order to preserve his self-esteem. Rather than encouraging growth, the result is reinforcement of the ineffective coping mechanisms. Good self-awareness and an understanding of the meaning of the client's behaviors are necessary to implement an effective treatment plan. Interventions in narcissistic behavior are presented in Table 27-11.

EVALUATION □ Narcissistic behavior as an ineffective coping mechanism embodies many immature qualities. Effective interventions by the nurse can be evidenced by the following behaviors:

1. Increased tolerance for frustration
2. Increased ability to delay need gratification
3. Increased ability to understand the feelings and needs of others
4. Increased maturity in relationships
5. Improved self-esteem
6. Decreased feelings of fear and anger

As a behavioral response to a situational crisis, there may be rather quick and dramatic changes. When the behavior exists as a lifelong pattern, the nurse is cautioned to remember change will be limited and occur over a long period of time. Recognizing any change, even the smallest, will be important if growth is to continue.

TABLE 27-11 *Intervening in Narcissistic Behavior*

Intervention	Rationale	Evaluation
Set firm limits with manipulative behavior (see care plan on manipulation)	Client must know limits to be able to comply with them	Client will comply with limits
Explore feelings motivating behavior (Client tells "better" story each time someone else talks) N: "Mary, you seem to have something worse to tell each time someone else talks." C: "What's the matter? Don't you believe me? That stuff really happened." N: "I'm not questioning the truth of what you're saying. I wonder if you could talk about how you feel when someone else is getting the group's attention."	Understanding the feelings motivating behavior can help increase the client's control with behavior— alternatives for meeting needs can be explored	Client will talk about feelings
Maintain a nonjudgmental approach C: "Sometimes I think my wife doesn't want me since she's got *that baby*." N: "It must be hard to feel you have to share her attention." C: "Yea, she should take half as good of care of me as that brat of mine." N: "Can you talk about your feeling of wanting to be taken care of a little more?"	The testing, "me-ness" of behavior distances others; a "shame on you" attitude will increase the client's need to preserve self-esteem	Nurse and client will remain positively involved
Present feedback in a clear, concrete manner N: "Tim, you are telling people you own the company and you are an employee there." C: "You just want to make me look small." N: "No, I want you to understand that distorting the facts can be deceiving to other people." C: "I could own the company if I wanted to." N: "We can talk about how you're feeling. First, I want to be sure you understand it can make others feel bad if you deceive them."	Any criticism, even positively stated can be crushing to this client—avoiding any judgment and presenting facts can help client to understand information with less fear and anxiety	Client will be able to relate a verbal understanding of behavior

WITHDRAWN/DETACHED BEHAVIOR

ASSESSMENT □ Withdrawn/detached behavior occurs in varying degrees. As a response to stress from a crisis situation, it is viewed as a defense mechanism which provides the individual with time to rest, restructure, and gather his resources in order to deal with the trauma. As a behavioral component of some of the major psychiatric illnesses, it is viewed as an example of ineffective coping. In behavior assessment, the key is to determine the degree of withdrawn/detached behavior being utilized by the client. A determination must be made when withdrawal becomes negative and destructive to the client's well-being.

Client Assessment □ Withdrawn/detached behavior that is health promoting occurs at a transitory period of emotional trauma in which the client may appear temporarily mildly stunned or shocked. Problems arise when withdrawal has not successfully relieved the tension and stress of a crisis event. For example, a client is diagnosed as being diabetic, yet after many weeks remains depressed and unable to follow the insulin and diet requirements. This client fails to keep appointments with the physician and begins to isolate

himself. In the client for whom this is a lifelong pattern of behavior, the isolation from the environment will be much more severe. The behavior is used in an effort to protect the self and create a "safe" environment. The withdrawn/detached behavior as an effort to cope can in fact become life-threatening as basic needs are increasingly ignored. Table 27-12 delineates withdrawn/detached behaviors.

A special need for this client may be for the nurse to recognize his presence since withdrawal and lack of demands on others can mean that he is in effect unnoticed. Assessment that these behaviors indicate a problem, rather than just a quiet, undemanding client, is necessary so that active treatment can be initiated.

Self-Assessment □ The withdrawn/detached behavior of the client poses a variety of problems for the nurse. The overall feeling response frequently is frustration and guilt. This can then result in accepting a hopeless stance or becoming angry toward the client for "not responding to treatment." Self-awareness is important when caring for the client.

This behavior can cause a desire for the nurse to try to become close to the client before he is able to accept the relationship. Attempting to push the client too fast will only cause increased withdrawal. The nurse's need to heal the client and "see" him get well can precipitate this behavior. His increased withdrawal will then serve to increase the nurse's sense of frustration.

When withdrawn/detached behavior appears vegetative, some nurses respond with a sense of hopelessness. It is easy to understand the confusion that is felt by the nurse who wants to instill hope yet feels hopelessly depressed about this client. The nurse's feelings can then motivate avoidance behavior. Such statements as "I can hardly stand to go into her room. I don't know why, she just makes me feel sad or down," can be a good clue to the nurse that she has been infected by the client's sense of hopelessness.

Another nurse reaction is anger at the client. The nurse has worked hard to help this client who "refuses" to respond. This can precipitate punitive behaviors. Such displays of anger include threatening ("If you don't get out of bed you can't have any visitors!"); refusing to give care ("If she doesn't want to help herself, why should I?"); judgmental behavior ("If you weren't so lazy you would do it"); and/or transferring the client to someone else's care.

TABLE 27-12 Examples of Withdrawn/ Detached Behavior

Behavior

Lack of spontaneity

Inattention to grooming and/or hygiene

Decreased or absent communication

Apathetic appearance: Slumped posture
                       No eye contact
                       Rapid shallow breathing
                       Decreased motor activity

Isolation: Remaining by self
            Spending a great amount of time in bed

Reduced body functions: Inadequate food and/or fluid
                              intake
                           Retention of urine or feces
                           Decreased or absent libido

Lack of problem-solving ability

Disturbance of affect and/or mood: Inappropriate
                                   affect
                                Depression

In severe forms: Muteness
                 Hallucinations
                 Delusions
                 Maintaining fetal position
                 Indifference to surroundings

■ *Point of Emphasis*

It is imperative that the client be allowed adequate time and support to begin to reengage with others. The nurse will need patience and the support of peers to be able to handle personal feelings and needs.

Family and Environment □ Because of the isolating nature of withdrawn and detached behavior, the client's support system may be greatly impaired. The extent of the disruption and its duration will greatly effect the availability of others.

As a response to a situational crisis, withdrawn/detached behavior will elicit many of the same responses in family members as in the nurse. They will speak of feeling frustrated, angry, powerless to help the client, and rejected by him. Help the family recognize that the behavior is used by the client to increase feelings of safety and assist them in coping with their feelings of rejection. One of the signs that the family is frustrated can be their attempts to push the client into recovery. As with the nurse, the family's demands for wellness will not produce positive results.

The client with long-standing withdrawn/detached behavior may be seriously devoid of a support system. The rejecting effect of this behavior may have created for him an environment of extreme isolation. The emphasis then is to assist family members in learning how they can begin to reengage with the client.

PROBLEM IDENTIFICATION □ Withdrawn/detached behavior is an example of ineffective coping. The client displays a general aloofness which is manifested by intellectualization, denial, regression, and projection. The behavior is employed in an effort to cope with stress. The client who exhibits this behavior in response to a situational stress will experience a variety of problems, including an inability to meet basic needs, decreased social activity, and an inability to meet role expectations. The withdrawal behavior becomes a passive stance in which the individual is immobilized. As the behavior becomes intensified, or, becomes a long-standing pattern, additional problems will be apparent. The communication pattern changes (does not spontaneously communicate, becomes mute, displays echolalia), self-concept changes, thought processes change (blames others, projects own feelings, hallucinates, manifests delusions). The client may be indifferent to the environment and become withdrawn.

INTERVENTION □ Nursing intervention must allow sufficient time for the client to accept the nurse without becoming overly anxious about the new relationship. Remember that his current behavior, though it may be basically unhealthy, does afford him some sense of safety. Table 27-13 sets forth interventions to be used in withdrawn/detached behavior.

PASSIVE-AGGRESSIVE BEHAVIOR

ASSESSMENT □

Client Assessment □ The key factor in assessing the client who displays passive-aggressive behavior is the resultant degree of impairment. The person may see no connection between his behavior and his difficulties with others, and may feel no need to make any alterations in relationships.

Self-Assessment □ Working with a passive-aggressive client can be frustrating to the nurse. The client's clinging manner can cause the nurse to feel overwhelmed and angry. It is not uncommon for staff members to say that no matter what they do for this client, it never seems to be enough. Or that the client complains about the nurse to other staff members no matter how great her efforts to please him.

As with other behavioral disorders, the nurse needs to be aware of how much anger the client may arouse by his behavior and guard against reacting in a similarly passive-aggressive manner.

Family and Environment □ The effects of the behavior on others in the client's life or in his work setting determine whether the behavior is merely annoying or constitutes a real problem. Inhibiting his anger and expressing it only in passive-aggressive behavior can cause the client to feel deeply depressed, and he may then turn to drugs or alcohol to numb his feelings of hurt and anger. He is most likely to seek treatment when he recognizes that his behavior is affecting his significant personal relationships or his job.

PROBLEM IDENTIFICATION □ Once the nurse has assessed the behavior as a problem for either

TABLE 27-13 *Intervening in Withdrawn/Detached Behavior*

Intervention	Rationale	Evaluation
Provide for meeting basic needs	Regressed behavior of client can interfere with basic functions which must be achieved if life is to continue	Client will receive food and fluid and elimination needs will be met
Meet client at present level of functioning (i.e., sit with client if mute; explain time frame you will be present; allow silence—don't overload with talk)	If regressed, the client may not be able to communicate in the usual way; offering your presence is necessary to convey a nonpressured way of relating	Client will spend time with others
Begin activities slowly and based on client's present level of functioning (include client in area with other people; begin with low numbers; gradually increase level of participation)	If pushed, fear and anxiety will increase causing more withdrawal	Client will spend time with others
Set clear expectations N: "I know it's uncomfortable for you to be out of your room. You will be expected to spend at least 1/2 hour each morning and each evening in another area of the unit."	Client must know what is expected of him if he is to comply with his treatment plan	Client will be able to identify the expectations
Assist client in verbalizing feelings N: "It must feel overwhelming to have to figure out how this unit works." C: "Yes, I'm really scared of all these people. I don't understand why they're here." N: "Can you tell me more about how you're feeling about being here? Do you feel confused as to why you're here?"	Talking about his feelings can increase the client's awareness of his behavior	Client will verbalize feelings
Emphasize daily living issues—limit intellectualizing N: "Mr. T., you haven't had your shower yet." C: "The world's falling apart and you're talking about showers." N: "The world is not something you can change right now. It is important you take care of your grooming." C: "But don't you care about nuclear war?" N: "Yes, but right now I care most about how you're feeling and how that keeps you from taking care of yourself."	Concrete, reality-based issues can help increase the client's control; broad philosophical discussions can be distracting and are not something from which the client can effect immediate change	Client will attend to daily issues increasing awareness of needs related to same
Set limits with manipulative behavior, that is, hostile, limit testing (see care plan for manipulative behavior)	Client must understand and know limits to comply with them	Client will comply with limits
Maintain a nonjudgmental approach	The withdrawn behavior may precipitate withdrawal by the nurse such as anger at client—she must keep mutual distancing at a minimum	The nurse and client remain involved in a positive manner
Reality-test the client's perceptions and thoughts (see care plan on schizophrenia)	Hallucinations and delusions are distortions of reality; self-image may be distorted as well for the client	The client will begin to express reality-based concepts

the client or others (for example, the nursing staff of a general hospital unit) she will be able to recognize that this behavior is yet another form of ineffective individual coping.

The client's adaptive behavior and problem-solving skills are impaired either because a crisis situation has occurred or because his behavior pattern has been maladaptive over a long period of time. His avoiding direct interaction or confrontation is an indication that he is unable to cope or openly ask for help. Against this background, he cannot meet role expectations, cannot effectively meet his basic needs, and finds social interaction difficult. He may also be ill frequently (an avoidance technique) or have "accidents" in order to win sympathy or make others feel guilty about their treatment of him. As such behavior evolves over a long period of time, the nurse should keep in mind that change will not come readily.

Nurses often encounter such a client in the work setting. He often attributes his noncompliant behavior to others. His motivation is basically the same as that of the client identified as requiring psychiatric care, thus, as with the psychiatric client, he needs consistency in his relationship with the nurse and needs to be able to express his feelings.

INTERVENTION □ It is generally helpful to begin treatment by focusing on those aspects of behavior that pose the greatest threat to the client, such as job-related problems. The client should be involved in identifying the problem.

The behavior is a protective shield for the fragile self-esteem, and giving up this self-protective behavior is frightening to the client because he feels extremely vulnerable in all aspects of his life. Appropriate interventions are outlined in Table 27-14.

EVALUATION □ Successful intervention is evidenced by a decrease in the target behaviors; The client is able to ask for what he wants, can validate and correct his perceptions of others' actions, and have his needs met in a direct and satisfying way. His ability to problem-solve will improve, as will the ability to verbalize a problem and ask for help because he now deals with facts rather than imagined fears. As his anxiety diminishes and he is better able to satisfy his needs, his self-esteem is enhanced and his interpersonal relationships improve.

HELPLESS/DEPENDENT BEHAVIOR

ASSESSMENT □ Dependent, helpless behaviors are very difficult to deal with. At various periods everyone is helpless and dependent on others. The nurse encourages clients to assume this behavior. She is taught to allow the client to be "as sick as he needs to be" and to anticipate and care for his needs. Helpless/dependent behavior can be viewed as positive for the client admitted to the medical-surgical setting, where he needs to assume a sick role and allow others to meet his basic needs. For example, the nurse is in control when the client responds to the presence of a thermometer by opening his mouth. He is not encouraged to decide whether or not to have his temperature taken. The message is "Let me decide what's best for you." Whether a helpless/dependent behavior assumes a negative force is thus a question of why it is exhibited.

Client Assessment □ Helpless/dependent behavior becomes a nursing problem when it is the primary way in which the client relates to others. The behavior appears to be rooted in feelings of inadequacy and helplessness. The client feels unable to change the outcome of events. As with other problematic behaviors, helpless/dependent behavior can occur in response to a crisis event or can persist as a lifelong pattern of functioning.

The client has many varieties of helpless/dependent behavior at his disposal: he can be hostile and demanding, whining, crying, can appear confused, can make frequent requests that underscore his weakness through physical and psychological means and through manipulative behavior. By his behavior he can create divisiveness within the nursing staff or can pit other clients against staff.

As stated previously, this behavior may occur in response to a crisis situation, be it admission to the hospital, an unfavorable diagnosis, loss of a significant person through death or divorce, and so on. When the behavior is manifested in response to a situational crisis, the client feels overwhelmed, anxious, and unable to solve his problems. He then displays helpless/dependent behavior to avoid the unpleasantness of the situation and control his anxiety. Recognizing that this behavior signals underlying unmet needs can assist the nurse in identifying those needs.

The client in whom this behavior has become a lifelong pattern may be exhibiting what is described by Seligman (1975) as learned helpless-

TABLE 27-14 Intervening in Passive-Aggressive Behavior

Intervention	Rationale	Evaluation
Give the client concrete, specific feedback on behavior ("John, you have an angry look on your face and you have stopped talking")	Concrete feedback increases the client's awareness of what the behavior communicates to others as well as increases the client's self-awareness of the feelings he or she is experiencing. Awareness of behavior must occur prior to change	Client is able to recognize feelings and resultant behavior
Ask client to express feelings and beliefs about the response of others toward the client (i.e., "George, tell me what you think will happen if you tell me how you feel.")	Feelings can be so intense for the client that there occurs an unrealistic fear that expression of these feelings can "destroy" others. The nurse assists the client to see that others won't die and that what the client fears is usually worse than what occurs in reality.	Client is able to express "negative" or feared feelings and see that this does not "destroy" people
Ask the client to identify both verbally and nonverbally, what he expects from others that meets the client's needs	Fear of rejection causes the client to constrain his behavior, rather than ask for what's needed. Dependence and need for acceptance motivate behaviors which in fact cause rejection to occur. Also, when the client becomes anxious, perceptions of others' behavior is distorted	Number of times client is able to state what he would like from others
Give client the expectation to ask others to validate or correct his perception of his behavior or feelings toward the client	Consistent reality testing of one's perception lowers anxiety	Number of times client asks others for validation or correction of client's perceptions ("Maggie, you are frowning. Are you upset with me?")
Assist client to identify alternate means (other than passive-aggressive behavior) to meet needs; enlist support from others in encouraging new behaviors (i.e., client may ask group members or significant others or client may join assertiveness group)	Alternative means are more direct and will elicit satisfaction of having spoken up for what one needs. Support is important because behavior change is difficult and risky. Changed behavior must be seen as meeting needs (for acceptance) in order for the client to persist.	Number of times client identifies and utilizes alternative behaviors. Number of times client can ask for support from others and spontaneously receives it
Give client expectation that he respond to feedback or input from others *at the time it is given*	Concrete factual information from others assists the client's understood effects of their behavior on others. Also, immediate response eliminates time for client to brood over and imagine "Exactly what did George mean by that?" By getting feedback at the time of the situation, anxiety is thereby decreased.	Number of times client responds to feedback or input from others. Number of times client is able to express negative feelings at the time of interaction rather than using a delayed response. Decrease in anxiety as evidenced by behavioral manifestations and client's subjective input

ness. He believes that certain outcomes will occur regardless of what he does or does not do, that nothing can be done to alter the outcome of any situation. The behavior becomes passive as he views himself as dependent on others who are seen as having control. The client cannot deal effectively with daily situations and may be repeatedly admitted to the hospital with various complaints, which may be evidenced through physical or psychological symptoms. Table 27-15 gives some examples of typical helpless/dependent behaviors.

Self-Assessment □ The helpless/dependent client will generally elicit two strong and opposing feelings within the nurse. As a student, the nurse learns to allow the client to be dependent and to assist him in assuming a dependent role. Yet she is also taught to promote independence and to encourage the client's utilization of his

TABLE 27-15 Examples of Helpless/ Dependent Behavior

Dependency on others for basic living skills	Client will request you do things for them that they can do themselves (i.e., feeding them, combing their hair, etc.)
Inadequate skills for daily living; poor judgment and problem-solving ability	Client will ask you to make decisions for them (i.e., "Should I take my shower first or make my bed first?"); will exhibit poor decision making
Feelings of inadequacy, worthlessness, hopelessness, or failure	Client expresses feelings that exhibit a low self-concept such as: "I never do anything right"
Depression—chronic or recurring with possible suicidal behavior	Client may have history of suicide attempts; will describe depression as a persistent problem
Repeated illness	Client may have long history of repeated admissions to the hospital or having someone "care for" him
Manipulative behavior (crying, clinging, flattery, threatening behavior)	Client may test limits, attempt to split staff in an effort to align someone with them; may attempt to induce guilt in others to secure their continued help
Repeated legal difficulties	Client may exhibit helplessness through stealing, writing bad checks, and so on
Substance abuse	Client may have used chemicals rather than people as a means to meet needs

strengths and "doing for himself." Because the traditional nursing role has been that of caretaker and "mother" she may find it difficult to define how much "doing for" the client can be helpful. Feeling needed by the patient can meet the nurse's personal needs. She needs to ask herself, "How much care does this person need and how much makes it possible for *me* to feel useful?"

The client's behavior can also elicit a sense of power in the nurse. If he consults her and seeks her opinion incessantly she begins to feel self-important. But as this behavior persists, she sees it as demanding behavior, and feels angry. The client may hold her responsible for decisions that do not work out well. The initial seeking of a "val-ued opinion" then becomes an accusation that the nurse is responsible for the client's problem.

It can be seen that the nurse must explore her personal needs and feelings when working with this client. Her frustration and anger when the client is unresponsive, resists treatment, and refuses to help himself is quickly conveyed, leaving both client and nurse feeling uncomfortable and distressed.

Family and Environment ☐ If the behavior is a response to a crisis event, the nurse can generally intervene to help the family manage the situation and remain involved with the client. The family needs to learn to set limits for the client, yet not withdraw support. For example, if the client telephones family members repeatedly during the day, assist them to set a limit on specific times in which calls can be made and support their following through.

If the client is manifesting the behavior as a lifelong pattern, his support system may be lacking—"burned out" due to the frequency and intensity of demands placed upon them. Those who remain involved in the relationship most often are having their own need to be needed met, or feel obligated to the client in some way. For example, an adult child who feels responsible for the welfare of his parent will appear to "sacrifice" his own life in order to provide the parent's care. It is unrealistic to expect dramatic changes in the situation. The nurse needs to help the family understand that change will come only slowly, while encouraging the family not to neglect their own well-being.

PROBLEM IDENTIFICATION ☐ Helpless/dependent behavior results from ineffective coping. It is employed in an effort to control the stress generated by a change or a crisis event. Although the behavior is often considered negative, it may serve to temporarily control the client's immediate anxiety. Yet, as the behavior persists anxiety increases. The client invokes this behavior to signal others that he is having difficulty dealing with stress. The two critical factors of ineffective individual coping identified in the *Classification of Nursing Diagnosis* (1982) can readily be seen in helpless/dependent behavior. The first, the client's verbalization of his inability to cope or inability to ask for help is caused by his confusion about what could help. Frequently he has a sense of hopelessness, believing there is nothing that will make a difference in the outcome of the crisis.

TABLE 27-16 Intervening in Helpless/Dependent Behavior

Intervention	Rationale	Evaluation
Provide a safe environment (see care plan for suicidal behavior)	Client will frequently exhibit suicidal behavior or ideation and will need help to avoid harming himself.	Client will not harm self
Encourage as much independent care as possible c: "I'm too tired to get my tray. Would you get it for me?" n: "I want you to get it; then let's sit down and have lunch together." c: (begins whining) "You don't care how I feel. I'm so tired." n: "If I believed you were unable to get your tray I would. I would like to talk about what it would mean to have me get it for you." c: (Stares at nurse sullenly) n: "Let's walk up together and we can talk if you want to."	Client will want you to do things for him because he feels insecure and helpless. Expectations need to be within realistic limits. Remaining with the client during the activity can provide support.	Client will do own care as able
Encourage problem-solving behavior by exploring available choices in a situation n: "What happened that made you start to cry and leave the group?" c: "John made me cry. He is so mean." n: "How did John make you cry?" c: "He always gets his way and he made me move out of my chair." n: "Is there any other way you think you could have handled this? For instance, could you have remained in the chair and told John how you felt?" c: "I've never throught about saying something to him."	The client frequently does not recognize the control he has in a situation. Helping the client to identify his control can increase his ability to problem-solve. This diminishes blaming behavior, which indicates others have control.	Client begins making active rather than passive choices If choices are not actively made, client will be able at least to identify other options in behavior
Avoid making decisions for the client c: "I don't know what to wear tonight. Should I wear the red or blue top?" n: "Which one do you like better?" c: "I don't know, which do you like?" n: "They both are pretty. Pick one and put it on, then you can see how you feel."	Relying on others to choose increases the client's feelings of dependence and helplessness. Making choices increases his self-esteem.	Client will begin to make choices rather than have others do it for him
Encourage the client to express the feelings he is having at the time of the behavior (Client is sitting in day hall by himself) n: "Is there a reason you're not at the activity?" c: "I don't know. Please don't make me go." n: "Can you tell me how you're feeling now?" c: "I don't like that group. The leader doesn't like me."	Understanding the motivation for behavior can help the client to define alternative ways to meet these needs.	Client will express his feelings in a more constructive manner

600

TABLE 27-16 *(continued)*

Intervention	Rationale	Evaluation
N: "Sometimes it's scary, getting to know new people."		
C: "I am scared. People never seem to like me."		
Keep client informed of what is expected in the hospital setting	Expectations must be clear to enable client to comply. Choices can be made effectively only if adequate information is available.	Client will use information available in decision-making process
Set firm, clear limits to manipulative behavior (see interventions in manipulation)	Limits must be clear and understandable in order for the client to comply.	Client will stay within limits

The second, the inability to problem-solve, is due to feelings of powerlessness. Since he believes that he has no control over life events, the client's helpless/dependent behavior avoids the need to make any decision. He decides "not to decide" and allows matters to "fall as they may."

If helpless/dependent behavior is a response to an immediate and identifiable stress rather than a lifelong pattern, other problems will become apparent. Among these are an inability to meet basic needs, an inability to meet role expectations, an alteration in social participation, destructive behavior toward self (such as suicidal behavior), and a change in usual communication patterns. Each of these behaviors may result from overwhelming feelings of stress and anticipated defeat or failure in constructively resolving the crisis.

The client whose helpless/dependent behavior has become a lifelong pattern will exhibit additional behaviors indicative of ineffective coping. These include much sickness (frequent and recurring episodes of physical or psychological complaints requiring the care of others), numerous accidents (recurring situations in which because of a lack of planning there is a traumatic outcome), and inappropriate use of defense mechanisms (overuse of denial and rationalization in which the client identifies himself as a victim of others or of circumstance). These helpless/dependent behaviors are also seen in passive aggressive personality disorder.

INTERVENTION □ Many of the commonly employed interventions are not helpful and can be destructive by reinforcing or increasing negative behaviors—for instance, avoiding, ignoring,

threatening, or responding in a judgmental manner.

Table 27-16 presents some constructive interventions. Nevertheless, even the most effective approach can fail if the nurse does not remain aware of her personal feelings and needs and is not able to use them as cues to the client's needs.

EVALUATION □ Helpless/dependent behavior is due to low self-esteem with its related feelings of frustration, depression, futility, hopelessness, and lack of control. Effective nursing interventions will be reflected in client behaviors evidencing an increased sense of control. Clients will begin to take an active role in relationships rather than seeing themselves as just being "swept along in the stream of life."

■ Enrichment Activities

DISCUSSION QUESTIONS

1. Discuss how values in our society may encourage the development of a personality disorder such as antisocial or histrionic personality.

2. Identify situations of violence that may be due to disorder of impulse control. Examine your feelings toward violence. In which situations do you feel physical violence is justified/unjustified? What values do you have that influence your answer?

LEARNING ACTIVITIES

1. Select a prominent personality trait in yourself. Ask a friend to help you identify a specific

trait. Discuss how this trait is harmful or helpful in your relationships. Decide if exaggeration of this trait would be helpful or harmful to your life-style.

2. Identify what a client in your clinical practicum feels are his "best" personality traits and ask him to explain his response.

3. Make a list of personality traits that you find desirable or undesirable. Explain how these choices might be influenced by your own moral, ethical, or religious values.

4. In working with a client who demonstrates a personality disorder (patterns of behavior that disrupt the life-style) identify specific nursing interventions and evaluations.

■ Recommended Readings

Aguilera, D., and Messick, J. *Crisis intervention: Theory and methodology*. 4th ed. St. Louis: Mosby and Company, 1982. This classic book about crisis theory and crisis intervention includes discussion of maturational and situational crises with case examples.

Alberti, R.E., and Emmon, M.L. *Your perfect right: A guide to assertive behavior*. San Luis Obispo, CA: Impact, 1974. Assertiveness is a skill that can be utilized to enhance one's personal life and to help others. This book describes the differences between assertive, nonassertive, and aggressive behaviors. A step-by-step process of development of assertive behavior is provided.

Chenevert, M. *Special techniques in assertiveness training for women in the health professions*. St. Louis: Mosby Company, 1978. Written for women health care professionals, this book addresses many problems and situations in health care from a societal, sexual, and health care issues view.

AUDIOVISUAL

Concept Media, *Personality Disorders*. Irvine, CA: 1980. (slides) These slides discuss the various types of personality disorders and how they affect the person's life-style.

Human Relations Media. *Overcoming Inferiority*. Part I and II. Pleasantville, NY, 1980. These filmstrips discuss, developmentally, the importance of self-image. A sense of inferiority can affect one's life-style dramatically. Overcoming these feelings result in healthier personal adjustment.

The Psychiatry Learning System, 3d ed., Part II, No. 13. *Personality Disorders*, Health Sciences Consortium Inc, Chapel Hill, NC, 1982. (2 videocassettes)

These two videocassettes present basic concepts in the development of and criteria for personality disorders. They closely follow the guidelines of the American Psychiatric Association's Diagnostic and Statistical Manual (DSM III).

■ References

Akhtar, S., and Anderson, J. Overview: Narcissistic personality disorder. *American journal of psychiatry*, 139, 1, 1982:12–19.

American Psychiatric Association. *Diagnostic and statistical manual of mental disorders*. 3d ed. 1981.

Baron, M.; Gruen, R.; Asnis, L.; and Kanes, J. Familial relatedness of schizophrenic and schizotypal states. *American journal of psychiatry*, 140, 1983:1437–1442.

Bursten, B. The manipulative personality. *Archives of general psychiatry*, 26, 1972:318–321.

Chodoff, D. Diagnosis of hysteria. *American journal of psychiatry*, 131, 1974:1073–1078.

Cicone, J.R., and Kaskey, G.B. Life events and antisocial behavior. *Bulletin of the American academy of law*, 7, 1979:63–68.

Cleckley, Hervey. *The mask of sanity*. 4th ed. New York: Mosby, 1974.

Dorpat, T.L. A developmental perspective on charater pathology. *Comprehensive psychiatry*, 20, 1979:548–559.

Graham, S.A. Psychotherapist's attitudes toward offender clients. *Journal of consulting and clinical psychology*, 48, 1980:796–797.

Grant, D.A. A model of violence. *Australia-New Zealand journal of psychiatry*, 12, 1978:123–126.

Horney, Karen. *Neurosis and human growth*. New York: Norton, 1950.

Hott, L.R. The antisocial character. *The American journal of psychoanalysis*, 39, 1979:235–244.

Hughes, J. Manipulation: A negative element in care. *Journal of advanced nursing*, 5, 1980:21–29.

Johansen, K.H. The impact of patients with chronic character pathology on a hospital inpatient unit. *Hospital and community psychiatry*, 34, 9, 1983:842–846.

Kendler, F.S., and Gruenberg, A.M. Genetic relationsip between paranoid personality disorder and "schizophrenic spectrum" disorders. *American journal of psychiatry*, 139, 1982:1185–1186.

Kim, M. and Moritz D. (eds.). Classification of nursing diagnoses: Proceedings of the third and fourth national conferences. New York: McGraw-Hill, 1982.

Kolb, L. *Modern clinical psychiatry*. 9th ed. Philadelphia: W.B. Saunders Co., 1982.

Link, N.F.; Scherer, S.E.; and Niall, P. Moral judgement and moral conduct in the psychopath. *Canadian psychiatric association journal*, 22, 1977:341–346.

Locke, R. Researchers debate whether criminality has a genetic factor. Report on work of Mednick, S.A. in Omaha *World-Herald*, May 30, 1982.

McMorrow, M.E. The manipulative patient. *American journal of nursing*, 81, 1981:1188–1190.

Perry, J.C., and Flannery, R.B. Passive-aggressive personality disorder: Treatment implications of a clinical typology. *The journal of nervous and mental disease*, 170, 1982:164–173.

Reid, W.H. The sadness of the psychopath. *American journal of psychotherapy*, 32, 1978:496–509.

Richardson, J. Managing the manipulative patient. *Nursing*, 81, 1, 1981:49–52.

Schlesinger, L.B. Distinctions between psychopathic, sociopathic and antisocial personality disorders. *Psychological reports*, 47, 1980:15–21.

Seligman, M. *Helplessness*. San Francisco: W.H. Freeman Co, 1975.

Stringer, A.Y., and Josef, N.C. Methylphenidate in treatment of two patients with antisocial personality disorder. *American journal of psychiatry*, 140, 10, 1983:1365–1366.

Tyrer, P., and Alexander, J. Classification of personality disorder. *British journal of psychiatry*, 135, 1979:163–167.

Valliant, G.E. Sociopathy as a human process. *Archives of general psychiatry*, 33, 1975:178–183.

Warner, R. The diagnosis of antisocial and hysterical personality disorders. An example of sex bias. *Journal of nervous and mental disorders*, 166, 1978:839–845.

Weiss, J.M.; Davis, D.; Hedlund, J.L.; and Cho, D.W. The dysphoric psychopath: A comparison of 524 cases of antisocial personality disorder with matched controls. *Comprehensive psychiatry*, 24, 1983:355–369.

Zuckerman, M., and Neeb, M. Sensation seeking and psychopathology. *Psychiatry resident*, 1, 1979:255–264.

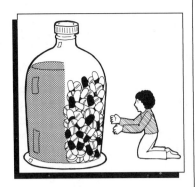

28

Substance Use Disorders

Joan Norris

Learning Objectives

Upon completion of this chapter, the reader will be able to:

1. Identify substance abuse as a significant health problem in the hospital and community.

2. Examine own beliefs and values concerning substance use and abuse to identify and correct any barriers to providing safe and effective nursing care.

3. Discuss physical and psychosocial aspects of substance abuse including social roles that promote and maintain substance abuse behaviors.

4. Describe phases in the development of patterns of abuse and the treatment methods available.

5. Use the nursing process to plan effective care at all levels of prevention for individuals, families, and community groups.

☐ *Substance Abuse*

The use of various substances to alter mood and perception is not a recent phenomenon. Ancient cultures discovered the process of fermentation to produce alcoholic beverages as depicted in biblical references to wine and the use of mead described in *Beowulf*. Freud experienced and described the pleasures and problems associated with cocaine use in Victorian times. Poets such as Coleridge and Poe struggled with the problem of opiate dependence. Straitlaced Victorian ladies indulged in tonics that were primarily alcohol. The original popularity of cola drinks was due in large part to the ingredient cocaine (subsequently caffeine was substituted). Many individuals may consider themselves untouched by substance abuse while in actuality being at least psychologically dependent upon the stimulant effects of beverages such as coffee, tea, and colas, or cigarette smoking.

Social attitudes toward substance use and abuse are highly ambivalent. Drunkenness is abhorred because of the destruction of family life and highway carnage that frequently ensues but is condoned as a "rite of passage" to adulthood and a form of celebration for holidays and other significant events. Public awareness of the hazardous effects of smoking is widespread, but tobacco use continues relatively unabated. Drug use, previously viewed as a problem of lower-class minorities, has become widespread and is frequently defended as being less problematic than alcohol or tobacco use. Myths and rationalizations abound for all forms of substance use.

A PUBLIC HEALTH PROBLEM

Various studies have attempted to estimate the prevalence of substance abuse. The difficulty of the task is increased by the illegal nature of most of the categories of substances used, the difficulty inherent in attempting to differentiate between use and abuse, and the tendency of users to use more than one kind of substance.

Investigations of substance use in high school students over the 1970s suggest that the majority of students have tried alcohol, 15 percent have tried cocaine, and 10 percent may use marijuana on a daily basis.

It is estimated that 8 million adult Americans have used cocaine at sometime. This drug has achieved widespread acceptance as a recreational chemical and status symbol of sorts in the middle and upper socioeconomic classes. The use of marijuana, prescription drugs, and alcohol is very common. Six hundred thousand Americans (about one in every 400 people) are believed to be heroin dependent and it is estimated that approximately 5 million are alcoholic. This represents a large financial cost in terms of personal income expenditure and becomes truly staggering in the context of the larger related costs (such as losses in productivity, health care costs, accidental death and injury, and necessary social programs). For instance, Berry and associates (1977, 75) attribute 20 percent of general hospital use to alcohol-related problems (e.g., injuries or diseases such as cirrhosis, gastritis, pancreatitis). Califano (1982) places overall economic costs of alcoholism including health care and lost productivity at $60 billion.

Aside from financial aspects, the social and emotional costs to the families of alcoholics and drug abusers are highly significant. Substance use disorders clearly are a major public health problem today. Health care professionals, families, educators, and employers all share a great need to be better informed in coping with this growing problem.

MYTHS AND ATTITUDES

Attitudes of health professionals, like those of the public in general, are formed through cultural learning and personal experiences. These attitudes may be moralistic, negative, punitive, ambivalent; and based on no real consensus of what constitutes responsible substance use (as opposed to abuse). Stereotypes, stigma, and lack of understanding inhibit the nurse's ability to recognize the problem in those who do not fit the stereotype and also create problems in relating to those who are identified as having a substance use problem. These beliefs and values are brought into the health care system and, if unchallenged, can be detrimental to client care. Some common myths and the factual information that refutes them follow.

Myth: Alcoholics are skid row bums.
Fact: Ninety-five percent of alcoholics do not fit this stereotype. They are lawyers, carpenters, health care professionals, housewives, and so on; and they come from all socioeconomic classes.
Myth: Information alone on the dangers of drug abuse will decrease the problem.

Fact: Physicians, pharmacists, and nurses—who are most knowledgeable about the dangers of drug abuse—have also traditionally been among the occupational groups with the highest rates of abuse. Accurate information is vital but not sufficient to deal with alcohol and drug abuse.

Myth: Substance abusers are weak and self-indulgent people who could stop if they really want to.

Fact: Although initial use is subject to voluntary control, once the individual is psychologically or physiologically dependent, "will power" is generally not sufficient to control or stop substance abuse.

Myth: Abusers must "hit bottom" before they are motivated to change.

Fact: Early treatment is as beneficial in substance use disorders as in any other physical or behavioral disorder.

Nurses' and doctors' attitudes can inhibit recognition and early treatment through avoiding the issue of substance misuse. This "conspiracy of silence" enhances denial of the problem and delays needed care. Moralistic and punitive attitudes frequently occur, and the substance abuser is seen as the cause of his or her problem thus meriting less time, attention, and concern than other clients. This barrier deprives the client of the quality and kind of care needed. Nurses have a professional responsibility to examine and recognize negative beliefs and values in the context of the influences that formed them and to strive for more positive attitudes in providing care.

ROLE OF THE NURSE

The nurse can serve as an agent of primary prevention throughout the health care system and community by providing accurate information pertinent to substance use and abuse and also by promoting healthy communication and family dynamics. The nurse as case finder in secondary prevention can assist parents, educators, and other health professionals to recognize and confront, in an effective way, the signs of substance abuse in both hospitalized patients and the larger community. The nurse's role in tertiary prevention (rehabilitation) may be short term in detoxification settings or long range in the community as the family and client cope with the struggle to maintain sobriety and repair the disrupted family roles and dynamics.

☐ Theoretical Concepts

The categories of substances commonly abused include tobacco, alcohol, marijuana, hallucinogens, PCP, stimulants, sedatives, narcotics, and inhalants. These substances share the property of altering mood or perception and the potential for creating psychological and, in some cases, physiological dependency.

TERMINOLOGY

Not everyone who uses these substances loses control over their use and becomes dependent. The majority of people, for instance, are able to drink socially in moderation. Acceptable use is voluntary and recreational in nature. Pathological use or *abuse* of substances is characterized by excessive use, a tendency to use during the day or on an almost daily basis, an inability to cut down or stop use, and impairment of social or occupational functions. *Dependence* includes a pattern of abuse and the development of *tolerance* (an increased amount of the substance is required to bring about the customary effects) or *withdrawal* (physical symptoms occur when use of the substance is stopped or markedly decreased).

The National Commission on Marijuana and Drug Use (1973) described *five patterns of substance use*. The first, *experimental*, is merely trying a particular substance out of curiosity or peer pressure. The second, *recreational*, is characterized by voluntary and social use. These two levels of use do not constitute abuse although, for many of these substances, possession and use are illegal. The third, or *circumstantial*, pattern of use merits concern because it involves use of a particular substance to cope with life problems such as loneliness, tension, or loss. The "chemical crutch" provides temporary solace but a potential danger if its use becomes a pattern and a substitute for problem solving. *Intensified use*, the fourth pattern, is heavy and frequent use which causes personal problems and is characterized as abuse. The fifth pattern, *compulsive use*, incorporates both the high frequency and high intensity abusive pattern, with dependence on the substance. Jellinek (1952) has described a similar pattern depicting the development of alcoholism as progressing from (1) a prealcoholic phase in which use is circumstantial (coping with problems); (2) a prodromal phase of intensified use in which blackouts occur (episodes of amnesia without loss of consciousness when drinking); (3) the compulsive or crucial phase in which loss of control over drinking and social withdrawal is experienced; and (4) the chronic phase characterized by physical and mental deterioration due to alcoholism.

PREDISPOSITION AND DYNAMICS

Studies attempting to define specific traits of the dependency-prone personality have not produced conclusive findings. It is generally believed that individuals who develop substance use disorders have low self-esteem and decreased ability to tolerate and cope with frustration and anxiety. This suggests a heightened vulnerability for individuals in both situational and developmental crises. It has also become evident that a person who has become dependent upon one substance is increasingly more likely to become dependent upon another. For this reason, alcoholics in remission (no longer drinking) are cautioned against use of tranquilizers or analgesics except under highly controlled medical situations.

Learning theory suggests that substance use provides positive reinforcement (reward) for use through the chemical mood-altering effects and negative reinforcement (also rewarding) through diverting attention and emotion away from life problems. Reinforcement then produces a conditioned response or habit formation. This theory suggests that the conditioned response can be unlearned, and many behavioral treatment approaches such as aversion therapy are based on this model.

Steiner (1971) in working with alcoholics applied concepts of *Transactional Analysis*. He saw alcoholism as a result of a tragic "life script" based in self-destructive decisions made in childhood. He believed that alcoholics, by disposing of this destructive script, could be cured and resume social drinking patterns. This belief is very controversial and not well validated by research. Long-term alcohol abusers particularly do not appear able to sustain a social drinking pattern without progressing to abusive levels.

The *disease model* of substance abuse is advocated by Alcoholics Anonymous and its related substance abuse treatment groups. In this view, substance abuse is described as a chronic and generally progressive disorder characterized by dependence on a particular substance and resulting in physical, mental, social, or economic disabilities. The cause of the disease is viewed as an underlying physical or psychological disorder which is demonstrated by the person's dependence upon

and inability to control the use of a particular substance. The cure is viewed as abstinence which is achieved through application of specific principles of living and group support. This model is a currently accepted view in America and is often credited as being the most successful approach to the problem now in use.

Research into predisposing factors has focused on both physiological and social factors. Findings have been of interest but do not indicate any single cause. Heredity has been studied with inconclusive results, though relatives of both clinically depressed and alcoholic patients tend to demonstrate higher rates of alcoholism and depression than the general population. Metabolic and endocrine theories are currently being investigated regarding possible genetic differences in ability to metabolize alcohol, endocrine imbalances, and the role of endorphins in mood and pain tolerance.

Cultural rates of substance abuse vary widely. High rates of alcoholism exist among the French, Irish, Swedish, and Polish. Chinese and Jewish orthodox populations experience low rates. Whether these differences are physically based or a result of ethnic religious and social values is not clear. Both the children of alcoholics and those of moralistic believers in total abstinence are at higher risk for alcoholism. The American Indian and the Australian Aborigine experienced dramatic rates of alcoholism with the loss of traditional cultural values and migration to urban living. Narcotic abuse was originally considered a problem limited to the socioeconomically disadvantaged. Some studies suggest that cultural attitudes that stress patterned social or religious use of substances while applying sanctions against intoxication or abuse offer social guidelines for substance use which decrease the likelihood of misuse. Americans vary widely in their attitudes and tolerance toward alcohol and drug use. American values which emphasize technology and scientific solutions do, however, contribute to the emphasis in the media on chemical solutions to human problems, both physical and psychological.

In general, current theories are incomplete and inadequate in describing causation. Most likely, individuals are predisposed to substance abuse through several physical, psychological, and social or situational factors acting together in the case of any one individual.

In the development of substance abuse patterns, the individual tends to associate with others who share similar attitudes and behaviors and also becomes involved with them in activities revolving around obtaining and using the substance. Peer pressure and life-style thus may serve to initiate and maintain the substance abuse pattern (Hofmann, 1983). Once a substance abuse pattern is established, the individual's time may be preoccupied in large part with obtaining and using alcohol or drugs.

□ *Nursing Process*

ASSESSMENT □

Individual □ A general assessment of substance use should be incorporated into any nursing history. This assessment includes the client's own report and also nursing observations of client behaviors, physical condition, family concerns, and other data that may relate to substance use. The interview should be formulated matter of factly without judgmental bias, and the questions should be ordered to progress from commonly used substances (cigarettes, coffee, tea, or cola) through alcohol, use of prescription and over-the-counter drugs, to use of other stimulant or relaxant drugs. The frequency, amount, and duration of use should be recorded for each substance the client indicates used, for example:

> Reports smoking since age 18, one pack of a non filtered regular brand per day for the past 20 years
>
> Drinks one or two cups of coffee and one bottle of diet cola per day
>
> Rare use of alcohol until 5 years ago, since then reports 3 to 6 beers per week with meals and an occasional mixed drink on weekends (approximately 1 to 2 per month)
>
> Reported using an over-the-counter diet aid product (state brand name) 2 months ago for 1 week but stopped because of "feeling shaky and weak;" uses aspirin or Tylenol™ approximately once or twice per month for headache or muscle soreness
>
> Denies past or current use of prescription drugs
>
> States "has tried marijuana" on two occasions in the past year but uses no other substances

If the individual indicates heavy or intensified use of alcohol or other substances, additional exploration should follow as to perceived factors related to use such as personal or occupational stress. Individuals who report a prior (but not current) problem with substance misuse should be encouraged to discuss the ways in which they coped with the problem and whether they have any further needs for support. Open-ended questions exploring the extent and impact of the problem and how it was resolved can lead into a focus on current problems and needs.

Heavy or long-term use of any substance indicates a need for careful assessment to check for tolerance, dependence, and related physical or psychosocial problems associated with use. Appropriate questions might be:

1. "Have you noticed it takes more of _____ to bring about the same effect?" or "Have you had to increase the dosage to get the same relief?" (tolerance)
2. "Have you tried to go without using _____ for any period of time?" "Were you successful?" "Did you experience any unusual physical symptoms?" (dependence)
3. "Has your use of _____ caused any problems for you with your family or at work?"

Assessment of objective data related to use of the specific substance is vital (see Table 28-1) since persons often deny or minimize use. The person with a substance use disorder may not be open about substance use in the general interview. The observant nurse gathers a variety of data from different sources in the assessment phase, recognizing the strong need of the substance abuser to deny, to minimize, and to rationalize the use of a substance over which voluntary control has been lost. This defense should be recognized as an attempt to preserve self-esteem and to avoid external pressure to stop using a substance which has come to be perceived as a real need by the client.

■ *Point of Emphasis*

Substance use assessment involves the subjective perception and recall by the client and family plus observation for physical and behavioral indicators.

Family and Environment Assessment □ Substance abuse disorders cause changes in family relationships, friendships, and life-style. These changes may provide cues to the presence of a substance use disorder as well as identifying stressors

TABLE 28-1 Information Related to Specific Types of Substance Use Disorders

Substance	Physical Findings	Behavior Cues
Alcohol Blood level of 0.1 percent: legally intoxicated Route: oral Metabolized and excreted in 12 hours	*Immediate intoxication* CNS depression: decreased cognition and inhibitions, relaxation, impaired neuromuscular coordination, shortened REM sleep with restlessness and early wakening	Poor judgment may result in financial losses, fights, accidents, child neglect, domestic violence
	Sequellae Tremors, fatigue and irritability, hangover (headache and GI upset)	Tardiness and absenteeism at work, decreased productivity
	Long-term abuse Nutritional deficiencies, especially B complex, gastrointestinal irritation (gastritis, diarrhea, GI bleeding) sexual dysfunctions, cirrhosis and pancreatitis, neuropathy and brain syndromes (Wernicke's, Korsakoff's), fetal alcohol syndrome (growth and mental retardation with cardiac, joint or cranial, and facial deformities in neonates born to mothers with heavy alcohol intake during pregnancy)	Tolerance manifested by high intake without visible comparable signs of intoxification
	Dependency Withdrawal tremors	Shakiness prior to resuming drinking
	Withdrawal-delirium tremens	Fever, diaphoresis, increased vital signs, tremors, disorientation and visual hallucinations following decrease or stopping intake of alcohol
Marijuana and hashish (Pot, grass, maryjane, weed, hash) Route: smoking Active ingredient: THC Excretion: may accumulate in fatty tissues for up to 1 month	*Immediate intoxication ("high")* Euphoria, relaxation, dry mouth, reddened eyes, increased heart rate, decreased coordination and reaction time	Poor judgment and coordination results in hazardous driving even after "high" subsides Occasional flashbacks (especially with young users) resulting in fear of "losing mind"
	Excessive doses Image distortion and anxiety, nausea, tremors and possible hallucinations	
	Sequellae Impairment in short-term memory, slowing of speech and thought patterns, lung irritation greater than with cigarette smoking of comparable frequency and amount	Impedes learning and retention
	Long-term abuse Males—lowered testosterone levels with gynecomastia and lowered sperm count Females—menstrual irregularities which may persist several months after stopping use	Tolerance results in heavy use, personality changes (loss of motivation and ambition, moodiness and irritability, apathy and academic impairment, neglect of appearance), impedes developmental task attainment

TABLE 28-1 (continued)

Substance	Physical Findings	Behavior Cues
Hallucinogens LSD (acid) Mescaline, peyote ("mushrooms") Scopolamine and atropine Route: oral Duration: 2–24 hours	*Immediate ("tripping")* Intense and distorted perceptions, impaired judgment and suggestibility, visual hallucinations, altered libido, synthesia (perceiving a sense stimulus in different modes), "bad trip" characterized by frightening perceptions *Sequellae* "Flashbacks" may occur—recurrence of perceptual phenomena without repeated drug use (may be precipitated by stress or antihistamine use)	Withdrawal and self-absorption Fear or paranoia Panicky and impulsive behavior, fear of "going crazy"
Phencyclidine PCP ("angel dust" or "hog")—an animal tranquilizer Route: smoking, oral, snorting, or injection	*Immediate* *Low dose*—euphoria and numbness *Higher dose*—excitement, confusion, visual disturbances and distorted body perceptions, delirium and panic *Sequellae* Possible schizophrenia-like or paranoia-like psychosis of days to weeks in duration	Accidents, ataxia, loss of concentration and memory, bizarre and violent behavior, loss of pain sensation, depression and withdrawal, or excited, incoherent and aggressive acts
Stimulants Cocaine ("snow," "crack," "coke") Route: nasal inhalation, smoking or IV Amphetamines ("speed") Route: oral or IV Duration: 1–14 hours	*Immediate ("speeding" or "high")* Increased alertness, increased activity, increased heart rate, decreased appetite, dilated pupils Injection or high dose produces a "rush" of euphoria *Sequellae* Damage to nasal mucosa from "snorting" coke *Long-term use* Heavy and intensified use due to tolerance, insomnia, malnutrition, and weight loss, hypertension and cardiac irregularities possible Acute paranoid psychotic state may occur with delusions and hallucinations Psychological dependence with no physical withdrawal syndrome other than exhaustion and depression	Hyperactivity, irritability Fatigue and depression as increased energy is derived from use of stored neurohormones (norepinephrine) Neglect of nutrition and appearance, paranoid and impulsive, assaultive behavior May feel unable to face a day without "uppers" Often need sedatives to sleep leading to polydrug abuse
Sedatives Barbiturates ("reds," "yellows," "christmas trees") Antianxiety tranquilizers such as Librium, Valium, Equinal Hypnotics such as chloral hydrate, Doriden, Dalmane	*Immediate* CNS depression with decreased cortical function, impaired coordination, decreased pulmonary function Additive effects of alcohol may lead to coma	Appearance similar to alcohol intoxication

(continued)

TABLE 28-1 (continued)

Substance	Physical Findings	Behavior Cues
Duration: 3–8 hours Excretion: slow due to accumulation—seizures may not occur in withdrawal for up to 1 week		
	Sequellae Fatigue, irritability similar to hangover *Long-term abuse* Intensification of use due to tolerance	Poor judgment and memory, incoordination, accidents, neglect of activities of daily living
	Dependency Withdrawal syndrome: muscle spasm, seizures, status epilepticus possible	Acute confusion state
Narcotics Opiates and synthetics such as morphine, codeine, heroin (H or "horse") Synthetics such as Demerol, Talwin, Percodan Route: oral, IM, IV Duration: 4–12 hours	*Immediate* Lethargy and euphoria, CNS depression with pupillary constriction, depressed respiration, needle marks evident with IV use	Social withdrawal, episodes of stupor May inject in areas normally covered by clothing or wear covering clothing even in hot weather
	Overdose Fixed pupillary constriction, respirations below 6 per minute	Coma
	Abuse Prone to hepatitis, AIDS (acquired immune deficiency syndrome), local abcess and subacute bacterial endocarditis secondary to poor injection technique and sharing of needles, physical debilitation and malnutrition	Uninterested in hygiene and appearance, preoccupied with obtaining and using drugs, cost may require prostitution, theft, and "dealing" to support habit
	Dependency Withdrawal syndrome occurs approximately 6–12 hours after latest dose with GI upset, restlessness, chills, insomnia, and upper respiratory symptoms (nasal mucus excess and sneezing) Neonatal narcotic withdrawal: hyperactivity, tremors, frantic sucking, regurgitation and poor weight gain 24–28 hours or more after delivery in infants of narcotic-dependent mothers	Craving results in desperate drug-seeking behaviors
Inhalants Aromatics, glues, spray can propellants, spray paint, paint thinner, hair spray (most commonly used by children and adolescents because of easy accessibility)	*Immediate* Feelings of euphoria and vertigo, incoordination and confusion	Poor judgment, accidents, drunken gait and behavior, impulsive behavior
	Risks Cardiopulmonary arrest, brain damage, liver damage, bone marrow depression, weight loss	Memory impairment

and problems that result for the client and the family.

The effects of alcoholism have been identified and categorized according to the stages families experience in adjusting to the problem. These stages also apply to other forms of substance abuse. Initially the family shares in the denial, minimization, and rationalization of the problem. In an attempt to protect the substance abuser and themselves from shame and humiliation, the family ignores the problem or attempts to place blame for the episodes on others, on circumstances, or on themselves. They may make excuses for behavior problems and attempt to conceal the real reasons for absenteeism from school or work. Promises are elicited from the substance abuser that further episodes will not occur. When these promises are broken, the family members feel angry, hurt, and unloved. Guilt and defensiveness (as well as the irritability common to many substance abusers) lead to belligerence and hostile outbursts. Communication deteriorates in the family and is often replaced with avoidance, nagging, and angry confrontations. Family members may attempt to exert control over substance use activity by threats, punishment, or attempts to control the environment. This may include locking up or throwing out liquor, cutting off access to peers who are seen as contributing to the problem, and assuming the role of watchdog over the abuser's activities. These efforts generally meet with frustration and failure. They also serve to focus major energy and activities of family members on attempts to control the abuser's activities, thus limiting the normal task role activities and social functions of the family.

Because of the stigma attached to substance abuse, family members decrease outside social contacts. Children are reluctant to bring friends home from school, and spouses may limit social activities to avoid shame and limit outsiders' knowledge of the extent of the problem. Friends may also withdraw out of frustration with the substance abuser's behavior, judgmental attitudes, or inability to cope with the problems evidenced in the family. Guilt and blame placing are shared and exchanged by the substance abuser and the family. They may alternately play the roles of persecutor, victim, and rescuer or enabler. Attempts by the substance abuser to manipulate the family may include blame placing ("If you wouldn't nag all the time, I wouldn't drink as much"), dependency (need for money and assistance in avoiding consequences of behavior), and frequent promises.

When family members or friends are manipulated into rescue or enabling types of behavior, they assist the substance abuser in maintaining the problem. If they do not permit themselves to be manipulated, they may feel guilty and uncaring.

■ Point of Emphasis

Substance abuse affects all members of the family and has been called a family disease.

Family roles and tasks are often reallocated as the substance abuser becomes unreliable and more isolated. The spouse of the abuser may assume all parental responsibility and often the role of breadwinner too. Children may respond by assuming parental roles and responsibilities in the family (often called the "super coper" or hero), running away, or by "acting out" at home and in school as a result of the emotional drain and inconsistent discipline often found in the home. The substance abuser often assumes a childlike role in the family. Scapegoating may occur. All family members share feelings of low self-esteem, frustration, anxiety about future events, shame, and guilt. Additional problems related to substance abuse in the family that may occur are neglect, abuse, and violence.

Changes in peer relationships and life-style are due to the increasing absorption of the substance abuser in substance-related activity. Former friends who do not participate in or approve of the substance abuse are avoided or dropped. Substance abuse activity fills in time formerly devoted to thought, communication, socialization, and leisure activities. Substance use masks awareness of feelings and problems and impedes personal growth, interpersonal relatedness, and realistic problem solving. Adolescents are impeded in developmental task attainments such as (1) the cognitive shift from concrete to formal (abstract) thought processes, (2) developing age-appropriate behaviors related to formation of a positive, stable identity, and (3) later aspects of interdependency and intimacy in young adulthood. Some peer groups of substance abusers form a subculture of sorts with a distinctive language, dress, and way of structuring time and activities which reinforces the group's sense of identity and belonging. This also serves to defend the individual from the disapproval and censure of outsiders.

Self-Assessment □ In order to provide effective care, the nurse must recognize attitudes and beliefs that impede identification of and intervention for substance abuse problems. This process includes:

> Awareness of own attitudes and values regarding substance use (See discussion questions in the Enrichment Activities at the end of this chapter.)
>
> Identification of influences in the formation of negative attitudes (Take time to identify the experiences on which stereotypic or emotional attitudes are based.)
>
> Recognition of "blind spots" based on one's own use of particular substances which makes it difficult to identify problem use in others (For instance, the nurse who regularly uses drinking to cope with anxiety and depression will fail to pick up cues to possible abuse when clients refer to "drinking to forget.")
>
> Examination of communication patterns with clients who have substance use disorders (Check for judgmental, moralistic, or "parental" comments.)
>
> Noting any tendency to avoid or minimize contact.
>
> Identifying any tendency to assume pathological roles such as: persecuting (judgmental, punitive approaches), playing the victim (permitting oneself to be blamed, used or manipulated, rescuing or enabling (seeing oneself as a "savior" or "mother" who assumes responsibility for managing behavior and its consequences for another).

Once self-awareness has brought about a realistic assessment of strengths and areas for further development, the professional responsibility for action includes (1) recognizing one's limitations and seeking appropriate assistance in caring for clients and families, and (2) striving to develop more helpful attitudes and behaviors in providing care.

Recognizing limitations involves acknowledging that prior learning and experiences may inhibit effectiveness in this area. It also requires that one seek help from others (nurses, instructors, supervisors) to assure safe and effective care. This may include having others provide care or asking someone else to serve as a consultant regarding the quality, objectivity, and effectiveness of the care provided.

Healthy attitudes to be developed include the following:

> Substance use disorders are complex and poorly understood diseases that bring about suffering in both the abuser and the family.
>
> The client with a substance use disorder is a person of worth who merits the same respect, acceptance, skill, and concern as any other client.
>
> It is possible to accept and respect a person without approving or assisting that person in self-destructive behavior.
>
> Substance abuse is preventable and treatable, and it benefits from early recognition and intervention.

Health care workers have a professional responsibility to work openly, objectively, and without prejudice to assist clients and families to confront, explore, and cope with substance use disorders. If the nurse has honestly and skillfully carried out this responsibility, the success or failure of the client outcome should not become an issue of personal involvement (feelings of failure or blaming the client).

Expectation of 100 percent success on the initial attempt is not always realistic. Relapses should be accepted, and encouragement offered to help the client continue efforts toward recovery and recognition of the progress made to date.

In addition to nurse-client relationships, the nurse needs to be aware of potential substance abuse problems in relationships with other health professionals. Currently physicians and nurses are becoming much more aware of professionally impaired co-workers with alcohol or drug problems. The same attitudes and behaviors that impair effectiveness in recognition and referral for clients frequently exist in relationship to these co-workers. Their problems may be denied and minimized; other workers may serve as enablers by "covering up" the problem and failing to confront the abuser or report the problem to supervisors.

PROBLEM AND NEED IDENTIFICATION □ Priorities will be based on the individual's physical and psychological status. In the acute care setting, physical needs are often most vital initially. These may be based on the need for (1) treatment of complications of substance abuse, (2) detoxification, and (3) withdrawal. (See Table 28-1.) Safety needs are also essential for the intoxicated client and those who are disoriented or hallucinating due to substance abuse or withdrawal. Recognition of the underlying issue of low self-esteem and the related feelings of worthlessness and guilt is basic to understanding the person's denial and defensiveness if the nurse is to work at building a trusting relationship. Only when physical and safety needs are met and trust is established is it possible to explore and confront the substance use disorder effectively. The clients' awareness of the physical consequences of substance use may actually make them more open to intervention at this point. Referral and initial contact with the substance treatment agency is best accomplished prior to dismissal.

Family needs and problems may be met either in the community setting or while the client is hospitalized (even if the client is not willing to acknowledge the problem and seek help). The concerned nurse will establish a relationship with significant family members to identify their problems in a climate of acceptance and caring. Needs for information and understanding of the problem can be met in any setting as can the exploration of need for referral to various community agencies.

The community nurse needs to be particularly aware of the need for family support following a successful treatment program. Many people feel that once the substance abuse has stopped, there will be no further problems or needs. This is unrealistic. Substance abuse is a long-standing problem with profound and lasting effects. The substance abuser in remission must alter a life-style and reestablish roles and relationships in the family and society. The family itself must learn new patterns of communicating and relating. The roles previously relinquished by the patient must be reestablished with the recognition and support of the family. The nurse can assist and support this long process and assess whether additional intervention and referral, such as marital or child counseling, is needed.

Particular problems associated with substance use disorders may arise as a result of life-style or circumstances related to use of illegal drugs. Variations in quality and strength of street drugs occur in the distribution process. Powdered substances such as heroin or cocaine are purchased and then are "cut" by the addition of similar appearing substances such as sugar or talc. This process may take place several times before the drug reaches the streets; the outcome may be variations in drug strength, as well as the pres-

ence of various contaminants which may include cheaper drugs such as LSD or nonpsychoactive substances. The user may inadvertently overdose by injecting a customary dose of "purer" substance, or may experience unusual side effects because of the contaminating substances. Sales of "look alike" products (which are over-the-counter substances marketed in forms resembling brand name amphetamines or sedatives) may also give rise to medical emergencies if, for example, an individual accustomed to injesting several caffeine-based "look alike" stimulants acquires and takes the same number of amphetamines.

Physical complications may also result from life-style aspects of drug use. Sharing of injection equipment and nonsterile technique may cause local abscess, systemic infection, and transmission of hepatitis and AIDS (autoimmune deficiency syndrome). Prostitution in order to maintain an expensive habit carries the high risk of sexually transmitted disease. General neglect of health is common in those dependent upon substance use since the drug-related activities become a priority and consume the time, energy, and resources required for health needs. Withdrawal symptoms, particularly following abrupt discontinuance of barbiturates or minor tranquilizers, may constitute a medical emergency (status epilepticus).

A particular problem of early adolescent drug abuse is the interference with attainment of developmental tasks. Cognitive development, physical health, social interactions, and identity formation are negatively affected by drug abuse and the associated life-style.

INTERVENTION □ Nursing intervention is appropriate at all levels of prevention for clients, families, and the community. The effectiveness of these interventions is dependent upon the willingness of the nurse to develop the attitudes, knowledge, skills, and interpersonal relationships required.

Primary Prevention □ The nurse as health educator has a dual focus in preventing substance use disorders: (1) providing accurate information about and promoting healthy attitudes toward substance use, and (2) assisting individuals and families to improve their ability to communicate and cope with the stress of living. These tasks are most often accomplished in the community as the nurse interacts with families and concerned groups of parents, educators, employers, and others. Theoretical principles and approaches are derived from a knowledge of developmental needs, techniques to facilitate open communication and acceptance of feelings, and crisis intervention (see relevant chapters). The nurse's knowledge of the actions, effects, and potential problems associated with use of varied substances is also a valuable source of information. (See Table 28.1.) A wealth of educational media is widely available including brief films that foster group discussion. These materials are targeted for a variety of age groups, cultures, and levels of knowledge ranging from school-age children through health care professionals. (A partial list of resource agencies will be found at the end of this chapter.) Before these materials are ordered, several types appropriate to the planned audience should be obtained and previewed so that the most effective presentation for that particular group may be selected. A comprehensive approach emphasizes the following pertinent aspects: accurate information; recognition and clarification of values and concepts of responsible substance use (age appropriate); discussion of peer and societal pressures on individuals; and ways of coping with stress through recognition of feelings, open communication, and seeking support.

The media play an important role in shaping attitudes and informing the public. The nurse can serve as an advocate through recognizing and supporting programming that enhances accurate community information and awareness or by protesting media presentations that are inaccurate or glamorize substance abuse. Legislation strongly affects the resources available for substance abuse education and treatment. Community nurses need to involve themselves in this process both as health educators and as client advocates.

Secondary Prevention □ The nurse as case finder and referral source can be a valuable agent of secondary prevention in hospital and community settings. In the hospital setting, awareness of the prevalence of alcohol and drug abuse should make the nurse alert to physical findings and cues suggesting the need for sensitive exploration with the client and family to determine whether a problem exists. The nurse in the community assists families, teachers, employers, and other concerned groups to become more alert to the signs of substance misuse. Parents and teachers can be helped to recognize drug-related paraphernalia; signs of use; and behavioral changes such as ap-

athy, irritability, social withdrawal, changing friends, and truancy and poor grades. Remember, however, that adolescence is a time when a certain degree of behavior change is normally expected as the teenager experiences a need for privacy and autonomy and responds to the physical and emotional changes of development. Physical and behavioral cues suggesting substance use should be viewed as signals indicating a need for open communication and exploration.

Women were formerly underrepresented in substance abuse statistics. The traditional housewife role permitted regular drinking or excessive use of pain killers and tranquilizers to be hidden from public scrutiny. Families concealed, denied, and rationalized the problem. Public attitudes toward drinking by women and drunkenness in women (less opportunity to drink) in the past may have served to inhibit both the development of alcoholism and the acknowledgment of alcoholism (hiding the problem) in women.

Current deemphasis on the "double standard," with greater freedom of life-style for women, and the increasing awareness of substance abuse in women that was brought about through public education and the efforts of former first lady Betty Ford, have served to narrow the statistical gap. Nurses need to be aware of the potential problem in both the housewife and the career woman.

Families of substance abusers are encouraged to seek help for themselves in understanding and coping with the problem whether or not the substance abuser chooses to seek treatment. The nurse should be knowledgeable about local sources for treatment and family support.

Many businesses have recognized substance abuse as an employee health problem and are taking steps to combat it more effectively. With the help of local mental health agencies, they have developed strategies for identifying and confronting affected employees, and providing treatment for them. Rather than avoiding the situation, the employer deals with it directly, and the threat of job loss often motivates the employee to deal with the problem at an early stage. The retention of valuable employees avoids the costs of replacement and training, thus providing business incentives.

Because of denial and the perceived or real need (based in dependence) to continue substance use, it is uncommon for the alcoholic or drug abuser to seek treatment voluntarily. Pressure from employers, the legal system, or families is generally the motivating factor. Alcoholism treatment groups have developed strategies for effective confrontation for families seeking to encourage a family member to enter treatment. Betty Ford has publicly discussed this approach as motivating her to seek help for misuse of alcohol and prescription drugs. Families can be helped by the nurse to try this technique rather than angry threats and recriminations which, more often than not, create increased family stress while accomplishing little. In a caring confrontation, family members are helped to plan an organized, concerned approach to the person needing treatment. Sources of treatment will already have been explored and evaluated in terms of their effectiveness and appropriateness for the patient and problem through contacts with the nurse, referral agencies, and the family physician. Family members are assisted to formulate their concerns using effective communication techniques so that they are able to:

Matter of factly describe the problem behavior and its effects on them using objective, non-blaming "I" messages

Indicate their genuine caring and concern for the person needing treatment

Present a united front in urging immediate entry into treatment

Preparation, family agreement, and timing are essential for effectiveness. The person should be confronted at a time when he is alert and responsive, not under the influence of substance use. The arrangements for treatment should be complete so there is no lengthy time period in which denial and defenses are reorganized. It is possible to arrange consultation and perhaps a home visit by a member of the treatment agency to smooth the transition and assist the individual in decision making and entry into treatment. Types of treatment and referral sources are discussed in the next section.

Tertiary Prevention □ Tertiary prevention includes interventions that stress the active treatment and rehabilitation of substance use disorders involving three phases: detoxification, short-term therapy (most commonly thirty days), and long-term supportive follow-up. Depending on the individual and the substance used, some or all of these will be used.

Detoxification is the process of assuring that the individual is free of substance use and any

related complications or withdrawal symptoms. It may be accomplished in either a social agency by counselors trained to provide physical and emotional support, or in a hospital setting. Patients with medical conditions, those with alcoholic delirium tremens, or those dependent upon antianxiety agents or barbiturates (and thus likely to experience repeated seizures during withdrawal) should be hospitalized so they can benefit from medical supervision and support. Barbiturates and tranquilizers are never abruptly withdrawn. The general focus of care during detoxification is concerned with the following:

1. Physical assessment and support:
   a. Assuring adequate hydration, nutrition, and rest
   b. Monitoring client condition during intoxication or withdrawal by assessing vital signs and mental status
   c. Supportive care to minimize withdrawal symptoms (this may include administration of decreasing amounts of prescribed drugs in the hospital setting)
   d. Treatment of medical complications in the hospital setting
2. Maintaining safety:
   a. Constant supervision necessary for intoxicated, stuporous, confused, and agitated clients
   b. Restraints to be used only if other measures are inadequate and client behavior poses a danger to self or others
   c. Environmental management to minimize stimuli that promote confusion or hallucinations and to exclude hazardous objects if patient is impulsive, agitated, or prone to self-injury
3. Preventing access to further substance use
4. Emotional support:
   a. Nonjudgmental acceptance of the person and matter of fact, open communication about the effects of substance abuse
   b. Exploration of the ways substance abuse has affected the person's life and caused problems
   c. Encouragement to seek further treatment

The duration of detoxification may range from 24 hours to several weeks depending on the client's physical condition and the presence of withdrawal symptoms or medical complications. (See Table 28-2 for general nursing care measures.)

Therapy of substance use disorders may include outpatient treatment or partial hospitalization but most commonly is a 30-day residential program in a substance abuse program or mental health center. Family members are usually included in treatment, either in the program itself or in a separate program emphasizing education, support, and coping. Self-help groups for family members may be recommended to afford additional support or if the treatment agency does not include family programming. The focus of therapy is a comprehensive approach to the problems of substance abuse.

1. Education—the development and physical and personal effects of substance abuse are presented and discussed in terms of the individual and family.

2. Confrontation—the individual is given active, continuing feedback about involvement in the program, interpersonal relationships, and communication in a reality based "here and now" approach. Confrontation is active and frequent, to break through the defenses of denial and avoidance. Many counselors in these programs are former substance abusers, which makes the confrontation more direct (e.g., "Don't try to con me—I've been there."), while also conveying that the problem can be dealt with successfully.

3. Emphasis on rebuilding skills of communication and interpersonal relatedness—this is important because of the previous pattern of relying on alcohol or drugs to deal with feelings and problems. Relating and seeking support from others is actively promoted.

4. Group cohesiveness and support—group approaches are used to enhance opportunities for confrontation, universality, and support. Recognition, honest sharing, and group acceptance of feelings are encouraged. Methods such as the group members' sharing of perceptions of the person's strengths and weaknesses (sometimes called "hot seat" or "caring and sharing") or graduation ceremonies in which a symbol of the program, such as a medallion, is passed by the group (accompanied by their expressions of encouragement for the person who is completing treatment) enhance group support and cohesiveness.

Follow-up care and support is encouraged. Options include halfway houses where individuals may reside while working in the community. They still derive the benefits of resident counselors and group meetings as they gain strength and confidence in their ability to cope without substance use. Outpatient groups or counseling may be continued, or the individual in the community may be referred to self-help groups such as Alcoholics Anonymous. Alanon, a support group for spouses of alcoholics, and its related Alateen and Alatot groups for children provide family support.

Alcoholics Anonymous, an organization based on self-help principles, provides the model and approach for a majority of alcoholism and drug abuse treatment programs. The philosophy of recovery is stated in the serenity prayer and twelve steps.

The Serenity Prayer: "God grant me the serenity to accept the things I cannot change, the courage to change the things I can, and the wisdom to know the difference."

AA's Twelve Steps*:

1. We admit we were powerless over alcohol—our lives had become unmanageable. (One must acknowledge the problem and give up the defense of denial.)

2. Came to believe that a power greater than ourselves could restore us to sanity.

3. Made a decision to turn our will and lives over to the care of God *as we understood him.*

4. Made a searching and fearless moral inventory of ourselves.

5. Admitted to God, to ourselves, and to another human being the exact nature of our wrongs.

6. Were entirely ready to have God remove all these defects of character.

7. Humbly asked him to remove our shortcomings.

8. Listed all persons we had harmed and became willing to make amends.

9. Made direct amends whenever possible except when to do so would injure them or others.

---

* The Twelve steps of Alcoholics Anonymous reprinted by permission of A.A. World Services, Inc.

TABLE 28-2 Withdrawal Syndromes and Care

Syndrome and Substance	Symptoms	Medical Treatment	Nursing Intervention
Alcohol withdrawal (Delirium tremens) (24–48 hours after decreasing or stopping intake of alcohol), commonly lasts 1–3 days	Fever and diaphoresis, increased vital signs, tremors and motor restlessness, disorientation, visual illusions and hallucinations	Maintain hydration (IVs commonly used), vitamin therapy, sedation with Librium, Valium, or Thorazine as ordered	*Maintain safety* constant supervision to prevent impulsive behavior and self injury; restraints if necessary *Monitor vital signs and intake* vital signs every 2–4 hours promote frequent high caloric-high vitamin feedings and fluids and assist as needed; record intake and output *Reorientation* orient frequently, maintain calm, reassuring manner *Control environment* adequate lighting to reduce visual distortion, decrease stimuli (noise, activity)
Opiate withdrawal (12–16 hours after most recent injection of heroin or other opiate)	Tremors, diaphoresis, running eyes and nose, chills, muscle aches and cramps, abdominal pain and diarrhea	Maintain hydration (IV if ordered); may administer decreasing doses of CNS depressants as ordered or methadone (a synthetic narcotic) for gradual withdrawal; antidiarrhea medication may be ordered if prolonged and severe diarrhea present	*Supportive care* Keep warm, maintain hydration by offering frequent fluids that do not increase GI irritation and motility; maintain calm reassuring manner; provide nonstimulating environment; methadone administration if ordered generally given in liquid form in juice to control and decrease dosage; methadone is a controlled substance which is addictive; client may be maintained on methadone in a community program as a less destructive form of addiction subject to careful control
Sedative withdrawal (24 hours to 1 week[a] after stopping use of barbiturates, anxiety agents or soporifics)	Tremors, confusion, and perceptual distortion, muscle spasms, seizures with possible status epilepticus	Maintain hydration (IVs commonly used); gradual withdrawal by decreasing dose of substance used as ordered; Dilantin or other antiepileptic commonly used	*Maintain safety* constant supervision, seizure precautions *Monitor vital signs and intake* vital signs every 2–4 hours, encourage food and fluids, record intake and output *Reorientation* orient frequently, maintain calm, reassuring manner *Control environment* adequate lighting to reduce visual distortion, decrease stimuli

[a] Antianxiety agents are cumulative—causing delayed withdrawal symptoms.

10. Continued to make personal inventory and when we were wrong promptly admitted it.

11. Sought through prayer and meditation to improve our conscious contact with God, praying only for his will and the power to carry it out. (God is defined by the individual and for some may mean a power greater than the person or a philosophy.)

12. Having had a spiritual awakening as the result of these steps, we tried to carry this message to alcoholics, and to practice these principles in all our affairs.

Alanon, an AA support group for spouses, is based on the twelve steps and these additional principles:

Alcoholism is a disease of the mind and body and not a moral fault or perverse whim of the alcoholic.

"Loving detachment"—the spouse cannot control the actions of anyone but self. By modifying one's self, surrounding conditions also improve. Changes in the self may or may not change the alcoholic's behavior.

"Selfishness"—reestablish self-esteem and independence through own self-improvement.

Reliance on a "higher power" is based on acceptance and implementation of the Twelve Steps.

"Tough Love"—truly loving the alcoholic means *not* being an "enabler" who assists the alcoholic in excusing or avoiding the consequences of his or her behavior.

Group support occurs through candid sharing of reactions and experiences to common problems. This provides sharing of feelings and also a variety of coping strategies that may be used.

Spouse's sobriety does not mean an end to marital and life problems.

Alateen and Alatot are Alanon-based programs to provide support and understanding to children of alcoholics. The emphasis is on assuming responsibility for self and personal growth. Families Anonymous emphasizes support of the family as a unit. Drug abusers may be incorporated into traditional AA programs or treated in separate but similar programs.

EVALUATION □ Evaluation of client and family progress in substance use disorders is most readily discussed in terms of short- and long-term goals. Short-term goals for the client in the acute care hospital setting often focus on relief or control of physical symptoms secondary to debilitation, complications, or withdrawal. Equally important to this treatment phase are the psychosocial goals aimed at promoting client and family recognition of the problem and providing support for healthy adaptation. Criterion measures might include acknowledgment of the problem, realistic discussion of options for referral, and selection of and initial contact with a treatment agency and a family support agency.

Long-term goals broadly stated are (1) the client's ability to function effectively without substance abuse and (2) the family's ability to function productively to meet the physical and emotional needs of its members. This latter goal is not necessarily dependent upon the substance abuser's goal attainment. The criteria for attainment of these goals are less readily stated. For the client, some theorists would accept a return to responsible, voluntary substance use while others, in the majority, would argue that only abstinence from substance use is a realistic measure. This discussion is further complicated by the person's tendency to relapse into substance abuse. Is the alcoholic who is able to function effectively once more for long periods of time, but who occasionally lapses into an episode of drinking, a success or a failure? Probably, in this case, a more flexible criterion of sustained, improved functioning would be applicable. The important issue about relapses is how they affect the individual's future attempts to avoid substance use. As in dieting, the relapse episode itself is less important than the decision that follows: (1) to return to healthy behavior or (2) to give up, feeling helpless and hopeless. The attitudes of others can be significant in influencing this decision.

In the event that the substance abuser does not seek or profit from treatment, several criteria for improved family functioning are appropriate. First is the ability to place the substance abuse in perspective and to relinquish feelings of self-blame and attempts to control the abuser's behavior. This frees energy to focus on the needs and development of self and others in the family. The second is to overcome the feelings of shame and embarrassment in order to seek and utilize needed resources. This includes resuming social contact and activities in addition to the use of support groups and social agencies for needed assistance. If these goals are met, the family is rechanneling its energies into healthy pursuits and is less likely to fall into persecuting, victim, or enabling roles. This has a secondary effect of making substance abusers more responsible for their own behavior and its consequences (which may or may not influence them in seeking treatment). It is important to understand and convey to families that the end of substance abuse behavior does not mean the end of family and life problems. The community nurse needs to evaluate the family's ability to reestablish healthy communication, to reinvolve the former substance abuser in family decision making and problem solving, and to deal with any legacy of anger and anxiety that remains.

■ Enrichment Activities

DISCUSSION QUESTIONS

1. Engage in small group discussions designed to clarify individual members' attitudes toward substance use. Include such personal beliefs as:
   a. Are some substances acceptable for recreational use? If so, which ones?
   b. How would each individual differentiate between responsible use and abuse of various substances?
   c. Are there parallels, for instance, between overeating compulsively, the smoking habit, and substance disorders?
   d. Describe personal experiences in trying to break a long-standing habit (e.g., dieting, giving up smoking, or nail biting).

2. Describe some myths about alcoholism or drug use which you have believed. Attempt to identify the source and effects of these beliefs.

LEARNING ACTIVITIES

1. Role-play a substance use assessment and obtain feedback on the comprehensiveness, clarity, organization, and matter-of-factness of your approach.

2. Role-play use of communication techniques in a caring confrontation designed by family members to motivate a middle-aged alcoholic to seek treatment.

3. Role-play acceptance, caring, and confrontation in a medical client-nurse relationship

when the client tells you he drinks only socially although he has cirrhosis and you have just observed him drinking from a bottle of bourbon hidden in the bedside stand.

4. Contact your local chapter of AA or Alanon for permission to visit an open meeting.

SUPPLEMENTAL SOURCES OF EDUCATIONAL MATERIALS

Department of Health and Human Services
Alcohol, Drug Abuse and Mental Health Administration
5600 Fishers Lane
Rockville, MD 20858
(Publications on alcoholism and drug abuse.)

Alcoholics Anonymous	Al-Anon Family Group
P.O. Box 459	Headquarters
Grand Central Station	P.O. Box 182
New York, NY 10017	Madison Square Station
	New York, NY 10010

(Free or inexpensive materials on alcoholism for various age groups.)

State and local councils on alcoholism and local Alcoholics Anonymous chapters are excellent sources for print media and film loans such as:

"The Life, Death and Recovery of an Alcoholic," narrated by Dr. A. Pirsch, describing the development of alcoholism and the influence of community attitudes.

"If You Loved Me" depicting the family effects of alcoholism and Al-Anon as support group.

"Dial A-L-C-O-H-O-L" a series of four 30-minute films on responsible use of alcohol for teenagers.

■ References

Abernathy, M.W. "Alcohol related problems—A perspective." In *The community nurse and alcohol related problems—A book of readings*. Washington, D.C.: U.S. Government Printing Office, 1978:5–24.

Ackerman, R. *Children of alcoholics—A guidebook for educators, therapists and parents*. Holmes Beach, FL: Learning Publications, 1978.

Bennett, G.; Vourakis, C.; and Woolf, D. (eds.). *Substance abuse—Pharmacological, developmental and clinical perspectives*. New York: Wiley, 1983.

Berry, R.; Boland, J.; Samrt, C.; and Kanak, J. *The economic cost of alcohol abuse—1975*. Prepared for the National Institute on Alcohol Abuse and Alcoholism. Contract No. ADM 281-76-0016, August 1977.

Butnaresco, G.F.; Tillotson, D.M.; and Villarreal, P.D. *Perinatal nursing.* Vol. 2, Reproductive risk. New York: Wiley, 1980:409–444.

Califano, Joseph. *Drug abuse and alcoholism.* New York: Warner Books, 1982.

Let's talk about drug abuse. DHHS. Publication No. (ADM) 80-706, 1979. National Institute on Drug Abuse.

Drug abuse in america. Report of the National Commission on Marijuana and Drug Use. 1973.

Fornaciari, S. *How to talk to kids about drugs.* Washington, D.C.: Potomac Press, 1980.

Goodman, L.M. "Support for the family of the person with alcohol related problems." In *The community nurse and alcohol related problems—A book of readings.* Washington, D.C.: U.S. Government Printing Office, 1978:83–102.

Hofmann, F.G. *A handbook on drug and alcohol abuse.* 2d ed. New York: Oxford Press, 1983.

Jellinek, E.M. "Phases of alcohol addiction." *Quarterly journal of alcohol studies,* 13, (December 1952):673–684.

Johnston, Backman, and O'Malley. *Drug use among American high school students.* University of Michigan Institute for Social Research, 1975–1977.

Kendal, E.M. "Effect of attitudes on delivery of health care." In *The community nurse and alcohol related problems—A book of readings.* Washington, D.C.: U.S. Government Printing Office, 1978:25–47.

Loebl, S., and Spratto, G. *The nurse's drug handbook.* 3d ed. Wiley, 1983.

McCoy, S.; Rice, M.; and McFadden K. "PCP intoxication: Psychiatric issues of nursing care." *Journal of psychiatric nursing and mental health services,* 19, 7 (July 1981):17–23.

Sckuchard, Marsha. "Adolescent marijuana use: Growing problem for parents and physicians," *Atlanta medicine* (May 1979):15–18.

Steiner, C. *Games alcoholics play.* New York: Grove Press, 1971.

Van Gee, Susan. "Alcoholism and the family: A psychodrama approach." *Journal of psychiatric nursing and mental health services* (August 1979):9–12.

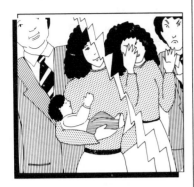

29

Interpersonal Violence

Patricia Mayer Ehrhart
Kathryn Murphy Schinker

Learning Objectives

Upon completion of this chapter, the reader will be able to:

1. Increase awareness and knowledge of the problem of violence in families.

2. Discuss internal and external factors involved in violent behavior.

3. Explore the generational cycle of family violence.

4. Utilize assessment factors in identifying physical and psychological signs of spouse abuse.

5. Discuss the myths that create obstacles to the therapeutic process in spouse abuse.

6. Discuss the need for immediate medical attention, emotional support, and legal assistance for the victim of sexual assault.

7. Understand the physical, emotional, and psychological trauma to a sexual assault victim and the long-term effects if not treated.

8. Recognize the physical, behavioral, and emotional signs of child abuse and neglect.

9. Describe the long-term effects of child abuse.

10. Understand elder abuse.

11. Evaluate personal attitudes toward working with clients who are victims of abuse or family members who are abusive.

12. Analyze data and formulate plans for referral and interventions at the primary, secondary, and tertiary levels.

Throughout recorded history, violence has been inflicted on individuals, groups, and nations, yet much of society has remained passive toward it. In recent decades two divergent forms of violence or potential for violence have raised the consciousness of people in industrialized societies—the potential for worldwide violence represented by nuclear arms and the personal violence among family members. This chapter deals with personal violence.

Statistics on family violence are gradually being gathered. As American society began to face the evidence of physical, sexual, and emotional violence perpetrated on infants and children by their caretakers, information began to emerge that women were being beaten and injured by their mates. Still more recently, investigations have been undertaken about sibling, adolescent, and elderly abuse. Both men and women are the victims of emotional and physical abuse. However, most men are larger, stronger, and more powerful than women, so women are more vulnerable to injury. Hence, the focus of this chapter is women, children, and the aged—those most likely to be abused.

☐ *Spouse Abuse*

BACKGROUND

Historical Perspectives

In times past, a woman had the same legal status as a child or a slave. She could not own or sell property. She was a legal minor, first "owned" by her father, who "gave" her away in marriage after which her legal existence was incorporated into that of the husband under whose legal protection she lived. A husband who beat his wife was usually protected by the courts. Ancient laws gave the husband the right to punish his wife with a whip or stick "no bigger than my thumb" in order to keep her in line (*Bradley* v. *State*, 1824). If no permanent injury was inflicted, it is better to "draw the curtain, shut out the public gaze, and leave the parties to forget and forgive" (*State* v. *Oliver*, 1874).

The marriage contract itself traditionally placed women in a disadvantaged position, and even today, no state in the U.S. provides for a woman to be paid for labor done in her own home. Through the marriage contract, she has a right to food, clothing, and a roof over her head. These rights were the same as those granted to slaves under the southern "Slave Code" (Washburne, 1975).

The subordination of women goes back at least as far as the early Judeo-Christian and classical cultures. Ruether (1979) explores the dualities of these religions and their effect on social conditioning over time.

All the basic dualities—the alienation of the mind from the body; the alienation of the subjective self from the objective world; the subjective retreat of the individual, alienated from the social community; the dominations or rejection of nature by spirit—these all have roots in the apocalyptic-platonic religious heritage of classical Christianity. But the alienation of the masculine from the feminine is the primary sexual symbolism that sums up all these alienations. The psychic traits of intellectuality, transcendent spirit, and autonomous will that were identified with the male, left the woman with the contrary traits of bodiliness, sensuality, and subjugation. Society, through the centuries, has, in every way, profoundly conditioned men and women to play out their lives and find their capacities within this basic antithesis (Ruether, 1979).

Family and Cultural Influences

Though by the 1940s women were becoming intellectually aware of their value, they still had to work through the "unconscious effects of training" and experiences that kept the attitudes of inferiority alive (Thompson, 1942). A conscious effort on the part of both men and women to free themselves from the belief that women are inferior is only now being exerted.

In one study, battered women were shown to have been more likely than a control group to have had poor relationships with their fathers, to have had fathers who were alcoholics, mentally ill, violent, and/or severe and controlling. They were also more likely to have observed violent behaviors in their husbands-to-be. These earlier experiences may have predisposed these women to expect and accept violence in marriage (Price and Armstong, 1978).

Results of another survey, involving 2000 couples, suggested that families often engage in power struggles. Superior strength and size as well as cultural conditioning give the advantage to men. The first beating a man gives his mate can set the balance of power in that relationship for life (Straus, 1978).

Goodstein and Page (1981) define a controlling husband as one who has a history of getting his own way; believes that persons other than himself are always to blame; has an interest in others only in relation to what they can do for him; and is lacking in emotional reciprocity. Violence occurs when he can no longer dominate, and feels out of control.

■ Point of Emphasis

The power of the male in the marriage relationship reflects social mores. "The state, the laws, the morality, religion, and the sciences are the creation of men" and are reinforced by women who socialize children (Horney, 1976).

Physical and Biological Influences on Aggression

Some ethologists have suggested that aggressive behavior is innate and simply an evolutionary extension of man's biological past. Bettelheim supports the belief that aggression is "basic to human nature." He believes that children should be taught about aggression in controlled situations so they so they will know how to handle aggressive feelings and thoughts (in Steinmetz and Straus, 1974). Certain genetic defects have been identified as possible determinants of violence. The XYY chromosome was thought at one time to predict violent behavior in males, but this idea has been fairly well dispelled (Sadoff, 1976). Abrupt onset of violent behavior in persons with no history of violence may stem from such physical conditions as epilepsy, subdural hematoma, drug reaction, and brain tumor (Goodstein and Page, 1981).

Psychodynamic Perspective

Psychological problems are often suggested as reasons for violent behavior. Symonds (1978), in his study of violent marriages, found three significant psychological profiles of the abusing husband:

1. The person who feels no guilt about the abuse. The violence is egosyntonic. He continually tries to restore his power by the use of force and is persistent in the use of violence based on pervasive inner feelings of powerlessness. He is impulsive, irritable, explosive, immature. He has a history of family violence and was probably abused as a child. This behavior is reinforced by a machismo attitude and grandiosity. The man is emotionally insulated and cannot relate to the suffering of his victims. His wife and children are objects for displacement of life's frustrations. To outsiders—those who are not objects of his violence—he can be pleasant and likeable.

2. The "Jekyll and Hyde" behavior. This man appears highly anxious. He is guilt ridden when confronted with the result of his violent behavior. He is generally compliant, but his aggression is released by alcohol consumption. He usually denies being abusive, begs forgiveness, and promises never to be abusive again. He may have resentment about being pushed into marriage. He is usually emotionally dependent upon others.

3. The overly controlling, compulsive, hostile man. This man is described as arrogant and vindictive toward his partner in order to maintain power. He keeps his partner off balance through being alternately critical and silent. He deliberately undermines the partner's confidence and mental health.

The wives of these violent and aggressive men are likely to feel profoundly terrorized and traumatized. This often leads to subdued, clinging, and submissive behavior toward the husband.

Situational Stressors

Some theorists believe that situational forces should be more seriously considered as catalysts of violent behavior (Straus et al., 1980). Circumstances such as poverty, job loss, job frustration, and personal or family trauma can trigger violent behavior. Situations that may give rise to abusive behavior include the following:

1. Single-parent households. These households are on the increase, with the majority resulting from divorce. Besides the obvious problems of coping with the emotional aspects of a broken family unit, there are additional stressors, for example, mothers going to work and attempting to make ends meet, or fathers who have custody trying to be homemakers and primary caretakers for the first time.
2. Working parents. These parents usually hold two jobs—one in the market place and one at home—out of financial necessity.
3. "Latch-key" children. The children must fend for themselves several hours a day. This causes worry and stress for the parents and some deprivation for the children.
4. Mobility. The mobile society in the U.S. has eroded the comfort and security of the extended family. Corporate and military needs require families to move from one place to another, so it is difficult for them to maintain close social ties with families, friends, and neighbors. In the past, neighborhoods were like extended families. Neighbors knew each other, cared for each other, and watched out for each other's children. The move away from these community units has placed additional stress on parents who now must cope largely alone.

■ Point of Emphasis

Social changes create the potential for stress and frustration that can lead to abusive behavior among family members.

Social Learning Theory

The concept most supported in the literature on spouse abuse is the social learning theory of violence. According to Bandura, "violence is a technique of adaptation which is systematically learned by the child through interaction with and observation of parents and others using violence" (in Steinmetz and Straus, 1974), corresponding to the generational cycle of violence in which those who were beaten as children will likely be abusive as adults, in turn abusing their children. Investigators found that among sons of violent parents, the rate of wife beating was 1000 percent greater than among sons of nonviolent parents; among the daughters of violent parents the rate of violent behavior toward their husbands was 600 percent greater than among daughters of nonviolent parents. (Steinmetz and Straus, 1974)

It is in the family setting where most people learn the emotional and moral meaning of violence. It is in the home where children are hit by those who love them, and here that children learn that they are spanked for "their own good." Some parents believe that "spare the rod and spoil the child" builds moral character, while others believe that it builds a new generation of violent people (Straus et al., 1980; Gelles and Cornell, 1985).

Owen and Straus (1975) studied three hypothetical aspects of the social learning concept pertaining to approval of violent behavior and the effects of this learning in adulthood: the child's observation of violence; the child as a victim of violent behavior; and the child who commits violent acts. The investigators wanted to learn how these violent learning situations (experienced in childhood) affected adult approval of violence in the following situations: interpersonal, national (war), and political ends (e.g., nuclear disarmament groups, civil rights demonstrations). The findings indicated that people who experienced violence as children in each of the three categories would approve of interpersonal and political violence, but not necessarily national violence. This is probably because children have excellent role models for hitting on a one-to-one basis and also for crowd and riot control violence; whereas war (national violence) deals with global issues.

The potential for humans to perpetrate violence on their fellow humans has been well studied. In one widely known study, volunteers were given roles as teachers and learners. The teacher was instructed to give an electric shock to the learner when the learner gave a "wrong" response. Voltage was between 75 (low) and 450 (high). The investigators assumed the role of authority figures. Signaling to the teachers to shock the learners, the investigators were amazed to note the extent to which the teachers complied. Sixty-five percent of the teachers inflicted the maximum of 450 volts (which they believed would cause maximum pain) and none inflicted less than 300 volts (intense shock). The 40 volunteers came from diverse occupations: skilled and unskilled, blue collar, business, and the professions (Raven and Rubin, 1976). This study is frequently cited as an example of human obedience to authority and also is claimed to indicate human willingness to inflict pain if there appears to be justification for it.

National Attitudes

The Owens and Straus (1975) study found that one of 10 Americans said they would participate in physical assaults "against a group of people who were blocking rush hour traffic as a means of political protest." In a different survey, one-half to two-thirds of American men approved of shooting by police in situations such as ghetto riots and campus disturbances. Twenty to thirty percent of these respondents would want police to "shoot to kill" in these circumstances (Blumenthal et al., 1972).

> **■ Point of Emphasis**
>
> *Violent behavior can be learned from observing the behavior of others, even though violence was not a part of the person's familial or cultural background.*

SCOPE OF WIFE ABUSE

Each year over one million American women are physically injured by their mates. This is a conservative estimate, as only about one in 10 episodes is reported to the police.

Ganley (1981) describes women as being subjected to two types of abuse:

1. Physical—punching, pushing, choking, burning, stabbing, clubbing, thrown objects, shooting.
2. Psychological—threats including the threat to kill, controlling the woman's social relationships or access to money, consistent attacks on her self-esteem through verbal abuse and denial of her feelings and ideas, and frightening her by behaviors

such as speeding through traffic or handling weapons.

The battered woman may also suffer because she does not know what it is she may say or do that will set her mate off to abuse her—she "walks on eggs." Abused women report feelings of shame, guilt, fear, and anger. She questions her worth, becomes depressed, and may feel psychologically helpless. When in desperation she goes to the emergency room, calls the police, or sees her physician, she often finds that her situation is met with skepticism.

Myths about Violence in Families

Certain myths about abused women have fostered negative attitudes, not only among police, the courts, and physicians but within the community at large. These myths contribute to the low self-esteem felt by the victim and hinder therapeutic intervention:

1. *The lower class myth.* The battered wife is of the working class or of a low economic status. *Fact*: Spouse abuse occurs at every level of economic strata. Poor persons often appear in greater numbers at shelters because they have fewer options and support groups. Poverty is only one stress factor that ignites violence.
2. *The provocation myth.* The battered wife asks for violent treatment. *Fact*: Most of these wives have done everything possible to try to please their husbands, but have found that nothing they did helped the situation.
3. *The "get-going" myth.* The victim can leave any time she wants to. *Fact*: It is often difficult for the victim to leave her spouse. She may still love him and believe that he will change. Many husbands are contrite after abusing their wives, and promise emphatically that it won't happen again. The wife may be fearful—she may have been threatened by her husband, she may have no means of support, she may have young children.

A woman of means may feel that she has too much to lose (e.g., her social position, her financial security). In such a situation, she may feel the benefits of the relationship outweigh the costs (Goodstein and Page, 1981). Some wives may come to believe, finally, that they have little worth; they become psychological prisoners, feeling they deserve the treatment they receive. Some who have observed violent behavior in their childhood believe that their adult situation reflects a natural way of life. Some women feel such deep humiliation that they do not want others to know about their situation. Many women, because of their religious affiliation, believe that their marriage vows hold until death, regardless of their circumstances.

Barriers to Seeking Help

Law Enforcement. Many abused women have unsatisfactory experiences with police officers. The officer often does not want to be involved in a family affair—yet if a stranger had caused the same injuries to the woman, the officer would not hesitate to make an arrest. Some officers become disinclined because the victim will not press charges against the spouse (often because of fear of reprisal). Finally, police do not want to become involved in domestic affairs because of what they perceive as danger to themselves. Close to 35 percent of police officers were killed while answering family disturbance calls (Kirkland, 1982), and some 40 percent of police injuries are sustained as a result of responding to calls in family disputes. Most police are not trained to give interpersonal services in domestic situations, though police departments in some cities have developed excellent training programs designed to help the police respond with skill and compassion to such crisis calls.

In one notable study, a specially trained unit consisting of nine white and nine black officers worked in conjunction with the psychology department of a local college. They responded only to domestic calls in a West Harlem community of 85,000 persons. In a 22-month period, the patrolmen were called by 962 families on 1375 occasions. During this period there were no homicides and only one officer received a minor injury (Bard and Berkowitz, 1967). Training of this sort is increasing. In some police divisions, clergy accompany police officers on domestic calls. These types of programs can go a long way to improve police-community relations in general, and to help relieve hostile family situations in particular.

The attitude of the courts is beginning to change, from the earlier one of supporting the male partner, to one of holding the abuser responsible—by arresting him—regardless of the wishes of the victim. The purpose of this act is to protect the victim by making it unnecessary for her to press charges. Thus her safety is not jeopardized nor is the possibility of reconciliation.

The Health Care System. Battered wives often report that health care professionals are not supportive. For example, Mrs. A., an elementary school teacher, had four young children, ages 1, 3, 5, and 7 years. At her second visit to her physician, when she again stated that she was depressed because her husband physically mistreated her, the physician again counseled her to be a "good wife" and not set up situations that might cause tension. Mr. A. was a respected business man, and the physician appeared embarrassed by the conversation with Mrs. A. Mrs. A.'s mother-in-law told her that her own husband was strict with her also, and she hoped Mrs. A. would not embarrass the family by talking about the husband's abusive behavior.

Mrs. A. subsequently became pregnant. One evening Mr. A. came home late, having stopped at a bar with some friends. To Mrs. A.'s reproaches, he responded by hitting her across the face with the telephone. It was this incident that led Mrs. A. to go to a Women's Shelter and eventually divorce her husband.

Had intervention occurred at an earlier time, treatment might have been effective. The health professional needs to examine personal biases and cultural mores before attempting to offer support and guidance to the victim of abuse.

The Shelter Experience

Erin Pizzey of Chiswich, England, opened the first shelter for abused women in the 1970s. Pizzey's book, *Scream Quietly or the Neighbors Will Hear,* called attention to battered women, and as a result of the growth of the women's movement, media coverage, and legislation, shelters have opened in many parts of the U.S. (McNeely and Jones, 1980).

Shelters vary from providing a temporary refuge for women and their children for a day or two, to offering board and room for 2 weeks, to providing a variety of services and housing the victims for up to 4 weeks. Shelters that provide a full range of service offer a safe and protected environment, education in family living, counseling by trained counselors, support groups, parent education (the longer period of 4 weeks gives the women an opportunity to practice what they learn), advocacy and referral within the courts, access to medical and nursing care, comprehensive services for children (including play therapy and counseling), and aftercare services to families that includes home visits, family counseling, and referrals.

THE ABUSIVE MALE

The emphasis on sex and violence as depicted in magazines, on television, and in advertising encourages a man to "take command" and be in control, do his "own thing," and be "strong." At the same time he is encouraged to be a good father, to share responsibilities with his wife in the care and raising of his children and care of the home, and to ask rather than to take. Boys are taught that only "sissies" hit girls, yet they may see their father hit their mother during an argument.

Abuse is a learned behavior, and it is learned at home. A child who witnesses threatening behavior on the part of an adult may learn that when he is big enough it will be all right for him to hit. Most children grow up to be the kind of parents their parents were.

Abusive men come from all walks of life and educational backgrounds. Various factors may predispose them to become violent. Ganley (1981) has identified such factors as abusive family background, poor communication skills (especially toward women) inferiority complex, high (unrealistic) expectations, low self-esteem, alcoholism, drug dependency, and inability to cope effectively with stress, conflict, and anger.

Since abusive behavior is learned, it can be changed. Many programs exist for this purpose. One, called Men and Domestic Violence, teaches communication skills, relaxation techniques, and alternative behaviors to physical violence, once the man accepts responsibility for his abusive behavior. Some of the strategies taught include the following:

1. Taking time out. This allows the man to remove himself from the situation, regain composure, deflate his anger, and try again to work toward resolution of the behavior.
2. Recognizing emotional red flags. The man becomes able to identify emotional surges before they become excessive and uncontrollable, so he can practice more appropriate behavior.
3. Building communication skills. The man

learns to identify and verbally express feelings such as rejection, anger, hurt, fear, anxiety, and inferiority, rather than acting out his violent impulses.

It is important that men learn that the discipline they experienced as children was, to some extent, abuse. The following examples will help the health professional understand how childhood perceptions affect adult behavior.

Vignettes

Joe related how, as a child, he hated his father for hitting his mother and despised his mother for not protecting herself (by leaving). He was severely disciplined and also felt unprotected by his mother. When, as an adult, he realized he was repeating his father's behavior by being abusive toward his wife, he contemplated suicide. In therapy, he became able to verbalize his self-disgust and anger toward a parent with whom he had severed connections long ago.

Frank remembered that chaos and turmoil were common in his family home, yet when his father abused his mother, calm and order were restored. Frank didn't judge whether it was right for his dad to hit his mother, only that order seemed to result. In the group program, he was dismayed, confused, and angry at first. Frank shared the information that he beat his wife only to "settle things down." The expected result—submissiveness—did not occur. Rather, his wife said she would leave him if he didn't seek help for his abusive behavior.

Marital Rape

Marital rape is defined as intercourse or other sexual activity forced upon the spouse in a display of domination, anger, or a drug-altered state, without any regard for feelings and shared affection (Fortune, 1983). If other manifestations of physical abuse occur, marital rape will tend to occur during a passive stage in the cycle of violence (Walker, 1979). The man may tender such signs of affection as flowers and gifts, then force himself upon his mate to prove how much he loves her. (An example of marital rape was portrayed in a television production that related an actual case of marital rape, which resulted in the wife killing the husband.)

☐ *Nursing Process*

Initially, it is the nurse's responsibility to identify the problem, relate empathically to the client, and make a referral to the appropriate community agency. Usually the health professional will encounter the battered spouse in a hospital emergency room, a community mental health center, or home care setting. The initial meeting may take place in a psychiatric hospital, to which the victim has been admitted with a different diagnosis.

ASSESSMENT ☐ It may be difficult to identify the problem because the victim feels fearful and ashamed. Most women do not fully disclose the cause or nature of their injuries. Hence the nurse in the ambulatory clinic or emergency room needs to be keenly aware of the physical and behavioral indicators of battering.

According to Goodstein and Page (1981) and Greany (1984) the following are important indicators of abuse that may be seen in the acute care setting:

Physical Signs and Symptoms. Bruises and lacerations of the face, neck, back, and arms may be visible or be present only on areas of the body covered by clothing. Pregnant women may have bruises in the abdominal area from blows or kicks. A broken arm accompanied by other bruises may have been the result of the woman's attempt to ward off blows to the face or body. Physical symptoms of anxiety and stress may be reported, such as chest pains, choking sensations, hyperventilation, claustrophobia, gastrointestinal upsets, and insomnia; Greany (1984) has noted that these may be symptoms of anticipated further abuse. Pelvic pain may be reported in response to related sexual assault. Complaints of chronic fatigue are common. Old scars or bruises in various stages of healing may be present.

Behavioral Clues. Inconsistent or irrational accounts of the causes for the injuries sustained are highly indicative of abuse. The wife and husband may describe different stories when asked what happened to cause the injury, or the event described seems unlikely to lead to the type and degree of injuries present. For instance, "running into a door" may explain a cut or bruise on one side of the face, but not bilateral bruises or bodily injuries.

A significant lapse between the time of the injury and the time of seeking medical attention is a clue to other indicators because it suggests a reluctance to expose the problem to outside scrutiny (unless there are other reasons why treatment had to be delayed). A client wearing sunglasses when indoors should be asked to remove them so that the nurse can determine whether she has a black eye. Interview data suggesting suicide attempts, accident proneness, drug and alcohol abuse, or child abuse should also be looked into.

Interviewing and Recording Aspects ☐ If abuse is suspected, the client needs a sensitive and caring approach. She should be interviewed alone so she can feel free to discuss the incident openly. The nurse should not berate the abusive spouse because this may cause the victim to feel she has to defend him.

The nurse should express genuine concern at the extent of the injuries and ask if these were the result of a beating (Walker, 1979). The client should be helped to understand that she has been the victim of a crime and given assurance that agencies are available to offer safety and support. If the victim is willing to press charges, photos of the injuries should be taken for use as evidence (Greany, 1984). If the woman is fearful or reluctant to admit to being beaten or refuses to take action against the abuser, it is essential for the nurse to remain nonjudgmental in manner and to reiterate the availability of help and protection when the woman is willing to avail herself of it. An accurate, objective record of the physical assessment and interview findings in the clients' own words must be made, as this may later be used as legal evidence.

When abuse has been validated, the nurse may wish to complete a crisis assessment of the abuser (Table 29-1) and the victim (Table 29-2) to determine the immediate and appropriate referral needs. The degree of danger to all parties is an important consideration in this situation.

Nurse Self-Awareness ☐ Nurses in all settings play a crucial role in identifying and referring abuse cases. The nurse may well be the first person to come in contact with the abused individual. For this reason, all nurses need to examine their bias toward the abused and the abuser in order to make a meaningful intervention. Judgmental or punitive behavior will not bring about a therapeutic outcome. Health professionals often feel anger toward the abused woman because of what

TABLE 29-1 Crisis Assessment—Abuser Profile[a]

Category	These questions are useful in determining the severity of the situation so that safety can be assured and referrals can be made
Presence of weapons	Are weapons available to assailant? Has abuser made previous threats with a weapon? Have weapons been used in previous episodes? Is abuser now threatening to use a weapon?
Presence of alcohol/drugs	Is abuser intoxicated and making threats? Has abuser been violent during intoxicated states in the past? Is abuser threatening to harm family members?
Suicide threats	Is there a threat to kill self? Is there a previous history of mental illness when there were episodes of violence? Has abuser made previous suicide attempts? Does abuser threaten to kill family members?
Intimidating behavior	Does abuser engage in threatening behavior? Does abuser frighten friends and family members? Does abuser make abusive telephone calls? Does abuser make verbal threats of violence against spouse?
Previous history of violent episodes	When did most recent incident occur? What was severity of episode? Outcome for assailant? Was abuser remorseful? Was legal action taken?
Violence outside the family	Has abuser assaulted extended family members? Has abuser assaulted friends? Has abuser assaulted strangers? Number of incidents, degree of injuries?
Previous history with court system	Does abuser have a record with courts, or has he been in prison? Was abuser previously charged with assault? Is abuser on probation? Is there a peace bond or restraining order?
Sophisticated knowledge of legal system	Does abuser know terms and degrees of court sanctions and how far he can go before court action can be taken? Has abuser manipulated legal system before? Does abuser respect the law?

[a] Source: U.S. Department of Health and Human Services. Family violence: Intervention strategies, May 1980.

appears to be her passive acceptance of her situation. If the nurse understands the dynamics of abuse and treats the victim in a nonjudgmental way, it will allay defensive behavior and allow the woman the freedom she needs to consider alternatives (Greany, 1984).

The nurse needs to evaluate her own attitudes and readiness to provide accurate, helpful information. An offer of assistance is very limited if the nurse does not have the information and ability to mobilize the necessary help. The phone numbers of the appropriate police service unit and the shelter agency need to be readily available to all emergency room and ambulatory clinic staff. In this way, immediate protection and an alternative to returning home is provided for the battered wife and her children.

PROBLEM IDENTIFICATION □ The abused woman will commonly have several nursing diagnoses. Generally, the physical injuries and the need for safety, to prevent future or potential injury, take precedence. The short-term goals are to address these physical problems and to make cer-

TABLE 29-2 Crisis Assessment—Victim Profile[a]

Category	These questions are useful in determining the severity of the situation so that safety can be assured and referrals can be made
History of abuse	Was victim abused previously? When did the last incident occur? Has victim been abused by current partner? Severity of past episodes? Degree of injury? Frequency of abuse?
Legal remedies	Has victim called police in the past? Has victim taken court action before? Has victim followed through on warrant? Has victim followed through with a court hearing?
History of separation	Has victim separated from current spouse? How many times? Outcome? Has victim separated from previous spouse?
Limited ability to function or make decisions	Is victim capable of making decision about how to avoid violence? Has victim developed a workable plan or is she immobilized? What barriers are preventing victim from making a plan?
Children at risk	Are children in danger? Has there been previous abuse? Has victim made a decision to take the children in the event of separation? What are the best plans for the children?
Victim's potential for violence	Does victim feel that in anger or rage she could use a weapon to harm the attacker? Does victim have access to weapons? Does victim plan to fight back? Has victim been violent in past?

[a] Source: U.S. Department of Health and Human Services. Family violence: Intervention strategies, May 1980.

tain that the client has sufficient knowledge of available resources to secure her safety.

Long-range goals for follow up in the community are to address the long-term nursing diagnoses. High levels of anxiety and specific fears of what the abuser may do next are likely and realistic. Self-esteem disturbance is common. Low self-esteem may play a role in the woman's willingness to remain in an abusive situation; it is one of the general effects of abuse, with resultant feelings of helplessness and powerlessness.

Role relationships in the family are dysfunctional. Social isolation may have occurred over a period of time as the woman attempted to avoid situations that might trigger an abusive episode and tried to conceal the problem. Marital rape may result in the rape trauma syndrome (mental anguish and somatic symptoms) if the spouse forces sex against the woman's will in conjunction

with or following a beating. Ineffective individual and family coping is clearly evident in the relationship, and the abuser is characterized by his continuing potential for violence. Many abusers share the low levels of self-esteem of their victims.

INTERVENTION □

Primary Prevention □ One focus of primary prevention assumes that abusive behavior is symptomatic of underlying psychiatric disorder and that general mental health promotion activities will reduce the incidence of abuse. Jayaratne (1977), for instance, advises that parents need to be educated to the fact that emotional deprivation, rejection, and excessive demands on children may lead to abusive behavior in adulthood. In a similar vein, Garbarino (1976) suggests teaching elementary school children communication and coping skills. Children can be assisted to set realistic goals, emphasize sharing over competition, and develop a sense of competence. These values enhance the child's ability to cope with stress and diminish reliance on less effective behaviors such as aggressiveness.

Another aspect of primary prevention reflects an awareness of attitudes toward women and violent behavior which are prevalent in American culture and have been transmitted in the family and by the media. Gelles and Cornell (1985) note that preventing domestic violence depends in part upon ridding the public of the notion that intrafamily violence is an acceptable form of discipline or control and that violence and sexism portrayed in television, books, and movies is legitimately glorified. Community-based efforts to reduce stressors, so that families can be integrated into social networks with resulting decrease in the cycle of family violence, are also advocated.

Secondary Prevention □ The nurse, policemen, welfare workers, and other health professionals need to acknowledge indications of abuse, validate the problem with the victim, and immediately refer her to the appropriate resources for protection, shelter, and recovery. Knowledge about the legal processes involved in separation and divorce, or court-supervised mediation and counseling, will be important as the woman begins to make decisions. Counseling is available for both the victim and the abuser.

Tertiary Prevention □ The rehabilitation process is best initiated in a supportive and protective environment in which the victim and her children feel safe and can build a supportive network. Personal counseling may be directed toward goals of

independence and increased self-esteem. Parent education is aimed at strengthening these skills so as to build the woman's competence and sense of confidence as well as to interrupt the cycle of abuse to prevent its occurrence in future generations—the children may have witnessed and may have experienced abusive incidents. Support groups emphasize the development of communication, coping, stress management, assertiveness, and daily living skills.

The abusive partner should receive therapy to help him to confront his problems, learn to express feelings verbally rather than act them out, and develop coping and stress management skills. Family therapy may help families who want to remain together to develop strengths and to rebuild a functional unit. Table 29-3 lists agencies and services that nurses may consult in the referral process.

EVALUATION □ The nurse in the acute care setting will need to determine (1) the effectiveness of care in meeting the client's physical care needs, (2) the adequacy of the medical record and any related evidence in the event of legal action, and (3) the accuracy and specific value to the client of the information provided for referral and support. Nurse self-evaluation efforts should focus on the ability to communicate genuine caring and concern without attempting to coerce the client into acting if she is unwilling to act.

Long-term evaluation criteria for the abused woman focus on changes relevant to improving self-esteem, communication, stress management, and independence. Goals for the abuser relate to similar changes with the overriding concern being to bring about sufficient behavior change to per-

---

TABLE 29-3 Agencies and Services to Which Families May Be Referred[a]

Criminal Justice System	Possible Services
Law enforcement agency	Crisis intervention Arrest of abuser Related assistance Referral
Magistrate	Warrant for arrest

Civil courts	Protective custody of child(ren)
	Psychiatric commitment
	Orders for medical and/or psychiatric care
	Hearings for assault, separation, divorce, child custody, visiting
	Protective orders
	  Injunctions and restraining orders
	  Peace bond
	  Court conciliation/mediation

(continued)

TABLE 29-3 *(continued)*

Criminal Justice System	Possible Services
Criminal courts	Arrest warrant Arraignment Preliminary hearing Plea bargaining Trial for assault Imprisonment Fine Probation
Legal services	Consultation regarding spouses' legal rights Advice about filing arrest warrants, petitioning the court for separation, divorce, child custody, and visiting Representation in court Advocacy with welfare and other agencies
Department of social services	Child protective services Financial assistance Child care Homemaker services Counseling Respite care for children Foster care and residential treatment Payment for emergency shelter Security deposits for apartments Transportation
Mental health agencies	Crisis counseling Family outreach Assessment for psychiatric care/commitment Individual, marital, family, group psychotherapy Therapy for children and adolescents Partial hospitalization (therapeutic day care)
Hospitals	Alcohol or drug detoxification Inpatient psychiatric treatment Emergency medical care for adults and children
Public health agencies/private physicians	Pre- and postnatal care Well-baby care Dental care Family planning Outpatient medical care
Employment agencies/services	Career counseling, job training and placement; vocational rehabilitation; adult education
Alcohol/drug treatment agencies	Residential treatment Outpatient counseling Services for other family members Self-help groups (AA, Al-Anon)
Volunteer agencies	Emergency food, clothing, shelter Transportation (emergency or support) Support groups Recreation Socialization Hot lines Women's advocacy and counseling groups
Housing services	Emergency shelter/crisis housing Second-stage housing (structured environment to assist during transition stage of separation from spouse Third-stage housing (group home or adult foster home setting) Assistance with securing affordable, permanent housing

[a] Source: U.S. Department of Health and Human Services. Family violence: Intervention strategies, May 1980.

mit self-control in situations that formerly evoked physical aggressiveness. The community nurse who may be following the family will need to be alert to cues of ongoing abuse as well as cues to growth and change in positive directions.

Sexual Assault

Sexual assault is not typically considered as intrafamily violence, although rape may occur within marriage, between couples who know each other casually (date rape), and as a crime of random violence in which rage, control, and degradation are the rapist's goal. Date rape tends to go largely unreported, just as courtship violence does, and only recently have surveys on college campuses reported its frequent occurrence. Men who force sex upon their dates are typically surprised to be categorized as rapists, believing that women who say no to sex on a date "don't really mean it." Their dates rarely report these cases of rape because of shame, embarrassment, and frequently feelings that they were somehow responsible for the attack by accepting the date and thus "leading him on." Nevertheless, victims of date rape commonly feel violated, shamed, and powerless. Future dating relationships can be colored by the experience.

The more typical rape is that by the stranger who assaults a woman on the street or invades her home. Threats, physical injury and domination, and a realistic fear of death terrorize the victim. After effects include physical injuries, fear and insecurity, diminished self-confidence, nightmares, insomnia, and feelings of humiliation and rage. If the police and emergency room personnel are not sensitive to the victim's emotional state, the victim may feel that the interrogation and examination procedures are further assaults. Rape victims who press charges may see their assailants go free because of insufficient evidence or may experience numerous delays while awaiting trial. Once the case is heard, the defense attorney may lead the victim to feel that her own credibility and behavior are on trial. Ultimately she may feel brutalized by the justice system and fear that the rapist will seek her out to further intimidate her or exact revenge. With this knowledge in mind, the nurse who cares for the rape victim must exhibit sensitivity and concern.

Client Assessment □ Before emergency care is given, the victim who contacts friends or a crisis line must be told not to shower, bathe, or change clothing. The urge to wash away feelings of being soiled is strong, but it will hamper evidence gathering. Most cities sponsor a rape crisis line; a volunteer will respond immediately to assist the victim through the medical and legal procedures and to provide support services such as a place to stay if the victim feels unsafe at home. If the woman appears in the emergency room without a supportive person the nurse should contact a rape crisis volunteer or a hospital-based counselor before initiating care. Most hospitals have available a "rape kit" and provide certain protocols that assure both careful attention to the evidence necessary for legal prosecution and sensitive treatment of the victim (Braen, 1981). Most victims are in a state of crisis or disorganization and need clear, direct, and reassuring communication. Procedures should be carefully explained and evidence handled according to hospital protocol. Physical injuries are described in the chart, the client's statements are accurately recorded in her own words, and photographs are taken of injuries. Victims commonly respond in either an expressive or a controlled style, in equal numbers. Expressive victims exhibit tension, restlessness, tears, fear, and anger openly, while controlled victims conceal the feelings or mask their feelings, to appear calm and composed. The nurse should accept either mode.

Nurse Self-Assessment □ It is important that the nurse accept the client's behavior and decision at this critical time. The nurse may be angered at the sight of the victim's injuries and want her to prosecute the rapist. The victim, in her disorganized state, may be fearful and reluctant. The nurse should not attempt to persuade the victim to change her mind at this time, but should assure her that the evidence and medical records will be maintained should she change her mind later.

PROBLEM IDENTIFICATION □ Rape trauma syndrome (Burgess and Holmstrom, 1975) is the name given to the acute phase and long-term reorganization process that evolves from either forcible or attempted rape. The behavioral, somatic, and psychological reactions represent an acute stress reaction to a life-threatening situation.

The characteristics of rape trauma syndrome include anger, fear, embarrassment, revenge, self-blame, and physical symptoms such as insomnia, gastric distress and genitourinary discomfort. If the victim had a history of physical or psychosocial difficulties along with the rape trauma syndrome, the earlier features are present, and symptoms of previous conditions or illnesses are reactivated (e.g., substance abuse, psychiatric disorders, psychosomatic illness). In the silent reaction, all of the reported features may be present but the victim conceals the rape and does not report it to anyone. Nightmares, phobias, and anxiety symptoms may be present and relationships with men may change abruptly (Gordon, 1985).

INTERVENTION □ Initial nursing actions in the emergency room are directed toward offering sensitive and caring concern for the woman. Crisis intervention (Chapter 22) should be initiated immediately through a rape crisis service or other counseling agency. Nurses who encounter rape victims in other settings or who are involved in rape crisis support services need to be aware of crisis intervention techniques and be able to provide anticipatory guidance and support throughout the recovery process.

Physical soreness, bruises, and abrasions generally heal first. The rape victim may gradually become less likely to be jumpy and easily startled. She may feel it necessary to move, to ask someone to stay with her for a time, and may change her phone number until fears gradually subside. Feelings of anger-rage-desire for revenge and fear of crowds, deserted places, being alone, or seeing a face like the rapist's will lessen but may be reawakened on occasions (e.g., reliving the event when testifying). Gradually the nightmares, phobias, and sleepless nights end. Some women may require specific psychotherapy if phobias or disrupted relationships persist. Family counseling may be necessary if the woman's boyfriend or husband has difficulty dealing with the situation and the couple's relationship is disrupted.

EVALUATION □ The nurse should be able to see a reduction of symptoms characteristic of the rape trauma syndrome. She should also evaluate the woman's long-term sexual adjustment and that of her mate.

Self-evaluation includes the nurse's ability to (1) be caring and supportive to clients, (2) maintain the evidence and accurate records, (3) obtain adequate support for the victim throughout the crisis and its aftermath, and (4) have knowledge sufficient to provide adequate anticipatory guidance and referral as needed.

□ *Child Abuse*

("Parent" is the word used throughout this section to identify the caretaker of the child whether that be father, mother, foster parent, relative, or other person.)

Child abuse is any physical, sexual, and/or emotional act by a parent, whether intentional or unintentional, that is injurious to a child.

Physical abuse is any intentional physical injury caused by the parent.

Neglect is passive conduct on the part of the parent that results in harm to the child. It is characterized by inattention to the child's basic needs. Neglect may be physical (malnutrition, lack of medical care) or material (insufficient housing or supervision due to parent substance abuse or absenteeism). Neglect occurs over time and does not carry the visible signs of physical abuse.

Emotional maltreatment is a continuing pattern that has harmful effects on the child and is difficult to pinpoint. The pattern within the family is one of chronic failure to provide psychological and emotional support to the child. Maltreatment includes belittling and rejecting.

Sexual abuse has been defined by the National Center on Child Abuse and Neglect as contact or interaction between a child and an adult in which the child is used for sexual stimulation of the adult or another person. Sexual abuse may be committed by a person under the age of 18 if he is either much older than the victim or is in a position of power or control over another child (e.g., a babysitter).

REPORTING

Suspicion or discovery of child abuse by friends, neighbors, teachers, or health professionals has created ambivalence and confusion. Most adults are reluctant to believe a child's word against that of an adult, particularly if the adult is of middle- or upper-class status. According to one study, approximately 4 percent of parents are abusive toward their children (Gelles and Cornell, 1985).

Every state requires reporting of child abuse. All health professionals who deal with children must report such incidents. The definitions of abuse, the procedures, and the decision-making processes vary widely from state to state. Nevertheless, each nurse, whatever her practice setting, needs to be acquainted with the state law, the agency or service to which the abuse should be reported, and the legal definition of abuse in the state where she practices.

Sexual exploitation of children by adults who are unrelated to them is another area of concern. In return for caring for the young child, the adult exacts a penalty—the child must participate in sexual activity instigated by the adult. Threats to hurt the child or his family members and other scare tactics may be used to force the child to engage in sexual activity.

PERSPECTIVES ON CHILD ABUSE

Some sociologists focus on the social environment in which child abuse occurs; others focus on intrafamily dynamics. David Gil (1975, 1979) describes the necessary conditions for child abuse as a social philosophy that fails to consider all individuals to be of intrinsically equal worth; the social expectation that children be obedient, submissive, and conforming; and a social belief in the use of force as a legitimate means for achieving goals. Garbarino and Gilliam (1980) theorize that isolation from support systems, cultural justification of the use of force against children, and the belief that children are the property of their parents are necessary conditions for child abuse.

Another group looks at child and adolescent abuse from a multicausal perspective. There are interacting variables both from within and outside the family unit (Belsky, 1980; Garbarino and Gilliam, 1980). These include violence in the family of origin of the caretaker, use of alcohol and other drugs, lack of awareness of child development and appropriate child-rearing practices, and high levels of personal or external stress.

According to the National Center on Child Abuse and Neglect, family factors may either cause or prevent child abuse, as outlined below.

1. Individual capacity. Physical and mental health, personality, intelligence, and previous life experiences all play a part. These reflect innate and experiential influences and are present in both child and parent.
2. Attitudes and behaviors. Parental attitudes toward children, changing family roles, violence, corporal punishment, and religion are significant factors in child abuse.
3. Specific life situations. There may be various situations, either chronic or acute in nature, that affect parent/child relationships. The quality of the marital relationship, employment situations, housing conditions, presence of extended family members, family economic stability, and isolation from social contact all play a role.

4. General community welfare. Social institutions affect all families on several levels—for example, churches, businesses, schools, radio, television. When positive, these forces can help families to grow and engage in healthy interactions; when negative, child abuse is likely.

Institutions such as mental health centers or drug and alcohol abuse programs deal with specific groups of adults. Other institutions deal directly with child abuse and neglect, such as child protective services and juvenile courts.

INCIDENCE

Studies differ widely in estimating the numbers of children subjected to abuse and neglect, though there is general agreement that the numbers increase yearly. According to the American Humane Society, there were 413,000 reported cases of child abuse and neglect in 1976; 851,000 in 1981; and more than one million cases in 1982. The National Center on Child Abuse and Neglect estimates that more than one million children are maltreated by their parents each year. Annually, more than 2000 children die in circumstances that point to abuse or neglect.

Gelles and Straus, in a controversial study reported in 1985, state that there has been a marked drop in violence over the past decade; their report is based on family self-reporting of violence against children. Other sociologists question whether parent self-reporting provides an accurate picture, and note that the available statistics do not reflect such a drop. Gelles and Straus attribute the changes in self-reporting of violent acts that ranged from slapping to punching or hitting with an object such as a belt to greater public awareness created by media campaigns.

The topic of child sexual abuse dominated the sessions at the Third International Congress on Child Abuse and Neglect which was held in Amsterdam in April 1981. A growing area of concern is the sexual exploitation of children by adults unrelated to them (Densen-Gerber, 1981).

The prevalence of child sexual abuse is unknown because it frequently is not reported, though 6.5 percent of overall child abuse reports deal with sexual abuse. The victims may be of any age, including infancy and early childhood.

EFFECTS OF CHILD ABUSE

The consequences of child abuse are seen on individual, family, and national levels. The immediate tragedy is the physical and psychological damage, sometimes even death, inflicted on the victim. The cycle of violence suggests that the potential for parent and elder abuse is increased among adults who were abused as children. It has also been noted that abused children are more likely than others to be involved in acts of juvenile delinquency, and that murderers of public figures have often reported being abused as children (Gelles and Cornell, 1985). The effects of abuse can be categorized as follows:

Developmental Effects. Learning problems and inadequate social functioning in school are attributed to child abuse and neglect. Developmental delays due to malnutrition, lack of social stimulation, and general deprivation may never be overcome, and this underdevelopment has its effects on language and perceptual skills, hindering the child's ability in all areas. Such a child may become a so-called juvenile delinquent and exhibit acting-out and aggressive behavior.

Physical-Emotional Effects. Physical damage to internal organs may be irreparable and can lead to retardation, blindness, or deafness. A limb may be lost due to excessive physical punishment. Permanent scarring from burns, cuts, and other wounds may be associated with emotional scarring as well. The emotional scars can leave the child aggressive, anxious, and self-destructive.

Long-Range Effect. Abused children tend to become abused or abusive adults and abusive as parents. As noted above, crimes of violence, such as assault and murder, are more likely to be committed by persons who were abused as children.

ENVIRONMENTAL FACTORS

Child abuse does not occur only in poor, deprived families. There is no such thing as a stereotypical family whose children are victims of abuse, neglect, incest, and other social problems. It is true, nevertheless, that environmental factors do play a part in family problems (Table 29-4). Unemployment may force a family into substandard housing or make it impossible for them to repair and maintain the home. Illness can wipe out a family's resources, and leave parents emotionally bankrupt and unable to cope with their children's needs. The isolation experienced by a family with an alcoholic parent deprives them of normal social contact with neighbors, participation in community groups such as church and school, peer relationships, and knowledge of the outside world. Sharing child-rearing practices and knowledge and comparing a child's progress with friends and neighbors helps a family become a part of the community. This community sharing assists a parent in verbally expressing feelings of frustration, anger, fear, and anxiety rather than "taking it out" on the child.

If a child's basic needs for safety, health, nutrition, clothing, and housing are not met and this impoverishment continues over extended periods of time, the resulting psychological effects will harm the child's emotional and mental health. An environment of constant criticism, devaluing, meanness and psychological cruelty, such as enforced and deliberate isolation and the withholding of affection and security, can severely damage the child's emotional and mental health.

Incest may occur if the family lacks adequate space to accommodate all members, or if extended family members are present. Incestuous fathers tend to believe in the older family model in which father is head of the household and the spouse and children are his subjects. He may have been abused as a child, and may see his "use" of the child as fulfilling a personal need; there is no regard for the possible harm to the child or to others in the family. Incest is known to exist in every socioeconomic stratum. However, it is more likely to be reported if the family is receiving assistance from a social agency such as Aid to Families with Dependent Children or welfare agencies. If the mother is absent regularly or is sick or separated from the family for any reason, the child is more accessible to the father. Chemical dependency also can create an environment conducive to incest. Families were often scrutinized to uncover the psychological problems of the parent that caused them to abuse their children. Newberger (1982) proposes that sociocultural factors influence responses to family stresses. Understanding these sociocultural factors and stresses on families will assist the helping professions form plans to assist families, change behavior, reduce stress, and move toward healthier family interactions. Parental stress factors are depicted in Table 29-4.

CLIENT ASSESSMENT □ How can the nurse assess whether injury to a child is due to an accident or to possible abuse? Table 29-5 describes physical and behavioral indicators of abuse and neglect.

TABLE 29-4 Factors Influencing Child Abuse[a]

Sociocultural Factors

- Values and norms about violence and force; acceptability of corporal punishment
- Inegalitarian, hierarchical social structure; imbalanced interpersonal relationships
- Values about competition versus cooperation
- Exploitative, alienating economic system; acceptance and encouragement of permanent poor class
- Devaluation of children and other dependents
- Institutional manifestations of the above factors in areas such as law, health care education, welfare system, sports, and entertainment

Family Factors

Child-produced Stresses	Social-situational Stresses	Parent-produced Stresses
Physical difference (e.g., handicapped)	*Structural factors:* poverty, unemployment mobility, isolation, poor housing	Low self-esteem
Mental difference (e.g., retarded)		Abused as child
Temperamental difference (e.g., difficult)	*Parental relationship:* patterns of discord-assault, domination-submission	Depression
Behavioral difference (e.g., hyperactive)		Substance abuse
Foster child	*Parent-child relationship:* attachment problems, perinatal stress, punitive child-rearing style, scapegoating, role reversal, excess or unwanted children	Character disorder
		Ignorance of child rearing; unrealistic expectations
	Triggering situation: Discipline	
	Argument; family conflict	
	Substance abuse	
	Acute environmental problem	
	Maltreatment	
	Injury	
	Inability to provide care	
	Poisoning	
	Psychological maltreatment	

[a] Newberger, Eli H. (ed.). *Child abuse.* Boston: Little, Brown & Co., 1982.

These indicators will aid the nurse in making an assessment and taking the necessary action.

Table 29-6 A and B outlines the behaviors of children and parents caught in the web of emotional maltreatment and provides a valuable tool for accurate assessment.

■ Point of Emphasis

Accurate assessment may mean the difference between further child abuse and intervention that helps the entire family.

If the nurse suspects abuse, additional risk factors should be investigated: Has the child been admitted previously? Were there previous emergency room visits? Do unexplained injuries appear at school? Is there reason to believe other hospital or emergency facilities have been used?

Interviewing the Child □ Interviewing must be appropriate to the age of the child. The child may feel fearful of potential punitive action from the caretaker if information about the abusive behavior is disclosed.

TABLE 29-5 *Physical and Behavioral Indicators of Child Abuse and Neglect*[a]

Type	Physical Indicators	Behavioral Indicators

Physical abuse	Unexplained bruises and welts:
	    on face, lips, mouth, torso, back, buttocks, thighs;
	    in various stages of healing;
	    clustered, forming regular patterns;
	    reflecting shape of article used to inflict (electric cord, belt buckle);
	    on several different surface areas;
	    regularly appear after absence weekend, or vacation
	Unexplained burns:
	    cigar, cigarette burns, especially on soles, palms, back, or buttocks;
	    immersion burns (socklike, glovelike, doughnut-shaped on buttocks or genitalia);
	    patterned (electric burner, iron);
	    rope burns on arms, legs, neck, or torso
	Unexplained fractures:
	    to skull, nose, facial structure, in various stages of healing;
	    multiple or spiral fractures
		Wary of adult contacts
		Apprehensive when other children cry
		Behavioral extremes: aggressiveness or withdrawal
		Frightened of parents
		Afraid to go home
		Reports injury by parents

Physical neglect	Unexplained lacerations or abrasions:
	    to mouth, lips, gums, eyes
	    to external genitalia
	Consistent hunger
	Poor hygiene
	Inappropriate dress
	Consistent lack of supervision especially in dangerous activities or for long periods
	Unattended physical problems or medical needs
	Abandonment
		Begging; stealing food
		Extended stays at school (early arrival and late departure)
		Constant fatigue; listlessness or falling asleep in class
		Alcohol or drug abuse;
		Delinquency (e.g., theft)
		States there is no caretaker

Sexual abuse	Difficulty in walking or sitting
	    torn, stained, or bloody underclothing
	    pain or itching in genital area
	    bruises or bleeding in external genitalia, vaginal, or anal areas
	    venereal disease, especially in preteens
	    pregnancy
		Unwilling to change clothing in gym or participate in physical education class
		Withdrawal, fantasizing or infantile behavior
		Bizarre, sophisticated, or unusual sexual behavior or knowledge

Emotional maltreatment	Speech disorders
	Lags in physical development; failure-to-thrive
		Poor peer relationships
		Delinquent or runaway
		Reports sexual assault by caretaker
		    Habit disorders (sucking, biting, rocking)
		    Conduct disorders (antisocial, destructive)
		    Neurotic traits (sleep disorders, inhibition of play)
		    Psychoneurotic reactions (hysteria, obsession, compulsion, phobias, hypochondria)
		    Behavior extremes: compliant, passive-aggressive, demanding
		    Overly adaptive behavior: inappropriately adult; inappropriately infant
		    Developmental lags (mental, emotional)
		    Attempted suicide

[a] Source: National Center on Child Abuse and Neglect. DHHS Publications, *Child Abuse and Neglect Series.*

TABLE 29-6A *Indicators of Emotional Maltreatment of Children*

Child Behavior		Parent Behavior
Adaptation		Abusive if Consistent
Low	High	Gross Failure to Provide
Psychosocial dwarfism, poor self-esteem, self-destructive behavior, apathy, depression, withdrawal	Passive-sheltered, naive, "over-self-esteem"	Love (empathy) (praise, acceptance, self-worth)
Academic failure, pseudomental retardation, developmental delays, withdrawal	Hyperactivity, driven	Stimulation (emotional/cognitive) (talking-feeling-touching)
Symbiotic, stranger, and separation anxiety	Pseudomaturity	Individuation
Lack of integrative ability, disorganization, lack of trust	Rigid-compulsive	Stability/permanence/continuity of care
Feelings of inadequacy, passive-dependent, poor self-esteem	Pseudomaturity, role reversal	Opportunities and rewards for learning and mastering
Autistic, delusional, excessive fantasy, primary process, private (unshared) reality, paranoia	Lack of fantasy, play	Adequate standard of reality
Tantrums, impulsivity, testing behavior, defiance, antisocial behavior, conduct disorder	Fearful, hyperalert, passive, lack of creativity and exploration	Limits (moral) guidance, consequences for behavior (socialization)
Impulsivity, inappropriate, aggressive behavior, defiance, sadomasochistic behavior	Passive-aggressive, lack of awareness of anger in self/others	Control for/of aggression
Interpersonal difficulty (peer/adults), developmental lags, stranger anxiety	Lack of familial attachment, excessive peer dependence	Opportunity for extrafamilial experience
Poor peer relations, role diffusion, (deviant behavior, depending on behavior modeled)	Stereotyping rigidity, lack of creativity	Appropriate (behavior) model
Gender confusion, poor peer relations, poor self-esteem	Rigid stereotyping	Gender (sexual) identity model
Night terrors, anxiety, excessive fears	Oblivious to hazards and risks, naive	(Sense of) (provision of) security/safety

With the very young child, nursing staff will need to document the presence of physical, emotional, and behavioral signs that point to abuse (Table 29-6 A and B). A family history must be obtained from the parent. Any inconsistency in reporting the accident and the injury should be noted.

A safe, protective environment and an accepting, caring staff set the stage to begin the interview with the verbal preschool child. Knowledge of developmental abilities will enable the nurse to stay within the boundaries of the child's verbal and comprehension skills.

As the child's age and ability to express him-

TABLE 29-6B Problematic Parent Behaviors [a]

Adaptive Behaviors in Children	Parent Behavior (Abusive If Present to a Severe Degree)
Poor self-esteem, depression	Scape-goating, ridicule, denigration
Lack of purpose, determination, disorganization, or rigidity	Ambivalence
Pseudomaturity or poor self-esteem, passivity	Inappropriate expectation for behavior/performance
Depends on parent behaviors while intoxicated. (Can lead to personality disorder and/or chemical dependency)	Substance abuse
Depends on parent behaviors/type of behavior/frequency)	Psychosis
Night terrors, excessive fears Self-destructive dangerous behavior	Threats to safety/health
Sadomasochistic behavior, low self-esteem, anxiety, passivity, antisocial behavior	Physical abuse
Anxiety, excessive fear, dependency	Threatened withdrawal of love

[a] Laurie, Ira S., and Stefano, Lorraine. On defining abuse: Results of an NIMH/NCCAN Workshop. Proceedings of the Second National Conference on Child Abuse and Neglect, Vol. 1, 1977.

self increase, so does the pressure on him not to disclose "family secrets." The child becomes more aware of the possibility that he may be punished for telling someone in authority what has happened. Keeping the family secrets is usually a very strong (sometimes unspoken) rule.

The use of anatomically correct dolls will help the very young child to clearly verbalize what has happened to him. A doll is especially helpful in cases of sexual abuse, because with it the child can pinpoint the areas where the abuse occurred.

Interviewing the Adolescent □ Adolescence is a difficult time, at best, for both children and parents. It can become immensely more difficult if abuse enters into the family picture. Slapping and spanking the child may escalate to hitting the adolescent with a fist or a belt. Problems grow when the youngster enters junior high school and then high school, and is attempting to establish his identity and a degree of autonomy.

The nurse interviewing the adolescent needs to be acutely sensitive to and aware of adolescent developmental concerns. Previous interviews may have brought in their wake parental abuse (when the parent learned of the interview) or may not have been felt to be helpful. An adolescent is more fully aware than a young child of the existence of family secrets as well as of the consequences of divulging them.

Signs of physical abuse are less visible in the adolescent than in the young child, while emotional abuse and physical neglect may leave their mark in the form of delayed completion of developmental tasks, low self-esteem, low motivation to learn, acting-out, or other problems such as drug abuse. The adolescent may become the family scapegoat, because he is going through a particularly difficult and vulnerable stage.

Interviewing the Parent □ Parents may use any number of ruses to cover up, deny, or explain their abusive behavior. Their expressions of shock or dismay that another person could entertain the notion of parental abuse as the cause of injury may engender doubt in the nurse's mind, especially if the parents appear to come from a comfortable socioeconomic environment. Nevertheless, the nurse must ask the necessary questions after putting aside her personal feelings, biases, and judgments. Encouraging the parents to talk about the family situation and any other problems and concerns is important in gathering the family history, helps the parent to feel understood, and may point the way to appropriate intervention strategies.

NURSE SELF-ASSESSMENT □ The nurse dealing with child abuse and neglect needs first to assess personal attitudes, values, and belief systems that

■ **Point of Emphasis**

Parental cooperation in the information gathering process can be facilitated or impeded by the nurse's behavior. Open, direct questions need to be asked in a nonjudgmental manner. The nurse can take advantage of her position as a non-threatening, helping professional to elicit parental cooperation.

may impede positive interaction with the child and the abusive parent. Merely thinking about the pain and suffering inflicted upon a child by a parent may arouse a deep sense of anger and rejection, and a desire to punish the parent. Nonverbal messages that imply anger, contempt, or revulsion will sabotage efforts to encourage parental participation in the interview/information gathering process, effectively foreclosing opportunities to involve the parents in any activities designed to stop the abusive behavior.

Personal feelings about sexual assault of children can inhibit the nurse's ability to ask questions and seek further information; a team approach therefore is helpful if the violence has been extreme or if the victim is a very small child. The nurse's intense feelings of anger and rage need to be diffused, yet burying such feelings and proceeding as though nothing is wrong will be harmful to the nurse. By ventilating her feelings with other team members, she can work through the personal issues and maintain her objectivity toward clients. Specially trained interviewers should conduct the interviews with the child, not only to ensure the proper atmosphere, but also to ensure that evidence will stand up in court.

The nurse's personal family experiences can either enhance or impede her work in child abuse cases. If she can call upon personal strengths and positive experiences, she will be in a better position to help. If, on the other hand, earlier events have left the nurse feeling angry and resentful—feelings that might be unleashed upon an abusive parent—she will need first to face her own feelings and deal with them.

■ **Point of Emphasis**

The problem of child abuse and neglect generates emotional and judgmental feelings in the nurse. These issues must be resolved in order for the nurse to develop a healthy interactive relationship with the child and the family.

Vignette

Sue, a second-year nursing student, was assigned to work in a shelter for abused women and children as part of her community nursing course. Sue related to a staff member her personal experience with an abusive boyfriend. She was a single parent and had little family support. After the first week in the shelter, she became critical of staff procedures and objected to interacting with the children. She received a negative evaluation, prompting the supervisor to discuss the situation with Sue. Sue revealed how angry she was with her parents, her frustration at attempting to raise her child herself and continue her education, and how ashamed she felt for allowing herself to be abused. It turned out that one of the children in the center reminded her of her own situation; her self-defense took the form of criticizing the entire program. Sue was referred to a counseling agency.

Questions the nurse needs to resolve include: What sort of family background did I have? Have I worked through parental alcoholism, rejection or abandonment, divorce, child or spouse abuse?

Physically moving away from the home situation will not automatically erase the past. She must deal with the emotional issues that influence her feelings. Ventilating her feelings to a counselor or other health professional will help her to cope with her pain, as will involvement in support groups such as Al-Anon Family Groups, Alateen, or Parents Anonymous.

Stereotypes must be identified. Child abuse does not occur only in poor families, or in families of minority groups. It is important to remember that most parents do not set out to intentionally harm their child; it usually is their lack of resources, lack of knowledge of alternatives, lack of understanding a child's needs or developmental processes that leads to abusiveness. A concern that the child learn "to do better" or "not to do that again" may be the underlying justification for the abusive act.

The nurse will encounter child abuse in various situations. For many parents, the encounter with the nurse will be the first one with an authority figure who may be involved in their child's life. The positive image of nurses and nursing confers a distinct advantage through which the nurse may have access to the family system. Her caring and nonpunitive approach encourages easy communication with the family; she is able to describe her role, what she can and cannot do to help them, and what she expects of them.

The nurse must guard against becoming too attached to a child. For example, if the nurse buys toys for the child and frequently visits him during her free time, the child may seek out the nurse over his parent. This behavior is threatening to parents and can contribute to their feelings of inadequacy. Any resulting hostility and unwillingness to participate further in treatment will negate progress and the child could be further abused.

PROBLEM IDENTIFICATION □ The abused child is likely to have suffered physical injury, pain, and self-esteem disturbance secondary to physical or sexual abuse; alterations in nutrition and potential injury secondary to neglect. The abusive caretaker commonly is diagnosed as experiencing ineffective family coping in response to stressors, parenting alterations, and potential for future violence/neglect.

■ Point of Emphasis

The needs of the child are primary in any setting.

NURSING INTERVENTION □

Primary Prevention □ Nurses have a role in primary prevention of child abuse. The maternal-child nurse assesses and promotes parent-infant bonding, referring at-risk families for further assessment and support in the community. Community nurses assess parent knowledge and teach skills such as the importance of good nutrition and adequate safety, positive growth and development patterns, and effective techniques to promote self-esteem and appropriate discipline. Identifying family stressors (Table 29-4) and referring the family to the appropriate agency will reduce the potential for child abuse.

On the social level, nurses can assist in efforts to increase public awareness of the extent of child abuse and to mobilize efforts to establish and enforce protective laws and services.

Secondary Prevention □ The community nurse and the school nurse share with the emergency room nurse the responsibility to identify clues to child abuse at the earliest possible opportunity. Teachers too can be helped to identify

the physical and behavioral indicators (Tables 29-5 and 29-6). At-risk adults, those who themselves were abused or under stress, should attend parent classes and should receive supervision and support.

The nurse's primary responsibility in cases of suspected abuse is for the child's safety. She needs to be familiar with the relevant state laws in order to obtain help promptly when it is needed.

Documentation □ All data about suspected abuse or neglect must be recorded immediately. Medical and psychosocial observations need to be charted in detail in the client's record. All procedural steps must be included in the appropriate medical forms.

Table 29-7 describes nine areas applicable to the assessment/documentation process. Assessment of the home environment will not be possible for the emergency room or inpatient nurse but will be a valuable resource for the community health nurse and the school nurse. Information about the home environment may be available from other resources such as social workers and case workers.

Many medical centers include a team trained to manage cases of child abuse and neglect. Their underlying philosophy is one of support for a family in crisis, by ensuring immediate safety for the child(ren) involved, and by providing immediate assistance for their parents.

The team approach is important. If the family is already involved in the situation, a united effort is beneficial for the child, the family, and the health professional. Observed interactions between parent and child give valuable pieces of information and need to be documented accurately in the record.

■ Point of Emphasis

The health professional must have up-to-date information about mandatory reporting laws in the state, make proper referrals, and keep accurate records that could be used in legal disposition of an abuse case.

Tertiary Intervention □ The decision whether to remove the child from the home and place him in foster care or to try to maintain the support and family is a controversial one. Both alternatives carry risks. Generally the decision is made

TABLE 29-7 Assessing and Documenting Child Neglect/Abuse[a]

Physical examination
Systematically inspect child's body

Document presence (including location and appearance) of anomalies and any cuts, bruises, burns, welts, or other signs of trauma
Document signs of hygiene (such as hair clean and not matted, body crevices free of caked dirt)

Physical growth
Measure height and weight (and head circumference for child under 2 years) and plot on standard growth chart

Document age, weight, height, and percentiles in which these fall on the growth chart
Document any changes noted in serial observations of height and weight

Nutritional status
Obtain 24-hour diet history and compare to basal caloric and fluid requirements; check food supplies in cabinets and refrigerator

Document caloric and fluid intake for 24-hour period and how it compares to basal caloric and fluid requirements recommended for age, weight, and body surface area
Document type and quantity of food supplies on hand for child and instructions to family regarding appropriate foods

Home environment
Note general home conditions: temperature, ventilation; cleanliness, sanitation facilities; condition of child's sleep and play areas, including child's access to poisons, open windows, and other hazards; child's clothing; home size and number of residents

Document presence or absence of basic facilities—water, light, ventilation, heat in winter, nature and appropriateness of child's clothing, sleep area, and play area

Family history
Obtain history of stressful life events in relation to family's ability to manage stress, interventions for stress reduction, and family progress in stress management

Document stressful life events

Task development
Obtain history of age at milestones (sitting, standing, walking, talking); note ability to perform age-specific behaviors identified in a recognized developmental screening tool

Document any diagnosis of mental retardation
Document age of milestones in relation to age-specific norms
Document inability to perform age-specific developmental tasks or their quality
Document reference used in determining norm

Child care
Identify primary and all other child caretakers; observe caretaker's handling of child and performance of child-care tasks; obtain verbal description of method and frequency of well-child care and plan for sick-child care from primary caretaker

Document knowledge of child care demonstrated by primary caretaker(s)
Document teaching provided and evidence of progress in child care

Parent-child and social interactions
Observe who initiates parent-child interactions and response of parent and of child; note other people or objects with which child has opportunity to interact; note any sign of unusual behavior

Document parents' responses to child-initiated interactions (ignores crying child?), child's response to parent-initiated interactions (shies away at mother's touch or glance?), and child's interactions with nurse, with others in home, with reachable objects (curious? reaches out? ignores?)

Health history
Obtain history of mother's prenatal course, neonatal health status, and child's illnesses

Document prenatal history that may be related to child's failure-to-thrive signs (prenatal infections, smoking, drug or alcohol abuse, toxemia)
Document neonatal history that suggests organic factor in failure to thrive
Document childhood illnesses that suggest underlying metabolic or organic problem versus illness that suggests neglect

[a] Helberg, June. Documentation in Child Abuse. *American journal of nursing.* 83, 2, 1983:237–239.

by the courts after review of the evidence and consultation with social workers and other professionals.

The nurse may be involved in tertiary care in many ways. Nursing care may be requested for follow-up home care for the abused child, whether the child is placed in foster care or returned to his parents. In the latter case, family follow-up and supervision may be requested so that indications of further neglect and abuse can be noted quickly. Also, the nurse can assist in parent education and community support groups.

Research suggests that abusive parents lack self-control, have chronically high levels of anger and aggressiveness, are socially isolated, and are deficient in interpersonal relationships and parenting skills (Goldstein, et al., 1985). Appropriate support groups address these specific problems as well as aspects of group dynamics. (See also Chapter 13.)

Self-control Skills. Learning self-control involves a sequence of basic skills. Initially, clients must learn to monitor and identify their own feelings. Useful techniques include modeling of real-life situations in which intense feelings arise and exploring ways in which the feelings can lead to either destructive or constructive actions. Roleplay may help clients to identify their behavior patterns and attempt alternative behaviors. Progress in everyday situations can be noted and related to the group for discussion. Skills in problem solving and stress management may be valuable in portraying effective ways to deal with feelings.

Expressing Anger. Skills in communication (e.g., "I" messages, assertiveness, and conflict resolution) are the basis for effectively expressing anger and coping with it. Learning to verbally express displeasure at another person's behavior rather than engaging in a physical or verbal assault on the person is the initial skill to be mastered, and mastery of this skill alone may significantly decrease the incidents of psychological abuse within the family. Learning assertiveness permits the person to become more effective in communicating needs rather than passively and resentfully repressing them until he "explodes." Conflict resolution skills then promote interpersonal exchanges based on awareness of the needs of both self and others rather than on power struggles and intimidation.

Social Skills. Increasing social contacts and skills serves to reduce the isolation that adds to family stress and increases the likelihood of

abuse. People may need assistance in mastering basic skills such as initiating a social conversation, listening, expressing appreciation, and asking for or offering help to others. The group is an effective arena in which both teaching and practicing can be carried out.

Parenting and Marital Skills. All the skills described above are pertinent to family living. In addition, anticipatory guidance about the growth and development needs of children and about common family stresses may correct misconceptions and promote more realistic expectations in the parent-child relationship. Other key factors, often overlooked, are empathy and positive reinforcement skills. Being able to listen and understand the other person's viewpoint generally brings about a greater degree of tolerance, support, and flexibility in family roles and relationships. The importance of affection and positive reinforcement cannot be overestimated; many families need help in expressing the positive feelings they have for one another. Strengths need to be acknowledged and people need to know they are valued. Families can be assisted to express positive feelings in many ways—such as hugging, kind or humorous expressions, and acts of kindness.

EVALUATION □ Evaluating changes in the lives of the abuse victim and the family is crucial to monitoring both the client's physical safety and the family's growth and effectiveness. The nurse needs to work closely with the designated social service agency to share observations and coordinate services. Criteria for evaluating progress need to be developed in the following areas: (1) The victim: careful physical monitoring and notation of changes in psychosocial behaviors. (2) The family: reduction in abusive behavior, increased parenting knowledge and skills, impulse control, better socialization and interpersonal relations. (3) The nurse: knowledge of the characteristics associated with abuse, awareness of legal requirements for documenting and reporting, attitudes and effectiveness in working with families, and knowledge of support services for referral and assistance.

□ *Elderly Abuse/Neglect*

As the population of older persons increases, so does abuse of that group. Though data are limited, the incidence of elderly abuse is believed to be comparable to child abuse, that is, one in 10 families is involved (Anderson, 1981; Beck and Phillips, 1983). It is projected that 30.6 million Americans will be above age 65 by the year 2000 (Sanders and Plumer, 1983), and by the year 2040, the number of those over 85 years of age will increase from 2.2 million to 13 million (Gelman, et al., 1985).

As the numbers of elderly increase, the numbers of adult children available as caretakers will decrease. Hence, an adult married couple may be in the position of having to care for two sets of parents. This may become a staggering responsibility for adults with dependent parents. Approximately 95 percent of the elderly population live at home, most of them independently. The frail elderly, however, depend on others for economic, emotional, or physical care. The caretaker is usually a family member, most frequently a spouse or a daughter. The frail elderly were defined in a 1976 Report to the President of the Federal Council on Aging as those older individuals, who because of problems related to health, economics, housing, or support systems, found it difficult to cope and are dependent on others for assistance in normal activities.

It is often falsely assumed that the majority of frail elderly who are bedfast and/or housebound are living in institutions—actually twice as many live at home than in institutions (Phillips, 1978; Shanas, 1979b). These persons receive care according to the following figures: 39 percent, spouse; 20 percent, children outside the household; 6 percent, others in the household; 3 percent, paid helpers; 6 percent, relatives outside the household; 11 percent, nonrelatives outside the household; 14 percent, self; less than 1 percent, social service agencies (Shanas, 1979b).

EVIDENCE OF ABUSE

Many frail elderly people receive safe, adequate, and loving care from their caregivers; but many others are not as fortunate. Phillips (1980) has identified four elements that support the belief that the abuse of elderly dependent persons is more widespread than statistics indicate.

1. The relevant literature reveals that intra-family violence is a significant phenomenon in the American culture.
2. The concept of the cycle of violence suggests that abused children often become abusive spouses and later become abusive to their parents.
3. Literature of child abuse and spouse abuse

reveals patterns that can readily be generalized to older persons. The elderly person may be perceived to be difficult, different, or troublesome.

4. Health care providers informally acknowledge the existence of elderly abuse. They believe that long-term illness and dependency provoke abuse and neglect, though why some families can cope well and others cannot is not known. Family relationships that existed before the person became dependent may play an important role.

The home health nurse sees clients with Alzheimer's disease in the home setting. Because of high costs, lack of third-party reimbursement, and the reluctance on the part of many nursing homes to accept these patients, many are living at home with spouses or children. Alzheimer's disease causes a severe drain on time, emotions, energy, and finances of the caretakers. Without community support and respite care, the burden could be unbearable. Yet, most family members whom we have observed have been incredibly loving, and provide safe, excellent care. These beneficial relationships may be a natural extension of the earlier family relationship and the family also may be adept in searching out effective support networks.

SITUATIONS THAT CAN LEAD TO ELDER ABUSE

1. The disappearance of the extended family unit (Podniek, 1983). In the past there was an expectation that the elderly parent would live in the home of an adult child. The aged parent often contributed greatly to family maintenance through caring for children and doing household tasks, thereby holding a respected place in the family. Today, with the loss of the extended family setting and the resulting community family life, elderly parents are often isolated from their children and grandchildren. Relationships deteriorate, and roles of respect are absent.
2. Role reversal (Ferguson and Beck, 1983). Adult children often must assume the role of parent to their aged parents. They may have responsibility for managing the parent's financial affairs, being the primary or only social contact for the aged parent, making decisions for the parent, taking

care of the physically dependent or mentally impaired parent on a day-to-day basis.

3. Living under the same roof (Ferguson and Beck, 1983). When frail elderly live with their children problems may follow: the elderly parent may invade the family's privacy; the family may resent taking on added financial responsibilities; and the constant care of the elderly person can cause fatigue, social isolation, and stress.

4. The personality/socialization of the caregiver. Individual personality or the socializing process may cause a person to feel no responsibility to the aged parent, and an adult child who had been abused by the parent when a child may retaliate in kind against the dependent parent. Either way, the parent may be neglected or his situation denied.

FORMS OF ABUSE

Lau and Kosberg (1978) define four categories of abuse toward the frail elderly person:

1. Physical neglect—lack of provision of nutrition, medication, and treatment. This form of abuse is seen with some regularity by home health nurses. Often the elderly person lives alone, trying to cope with a chronic illness, such as diabetes or congestive heart failure. His memory may be impaired to the degree that he remembers some events, but cannot remember to take his medication. The person may have physical problems, such as leg ulcers, for which a family member has agreed to provide care, but then missed visits to bathe and dress the wounds. The parent's diet may be dangerously inadequate. These situations may lead to catastrophic outcomes, such as losing a limb.

2. Emotional neglect—lack of love, interpersonal relationships, and esteem. The elderly person may be isolated from the family, receiving no phone calls, visits, or letters. Physical needs may be attended to, but the elderly person has no one to relate to or confide in on a personal level. Elderly persons who have telephone contact with friends or neighbors fare better than those who depend solely on family for emotional support.

Emotional abuse can also take the form of verbal tirades on the part of the caretaker. Blaming and devaluing occur. The older person may also suffer acutely because he is never touched. Adult children, caretakers, and nurses are often unaware of the need the aged have to be touched. Persons of all ages need and respond to the warmth that goes with holding, touching, and hugging. Persons living alone in their houses or living in nursing homes are most likely to suffer from this form of neglect.

3. Physical abuse. An elderly person suffers the same types of abuse that children and victims of spouse abuse endure (e.g., being slapped, knocked down, kicked) and often remains silent for fear of losing the caretaker.

4. Material abuse—unjust use or manipulation of the elderly's persons income or property, which may be "stolen or converted" by the caretaker, by force or misrepresentation (Giordano and Giordano, 1984).

CHARACTERISTICS OF ABUSED PERSONS

The majority of abused elders tend to be caucasian women over 75 years of age. They have at least one significant physical or mental handicap, are widowed, and live with relatives (Lau and Kos-

---

Vignette

Mrs. J. exemplified a problem seen by home health care nurses. When then nurse entered the home to give routine care, she found Mrs. J. with a cut on her forehead, a cut and a bruise on her eye and cheek, and a leg that was black and blue and swollen. Mrs. J., who was 89 years old, told the nurse that she had fallen. However, she was nervous and evasive, and did not make eye contact with the nurse. Mrs. J.'s caretaker was her 50-year-old nephew, unemployed due to a chronic mental illness. He was known to be intimidating and verbally abusive. Mrs. J. was dependent on him for food, medication, and transportation, and he responded to those needs. The nurse was disturbed and returned later in the day to talk to Mrs. J. When questioned with sensitivity about her injuries, Mrs. J. admitted that her nephew hit her and knocked her down when she irritated him by interrupting some activity. She later protected the nephew because she feared having her living situation changed.

berg, 1978; Block and Sinnott, 1979). Daughters were the perpetrators of abuse twice as often as any other relative, followed by sons, granddaughters, husbands, and siblings (Lau and Kosberg, 1978).

NURSE SELF-ASSESSMENT □ One barrier the nurse may need to overcome in order to effectively prevent or detect elderly abuse is to recognize that the problem does exist. Many professionals who accept the possibility of wife battering and child abuse deny that anyone would abuse an aged, helpless parent (Rathbone-McCuan and Voyles, 1982). Once abuse is identified the nurse must face her personal beliefs and feelings about aged persons. If she believes elderly people are worthy of dignity and respect, she will see that their rights are attended to.

The nurse must remember that the elderly person's concerns must be taken into account. A hasty referral, as by removing the aged person from the home, could lead to greater dissatisfaction and unhappiness. The nurse needs to deal objectively with the abuser so she can determine whether counseling, respite care, and referrals (such as day care) would ease the family situation and perhaps help the elderly person remain where he desires.

Signals of Elder Abuse □ Some warning signs have been identified to help the nurse recognize possible abuse situations (Sanders and Plumer, 1983; Ferguson and Beck, 1983): the person offers an illogical account of how the injury occurred; has poor self-esteem; has multiple contusions or abrasions; is reluctant to give information; seeks treatment many days after being injured; is treated as a child by the caregiver; is passive and withdrawn; or shows signs of inadequate nutrition or of dehydration.

It is important to take a careful history in helping the elderly person who presents with an injury in the clinic, emergency room, physician's office, or home setting. A comprehensive form is helpful in classifying the type of abuse that occurred so that help and referral can be offered. Table 29-8 gives an example of an Abuse Report Form (ARF) devised by Block and Sinnott (1979). Phillips has added some specific types of abuse to this form, and they are included in the table. Such a form is an aid to the nurse in determining if abuse has occurred and judging its severity (Phillips, 1980).

Legislation and Reporting □ Laws on elderly abuse are defined by state legislatures. The laws may be limited in describing types of abuse as well as in defining the abused person.

PROBLEM IDENTIFICATION □ Nursing diagnoses include actual and potential injuries related to physical abuse; malnutrition and fluid deficit related to neglect; impaired skin integrity and joint contracture related to being tied to a chair or bed for prolonged periods (often in wet or soiled linens); self-esteem disturbances secondary to physical and/or psychological abuse. Related elder conditions which may predispose the caretaker to elder abuse include self-care deficits, cognitive impairment, impaired communication and sensory deficits, and social isolation.

Diagnoses commonly found in abusive caregivers include violence and potential for violence, ineffective individual coping, and ineffective family coping with stress. These coping deficits may be related to isolation from support systems or an unfair distribution of responsibility and a perception of being overburdened on the part of the primary caregiver.

INTERVENTION □ The nurse who has reasonable cause to believe that abuse is taking place has a moral responsibility to report it. Others who are likely to observe an abused elderly person are doctors, nurses, social workers, administrators of nursing homes, persons in charge of nutrition sites, senior centers, adult day care centers, funeral directors, dentists, home aides, family members, relatives, neighbors, and friends (Ferguson and Beck, 1983). The report can be made to the police department or the local department of public welfare, usually to the Adult Protective Service (APS) branch.

Primary Prevention □ Primary prevention really begins at birth! Ideally, nonviolent coping mechanisms should be taught through the life span. Present strategies include the following:

1. Increase outside activities and socialization for the elderly person in order to promote self-esteem and independence and decrease dependence on the caregiver.
2. Facilitate opportunities for caregivers to ventilate feelings of anger, frustration, guilt, hopelessness, and fatigue toward the care of their elderly charges (Podniek, 1983).
3. Educate family members about the normal aging process and help change negative at-

TABLE 29-8 Abuse Report Form (ARF)[a]

	Degree of Severity Mild Moderate Severe				
	1	2	3	4	5
Physical					
Bruises, welts	___	___	___	___	___
Sprains, dislocations	___	___	___	___	___
Malnutrition, dehydration	___	___	___	___	___
Freezing or excessively hot	___	___	___	___	___
Burns, scalding	___	___	___	___	___
Wounds, cuts, punctures	___	___	___	___	___
Internal injuries	___	___	___	___	___
Dismemberment	___	___	___	___	___
Bone fractures	___	___	___	___	___
Skull fractures	___	___	___	___	___
Direct beatings	___	___	___	___	___
Lack of personal care	___	___	___	___	___
Lack of food, inappropriate food	___	___	___	___	___
Lack of medical care	___	___	___	___	___
Lack of supervision	___	___	___	___	___
Tied to chair	___	___	___	___	___
Tied to bed	___	___	___	___	___
Decubitus ulcers	___	___	___	___	___
Perineal excoriations	___	___	___	___	___
Physica force used in care	___	___	___	___	___
Inappropriate clothing	___	___	___	___	___
Other (describe) _____	___	___	___	___	___
Psychological					
Verbal assault	___	___	___	___	___
Threat	___	___	___	___	___
Fear	___	___	___	___	___
Isolation	___	___	___	___	___
Refusal of reasonable requests for diversion	___	___	___	___	___
Use of derogatory terms to describe subject	___	___	___	___	___
Usurping attention of health professional	___	___	___	___	___
Other (describe) _____	___	___	___	___	___
Material					
Theft of money or property	___	___	___	___	___
Misuse of money or property	___	___	___	___	___
Income withheld	___	___	___	___	___
Other (describe) _____	___	___	___	___	___
Rights					
Forced from home	___	___	___	___	___
Forced into nursing home	___	___	___	___	___
Forced to stay in home not desired	___	___	___	___	___
Other (describe) _____	___	___	___	___	___
Medical					
No medication purchased when prescribed	___	___	___	___	___
No false teeth when needed	___	___	___	___	___
No hearing aid when needed	___	___	___	___	___
No glasses when needed	___	___	___	___	___
No assistive devices that would improve functioning	___	___	___	___	___
Inappropriate medications (too much or too little), substance abuse encouraged	___	___	___	___	___
Other (describe) _____	___	___	___	___	___
Environmental					
Dirt in house	___	___	___	___	___
Vermin in house	___	___	___	___	___
Odor of urine	___	___	___	___	___
Inadequate heating or cooling	___	___	___	___	___
No food in house	___	___	___	___	___
No means of summoning help	___	___	___	___	___
No transportation for essential needs	___	___	___	___	___
Other (describe) _____	___	___	___	___	___

[a] Block and Sinnott, 1979. (Additions by Phillips, 1980.)

titudes toward the elderly (Ferguson and Beck, 1983).

4. Counsel families to involve other relatives, friends, and neighbors in some aspects of socialization and care needs of the elderly person so care can be shared by many caregivers (Ferguson and Beck, 1983).

5. Inform family members and the elderly person about helpful resources that could reduce family stress. Examples of resources are home health aides, meals-on-wheels, adult day care services, elderly transportation services, and companions provided through an office or agency on aging.

6. Facilitate increased public awareness and legislative involvement in providing economic aid in caring for the frail elderly person.

Secondary Prevention □ The nurse needs to make thorough assessments of high-risk and actual abuse situations in order to secure prompt treatment. If abuse is identified, Adult Protective Services (APS) should be called. Most states sponsor agencies that follow specific guidelines relating to elderly abuse and neglect. If APS intervenes they may be expected to respond within 24 hours of the report. They will interview the elderly person, family members, and the reporting nurse or agency; can offer supportive services, such as providing meals and medical transportation; and will work with the family for 60 days. If the aged person is in immediate danger, APS will refer him to a hospital or make other living arrangements. It may be necessary to seek the help of a law enforcement agency or legal aid services (Johnson, 1979).

Tertiary Prevention □ If the patient remains with the abusive caretaker, the community nurse or social worker must provide supportive care and continually evalute the situation (Johnson, 1979). Respite care is valuable for aged persons and families to enable the caretaker to regain the energy needed to continue caring for the elderly (Ferguson and Beck, 1983). Many of the interventions identified for primary prevention are also effective in reducing stress and the potential for abuse, in combination with careful monitoring by community nurses or service workers. Careful physical assessment to detect signs of abuse or neglect is needed.

■ Enrichment Activities

DISCUSSION QUESTIONS

1. Most married couples engage in conflict at one time or another. How do you distinguish between conflict and violence?

2. Discuss the following marital situations:

   a. Henry had had a very difficult day at work on Friday. The boss criticized him for turning in some reports late. A bill collector called him at the office. (Henry has long since given up his weekend golf since he took a second job to help pay the mortgage.) When Henry came home from work, his wife, Mary, met him at the door and related her problems: the washer broke down; the baby has diaper rash; the 2-year-old ate some aspirin and had to be rushed to the poison control center. Dinner was not yet started. Mary began to cry, "Why can't you help more? If you asked for a raise we could get some help." Henry entered his home hoping for some solace. Mary needed to share her frustration. Henry felt enraged. He wanted to scream, hit out. Discuss ways that Henry might handle the conflict without the use of verbal or physical violence. Discuss ways that Mary could have handled her frustration.

   b. Mike comes home from work and starts to complain about Jane's housekeeping. He criticizes the way she takes care of the children. At dinner, he complains that the meat is too well done. Jane works very hard to please Mike, but it seems that no matter what she does, he complains. She also knows that when he is in a certain mood he will hit her or shove her around. Jane has lived under this tension for 8 years. Discuss some reasons why Jane may still be living in this stressful situation. Discuss alternatives she might explore.

3. A majority of people believe that it is all right to spank or hit children to discipline them. How do you feel about this? Can you think of alternative methods of discipline?

4. Have you ever thought about becoming a parent? Have you thought about the frustration of that role as well as the joys? Have you thought about the responsibility? If you are a woman, what portion of responsibility do you expect

your mate to take in childrearing? If you are a man, how involved do you intend to be in raising your children? If you are about to be married, have you discussed these issues with each other? You and your future spouse may come from different backgrounds with different parental behaviors toward childrearing. With this in mind, how will the two of you respond to childrearing?

5. What is it about the stage of adolescence that causes family conflict? Name three teenage behaviors that upset parents. Role-play them. One student takes the part of the teen and another the part of the parent for each of the three situations.

6. An elderly parent who is partially disabled has moved into the home of one of his adult children. The adult caretaker's spouse and two teenage children also live in the household. Discuss some preventive measures the family can take to avoid frustration in caring for the elderly parent.

LEARNING ACTIVITY

Check with your local child and adult protective services for the reporting laws in your state and the procedures for reporting suspected child and elder abuse and neglect.

SUPPLEMENTAL MEDIA

IBIS Media, *Violence in the Family*, slide presentation, 175 Tomkins Ave., Pleasantville, NY, 10570, 1978.
    Part I: Dynamics of Family Violence, 10 min.
    Part II: Child abuse and Neglect, 12 min.
    Part III: Battered Wives, 12 min.
    Part IV: Adolescent Abuse, 10 min.

Soft in the Heart of a Child, 16 mm., Available through a chemical dependency program in your community or a medical film library.

■ Recommended Readings

Davis, James. *Help me, I'm hurt: The child abuse handbook*. Dubuque, IA: Kendall/Hunt Publishing Co., 1982.

Fortune, Marie, and Horman, Denise. *Family violence: A workshop manual for clergy and other service providers*. 1914 N. 34th St., Suite 205, Seattle, WA, 98103: The center for the Prevention of Sexual and Domestic Violence, 1980.

■ References

Anderson, C. Abuse and neglect among the elderly. *Journal of georontological nursing*, 7, 2 (February 1981):77–85.

Bandura, A.; Ross, D.; and Ross, S.A. Transmission of aggression through imitation of aggression. *Journal of abnormal and social psychology*, 63, 1961:575–582.

Bard, M., and Berkowitz, B. Training police as specialists in family crisis interventions: A community psychology action program. *Community mental health journal*, 3, 1967:315–317.

Beck, C., and Phillips. L. Abuse of the elderly. *Journal of gerontological nursing*, 9, 2 (February 1983): 96–101.

Belsky, Jay. "Child maltreatment: An ecological integration," *American psychologist*, 35, 4 (April 1980):320–335.

Block, M.R., and Sinnott, J.D. *The battered elder syndrome: An exploratory study*. College Park, MD: Center on Aging, University of Maryland, 1979.

Blumenthal, M.; Kahn, R.L.; Andrews, F.M.; and Head, K.B. Justifying violence: The attitude of American men. Ann Arbor, MI: Institute for social research, 1972:243.

Bradley v. *State*. Walter, 158, Miss. 1824

Braen, Richard G. *The rape examination in hospitals*. American College of Emergency Physicians, Dallas, TX: Abbot Laboratories, Abbot Park, 1981.

Burgess, Ann W., and Holmstrom, Lynda L. "Rape trauma syndrome," *Nursing Digest*, May-June, 1975:17–19.

Densen-Gerber, Judianne. 3rd International Congress on Child Abuse and Neglect. Amsterdam, The Netherlands, April 21–25, 1981.

Feguson, D., and Beck, C. "H.A.L.F.: A tool to assess elder abuse within the family," *Geriatric Nursing*, Sept.-Oct., 1983.

Fortune, Marie M. *Sexual violence: The unmentionable sin: An ethical and pastoral perspective*. Chapter 1. New York: Pilgrim Press, 1983.

Ganley, Ann. Court mandated counseling for men who batter. A three-day workshop for mental health professionals. Washington, D.C.: Center for Women's Policy Studies, 1981.

Ganley, A., and Nickles, N. Counseling men who batter their mates. Workshop sponsored by the Center for Women's Policy Studies, Coral Gables, Florida, February 1981.

Garbarino, J. The family: A school for living. *National elementary principal*, 55 (May-June 1976):66–70.

———. The meaning and implications of school success. *The educational forum*. 40, 1976:178–185.

Garbarino, James, and Gilliam, Given. *Understanding*

abusive families. Lexington Books, Lexington, Mass, 1980.

Gelles, R.J., and Cornell, C.P. *Intimate violence in families.* Beverly Hills, CA: Sage, 1985.

Gelles, R.J., and Straus, M. Report to the National Conference on Child Abuse and Neglect. Chicago, Oct. 18, 1985.

Gelman, David; Hager, Mary; Gonzalas, D.; Morris, H.; McCormick, J.; Jackson, T.A.; and Karageanis, E. Who's taking care of your parents? *Newsweek*, May 6, 1985.

Gil, David. Unraveling Child Abuse: A holistic perspective on child abuse and its prevention. *American journal of orthopsychiatry*, 45, 3 (April 1975):346–356.

————. *Beyond the jungle: Essays on human possibilities, social alternatives and radical practices.* United Kingdom, Hall Co., London, 1979.

Giordano, N. and Giordano, J. Elder abuse: A review of the literature. *Social work* (May/June, 1984):232–236.

Goldstein, A.; Keller, H.; and Erne, D. *Changing the abusive patient.* Champaign, IL: Research Press, 1985.

Goodstein, Richard K., and Page, Ann W. Battered wife syndrome: A review of dynamics and treatment. *American journal of psychiatry*, 138, 8 (August 1981):1036–1044.

Gordon, Marjory. *Manual of nursing diagnosis.* New York: McGraw-Hill, 1985.

Greany, Geraldine. Is she a battered woman? A guide for emergency response. *American journal of nursing*, 84, 6, 1984:725–727.

Helberg, June L. Documentation in Child Abuse. *American journal of nursing*, 83, 2 (February 1983): 237–239.

Horney, Karen. The Flight from Womanhood. *International journal of psychoanalysis.* 7, 1976:324–339.

Jayaratne, S. Child abusers as parents and children: A review. *Social work*, 22, 1977:5–9.

Johnson, Douglas G. Abuse and neglect—not for children only. *Journal of gerontological nursing*, 5, 1979:11–13.

Kempe, C. Henry, and Helfer, Ray E. (eds.). *The battered child.* 3d ed. Chicago: The University of Chicago Press, 1980.

Kirkland, Karl. Assessment and treatment of family violence. *The journal of family practice.* 14, 4, 1982:713–718.

Lau, E., and Kosberg, J. Abuse of the elderly by informal care providers: Practice and research issues. Paper presented at the 31st Annual Meeting of The Gerontological Society, Dallas, Texas, 1978.

Laurie, Ira S., and Stefano, Lorraine. On defining emotional abuse: Results of an NIMH/NCCAN work-shop. Second National Conference on Child Abuse and Neglect, Vol. 1, 1977.

McNeely, R., and Jones, J. Refuge from violence: Establishing shelter services for battered women. *Administration in social work*, 4, 4 (Winter, 1980):71–82.

Newberger Eli H. (ed.). *Child abuse.* Boston: Little, Brown & Co., 1982.

Owens, David J., and Straus, Murray A. The social structure of violence in childhood and approval of violence as an adult. *Aggressive behavior*, 1, 2, 1975:193–211.

Phillips, Linda R. Neglect, abuse and feelings of neglect among a sample of elder individuals. Manuscript, Tucson: University of Arizona, 1978.

————. Family relationships between two samples of frail elderly individuals. Doctoral dissertation, University of Arizona, Tucson, 1980.

Pizzey, E., *Scream quietly or the neighbors will hear*, London: Anchor Press, 1974.

Price, John, and Armstrong, Jean, Battered wives: A controlled study of predisposition. *Australian and New Zealand journal of psychiatry*, 12, 1 (March 1978):43–47.

Podniek, E. Abuse of the elderly. *Canadian nurse*, 79, 5 (May 1983):34–35.

Rathbone-McCuan, E., and Voyles, B. Case detection of abused elderly parents. *American journal of psychiatry*, 139 (February 1982):2.

Raven, B., and Rubin, J. *Social psychology: People in groups.* New York: John Wiley & Sons, 1976.

Robitscher, Jonas. Battered wives and battered children. Symposium B.W. and B.C. Annual Interdisciplinary Symposium in Law and Behavioral Sciences, 1977:374–379.

Ruether, R. Motherearth and the megamachine: A theology of liberation in a feminine, somatic and ecological perspective. In *Woman spirit rising* (Christ, C., and Plaskow, J., ed.). New York: Harper & Row, 1979:44.

Sadoff, Robert L. Violence in families: An overview. *The bulletin*, 1976:292–296.

Sanders, F., and Plumer, E. Assault on the aged—Is your patient a secret victim? *Registered nurse*, (July 1983:21–25.

Shanas, Ethel. The family as a social support system in old age. *The gerontologist*, 19, 1979a:169–174.

————. Social myth as hypothesis: The case of family relations of old people. *The gerontologist*, 19, 1979b:3–9.

State v. *Oliver*, 70, N.C., 60, 61, 1874.

Steinmetz, Suzanne. *The cycle of violence: Assertive, aggressive, and abusive family interaction*, New York: Praeger, 1977.

Steinmetz, Suzanne K., and Straus, Murray A. (eds.).

Violence in the family. New York: Dodd, Mead and Company, 1974.

Straus, Murray. Wife Beating, How Common and Why? *Victimotology: An international journal*, 2, 3–4 (November 1978):443–458.

Straus, Murray A.; Gelles, Richard J.; and Steinmetz, Suzanne K. *Behind closed doors*. Garden City NY: Anchor Press/Doubleday, 1980.

Symonds, Martin. The psychodynamics of violence-prone marriages. *The American journal of psychoanalysis*, 38, 3, 1978:213–322.

Thompson, Clara. Cultural pressures in the psychology of women. *Psychiatry*, 5, 1942:147–155.

U.S. Department of Health and Human Services Publication. Family, violence: Intervention strategies, Washington, D.C., May 1980.

Walker, L. *The battered woman*, New York: Harper & Row, 1979.

Washburne, Carolyn (Coordinator); Backiel, Linda; Daily, Susan; Washborne, C. (Eds.). *Women in Transition: A feminist handbook on separation and divorce*. Charles Scribner's Sons: New York, 1975.

PART SIX

Nursing Process and Major Psychiatric Disorders

All levels of prevention are addressed in nursing care for identified psychiatric disorders of childhood, adolescence, and adulthood. Emphasis is placed on understanding and acknowledging persons and their comprehensive needs for care. Both DSM III and nursing diagnosis terminology are incorporated.

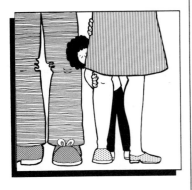

30

Disorders of Childhood

Stephanie Stockard

Learning Objectives

Upon completion of this chapter, the reader will be able to:

1. Identify five major categories from which emotional disorders originate.

2. Describe emotional and behavioral disorders that may develop at various developmental stages of childhood.

3. Identify problems pertinent to specific disorders of childhood.

4. Develop nursing interventions specific to emotional disorders of childhood.

5. Recognize the influence of familial or environmental factors on development, progress, and treatment of emotional disorders of childhood.

6. Identify specialized nursing skills essential in working with an emotionally disturbed child and his/her family.

7. Describe various types of treatment modalities used for emotionally disturbed children.

The Joint Commission on Mental Health in Children (1969) distinguishes five major categories from which emotional disorders originate. These are (1) faulty training and faulty life experiences; (2) surface conflicts between children and parents during adjustment to siblings, school, social, and sexual development; (3) deeper conflicts internalized within the self that create emotional conflict; (4) difficulties associated with physical handicaps and disorders; and (5) difficulties associated with severe mental disorders.

An emotionally disturbed child is one whose progressive personality development is interfered with or arrested, resulting in impairment of a reasonably accurate perception of the world around him, impulse control, the ability to establish satisfying and satisfactory relations with others, learning, or any combination of these. Disturbances in intellectual, emotional, behavioral, physical, or developmental areas signals a troubled child.

The numbers of children and families who need mental health services continue to outweigh the current treatment facilities and trained professionals. Societal, biological, economic, familial, and racial factors individually or in combination may place a child at risk for emotional disorders. Political and economic climates have a strong influence on preventive services, such as prenatal screening, nutrition, genetic counseling, and parenting education, which are primary to healthy child development.

The child's development is marked by both spurts and plateaus, yet optimally progresses daily, sometimes, it seems, hourly. The child is engaged daily in processing a new world of strange, joyful, frightening, and awesome sensations. In most children this complex activity proceeds with little fanfare—it's just part of growing up. (See Chapter 1.) For others, however, interferences and obstacles from a variety of sources may cause a lag in, inhibition of, or permanent damage to the realization of a positive sense of self, an awareness of who the child is, and where he fits into the world around him.

☐ Problems of Infancy and Early Childhood

REACTIVE ATTACHMENT DISORDER OF INFANCY: Trust versus Mistrust

According to the Diagnostic and Statistical Manual of Mental Disorders (DSM III) reactive attachment disorder of infancy may be recognized as early as 1 month after birth but not later than 8 months, since attachment would have occurred before 8 months had the infant received adequate care.

The disorder, sometimes known as nonorganic failure to thrive, is due to deficient caretaking. As early as 2 months of age, the infant seems apathetic, not responding to voices or reaching out to the mother. A weak cry, poor muscle tone, weak rooting response, and low activity level characterize the infant's behavior. Before 8 months of age, the child fails to demonstrate social responsiveness, smiling response, and reciprocal gazing. He does not visually track eyes and faces. By 7 or 8 months, the baby might not crawl or express vocal or visual communication with the caretaker. Observation may be done in the pediatrician's office or the well-child clinic. Observation of mother-infant interaction at home provides the most accurate picture, though.

> ### ■ *Point of Emphasis*
> *Any interference with bonding can predispose an infant to reactive attachment disorder of infancy.*

Illness, indifference, neglect, severe depression, psychosis, lack of support or parenting information, and fears of hurting the baby are frequent in disturbances of bonding. The mother may have been extremely deprived herself and unable to convey a caring attitude or may not have learned maternal behaviors. The infant's temperament may elicit maternal frustration or rejection, or the infant may be unwanted or regarded as less than a human being. Other contributing factors are lack of tactile stimulation and early separation from the mother or caregiver.

Fischhoff (1979) outlines five indicators of a severely disturbed mother-infant relationship (when no organic problem exists): (1) marasmus (wasting and illness); (2) extreme irritability, difficult to soothe; (3) lethargy, unresponsiveness; (4) diminished or absent vocalization and (5) marked developmental arrest.

Obviously, if the situation giving rise to the disorder continues, the baby could die from malnutrition and/or infection. The lack of psychosocial stimulation may be evidenced in feeding disorders which may eventually cause starvation.

The mother may avoid the baby, may neither touch, stroke, nor cuddle him, and may even avoid providing routine care to the baby. Conversely, she may feel anxious and irritable toward the baby, may insist on feeding him even when he rejects the food, or may handle him roughly and overstimulate him, so that he vomits or spits up (Fischhoff, 1979).

Table 30-1 summarizes key elements involved in nurse/family interaction. The outcome is hopeful if intervention is immediate. Although the situation seems to be reversible, it is not yet established whether early deprivation can affect the child's long-range potential.

PERVASIVE DEVELOPMENTAL DISORDERS

As the phrase suggests, pervasive developmental disorders are characterized by concurrent difficulties in multiple areas. The DSM III distinguishes between *pervasive* disorders—those simultaneously affecting language, perception, reality testing, social skills, and motor development—and *specific* developmental disorders—such as a receptive language disorder.

Infantile Autism

Probably the most prominent among these disorders is infantile autism. Approximately 1 to 2 percent of infants are affected, the ratio of boys to girls being 3:2. In the past, autism, childhood schizophrenia, profound retardation, and brain damage have been considered together with no clear distinctions made. The DSM III, however, describes infantile autism as a separate disorder.

The behaviors of the autistic baby are evident in the first months of life, and are full-blown before 2-½ years of age. Four areas are most obviously affected: relatedness, communication, environmental response, and physical and motor responses. Most prominent among these is the inability to develop interpersonal relationships.

The infant does not "mold" when picked up, lacks eye contact, and appears apathetic to expressions of affection or to physical contact. Normal attachment behavior, such as anticipatory reaching out and gazing and smiling at familiar faces is absent. The older baby may demonstrate awareness of others, but does not advance to cooperative play, and exhibits only superficial social responses.

Communication, both verbal and nonverbal, is impaired. Facial expressions and gestures may be bizarre or absent. Language may be delayed or absent. The child may be unable to name objects, may demonstrate echolalia, and often responds to statements with merely a querulous grunt. His grammar is faulty and unstructured. He may refer to "you" when he means "me" and may have speech idiosyncracies. It is difficult to establish the presence of language retardation, however, before 18 months of age. At 6 months the infant's babbling, which may have been delayed, stops altogether, and by 2 years, the child is mute or echolalic (Fish, 1979).

Response to the environment varies among autistic children, but it is usually bizarre. Some children demonstrate great distress about environmental changes such as rearranged furniture, retracing steps, going in reverse in a car, or a change in routine. The child often displays his dis-

TABLE 30-1 Caring for the Child with Reactive Attachment Disorder: Key Concepts	
Self-awareness	Tendency to blame mother; rescue feelings interfere with intervention.
Support	Mother needs support, not blame; may not know how to nurture or may be unable to do so. Economic support often needed.
Education	Teach mother or caretaker importance of touching baby and talking to him; how to give physical care. Role model how to care for baby, but don't "take over." Give mother encouragement and praise.
Legal	Contact protective services—situation may warrant temporary or permanent removal from home.
Therapeutic	Severe maternal emotional disorders warrant psychiatric intervention. Family therapy may be indicated.

Vignette

Peter, age 4, was diagnosed as demonstrating infantile autism. Aside from other behavioral manifestations, Peter had an unusual speech pattern. He liked the characters Bert and Ernie of the television show "Sesame Street" and talked to them, using Bert and Ernie puppets. Frequently when he spoke about himself, it was as though Ernie or Bert was talking. "Look, Bert's hungry" or "Ernie sleeps now. Let Ernie sleep."

Vignette

Roger, age 3, had no relationships with others and could not interact verbally, but he could recite from memory books and articles read to him. His remarkable recitations were in marked contrast to his interpersonal communication. He might be heard quoting from his bird book, "The osprey is a bird of the genus *Pandion haliactus* and is a large brown-and-white fish-eating hawk."

---

tress by screeching, growling, and/or flapping his hands in panic. For no apparent reason, he may become attached to a certain object such as a stick, a game piece, or part of a toy.

Motor behavior is abnormal. He may rock, may spin objects repeatedly, and may appear fascinated by fans, tops, and the like. There may be ritualistic behavior as shown in hand or facial movements or insistence on certain sequences of events. The child may be fascinated by music and may possess excellent rote memory.

Fish (1979) described the autistic child as overly quiet and apathetic, irritable, rigid, and tense. Sleep habits may be irregular. Vasovegetative functions are underresponsive or extremely labile, for example, a minor illness might give rise to very high fever while a severe illness may have no associated fever.

Campbell, et al. (1980) examined physical parameters of a group of 101 autistic children. They found no difference in birth weights, and no significant differences in height or weight or bone age. The IQs of the majority, when compared with the normal groups, revealed profound to moderate retardation, only 3 percent tested as normal to bright. Fish (1979) noted that many autistic children were able to do advanced tasks on developmental tests, yet failed in simple ones. She noted developmental fluctuations over time, with transient losses followed by transient acceleration.

According to the DSM III, certain illnesses may predispose the infant to autism, such as maternal rubella, encephalitis, meningitis, and tuberous sclerosis. Finegan and Quarrington (1980), studying 23 autistic children, found seven potentially neuropathogenic factors more prominent in autistic children than in siblings or controls. These were: (1) breech delivery, (2) amniotic meconium, (3) low birth weight, (4) low Apgar score, (5) elevated serum bilirubin, (6) hemolytic disease, and (7) respiratory distress syndrome. Any of these, along with hypoxia, may, it is believed, have caused brain damage.

Studies do not support the view that autism is due to psychodynamic factors, such as maternal rejection. Infantile autism is seen 50 times more often in siblings of autistic children than in normals, suggesting a genetic predisposition.

Table 30-2 outlines some theories and research findings about infantile autism.

Pervasive Developmental Disorder, Childhood Onset

Although the behaviors are similar to those seen in infantile autism, this disorder differs mainly in the time of onset, which is after age 2-½ or before age 12. Besides displaying the behaviors described under infantile autism, the child may have bizarre or morbid fantasies, preoccupations, or thoughts. This disorder, which is chronic, appears to have a somewhat better outcome than infantile autism though special education and support are needed. Usually language ability has developed to some degree.

Nursing Process in Pervasive Developmental Disorders

ASSESSMENT □

Client Assessment □ Utilizing the assessment guidelines presented in Chapter 17, the nurse should gather information about the child. Most often, the child will be presented for diagnostic testing because of speech delay or regression and/or withdrawal, and will be 18 months to 3 years of age. However, the nurse who sees infants in the clinic or community health setting should be alert to early symptoms before 18 months, especially as regards the following factors:

1. Relationships. This can be assessed by observing mother-infant interaction such as molding or cuddling, gazing, visual tracking, and responsiveness to sound and presence of others.
2. Communication. Observe the infant's random babbling, crying (in response to hunger, wetness, and so on), and ability to respond to communication by smiling, squawking, or babbling.
3. Motor impairment. Observe for signs of ritualistic behaviors; unwarranted panic; hand flapping, persistent rocking or rhythmic movements; over- or underresponsiveness to light, pain, sound; failure

---

TABLE 30-2 Infantile Autism: Theories of Causation

Psychological origin. One of the earliest theories attempting to explain the autistic nature of the disorder was that the extreme withdrawal was due to maternal rejection. This theory is no longer espoused by most mental health professionals.

Biological origin (research proceeds in several areas);

Physical deviations. Minor physical anomalies that developed in embryo stages have been noted. Deviations in nervous system development are suspected. Both embryonic development and birth hypoxia may contribute to autism.

Neurophysiologic studies. EEG differences suggest variations from the norm; sleep studies indicate possible CNS maturational deviations; differences in auditory evoking response; disruption in autonomic functions (arrhythmias, vestibular deviations).

Biochemical. Catecholamine and indoleamine (dopamine B hydroxylase and serotonin levels differed in autistic children). Tryptophan levels in autistic children differ from those in normals. Serotonin levels differ from normals. Enzyme and immunologic studies suggest need for further investigation.

Neurosensory. Ney (1979) proposed hypothesis that autism is due to excessively sensitive hearing and that the withdrawal is a conditioned avoidance to sound, a source of pain. He theorizes that pain causes anxiety and withdrawal, with consequent information deprivation. The stereotyped behavior and self-stimulating spinning are seen as attempts to control the level of arousal and anxiety giving rise to developmental delays and irreversible retardation. Ney's belief may be supported by the fact that boys, whose hearing is more sensitive in frequency range, are more often autistic than girls.

---

to master developmental milestones, or erratic learning followed by loss of these abilities (e.g., turning over, sitting up).

Environmental Assessment ☐ The child's environment may be of any type; however, for reasons that are unclear, the disorder is more common among upper socioeconomic groups. Parents and family must be assessed as to their understanding of the disorder and their ability to support, emotionally and financially, the child's multiple disabilities.

Self-Assessment ☐ The nurse may experience feelings of frustration and helplessness. Progress is minimal because autism is chronic. Since so little is yet known about the cause, neither prevention nor cure is possible. Meeting the child's needs is complex and exhausting. About 65 percent of these children are incapable of independent living; among the remaining children, the range is from minimal residual disability to partial independence. Recognizing the chronicity of the disorder, the nurse should set realistic goals for the child.

The child's inability to form relationships may be extremely frustrating to the nurse, who gains little emotional feedback. Often she will rejoice in the child's progress only to find that he cannot do the same task the next day. The danger is that the nurse may give up on the child.

PROBLEM/NEED IDENTIFICATION AND INTERVENTION ☐ The multiple needs of the child with pervasive developmental disorder can be overwhelming. Identification of problems, interventions, rationale, and evaluative criteria are outlined in Table 30-3.

EVALUATION ☐ Evaluation is based upon highly individualized behaviors, such as the reduction of an undesirable behavior, (e.g., head-banging) or increases in desired behavior (e.g., speech, eye contact, learning). These behaviors should be specific and should be evaluated on a regular basis.

In most treatment facilities, a strict behavior modification program is instituted based on the child's individual needs. Evaluation is done on the basis of increased number of specifically noted desired behaviors and decreased number of undesirable behaviors. Fewer than 25 percent of autistic children are helped by therapy.

Differentiation of Pervasive Developmental Disorders and Childhood Schizophrenia

The diagnosis of schizophrenia currently is reserved for onset during adolescence or adulthood. (In the past, the term childhood schizophrenia was synonymous with autism.) The characteristics of true childhood schizophrenia, as described by Fish

TABLE 30-3 Nursing Process in Pervasive Developmental Disorder

Problem #1

Disruption in interpersonal relatedness secondary to altered thought processes and sensory perceptual alterations (visual and auditory) and impaired communication.

STG: The child will evidence increased social behavior (specific to individual) and decreased autistic behaviors (specific to individual).

LTG: The child will develop interpersonal relationships according to individual potential within a sheltered environment (home, school, residential treatment center).

Intervention	Rationale	Evaluation
Assign one person to work with child, as often as possible.	The autistic child has difficulty with change.	Consistency of caretaker.
	Multiple caretakers create confusion.	Child's increased responsiveness to caretaker (specific behaviors of individual child, increased eye contact, others).
Explain the child's lack of responsiveness to parents and siblings and support their interactions with the child.	Lack of affectional response is discouraging to parents and they may cease interacting.	Continued verbal and nonverbal involvement with chid.
Include the child in group, and age-appropriate activities. Be alert to signs of overstimulation. One or two other children desirable.	Although ability to relate is impaired the child is aware of others and should have a developmentally stimulating environment, to the extent possible.	The child remains in a group with decreased signs of autistic behavior (individually determined) and increased social behaviors (individually determined).

Problem #2

Impaired verbal communication secondary to altered thought processes and sensory perceptual alterations (visual and auditory).

STG: The child will increase verbalization.

LTG: The child will demonstrate increased ability to communicate as evidenced by verbal and nonverbal behavior.

Intervention	Rationale	Evaluation
Encourage verbalization by naming objects each time they are used or stating to the child what is happening.	Although child may appear unresponsive at times, good communication is modeled.	Increased verbalization.
Provide specialized educational or behavioral treatment settings in private or public facilities.	The special needs of each child require an individual and/or behavior modification approach designed specifically for him.	

Problem #3

Alterations in nutrition (less or more than required) secondary to alteration in thought processes and sensory perception.

STG and LTG: The child will eat a nutritonally balanced meal.

Intervention	Rationale	Evaluation
Provide nutritious foods that are easily eaten (e.g., fruit, milkshakes, vegetables, hotdogs).	Provides balanced diet to child who may be unable to meet nutritional needs.	Maintenance of optimal weight and growth.
Offer the food or place it where it will be accessible, if low intake is problem.	Allows the child to have food when hungry. May be unable to communicate sensation of hunger.	As above.
Provide quiet, predictable mealtime environment.	Noise may distract or overstimulate the child at mealtime.	Participation in mealtime.

TABLE 30-3 (continued)

Problem #4

Alterations in urinary and bowel elimination secondary to cognitive perceptual alterations.

STG and LTG: The child will maintain adequate urine and bowel elimination.

Intervention	Rationale	Evaluation
Monitor urine output and bowel movements on daily basis.	Child's perception alteration may cause inattention to bodily signals to urinate or defecate.	Regular urine and bowel output.
Be alert to potential for constipation/diarrhea or impaction.	Drugs may increase side effects of constipation/diarrhea and child's inattention to body signals may cause retention of stool.	Maintenance of normal bowel elimination pattern.
Provide adequate fluid intake.	Child may not be able to meet fluids needs through inability to communicate.	Normal intake and output.

Problem #5

Potential self-care deficit (feeding, bathing/hygiene, dressing/grooming/toileting) secondary to altered thought process and sensory perceptual alterations.

STG: The child will perform two basic skills of self-care.

LTG: The child will be self-caring according to appropriate age level.

Intervention	Rationale	Evaluation
Assist child with self-care needs according to level of skill.	Child may be unable to recognize need for self-care or communicate these needs.	Child performs self-care tasks.
Plan a behavior modification program to reward the child for performing self-care.	Child receives positive reinforcement for self-care.	Child performs designated self-care tasks routinely.

Problem #6

Sleep pattern disturbance secondary to altered cognitive perceptual pattern.

STG: The child will sleep 6 to 8 hours per night.

LTG: The child's sleep pattern will be adequate for rest and will not be disruptive to the family.

Intervention	Rationale	Evaluation
Provide structured time periods for naps and rest.	Decreased stimulation and routine nap will encourage rest.	Child sleeps.
Provide comforting bedtime routine (story, warm bath).	Structure is helpful to the child.	Child participates in routine and goes to sleep.
If child is disruptive at night, remove him so he will not disturb others or distract him with toy or activity.	Others' sleep should not be disrupted.	Child able to sleep on same schedule.

Problem #7

Potential for injury secondary to alterations in thought processes and sensory perceptual alterations.

STG: The child will not endanger self or others.

LTG: The child will learn to control outbursts of rage, self-destructive behavior, or violence.

Intervention	Rationale	Evaluation
Restrain the child from engaging in self-destructive or violent behaviors by physically holding him or by other nonpunitive means.	Protect child and others from physical injury.	Decrease in rage or panic attacks and violent behavior.
Provide calm, routine environment.	Light, sound, smells, or activities may trigger outbursts.	Decrease in behavior with potential for injury to self or others.
Interrupt disruptive behavior by offering toy, new activity, or removing child from group.	Prevents buildup of stimulation causing outbursts.	Building signs of overstimulation (handflapping, head banging) are decreased.

(continued)

TABLE 30-3 *(continued)*

Problem #8

Potential alterations in parenting (e.g., self-blame, lack of involvement) secondary to child's unresponsiveness, unusual behavior, and chronic nature of disorder.

STG: Parents will understand theories of etiology of autism and available treatment modalities.

LTG: Parents will support and remain involved in child's treatment and will help to promote research and treatment efforts.

Intervention	Rationale	Evaluation
Provide accurate, current information on autism. The National Society of Autistic Children (NSAC) provides support for parents of autistic children and professionals involved with autistic children.	Parents may blame themselves for the child's disorder whereas cause is not known.	Parental knowledge and involvement in child's treatment.
Encourage parents to seek genetic counseling.	Incidence of autism 50 times greater in siblings of autistic children.	Participation is genetic counseling.
Encourage parents to join parental support groups.	Support groups offer specific solutions from other parents, offer hope, and allow for ventilation of feelings and experiences.	Participation in support groups.
Encourage parents to take breaks from child care through babysitters or community respite care.	Autistic child's care is draining and 24-hour job. Parents need to maintain their mental and physical health.	Parents regularly plan "rest breaks."
Emphasize importance of treating child as a family member when at home.	Although special needs will be evident, the child should be treated as normally as possible.	Child is considered part of family verbally and nonverbally and is included in activities.
Assist parents in explaining disorder to siblings and point out importance of other childrens' needs.	Siblings will be better able to deal with autistic child and understand differences in parents' expectations.	Siblings include autistic child and can care for him.
Encourage active participation in federal and state funding for research and treatment.	Long-term, expensive care for the child will require disability assistance.	Parents are able to provide responsible care.

STG: Short-term goal, LTG: Long-term goal.

(1979), are included under pervasive developmental disorder (childhood onset). It is not clear whether there is a true psychotic state in childhood that is distinct from pervasive developmental disorders.

☐ *Problems of the Toddler and the Preschool Child: Autonomy versus Shame and Doubt and Initiative versus Guilt*

ATTENTION DEFICIT DISORDER

Attention deficit represents a confusing complex of behaviors. It is known also as minimal brain dysfunction (MBD), hyperkinesis, hyperactivity, and minimal cerebral dysfunction. The affected child generates frustration and irritation in family and friends.

The lack of attention, which is characteristic, may or may not be accompanied by hyperactivity. However, it is the hyperactive child who is most frequently seen by the nurse because the parents feel frustrated in their efforts to understand and cope with the behavior.

Three is the usual age at which the disorder may appear, but frequently it is not reported until the child attends preschool or grammar school and then is expected to follow a certain routine, to concentrate, and to interact with others.

The DSM III describes three prominent behaviors seen in attention deficit disorder with hyperactivity.

1. Inattention. The child has difficulty in following through with tasks and concentrating on schoolwork, games, hobbies, or

play activities. He is distracted easily by noises, other children, or nearby activities and appears to totally ignore instructions, requests, or other communications directed toward him.

2. Impulsivity. The child displays rapid changes of activity, difficulty in "settling down" to a task, and low frustration tolerance. He gets into trouble by acting without thought for the consequences, demanding attention by calling out in class, or pulling on the adult's hand, clothing, or leg. If given several tasks at once, the child becomes overstimulated and cannot organize himself to deal with them. He does not wait his turn, he grabs toys, and he upsets games. He then is rejected by the other children.

3. Hyperactivity. This aspect causes the greatest distress to the child's parents and teachers. The child is constantly "on the go," up and down, in and out, talking constantly, tapping a pencil, kicking the desk in front of him, seemingly inexhaustible. Even in sleep the child is "all over the bed," tangled in bedclothes, often finally asleep under the bed rather than in it. Even the hardiest adult is worn out after an hour with this human dynamo! It also seems that when the child is "wound up," rather than becoming exhausted as most children do, his disorganization and motor activity become even more frantic.

Attention deficit with hyperactivity is manifested variously according to age. Weiss and Hechtman (1980) point out that this behavior is present from early life and is not a temporary reaction to environmental stress. During infancy, irregular sleep, colic, feeding problems, and a dislike of or "impatience" with cuddling are early signs. Toddlers run constantly, are "into everything," and are absolutely fearless. A preschooler may appear to be demanding, not listening, unable to play well alone, yet rejected by playmates. In school, where the behaviors generally prompt first referral, the child may do well on a one-to-one basis but have difficulty in a large classroom or in unstructured play with peers. The adolescent is fidgety and restless, and may become involved in antisocial behavior.

It is estimated that 5 to 10 percent of children have attention deficit disorder (Backman and

Firestone, 1979); the sex ratio of boys to girls is 10:1. The cause of this disorder is unknown though Weiss and Hechtman (1980) address some possible factors:

1. Gentic brain dysfunction. This disorder appears to be more common in families; a father may describe himself as having had similar problems in school and with peers.

2. Biochemical. Research suggests that dopamine turnover is decreased, and decreased levels of norepinephrine have been found.

3. Food allergies. Many people believe that food allergies, particularly additives, are the basis of attention deficit behaviors. Some parents have found that modification of the child's diet has had positive effects on behavior but research is not yet conclusive.

4. Environment. Some theorists believe the environment gives rise to behavior, affecting each individual child differently from others. If a parent describes similar behaviors in himself as a child, this may also suggest that parenting practices and attitudes have been transmitted.

It is unlikely that there is a single causative factor. Research points to probable biochemical and neurological reactions, possibly familial, and perhaps triggered by such factors as allergies and/ or environment. The preponderance of the disorder in boys suggests a neurological origin, as their neurological development tends to be slower.

Associated problems that arise have a bearing on the child's emotional well-being. The most significant feelings displayed are low self-esteem, inadequacy, and worthlessness. The child spends the greater part of the day in school, where he experiences little success. Then, at the stage when learning about group play, rules, and sharing is of primary importance, the child has trouble waiting for turns, staying at a task, and sitting quietly. This behavior leads to peer rejection and teasing. The child who feels worthless may attempt to attract attention by acting as "class clown" or by getting into trouble. He may allow peers to "set him up" for trouble or carry out their plans for mischief in order to gain acceptance. On the other hand, he may withdraw, using somatic complaints or daydreaming to protect himself from the critical eyes of others.

The child often utilizes the defense mechanism of denial. He may be given information about his behavior, and yet claim that the teacher lied or may deny doing whatever he was said to have done. Often he appears behaviorally as well as developmentally immature. Baby talk, whining, giddy behavior, and clinging dependence may sometimes be observed. Parents may respond by overprotecting the child and discouraging age-appropriate behaviors because they fear the child will fail (Gardner, 1979).

Therapeutic intervention involves four areas: parental guidance, special education, psychotherapy, and psychopharmacology. The first two of these are described in Table 30-4. Types of psychotherapy include structured and organized play therapy and behavior modification—the latter will help parents to cope with the child's impulsivity and hyperactivity.

Psychopharmacology includes the use of stimulant drugs such as methylphenidate (Ritalin) and dextroamphetamine, which have been helpful to some children, ages 6 through 12, with attention deficit disorder accompanied by hyperactivity. The drugs allow the child to concentrate better, decrease his activity level, and enhance his ability to pursue tasks. The child experiences improvement in school and social behavior, and ultimately gains in self-esteem and acceptance.

Stimulant drugs should be used conservatively as it is uncertain whether they cause tolerance, long term. The nurse should be alert to adverse effects such as anorexia, weight loss, irritability or dejection, complaints of stomach or headache, and urticaria. Heart rate and blood pressure may increase. Contrary to popular belief, these drugs do not have paradoxical effect—they stimulate certain areas of the brain, resulting in decreased activity and improved concentration and organization (Weiss and Hechtman, 1980).

Nursing Process and the Child with Attention Deficit Disorder

ASSESSMENT □

Client Assessment □ Particular attention should be directed to the pregnancy, labor, and delivery. Specific behavioral symptoms of the child, their severity, frequency, duration, and background are relevant. A complete neurological assessment should precede any planning and intervention. A family history of similar behavior may be revealed.

Environmental Assessment □ The child with attention deficit disorder is strongly influenced by his environment. In many instances the family's temperament is such that the child's behavior is viewed as being acceptable, and it is the school environment that ultimately brings about referral for study.

> ■ **Point of Emphasis**
>
> *Environmental influence is pervasive and may enhance or diminish the child's behavioral problems.*

Self-Assessment □ The nurse who works with the child must possess both patience and persistence. The child will very likely be eager to form a therapeutic relationship, while the nurse often finds the child's impulsivity and hyperactivity difficult to deal with. She needs to realize that the child's neurological and developmental deficits contribute to these difficult behaviors. It is essential that the nurse be consistent and firm so that the child will learn that the relationship has a definite structure.

In dealing with the parents, the nurse may be unable to convince them of the importance of a structured environment or to see that the home environment is unlikely to meet the child's needs. This can create in her feelings of anger and frustration, leading to a tendency to blame the parents for the problems. The nurse must be aware that such feelings can arise, and be prepared to discuss them with a colleague or supervisor.

Problem/Need Identification □ The child's problems are complex because so many areas of his life are affected. Four overall areas can be identified: child, peers, school, and family. Table 30-4 illustrates use of nursing process in attention deficit disorder.

ANXIETY DISORDERS OF CHILDHOOD

Three types of anxiety disorder may occur in childhood: separation anxiety, avoidant disorder, and overanxious disorder. The first two may occur as early as preschool age, when the child begins to experience inner conflicts leading to anxiety. Overanxious disorder, which is a more pervasive type of anxiety disorder, is seen more often in latent and early adolescence.

TABLE 30-4 *Nursing Process in Attention Deficit Disorder*

Problem #1

Difficulty maintaining attention and persistence secondary to attention deficit disorder (etiology unknown).

STG: The child will demonstrate an increase in attention and persistence in structured environment.

LTG: The child will demonstrate increased attention and persistence outside the structured environment.

Intervention	Rationale	Evaluation
Give the child tasks that can be completed in a short time. Avoid tasks that involve many directions or multiple complex steps.	This allows the child with a short attention span to feel successful at completing projects.	Ability to pay attention improves as evidenced by increased completion of tasks, games, or hobbies.
Give simple, short directions, one at a time. ("Take a seat." "Get the game." "Choose your playing piece.")	The child's attention span is so short he cannot remember several directions at once.	Same as above.
It is helpful to gently touch the child's face to elicit eye contact and attention.	Touch focuses the child's attention.	Same as above.

Problem #2

Difficulty controlling impulses secondary to attention deficit disorder (etiology unknown).

STG: The child will demonstrate decreased impulsive behavior in a structured environment.

LTG: The child will recognize impulse behavior and be able to control it himself.

Intervention	Rationale	Evaluation
To decrease impulsivity provide a structured environment and predictable routine (e.g., get dressed, make bed, eat breakfast, go to school).	Structure limits overstimulation and gives the child a sense of knowing what to expect and how to act in the situation. "Free" time should be free from "work" but include activities from which to choose, so that the child is not "at loose ends."	Impulsivity decreases as evidenced by ability to wait turn, fewer interruptions.
When impulsive behavior occurs, remind the child quietly (away from others) what's expected.	Touch provides a sense of extenal control, which the child may not sense internally.	

Problem #3

High level of motor activity secondary to attention deficit disorder (etiology unknown).

STG: Child's activity level will decrease in structured setting.

LTG: Child will recognize when he is becoming overly stimulated and hyperactive and remove self from setting.

Intervention	Rationale	Evaluation
Allow time for discharge of energy in running, ballplaying, vigorous exercise.	This allows outlet for child's high level of motor activity.	Motor activity is decreased as evidenced by staying in seat, less fidgeting.
Assist child to control motor activity by reminders to raise hand, stay in seat—using touch as necessary.	Encouragement and support of the child's efforts to control self are important.	

Problem #4

Disruption in cognitive perceptual pattern and motor activity secondary to sugar, caffeine, and food additives intolernce.

STG: Child will eliminate these foods from diet.

LTG: Child's diet will contain foods that do not promote high activity and impulsivity.

Intervention	Rationale	Evaluation
Decrease sugar, caffeine, and foods with additives.	This therapy appears to have helped some children.	Nutritional intervention should be correlated with changes in behavior.

(continued)

TABLE 30-4 (continued)

Problem #5

Social isolation secondary to peer rejection of child's impulsive and disruptive behaviors.

STG: The child will be able to play with one other child.

LTG: The child will improve control of impulsive or disruptive behaviors thereby becoming more acceptable to peers.

Intervention	Rationale	Evaluation
Assist the child to recognize the social behavior that provokes others and discuss more acceptable ways to approach others.	In the relationship the child feels safe and may try out new behaviors with less threat of rejection.	Child able to get along with others (chosen for teams, sought by others for games).
Role-play or discuss with the child better ways of handling situations at home or school.	This helps the child see how his behavior appears to others and understand their feelings.	Decreased use of defensive behavior such as "clowning," denial, negativism.

Problem #6

Disturbance in self-concept, lowered self-esteem secondary to peer rejection and school failure.

STG: The child will be able to name one good thing about self.

LTG: The child will exhibit behaviors indicative of healthy self-esteem, such as ability to name strengths, make a friend, and decreased defensive behaviors.

Intervention	Rationale	Evaluation
Discuss honestly with the child the reasons for his difficulties, and encourage questions.	The child must realize that this problem may be an illness but that he can do things to overcome it.	Child can state ways to help self and does them.
Praise the child's behavior, as closely as possible to the time it occurs. ("You did a good job." "I'm proud of the way you handled that." "You were able to wait your turn.")	Praising behavior rather than the person contributes to the acceptance of the self, even if behavior is unacceptable. A person isn't good or bad. The child's short attention span makes immediate feedback more meaningful.	Child able to say good things about self.
Focus on strengths the child may possess.	Encouragement in these areas contributes to self-esteem.	Child does not denigrate self.
Ignore negative behaviors if possible. If the behavior is harmful to self or others, is disruptive, remove the child to a less stimulating environment and talk in a quiet voice. As much as possible set limits away from others.	If the behaviors are practiced to gain attention, ignoring them will not obtain the desired goal. Protection of the child or others is essential. A quiet voice and calm environment is less stimulating. Setting limits away from others protects the child's self-esteem.	Decrease in specified negative behaviors.

Problem #7

Knowledge deficit (academic skills) secondary to attention deficit disorder.

STG: Child will be evaluated by qualified educational professional.

LTG: Child will be placed in educational setting most appropriate to his needs.

Intervention	Rationale	Evaluation
Interventions are done by a qualified educational therapist but usually include a structured classroom, short assignments which take into consideration the child's disabilities, remedial lessons, and social learning for activities of daily living.	Provides an environment of learning and success for child.	Improved grades and school performance.

TABLE 30-4 (continued)

Problem #8

Potential alterations in parenting secondary to attention deficit disorder (etiology unknown).

STG: Parents will become aware of child's problems, socially and academically.

LTG: Parents will understand child's problems and provide support and involvement in treatment.

Intervention	Rationale	Evaluation
Teach the family about the child's disorder. Differentiate child's behavior from other family problems.	This reduces parental guilt and sibling jealously if they realize much of this behavior is not deliberate or caused by parenting.	Parents report feeling better about child; may include child more, seek him out for praise.
Assist the family to design a structure for the child that fits their life-style.	Each family is unique, and the family needs to decide how they can best help the child.	The child is successful in structure at home based on specific criteria (e.g., does chores).
Expect the child to do certain chores that siblings do.	This decreases jealousy and promotes responsibility.	Siblings able to assist child to handle situations.
Involve the child in sports, hobbies, or activities (e.g., Scouts) in which he can succeed.	Enhances self-esteem and provides growth experiences.	Child states he likes outside activities and attends regularly.
Provide opportunities for parents to ventilate anger and frustration.	The child is difficult to live with, and behavior can be extremely frustrating. The nurse can provide an outlet by listening to parents rather than having the child become the scapegoat.	Parents ventilate to nurse or support group.
Encourage the parents by praising efforts to spend time and effort with their child and pointing out improvements.	Often, day-to-day improvements are missed by people close to the child. The nurse can provide objectivity.	Parents able to praise child and name improvements.

STG: Short-term goal, LTG: Long-term goal.

Separation Anxiety Disorder

The child appears extremely anxious when a threatened or actual separation from persons to whom he is significantly attached occurs. In contrast, separation anxiety is a normal occurrence in young children, arising from their dependence on and need of the caretaking person. Separation anxiety *disorder* develops from the child's unrealistic fears about harm coming to his parents, caretaker, or himself.

According to the DSM III, the child may display a variety of stress-related behaviors, at least three of which must have persisted for 2 weeks:

1. Fears that the parent or major attachment figure will be injured or will leave and never return

2. Fears that the child himself will be somehow separated from the significant person (e.g., accident, kidnapping, getting lost)

3. Continued reluctance or refusal to attend school, due to fear of leaving significant person at home

4. Fears of sleeping away from home or away from the significant person

5. Fear of being alone at home, with signs of emotional distress if unable to follow the significant person around the house

6. Persistent nightmares having a theme of separation

7. Physical complaints on schooldays (headache, stomach ache, nausea, vomiting)

8. Extreme emotional distress when separated from significant person(s) or if separation is anticipated (may be exemplified by temper tantrums, crying, begging parents not to leave; child may become panic-stricken, may throw himself at the adult, may cling tenaciously and refuse to let the adult leave).

9. Child appears apathetic, sad, withdrawn, and unable to work or play unless the significant person is nearby

■ *Point of Emphasis*

The child's fears are unrealistic and persistent. Most children see movies or news stories that highlight acts of violence or accidents that are truly frightening, but normally the fears do not persist.

The disorder is not uncommon. The child's school life and social life are impaired. He is afraid to visit friends or relatives for a "sleepover," or to go to camp. He is frequently fearful of the dark and envisions monsters, killers, witches, and the like lying in wait for him. Concerns about dying, accidents, and kidnapping may cause panic at the thought of separation. Since the preschooler stays closer to home, these fears may not be readily apparent until the child starts school and is expected to become involved with peers.

The fears may be so overwhelming that the child refuses to attend school despite the consequences. School refusal is a symptom of separation anxiety disorder and is usually seen at around 11 to 12 years. Generally there is a precipitating factor such as illness, loss of relative or pet, a move, a new school, or a change in the family.

The social and academic consequences may severely impair emotional growth, because he has only limited interaction with peers and the learning environment. Energy that should be utilized in socializing and intellectual development is channeled into efforts to control anxiety.

Both sexes appear to be equally affected, and there appears to be a familial tendency in the disorder. Affected families tend to be close and caring.

The underlying cause of separation anxiety disorder is thought to reside in the caretaker, usually the mother/child relationship. The mother (or caretaker) is the person who is actually anxious about separation; the child senses this anxiety and becomes fearful of separation. The child, who sees the parent as strong and protective, on an unconscious level might be said to think "Well, if she's so worried, I should worry too. Who knows what can happen?" Imagination does the rest. Often, the mother treats the child as an adult, confiding to him her marital problems and concerns—she seeks to meet emotional needs through the child. If both parents are at home there are likely to be marital problems and disharmony, which bring the problem to a head.

Vignette

John S., 3 years old, began preschool when his mother obtained a part-time job. Upon arrival at preschool, he would kick, scream, and beat upon his father or mother (whoever brought him) and plead to be taken home. He continued to sob and withdraw after his parents left. The behavior continued far longer than was normal, while at home this behavior did not occur. His father became especially concerned when John at times held his breath until he lost consciousness.

Several factors were at work in this situation. First, John's mother started to work outside the home over his father's vehement objections. Mr. S.'s ethnic background was such that he viewed the idea of women working outside as an insult to his masculinity and role as provider. He also had unfounded fears that working outside would cause his wife to be unfaithful. Second, his culture focused on strong family "togetherness" and indulgence toward the children, especially boys. Mrs. S., on the other hand, did not share her husband's cultural background, but viewed her job as meeting a financial need and John's preschool as providing an important social experience for him.

John sensed the parental discord, and become worried about what would happen to his parents as they argued, freely and explosively, at home. John's tantrums and breath holding elicited tears, agitation, and fear in his father, who then would not force him to stay at school, but would bring him home or take him along to his various jobs.

The nurse discussed the problems with both parents. She helped them to appreciate their different cultural values. Mr. S. was assured that John's breath holding was not life threatening and that his wife remained faithful to him.

Mr. and Mrs. S. were able to agree that Mrs. S. would continue to work outside and take John to preschool. John's distress ended after 3 days, and he then adjusted to preschool quickly.

Avoidant Disorder of Childhood

The predominant behavior of a child with avoidant disorder is "persistent (at least 6-months' duration) and excessive shrinking from contact with strangers" (DSM III, 1980). The avoidance is a cause of poor peer relationships and other situations in which social skills are necessary. Nevertheless, the child is desirous of warmth and acceptance from family and other familiar people.

The behavior may be seen as early as age 2-½ but is not to be confused with normal stranger anxiety or the slow-to-warm child, because in those situations, the child eventually warms up to the person as his familiarity with the person increases.

The younger child may speak only in whispers and hang behind the caretaker, clinging to her clothes or her leg. If asked to do something that involves interaction with a stranger, he becomes extremely anxious and tearful. An older child may be extremely withdrawn in the presence of strangers. If the child goes to school, he may appear to ignore the teacher and other students and, by shrinking from activities, try not to attract notice. When asked to recite, he becomes anxious, and unable to communicate. He is timid, embarrassed, and inhibited of movement and initiative. When the anxiety level is high, the child may appear mute and immobilized.

Thought disorder is not present. The child has satisfying relationships with close, familiar peopll, but his low self-esteem makes exposure to strangers frightening to him. Shrinking from others, the child fails to become involved in activities that enhance development. He feels isolated and depressed because he lacks friends and lacks a sense of satisfaction about his accomplishments.

Overanxious Disorder

Worrying, fearfulness, excessive conformity, lack of risk taking, and extreme need for approval characterize the child with overanxious disorder. He appears tense, nervous, and often physically rigid. The behavior is persistent, and cannot be traced to a single precipitating event or life stressor.

Physically, the child may have many anxiety-based somatic symptoms such as stomachache, headache, tingling, dizziness, hyperventilation, and insomnia. The nurse may first meet this child when the parents become concerned about his physical complaints.

The child worries inordinately about what others think, about being accepted, about performing well at school and in social activities, and about meeting expectations. He may be perfectionistic, believing that being less than the best equals total failure and that a failure or a mistake is disastrous. He may be preoccupied with the belief that a teacher or another significant adult is "mean" and has singled him out for particularly severe treatment.

Often the family is of the upper middle class and expresses, directly or indirectly, high expectations, which may be unrealistic in light of the child's talents and abilities. The oldest child of a small family—especially a boy—is most likely to be affected. The child may believe acceptance by the family hinges on his giving a superior performance in various realms, such as school, social sitautions, and sports.

Vignette

Nancy B., a 10-year-old fourth grader, became known to the school nurse because she complained of repeated stomachaches and headaches. No physical basis was found. The nurse engaged Nancy in conversation during these times.

Nancy was a precocious girl. Her vocabulary was more advanced than that of the average fourth grader. Nancy told the nurse that arithmetic was not her "best" subject. Nancy's teacher was surprised to learn this, because Nancy was an average student who had never received a failing grade in arithmetic. The teacher added the observation that Nancy's physical symptoms occurred most often during the arithmetic period and that she became tearful if asked to recite. The teacher tried through various means to help Nancy but her efforts failed. She suggested that Nancy continue to visit the nurse. During the next two meetings with the nurse, Nancy related that her father, a physician, and her mother, an attorney, were very "smart," as were her two older brothers. The brothers attended the same school, were excellent students and popular athletes. Nancy then burst into tears and exclaimed, "Everyone's smart but me!" In her perception of herself, she was stupid and unpopular, although her grades were average or above average, and she had several girl friends.

After assessing Nancy's difficulties, the principal and teacher met with the family, whom they knew well, relating Nancy's problems and their concerns. The parents were eager to remedy the situation, and were able to identify some of the things they said or did that indicated to Nancy that failure was a disgrace. They thought of how they might praise Nancy for her achievements without implying that she could have done better. Within a month, Nancy was able to participate in the arithmetic class and her grades improved. The physical symptoms ceased almost immediately.

Nursing Process and Anxiety Disorders of Childhood

ASSESSMENT □ In the assessment phase, the nurse first obtains a clear picture of recent events and possible stressors in the child's life and the family environment. When interviewing family and child, she notes their interactions, as well as their nonverbal expressions indicating warmth or its absence.

In assessing self, the nurse needs to be alert to any tendency to blame the parent or caretaker. Although the child's anxiety is usually related to family anxieties, it is not helpful to place blame. The nurse needs to recognize the child's signals of anxiety, and respond with warmth, acceptance, and support when the child fears a new situation or person.

INTERVENTION □ Interventions that are helpful in adult anxiety apply to children also. The nurse must remember that a child may be unable to verbalize the anxiety, thus behavioral clues must be observed. Touching a child who is panicky because of impending separation is not recommended—it tends to increase his fears and may cause him to strike out. When talking with a child, she should use language that the child understands. For example, "Sometimes children have lots of worries." "Kids sometimes worry about moms and dads." "It's scary when mom is away."

■ *Point of Emphasis*

A small child's fears are real—his power over life events is nearly nonexistent. Being among strangers can be a frightening experience.

Family or marital counseling is essential if the source of the problem is to be discovered and resolved. The child who is old enough to understand needs verbal reassurance that no harm will befall the parents when he is separated from them but will also need to see less anxiety in the parents. If he has nightmares and crawls into the parents' bed, it is better that he be comforted and returned to his own bed. Sleeping with parents can intensify existing marital problems.

School attendance should be reinforced as an environment that will help the child develop. He needs the supportive presence of familiar figures,

and at the same time firmness and persistence, in the expectation that he will participate in various activities. The child needs to learn that a mistake is not catastrophic. The adult can be a desirable role model who makes a mistake and works out a solution, at the same time expressing natural feelings of disappointment or frustration.

The child with an anxiety disorder is especially sensitive to ridicule. The friendly banter of other children or the loving teasing of significant adults often is misinterpreted. This behavior is best minimized; when it does occur the nurse points out that she really likes him. As the nurse-client relationship develops, it is less likely that gentle teasing or humor will be misperceived. The child feels more relaxed with himself and may be less bothered by teasing.

Parental guidance and teaching is essential to prevent or alleviate these childhood disorders. Ways of building self-esteem and indicating acceptance may need to be taught. As the parents and families are helped to increase control over their problems, the child's problems will diminish.

EVALUATION □ The nurse evaluates her interventions by observing fewer identified problem behaviors, an increase in developmentally appropriate interactions, the child's own report of feeling less worried, and reports from parents and teachers.

SCHIZOID DISORDER OF CHILDHOOD

The child with schizoid disorder is isolated, aloof, withdrawn, and seclusive. Most prominently, the child seems unable to form social relationships. A "loner," he does not have any interest in making friends, is awkward in social situations, and avoids cooperative activities such as scouting or group play. There is usually attachment only to the parent and possibly to one other child who is equally withdrawn or is much younger.

The child responds unpredictably to demands made of him; there may be outbursts of aggression and hostility that may be bizarre or sadistic. He is the class or neighborhood scapegoat. Although he is detached and absorbed in fantasy and daydreaming, the child is not out of touch with reality. He may be preoccupied with certain topics such as ghosts, robots, science fiction, and aggressive violence. One senses the child's emotional distance and vagueness.

This disorder is not common, occurs most often in boys, and becomes evident when the child is around 5 years of age. There is little information about the cause of this behavior, but it is reasonable to suspect that the child has not experienced the trusting environment that is necessary for the development of a sense of self.

☐ *Problems of the School-Age Child: Industry vs. Inferiority*

Table 3-5 gives a behavioral checklist of signs of emotional disturbances in the school-age child (Hammer, 1970). The behaviors are significant if they persist.

CONDUCT DISORDER OF CHILDHOOD

Conduct disorder has become relatively frequent. It is more common in boys, though it is now seen with increasing frequency in girls since they are less protected and sheltered than in earlier decades (Meeks, 1979). (See Chapter 31.)

OPPOSITIONAL DISORDER

A pattern of behavior that is negative, self-defeating, and contrary to authority is termed oppositional disorder. In general, the rights of others and rules are not violated. Instead the child does the opposite of what has been suggested or argues against it, carries out activities from which he has specifically been asked to refrain, and annoys everyone by his uncooperative and defiant behavior. This behavior is demonstrated toward parents and teachers as early as age 3 but most often is seen in the school-age child. At the younger age, this form of resistance is a part of autonomous development. However, in later years, its self-defeating nature causes difficulties.

Dawdling, procrastination, and stubborness are passive forms of resistance. Temper tantrums may result when the child's desires are thwarted. He appears to feel compelled to provoke others by arguing, resisting, or acting oppositely. He believes others are making unreasonable requests and that it is not he who has the problem, and he

---

TABLE 30-5 Warning Signs of Emotional Disturbance[a]

Disturbed classroom behavior

  Daydreams constantly and shows little interest in activities

  Very impulsive or hyperactive; appears "driven"

  Short attention span, poor concentration, rarely finishes task

  Cannot tolerate frustration, can't wait turn

  Asks to go to bathroom frequently

  Impatient for snacks and lunchtime; asks frequently

  Destructive of property

  Will not or cannot abide by rules

  Constantly seeks attention

  Ritualistic or compulsive about work or behavior

  Rigid about performance of tasks; bothered by that which he believes misplaced or
    unbalanced

  Resists changes and adjusts poorly to new activity or situation

  Unable or unwilling to handle minor responsibility, excessively doubtful and indecisive

  Chronically fearful, worried, or depressed

  Denies wrongdoing vehemently even if caught

Disturbances in attitude toward self

  General sense of inferiority and worthlessness; unrealistic about strengths and limitations;
    self-critical or ridiculing

  Overestimates abilities and adequacies—believes should be treated as special or
    privileged

  Feels desires or impulses are bad, therefore he is bad; may insist on punishment or act
    out in order to receive it even though undeserved

  Either overly guilty or lacks remorse

  Preoccupied with ugliness of body or idea he is crazy or retarded

  Feels unable to love or be nice to anyone

  Wishes he were a member of the opposite sex

(continued)

TABLE 30-5 (continued)

Disturbed behavior toward teacher

    Extreme rebelliousness, resistance to requests or suggestions, feels every request a demand; may be active or passive in resistance

    Easily hurt or rejected; cannot tolerate criticism

    Monopolizes teacher

    Extremely dependent on teacher and tries to be "teacher's pet"

    Overly shy with teacher or other adults

    Steals from teacher or peers

Disturbed relationships with peers

    Overly aggressive; bullies, teases, tattles frequently

    Boastful and brags about achievements

    Very competitive and upset when others are praised

    Overly shy and fearful of peers

    Scapegoated by peers

    Lack of concern for the group

Inappropriate infantile behavior

    Unable to separate from parent

    Whining, crying, tantrums without provocation

    Thumb or finger sucking

    Enuresis or encopresis

    Unable or unwilling to dress self

    Doesn't know age or birthday

Disturbed physical functioning or appearance

    Chronically tired

    Frequent vomiting in class

    Frequent and severe skin eruption, or picking at skin or sores

    Chewing fingernails constantly

    Obesity or overly thin with no organic cause

    Tics

    Accident prone

Disturbances of speech

    Baby talk

    Afraid to recite; stutters or barely audible

    Selectivity mute, talks at home but not at school

Sexual disturbances

    Frequent masturbation, overt or covert

    Exposes genitals deliberately and/or makes sexual advances to classmates

    Curses and uses vulgar language frequently

    Preoccupied with sex or birth process and constantly asks peers or teacher about them

Difficulties in learning

    Discrepancy between test scores and performance

    Discrepancy in ability or performance in certain tasks (good in one area very poor in another)

    Lacks motivation to learn or try

[a] Adapted from *Journal of learning disabilities*, A Teachers Guide to the Detection of Emotional Disturbances in the Elementary School Child, 3, 1970:36–37.

may use alcohol and other drugs in deliberate defiance of parental control. Of course this behavior interferes with social relationships and learning. The disorder may progress into passive-aggressive personality disorder.

The child's stubborn persistence can be channeled into constructive activity through appeals to self-esteem: "Jimmy, you're good with cards. You deal." Asking the child to help a younger child also increases self-esteem.

Parents need to be counseled also. Many times the behavior becomes worse as power struggles build. A pattern of negative interaction between parent and child develops that must be broken.

FUNCTIONAL ENURESIS

Enuresis, or bed-wetting, is a common problem. Enuresis not due to a lack of toilet training is called secondary enuresis. Most children are toilet trained by age 3 and have good nighttime control by age 4. Overexcitement, too much fluid, and staying up late often cause a young child to have a bedtime "accident."

The school-age child who wets the bed consistently should be examined to rule out organic causes. Enuresis is more common in boys and has familial links—fathers of these children were frequently bed wetters. A slower neurological development that signals the brain to "wake up" when the bladder is full seems to be the cause.

The child's self-esteem must be protected. In counseling parents, the nurse emphasizes that shaming is ineffective and that a matter-of-fact attitude works best. The child can change his bedclothes. Parents can limit fluids before bedtime and awaken the child several hours later when they go to bed so he can urinate. Rewards for keeping the bed dry sometimes motivate the child. If a child sleeps over at a friend's house, the friend's parents can be alerted to how the bed wetting is handled.

If the child has other behavioral problems or if there are family problems, the family should be referred for counseling. Enuresis frequently is associated with learning problems, hyperactivity, conduct disorders, and fire setting.

Drug therapy has proved fairly useful. Imipramine appears to exert anticholinergic effects that allow the child to awaken in response to the urge to urinate (Anders and Freeman, 1979). It is thought that the drug lightens sleep stages so that the child senses the micturition reflex.

FUNCTIONAL ENCOPRESIS

Secondary encopresis, or fecal soiling, is a problem in the 4- to 8-year-old who has been bowel trained and continent for a year or more and reverts to willful or involuntary soiling of clothing or other inappropriate articles. The child with primary functional encopresis has not been bowel trained.

A combination of obstipation, punitive or too-early toilet training, stressful family life, and possibly motivational lag due to immaturity of the nervous system are causes of encopresis. Affected boys outnumber girls in a ratio of 3 to 1, suggesting neurological influence.

When involuntary, encopresis is often related to constipation, retention, or impaction. Deliberate soiling, sometimes accompanied by smearing of feces, often is associated with other symptoms of disturbed behavior, such as severe language disorders, withdrawal, and near-psychotic behavior (Bellman, 1966). The child will attempt to hide underwear or clothing that has been soiled, usually near the bathroom or his own room. Shame and ostracism by peers (because of the odor) cause the child to withdraw from social activities.

Parental responses are usually angry and punitive. The child's seeming indifference to his soiling tends to greatly aggravate the parents (usually mother). The child may be a few feet from the bathroom and soil, even sitting in soiled pants until the odor is apparent to others.

Associated behaviors include nail biting, language disorders, petty stealing, negativism, food refusal, sleep disturbances, stomachaches, withdrawal, and stubbornness. Also frequently found are poor body image expressed in immature drawings of the human figure and delayed language facility (Fisher, 1979).

The child seems overdependent on the mother, passive but quietly agressive. Fathers are often absent or uninvolved and mothers often seem angry and ungiving (Fisher, 1979).

Nursing intervention should be preceded by a thorough physical examination to rule out organic disease. Parents are advised to ignore the soiling as much as possible, not to discuss it, and not to focus any attention on it. The child should take responsibility for changing underwear and putting the soiled clothes where they belong. Positive reinforcement for successful toileting (small toy, stickers, stars) can be offered. Play therapy helps him release his aggressive feelings, and family therapy is also most helpful.

Useful drugs include stool softeners or mild laxatives to prevent impaction. Imipramine has been given with positive results in conjunction with psychotherapy.

EMOTIONAL DISORDERS OF CHILDHOOD

Table 30-6 summarizes other common emotional disorders of childhood

Childhood Depression

Until the 1970s, children were regarded as being incapable of experiencing depression in a clinical sense because of the absence of superego development. The Freudian view was that children had not developed the inner processes necessary to feel depressed.

At least three other views now exist (Cantwell and Carlson, 1980). The first claims that childhood depression exists but has characteristic symptoms unique to childhood, such as encopresis, phobias, or simple depressive symptoms (sadness, irritability, crying). The second theory holds that childhood depression is "masked"—it is hidden by such behaviors as hyperactivity, somatic complaints, or conduct disorders. The third view is that children exhibit depressive symptoms similar to those of adults.

The existence of these divergent views is reflected in the lack of a diagnostic category for childhood depression in the DSM III. The diagnosis that most closely approaches childhood depression is dysthymic disorder of adulthood, which usually begins in early adult life. It seems likely that children can in fact feel depressed in the sense of experiencing feelings of sadness, loss of pleasure in activities, fatigue, and low self-esteem. These feelings may be exhibited in a variety of behaviors ranging from withdrawal, tearfulness, boredom, low activity level, and poor con-

centration, to hyperactivity, irritability, aggressiveness, anger, restlessness, and preoccupation with health or death. This diversity makes it difficult to estimate the prevalence of childhood depression.

In infancy, depression may be displayed by poor appetite, slow response to stimuli, flaccid body tone, sadness, or apathetic expression. The toddler or preschool child may communicate depression through unhappy behavior, irritability, and withdrawal. The child conveys a sense of discontent, boredom, feelings of rejection, or being unloved. Often overactivity, rocking, sleep and appetite disturbances, nail biting, bed-wetting, and encopresis signal depression (Katz, 1979). As Phillips (1979) points out, the preschool child, with his greater cognitive development and learning through observation and imitation, may also identify with a depressed parent.

The school-age child, understanding the world in more operational and concrete terms, may exhibit depression in provocative or aggressive behavior which elicits punishment rather than consolation. Schoolwork suffers, the child may withdraw or constantly annoy others, or may complain of physical ills. Easily hurt and overly sensitive to rejection, the child may view himself in a depreciating manner: "I'm no good (rotten, lousy, bad.)" Teachers and parents may not recognize the child's desperate bids for attention as depression (Phillips, 1979).

Etiology of Childhood Depression. A single cause of depression is not readily evident and current research suggests multiple causative factors. Lewis and Lewis (1979) reviewed current concepts according to the three areas: psychological, genetic, and biochemical.

Loss and deprivation in early childhood are also thought to be causative factors. Deprivation as a factor in depression can occur in four major ways (Langmeier and Matejcek, 1975): (1) Stimulus deprivation—in early life there is a lack of sensory and/or motor stimulation. (2) Cognitive deprivation—the environment does not offer reasonable and understandable feedback and its structure is such that the child has difficulty making sense out of that environment and his own behavior. (3) Attachment deprivation—there is not a caring, responsive, and reliable person to whom the child can attach. (4) Social deprivation—inadequate or absent social experiences impair the child's ability to function in the larger social arena (e.g., school, neighborhood).

TABLE 30-6 Emotional Disorders of Childhood

Emotional Disorder	Stage of Development	Possible Causes	Therapeutic Intervention
Speech Disorders Elective Mutism: continuous refusal to talk in social situations	Autonomy vs. doubt Initiative vs. guilt Seen before age 5, more girls than boys	Maternal overprotection Psychological trauma at the age of speech development.	Assessment of family relationships Child may be removed from home and hospitalized to decrease overprotection Counseling for parents Support of child and one-to-one therapy Avoid power struggle to force speech; let child take the lead
Stuttering: repetition or prolongation of sounds or hesitations that disrupt the word flow	Initiative vs. guilt Industry vs. inferiority 2-½–3 years or 5–7 years Four times more common in boys	Familial link Anxiety based Neurological dysfunction	Referral to speech clinic
Movement Disorders Tics: involuntary rapid movement of skeletal muscles or involuntary production of noises or words—chronic or transient	Autonomy vs. doubt through adolescence—usually between 4 and 10 More common in boys	**Organic** Heredity Neurological Biological Mechanical irritation Infection **Psychodynamic** High intelligence, emotional immaturity, temper tantrums **Behavioral** Learned behavior as avoidance response	Watch for side effects of phenothiazines if used in treatment Prevention of secondary emotional problems such as low self-esteem, isolation, depression, and academic failure (Lucas, 1979)
Atypical Stereotyped Movement Disorder: voluntary movements such as head banging, rocking, repetitive hand motion	Infancy through adolescence	Grossly inadequate social stimulation Also seen in children with mental retardation, pervasive developmental disorder	Protect the child from injury by removing dangerous objects or by restraint
Sleep Disorders Sleepwalking Disorder: getting out of bed during sleep and walking around (usually 30 minutes to 3-½ hours following onset of sleep)	Industry vs. inferiority (6–12) also in adulthood More common in boys than girls	Fatigue, stress, hypnotics, or sedatives Some familial link in regard to deeper sleep	Reassure parents child will outgrow Explore current stressors in child's life Counsel parents to secure child's environment to avoid injury while sleepwalking
Sleep Terror Disorder: abrupt awakening from sleep preceded by piercing scream (usually 30 minutes to 3-½ hours after onset of sleep); episodes last 1–10 minutes, child is intensely anxious, agitated, perspiring, and hyperventilating; no recall next morning	Initiative vs. shame and doubt through industry vs. inferiority More boys than girls	Fatigue Stress Antidepressants or neuroleptics Family link	Reassure parents child will outgrow; encourage them to comfort the child Not the same as a nightmare which is usually less anxiety provoking, and the child can remember it Explore current stressors in family, at school Parents should be discouraged from taking the child into their bed Child should be comforted and reassured until he falls asleep again

(continued)

677

TABLE 30-6 (continued)

Emotional Disorder	Stage of Development	Possible Causes	Therapeutic Intervention
Eating Disorders Pica: consumption of nonnutritive substance such as dirt, hair, cloth, sand, bugs, leaves, and paint chips	Trust vs. mistrust through initiative vs. guilt	Distorted oral gratification in response to psychological stress Contributing factors—Frequent moves, Poor housing, Irregular employment, Major emotional problems in the family, Disorganized family life, Cultural traditions, Mineral deficiency	A multidisciplinary approach of pediatrician, visiting nurse, and social worker, plus mental health professional Screening for lead poisoning is essential and assessment and intervention with physical and emotional needs of the family Education of parents With more severe cases, child should be hospitalized for individual psychotherapy
Rumination Disorder of Infancy: repeated regurgitation of food resulting in weight loss or failure to gain after normal eating Child strains, arching back and holding head back, bringing up partially digested food	Trust vs. mistrust (3–12 months) Equally common in boys and girls	Severe disturbance of the mother-child relationship (potentially fatal due to possible malnutrition)	Physical causes must be ruled out The nurse should take a complete nursing history and observe the mother's way of relating to the child, especially during feeding If child is hospitalized, consistent personnel should be assigned Avoid blaming mother but reeducate by role modeling and suggestion and performance of helpful strategies If mother is severely disturbed, therapy should be instituted
Specific Developmental Disorders (May or may not be accompanied by others such as conduct disorder; lack of education and chronological mental age are not reasons for the impairment) Reading (dyslexia): characterized by omissions, additions, and distortions; comprehension reduced Arithmetic: arithmetic skills impaired and performance on arithmetic tasks below intellectual capacity Developmental Language Disorder (three types): 1. Failure to acquire language	Stage at which each area of function should develop Industry vs. inferiority Males outnumber females 2:1 Industry vs. inferiority Autonomy vs. doubt Initiative vs. guilt Males outnumber females 2:1	Biological Neurological 1. Mental retardation 2. Trauma or neurological impairment 3. Neurological More common in families; about 1 in every 1,000 children have this disorder	Refer the child for testing and evaluation by educational specialist and/or speech and hearing specialist Educate parents about the disorder—emphasize the child is not "retarded" Provide emotional support to child, who frequently, expresses low self-esteem and isolation due to failure in the academic setting and teasing by peers Involve child in activities that utilize strengths and in which he will experience success

TABLE 30-6 (continued)

Emotional Disorder	Stage of Development	Possible Causes	Therapeutic Intervention
2. Acquired language disability			
3. Delayed language acquisition—receptive or expressive			
Developmental Articulation Disorder: failure to develop consistent pronunciation of later acquired sounds like r, sh, ch, z, or f	Industry vs. inferiority Males outnumber females 2:1	(same as specific developmental disorders)	

The genetic factor is more evident in adult bipolar disorder, but there is no conclusive evidence that childhood depression is predisposing to adult depression.

Another factor in childhood depression is parental influences. Poznanski (1979) reported that studies of childhood depression reflected considerable parental depression. In addition, obvious rejection of the child was evident in situations where the parent was depressed.

Hughes (1984) reported on the relationship of recurrent abdominal pain and childhood depression. In 23 schoolage children, hospitalized because of abdominal pain for which there was no organic basis, Hughes found the children to be healthy looking, but timid, lethargic, withdrawn, and irritable. They were described as self-sufficient, considerate of others, and "constant worriers". Depressive themes were evidenced in their stories, play, drawings, and fantasies. All the children were acutely aware of family worries, illnesses, losses, and deaths. Their anxiety took the form of morbid preoccupation with fear of loss and death.

The children's mothers, five of whom fit the clinical picture of adult depression, all had depressive concerns and worries about themselves and family members. The mothers tended to be preoccupied with their own needs and often the child was seen to attempt to comfort them. Usually, the mothers could not describe their child's thoughts and feelings and related to them on the basis of their physical symptoms.

Nursing Process and the Depressed Child

In light of the difficulty in defining and understanding the cause of childhood depression, the nurse faces quite a challenge. (See Table 30-7).

ASSESSMENT □

Client □ Assess the child's current behaviors and ascertain if there has been a sudden change in behavior. Areas to be assessed:

Mood. The child seems sad, blue, hopeless, or irritable. A sad facial expression, tearfulness, and lack of confidence are present.

Physical Signs. Weight loss or failure to make expected gains, poor appetite, inability to sleep or sleeping too much, slowed activity level, boredom, or restlessness may be evident. Somatic complaints such as headache, stomachache, nausea, bodily pains, and actual vomiting may occur.

Feelings. The child may report feeling "tired all the time," worthless, "no good," or excessively guilty. He may be preoccupied with death, illness, suicide, or other family worries. The child may express apathy and feel "nothing is fun."

Cognition. Concentration is poor, and the child may appear slow or indecisive.

> ■ *Point of Emphasis*
>
> *Each child is unique in his expression of depression. One may appear slow, apathetic, sad; another may be anxious, hypervigilant, worried, and overactive.*

Environment □ A thorough assessment of the child's family and environment is essential. The frequent finding of actual or threatened loss or illness at home is an important causative factor in their depression. Often the child attempts to comfort the parent and feels helpless in these efforts. The family needs to be assessed for its ability to nurture the child and handle family crises in a growth-promoting way.

TABLE 30-7 Nursing Process in Childhood Depression

Problem #1

Disturbance in self-esteem resulting from perceived or actual loss or rejection by significant other.

Intervention	Rationale	Evaluation
Establish a one-to-one relationship for specified time period	Indicates to child he is worthwhile	Child participates in sessions and develops trust
Listen to child's expression of feelings about self and significant others and encourage expression of feelings	Allows for release of tension and understanding of child's self-perception	Increased ability to say positive things about himself and his activities
Correct misperceptions		
Initiate activities that child can complete successfully	Allows child to feel competent	Child completes task and seeks involvement in others
Praise child when he accomplishes tasks—be genuine, not gushy	Reinforce good feelings and positive activities	Child can accept praise without "putting self down"
Initiate counseling with parent(s) and family or refer for family counseling	Entire family needs counseling to better handle family situations causing child's depression	Family enters treatment
Teach parents positive ways to communicate with their child and give support, or have parents attend parenting classes	Parents may have had inadequate parenting and need to learn effective parenting skills	Parents seek education and begin using new skills

Problem #2

Helplessness and isolation due to environmental stresses resulting in apathy, withdrawal, and preoccupation.

Intervention	Rationale	Evaluation
Encourage development of trust by meeting consistently and carrying out planned activities	Child needs to feel secure and trust adult	Child responds positively to meetings and seeks out nurse
Involve child with other children, gradually if necessary (e.g., pairs, then three or more)	Needs developmentally appropriate peer interaction	Child participates actively with others
Use warm, caring approach, express interest in the child's ideas and thoughts	Feeling of warmth encourages trust and decreases anxiety	Child better able to verbalize and shows interest
Reassure child about unrealistic fears such as dying, being ill, or being the cause of other's illness or death	Children often imagine themselves as cause of, or take responsibility for, misfortunes in the family	Child able to realistically look at his role in these occurrences
Convey a sense that the child's problems are not hopeless and can be worked out	Relieves child of fears he must be able to handle all his problems	Child learns new ways of coping

Self □ The nurse may experience rescue feelings toward the child, especially if the parents find it difficult to give support and nurturance. She may feel angry about the parent whose own needs are so great that the child's needs are not recognized. She may also feel frustrated when the child improves in a warm supportive atmosphere, then is returned to the unchanged environment.

PROBLEM/NEED IDENTIFICATION □ The child's needs and his family's needs are interrelated. Usually the child's depression is a reaction to the family's problems and his sense of helplessness in resolving them.

Prominent in the depressed child are mild to moderate anxiety, fear, disturbance in self-esteem, grieving, either anticipatory or dysfunctional, and social isolation. Physical problems may include disturbance in sleep patterns and alterations in nutrition. Family problems typically involve inattention to the child's needs, parental illness, and inadequacy. Often the parent is in a state of grief that has become dysfunctional, or suffers from a major depressive illness. Ineffective family coping may be the resulting problem.

INTERVENTION ☐ Table 30-7 illustrates nursing intervention, rationale, and evaluation for selected problems.

EVALUATION ☐ Physical problems diminish as mood improves, and can be evaluated by weight gain and reports of better sleeping. The child should exhibit greater confidence and less preoccupation with fears. He will look more relaxed, play more easily, and improve in attention and concentration. Involvement with same-age peers will increase and there will be less focus on morbid thoughts.

☐ *Suicide and Suicide Attempts in Childhood*

Although suicide attempts in preadolescent children are not common, the lack of statistical evidence is not proof of infrequency of attempts and completed suicides in this age group. Ackerly (1967) reported that 1 to 5 percent of children under 10 years of age admitted to psychiatric facilities had a history of threatened or attempted suicide.

It is questionable, especially in the younger child, whether the child understands the consequences of actions, because he does not view death as a permanent situation. At the age of magical thinking he believes he has power over situations. Therefore, the intent of childhood suicide attempts does not include full comprehension of death as permanent.

Teicher (1979) noted that childhood suicide attempts generally are impulsive and motivated by the desire to punish those whom the child perceives as treating him badly. "You'll be sorry when I'm dead" expresses rage, usually toward a parent. Jumping from heights, running in front of cars, hanging, or taking pills are modes of suicide attempts.

A significant factor preceding actual suicide attempts was loss of a parent due to divorce, desertion, death, or other separation, according to Teicher (1979). A move, loss of friends, or change in neighborhood may cause a child to consider suicide. Children who attempt suicide usually appear isolated, sad, and tearful. There may be a change in customary activities or school performance. The child may view the attempt as an escape from problems and pain. It represents a desperate wish to change an environment the child finds intolerable.

Children also may verablize their intentions; "I'm no good anyway." "No one likes me. I might as well be dead." "I feel like killing myself." These words couldn't be anymore direct in their message of sadness, low self-esteem, and sense of worthlessness.

Orbach, et al., (1983) found that it was possible to identify suicidal tendencies in young children using a tool that measured attitudes toward life and death. Suicidal children demonstrated more awareness of different aspects of life and death and had more inner conflicts about life and death than did a control group.

The nurse should take suicide attempts very seriously, keeping in mind differences between the child's and adult's perception of death.

■ *Point of Emphasis*

Safety measures should be instituted to prevent injury. A one-to-one relationship should be initiated immediately to begin building trust, facilitate verbal and nonverbal expression of feelings, and provide warmth and acceptance.

☐ *The Nurse-Client Relationship When Client Is a Child*

Special skills are needed to establish a therapeutic relationship with an emotionally troubled child. Because the client is a child it is especially important that the relationship be growth enhancing.

ESTABLISHING THE RELATIONSHIP

The establishment of a therapeutic relationship with a child demands patience, sensitivity, and a willingness to assist the child to learn and grow. Building a foundation of trust is an integral part of the relationship. The nurse must be reliable in keeping appointments, honest about limits of her knowledge, and consistent in the setting of limits. Structuring of time and place of the sessions is helpful in building a sense of security in the child.

Should the nurse be ill or absent, the child should be notified, given the general reason, and reassured about the next meeting. If the reason has to do with illness, the child must be reassured that the nurse will recover.

Acceptance and Understanding

A first principle is acceptance of the child's feelings and level of maturity. Feelings are not right or wrong—they simply *are*. Behaviors that express those feelings may, however, be destructive. The child should be clearly told what is unacceptable, and appropriate limits should be set.

Often, one hears an adult say to a child, "Act your age!" or "Stop being a big baby!" If the child is behaving in a way that is less mature than would be expected for his chronological age, there is usually a good reason. Any number of factors may underlie the child's regressed or immature behavior—anxiety, low self-esteem, hurt, anger, need for attention, and other uncomfortable feelings. Such remarks are not helpful and do not produce the desired behavior.

The nurse must know the expected behaviors for the child's chronological developmental stage, but also recognize when the level of functioning is at an earlier stage of development. Accepting the child at his level allows the nurse to set realistic goals and provide interventions that will be growth promoting.

Often it is difficult to understand the child and his behavior. He cannot verbalize feelings, so he expresses them through other means. The child in his magical and fantastical thinking, may interpret facts differently from adults and therefore is often confused and bewildered by the actions of adults.

Adults often lie to children "to protect them" when it is perfectly obvious to the child that something is wrong. Although intimate details and painful truths that don't involve the child need not be shared, a child may be told, "Yes, Mom's worried about her job, but she can handle it. You don't need to worry."

■ **Point of Emphasis**

Genuineness and warmth are essential in building a relationship with a child. He senses phoniness and a patronizing attitude.

Verbal Aspects

A child gains verbal mastery as he grows older, increasing in ability to put abstract concepts and feelings into words. However, many children do not learn to verbalize except to express concrete needs. These children may live in a family where people do things instead of talking about them. If someone is angry, he may slam a door, break a vase, or hit a wall or person. In this environment, the child learns to act rather than talk, so he may never learn to express his feelings verbally.

As all children are less skilled at verbal expression than adults, the nurse needs to consider the following:

1. Use language the child understands (e.g., an angry child would probably use the word "mad").
2. Avoid asking the child numerous questions that can be answered with "Yes," or "No," or by nodding. Try making open-ended statements such as, "Tell me about your Mom" or "Jim sounds like a good buddy."
3. Avoid asking *why* a child did something. Usually his reasons are unconscious and he cannot say why he did something.
4. Clarify words or statements the child uses that you don't understand (e.g., "Tell me what that word means" or "She was 'bugging' you? What do you mean?"
6. Avoid moralizing or preaching to a child—he will practice denial. It is more effective to help him see how an action affected him or others, and facilitate his expression of feelings.

Nonverbal Aspects

Touch. Touch is an essential means of communication in all aspects of human relationships. Indeed, from the first moment of life, development depends upon the communication of caring through touch. With a child who is experiencing emotional stress, touch must be used judiciously and individually. Spontaneity is commendable but can often frighten a child who may perceive touch negatively. A hug, a pat on the back, and other expressions of nonverbal support and praise are appropriate. When talking with a child, the nurse might touch the child's arm, shoulder, or face to gently communicate caring. A way to calm a child is to rub his back slowly and rhythmically.

Not all children, however, should be spontaneously and casually touched. An autistic or psychotic child may be overstimulated by too much touching; a panicky child may react with terror to a well-intentioned touch; an abused child may cringe at an attempted hug; a child with sexual concerns and fears may misinterpret a benign gesture. It is therefore important to be aware of the child's needs and concerns and utilize touch therapeutically.

Eye Contact and Movement. Eye contact is as important in children as in adults. Shyness, discomfort, or anxiety may be revealed by infrequent eye contact. The nurse should be aware of topics that cause the child to avoid or reveal eye contact. Her eye contact should be direct, but she should avoid staring at the child. To a small child, the adult looms very large, so it is helpful to stoop or squat to the child's eye level when talking to him.

Play. Play has been termed a child's work and "work" in this case is his daily activity. (As a form of therapeutic intervention, play is discussed later in this chapter.) Play is the nonverbal expression of thoughts, feelings, worries, and concerns of every child. Play provides a means of mastering experiences that confuse, overwhelm, and cause anxiety, and contributes to learning and growth in sensorimotor skills. It is indeed "serious business" in that it is a necessary activity of a child's day. Nevertheless, play should afford fun and relaxation, and serve as an outlet for the child's energy.

The nurse observes carefully when assessing a child's ability to play and the content of his play. Themes are often evident, such as "house," "dressing up," and "school,"—daily activities in which the child tries new roles and behaviors in attempts to learn more about self and larger world.

A child's play and flights of fantasy should not be ridiculed or belittled. Adults should make sure that the child has free time for play, and the appropriate play (Table 30-8) materials.

SETTING LIMITS

The purpose of a limit is to provide safety and a secure boundary. The child knows what is expected and what is allowed in various settings. The resulting sense of security communicates caring from the nurse and helps diminish anxiety.

Directional limits provide clear expectations about behavior in a given environment (e.g., play ground rules, dining rules). *Disciplinary* limits include restraint, restriction, and physical intervention when an expectation is not met or a rule is violated.

Limits should be clear and consistent and are important for several reasons.

1. Emotional energy (anxiety, aggression) is directed into symbolic channels. The emotional catharsis is constructive. For example, punching a pillow or pounding clay affords positive channeling of anger.

2. Limits help the nurse to remain accepting of the child. Limits define the boundaries of another person—the child may not hit the nurse, destroy property, or hurt others. If the nurse does not set limits she may become angry and punitive toward the child, and this will decrease the effectiveness of the therapy.

3. Limits strengthen the child's inner control. All children learn self-control or inner control by the imposition of limits at an early age. Parental definitions of right and wrong, of what's allowed and what's not allowed, are integrated into the child's growth.

If the child does not learn acceptable behavior and its boundaries, he is burdened with unnecessary anxiety stemming from his strong feelings and desires. This anxiety is often discharged in impulsive, destructive behavior, affording temporary relief; but because the behavior is negative, the child loses in self-esteem and a cycle of anxiety, inappropriate discharge, and lowered self-esteem is begun.

A child who feels "bad" often feels obliged to break limits, because this is one thing he can do well. When this happens, the nurse deals with the behavior while accepting the feelings underlying the behavior "I can see you're angry, but breaking toys is not allowed."

Techniques of Limit Setting

1. Recognize the child's feelings or wishes and help him express them as they are; "You look very angry." "I'll bet that made you mad." "Sometimes the things people say hurt our feelings."

TABLE 30-8 Types of Therapy with Children

Play Therapy	Used almost exclusively with children. Based on the idea that a child's play reflects feelings and concerns and that play is an attempt to master those feelings. Through play, a child works out problems he can't verbally discuss.
	Equipment needed: Playroom with creative materials such as sand, clay, paints, water, family dolls and doll houses, puppets, and punching Bobo.
Family Therapy	Aim is to assist the entire family to establish a new, satisfying life-style. The child is viewed as a symptom bearer of a troubled family. The family becomes the identified client. The family therapist has a master's degree and specialized training in family therapy.
Group Therapy	With young children, a play group helps the child learn to relate to others and express feelings through games and pictures. Children learn to identify their own feelings and how feelings may be expressed by others. Stories relating how other boys and girls solve problems may be the focus of the group. Older children may benefit by sharing their feelings and helping others solve problems. Ideally, six to eight children are in the group. Initially, the nurse needs to be directive and structure the activities. Group is helpful in any setting.
Art Therapy	Art is a natural medium for children to express feelings. Children enjoy painting, drawing, coloring, and using clay. The occupational or art therapist or nurse directs the art according to the individual child's needs.
Behavior Modification	Behavior is learned and, by either positive or negative reinforcement, continues or ceases. Behavioral therapy is not concerned with underlying motivation, only the behavior; it advocates a change in the behavior to change underlying attitudes. The aim is to change harmful behavior to constructive behavior. This type of therapy is helpful in working with children because they act rather than talk and behavior can be identified easily. Although unable to verbalize feelings child can show a change in behavior. This method requires the child to be responsible for the consequences of his behavior.

---

2. State *clearly* the limit; "You may not hit other people." "I won't allow you to break toys." "If you try to break that toy, I will have to put it away for today."

3. Provide alternative channels through which the child can express his wishes: "You may not hit me, but you can hit the Bobo or pound the pillows." "Draw a picture of how mad you are."

4. Help the child bring out feelings of resentment that are bound to arise when restrictions are involved. "Draw a picture of how you feel. You can pretend the Bobo is the one you're maddest at!"

5. Make the limit realistic and fit the behavior: typical limits are loss of privileges or sitting away from other children.

Modes of Limit Setting

There are four basic modes of limit setting.

Verbal. In verbally setting a limit, the nurse should state what is expected, in what way the child is not meeting the expectation, and the available choices. For example, "In line, we're quiet—you're hitting Joe—you may stop or stand alone with me." (Child has the choice to stop misbehaving or stand away from group.) When offering choices, make sure they are actually choices (e.g., "You may play cards or read.").

Touch. As noted earlier, touch may be used to offer encouragement and praise. It may also be used to calm a child who is frightened or upset. It is important to know what works best for a particular child. A gentle hand on the shoulder may calm an anxious child. Learning the best method develops from accurate assessment of the child and from experience.

Physical restraint, when necessary, should be nonpunitive and used in extreme situations. A very small child can be picked up and removed from a dangerous situation or held firmly for protection of self or others. A bigger child should be restrained in the same manner as an adult, if such intervention is absolutely necessary. It is important that the child be allowed to verbalize or play out his feelings about the incident following his restraint.

Eye Contact. A child with whom the nurse has established a relationship may respond to a meaningful look when violating a limit. Often a child will look at the nurse to see whether she responds to what he is doing. A responsive look may indicate that the behavior is not allowed and the child may stop without needing verbal intervention.

Removal of Interaction. Removing self from interaction with the child is a very effective modifier when the nurse has an established relationship. Every child wishes to have social interaction with a significant adult, and removal of this interaction means the loss of positive reinforcement. Parents use this technique daily, and it is also an effective tool for the therapist with certain children. "I will come back when you stop the tantrum." "We can talk again when you stop swearing" are examples of ways to remove self from interaction. It is important that this technique be utilized carefully, because a child who mistrusts relationships and acts out to keep people at a distance may not be a candidate for this mode of limit setting.

Removing a child from activities and peers is also effective. It not only gives the child a chance to "cool down," it also removes the positive reinforcement of socializing and the secondary gain from peers that a child may achieve when acting out.

☐ Problems in Therapeutic Relationship with a Child

THE NURSE'S NEEDS

The most critical aspect of the therapeutic relationship with a child is the nurse's own self-awareness. Understanding self and her own needs, along with having knowledge of child development and emotional disorders, is important in the nurse's ability to work therapeutically with the child.

The nurse may become aware of such needs as mothering, rescuing, or authority. The first two, mothering and rescuing, generally arise in relation to the child and family. The nurse may become aware of her anger toward the child's family, most often in cases of obvious neglect or abuse, or in situations where the parents attempt to abdicate responsibility for the child.

The nurse is not, however, the rescuer of the child, saving him from the "evil" intentions of the family. Nor is it the nurse's role to "mother" the child—instead she should strive to help nurturance develop in the child's own family.

If the nurse becomes aware of her own growing lack of objectivity she should examine her own needs. What she believes to be best for the child may actually be a reflection of her own moral values and attitudes toward children and families. Rescue feelings may be very strong and often reflect the nurse's own needs to "save" the child.

Blame

It is nonproductive and often counterproductive to waste time blaming the child's family, the system, or whatever seems to have contributed to the situation. Angry feelings that may arise must be dealt with through sharing them with a supervisor, an instructor, or one's peers. Many situations are unjust and the nurse will respond with human compassion. It must be remembered, however, that many times families have problems because they have few alternatives and skills in problem solving. They may also lack the basic necessities of life. Parents, who in general do not wish to hurt their child, nonetheless may lack knowledge of child development and skills in parenting. Parents may lack the capacity to provide nurturance and firmness for their children because they themselves were not nurtured. The old adage, "You cannot give what you do not have," applies very meaningfully.

The nurse assesses the child and the family to provide education in parenting, and support and guidance. Often the parents are desperately in need of therapy also. Most parents feel guilty if their child needs therapy, and believe they have failed. The nurse must be sensitive to these feelings and communicate to the parents the importance of their involvement as well as the confidence in the parents' ability to learn and change.

In situations where obvious danger to the child exists such as physical abuse, sexual abuse, neglect, and emotional trauma, the nurse must work with appropriate resources in the community, including the legal system, to insure the child's safety.

The Unlikeable Child

Although many people believe all children are "cute" and carefree, there are, realistically, children the nurse will not like. Children who are physically attractive tend to elicit a positive response from everyone. This is a fact of life. Many children who have emotional disorders reflect in their appearance feelings of sadness, "badness," and low self-esteem. Though this is a superficial aspect, the nurse must be aware of it.

The child's behavior may give rise to the nurse's dislike. The nurse may work better with a child who is withdrawn than with a child who is hyperactive. Usually, an established relationship makes the nurse feel she has met some of her own needs (e.g., to feel successful in working with the child). If the child's behavior causes the nurse to feel frustrated, angry, or disgusted, she may then dislike the child.

> ■ **Point of Emphasis**
>
> *If the nurse is unable to resolve her feelings toward the child, another therapist should be assigned to work with the child.*

The inexperienced nurse may be distressed and embarassed by a child's obscene words or gestures, or descriptions of sexual subjects. Many times this behavior is tried simply to test the nurse's reaction. The nurse may say, "I don't like that language and I'd like you to stop." If the child continues she may say, "I think you might be trying to embarrass me. I'd like to spend time with you, but I won't if you continue." Usually the child will comply because he would like to spend time with the nurse. Often the child has heard this language at home or school and does not realize it is offensive. A younger child may not really understand what he is saying.

The client may remind the nurse of someone she dislikes, and this could cause negative trans-

ference. The nurse needs to realize that the child is a different person from the one she dislikes.

If the family is threatening, or appears to be lacking in concern about the child, the nurse may become angry and defensive, and she may become unable to work therapeutically with the child. The nurse must be aware of these feelings and not allow them to affect the relationship with the child. Usually, conflicts about her own values and attitudes give rise to such problems.

Physical Affection

Physical affection plays an important role in working with children. Touch communicates caring and concern. Yet the nurse may wonder when hugs and kisses are appropriate. If the child is hospitalized or resides in a group home or other institution, a homelike atmosphere is one of the goals. Goodnight kisses and hugs just as most children experience at home, may be part of the routine. The nurse should consider the following: (1) Meaning of the gesture to the child. Will it be perceived as threatening? Will the child see it as a sexual overture? (this may occur when the client is preadolescent and the nurse is of the opposite sex). (2) The nature of the disorder. Has the child experienced sexual abuse? Would the physical stimulation prove upsetting?

In general, physical affection may be sought by the child and can usually be taken at face value—a hug is nice. In the one-to-one relationship with a child, again, the appropriateness of the gesture should be considered. Does the child need to be comforted? If so, a hug is an appropriate gesture toward a young child. Is the nurse meeting her own needs? If so, a hug is nontherapeutic. Each situation and child should be judged individually.

Feelings of Pessimism

The nurse may feel sad and discouraged because her young client is experiencing so much distress, yet he has so little control of his environment. Initially, the child did not choose his family, en-

> ■ **Point of Emphasis**
>
> *It is not possible to change the child's entire past life—but it is possible to institute interventions that will improve the child's chances for a better future.*

vironment, or his behavior. The child's problem developed in most situations as a way of coping with an environment he did not choose.

When the nurse becomes aware of her feelings of pessimism, she needs to reassess the goals of the relationship.

Termination

Termination of the therapeutic relationship may be problematic if the child withdraws abruptly or one of the parties needs to end the relationship. If this occurs the child may not be able to resolve his feelings of loss, and the nurse may also feel frustrated at a time when she felt therapy was proving helpful.

Continuing the relationship after termination is usually inadvisable. The child naturally may wonder why the sessions have ended, and the nurse should be able to tell him. The nurse who wishes to continue the relationship outside of the therapeutic setting may be meeting personal needs. However, genuine interest in the child's welfare, reflected in an occasional phone call may be completely appropriate following termination.

☐ Therapeutic Modalities for Children

A brief description of therapeutic modalities and their purpose is presented below. These modalities are discussed in greater depth in other chapters.

ENVIRONMENTAL THERAPIES

Environmental therapies are those in which the child's surroundings are manipulated to produce a desired therapeutic effect. These encompass a wide variety of setttings including residential, hospital, and day treatment.

Residential

A residential setting is a place where the child lives 24 hours a day. It may be a school, a group home, a private or public treatment facility, or a camp. The purpose is to produce "specified results for a defined group of problems" (Stone, 1979). Treatment is generally long-term.

Stone (1979) outlines general criteria for the consideration of residential treatment for children and adolescents. These include severe in-

trapsychic disorder, serious developmental disturbances, and significant disturbances in environmental relationships.

Hospital Treatment

The hospital setting is often a short-term, acute care unit designed especially for children. The program usually includes diagnostic services in the psychiatric, psychological, physical, occupational, educational, social, and environmental fields. The child usually is evaluated and either treated on a short-term basis or referred for residential treatment. The hospital setting may also be used in a crisis situation, or to defuse family tensions by providing separation while the family is assessed.

Day Treatment

In day treatment, as the term suggests, the child attends a special program during the day and returns home at night. Westman (1979) describes general criteria for the child who may benefit from day treatment: those unable to function in special education programs in regular school and those with academic or behavioral disabilities due to faulty ego development or very high anxiety.

Foster Care

Foster care whether in a family or an institution may be helpful to a child whose difficulties are reactive in nature, rather than severe intrapsychic problems. (The foster family setting is discussed in Chapter 17.)

Other Environmental Resources

Boarding schools may help to resolve persistent family problems, although these may be economically unfeasible for some families (Schulman, 1979). Most larger communities offer resources such as boys' clubs, girls' clubs, Big Brothers, Big Sisters, and volunteer grandparents who provide a supportive presence to the child experiencing situational stress.

PSYCHOPHARMACOLOGICAL INTERVENTION WITH CHILDREN: NURSING IMPLICATIONS

At the present time, no specific drug is available to treat any of the emotional disorders of child-

TABLE 30-9 Psychopharmacological Agents

Category	Use	Special Side Effects

Neuroleptics
  Phenothiazaines
  Thioxanthenes
  Butyrophenones
  Dihydroindolones
	Adjunctive therapy in pervasive developmental disorder, organic brain dysfunction, mental retardation with psychomotor agitation, some adolescent character disorders
	Thioridazine with seizure disorder, attention deficit disorder
		Allergic reactions
		Extrapyramidal symptoms
		Impaired liver function

Antidepressants No definite evidence of efficacy	Moderate to severe depression in adolescence	Same as in adults

Psychomotor stimulants
  Amphetamine
  Dextroamphetamine
  Methylphenidate
  Magnesium pemoline
	Symptoms of hyperactivity, impulsivity, inability to concentrate, and aggressiveness	Anorexia, weight loss insomnia, lethargy, a drowsiness; drug "holidays" recommended to prevent tolerance and increase of dose.

Sedatives, megavitamins, hypnotics, anticonvulsants, anxiolytics	No evidence of efficacy; only use as antiepileptics Not recommended; may precipitate psychosis in borderline adolescent	

hood. In attention deficit disorder due to minimal brain dysfunction, stimulants are often effective. However, many drugs are available to reduce certain symptoms such as aggression, impulsivity, and psychotic thought (Campbell, 1979). The nurse should be familiar with the various types of drugs used with children, the desired outcome, the side effects, and the nursing implications.

A child who is to receive medication should be told what the medication is and how it is expected to help. Parents also should be informed and should understand the place of the drug in the entire treatment plan.

Children are able to tolerate higher doses of psychoactive drugs than adults or adolescents and usually addiction is not a problem. Long-term therapy may affect growth, reproduction, and the central nervous system (Campbell 1979). Drugs given to children therefore should be viewed with extra caution.

Psychopharmocological agents prescribed for children are presented in Table 30-9.

■ Enrichment Activities

DISCUSSION QUESTIONS

1. Discuss various environmental stresses that contribute to emotional disorders in children.

2. Discuss ways in which the nurse in the community can assist families of emotionally disturbed children.

3. Compare and contrast the nurse-child client relationship with the nurse-adult client relationship.

4. Describe common reactions on the nurse's part in relation to the emotionally disturbed child.

5. Discuss the role of nonverbal interaction in therapy with children.

6. List ways in which the nurse can assist the family in improving parenting skills.

LEARNING ACTIVITIES

1. Attend a community meeting of an organization that provides education and/or support for children or families with emotional disorders (e.g., National Society for Autistic Children [NSAC]).

2. Spend some time with local child protective services, social services, and/or the juvenile court system in order to understand the functioning of the legal system and its impact upon children.

3. Observe various types of treatment settings for emotionally disturbed children such as residential care, group homes, foster care, day care, and acute inpatient care.

4. Observe a psychological and/or educational diagnostic session with a child and learn the purpose of various tests.

5. Observe individual play therapy, family therapy, or group sessions with a child in a mental health setting.

6. Co-lead a parent support teaching group for parents of children with emotional disorders.

ACTIVITIES WITH CHILDREN

1. Help the child identify feelings expressed on the faces of pictures. (Many games are available for this purpose.)

2. Draw family pictures with the child, noting who is included and what the person is doing. Ask the child to tell you about it.

3. In order to begin forming a relationship, ask the child to draw pictures of things he likes.

4. In a box, place slips of paper with words such as *family, sister, brother, mother, father, school, teacher, sad, happy, fun, scared, fight,* and let each child in a group take a turn choosing a slip of paper. Let each child talk about the topic on his slip.

5. Individually or in a group, ask the child to write three good things about himself and tell you about them.

6. Initiate/develop a therapeutic relationship with a child with emotional problems.

7. Role-play the following situations, with child and nurse trading roles:

   a. A mother telling her child she is very angry because he broke a dish.

   b. A teacher telling the child his work was good/bad.

   c. A child feeling sad because the dog died.

   d. A child whose parents are getting a divorce.

   e. A younger brother/sister who gets into the child's belongings.

   f. How I feel when another child teases me.

   g. How to give someone a compliment.

   h. How and when to say "I did a good job."

■ Recommended Readings

Axline, V. *Dibs: In search of self.* New York: Ballantine, 1964. Describes the author's relationship with an emotionally disturbed child. It highlights the child's perceptions and the author's sensitivity to him. Highly recommended for the beginner in child psychiatric nursing.

Axline, V. *Play therapy.* Boston: Houghton Mifflin, 1947. The basic handbook and guide to utilizing this type of therapeutic intervention with children. Discusses materials, setting, techniques, and the therapist. Case examples highlight the various uses of play for therapeutic benefit.

Bettelheim, B. *The uses of enchantment: The meaning and importance of fairy tales.* New York: Alfred Knopf, 1977. Provides an engrossing analysis of the purpose of myths and fairy tales in a child's life. Dr. Bettelheim illustrates the importance of fantasy in solving developmental and situational problems that children encounter. Absolutely fascinating.

DiLeo, J.H. *Children's drawings as diagnostic aids.* New York: Brunner/Mazel, 1973. The messages that the child sends in his drawings can be utilized to understand and treat a troubled child. This book includes examples and commentary on various problems including neurological deficit.

Green, H. *I never promised you a rose garden.* New York: Signet, 1965. Hannah Green's autobiographical account of a young psychotic girl is absolutely required reading for the nurse interested in psychiatric care of any age group. Told from the young girl's perspective, her fear, terror, isolation, and confusion are gradually lessened by the care of a sensitive psychiatrist.

Moustakas, C. *Psychotherapy with children.* New York: Ballantine, 1970. This book discusses essential aspects of therapy with children and is useful for the beginning practitioner. Case studies illustrate various childhood emotional disorders and methods of intervention.

Simmons, J.E. *Psychiatric examination of children.* Philadelphia: Lea & Febiger, 1969. Provides clear and easy-to-follow steps in history taking and assessment of a child and his family.

■ *References*

Ackerly, W.C. Latency age children who threaten or attempt to kill themselves. *Journal of the American Academy of Child Psychiatry*, 6, 1967:242–261.

Anders, T.F., and Freeman, E.D. Enuresis. In *Basic handbook of child psychiatry*. Vol. 2. 1979.

Backman, J., and Firestone, P. A review of psychopharmacological and behavioral approaches to treatment of hyperactive children. *American Journal of Orthopsychiatry*, 49, 1979:500–510.

Bellman, M. Studies in encopresis. *Acta pediatrica Scandinavia*, 170 1966:1–151. (Supplement)

Bower, E.M. Primary prevention of mental and emotional disorders. *American journal of orthopsychiatry*, 33, 1963:832.

Campbell, M. Psychopharmacology. In *Basic handbook of child psychiatry*, Vol. 3. New York: Basic Books, 1979.

Campbell, M.; Petti, T. A.; Green, W. H.; Cohen, I.L.; Genieser, N.B.; and David, R. Some physical parameters of young autistic children. *Journal of the American Academy of Child Psychiatry*, 19, 1980:193–212.

Cantwell, D.P., and Carlson, G. Problems and prospects in the study of childhood depression. In *Annual progress in child psychiatry and child development* (Chess, S., and Thomas, A., eds.). New York: Brunner/Mazel, 1980.

Crisis in child mental health: Challenge for the 1970's. Joint Commission on Mental Health in Children, New York: Harper & Row, 1970.

Diagnostic and statistical manual of mental disorders. 3d ed. Washington, D.C.: American Psychiatric Association, 1980.

Finegan, J., and Quarrington, B. Pre, peri, and neonatal factors and infantile autism. In *Annual progress in child psychiatry and child development* (Chess, S., and Thomas, A., eds.). New York: Brunner/Mazel, 1980.

Fischhoff, J. Failure to thrive. In *Basic handbook of child psychiatry*. Vol. 4, New York: Basic Books, 1979.

Fish, B. The recognition of infantile psychosis. In *Modern perspectives in psychiatry of infancy* (Howells, J.G., ed.). New York: Brunner/Mazel, 1979.

Fisher, S.M. Encopresis. In *Basic handbook of child psychiatry*. Vol. 2., New York, Basic Books: 1979.

Gardner, R.A. Helping children cooperate in therapy. In *Basic handbook of child psychiatry*. Vol. 3. New York: Basic Books, 1979.

Psychogenic difficulties secondary to MBD. In *Basic handbook of child psychiatry*. Vol. 3. New York: Basic Books, 1979.

Hammer, M. A teachers guide to the detection of emotional disturbances in the elementary school child. *Journal of learning disabilities.*, 3, 1970:36–37.

Hughes, M. Recurrent abdominal pain and childhood depression: Clinical observations of 23 children and their families. *American journal of orthopsychiatry*, 54, 1984:146–155.

Katz, J. Depression in the young child. In *Modern Perspectives in the Psychiatry of Infancy* (Harvells, J.G., ed.) New York: Brunner/Mazel, 1979.

Langmeier, J. and Matejcek, Z. *Psychological Deprivation in childhood*. Brisbane: Queensland University Press, 1975.

Lewis, M., and Lewis, D.O. A psychobiological view of depression in childhood. In *Depression in children and adolescents* (French, A.P. and Berlin, I.N., eds.). New York: Human Sciences Press, 1979.

Lucas, A.R. Tic: Gilles de la Tourette syndrome. In *Basic handbook of child psychiatry*, Vol. 2. New York: Basic Books, 1979.

Meeks, J.E. Behavioral and antisocial disorders. In *Basic handbook of child psychiatry*. Vol. 2. New York: Basic Books, 1979.

Ney, P.G. A psychopathogenesis of autism. *Child psychiatry and human development*, 9, 1979:195–205.

Orbach, I.; Feshbach, S.; Carlson, G.; Glaubman, H.; and Gross, Y. Attraction and repulsion by life and death in suicidal and in normal children. *Journal of consulting and clinical psychology*, 51, 1983:661–670.

Phillips, I. Childhood depression: The mirror of experience, interpersonal interactions and depressive phenomena. In *Depression in children and adolescents.* (French, A., and Berlin, I., eds.). New York: Human Sciences Press, 1979.

Piggott, L.R. Overview of selected basic research in autism. *Journal of autism and developmental research*, 9, 1979:199–215.

Poznanski, E. Childhood depression: A psychodynamic approach to the etiology of depression in children. In *Depression in children and adolescents.* (French, A., and Berlin, I., eds.). New York: Human Sciences Press, 1979.

Schulman, R. Environmental interventions. In *Basic handbook of child psychiatry*. Vol. 3. New York: Basic Books, 1979.

Stone, L.A. Residential treatment. In *Basic handbook of child psychiatry*. Vol. 3. New York: Basic Books, 1979.

Teicher, J. Suicide and suicide attempts. In *Basic handbook in child psychiatry*. Vol. 2. New York: Basic Books, 1979.

The psychiatric nurse's guide to therapy with stelazine, thorazine & eskalith. Smith, Kline and French Co., 1980.

Weiss, G., and Hechtman, L. The hyperactive child syndrome. In *Annual progress in child psychiatry and child development.* (Chess, S., and Thomas, A., eds.). New York: Brunner/Mazel, 1980.

Westman, J.C. Psychiatric day treatment. In *Basic handbook of child psychiatry.* Vol. 3. New York: Basic Books, 1979.

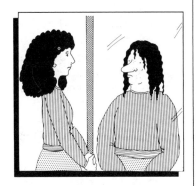

31

Adolescent Disorders

Mary Kunes-Connell

Learning Objectives

Upon completion of this chapter, the reader will be able to:

1. Discuss the influence of the milieu in the development of maladaptive behaviors in adolescence.

2. Describe theories of etiologies for borderline disorders, eating disorders, and conduct disorders.

3. Utilizing nursing process as a framework, discuss self, client, and environmental assessments; interventions; and evaluation criteria for borderline disorders, eating disorders, and conduct disorders.

4. Utilize nursing process to design plans of care for adolescents experiencing borderline disorders, eating disorders, and conduct disorders.

As a child reaches puberty, a number of complex physical, cognitive, and emotional changes begin to occur. These changes help to signify to the child, his family, and society a moving away from childhood and toward adulthood. As a result of these changes, the interpersonal and physical environment begins to place increasing demands on the adolescent. The new demands give rise to internal dissonance, because the childhood ego is no longer adequate to analyze the complex situations and decisions required in the new role. Dissonance furthers the process of ego maturation, preparing the ego to effectively (1) reevaluate and clarify feelings and thoughts; (2) develop more complex problem-solving and coping behaviors; (3) gain an increasing sense of control over impulsive behaviors; and (4) consolidate various aspects of personality to facilitate healthy adaptation to adulthood. A number of variables work together during this process and affect the adolescent's responses. These variables (intrapersonal, interpersonal, environmental, and sociocultural) can serve as enhancements to or inhibitors of the development of adaptive responses. If the variables serve to validate the positive, mature responses, the adolescent most likely will develop a set of ego behaviors capable of meeting the challenges of adulthood. This is a healthy progression toward adulthood. However, should these influences hinder the adolescent's efforts, he may display maladaptive responses that could lead to emotional disorders, limiting the capacity for effective entry into adulthood (Figure 31-1).

Emotional disorders require the use of secondary prevention techniques, the goals of which are threefold:

1. To identify adolescent emotional difficulties at an early stage in order to prevent further problems
2. To promptly refer the adolescent experiencing the difficulty to therapy (counselors, psychologists, outpatient psychiatrist, other health professionals, or in-hospital services) in order to prevent further difficulties
3. To initiate prompt in-hospital treatment for adolescents with severe emotional difficulties in order to provide corrective treatment, supervision, and a supportive milieu in crisis situations

To successfully accomplish these three goals the nurse must have not only a knowledge of normal growth and development; she must also have

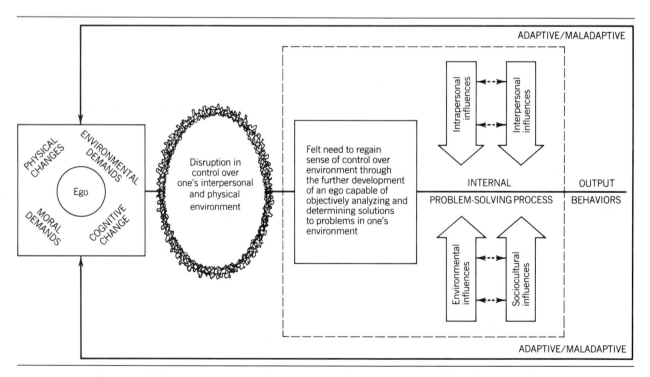

Figure 31-1 *Systems theory relating adolescent ego development to behavior development.*

a working knowledge of the signs and symptoms and treatment of emotional disorders that affect the adolescent population. To meet the goal of early identification of these disorders, the nurse must utilize an assessment guide comprehensive enough to afford a comparison between the normal and abnormal behaviors of development (Chapter 18). The guide offers a means for judging the level of wellness or illness. The goal of early referral requires casefinding abilities as well as knowledge of community resources. The third goal involves broad knowledge of specific dynamics associated with various disorders and the corresponding treatments and nursing interventions.

Even though hospitalization often alleviates the acute episode, some form of follow-up is often essential if the adolescent is to remain functional. There are times when the adolescent, on return to the community, finds it difficult to adjust to the outside environment. To prevent rehospitalization, the nurse may practice tertiary prevention, which includes both in-hospital and outpatient interventions. In-hospital treatment involves interventions that promote increasingly adaptive responses to the outside environment: the one-to-one relationship, group therapy, and milieu therapy. Community treatment occurs in such diverse settings as day hospitals, boarding houses, foster homes, half-way houses, and outpatient clinics. These facilities use a wide variety of treatment modalities similar to those employed in the hospital setting, for example, one-to-one therapy, group therapy, and family therapy—that emphasize the strengths of the individual while promoting a healthy interaction between him and his home, school, and leisure environment. This chapter discusses the nurse's role in secondary and tertiary prevention in borderline disorders, eating disorders, and conduct disorders.

☐ *Borderline Disorders*

The adolescent with borderline personality presents a definite challenge to the mental health nurse. Because of his difficulty with object relations, he is unable to express his feelings, to problem solve, and to maintain healthy interpersonal relationships. Though the nurse may first observe the manifestations of borderline personality or borderline-type behavior in the adolescent, she should keep in mind that its foundations arise in the toddler stage of development—the stage of au-

Vignette

Mary is a 15-year-old high school student who is being evaluated following self-destructive behaviors (overeating, sexual promiscuity, and self-mutilation). On admission, Mary stated that she did not understand why she was admitted nor could she identify reasons for her behaviors. Mary recently developed a boyfriend-girlfriend relationship with a boy at school. The boyfriend abruptly ended the relationship about 1 week prior to admission. In a further interview, Mary stated that she often felt lonely and depressed during the preceding two years (since the beginning of high school). When asked to describe herself, Mary was unable to do so. Her only statement was, "it depends on who I hang around with." When asked to clarify the statement, Mary said that she is "who others want me to be—I want to be liked." On interview (and through observations on the unit) it was noted that Mary demonstrated extremely manipulative behavior toward staff, (e.g., gossiping to one member about another one). When peers and staff personnel do not pay attention to Mary's clinging behaviors, she engages in self-destructive attempts.

The family interview revealed that Mary was heavily dependent on her mother, whom she described as "her best friend" and "the only one who understands me." On the other hand, Mary seems to relate poorly to her father, who describes their relationship as "stormy"—frequently fighting over even the most trivial matters.

tonomy vs. shame (Erikson, 1968) or separation-individuation (Mahler, 1975). To have a clear understanding of the borderline adolescent she must relate the tasks of toddlerhood to the tasks of the adolescent (Figure 31-2).

THEORETICAL FRAMEWORK FOR BORDERLINE PERSONALITY

Two fundamental tasks of toddlerhood are to establish an identity or sense of self separate from significant others, and to understand (at a basic level) that separateness does not result in abandonment by the significant other (Mahler, 1975; Mark, 1980).

To facilitate the toddler's accomplishment of these tasks, the significant others must reinforce appropriate behavior, allowing the toddler to form an identity apart from them, for example, allowing the toddler to make minor decisions or limited

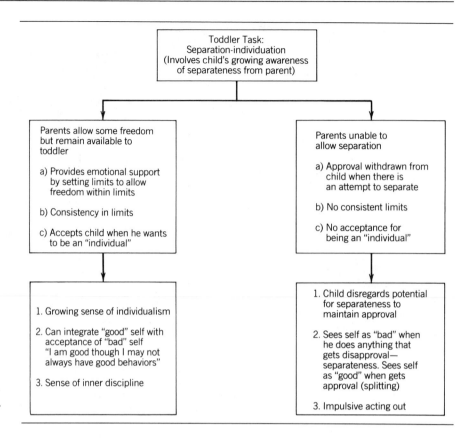

Figure 31-2 *Toddler task: Separation-individuation.*

choices with the help of the parent. Second, the parent must facilitate the integration of positive/negative (good/bad) aspects of self into a whole identity (Adler, 1981). A statement such as "Joey, it is okay to be angry at your brother, but you will not be allowed to hit him," is an example that illustrates acceptance of the person and his feelings along with an acknowledgment that the impulsive behaviors must be controlled. The parent needs to be able to exhibit both positive and negative feelings toward the child, for example, "I still love you, but I don't like your behaviors." Third, the parent must provide external controls in the form of clear rules and clear consequences so that the child can learn to problem-solve through verbal expression of feelings, needs, and concerns rather than through acting out impulsively to meet needs (Erikson, 1968; Mark, 1980; Platt-Koch, 1983). Successful parent-child interaction during the toddler phase will result in (1) a differentiation of self—an unfolding sense of individuality while simultaneously sensing acceptance by the caretaker, (2) an integrated self-concept incorporating both the good and the bad aspects of self into the personality and the capacity to hold both good and bad feelings toward others, and (3) a start at developing impulse control.

If the parent cannot respond in ways that foster an independent sense of self while maintaining a sense of security in the parent-child relationship, dysfunctional patterns of role relationships will arise, inhibiting the individual's potential for personal and social growth. Dysfunctional communication patterns involve consistently inappropriate responses to the child's attempt at individuation. For instance, a common response by a caretaker is to withdraw approval (verbally/nonverbally) for any independent decision. Autonomous behavior (decision making, separation from family) is perceived as a threat to family authority and is considered "bad." "Bad" behaviors are negatively reinforced by the family, for example, through rejection or manipulation of the child's thoughts ("Your mother will leave if you act like this"). Submissive behaviors are perceived as "good" and reinforced by the family (Green, 1983). Three responses tend to develop from such a family pattern: (1) Confused sense of self; the child fails to develop an identity apart from significant others and believes that he cannot function without them. Severe anxiety and depression may be associated with separation from a significant other. (2) Overuse of the defense mechanisms of denial and splitting accompanied by devaluation and idealization, and projective identification (Table 31-1) (Danziger, 1982). (3) Impulsive, acting-out behaviors because of the inability to express feelings.

Figure 31-2 illustrates successful and unsuccessful responses to the toddler's task of separation/individuation. If individuation was not achieved during childhood, the adolescent will be extremely vulnerable to crises in later life, because he is now confronted with more complex issues of separateness and relationship development. He is struggling to redefine his identity independently from the family, to develop successful peer relationships and other-sex relationships. These crises, difficult even for the healthy adolescent, become more frustrating for the ado-

---

TABLE 31-1 *Defense Mechanisms of the Borderline Client*

Defense Mechanism	Purpose	Behavioral Manifestation
Denial	Unconscious attempts to "push away" feelings that are unacceptable to the self or perceived as possibly endangering a relationship	Because the adolescent is unable to express feelings he will often act out these feelings in a variety of behaviors: Drug use Sexual promiscuity Overeating Self-destructive behaviors (Chethik, 1979; Danzinger, 1982)
Splitting	Unconscious attempt to separate the "good" and "bad" in both self and others based on inability to accept that the personality can have both "good" and "bad" selves	Splitting is often accompanied by two defense mechanisms: *idealization* and *devaluation.* There is a tendency to idealize those perceived as "all good" and consistently devalue those considered "all bad." The teen will try to form an exclusive relationship/alliance with those who are "all good" and blame the "all bad" person for all that goes wrong. When the "all good" person disappoints the teen he will: 1. Blame others in order that the idealized object remains idealized 2. Blame self for other's behavior and, to punish self, engage in self-destructive behavior 3. Devalue the idealized person (Chethik, 1979; Danzinger, 1982)
Projection	Unconscious attempt to project onto others what the individual perceives as unacceptable/bad in the self	Projection often results in "blaming" others for one's own actions. There is a marked inability to admit to one's actions (Chethik, 1979; Danzinger, 1982). Rather, the individual maintains an external locus of control—others are responsible for behavior. This may result in a learned helplessness—that is, the individual feels he is a "victim," powerless to take action over his own life (Murphy, 1982).

lescent who has not been able to achieve and maintain healthy relationships in childhood, so he responds in a maladaptive fashion.

■ *Point of Emphasis*

The behaviors exhibited by the borderline personality center on two primary issues: the inability to develop a cohesive sense of self and the inability to form healthy interpersonal relationships with significant others.

NURSING PROCESS IN BORDERLINE DISORDERS

Implementation of nursing process is essential in both case finding and treatment for the borderline adolescent. A consistent approach depends upon a thorough assessment of the client and his environment. Identification of problems and formulation of interventions is based on knowledge of developmental issues as they relate to the borderline adolescent.

ASSESSMENT □ Assessment involves collecting data about the client's pattern of relating, his attitude toward himself, and his responses to environmental demands. The nurse also must assess her own responses to personal relationships and her responses to feelings of loneliness, boredom, anxiety, and frustration. She needs to be self-aware because many feelings can have a negative effect on relationship development and problem solving.

Client Assessment □ The comprehensive assessment guide (Chapter 18) serves as a foundation for an overall client assessment. The following questions and observations deserve emphasis in the assessment:

1. Tell me how you describe yourself. Your strong points/weak points?
2. Complete the following:
   I view myself as _____.
   When I feel good about myself I _____.
   When I feel bad about myself I _____.

Questions 1 and 2 assist in the analysis of the adolescent's self-esteem and identity needs. They may begin to identify his use of splitting as a way to view himself, for example, "I view myself as a bad person."

3. We all experience feelings of sadness/anger/boredom/loneliness/emptiness.
   Have you experienced this feeling? If so, when?
4. How do you deal with this particular feeling?

Questions 3 and 4 assist in analyzing the adolescent's response to various feelings. These questions may facilitate assessment of the degree to which the adolescent uses defense mechanisms and the behaviors resulting from their use.

The interviewer will want to focus on the client's specific behaviors, (e.g., self-destructive behaviors, drug use, or other maladaptive behaviors). Table 31-2 depicts the DSM-III (1980) criteria for borderline disorders. The criteria also provide guidelines for behavioral assessments of borderline disorder.

5. What is a friend?
6. Tell me about the individuals that you call friends?
7. Whom can you confide in?
8. Do you have a boyfriend/girlfriend?
9. Describe your sexual activity as a teenager.
10. How do you respond when your friends do something that you consider wrong or that you don't want to do?
11. Describe your relationship with your family?
    a. Do you feel close to anyone in your family? If so, who?
    b. Do you argue with any member of your family? If so, who? How do you respond during/following an argument?
12. Are you allowed to make decisions in your family? If so, what kind? What responsibilities do family members have?

Questions 5–12 facilitate the analysis of relationship development with family and peers and response to disruptions in relationships.

Nurse Self-Assessment □ The behaviors of the adolescent with a borderline personality evoke strong feelings of frustration, anger, and rejection in nurses who interact with them on a daily basis. Frustration is a common response to the client's impulsiveness, unpredictability, and manipulation. Because of his distorted view of relation-

---

TABLE 31-2 Diagnostic Criteria for Borderline Personality Disorder[a]

The following are characteristics of the individual's current and long-term functioning, are not limited to episodes of illness, and cause either significant impairment in social or occupational functioning or subjective distress.

At least five of the following are required:

Impulsivity or unpredictability in at least two areas that are potentially self-damaging (e.g., spending, sex, gambling, substance use, shoplifting, overeating, physically self-damaging acts)

A pattern of unstable and intense interpersonal relationships (e.g., marked shifts of attitude, idealization, devaluation, manipulation—consistently using others for one's own ends)

Inappropriate, intense anger or lack of control of anger (e.g., frequent displays of temper, constant anger)

Identify disturbance manifested by uncertainty about several issues relating to identity, such as self-image, gender identity, long-term goals or career choice, friendship patterns, values, and loyalties, (e.g., "Who am I?" "I feel like I am my sister when I am good")

Affective instability: marked shifts from normal mood to depression, irritability, or anxiety, usually lasting a few hours and only rarely more than a few days, with a return to normal mood

Intolerance of being alone (e.g., frantic efforts to avoid being alone, depressed when alone)

Physically self-damaging acts (e.g., suicidal gestures, self-multilation, recurrent accidents or physical fights)

Chronic feelings of emptiness or boredom

If under 18, does not meet the criteria for Identity Disorder

---

[a] Reprinted with permission of American Psychiatric Association, Diagnostic and Statistical Manual of Mental Disorders, 3d ed. Washington, D.C. © American Psychiatric Association, 1980.

---

ships, he frequently protects himself from the anxiety associated with the relationship by devaluing and manipulating the other individual. The nurse is often the target of this behavior because of her reluctance to reinforce such unhealthy behavior. It requires a strong individual with positive self-esteem and a sense of inner security to interact with the borderline adolescent and maintain a neutral approach. However, even the strongest nurse can become frustrated with the seeming lack of progress. Frustration leads to anger, which has the potential to lead to rejection or aggression on the part of the nurse. Feelings of rejection are often demonstrated in avoidance behaviors. The nurse may begin to find other things to do rather than spend time with the client. She may assign herself to other clients or other duties in order to avoid communicating with the teenager. Anger might lead to aggressive responses that may force power struggles between them. The nurse may focus on the most trivial behavior, with limit setting giving way to arguing. Therefore, it is important that the nurse ask herself:

1. How do I view my own sense of self? Do I accept both my good and my bad characteristics?
2. What can I accept/not accept in others?
3. How do I deal with feelings of sadness/anger/boredom/loneliness/emptiness/frustration?
4. How do I cope when I have problems in relationships?
5. Do I have a tendency to devalue others to make myself feel good?

Environmental Assessment □ Questions related to family, school, and leisure-time activities identify the response to authority, responsibility, and the ability to experience pleasure and enjoyment in one's environment.

1. Who makes up the family in this household? This question identifies the family makeup, (e.g., nuclear, extended, nontraditional).
2. Who makes the decisions in the family?

This question could be further qualified by asking: Who makes the rules in the family? It becomes important to identify the process of decision making in the home especially as the adolescent becomes more responsible and capable of making decisions.

3. On an average day approximately how much time does the family spend together? Is there any special time set aside each day for the family to be together? What activities does the family do together? These questions are designed to determine the personal contact time that exists between family members in the home atmosphere.

4. Does each family member have a place in the house where he can go for privacy? Since the adolescent often seeks solitude, it is necessary to learn whether privacy is possible in the home setting.

5. Describe ways in which your family demonstrates their respect (or lack of respect) for you?

6. Describe ways that your family allows you to take control over situations?

7. Do you think your parents trust (mistrust) you? How do your parents show their trust or lack of trust?

8. What are the general rules in your home?

9. Are there different rules for different children? (If so, describe these different rules.)

10. Are the rules adhered to at all times and for all situations? If not, when aren't they?

11. What is the family's form of discipline for the children?

12. Who is the main disciplinarian within the family (or is discipline shared)?

Leisure Activities

1. Have the adolescent tell you where these activities take place, and with whom leisure time is spent.

2. Determine if these leisure activities are acceptable to the parents.

3. Determine how much time and money per week is spent in recreational (as perceived by the adolescent) activities.

PROBLEM/NEED IDENTIFICATION □ The nurse should now be in a position to identify a number of problems and concerns. Problem identification for the adolescent with borderline tendencies can be frustrating for the nurse because the problems tend to overlap, making it difficult for her to rank the needs and formulate a realistic care plan. It is helpful for the nurse to remember that there are three primary problems in the client with a borderline personality, and from these three problems stem other issues and concerns that must be taken into account. The three problems can be summarized as follows:

1. Independence-dependence conflict related to anxiety surrounding actual or perceived changes in relationship (the genesis being unresolved separation-individuation issues during toddlerhood). This results in the development of deficient or ineffective problem-solving skills in issues that might affect the relationship patterns between the adolescent and his significant others. These ineffective coping skills give rise to avoidance, regression, denial, poor verbal communication of feelings that the client believes will negatively affect relationship patterns, and acting out feelings through self-destructiveness or destructiveness toward others.

2. Self-esteem disturbance related to the inability to integrate one's "good" and "bad" selves into the personality. This disturbance creates behaviors used to avoid confusion when confronted with both good and bad in self and others: splitting, devaluation, idealization, violence when one's view of self is "bad." Acting out a sense of powerlessness over situations in one's life is manifested in indecisiveness, blaming others for one's behavior (external focus of control), and personal identity confusion often manifested by a sense of depersonalization (sense of unreality about oneself or one's body, such as feeling that one is outside of oneself and viewing one's own actions).

3. Perceived sense of social isolation or rejection related to constant anxiety over actual or perceived changes in relationship patterns. This causes feelings of "aloneness" and boredom and rigid use of transitional objects for security.

Figure 31-3 conceptualizes the relationship among the three primary nursing diagnoses and the resulting problem behaviors that can occur in the adolescent with a borderline disorder.

NURSING INTERVENTIONS □ Two goals form the framework for nursing intervention. They are: (1) The client will develop effective coping behaviors in independence-dependence issues with significant others as evidenced by: (a) an increased ability to express feelings of anger, frustration, and disillusionment verbally, rather than acting out feelings; (b) an increased ability to verbally identify expectations of others in a relationship and differentiate between realistic and nonrealistic expectations.

The client will demonstrate increased self-esteem as evidenced by: (a) a verbal awareness and acceptance of strengths and weaknesses; (b) a decrease in blame-placing behaviors and an increase in accepting responsibility for own actions; (c) an increase in decision-making skills.

To facilitate the accomplishment of these goals the nurse must provide an environment that

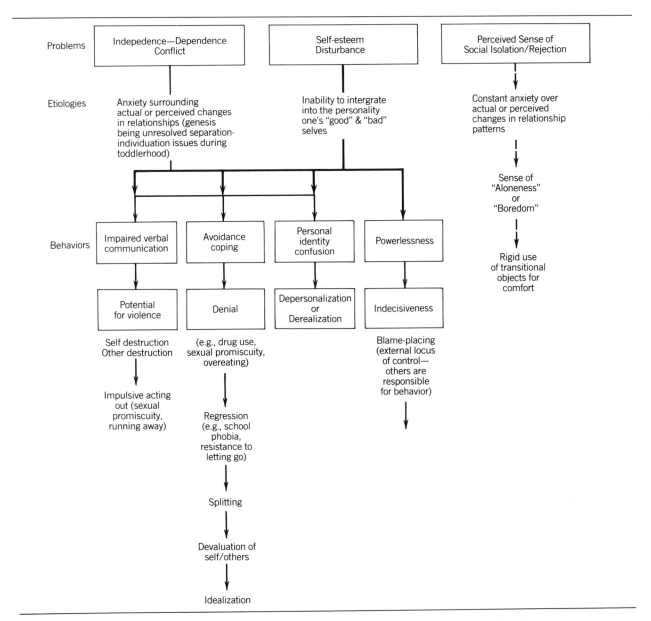

Figure 31-3 *Interrelationship of problems: Adolescent with borderline disorder.*

is simultaneously safe and therapeutic. A safe environment is one that provides the adolescent with consistent external controls (limits) in order to decrease the acting-out behavior. A therapeutic environment is one that provides the adolescent with a sense of support and acceptance as he attempts to test new behaviors (Castelli and Delaney, 1985).

Acting Out □ Because the adolescent has had a history of being negatively reinforced for expressing certain feelings (anger, frustration, anxiety), he has learned to deny the existence of these feelings for fear of rejection. This denial often manifests itself in acting-out behaviors that are self-destructive (drug use, sexual promiscuity, self-mutilation) or other destructive behaviors (violent fights, vandalism). Because the adolescent has never developed control over these behaviors, other individuals must impose external controls until he can set limits on himself. Limit setting defines reality while simultaneously providing safe boundaries for testing behaviors. Limits inform the adolescent that acting out his feelings in destructive ways is not acceptable and will not be tolerated as a form of problem solving. Providing safe limits can enhance the teen's ability to test new behaviors since he has been given guidelines for acceptable and unacceptable behavior. (Guidelines for setting limits have been identified in the chapters on childhood disorders.) When working with the borderline adolescent it is important to remember the following:

1. The limits must focus solely on the behavior and not on the adolescent as a person. This conveys that he is accepted even though the behavior may not be. If the limit focuses on the feeling, the adolescent senses that the feeling is not accepted and, therefore, that he is not accepted when he expresses this particular feeling.

(Wrong) ADOLESCENT: (angry tone) "I hate you" (shakes fist at nurse).
NURSE: "If you continue this, you will go to your room."
(Right) NURSE: "It's okay to be angry with me, but I will not allow you to threaten me. If this behavior continues you will need to be separated from the others. Let's talk about what's making you angry."

2. The adolescent must be allowed to express his feelings about the limit, how it affects his view of self, and how it affects the relationship with the nurse (Lyon, 1985). He may perceive the limit as a message that the nurse no longer likes him, or it may engender further feelings of anxiety and danger because he is not used to responding to these types of controls. Therefore, it is important that the nurse have the foresight to spend additional time with the adolescent and thereby elicit his thoughts and feelings about what the limit means to him.

ADOLESCENT: (Limit has been set). Pouting and teary-eyed. Will not maintain eye contact with the nurse.
(Wrong) NURSE: Lets client go to his room and does not follow through by later discussing the situation with him.
(Right) NURSE: Returns to client's room later to discuss the situation. If he is unable to express his feelings the nurse may use the communication techniques of reflection ("I noticed that when I told you to go to your room, you looked sad. Can you tell me how you were feeling at that time?") or giving permission ("I might be angry if I got sent to my room. How were you feeling at this time?").

3. The limit must be immediately communicated to other staff. If this is not done, the overall approach will be inconsistent. This will feed into the adolescent's use of splitting staff into "good staff" and "bad staff," so he can manipulate staff and stall confrontation and problem solving of relationship issues (Lyon, 1985).

(Wrong) NURSE: Sets limit but does not inform the others. She goes to lunch, and a second nurse, unaware of the limit setting does not follow through. The adolescent now states that only the second nurse understands him so he will talk only to her.
(Right) NURSE: Sets limit informs a second nurse, and goes to lunch. The second nurse follows through on the limit. The client will have difficulty manipulating and splitting staff.

Limit setting is important not only when intervening with the adolescent, but also when working with the family. Families of borderline adolescents have developed ineffective patterns of limit setting. They need to know that limit setting will not precipitate rejection if done in a way that communicates love, caring, and acceptance of the teen. Therefore, the nurse has to help the family develop good limit-setting strategies.

Expression of Feelings □ A supportive individual and group environment must be established so the adolescent can express his feelings. In the one-to-one relationship and in group therapy, the nurse may often have to take an active role in facilitating the expression of feelings. If she sits back and expects the adolescent to initiate a feeling discussion, very little work will be done. Rather, she must use her communication techniques skillfully to enhance verbalization. Techniques that are effective in working with the client include: giving permission to express feelings, reflection, focusing, nonjudgmental remarks, verbalizing the implied, and validating. The following statements represent examples of these techniques:

Sharing Observations: "I've been noticing that you have been pounding your fist on the table throughout the morning. Can you tell me what feeling you might be experiencing as you do this?"

Focusing: "When I ask you to tell me your feelings, you tell me your thoughts. I would like to know how you are *feeling* right now."

Nonjudgmental verbal or nonverbal language: Avoid such statements as "You shouldn't feel that way." Be aware of body language such as frowning or pulling back from the client when he states that he is angry.

Verbalizing the implied: Adolescent: "When I get into an argument with my boyfriend, I just want to hurt myself." Nurse: "I'm wondering if you would hurt yourself rather than tell your boyfriend that you are mad because you are afraid that he might leave you?"

Validation: "You look angry to me, tell me how you are feeling."

No matter which techniques are used, there are times when the adolescent will be unable to discuss his feelings. At such times it may be helpful to try some other form of communication. Writing may be effective. Encouraging the client to keep a diary may help. The diary may be the focus of the one-to-one relationship, especially if the client is willing to share the contents. This can happen because the diary is somewhat removed from the adolescent himself. Music and art may become vehicles for feeling expression (e.g., give him directions to use colors that express how he is feeling or identify or play a piece of music that expresses a certain feeling for him).

Self-Esteem □ Interventions revolve around increasing the client's ability to accept his "bad" as well as his "good." The teen will not accept himself just because the nurse tells him he should or says everyone has strengths and weaknesses. It is more effective for her to role-model acceptance behaviors. Not only does she accept the client when he has his good days but also when he has "bad" days. For instance, it would be inappropriate for the nurse to tell the client that she won't talk to him until he "shapes up." This message is perceived as rejection and merely serves to reinforce his self-defeating behaviors. Give him opportunities to succeed and to fail gracefully. For example, allow him to decide what he will do to avoid arguing with his mother while on pass. If he returns and reports that he did have an argument, do not belittle him; reiterate that there will always be a next time to develop better behaviors and it is more important that he learn from the most recent argument.

A second area related to self-esteem is the client's sense of control over his environment. His confidence in his ability to make decisions must be increased. Depending on his anxiety level, a variety of techniques may be used to enhance decision-making. If self-esteem is very low and the anxiety level high, the nurse may temporarily have to make most decisions in order to give the adolescent a sense of security. As the anxiety level decreases, he may be allowed to make simple choices. Later, more complex decision-making opportunities may be added. With more complex decisions, the nurse must support the adolescent by helping him sort out the decisions, promoting an understanding of the consequences of each decision and its effects on others. Thus the nurse validates reality for the client as he makes decisions.

For example, a 15-year-old girl states that if she runs away, she can get a job and rent an apartment. The nurse must help to validate reality about the ability of a 15-year-old to find a job that would not only support an apartment, but would enable her to buy food, and pay for clothes, utilities, and recreation. The nurse can also reality-test the effects that her running away would have on her family and friends.

■ **Point of Emphasis**

To successfully intervene with the client experiencing borderline behavior, and to promote social learning, the nurse must provide an environment that is simultaneously safe and therapeutic. She sets limits on inappropriate actions while allowing the client the freedom to experiment with new behaviors. Limit-setting inappropriate behaviors while role modeling acceptance of the client and his attempt to test new behaviors are the two most effective strategies.

EVALUATION □ Evaluation centers on the client's ability to verbalize feelings without fearing rejection. This ability often correlates with less avoidance and acting-out behaviors. Evaluation also centers on the client's level of self-esteem and corresponding feelings of powerlessness and rejection. Therefore, developing a relationship and the ability to communicate in both authority and peer relationships are important in measuring progress.

□ *Conduct Disorders*

Conduct disorders represent a maladaptive attempt by the adolescent to gain a sense of mas-

Vignette

Jerry, a 15-year-old boy, was admitted to a local mental health unit following a court referral. This is Jerry's fourth brush with the law; his first three arrests were for vandalism. This time he was arrested for stealing and vandalism. Jerry admits to daily use of marijuana and occasional use of drugs ("speed" and "downers"). He also admits to alcohol use. The interview with Jerry's mother and stepfather revealed that Jerry's natural father left his mother when Jerry was 3 years old. His mother remarried when Jerry was 8. Jerry's mother states that he has always been a difficult child: "He just never seems to be able to follow the rules that I set." She also states that Jerry has had a history of runaway behavior. He has been running away since he was 10 years old and has been away from home for as much as 11 days. Jerry's mother says that it is difficult to enforce rules because she works full-time, as does Jerry's stepfather. She states that she is very strict but Jerry doesn't seem to care and "does what he wants to do regardless of others."

tery and control over his environment. Remember that all adolescents experiment with a variety of behaviors, some of which are maladaptive, as a way of resolving the stresses that confront them. These behaviors are temporary responses to the "stormy times" of adolescence. In conduct disorders, however, the teen displays behaviors that are consistent in their disregard of the rights of individuals, groups, or society at large. These behaviors tend to be of longer duration and to be repetitive (DSM-III, 1980).

To effectively intervene, the nurse must understand that these behaviors are often symbolic of the teen's underlying problem. She must understand the individual and family dynamics that lead to the development of such behaviors.

ETIOLOGICAL FACTORS IN DEVELOPMENT

From a developmental perspective conduct disorders are manifestations of ego and superego deficits rooted in both toddlerhood and childhood. To effectively problem-solve crises there must be a balance between the superego (sense of right and wrong), ego (objective decision-maker), and id (impulsiveness). A balance of these aspects of the personality will prevent the adolescent from impulsively acting out the anxieties and frustrations that he often encounters with family members, peers, teachers, and others in his environment. This balance affords him the opportunity to think through his behaviors and realize their consequences (e.g., "If I do this . . . then this will happen . . .") as well as gain an awareness of their effects on others.

The superego, ego, and id formation of the child and adolescent tend to be closely tied to family structure, communication patterns, role modeling, and disciplining techniques (limit setting). Figure 31-4 demonstrates the interplay of those four factors and their impact on the development of id, ego, and superego.

Healthy development and adaptive responses of id, ego, and superego tend to be the product of a family structure that gives the child boundaries through firm, consistent limit setting in an atmosphere of love and acceptance, keeps the lines of communication open so that feelings can be freely expressed without fear of provoking rejection and shame, and role-models a value system that does not conflict with the social norms but conveys an appropriate sense of right and wrong along with a sense of responsibility for the rights of others (Figure 31-4). Thus the child develops an adequate superego, an ability to discipline his own inner urges to act out, and an ability to reality-test his environment in a way that meets his needs and simultaneously does not violate the needs of others.

Most teens with conduct disorders are not lucky enough to live in this type of family environment. Stierlin (1973) identifies three types of parent-child interactions that can have a negative effect on the development of behaviors needed to effectively cope with crises. Though the family

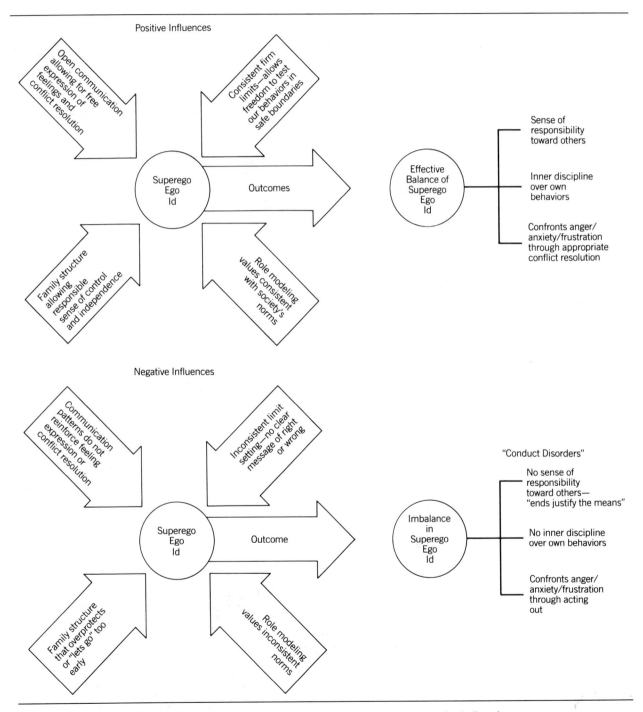

Figure 31-4 *Factors influencing the development of conduct disorders.*

modes are discussed in relation to the runaway, they are relevant to the understanding of other behaviors associated with conduct disorders. The first of these family patterns is described as "binding." In this transaction, the parents' communication seems to be designed to keep the child dependent on the family. Both verbal and nonverbal interactions convey the messages that separation and individuation will not be accepted or tolerated. The child receives reinforcement for dependent behaviors. This creates considerable conflict in the adolescent because he has a strong natural urge to crave some independence from the family. Because as a child he was not taught appropriate ways to be independent, in adolescence he tries to achieve freedom through persistent rebellious behaviors such as running away, stealing, drinking, and drug use. It is the only way that seems to offer emancipation from the family.

A second type of family structure that can lead to ego and superego deficits is the "expelling" family that communicates a lack of caring and concern for the child. Thus there is a laissez-faire attitude toward limit setting and disciplining. The child is allowed to do what he wants, whenever he wants. The parents tend to be so consumed by their own needs and concerns that they do not have time for their children. The absence of limit setting combined with the lack of role modeling can give rise to superego and ego deficits. Then, the teen's behaviors are inconsistent and erratic.

The third type of family structure is the "delegating" family, which delivers a very confusing message to the child. On the one hand the teen is verbally given messages not to act out and to behave appropriately in all situations; on the other hand he is given a covert message that he can do whatever he wants as long as it fulfills the fantasies or impulses of the parents. An example is parents who constantly worry that their son will "get in with a bad crowd and try drugs, steal, or vandalize" yet covertly give him permission to do these things by not discussing with him their finding in his room an expensive stereo set that he could not afford or their finding a supply of "pot" in his closet. These parental attitudes send a confusing message to the teen. Such parental behavior may meet the parents' underlying need to "get away" with thrill-seeking behaviors that they could not do with as teenagers.

Finally, there is a type of family that could be termed "disorganized" (Meeks, 1979). Here, the communication patterns between the parents are not organized, and this leads to confused communications in the child. Examples of such family situations include separation, divorce, and remarriage, and families in which one or both parents tend to exhibit impulsive, acting-out behaviors. In these families it is difficult to establish consistency in limit setting either because the parents do not communicate adequately with each other, or because they are too far apart in their thinking.

In a family where the parents are divorced and the mother has custody of the children, she may have a set of rules that are completely different from those that the husband has for the children when he takes care of them. If the two parents do not communicate well, the children can easily learn to manipulate each parent, (e.g., "When I'm with dad, he always lets me do . . . I don't like you any more.").

A stepparent may have an entirely different view of disciplining than the natural parent, and may subtly undermine the latter's attempt at limit setting (e.g., "Don't tell your mother I'm letting you stay up late, it will be our little secret.").

In such families as those described, the effect on the teen's superego, ego, and id may be profoundly negative. The adolescent's sense of right and wrong, his ability to reality-test behavior and consequences, and his ability to control impulses when feeling frustrated, angry, sad, and anxious can be seriously affected.

■ *Point of Emphasis*

Four family structures may influence the development of certain behaviors associated with conduct disorders: the "binding" family, the "expelling" family, the "delegating" family, and the "disorganized" family (Stierlin, 1973).

ASSESSMENT □ The nurse needs to understand the categories of conduct disorders in order to assess appropriately. According to the DSM-III (1980) there are four categories of conduct disorders: socialized, undersocialized, aggressive, and nonagressive. Socialized disorder categorizes a set of behaviors that demonstrate some degree of social attachment. The adolescent displays attachment behaviors to those that he considers his "ingroup." But he shows no concern or care for those not in this group. An example of socialized disorders is gang behavior. A gang member would never think of hurting anyone within his own

TABLE 31-3 DSM-III Criteria for Conduct Disorders

Conduct Disorder, Undersocialized, Aggressive

Diagnostic criteria

A. A repetitive and persistent pattern of aggressive conduct in which the basic rights of others are violated, as manifested by either of the following:
  1. Physical violence against persons or property (not to defend someone else or oneself), for example, vandalism, rape, breaking and entering, fire-setting, mugging, assault
  2. Thefts outside the home involving confrontation with the victim (e.g., extortion, purse snatching, armed robbery)

B. Failure to establish a normal degree of affection, empathy, or bond with others as evidenced by no more than one of the following indications of social attachment:
  1. Has one or more peer-group friendships that have lasted over six months
  2. Extends himself or herself for others even when no immediate advantage is likely
  3. Apparently feels guilt or remorse when such a reaction is appropriate (not just when caught or in difficulty)
  4. Avoids blaming or informing on companions
  5. Shares concern for the welfare of friends or companions

C. Duration of pattern of aggressive conduct of at least six months

D. If 18 or older, does not meet the criteria for Antisocial Personality Disorder.

Conduct Disorder, Socialized, Nonaggressive

Diagnostic criteria

A. A repetitive and persistent pattern of nonaggressive conduct in which either the basic rights of others or major age-appropriate societal norms or rules are violated, as manifested by any of the following:
  1. Chronic violations of a variety of important rules (that are reasonable and age-appropriate for the child) at home or at school (e.g., persistent truancy, substance abuse)
  2. Repeated running away from home overnight
  3. Persistent serious lying in and out of the home
  4. Stealing not involving confrontation with a victim

B. Evidence of social attachment to others as indicated by at least two of the following behavior patterns:
  1. Has one or more peer-group friendships that have lasted over six months
  2. Extends himself or herself for others even when no immediate advantage is likely
  3. Apparently feels guilt or remorse when such a reaction is appropriate (not just when caught or in difficulty)
  4. Avoids blaming or informing on companions
  5. Shows concern for the welfare of friends or companions

C. Duration of pattern of nonaggressive conduct of at least six months

D. If 18 or older, does not meet the criteria for Antisocial Personality Disorder

Conduct Disorder, Socialized, Aggressive

Diagnostic criteria

A. A repetitive and persistent of aggressive conduct in which the basic rights of others are violated, as manifested by either of the following:
  1. Physical violence against persons or property (not to defend someone else or oneself), for example, vandalism, rape, breaking and entering, fire setting, mugging, assault
  2. Thefts outside the home involving confrontation with a victim (e.g., extortion, purse snatching, armed robbery)

B. Evidence of social attachment to others as indicated by at least two of the following behavior patterns:
  1. Has one or more peer-group friendships that have lasted over six months
  2. Extends himself or herself for others even when no immediate advantage is likely
  3. Apparently feels guilt or remorse when such a reaction is appropriate (not just when caught or in difficulty)
  4. Avoids blaming or informing on companions
  5. Shows concern for the welfare of friends or companions

C. Duration of pattern of aggressive conduct of at least six months

D. If 18 or older, does not meet the criteria for Antisocial Personality Disorder

(continued)

TABLE 31-3 (continued)

Conduct Disorder, Undersocialized, Nonaggressive

Diagnostic criteria

A. A repetitive and persistent pattern of nonaggressive conduct in which either the basic rights others or major age-appropriate societal norms or rules are violated, as manifested by any of the following:

    1. Chronic violations of a variety of important rules (that are reasonable and age-appropriate for the child) at home or at school (e.g., persistent truancy, substance abuse)

    2. Repeated running away from home overnight

    3. Persistent serious lying in and out of the home

    4. Stealing not involving confrontation with a victim

B. Failure to establish a normal degree of affection, sympathy, or bond with others as evidenced by no more than one of the following indications of social attachment:

    1. Has one or more peer-group friendships that have lasted over six months

    2. Extends himself or herself for others even when no immediate advantage is likely

    3. Apparently feels guilt or remorse when such a reaction is appropriate (not just when caught or in difficulty)

    4. Avoids blaming or informing on companions

    5. Shows concern for the welfare of friends or companions

C. Duration of pattern of nonaggressive conduct of at least six months

a Reprinted with permission of American Psychiatric Association, Diagnostic and Statistical Manual of Mental Disorders, 3d ed. Washington, D.C. © American Psychiatric Association, 1980.

group; however, a rival gang, to which he has no attachment, could be the object of physical attacks, vandalism, or other forms of violence. The teen exhibiting undersocialized disorder seems to lack the ability to form social attachments and is a loner. The adolescent demonstrating aggressive disorders displays destructive behaviors toward others. Violent behavior can include thefts, vandalism, and assaults (muggings, rapes). The nonaggressive teen practices avoidance behavior—drug use, running away, stealing (avoiding direct confrontation with the victim), lying, and truancy. There are four disorders that have their roots in the categories mentioned: undersocialized nonaggressive disorder, undersocialized aggressive disorder, socialized nonaggressive disorder, and socialized aggressive disorder (Table 31-3).

Client Assessment □ As stated earlier, the comprehensive assessment guide presented in Chapter 18 serves as a foundation for an overall client assessment. When a conduct disorder is evident the questions and observations that deserve emphasis in the assessment are the following:

1. What purposes does (name behavior) serve for you? This question might enable the teen to look beyond the behavior and discuss the circumstances and feelings associated with it.

2. How do you feel when you (name behavior)? Does doing this make you feel better, worse, numb?

3. How often do you (name behaviors)? Also, when do you find yourself doing this?

Questions 1 to 3 might serve as a guide to help the nurse determine the meaning of the behavior for the adolescent and whether or not it serves as a coping mechanism. It also helps the nurse to determine whether or not the behavior relieves the confusion and frustration associated with the crises of adolescence.

4. Describe your relationship with your parents. Do you have conflicts with your parents? If so, describe them.

5. Describe the rules set up in your home. Do you think that these rules are fair? How well do you follow through? What happens when you don't follow the rules? What do you do when you don't agree with the rules?

6. Do you have a problem in any other areas of your life (school, friends, work)? What do you do about it?

Questions 4 to 6 help the nurse to determine the adolescent's perception of the family rules and relationships and his interpersonal problems.

Nurse Self-Assessment □ The adolescent with conduct disorders often evokes a strong sense of anger in the nurse. This may be because the adolescent violates the rights of others and seems not to care. His lack of responsibility toward others is not congruent with the nurse's sense of responsibility. To prevent those feelings from getting in the way of the nurse's objective understanding of the relationship with the teen, she might ask herself these questions:

1. How do I deal with personal problems and conflicts?

2. How do I deal with anger and frustration (especially as they are related to conflicts in my life)?

3. As an adolescent did I ever act out like my client? If so, for what purposes? Will this cause me to relate differently to the adolescent? Will I overidentify? How can I prevent this from occurring?

4. What is my view on limit setting? How do I set limits? Do I ever back down after I set a limit? If so, why?

Environmental Assessment □ The family situation is an important element. Questions about parent-teen interactions, rule setting, and discipline help to clarify the family relationships. The parents can be asked:

1. When you have a conflict with your teen, how do you deal with it?

2. What kinds of conflicts do you have with your teen?

3. What kinds of rules do you set in your home? What type of discipline do you use when your child does not obey?

4. Do you and your spouse set the rules together? Do you agree on the type of discipline to be used in the home?

5. What do you think your teen's behavior means? How have you dealt with this behavior in the past? What has been effective/ineffective?

The above questions merely serve as a guide for the nurse in assessing individual and family dynamics. The questions must be individualized depending on the behavior displayed by the client and the family.

PROBLEM/NEED IDENTIFICATION □ The teen's expectation that he will begin to mature and become more independent is difficult if he has not gained some mastery and control over his environment and has not been given the opportunity to verbally express feelings of anger, frustration, and confusion when facing new situations. This adolescent has a difficult time coping with the demands of adolescence. This inability to cope often leads to a persistent pattern of acting out that gets him into trouble with parents, teachers, or the law. Based on this knowledge, the nurse will realize that the major problem facing the adolescent is ineffective individual coping related to lack of developing a sense of responsibility toward others in meeting his own needs of control and mastery, and inability to appropriately express feelings of frustration, anger, and anxiety when faced with the demands of adolescence. Acting out behaviors may take the form of physical violence (property/person), thefts, running away, lying, substance abuse, truancy, and inability to follow rules. Such behavior is a consequence of family structure, role modeling, and limit setting that were established when the teen was a child.

INTERVENTIONS □ To effectively intervene with the adolescent displaying a conduct disorder, the nurse must focus her interventions not only on the overt behaviors, but also on the feelings and underlying problems that foster these behaviors. The overall goal is to develop more effective coping by: (a) identifying and connecting the coping behaviors with particular feelings and situations; (b) identifying alternative behaviors when the present behaviors prove ineffective or maladaptive; (c) verbally and nonverbally demonstrating appropriate behaviors when faced with anxiety/anger-provoking situations.

Maladaptive Behaviors □ A combination of limit setting and behavior modification is generally effective in maladaptive behaviors, and a highly effective tool combining these strategies is the contract. According to Croghan and Frutiger (1977), the contract serves several purposes:

1. It fosters a sense of inner responsibility to change behavior. Because the contract is mutually determined, the adolescent becomes an active participant in determining the behaviors to be changed and how to change them. He has input into his plan of care, so he tends to be more amenable to altering his behavior.

2. It facilitates the development of a sense of inner control over one's behavior. Through the repeated externalization of limits and controls and through the use of positive reinforcement, the adolescent is able to effectively control his behavior. As he learns to increase self-control over behaviors, the external positive reinforcements are gradually eliminated and he finds that he can maintain the behaviors without the use of the contract.

3. It provides for consistency in staff and parental behavior toward the adolescent. It also decreases the manipulative tendencies on the part of the adolescent. Because the contract is mutually determined between staff, parents, and the adolescent and because it is in written form, it facilitates consistent communication among them. It also serves as a diagnostic tool for assessing possible conflicts in following through with consequences.

The elements of an appropriate contract are:

1. Identification of the problem behavior.
2. Identification of goals for the development of appropriate behaviors. These goals should carry a positive tone and should be limited to one or two per behavior so as not to overwhelm the adolescent.
3. Identification of specific approaches to be used in accomplishing the goals.
4. Identification of rewards for accomplishing the goals. The rewards should provide the adolescent with incentive to try the new approaches, yet they must be realistic in relation to the adolescent's age and level of independence.
5. Identification of evaluation methods involving parents, staff, and adolescent. Timing of the evaluation may depend on the adolescent's level of impulse control. Initially, evaluation may have to be done every couple of hours, then every shift, daily, and weekly until the teen gains sufficient control of his behaviors.

The nurse plays a key role in helping the adolescent to examine his own feelings and behaviors and take responsibility for both. Often the adolescent is unaware of the feelings that accompany his action, and the nurse can help him to gain an awareness through both individual and group therapy. In the one-to-one relationship the nurse can facilitate the teen's awareness of his anger, how he communicates it, and the effects of this communication on others. The first step is to work with him to identify cues that indicate early anger. This is best accomplished if the nurse takes time to assess his behavior patterns. Once she identifies behaviors that may indicate anger, she must reflect to the adolescent when she sees these behaviors occurring.

For example, the nurse observes that Jerry is becoming increasingly anxious. He is pacing, clenching his fists, and mumbling under his breath. It is the nurse's responsibility to reflect these behaviors to Jerry (e.g., "Jerry, I notice that you've been pacing and talking under your breath. This tells me that you *might* be getting angry. Could you tell me how you are feeling right now?").

Such feedback heightens the adolescent's awareness of his behaviors. The next step is to help him connect his behaviors with the feeling of anger. In the third step, the nurse works with the teen to identify reasons that he may be feeling angry. A technique that might be used is to place the event in sequence: "Tell me what has been going on with you over the last couple of hours." In this way she can encourage him to review situations that may be causing these feelings. Concreteness and summarization may be needed to get the adolescent to clarify his thoughts and connect situations with feelings.

NURSE: "Tell me what has been happening with you during this past hour." (Placing events in sequence)

CLIENT: "I had a conference with my parents."

NURSE: "What went on in this conference?" (Concreteness)

CLIENT: "They told me that I have to go to a group home."

NURSE: "What did you do after the conference?" (Placing events in sequence)

CLIENT: "I left the room and have been out here in the hall ever since."

NURSE: "Your behaviors tell me that you might be angry. Could you tell me some of the feelings that you have had since the conference?" (Reflection)

CLIENT: "I don't know. I don't want to go to a group home."

NURSE: "I'm hearing two things—first of all, I hear you telling me that you weren't expecting this response from your parents and, secondly, I hear you saying that you don't want to go to a group home." (Summarization) "I would be angry if I didn't know what would be happening to me or if I wasn't expecting something like this to happen. I'm wondering if you're feeling angry right now."

The nurse then helps the adolescent determine what would happen if he allowed his anger to get out of control. Finally, she helps him find more appropriate ways to deal with his feeling. This may involve substituting behaviors, for example, expressing his feelings in written form rather than acting them out or using some physical activity to sublimate the anger (running, swimming, or other activities). It may also involve role playing the situation with the adolescent so that he can practice communicating his feelings to those involved in the conflict.

Group therapy calls for a similar strategy. The one significant difference between group therapy and individual therapy is that in group therapy peer pressure is exerted to promote change. It is often effective because the adolescent is more apt to listen to those who he believes have faced the same problems. Change comes slowly, since the maladaptive behaviors did not develop overnight and will not be changed overnight.

EVALUATION □ Evaluation criteria emphasize a decrease in negative behaviors and an increase in verbal expression of feelings. It is important that the evaluation be done by both the nurse and the client so that the client senses some control and responsibility for change. Initially, the evaluation should be done frequently (e.g., every shift) since the adolescent requires a great deal of feedback to become aware of his behaviors and their effect on others.

□ *Eating Disorders*

An example of an increasingly frequent eating disorder is the case of Sally (see Vignette).

Anorexia nervosa and bulimia are two eating disorders commonly affecting the adolescent population. Though they are different, both may occur together, a combination known as bulimarexia. Anorexia is starvation, bulimia is an overwhelming urge to binge followed by an urge to purge what has been eaten (DSM-III, 1980). Though both have been known to occur in males they predominate in adolescent females. Eating

---

Vignette

Sally is an emaciated 16-year-old high school student who is being evaluated at the insistence of her parents. She is 5'5" and weighs 95 pounds. Sally began to lose weight about 1 year previously. She states that she "felt fat" and knew that everyone would like her better if she lost some weight. She first eliminated all fat and carbohydrate-rich foods and now eats only vegetables. Sally's mother is concerned because Sally spends "hours preparing gourmet foods" but will not eat any. Her mother has found uneaten food hidden throughout the house. Her parents note that Sally "stays up all night," exercises 3 to 4 hours a day, and sees no problem with this behavior.

During the first few days after admission, the following assessments were made:

Sally eats 200–300 calories per day. She gives many excuses for not eating.

Following each meal Sally spends approximately 45 minutes in her room.

At room check, uneaten but chewed food is found under the bed, in pillow cases, and behind the radiator. There is evidence that Sally may be vomiting after meals.

Sally does 200–250 sit-ups every night.

When she is confronted about her behaviors by peers, staff, and family, Sally will not eat the next meal.

Sally views herself as "ugly."

She has amenorrhea, and her skin is dull and rough.

During the family interview Sally's mother describes her expectations for Sally. The mother frequently states that she has always wanted for Sally what she herself could not have. This included sending Sally to the best college, buying her the best clothes, and hoping that she would become a lawyer. Sally has been overprotected by both parents. Sally's mother states that she likes to help Sally make decisions so that her daughter will not make the same mistakes that she had made. Sally is a straight-A student and is on both the debating and volleyball teams. She is the youngest of three children. The older children are very successful in high-paying, prestigious jobs.

---

disorders are very challenging to the nurse because of the complexity of the physical and psychosocial problems they connote.

ETIOLOGICAL FACTORS

The etiology of eating disorders seems to be multifaceted. No single theory adequately explains these disorders. The nurse needs to understand the interplay of individual factors, family factors, and social/cultural factors when working with the affected teen.

Individual Factors

Some theorists believe that anorexia is due to an individual's inner conflicts about growing up. The conflict may exist at an unconscious level, while, it is believed, the teen has a strong desire to remain a little girl so as to avoid the sexual changes that accompany adolescence. The adolescent is thought to believe that if she does not eat she will remain a child and not have to confront the issues of identity, sexuality, and independence. The fear of these developments causes the adolescent to have a distorted sense of control about her ability to grow up. She feels that she can control growth and sexuality by controlling her body. The ultimate discipline requires controlling what one eats. Though she may be hungry, she refuses to eat—she feels that she has control over her life and her ability to grow (Bruch, 1982a; Swift, 1983).

It is possible that bulimia does arise from internal impulse-control conflicts. At times the bulimic develops an uncontrollable urge (impulse) to eat; it may be precipitated by stress, depression, boredom, and anger, among other feelings. The impulse gives way to bingeing or gorging to relieve the feelings. Bingeing leads to a strong sense of guilt and anxiety over the loss of control. Then, to alleviate this anxiety, the girl may purge herself, to temporarily restore a sense of control over herself (Worthington-Roberts, 1985). Purging can take many forms—self-induced vomiting, excessiver exercise, fasting, and use of diuretics and cathartics (Rickarby, 1979; Bruch, 1982b; Johnson, 1982; and Swift, 1983).

Family Factors

The family plays a crucial role in the development of anorexia. It is believed that during toddlerhood and childhood the family was overprotective. This overprotectiveness is stifling; the child is not allowed even the semblance of autonomy. As with the development of the borderline personality, the early anorexic is not allowed to separate from the family, but is led to believe that all needs and wants can be met through the family. Therefore, the child's behavior is based entirely on pleasing the parents and meeting their expectations—which tend to be quite high. The child, in trying to meet them, becomes obsessed with perfectionism, which is positively reinforced by the family, while lapses are punished.

Such dysfunctional family patterns precipitate a crisis situation in the adolescent. She yearns to become more independent. But this independence cannot be realized and she begins to feel ineffective and powerless. She believes that she is unable to control any aspect of her life, except her body. The ultimate discipline is to control what she puts into her mouth—a distorted sense of control that leads to anorexia.

Social/Cultural Factors

A theory gaining ground is rooted in the preoccupation with becoming and staying thin that is prevalent in American society. The message conveyed by the media is that the thin woman gets the best jobs, richest clothes, most expensive cars, and most successful and good-looking spouses or dates—life is perfect if you are thin. Furthermore, American society encourages dating at an early age. Hence the younger adolescent becomes increasingly concerned about her body image. Losing weight is an obsession with many adolescents, who will often go to extremes to lose weight or maintain the "perfect" body. The adolescent begins to believe that if losing 5 pounds is good, losing 10 is better (Schwartz, et al., 1982).

At the same time, American society is also preoccupied with food. Both work and social situations often involve eating—business meetings, cocktail parties, after-school get-togethers. Snacking is so prevalent that the teen may feel she has to eat so that she will be accepted by her peer group. Therefore, she must find a way to stay thin while eating. Rather than eat moderately the adolescent often resolves this situation by bingeing and then secretly purging. Thus she is a part of the group but stays thin (Schwartz et al., 1982). Table 31-4 lists the DSM-III criteria for anorexia nervosa and bulimia.

ASSESSMENT □ Assessment in anorexia nervosa or bulimia in a complex process, because the nurse must thoroughly assess both the psychosocial status and the physical status. She also must have a working knowledge of the interplay between the psychosocial and the physical in

---

TABLE 31-4 Diagnostic Criteria for Anorexia Nervosa and Bullimia

Diagnostic Criteria for Anorexia Nervosa

Intense fear of becoming obese, which does not diminish as weight loss progresses

Disturbance of body image (e.g., claiming to "feel fat" even when emaciated)

Weight loss of at least 25 percent of original body weight or, if under 18 years of age, weight loss from original body weight plus projected weight gain expected from growth charts may be combined to make the 25 percent

Refusal to maintain body weight over a minimal normal weight for age and height

No known physical illness that would account for the weight loss

Diagnostic Criteria for Bulimia

Recurrent episodes of binge eating (rapid consumption of a large amount of food in a discrete period of time, usually less than two hours)

At least three of the following:

1. Consumption of high-caloric, easily ingested foods during a binge
2. Inconspicuous eating during a binge
3. Termination of such eating episodes by abdominal pain, sleep, social interruption, or self-induced vomiting
4. Repeated attempts to lose weight by severely restrictive diets, self-induced vomiting, or use of cathartics or diuretics
5. Frequent weight fluctuations greater than ten pounds due to alternating binges and fasts

Awareness that the eating pattern is abnormal and fear of not being able to stop eating voluntarily

Depressed mood and self-deprecating thoughts following eating binges

Bulimic episodes not due to anorexia nervosa or any known physical disorder

---

Reprinted with permission of American Psychiatric Association: Diagnostic and Statistical Manual of Mental Disorders, 3d ed. Washington, D.C., © American Psychiatric Association, 1980.

---

order to implement an effective treatment plan. This assessment involves collection of data about the adolescent's feelings and attitudes toward herself, her perception of her role within the family, and her response to the new demands placed on her. The nurse needs to confront her own feelings about control issues, food, and body image.

Client Assessment □ When the nurse suspects the presence of anorexia or bulimia she concentrates on the adolescent's attitudes toward her body and herself, her attitudes toward food, her eating habits, and her ability to relate to family members and friends. (See Chapter 18.) Self-esteem and body image are key elements in assessment. Questions might include:

1. Tell me about yourself (focus particularly on the physical self).
2. How do you see yourself physically? (What do you like best about yourself? What do you like least about yourself?)
3. Have you lost weight? If so, how much? (Would you like to continue to lose weight?)

4. Have you had significant fluctuations (more than 10 pounds) due to episodes of bingeing and purging?
5. What are your strengths?
6. What are your weaknesses?
7. If there were any part of you that you could change, what would it be?
8. Have you ever had periods when you have eaten uncontrollably? If so, describe some of these episodes?
9. If you have ever had episodes of bingeing, what might stop these episodes (e.g., abdominal distress, guilt, tiredness)?
10. Many people who eat too much at one time feel guilty. How do you feel when (if) you eat too much?

The above questions increase the nurse's knowledge of the perceptual distortion that is often present in these states. Most anorexics perceive themselves as "fat" even though emaciated. They will often focus on one part of their body, becoming obsessed with the "ugliness" of this part. Regardless of what others may say, they hold fast in their belief that they are overweight. They tend to be perfectionists. They seem to be obsessed with having to do everything "just right." This striving for perfectionism extends to their body and the need to be perfectly thin. Because the focus of anorexia and bulimia is food it is essential that the nurse understand the client's attitudes toward eating and eating patterns. Assessments might include a 24-hour dietary recall, observations of eating habits during meals, and observations of the client's conversation about food. Many anorexics will pick at their food and hide it in any conceivable place (napkins, clothes, plants). Bulimics may eat a normal meal, but following the meal will need to find a way to purge by immediately going to the bathroom and vomiting, taking laxatives, or taking diuretics. Conversation can be a clue to the preoccupation with food. Anorexics in particular talk endlessly about food. They can tell the nurse the calorie count of almost any food and recite the menus of the best restaurants.

A third element of assessment is to understand the adolescent's perception of her role in the family. Most anorexics perceive themselves as passive members of the family. Their obsession with food may stem from their perceived lack of control within the family. They feel overprotected to the point where they believe they are unable to make decisions for themselves. Thus they see themselves as victims of their environment—that is, they seem to have an external locus of control. They "take control" of their lives by controlling what they put into their mouths. Thus the nurse needs to inquire into their perception of their role. Questions might include:

1. Tell me about your relationship with your parents?
2. Who makes decisions in your family? Do you see yourself as being able to participate in making some decisions in the family?
3. Do you argue with your parents? (If so, how often and about what kinds of things do you argue?)
4. Tell me about happy times that you spend with your family.
5. How has your family responded to your weight loss?

A complete physical assessment is mandatory since the anorexic may have imbalances in oxygenation (hypothermia, bradycardia, and hypotension); fluids and electrolytes (such as hypokalemia and hypercarotenemia); nutrition (weight loss, emaciation); elimination (constipation); sexuality (amenorrhea, loss of pubic and axillary hair); sensory perception (photophobia); and sleep (insomnia). In bulimia the nurse may see elimination problems (pink urine due to laxative overdosing, diarrhea/constipation); alterations in oral mucous membranes (dental caries and mouth sores due to acid content of vomitus).

Self Assessment □ In a society that places great emphasis on being thin, being fit, and eating the "right kinds" of food, the nurse faces issues about her own body image and her attitude toward food and exercise. If a nurse is not comfortable with her own body image and sense of control over herself and her environment, she will be unable to effectively work with the client. Questions that the nurse might ask herself include:

1. Am I satisfied with my physical self?
2. If I could change any part of myself, what would it be?
3. Am I always on a diet? (Do I believe that being thin will solve all my problems? Do I feel out of control in regard to my own eating habits?)
4. How would I describe myself to others?
5. In what areas do I have control over my life? What areas of my life am I unable to effectively control?

Family and Environment Assessment □ Because the issue of control may be key to understanding the anorexic and bulimic, questions related to family structure and family roles are a necessary part of the nurse's assessment. Questions may include:

1. Tell me about your relationship with your child.
2. In what areas do you and your child have problems communicating with each other?
3. Do you argue with your children? (If so, about what and how often do you argue?)
4. How have you responded to your child's weight loss?
5. What expectations do you place on your child? What if your child does not meet these expectations?
6. What decisions do you allow your child to help make?

PROBLEM/NEED IDENTIFICATION □ The task of problem identification may be overwhelming for the nurse because the physical and psychosocial problems are so closely interrelated. The nurse may feel that she needs to deal with all problems simultaneously to effect a change. Figure 31-5 depicts the problems, etiologies, and resulting symptoms related to anorexia; Figure 31-6 depicts the problems, etiologies, and resulting symptoms related to bulimia.

INTERVENTION □

Anorexia □ Based on all the nurse has learned about the anorexic, she will plan the following goals:

1. Attain/maintain normal physical status as evidenced by an increase in weight to the norm appropriate to the client's height.
2. Enhance sense of healthy control as evi-

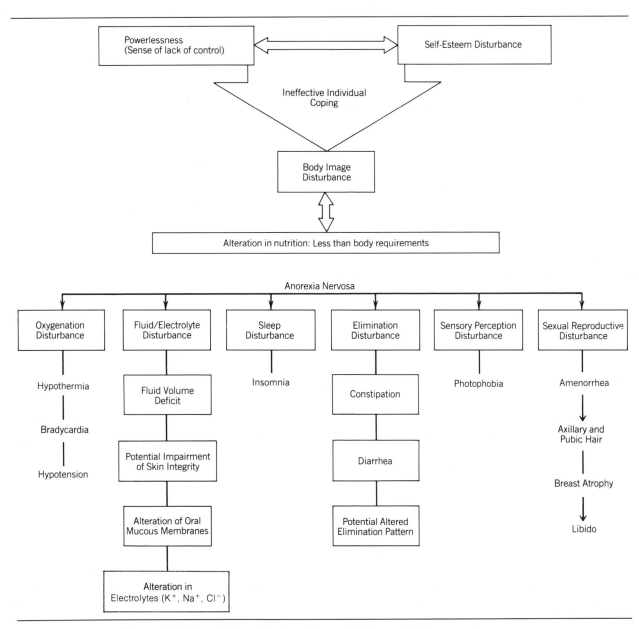

Figure 31-5 *Interrelationship of problems: Adolescent with anorexia nervosa.*

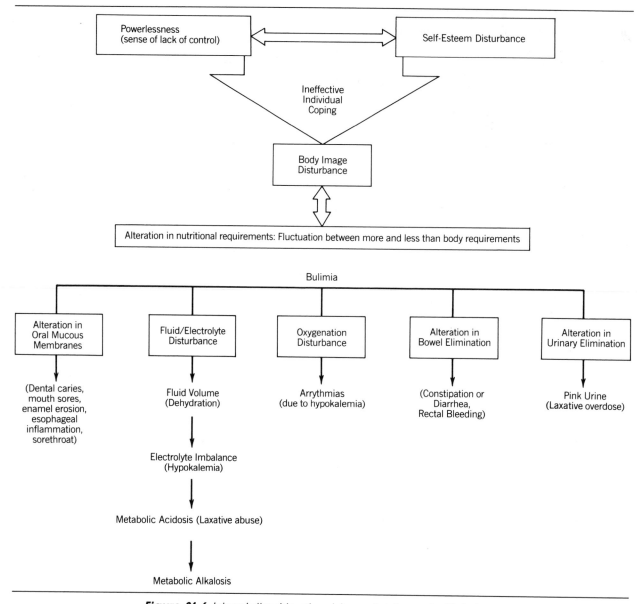

Figure 31-6 *Interrelationship of problems: Adolescent with bulimia.*

denced by a decrease in the adolescent's perception of herself as a victim, and by her taking responsibility for her own actions.

3. Establish healthy parent-child interactions as evidenced by a decrease in the use of symptoms to communicate and problem-solve family conflicts.

While helping the client to gain weight, the nurse also allows her to exercise some control and make some choices. Safety plays a key role—should starvation pose a danger to the client's life, it becomes necessary for the physician and the nurse to take control (e.g., by force feeding). How-

ever, it is hoped that the client herself will increase her food intake. A contract may be made with the adolescent (Sanger and Cassino, 1984), as part of the admission process. Rewards and privileges are spelled out in the contract, which can work successfully, especially if it encompasses the following elements:

1. Mutuality. The adolescent must feel that she has input into the planning of approaches and rewards. This enhances a healthy sense of power and control over both herself and her environment, so she is more likely to adhere to the treatment regimen.

2. Low-key communication approach. The contract should be presented in a nonpunitive, nonpatronizing fashion. Wording is all-important. A negative or punitive approach—if you don't eat you will lose (the reward)—allows the client no control. A positive approach enhances the client's sense of control—When you eat . . . then you will earn. . . . This is your choice. In other words, the choice is the client's, and if she chooses not to eat, the privilege is withdrawn in a matter-of-fact manner.

3. Consistency in follow-through. Without consistent follow-through the teen continues to practice manipulating others, using food and weight as her weapons. She has no opportunity to assume effective control over her life and her environment.

It may be necessary to insert a clause in the contract covering provisions that should be carried out if weight or laboratory values fall below a certain level. Various measures may be needed to ensure the safety of the client. This need for safety should be explained to her at the time the contract is drawn up.

Remember that in family therapy, conflicts between the teen and the parents, especially those centering on the issue of independence vs. dependence and the use of food as a manipulative device, can be identified. Family therapy is a vehicle for dealing with conflicts and developing healthier patterns of relating to one another.

Bulimia □ The goals for the bulimic client are similar to those for the anorexic. Apart from the goal about weight loss (bulimics may not lose weight) it is hoped that the bulimic (and anorexic) will gain a healthy sense of control over herself and her use of food and will change her attitudes and feelings about herself and her body image (Potts, 1984).

One method involves a restructuring of the individual's thoughts and attitudes in an attempt to alter maladaptive eating patterns. It is based on the premise that the individual often eats, not out of hunger, but because of irrational thoughts and feelings about herself and her interactions with the environment. A diary or journal is kept (Table 31-5) to heighten the adolescent's awareness of how and when she uses food. What and how much was eaten, when it was eaten and where, any significant circumstances before eating, and thoughts and feelings before and after eating are all included. These items are essential if the adolescent is to gain insight into her eating habits. The diary or journal is a foundation for one-to-one and group sessions in order to identify

TABLE 31-5 Sample Diary Format for a Bulimic Client							
When do I feel like bingeing?	What I ate	Where I ate	How much I ate	Feelings/thoughts/ situations prior to bingeing episode	Feelings/ thoughts during bingeing	Behaviors, for example, purging behaviors	Feelings/ thoughts after purging

patterns of eating and to differentiate appropriate from inappropriate reasons for eating. The diary also facilitates the restructuring of irrational thought patterns that lead to bingeing and purging.

Depression is thought to be a factor in many cases of bulimia. If depression is present, the physician may prescribe an antidepressant medication to supplement the other therapies (Worthington-Roberts, 1985).

EVALUATION □

Anorexia □ The nurse evaluates the physical and psychosocial status since each impacts the other. The desired physical outcome is an increase in body weight through proper nutritional intake. With weight gain come increasingly normal findings in other areas of physical assessment including blood and laboratory values (potassium, hemoglobin, hematocrit, urine specific gravity); increasingly normal vital signs (temperature, blood pressure, pulse, respiration); return to normal of secondary sexual characteristics (axillary and pubic hair) and sexual reproductive functioning (menstruation). It is also believed that a return to normal weight has the added benefit of returning the adolescent to more normal cognitive function. This is based on the premise that very low weight and poor nutritional level negatively affect the fluid and electrolyte balance which, in turn, affects cognitive function.

Psychosocially, the desired outcome is for the adolescent to be able to control her own life, make decisions, take responsibility for those decisions. The hope is that enhancing the adolescent's healthy sense of control will diminish her perceived need to manipulate her environment by losing weight.

The family's communication patterns also are evaluated. The desired outcome is for the family to deal openly with conflicts. Parents need to allow the teen a degree of autonomy—they need to relinquish some control and stop overprotecting.

Bulimia □ A change in how the teen thinks and feels about herself and her ability to control her environment is the goal (Potts, 1984). Evaluation criteria include positive verbalization about herself and her ability to take a healthy control over her life. Evaluation also includes realistic verbalization about the use of food, that is, the teen is able to verbalize how and why she has

used food in the past and to describe more effective ways of attaining control. Also included in evaluation is physical observation of decreased bingeing and purging.

■ *Enrichment Resources*

DISCUSSION QUESTIONS

1. Discuss factors (family structures, media, economic) in society that may influence the development of the adolescent's response to environmental demands.

2. What adolescent problems seem to predominate in your community? How is your community dealing with these issues? (Each group of four students could identify a problem in their community and report on the community's efforts to alleviate these problems.

LEARNING ACTIVITIES

1. Work alone or in groups of two or three. Choose one of the examples that were presented in this chapter (conduct disorders, borderline disorders, eating disorders) and identify the priority problems in each example. Formulate care plans for two problems (from each example). The care plans must take into account the one-to-one relationship, group therapy, and milieu therapy.

2. Tour an in-patient adolescent unit and interview nurses on the unit about the philosophy of the unit, the types of client problems, age range of clients, the daily structure, treatment modalities on the unit, and the type of limit setting used. Following this interview answer the following questions:

   a. How is the staff's philosophy implemented?

   b. How does the unit promote (or not promote) normal developmental tasks while modifying negative responses?

   c. What is the staff's philosophy on limit setting? Does limit setting promote a sense of responsibility on the part of the adolescent or does it serve merely as a method of behavioral control?

   d. What are the strengths and weaknesses of the physical environment where the care is delivered?

   e. What are the strengths and weaknesses of the interpersonal environment (staff)?

f. Are there mechanisms by which the staff can air their frustrations and concerns about working with adolescents?

3. Role-play (and if possible, videotape the role-play) a situation using the examples in the chapter. One student should portray the nurse, the other, the client.

a. Borderline disorder: The nurse is having a one-to-one session with the adolescent who has just made a self-mutilation attempt when she learns that the nurse is going on vacation for 2 weeks.

b. Conduct disorder: The nurse is helping the client establish a contract to decrease his impulsive behaviors when angry.

c. Eating disorder: The nurse is about to have a one-to-one session with a client who has just returned to the unit following dinner. The client has not eaten.

Following the videotape, have each student analyze the transaction, identify strengths and weaknesses in the transaction, and modify any communication techniques.

4. Identify community resources in eating disorders and conduct disorders.

■ Recommended Readings

Garfinkel, Paul, and Garner, David. *Anorexia nervosa: A multidimensional perspective.* New York: Brunner/Mazel, 1982. This book presents a comprehensive treatment plan for anorexia nervosa. It covers research, theory, and practice techniques for intervention.

Danzinger, Sharon. Major treatment issues and techniques in family therapy with the borderline adolescent. *Journal of psycholsocial nursing and mental health services,* 20, 1, 1982:27–34. Presents a concise but thorough overview of the treatment issues involved in working with the borderline adolescent and the family. Includes excellent client-family interactions and the nurse's response to the interactions.

Meeks, John. Behavioral and antisocial disorders. In *Basic handbook of child psychiatry. Vol. 2* (Noshpitz, Joseph). New York: Basic Books, 1979:482–530. Provides a comprehensive view of delinquent behaviors and their etiologies. The author discusses the individual and family dynamics that may precipitate these behaviors. Delinquent behavior is discussed in depth (e.g., vandalism, sexual promiscuity, cruelty to animals, sexual assault, lying, running away, stealing, and other forms of defiance).

■ References

Adler, Gerald. The borderline—Narcissistic personality disorder continuum. *American journal of psychiatry*, 138, 1, 1981:46–49.

American Psychiatric Association. Diagnostic and statistical manual of mental disorders, 3d ed. Washington, D.C.: The Association, 1980.

Bruch, Hilde. Anorexia nervosa: Therapy and theory. *American journal of psychiatry*, 139, 12, 1982a: 1531–1535.

——— Psychotherapy in anorexia nervosa. *International journal of eating disorders*, 1, 4, 1982b.

Castelli, Carolyn C., and Delaney, Jeanne R. In-hospital nursing care of the borderline client. In *Psychiatric/mental health* nursing: Contemporary readings (Backer, Barbara et al.). Monterey, CA: Wadsworth Health Sciences Division, 1985:159–167.

Chethik, Morton. The borderline child. In *Basic handbook of child psychiatry* (Noshpitz, Joseph). Vol. 2. New York: Basic Books, 1979:304–321.

Croghan, Leo, and Frutiger, A. Dewane. Contracting with children: A therapeutic tool. *Psychotherapy: Theory, research, and practice*, 14, 1, 1977:32–40.

Danzinger, Sharon. Major treatment issues and techniques in family therapy with the borderline adolescent. *Journal of psychosocial nursing and mental health services*, 20, 1, 1982:27–34.

Erikson, Erik. *Identity: Youth and crisis.* New York: Norton, 1968.

Green, Maurice. Treatment of borderline adolescents. *Adolescence*, 28, 7, 1983:729–737.

Johnson, Martha. Anorexia nervosa: Framework for early identification and intervention. *Issues in mental health*, 4, 1982:87–99.

Lyon, Glee G. Limit setting as a therapeutic tool. In *Psychiatric/mental health nursing: Contemporary readings* (Backer, Barbara et al.). Monterey, CA: Wadsworth Health Sciences, 1985:181–193.

Mahler, Margaret. *The psychological birth of the human infant.* New York: Basic Books, 1975.

Mark, Barbara. Hospital treatment of borderline patients: Toward a better understanding of problematic issues. *Journal of psychosocial nursing and mental health services*, 18, 8, 1980:25–31.

Meeks, John. Behavioral and antisocial disorders. In *Basic handbood of child psychiatry*. Vol. 2 (Noshpitz, Joseph). New York: Basic Books, 1979:482–530.

Murphy, Shirley, Learned helplessness: From concept to comprehension perspectives in psychiatric care, 20, 1982:27–32.

Platt-Koch, Lois. Borderline personality disorder: A therapeutic approach. *American journal of nursing*, 1983:1666–1667.

Potts, Nicki Lee. Eating disorders: The secret pattern of binge-purge. *American journal of nursing*, 1984, 32–35.

Rickarby, Goeffrey. Psychosocial dynamics in anorexia nervosa. *The medical journal of Australia*, 1, 1979:587–589.

Sanger, Eldine, and Cassino, Threse. Eating disorders: Avoiding the power struggle. *American journal of nursing*, 1984:31–32.

Schwartz, Donald; Thompson, Michael; and Johnson, Craig. Anorexia nervosa and bulimia: The socio-cultural context. *International journal of eating disorders*, 1, 3, 1982:20–35.

Stierlin, H.W. A family perspective on adolescent runaways. *Archives of general psychiatry*, 29, 1, 1973:56–62.

Swift, William, and Stern, Steven. The psychodynamic diversity of anorexia nervosa. *International journal of eating disorders*, 2, 1, 1983:17–33.

Worthington-Roberts, Bonnie. Eating disorders in women. *Focus on critical care*, 12, 4, 1985:32–41.

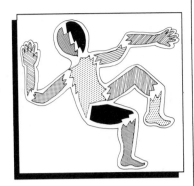

32

Disordered Behavior Patterns Related to Anxiety

Stephanie Stockard and Susan Cullen

Learning Objectives

1. Differentiate patterns of disordered behavior related to anxiety from those of psychotic disorders.

2. Explain the importance of anxiety as an underlying dynamic.

3. Describe disordered behavior patterns in which the individual engages to release anxiety.

4. Assess impairment in daily functioning.

5. Identify problems created in the client who displays disordered patterns of behavior due to anxiety.

6. Identify nursing interventions to assist the client toward healthier coping behaviors.

7. Discuss the nursing implications of psychopharmacological interventions in anxiety, somatoform, dissociative, and factitious disorders.

8. Evaluate nursing interventions for the client demonstrating specific behaviors.

☐ *Anxiety, Somatoform, Dissociative and Factitious Disorders*

The person who demonstrates a disordered pattern of behavior due to severe anxiety often is not considered as severely ill as the client with an affective disorder. Frequently, he is not admitted to a psychiatric facility, but attempts to cope with chronic, painful feelings of anxiety that constrict and narrow his emotional life and prevent or imperil close interpersonal relationships and the subsequent meeting of basic emotional needs. As a direct result, persons who experience an anxiety disorder often suffer much psychic pain and depression. Anxiety disorders affect about 5 to 7 percent of the general population and are frequently seen initially by the nurse in the general hospital setting. There are associated physical manifestations such as hypertension, peptic ulcers, tachycardia, palpitations, blackouts, and fainting episodes. Although the person may appear to function effectively in his daily activities, the drain on his ability to derive satisfaction and inner peace from daily life is extremely high.

Research indicates that prevalence of anxiety states with accompanying depression (Murphy, et al., 1984) has remained constant over the years despite positive or negative social changes. These researchers found a surprising stability in depression and anxiety disorders when studying a community in 1948 and that same community in 1970. At midcentury the rate was 12.5 percent and in the third quarter of this century, 12.7 percent. The researchers found slightly increased prevalence of anxiety and depression in women in their 30s and men in the 40 to 60 age group. It was suggested that increased complexity in women's social roles and the increasing technology leading to retraining for men were possible causes, but they concluded that depression, and anxiety, with biogenetic, personality, and psychosocial causes, was too complex to be attributed to any one source.

A review of Chapter 11 will help the reader understand the four categories of disorders to be discussed below—anxiety, somatoform, dissociative, and factitious. In the past, these disorders were known collectively simply as neuroses or psychoneuroses. If a person's behavior were labeled neurotic, this could mean any number of things to different people. The only message communicated by the word "neurotic" was that the person was not out of touch with reality as he might be if he were psychotic. It also communicated that this person probably was experiencing a great deal of anxiety or nervousness. Many other behaviors and feeling states were included in the collective term "neuroses."

Diagnoses make it easier for nurses and health care professionals to communicate in a common language regarding the difficulties a client is experiencing. However, there are limits to the value of describing or "labeling" a client. The diagnosis provides a general understanding of the situation in terms of common behaviors, feelings, and outcomes. Beyond this, it is essential to remember that a particular disorder represents only one aspect of the client. No person *becomes* a "neurotic" or an "obsessive compulsive" person. He remains a person who is experiencing certain feelings and certain behaviors that arise from his life situation. To limit a person to a descriptor is as dehumanizing as referring to "the upper G.I. in 405" or the "gallbladder in 680."

The most important common denominator in all of the disorders to be discussed is *anxiety*. Each disorder is characterized by the development and maintenance of a strong, often overwhelming, sense of anxiety, which may be demonstrated in three ways: (1) in its classical symptoms as in panic disorders; (2) in behaviors that have personal meaning to the individual (obsessive-compulsive or phobic disorders); (3) as an underlying feature creating a distinct set of behaviors (conversion disorder, somatization disorder, psychogenic pain, dissociative, and factitious disorders).

The distinctions among anxiety, somatoform, dissociative, and factitious disorders and the more severe or bizarre behavioral manifestations of disorders commonly termed "psychotic" are depicted in Table 32-1 (Kolb, 1982).

LEVELS OF PREVENTION

Primary prevention of anxiety-related disorders appears to be linked to the avoidance of traumatic separation or severe blows to self-esteem in early childhood, when the sense of security and need for acceptance is developing. Reliable child development information, parenting classes, and parental readiness and caretaking ability are essential for healthy emotional development.

Secondary prevention, aimed at early intervention, can be best accomplished by alertness to distress signals noticed by parents, peers, or significant others. When a person's anxiety begins

TABLE 32-1 Anxiety, Somatoform, Dissociative, Factitious Disorders[a]

	Anxiety Related Disorders	Psychotic Disorders
Behavioral manifestations	Apprehension, anxiety attack, phobias, obsessions, compulsions, conversion, fugue, amnesia, confabulation, repetitive actions	Overactivity, impulsivity, motor and intellectual retardation, suspiciousness, idiosyncrasies, withdrawal
Defense mechanisms	Repression, displacement, isolation, reaction formation, undoing, substitution, conversion	Denial, regression, introjection, projection, pathological identification (believing self to truly be another)
Emotional and behavioral affect	Responsive to external world and inner feelings, frequently stiff or rigid facial expression or body posture	Elation, depression, apathy, ambivalence, inappropriateness (i.e., laughing while telling a sad story)
Ego functioning	Still functioning but restricted, in touch with reality	Impaired, distortion of reality, confused
Relations with people and objects	Able to maintain relationships but frequent conflict present, erratic emotional swings, overdramatization or restriction of feelings, problems in sexual relations	Serious impairment of object and person relationships, often due to lack of feeling or relatedness with people, confusion about sexual relationships and sexuality

[a] Adapted from Kolb (1982).

to affect his socialization or school or job functioning, immediate counseling should be sought. School counselors or employee assistance programs may provide initial screening or referral to private or community mental health resources.

When the anxiety-related disorder has proven disabling for the client, tertiary prevention in an acute inpatient or long-term psychiatric setting may be necessary. Assistance in chronic psychiatric conditions may be needed temporarily or permanently; with proper treatment, however, the client need not be rendered totally disabled.

ANXIETY AND DEFENSE MECHANISMS

The client's behavioral symptoms and awareness about his anxiety may vary, but anxiety is always present. Many of the behaviors are in fact expressions of his effort to control and repress the anxiety and thereby defend his ego.

■ **Point of Emphasis**

The most important factor underlying the development of any of these disorders is anxiety.

Everyone uses defense mechanisms to defend himself against hurt, insults, emotional pain, and unbearable anxiety. Most people, however, recognize that they are protecting themselves emotionally, and do not invoke a particular defense mechanism exclusively and in all situations.

For example, a high school boy who greatly desires a place on the football team does not make final tryouts. He may *rationalize* (defense mechanism) by saying, "Oh, the coach had his mind already made up. I never had a chance" or "I don't want to go through all that work anyway." He may *project* (defense mechanism) the blame onto someone or something. "It's Ted's fault, he's such a grandstander he made us all look bad." He may *deny* (defense mechanism) by refusing to face the fact that he has failed, perhaps even telling others he made the team.

Most people have utilized these and other defense mechanisms at some time. Eventually, of course, most people realize that this does not change the facts. Defense mechanisms are temporary tools and serve a useful purpose by making it a bit easier to face the vicissitudes of life.

Defense mechanisms can be overused to the point of being ineffective or detrimental. In the example above of the high school boy, overuse of

TABLE 32-2 *Defense Mechanisms Characteristic of Anxiety, Somatoform, Dissociative, and Factitious Disorders*

Defense Mechanism	Definition	Examples in Daily Life
Denial	Some aspects of reality not allowed into consciousness of the self. Reality is transformed so that it is no longer unpleasant or painful. In the psychiatric sense, denial is not deliberate.	"Forgetting" an important but unpleasant appointment. Refusing to believe a loved one has died. Refusing to act on the basis of realistic factors (e.g., spending money one does not have).
Repression	The process of repression excludes desires, thoughts, impulses, or strivings from consciousness that are not compatible with the individual's ideas about the self. These drives remain at an unconscious level, causing anxiety. Experiences involving guilt, shame, or lowering of self-esteem are most likely to be repressed. Repression is an involuntary, unconscious process.	Viewing situations thought to be "wrong" and having no recollection of them. Being scolded or punished for certain behavior and not remembering it. Failing a test and "forgetting" that the test was taken.
Isolation	The facts of an experience are allowed to remain in the consciousness, but the feelings and emotions aroused by it are separated from the experience. Though aware of the facts, the person shuts out his feelings about them or does not relate his feelings to the specific incident.	A man loses his job, and finds another but does not associate his depression and nightmares as related to loss of self-esteem in his earlier job loss. A person who has lost a spouse and experiences "no feelings" or numbness.
Undoing	An act performed (unconsciously), that is the opposite of an earlier unacceptable action (or wish). The second unacceptable action is an attempt to neutralize, make up for, or "undo" the first action.	An individual makes an unkind remark about a person to a third person, then calls the person about whom the remark was made and invites him to lunch. A child says "I hate you" to a parent, then brings flowers to the parent.
Suppression	Suppression is a conscious attempt to deny the expression of a thought or an impulse. The individual knows he is deliberately trying not to think about it.	"I don't even want to think about it." Keeping busy to avoid thinking about a problem.
Projection	The person's feelings, wishes, and thoughts are attributed to another person or object.	A person dislikes a co-worker but says, "Oh, she doesn't like me at all."

denial might lead him to show up for practice, even though he was not on the team, or tell his parents he has daily practice. At this point, the defense mechanism no longer helps, but hinders his acceptance of his failure. His fellow students may tease him or his parents may learn the truth and lose trust in his word. If he continues denying, he will fail to seek other ways in which to achieve success and recognition, and this will limit his development as a person.

This discussion of defense mechanisms is limited to those most commonly used to control the extreme sense of anxiety. It is important that the nurse be able to recognize these defense mechanisms as part of the dynamics of the disorder, as they frequently cause her to feel frustration and anger toward the client. Table 32-2 presents these defense mechanisms with examples of how they might be utilized.

☐ *Theoretical Viewpoints*

THE FREUDIAN VIEW

Perhaps the most basic understanding of this group of disorders was developed by Sigmund Freud. Freud is considered the father of modern psychiatry because it was he who first began systematic observation of and theorizing about the human mind. In his writings, Freud describes the "neurotic personality" as a person who displays what we now consider symptoms of anxiety, dissociative, factitious, or somatoform disorders. Freud postulated that anxiety was the underlying factor in these disorders. He believed anxiety to be a converted form of libido (life force). He also postulated that human experience is based in the unconscious mind, a theory that had never before been considered.

A second basic idea necessary to understanding Freud's views is that the driving force of a person has three components—the id, the ego, and the superego (see Chapter 1). The ego may be thought of as a monitor, a reality force or controller that not only controls or modifies the passions (or drives) of the id, but also deals with the ideas of the superego, which dictate how the ego "ought to" or "should" perform. Freud then applied these basic principles to his theory of neuroses as we know them (i.e., anxiety, somatoform, dissociative, and factitious disorders).

Freud believed that events of the first few years of life were extremely important to the whole of the person's later life. Because of the pervasive influence of the Victorian era in which Freud did his work, much of his material focuses on masculine sexuality and the development of the personality from a male dominance viewpoint.

Freud postulated that the ego is weakened during its early developmental stages by conflict between the demands of the id (the passions) and the demands of the superego which are not in harmony with the ego. Freud's classic example was the case of Little Hans. Freud believed his small client, who had a fear or phobia or being bitten by horses, had unconscious feelings of sexual desire toward his mother, deriving from the id. These unconscious feelings of sexual desire conflicted with the small boy's developing superego values (morals and standards of the external world). This id and superego conflict created fear and anxiety about what would happen if his father knew of his feelings. Freud postulated that little Hans's fantasy about his mother was universal and that the anxiety about his feelings was translated into a fear of castration by his father (the penis being the symbol of erotic feelings). Jealousy and hostility toward his father because of his fears was not an acceptable solution either, so Little Hans's ego used the defense mechanism of repression. Hans repressed his anxiety about his hostility toward his father and instead developed a phobia about horses. His ego thus was forced to use the extreme defense of repression resulting in the behavioral symptoms of phobia.

In a simplified summary of Freud's view, the anxiety-related disorders (neuroses) are caused by the ego becoming overwhelmed by id drives and superego conflict. As the monitor of reality, the ego is forced to develop defenses to control the anxiety arising from these conflicts. Symptoms such as phobias, panic attacks, conversion, and amnesia are then displayed. The severe effects of such symptoms on the client's life-style and future growth are examined in the discussion of each disorder.

HORNEY'S VIEW

Perhaps one of the most important theorists following Freud was Karen Horney. Dr. Horney postulated that every symptom of these disorders grew out of a basic conflict within the person. This basic, or core, conflict is unconscious but at times can manifest itself vaguely in conscious ways. For example, when facing a major decision, such as getting married, a person may be indecisive and call upon others to resolve the issue. The person is aware of a conflict (e.g., whether to marry), yet unaware of the basic conflicts that cause such agonizing indecision. Or the inner conflict might be manifested in a person's awareness of an incompatibility between the self and the environment.

How did this basic conflict evolve? Horney saw the basic conflict arising from fundamentally contradictory attitudes that the person acquired toward others. This conflict evolves from basic anxiety—the feeling a child has of being isolated in a potentially hostile world characterized by indifference, lack of guidance, lack of warmth, hostility, erratic behavior, or lack of respect, or disparagement. Given such unfavorable conditions, a child tries to cope by developing various strategies that become part of his personality. Horney believed these coping strategies could be seen in the development of certain predominant attitudes (Table 32-3).

The first two coping strategies seem to represent extreme opposites. The first strategy includes a liking for everyone, the second sees all as enemies. The first avoids fights at all costs, the second relishes battles. While fear and helplessness characterize the first attitude, the second strives to conquer fear by striking out at others.

In the third attitude, feelings are suppressed and denied with neither overly dependent nor hostile feelings emerging. The person uses detachment to keep his basic conflicts out of conscious awareness, but this creates only an artificial harmony.

In Horney's view, an element of basic anxiety is overemphasized: first, helplessness; second, hostility; and third, isolation. The dominant attitude is the one that determines the person's conduct, although it contains elements of each of the other attitudes. These three attitudes create conflict within the person who behaves in the predominant way rigidly and inflexibly, whether his behavior is appropriate to the situation or not. If the individual tries to behave in any way other than his severely restricted ("neurotic") attitude, he will experience severe panic. Because this coping strategy developed early in life as a protective device for relating to the world, attempts to change, while not impossible, cause a severe threat to the individual's sense of inner security.

Horney recognized that not only did these three attitudes involve the way in which the person relates to others, but also how he thinks and feels about himself and his role in life. In the process of therapy, he can gradually come to under-

---

TABLE 32-3 Horney's Theory of Neurotic Coping Attitudes

Moving toward Individual
  Child is resigned to helplessness
  Constantly tries to win affection
  Overly dependent on others to feel safe
  Compliant, overly considerate, overly appreciative and generous
  Unconsciously cares little for others, but consciously believes he likes everyone
  Overidealizes others
  Evaluates self based solely on others' opinions of him
Moving against Individual
  Believes world is hostile and consciously or unconsciously decides to fight it
  Distrusts others
  Must be stronger and better, and defeat others
  Life is a struggle, but won't acknowledge feeling fear
  Must excel, achieve, gain prestige and recognition
  Often exploits others
  Relates to others based on status, benefit, or power they can give him
  "Soft" or "tender" feelings are abhorrent—may ridicule these in others
Moving away from Individual
  Intolerable stress in associating with others causes detachment and isolation
  Views self with detached objectivity, like a painting or piece of sculpture
  Appears to be a spectator of life, not a participant
  Needs to be completely self-sufficient and resourceful
  Avoids obligation, influence, or ties with others
  Restricts needs in order to be self-sufficient
  Advice or help from others seen as an attempt at domination
  Strong need to appear superior, recognized (with no personal effort), and unique
  If superiority threatened, may break isolation by frantic pursuit of affection or protection, often with disastrous results

---

stand his attitude and learn to replace distorted ways of thinking and feeling with healthier mental attitudes.

SULLIVAN'S VIEW

A basic tenet of H.S. Sullivan's theory is that the behavior of persons with mental disorders is not manifestly different from the norm. In emotional disorders, however, there is the reappearance of dynamic processes that normally appear in infancy and childhood. These early processes recur to normal adults only in dreams or in anxiety states.

According to Sullivan, the primitive processes of infancy and childhood recede from awareness as the self-system develops. The self-system is a collection of processes, selected memories, and knowledge of relationships that control awareness; it develops out of the human personality based on the need to feel secure with others. Thus, the interpersonal basis of Sullivan's theory.

The self-system develops long before the child can analyze or make sense of why he does this and not that, what is right or wrong, or what is said and done. As the self-system develops, one is cut off from awareness of earlier methods of thought (referential operation) when, as a child, one learns to think logically by means of language. As the child learns what behaviors bring social approval or disapproval, impulses for direct satisfaction of needs are sublimated in order to achieve partial satisfaction of needs that meet with social approval. For example, it is natural for a 2-year-old to soil his pants, but social approval, which meets his need for security, comes as he learns to use the toilet.

The self-system, that is, awareness of self, is the active self. Sullivan describes two other parts of the system: one part not readily accessible to awareness, the other spent in sleep, in which what occurs cannot occur to the active self. Often, a person will say "I'll sleep on it," when confronted with a problem; after a night's sleep a solution will present itself. In Sullivan's view, the self-system, or awareness, has been inactive, allowing earlier, referential operation thinking, which can be creative, to occur.

The self-system struggles to protect itself from the referential or early processes that cannot be admitted into awareness (lest security and satisfaction needs be threatened). To avoid or minimize anxiety during this struggle various specific processes are activated. These are known as *dynamisms* and are somewhat similar to the intrapersonal or Freudian concept of defense mechanisms. However, interpersonal relations are dynamic, not static; Sullivan emphasized that these processes to avoid or minimize anxiety are also dynamic, have energy, and will go on until some goal is reached.

Sullivan believed that everyone uses dynamisms in his self-system's struggle to protect itself and that mental illness is caused by the difference in degree, intensity, or timing of the dynamisms. He referred to dynamisms as "universal human equipment, sometimes represented almost entirely in dreadful distortions of living, but still universal" (1953, 305). When the dynamisms are activated but fail to achieve a goal, or achieve an unsatisfactory goal, they are misused and may go on indefinitely, becoming destructive rather than helpful to the individual. For example, a woman whose husband dies continues to deny his death long after the normal denial response of grief. She does not settle business affairs, still sets his place at the table, keeps all his belongings, and behaves as though he were still alive.

Dynamisms that recur frequently or for protracted periods are regarded as "dynamisms of difficulty," which distinguish those who are mentally ill from those who are well. This is similar to the concept of overuse of the defense mechanisms of intrapsychic theory. Overuse of defense mechanisms or dynamisms to protect the self from anxiety cause what are seen as symptoms of mental illness.

The discussion of each dynamism is beyond the scope of this chapter. Sullivan's theories, nevertheless, can be applied to anxiety-related disorders. When a dynamism is misused or overused so that reality is distorted, problems arise in daily living and personal relationships. For example, obsessional dynamism may be seen in a song, jingle, slogan, or sign that catches the attention and holds it, though why this is so is not within the person's awareness. However, beneath the level of awareness (the self-system) that which riveted the person's attention is related to an earlier referential process that is not understood during the waking state. Often, this distraction to awareness allows other processes outside one's awareness to do useful work at clarifying a problem or reducing anxiety.

Misuse of obsessional dynamism occurs in obsessive compulsive disorder, where goals are not achieved as hoped for. Using Sullivan's interpersonal theory, anxiety-related disorders can be viewed as distortions of universal human dynamisms, exaggerations of "normal" human states in which a person strives to meet needs while protecting the self.

Sullivan discussed many dynamisms that are part of daily life; those most pertinent to the anxiety-related disorders are sublimation, obsessionalism, selective inattention, and dynamisms of emotion—fear, anger, rage, hatred, grief, guilt, hysteria. When these are misused or overused, symptoms of a specific anxiety-related disorder or other mental illness may arise.

There are many other views as to how anxiety-related disorders may develop. The intrapersonal and interpersonal views presented here afford some notion of the dynamic nature of the individual and emphasize the importance of his inner processes and/or life experiences. Some theorists view these disorders as learned patterns of behavior which can be unlearned, or for which healthier patterns may be substituted. Review of Chapter 1 will help the reader appreciate the great variety of psychiatric and psychological theories.

Categories of Disorder Related to Anxiety

The major disorders related to anxiety are as follows:

1. Anxiety states
   a. Panic disorders
   b. Generalized anxiety disorder
   c. Phobic disorder
   d. Obsessive-compulsive disorder
   e. Post-traumatic stress disorder
2. Somatoform disorders
   a. Conversion disorder
   b. Somatization disorder
   c. Psychogenic pain
   d. Hypochondriasis
3. Dissociative disorders
   a. Psychogenic amnesia
   b. Psychogenic fugue
   c. Multiple personality
   d. Depersonalization disorder
4. Factitious disorder
   a. Factitious disorder with psychological symptoms
   b. Factitious disorder with physical symptoms

The general category of anxiety disorders is so named because the outstanding behavioral feature is that of anxiety or symptoms that are attempts to master anxiety. It is estimated that these disorders occur in 2 to 4 percent of the general population.

☐ Anxiety States (Anxiety Neuroses)

Two disorders the nurse should be familiar with are panic disorder and generalized anxiety disorder (DSM III). The predominant feature of both of these states is anxiety. (See Chapter 11.)

PANIC DISORDER

A person with panic disorder experiences recurring panic attacks which are characterized by a sudden feeling of fear, terror, or doom. Physical symptoms may include a sense of choking or being smothered, heart palpitation, difficulty in breathing, dizziness, unsteadiness, shaking, trembling, flushing or sweating or coldness, and a tingling sensation. The person may experience a sense of unreality, fear of losing control, dying, or "going to pieces." Most attacks last only a few minutes, but leave the person shaken, fearful, and often physically exhausted.

These series of attacks may be brief, may occur several times, or may become chronic. In severe cases, the person may be totally incapacitated (afraid to leave the house, go to work, buy groceries, and so on). Panic disorder generally does not begin until late adolescence or adult life, and often develops in response to a sudden loss. In early childhood, the basis for panic disorder is thought to be generated by severe separation anxiety experiences. There is growing evidence that panic disorders may occur due to individual differences in biochemical function of the brain; this causes some persons to be extremely sensitive to chemicals in the body and the sensitivity increases at higher levels of anxiety (Rainey, et al., 1985).

Care of clients in panic or generalized severe anxiety states is similar—therefore it is presented in combination later in the chapter. Anxiety progresses from mild, to moderate, to severe, to panic, so that interventions must occur in the early stages to prevent severe and panic levels of anxiety (see case study on page 729).

GENERALIZED ANXIETY DISORDER

Generalized anxiety disorder is different from panic disorder in that the individual experiences a generalized, persistent anxiety rather than discrete attacks. The former is rarely more than mildly incapacitating to work or social functioning. The person feels severely anxious all the time. According to DSM III, there are four areas in which the person experiences the symptoms:

1. Motor tension. Behaviors indicating motor tension include fidgeting, jumpiness, easy startle, muscle twitching, trembling, and shakiness. The person may present a strained expression and may report fatigue and inability to relax.

Case Study

Michael, a 32-year-old construction supervisor, lost his job because of a slowdown in the industry. He had a 3-year-old daughter, and he and his wife were expecting their second child in 4 months. His wife, a nurse, worked part-time. He had recently begun to experience episodes of shaking, profuse sweating, then chills, rapid breathing, and heart palpitations. The episodes were of 5 to 10 minutes in duration. His family doctor could find no physical basis for the experience, and Michael was referred for therapy.

Michael described that along with the physical symptoms during the attacks, he felt "like I was dying" and after the chills felt "like I'm paralyzed" for a few minutes. The nurse therapist found that the attacks occurred most frequently when his wife left for work and he had responsibility for their daughter. These attacks were exceptionally frightening because he was unable to care for his daughter while he was experiencing them.

When Michael was a child, his father had held a very important place in his affections; he died of a heart attack when Michael was 16. Both his parents had worked very hard running a business and raising six children. Michael was the oldest. He had always been taught that a man's job was to work hard and take care of his family. Although his college major was art, he had been unable to find a suitable job that afforded a salary sufficient for family needs.

After obtaining the background information, the nurse focused on Michael's present feelings. She helped Michael identify his feelings of frustration with his construction job. she also helped him acknowledge that he felt out of control of his life and how frightening this had become for him. In discussing his view of his life at this point, Michael realized how much he had idealized his father as a "real man" and how he compared himself in a self-denigrating way to his dad. He felt like a failure as a son, husband, and father, and felt he had failed to live up to this idealized concept of "a man."

One of his greatest difficulties in therapy was identifying and acknowledging his feelings, especially his anger. The nurse therapist helped him by naming what the feeling sounded like to her. For example, Michael would say he was "frustrated" when describing an incident in which he was clearly angry. He still had many feelings of unresolved grief and anger about his father's death and this anger was particularly difficult for

him to express, as he both loved his dad and was angry at him for dying. The nurse therapist used other ways to help him talk about this difficult emotion, such as discussing anger as a normal human emotion that is neither positive nor negative in itself, but only in its expression. It was also helpful for Michael to understand that everyone has both positive and negative feelings at times, even toward loved ones, and that he was not evil because of his feelings.

Another helpful intervention was "mirroring" his nonverbal signals of anger, of which he was unaware, such as frowning, turning red, and tensing his body. In the working phase of the relationship, the nurse also used humor to help him recognize when he was denying a feeling. Because trust had been established, he did not see this as being ridiculed, but could admit to his feelings.

Another feeling that Michael found difficult to examine was dependency, which he viewed as "weak and unmanly." Michael realized that he was afraid his wife would not return from work and he would be left alone, unable to cope—this despite her reassurances that she did not object to working and felt it was her contribution to the family. She was optimistic about making ends meet until he was able to obtain suitable employment. The nurse helped Michael to look at unhealthy types of dependency and the normal dependency–interdependency shared by couples. Michael was able to realize that "doing everything himself" didn't necessarily mean total independence.

Because of his father's early death, Michael had had no opportunity to know his father as a human being instead of the idealized parent of childhood. The nurse helped Michael understand that when one loses a loved one (especially as a child), it is common to attribute perfection to him. One of the goals of therapy was to help Michael distinguish between the real and the idealized versions of his father and how he himself differed from his dad.

As Michael became aware of his feelings, his panic attacks subsided. At the outset of therapy, imipramine was prescribed, and this soon alleviated the symptoms. As he continued in therapy, he obtained work in the graphic arts field, for which he had trained, and though the pay was less than he had been earning, the work was more enjoyable.

2. Autonomic hyperactivity. Observable behavior includes sweating, flushing or pallor, high pulse and respiration rate, and cold clammy hands. There may be diarrhea or a need to urinate frequently. The person may describe a pounding heart, upset stomach, lightheadedness, dizziness, hot or cold spells, and tingling of hands or feet.

3. Apprehensive expectation. The person experiences fear, worry, anxiety, and repetitive thoughts. Frequently, a fear of grave misfortune, doom, or fear of dying (self or others) permeates the thinking.

4. Vigilance and scanning. The individual is overly attentive to his surroundings, a hypersensitivity that causes distractibility, inability to concentrate, edginess, impatience, and irritability.

In order to be considered a true generalized anxiety disorder, this anxious state must persist for at least 1 month and be unrelated to any other mental disorder. The person must be at least 18 years of age. Overanxious disorder manifests similar symptoms in early adolescence.

Depression is a major disabling side effect in both panic disorder and generalized anxiety disorder. One study indicated that 50 percent of clients with anxiety disorders suffered from accompanying depression (Clancy, 1978). If the depression had been present for 3 months or less, it tended to be mild and reactive to positive changes in the environment. The client with more severe and chronic panic or generalized anxiety disorder was more frequently depressed and less responsive to improvements in his environment.

The client who experiences panic or generalized anxiety disorders because of a sense of hopelessness about getting better is vulnerable to depression and attempts at suicide. As well as maintaining awareness of these possibilities, the nurse must carefully assess the client's environment. An anxious client may stay home all or nearly all of the time, which will only exacerbate his depression.

Noyes (1980) found the median age of onset of anxiety states to be about 25 years. Older clients reported more severe symptoms, took more medication, and visited their physicians more frequently—a logical outcome in a client who has experienced such symptoms over a longer period of time. The prognosis was more favorable if the anxiety state was less than 5 years in duration. Clients of lower socioeconomic classes reported more severe symptoms and greater impairment of routine function.

Weiss and Rosenberg (1985) studied a population being treated for alcohol detoxification. In this group, the incidence of anxiety disorders was higher than expected, and generalized anxiety and phobic disorders were most common. Steady drinking usually began when the person was in his 20s; the anxiety state when he was approximately 25; alcoholism was an identified problem when he entered the 30s; and detoxification was begun in the mid-30s. This research indicated not that anxiety disorders are the cause of the alcoholism, but that a significant number of alcoholics have concurrent anxiety disorders. Early treatment of the anxiety disorder was believed to prevent alcoholism in some cases.

PHOBIC DISORDERS

The phobic disorders, or phobic neuroses, include agoraphobia with or without panic attacks, social phobia, or simple phobia. DSM III describes the essential features of a phobia which apply to all types.

A phobia is an irrational, persistent dread or fear of a specific person, object, or situation that causes the affected person to use any available means to avoid that person, object, or situation. The person knows that the fear is out of proportion to the actual threat posed by the object of the phobia. Many people experience an irrational fear of mice, spiders, and so on, but this causes no impairment in their daily lives; however, when avoidance behavior engendered by fear is so distressing as to cause disruption in social or work life, then the person may be considered to have a phobic disorder.

1. Agoraphobia. Agoraphobia is an extreme fear of being alone in or of being in a public place from which one cannot escape. Being in a tunnel, being part of a crowd, riding in an elevator, or riding in a bus is a common situation eliciting this fear. Because the person experiences panic attacks, and fears them, he refuses to leave his home alone, or may refuse to leave it at all times, obviously severely restricting his functioning. The focus of the phobia may change from day to day, depending upon the day's schedule. Agoraphobia is more frequent in women than in men and is the phobia for which treatment is sought more often than any other phobia.

2. Social phobia. The person with social phobia experiences an irrational dread of situations in which others might criticize his actions or in which he may be socially humiliated or embarrassed. Because of the anxiety aroused, the individual attempts to avoid such situations, yet recognizes the fear to be out of proportion to the event. Some examples include speaking or eating in public, or using public toilet facilities. Career advancement may be impaired should career involve travel, attendance at banquets, or speaking engagements.

3. Simple phobia. Included in the diagnosis of simple phobias are those that refer to particular fears, such as of heights (acrophobia), of closed places (claustrophobia), or of animals (zoophobia). Only when these fears sufficiently impair daily living will the individual seek treatment.

Most phobias originate in childhood, when anxiety about possible loss of nurturing and guilt about feelings of anger and sexuality may be generated. The development of the phobic disorder is a symptom of the underlying anxiety. A rising anxiety level, experienced as a threat from within, causes the person to displace, or project onto something else, the fear within. This object, person, or situation symbolizes the internal anxiety, although there may or may not be an obvious connection to a specific event. For example, a person experiencing guilt and anxiety about sexual feelings may develop a phobia about elevators or tunnels. These neutral objects have little to do with sexual feelings, but with each encounter feelings of anxiety or guilt arise.

As with other anxiety-related disorders, the person with a phobic disorder is at risk for abusing drugs and alcohol in an attempt to relieve the associated feelings.

Insight-oriented therapies have not been notably successful in treating phobias. The client avoids confronting the original anxieties and experiencing the feelings, since avoidance is his primary response. Greater success has been achieved through behavioral modification in the form of desensitization and reciprocal inhibition.

In desensitization, the individual encounters a predetermined group of anxiety-provoking situations in a continuum of least provoking to most provoking. Progressive relaxation techniques to promote desensitization to each situation are practiced until the continuum is completed. Even-

tually the provoking stimulus will no longer cause the anxiety response.

Reciprocal inhibition pairs the anxiety-provoking stimulus with another stimulus which is associated with a pleasant feeling strong enough to suppress the anxiety. This is usually achieved through the use of tranquilizers, biofeedback, meditation, or hypnosis.

It is important to remember that forcing the client to "face the phobia" will often give rise to a panic state or the development of another phobia. Learning healthier ways of coping with anxiety is essential. Antidepressants coupled with supportive group therapy are beneficial (Sheehan, 1980).

OBSESSIVE-COMPULSIVE DISORDERS

Two components make up the obsessive-compulsive disorder. The first, obsession, is defined as persistent, ritualized thoughts, images, words, or desires that intrude against the person's will. The person is not able to consciously stop these recurring thoughts, which often seem distasteful and frightening. The obsessive personality is orderly, stubborn, perfectionistic, rigid, frugal, and overly conscientious. His personal and moral standards are high, and his tolerance for anxiety is low.

The second component, compulsion, consists of persistent, ritualized behavior, which may be bizarre or irrational, but which is performed purposefully according to a set of rules or stereotypes. Usually the activity has no connection in fact with the desired outcome. The individual feels compelled to carry out the activity even though he may wish to avoid it. Generally, the activity does not generate enjoyment, but does provide a release of tension or anxiety. A harmless childhood compulsion is "Step on a crack, break your mother's back" in which cracks in the sidewalk are scrupulously avoided.

The compulsive person tends to exhibit tight control over his emotions, which may cause a tense body posture, inflexibility, stubbornness, and a flat, unemotional affect. The need for perfection, certainty, and guarantees is highly evident in his daily life-style.

Salzman and Thaler (1981) describe the elements of obsessive-compulsive disorders as follows:

1. Purposeless and useless behaviors and thoughts which persist despite conscious

attempts by the person to discard them. The person may ruminate about death, a moral issue, or somatic complaints.

2. General anxiety, or somatic distress, occurs because the nature of the thoughts and behaviors is foreign to the individual's perception of self. For example, a mother may have recurring thoughts of killing her child, or a successful executive may have an impulse to scream obscenities at his employees.

3. Though the illogical and unreasonable nature of the thought is recognized by the individual, he feels unable to stop it.

The Meaning of Obsessive-Compulsive Behavior and Defense Mechanisms

Obsessive-compulsive behavior was regarded in early times as possession by the devil which required exorcism. Much later, Freud and others recognized the usefulness of obsessive-compulsive behavior, in that the sudden occurrence of a distasteful or bizarre thought served to distract attention from another possibly more upsetting thought or feeling.

Theories about the etiology of this disorder range from genetic to psychodynamic to learning theory. Freud describes the disorder as a result of conflict between the ego and the id, in which id wishes that were repugnant to the ego were controlled by isolation, repression, suppression, denial, displacement, undoing, and reaction formation. Research into childhood obsessive-compulsive disorders has indicated that the affected children displayed pseudomaturity, excessive conformity, and extreme efforts to avoid displeasing adults. They were often characterized as "teacher's pet" or "goody-two-shoes" (Hollingsworth, 1980).

Learning theorists see the behavior as a conditioned response to anxiety-provoking events. In the past, the behavior helped control anxiety so it is practiced again, even though it is not helpful. Associating the anxiety with a neutral object or event results in obsessional preoccupation while the compulsive behavior reduces anxiety.

Researchers disagree on the prevalence of this disorder, because many people do not seek treatment until their daily functioning has become severely impaired. Men and women appear to be affected in equal numbers.

It is important that the nurse recognize the seriousness of compulsive behaviors. Besides interfering with job, family, or social functioning, these behaviors may adversely affect health or safety. For example, the person who compulsively washes his hands may contract a severe infection because of the breakdown of skin integrity. A mother obsessed with a fear of killing her baby may neglect the child completely because she is afraid that touching him will trigger violence on her part.

Table 32-4 lists examples of common compulsive behavior and persistent repetitive thoughts. Care of the client with these behaviors is presented later in this chapter.

POST-TRAUMATIC STRESS DISORDER

Post-traumatic stress disorder is of great significance to the nurse who is frequently involved in the care of accident, trauma, or disaster victims. It is characterized by symptoms arising from a traumatic event that is outside the range of normal experience.

Unlike the other anxiety disorders that have been discussed, post-traumatic stress disorder is clearly related to stressors in the actual experience of the individual. The traumatic event may be rape, assault, or burglary, may be related to military service (combat, prisoner of war, concentration camp), to flood, tornado, or other natural disasters.

TABLE 32-4 Common Behaviors and Thoughts in Obsessive-Compulsive Disorder

Ritualistic Behaviors	Persistent, Repetitive Thoughts
Starting a task repeatedly	Thoughts occur regardless of environmental stimuli
Repeated handwashing	
Repeated cleaning of an area	Fear of hurting someone or something
Repeated checking of items	Fear of losing control (of bodily functions or proper behavior)
Rigidity of structure (assigning special places for things and feeling distressed when they are "out of order," or needing to perform tasks in a specific sequence)	Fear that one's work or performance will be unacceptable to others

The person "experiences" the event again, in flashbacks, dreams, or nightmares; he is numbed emotionally (emotional anesthesia), and is detached or estranged from others. He may startle easily, may appear vigilant and tense, and may experience insomnia or difficulty in concentrating or remembering. Many survivors of life-threatening trauma (such as concentrations camps) experience guilt because they survived while others died.

The person is aware of the symptoms of numb detachment. The traumatic experience may be accompanied by physical problems related to the situation, such as malnutrition or injury.

Bloch (1978) found symptoms of post-traumatic stress in inner-city teachers who faced violence on a daily basis or had been directly endangered by growing urban school violence. Depression and anxiety are associated symptoms.

The disorder may be acute, lasting less than 6 months; chronic, lasting more than 6 months; or delayed, occurring 6 months after the trauma. The nurse in the emergency room or acute care facility should be especially alert when she encounters a victim of rape or accident and be prepared to direct the victim to the appropriate agency. In most cities, there are facilities organized to deal with the effects of natural or manmade disasters.

The relationship of post-traumatic stress disorder to external stressors requires careful history taking. The experience is not imagined; it can be identified through careful attention to details furnished by the client and family. The nurse should keep in mind that the event may have occurred as long as 6 months before symptoms appeared. The nurse may find it difficult to attach the same importance to the event that the client does, and therefore not realize how traumatized the client feels. She may then subtly and unconsciously convey the notion that the client's feelings are trivial, thereby limiting free sharing of feelings.

If the response to the event was intense, the client may be in a state of panic when he sees the nurse. After this panic phase has ended, the client

---

■ *Point of Emphasis*

The nurse must explore the meaning of the event to the client: it may have been objectively traumatic, such as a crime or an environmental disaster, or may have been subjectively traumatic, such as the death of a significant other.

Vignette

Terri Moore was referred to a mental health center by her physician because she complained of fatigue, anxiety, a decrease in appetite, and sleep disturbance. Terri had been having recurring nightmares of an assault by a man that took place 1 month earlier. She had been out with friends and stopped to have a cup of coffee before returning home. She was attacked as she left the restaurant to go to her car. Terri was robbed, and the attempted sexual assault was interrupted by the approach of other customers who were leaving the restaurant.

Terri's guilt centered around her feeling that she should have "had more sense" than to stop at the restaurant. She also identified feelings of helplessness toward being able to control her own life if she could be so easily overcome. Terri was concerned that these feelings were intensifying and were affecting her daily life; she was fearful of going out after dark, and at times was fearful of staying alone in her apartment.

A sample care plan for Terri is presented in Table 32-5. Other goals of the treatment plan included the following:

1. Exploring the client's feelings of guilt in a supportive climate so that she could begin to accept that she had not done something to "warrant" the attack.
2. Helping her to identify realistic ways in which she could plan to increase her own safety when out in the evening, such as parking her car in well-lit areas and leaving public places along with others. This increased her sense of control over herself.
3. Helping her to appreciate that her feelings were normal by involving her in a group of others who had similar experiences.

After about 6 weeks of therapy, Terri felt relief of her symptoms.

---

will be able to participate in problem solving. Treatment is generally of short term and does not require hospitalization unless there are accompanying physical injuries.

□ *Somatoform Disorders*

As defined in DSM III, somatoform disorders are characterized by physical symptoms that suggest an organic disorder; however, there is no physical

---

TABLE 32-5 Sample Care Plan, Post-traumatic Stress Disorder

Problem 1: Ineffective coping secondary to anxiety and fear, related to a sense of loss of control over life events and resulting in client withdrawing from activities of daily life.

Short-term Goal: Client will express feelings of anger about the assault in order to reduce sense of anxiety and guilt.

Long-term Goal: Client will be able to resume normal daily activities and social life without experiencing exaggerated anxiety and/or fear.

Interventions	Rationale	Evaluation
Client was encouraged to verbally explore her response to the assault. Identification of feelings was achieved through statements such as: "You sound angry when you say that. Are you aware of feeling that way?" "I notice you cry when talking about the assault. Can you tell me what your feelings are that cause you to cry?"	Clients have difficulty verbalizing their feelings. Awareness of the physical manifestations of the feelings (crying, tone, affect) can help the client to express the feeling in an identifiable fashion.	Evaluation of goals and interventions was based on the following: Statements by the client indicating an increased understanding of her own behavioral responses to her feelings. Expression of feelings in understandable terms. Statements by the client indicating increased acceptance of her own feelings. Increased comfort in performing daily activities as reported by the client.
Verbal support was given to allow the client to accept her own negative feelings (e.g., "Intense feelings are frightening but normal in response to an event as bad as that one was for you."). The client was reassured that allowing the feelings to surface would not cause loss of control (e.g., "Feeling that you want to hurt someone and saying so doesn't mean you will do it.").	Intense feelings can be frightening to the client, who may regard them as equal to loss of control of self. The client needs to learn that the feelings can be expressed and managed behaviorally, bringing relief from discomfort rather than loss of control.	

---

basis for the symptoms. The symptoms of somatoform disorders are believed not to be under voluntary or conscious control, and point to a relationship to a psychological factor or an emotional conflict of some sort.

CONVERSION DISORDER

Conversion disorder was formerly called hysteria, hysterical neurosis, or conversion reaction. The person experiences a loss of or alteration in physical functioning which appears to be physical, but which actually expresses an emotional conflict or need.

Neurological symptoms are common. There may be paralysis, loss of hearing (aphonia), blindness, tunnel vision, seizures, anesthesias or parasthesias, disturbances in coordination, or loss of smell (anosmia). Symptoms arise abruptly, usually when the person is under extreme psychological stress. Typically, the disorder is seen in adolescence or early adulthood though it may appear at a later time.

Women have presented with conversion

symptoms more frequently than men. These women have been labeled "hysterical." The word "hysteria," from the Greek work for "uterus," came from the notion held by the ancient Greeks and Egyptians that the "wandering uterus" was the cause of the disorder. However, cases of conversion disorder (hysteria) are well documented in men as well as in women. The term hysteria is archaic as a diagnostic term, and conversion disorder is more descriptive and appropriate.

The term "hysterical personality" describes a personality type rather than a specific disorder and is often confused with conversion disorder. Some theorists believe the hysterical personality (dramatic, demanding, suggestible, colorful) exists prior to the appearance of conversion disorder.

The DSM III established specific criteria for identifying conversion disorder:

1. Symptoms produce the loss or alteration of physical function.
2. Symptoms are not under voluntary (conscious) control.
3. Pathophysiological mechanisms do not explain the symptoms.
4. Although symptoms suggest a physical disorder, psychological factors seem to be involved, based on the following: (a) physical symptoms appear or are exacerbated by an environmental stress related to an emotional conflict or need; (b) the symptom allows the individual to avoid an activity or situation that is distasteful (primary gain); (c) the symptom allows the individual to gain environmental support (secondary gain).
5. The symptoms are not limited to pain or sexual dysfunction.

Dynamics of Conversion Disorder

In Freud's theory of hysterical neurosis, the symptom was caused by unresolved oedipal feelings (the preschooler's love for the parent of the opposite sex). Freud theorized that the normal sexual feelings were tainted by "incestuous feelings" because of failure to resolve this "mother love" or "father love" stage. This *unconscious* conflict resulted in anxiety related to sex drives, with development of a physical symptom that prevented the client from carrying out the anxiety-producing sexual drives (primary gain). Also, the symptom aroused sympathy on the part of friends and relatives (secondary gain).

Freud's theories were developed during Victorian times of repressive sexuality. One might conjecture to what extent a conversion symptom provided a convenient release from "marital duties" for women in an arranged or unhappy marriage from which no release in the form of separation, divorce, or sexual counseling could be obtained.

Engel (1970) believed conversion symptoms developed under conditions of deprivation or frustration and represented a regressive manner of fulfilling a need and relating to others. The inner conflict was said to be triggered by a frustrating life situation which gave rise to repugnant desire. The ensuing repression prevented conscious awareness of the wish. Engel believed the physical symptoms represented a symbolic wish that could not be fulfilled. For example, after a young woman observes her fiance embracing and kissing another woman, she loses her vision—literally, she does not see what she does not want to see.

In past times, the client with conversion disorder was said to exhibit "la belle indifference"—a seeming indifference to symptoms; however, this attitude is not universally present.

Although seen less frequently today than in past years, conversion disorder is found at all levels of cultural and socioeconomic groups (Jones, 1980). Nursing care of this disorder is presented in the section on somatic symptoms due to psychological disorders.

SOMATIZATION DISORDER

Somatization disorder, also known as Briquet's syndrome, is characterized by frequent and multiple somatic complaints, often described by the client in a colorful, dramatic fashion. The client usually is younger than age 30 and probably has sought frequent medical attention, and has had multiple surgeries. The client complains of pain (back pain, neck pain); gastrointestinal distress (abdominal pain, cramping, bloating); urinary and reproductive system distress (pain, cramping); cardiopulmonary problems (dizziness, dyspnea, hyperventilation); neurological dysfunction (blurred vision, memory loss, muscle weakness, loss of voice) (Zisook, 1979). Yet no physiological explanation can be found.

Anxiety, depression manifested in crying, sad feelings, "nervousness," sleep disturbances, and suicidal thoughts are common. Marital, interpersonal, and job-related difficulties as well as antisocial behaviors may be apparent in the client's history. Actual or potential complications include the frequent unnecessary surgeries, with the possibility of substance abuse due to the variety of prescribed medications, and attempted or completed suicide due to depression.

It must be emphasized that symptom formation is *unconscious* and not under the client's control. It is important that the nurse distinguish somatization disorder from malingering, which is the purposeful production of exaggerated symptoms (physical or psychological). In malingering, the client's symptoms are calculated to achieve a certain goal, for example, avoiding work or school, gaining financial rewards, obtaining drugs. In contrast, the client with somatization disorder achieves no identifiable gain. The nurse is cautioned not to label the latter as a malingerer.

Approximately 1 percent of the general population has experienced somatization disorder, and nearly all are women. It may be that society deems physical illness to be more acceptable in women than in men, or because women are believed to be less likely than men to express anger openly. Another factor may be that because the majority of physicians are men, they may prefer not to attach the label of "hysteria" to other men. Care of the client is discussed in the section on somatic symptoms due to psychological disorders.

PSYCHOGENIC PAIN

The chief symptom in psychogenic pain is severe and prolonged pain. In assessment, either an organic pathology is not found, or if found, the pain is out of proportion to the pathology. Psychological factors are also present, and they play a role in the onset of pain or its exacerbation. The individual usually refuses to believe that psychological factors may be involved; however, the pain serves the client by providing primary gain (avoidance of some undesirable activity or situation) and secondary gain (support from friends and family).

In working with the client, the nurse must be conscious of the latter's need to maintain the symptom. Attempting to force the client to gain insight into the underlying reason for the pain will only increase anxiety and therefore heighten the client's need to resort to defensive behavior. Guidelines for working with this client include the following:

1. Form a relationship in which the client feels free to express both negative and positive thoughts and feelings. Avoid creating a need for defensiveness in the client.

2. Minimize attention to the physical symptom, thereby decreasing secondary gain, and attend to the client as a person, rather than to the symptom.

3. Be alert to increasing dependence on or abuse of tranquilizers or narcotics that may have been prescribed by the client's various doctors.

4. Encourage the client to explore alternative methods of pain relief such as biofeedback, hypnosis, or meditation.

Vignette

Jane, a 34-year-old mother of three, was admitted to the inpatient psychiatric unit following a 2-month period of recovery from a truck accident. Jane was employed as driver of a semitrailer. To avoid hitting a car that had cut in front of her, she had crashed into the road shoulder. There were no serious injuries, and Jane recovered rapidly, except for prolonged pain in her right shoulder. No medical explanation could be found for this and a psychiatric consultation was recommended by her physician.

It was learned that Jane loved her job and strongly identified with the subculture of truck drivers. She expressed a strong sense of camaraderie with her fellow drivers. She was particularly proud of her driving skills and of her acceptance as one of a small number of female drivers. Sometimes she carried oil and gasoline in her truck—a job assigned only to the most careful and skillful drivers. Jane was accustomed to following the drivers' "rule" never to ditch the truck, even if this involved a crash or injury to oneself or to others. Jane remarked that it takes a few minutes to bring a fast-moving semitrailer to a complete stop, and that it was not unusual for a car to cut in front of the truck as it was slowing down.

For the first time in her career, Jane had ditched her truck, and as a result she lost her job. It was difficult for her to see a relationship between her continued pain (as a result of which she was held on disability status and could not look for a new job), and her sense of shame and guilt about violating a rule of her work culture. Jane was able to discuss her feelings of embarrassment, fear, and depression about the accident but unable to relate these to her persistent pain.

Jane's father, stepfather, and brother had died when Jane was a child, and her mother had died recently. Nursing assessment should take such multiple stresses into account.

HYPOCHONDRIASIS

The designation of hypochondriasis is sometimes carelessly assigned to multiple illnesses related to psychological factors, such as malingering, psychogenic pain, factitious disorders, and even the normal somatic symptoms of anxiety that may be experienced by a hospitalized client.

The diagnosis of hypochondriasis (or hypochondriacal neurosis) is made only when the individual is preoccupied with the fear or belief that he is experiencing a serious disease and interprets every physical sign or sensation as being abnormal. When he is given a thorough physical evaluation, no evidence of disease related to the symptoms can be found (although an actual physical disease may be present). For example, a person who has been successfully treated for peptic ulcer

disease may manifest a fear that the disease is cancer of the stomach.

Despite receiving reassurance as to his physical health, the person persists in his misguided belief, with impairment in his job performance, as well as his social functioning. He becomes preoccupied with bodily functions (e.g., pulse, peristalsis) or minor problems (e.g., a cut, a sore, a cough). Hypochondriasis usually becomes chronic, because most affected persons are offended at the implication that their fears are unfounded, and refuse to seek therapy.

Because of the nature of the disorder, therapy is lengthy; in many cases, however, it can be managed on an outpatient basis—the client is able to function intellectually and his ego is marginally functional. If the client is admitted to a general hospital for investigation of his physical symp-

---

Case Study

Marie M. was encouraged to seek psychiatric help following a number of hospital admissions and visits to emergency rooms and was seen on an outpatient basis. She complained of a variety of physical symptoms—feeling her throat had "shrunk" so that she could not swallow solid foods, intestinal pains due to "cancer," and back pains related to a disorder of the spine. The client claimed to have experienced several physical discomforts to which she could not or would not assign a specific cause. She was extremely angry and distrustful of all health care professionals. Marie complained that no one "understood" her or believed her and that she "suffered constantly."

Marie joined an outpatient therapy group while continuing individual therapy. Here, she was able to work on establishing relationships not centered around her physical complaints. Her treatment consisted of participating in this group for 1 year, and attending individual sessions for 2 years. At the end of this time, while still very sensitive to bodily concerns, Marie was able to distinguish organic illness from physical stress of fear and anxiety. She used biofeedback as a method of relaxation to reduce the physical symptoms of anxiety. She also had begun establishing friendships and improved her job performance and attendance record. In the first 6 months of therapy, her frequent trips for medical care ceased.

The nurse's first task with Marie was to establish trust. Since Marie's physical examinations revealed no organic basis for her complaints, the nurse listened to her somatic complaints, but did not argue with Marie about them. Instead, the

nurse focused on Marie as a person, rather than a "complaining patient," asking about her lifestyle, likes, dislikes, job, friends, and so on.

It soon became evident that Marie had felt rejected and "let down" by others since early childhood. She was able to recall early events that demonstrated maternal rejection. By engaging in narcissistic concern about herself and her bodily functions, Marie became disengaged from her immediate situation and also was able to focus attention on herself.

As the relationship progressed to the working phase, the nurse introduced the idea that unhappiness and anxiety often created physical discomfort. Marie trusted the nurse enough to consider this a possibility without becoming defensive. Because of past sessions, Marie was becoming more aware of her feelings about past incidents that had been painful to her; the nurse encouraged Marie to express those angry feelings and did not censor her for expressing them.

Marie was also able to look at the rewards she derived from her illnesses. The concern and attention from others, while initially present, soon dissolved when people lost patience with her repeated and excessive concerns. This left Marie feeling more abandoned and isolated. The nurse encouraged Marie to express the need for attention in healthier ways, such as making a direct request. The nurse also encouraged appropriate interactions between Marie and the other clients that were not centered on her physical complaints. She was encouraged to become involved in the activities of the group.

toms, the nurse may be tempted to try to "prove" to him that there is nothing physically wrong and that it is "all in his head." A complete physical examination should be done to determine that no organic disease is present. The nurse must convey by her attitude that although no physical cause has been found to account for the symptoms, she acknowledges that the symptoms are real to the client.

☐ *Dissociative Disorders*

Dissociation is an unconscious defense mechanism by which certain thoughts or feelings are kept out of awareness. As with all defense mechanisms, the purpose of dissociation is to control or block the anxiety arising from those feelings that threaten the person's sense of self. The result is an abrupt temporary alteration in integration of either consciousness, identity, motor behavior, or a combination of any of these. The person is then unable to recall important experiences. He becomes unable to recognize his true identity, and assumes a different identity, or feels the loss of the sense of reality, and experiences a sense of unreality. He may wander aimlessly, as a result of this loss.

PSYCHOGENIC AMNESIA

The DSM III describes psychogenic amnesia as "a sudden inability to recall important personal information." It must be emphasized that this form of amnesia is not due to an organic problem, or to drugs or alcohol, and is too all-encompassing to be regarded as forgetfulness.

There are four types of psychogenic amnesia:

1. Localized. In localized amnesia, the person is unable to describe events during a certain period of time, usually several hours following an emotionally traumatic event. For example, the lone survivor of a tornado in which the members of his immediate family die cannot recall any of the surrounding events for several days.
2. Selective. Selective amnesia involves the recall of only certain portions of a specific experience. For example, the person may recall making funeral arrangements after the death of a family member, but remembers little about the persons who were present at the funeral.

3. Generalized. One of the less common types of amnesia, generalized amnesia renders the affected person unable to recall any events—his life seems to be a "blank."
4. Continuous. In continuous amnesia, the person cannot remember any events that followed a specific occurrence.

In most cases, psychogenic amnesia follows a severely stressful event, although it may occur after a *threat* of injury or death (e.g., accident, assault, natural disaster). Feelings or actions that create unbearable stress (e.g., a homosexual affair, premarital sex, disobedience to a strict parent, a perceived religious transgression) may also trigger the amnesia. The stressor may be due to the perception that life is intolerable (e.g., sudden death of the spouse, loss of a business or job). In wartime, amnesia is more frequent in young men; in normal times, it is most frequent in adolescents or young women.

Usually, recovery is rapid, the impairment of function during the amnestic period varying according to the impact of the events on the person's overall functioning.

PSYCHOGENIC FUGUE

Psychogenic fugue is similar to amnesia and also involves a sudden trip away from home and the assumption by the person of a new identity. The person may be disoriented and confused, but once he recovers from the fugue, he cannot recall the events of the fugue period. He may assume a new identity, job, and residence, and have new social experiences, yet not appear to be suffering from an emotional disorder. In most instances, however, the person merely travels for a brief period without assuming a new identity. He may occasionally give way to an outburst of violence that causes social or legal difficulties.

Fugue states generally are precipitated by severe psychosocial stress (e.g., family arguments, rejection by loved ones or by an employer, war, natural disaster). Like amnesia, fugue states are not due to organic problems or to use of drugs, though heavy alcohol use can predispose the person to the disorder.

Nursing Care in Psychogenic Amnesia and Fugue States

The client enters treatment through the emergency room. The nurse's chief concern in that setting is to ensure client safety and referral to a safe environment (whether home or hospital). The initial aim is to determine the underlying cause, thus the client's physical condition must be assessed to rule out organic causes such as a brain tumor, injury, or ingestion of a toxic substance. The duration and frequency of the dissociative reaction are other important considerations.

Once organic causes have been ruled out, the source of the anxiety is sought. Some measures employed to identify the source include free association, dream description, hypnosis, intravenous administration of sodium thiopental (Pentothal), and psychometric tests such as the Rorschach test. If family members or close friends are available, they should be involved in the plan of treatment. This element is important, because the client may be receiving secondary gain in order to escape responsibilities that seem overwhelming. (Specific responses in anxiety states are discussed in the section on anxiety disorders.)

MULTIPLE PERSONALITY

Multiple personality disorder (MPD) is a relatively rare form of dissociation in which two or more distinct personalities coexist within an individual at the same time. Although reliable statistics are lacking, MPD is diagnosed more often in women than in men.

Each of the personalities consists of a set of behaviors, social relationships, and memories that differ from those of the other personalities. The person's behavior will be controlled by whichever personality is dominant at the moment. Researches have found distinct physiological differences in the various personalities (Putnam, et al., 1984). Some examples of multiple personality may be seen in the popular literature such as *Sybil* and *The Three Faces of Eve*.

The original personality generally is unaware of the existence of the other personalities. If there is more than one other personality, the "subpersonalities" may or may not be aware of the existence of the others.

The MPD client may initially present with chronic illness that mimics such psychiatric disorders as psychosis or anorexia/bulimia, or somatic problems, especially neurological, gastrointestinal, and cardiac disorders. Because the clients tend to be secretive about their psychiatric symptoms, diagnosis is difficult, with the result that the wrong sort of therapy may be given.

The critical factor in MPD is disturbance of memory and identity, along with multiple amnesic episodes involving alternating separate and distinct identities (Putnam, et al., 1984). Despite his memory deficits, the client's neuropsychological functioning is normal. He is often unable to account for certain periods of time; he denies personal behavior to which others can attest; and he has only a fragmented recall of his childhood.

Psychosocial stress causes the change from one personality to another. Headaches may signal the switch in personalities. Multiple personality usually begins in childhood, but usually is not diagnosed until adolescence. The normal adolescent is striving to achieve a clear identity, but in the MPD this is impossible because he is not one self, but several selves.

A way of viewing the dissociation that gives rise to multiple personality is to consider it a means of preserving aspects of personality that are threatened by inner anxiety or the external environment. For example, in *Sybil*, the child was abused and emotionally traumatized by a severely emotionally ill mother. To protect herself from the overwhelming anxiety, Sybil dissociated into sev-

---

Vignette

Carol, a 28-year-old legal assistant, had been diagnosed as having a multiple personality. As a child, she had been severely abused by being starved, being locked in a closet, and being verbally abused. Carol developed two distinct personalities, one, that of a responsible professional person, the other that of a 10-year-old child. The child spent money buying various things for her abusive family in a futile effort to win parental approval. At times, she thought, behaved, and played like a 10-year-old. She was aware of the existence of the two personalities and, on her days off, was a client in a day-hospital setting. At this point Carol was able to control the 10-year-old personality while she was at work, allowing it to emerge in the "safe" environment of the hospital, where her therapist was a primary nurse.

The goals of nursing intervention were: (1) to provide a safe environment in which Carol could regress; (2) to support the strengths of her "adult" personality; (3) to intervene when the whims of the approval-seeking child (giving money to family) would interfere with adult functioning.

Carol's family was a destructive force rather than a supportive one. The goal of hypnosis and long-term psychiatric treatment was to gradually integrate Carol's personalities

eral personalities, each exemplifying some part of herself.

Depression and suicide ideation or attempts are potential complications, and the client may seek help for these symptoms. Anxiety and panic attacks may also occur.

Treatment of this disorder is a long-term process. Hospitalization may be necessary, depending upon what the individual personalities may do. Psychotherapy and hypnotherapy are most often used to determine whether more than one personality is present.

DEPERSONALIZATION DISORDER

Depersonalization disorder is characterized by episodes in which feelings of unreality, estrangement, and separateness from one's self and one's actions emerge. Depersonalization often is associated with derealization (a sense of unreality) toward the environment.

The individual may feel that he is "mechanical" or as if "in a dream." A sense of numbness and a lack of complete control over his actions are frequently present. The person is aware that this estranged feeling is unusual and is disturbed by it.

According to the DSM III, factors predisposing to depersonalization disorder include fatigue, physical pain, altered states of consciousness (e.g., hypnosis, meditation), anxiety, depression, or severe stress. Lehmann (1974) presented three possible causative theories of depersonalization:

1. Organic theory. Depersonalization may be triggered by a physiological source, possibly a specific locus in the brain, as occurs in a temporal lobe seizure.
2. General psychiatric theory. Depersonalization results from anxiety, dysphoric affect, and disorganized thinking.
3. Psychoanalytic theory. Freud saw depersonalization as a struggle between conflicting identities and self-images. During the toddler phase, when the child begins to recognize that he is separate for his mother, he also starts to imitate and identify with the parents (separation-individuation phase of development). Freud theorized that depersonalization occurred because in early life, the child had no suitable parent with whom to identify, giving rise to difficulty in creating a strong self-image. Be-

cause of this shaky sense of self, when faced with loss (real or perceived), the person regresses to avoid anxiety (becomes unable to function normally), while at the same time remaining an "outside" observer of himself.

Torch (1978) viewed the process of depersonalization as a form of obsession wherein the person "sits back" mentally and observes himself. He described the depersonalized individual as one who tended toward obsessional thinking, held high standards for acceptance of self, and had low self-esteem. The person frequently experienced doubt and uncertainty, and was introspective. Constant refocusing on his insecurities and doubts created deeper anxiety, causing him to feel that he was a failure and in turn giving rise to depression and still greater anxiety. The greater the depression and anxiety, the greater the sense of unreality and estrangement from self and environment.

> ### ■ Point of Emphasis
>
> *The sense of depersonalization in true depersonalization disorder is different from the depersonalization of schizophrenic disorders in that the person is aware that his feelings are strange and bizarre.*

Treatment centers around working with the client to decrease the pattern of negative introspection that results in anxiety and depression. Having the client stop thinking when a negative idea occurs to him and replace the negative thought with a positive one may be helpful. Tranquilizing agents have not proven fruitful, and the phenothiazines only increase the sense of depersonalization. Depersonalization feelings are not transient. They are associated with specific anxiety-provoking events (see vignette, Mrs. M, on page 741).

As often occurs, insight does not progress in distinct phases, but tends to flow in a continuum. Nursing interventions must be geared to the needs the client exhibits at a given time.

☐ Factitious Disorders

Factitious, that is, not genuine, is the crucial word in descriptions of these disorders. There are two

---

Vignette

Mrs. M.'s son had had psychiatric treatment at various times since the age of 5, and had been arrested and required to appear in juvenile court many times. At the age of 14 he strangled another child, and Mrs. M. discovered the tragedy.

Mrs. M. also had been receiving therapy for some time before that event. Previously, she had reacted appropriately to stressful situations, but when talking about the strangling, she demonstrated a flat affect, and denied great distress about the event. Mrs. M. was not immediately able to recall how she felt when the nurse tried to discuss it with her.

In treatment, Mrs. M. was helped to gain insight into her feelings surrounding the event. The nurse's supportive attitude allowed Mrs. M. to gain understanding gradually. Over a period of time she became able to express and accept her sense of intense guilt and anger about the tragedy and to deal more effectively with those feelings.

The sample care plan shown in Table 32-6 provides two examples of goals for Mrs. M. In the initial phase, treatment focused on decreasing her denial and permitting awareness of her feeling to increase. Once the initial awareness occurred, much reassurance and support was offered Mrs. M. so that she felt free to express her feelings without having a sense of "going crazy" as she feared would happen. Also during this time, Mrs. M.'s need to express her intense feelings of anger and guilt were acknowledged in order to ensure that her feelings were directed outward rather than inward (which could have caused unnecessary self-punishment). Reality testing was done to help her define her role in the event more realistically. She had been expressing the unrealistic quality of her beliefs through statements such as "I may as well have been the one to strangle that boy."

---

types of factitious disorders, one physical and the other psychological, and the symptoms of both are under voluntary control; that is, the person is able to produce, direct, and terminate the symptoms.

Although the word voluntary implies that the behavior is seen to be deliberate and purposeful, the person may carry out these actions in a compulsive manner, so that the actions are not under his control. The goal of the person experiencing factitious disorder is, apparently, simply to be a client of professional health care, unlike the malingerer, whose goal is to be relieved of a troubling situation through his symptoms.

FACTITIOUS DISORDERS CHARACTERIZED BY PSYCHOLOGICAL SYMPTOMS

The person's symptoms and behaviors suggest the presence of a mental disorder, frequently a psychosis. Behaviors include apparent memory loss, hallucination, suicidal ideation, and conversion symptoms. These may appear more marked when the person is aware he is being observed. Usually the symptoms that the person presents are based on the way he thinks a psychotic or a suicidal person would behave.

FACTITIOUS DISORDERS CHARACTERIZED BY PHYSICAL SYMPTOMS

The disorder is characterized by imaginary or self-devised physical symptoms. The manifestation may in fact be nonexistent, such as complaint of severe pain where none exists; may be self-inflicted, such as deliberate infection of cuts or sores; or may be an exaggeration of an actual physical condition. The nurse needs to distinguish this form of factitious disorder, formerly called "Munchausen's syndrome," from malingering and hypochondriasis (see Table 32-7).

According to Stern (1980) the client is evasive and hostile, frequently threatening the staff. He may have multiple scars at various body sites, and may relate a medical history that indicates some serious physical problems but is usually not entirely convincing. He appears to be in pain, is well versed in medical jargon, and demands immediate attention, becoming bitterly distressed if attention is not forthcoming at once. A complete history would reveal that he was emotionally deprived as a child; his parents were sadistic or may have been alcoholics, or chronically ill; his self-image and ego ideal are distorted; he may be a substance abuser.

The self-destructive nature of this factitious disorder represents a pathological attempt to be loved. Because of his hostility and demanding behavior, the client presents a challenge to the nurse. She must remain firm, at the same time that she projects warmth and kindness.

The prognosis in factitious disorder is poor because of the long-term presence of unhealthy adaptation to a painful emotional past. The client also lacks insight into his emotions, which makes change difficult. His behavior was developed precisely to deny painful emotions, and it interferes

---

TABLE 32-6 Sample Care Plan, Depersonalization Disorder

Problem 1: Ineffective individual coping secondary to intense anxiety related to a stressful event resulting in estrangement of self from feelings and mental awareness of the event.

Short-term Goal: Client will identify her feelings about the event.

Long-term Goal: Client will be able to accept her feelings about the event and relate to her experience in an appropriate manner.

Interventions	Rationale	Evaluation
Client will be encouraged to explore her feelings surrounding the event by: Supportive statements such as: "It must have been very hard for you to learn that your son strangled another person." "I'm wondering if you can remember how you felt at the time."	The overwhelming nature of intense feelings can cause the client to block them off from awareness. Allowing time and providing a supportive environment rather than forcing the client to feel a certain way can facilitate the lowering of defenses.	Evaluation was based on: an increase in identification of feelings by the client. An increase in behavioral manifestations of feelings such as crying.
Use of videotaping allowing the client to see herself and the change in affect when discussing the event. She was encouraged to explore what she thought this difference in behavior might mean.		
Client was given the expectation to identify the actual controls she had in the situation and to reality-test through discussion with her therapist her fantasized controls.	Seeing the child as an extension of self can cause overresponsible feelings for the parent who sees himself as a direct causative factor for the child's behavior.	Evaluation was based on: A decrease in selfpunitive statements. Expression of parental responsibilities in a realistic way.
Client was asked to identify the steps she had taken to assist her son in treatment.	The separate identities of each needs to be identified and recognized. Intense guilt can cause the client's focus to remain only on a perceived negative image. Recognition of strengths in a matter-of-fact way can improve the self-image by reality testing the self-perception.	

---

with a therapeutic relationship because therapy aims to bring into awareness the feelings to be dealt with. The nurse must remember that this is a very severe emotional illness (See case study on page 743).

Because the factitious disorders are under voluntary control, the nurse often finds it difficult to keep her anger in check. Anxiety and stress motivate the client's behavior because he lacks effective coping mechanisms. Secondary gain can be prevented by focusing on healthy coping mechanisms rather than on the client's complaints. The nurse needs to assess the possible benefit to the client from a particular behavior, so she can identify the stressors and treat the resultant behavior. A consistent team approach is essential in working with this client. (See Chapter 27 for a discussion of intervention in manipulative behavior.)

TABLE 32-7 Differentiation among Disorders Manifesting Physical Symptoms

Disorder	Onset	Symptoms	Associated Features
Factitious Disorder with Physical Symptoms	Early adult life	Voluntary No goal evident	Severe personality disorder
Malingering	Adulthood	Voluntary Obvious goal	Antisocial personality Medicolegal aspects Discrepancies in distress and actual findings Lack of cooperation in treatment
Hypochondriasis	Adolescence Early adulthood	Based on unrealistic fear of illness Involuntary	Anxiety Depression Compulsive personality traits
Conversion Disorder	Adolescence Early adulthood	Unconscious Involuntary	Environmental stress "trigger" Primary gain Secondary gain

Case Study

Sally was 34 years old, married and the mother of four children. Her husband was a "career army man," and the family moved frequently, sometimes living abroad; the father was often away on assignment.

Sally was transferred from the general hospital to the inpatient psychiatric unit because no organic basis could be found for her admitting complaints of lower back pain, "bleeding" from her kidneys, and "breathing problems." Upon arrival, she appeared barely able to walk, and went to bed immediately. After Sally used a bedpan, the nurse noted blood in the urine and asked Sally if she was menstruating. Sally stated that she was not menstruating but that her kidneys "were bleeding and the doctors won't listen to me." She also claimed to be subject to grand mal seizures and respiratory arrest, and she displayed both convincingly. Initially, diazepam (Valium) was administered intravenously to control the seizures, though no organic cause for them could be found. Sally was addicted to this drug, and had been addicted to others, and the extensive scar tissues visible on her skin attested to the many injections she had received.

At one point, a nursing student was asked to remain with Sally so that the professional nurse on duty could give care to another client. Sally perceived this act as a lowering of her status, and promptly feigned a grand mal seizure. Both nurse and student, alerted to what was happening, came to her aid promptly. Sally was seen to deliberately reposition the tongue blade they had placed in her mouth. Another time, Sally feigned a seizure because the toast she had ordered was late in arriving and Sally regarded this delay as a rejection of her.

Sally suffered factitious respiratory arrests in the corridor connecting the general hospital and the psychiatric facility—a high traffic area. Each time an arrest occurred, a code was called, but the code team became increasingly skeptical and angry with the client.

Sally questioned the credentials of the medical/nursing team, pitted one member against another, and created confusion among other clients. She claimed to be both a nurse and a physician, and told the other clients to ignore their doctors' advice. Because Sally was extremely well versed in medical knowledge and medical terminology, her advice seemed genuine.

The staff developed several strategies for helping Sally:

1. The staff members ventilated their anger and frustration about her manipulative behavior and her hostile remarks.
2. They set firm limits on their interactions with Sally, with one staff member per shift assigned to her.
3. In the absence of physical findings, Sally was gradually weaned from her various drugs.
4. Safety measures were provided during Sally's "seizures" and "arrests" but any secondary gain after an episode was limited.

With these measures, Sally's behavior slowly improved, while she was hospitalized. She later signed herself out of the hospital to seek a new doctor.

PHARMACOLOGICAL INTERVENTION IN ANXIETY-RELATED DISORDERS

Treatment is based on the premise that decrease or relief of anxiety will enable the client to gain insight and with it, some degree of control over his unhealthy coping patterns. Five groups of drugs are currently prescribed as part of treatment. A detailed discussion of drug therapy is presented in Chapter 15. The presentation below is meant to provide only a general picture of drugs currently in use.

The benzodiazepines are the most widely used antianxiety drugs. They are safe unless taken in conjunction with alcohol. These drugs are effective muscle relaxants and do not disrupt sleep patterns—an important point in treating the severely anxious client who is rigid and finds it difficult to sleep. Like many other drugs, the benzodiazepines carry the potential for abuse, and the client must be given careful instruction in their use.

Antihistamines are less likely to cause dependency than the benzodiazepines and are helpful in anxiety secondary to a physical disorder. In the elderly client, these drugs may cause a paradoxical increase in anxiety. They may give rise to a sense of depersonalization in a client of any age, and thus are not prescribed in depersonalization disorder.

Phenobarbital is the most widely used barbiturate. It has the disadvantage of being habit forming, as well as lowering the blood level of other drugs the client may be taking.

Propanediols such as meprobamate are effective muscle relaxants but are highly addictive. In short-term use, they relieve tension headaches and other manifestations of tension.

The beta-adrenergic blocking agents such as propranolol (Inderal) decrease such symptoms of anxiety as tremor and hyperventilation and are not addictive.

The group of drugs known as tricyclic depressants (imipramine), and those included among the MAO-inhibitors (Phenelzine) may be administered in panic disorders.

General Guidelines in Nursing Care

1. Assess both subjective and objective symptoms of anxiety.
2. Note changes (increase or decrease) in symptoms before and after drugs are given.
3. Anticipate the need for medication before an anxiety attack becomes full blown by assessing the client's usual behavior pattern and maintaining alertness to indications of increasing anxiety, such as pacing, chain smoking, rapid speech, frequency of urination, withdrawal.
4. Spend time with the client in order to ensure verbal and physical release from anxiety (talking, walking, handiwork, physical exercise).
5. Be alert to signs of increased dependency or overuse of medication (sleepiness, slurred speech). The client will often request drugs in the absence of overt signs of anxiety.
6. Because the drugs are potentially lethal, especially when taken in conjunction with alcohol, medication teaching should be thorough. A client expressing suicidal ideation should be carefully observed to ensure that he does not hoard medication.

□ Nursing Process in Anxiety-Related Disorders

CARE OF THE CLIENT DISPLAYING PANIC AND SEVERE ANXIETY BEHAVIORS

ASSESSMENT □

The Client □ Age of onset is an important factor in the client's history. Panic disorder does not usually occur until late adolescence or adult life. In both panic and generalized anxiety states, a description of precipitating factors and of the physical, behavioral, and psychological manifestations should be obtained. The duration of the attacks and the client's feelings after them should also be assessed. Note any indications of depression and use/abuse of prescription or nonprescription drugs or alcohol. If the client is experiencing a panic attack or severe anxiety state at the time of the interview, intervene immediately to lower his anxiety level. Signs and symptoms of panic and severe anxiety are present in Table 32-8.

■ *Point of Emphasis*

During a panic attack, the client's intellectual and perceptual field is severely impaired. Limit the assessment to what is currently happening and gather additional data later when the client's anxiety level decreases.

TABLE 32-8 Signs and Symptoms of Panic and Severe Anxiety States

Panic Disorder	
Physical Signs	Behavioral Signs
Elevated blood pressure	High level of physical activity
Increased respirations	Striking out at others
Flushing or pallor	Pacing
Profuse perspiring	Rocking
Insomnia	Tremulousness
Anorexia	Clinging physically to others
Headaches	Pressured speech
	Crying
	Irritability

Generalized Anxiety Disorder	
Physical Signs	Behavioral Signs
Elevated blood pressure	Increase motor activity
Increased heart and respiratory rate	Fidgeting, inability to sit still
Headaches	Irritability
Urinary frequency	Poor concentration
Diarrhea	Lack of initiative
Gastrointestinal upset	Cries easily
Tightness of neck, pains in head or back	Inability to get along with others
	Withdrawal
	Indication of low self-esteem (poor grooming, hygiene)
	Depressed affect and body posture

Verbal Signs
"I feel so helpless."
"All I ever do is worry."
"I just can't get interested in anything."
"I feel so tired."
"Everything's out of control."

The Nurse □ When working with an individual experiencing either panic or severe anxiety disorders, self-awareness is essential. The client's anxiety is communicated to and easily arouses anxiety in others. The nurse may frequently experience tension and/or uneasiness when spending time with an anxious client or afterward. She must effectively manage her own anxiety so she can facilitate the client's growth. Questions such as "How am I feeling now?" "What feelings do I have now?" help the nurse keep a check on her own anxiety. If she recognizes a rise in her own level of tension, the question becomes "What do I see happening between the client and me?" "What am I telling myself *should be* happening here?" The nurse's need to reduce her own anxiety often causes her to try to hurry the client into

problem solving. The primary goal is to provide a warm, calm environment and not to try to solve the client's problems for him.

Despite all her efforts, there are times when the nurse's anxiety level will continue to rise because of the intensity of the client's anxiety. If her anxiety is conveyed to the client, her presence becomes nontherapeutic. At this point, she should take some time away from the client and seek other supervision of him.

> **■ Point of Emphasis**
>
> *Monitoring one's own anxiety level is essential. If client anxiety causes the nurse's anxiety to rise, the latter may respond with fear, impatience, or client avoidance. Remember that the client is experiencing such intense fear that he is not able to control his behavior.*

Environment □ The client's family or living situation should be assessed. Often the precipitating cause is some change in the environment or a personal crisis. For example, a spouse's taking a new job that requires travel may precipitate a panic attack or the gradual development of generalized anxiety disorder. Family or significant others may be able to identify and describe the onset of symptoms and their effects on the client.

PROBLEM IDENTIFICATION □

Panic Disorder □ The first priority in caring for this client is to protect him and others and to understand the cause of the panic. The first problem is the potential for injury (to self or to others) resulting from overactivity, pacing, tremulousness, or striking out at others. The short-term goal is to protect the client and others when the client himself is unable to control his behavior.

The second problem is the alteration in thought and sensory processes due to extreme anxiety, resulting in pressured speech, irritability, crying, and other manifestations of anxiety. The short-term goal here is to allow the client to freely express fears and feelings.

The long-term goal in both cases is to reduce anxiety to a mild to moderate level where problem solving can occur.

Anxiety Disorder □ The primary problem in generalized anxiety disorder is ineffective coping secondary to chronic disabling anxiety. Complications such as drug or alcohol abuse may be the presenting problem. The client's gestures, thoughts of suicide, or feelings of depression may further disable him.

The short-term goal is to help the client become aware of and identify the anxiety, while providing for his safety. Over the long term, the aim is to help the client decrease his anxiety and develop healthier coping skills.

INTERVENTIONS □ Interventions and rationale in both panic and generalized anxiety disorders are outlined in Tables 32-9 and 32-10. Many of the interventions described are equally useful in both disorders.

EVALUATION □ Interventions are evaluated by monitoring changes in the behaviors assessed and receiving verbal feedback from the client. Motor and verbal activity decrease; the client will be able to rest quietly or possibly sleep. The episodes of panic attack may physically exhaust the client. Evaluate which interventions increased or decreased the panic state. For example, did touch calm him, or did it cause increased fear and restlessness? Did pacing help? Did anxiolytic medication help?

CARE OF THE CLIENT DISPLAYING PHOBIC BEHAVIORS

ASSESSMENT □

The Client □ Phobic behavior, as a response to anxiety, can be highly restricting. Several factors must be considered in assessment.

1. Degree of impairment. If the phobia does not appreciably affect work, school, or per-

---

TABLE 32-9 Intervention in Panic Disorder

Intervention	Rationale
Remove client from large open areas to a more confined quiet space.	Patient is experiencing "flight or fight" behavior and feels out of control.
Allow client to move about room or pace unless he is physically assaultive.	Physical activity such as pacing and crying helps spend some of the client's energy.
If physical restraint is necessary, remember to remain with client.	External controls needed so client can feel safe.
Dim bright lights or raise dim lights to normal level.	The perceptual field is narrowed and stimuli bombard client, causing him to feel overwhelmed.
Assure client you are in control of the immediate situation (e.g., "I won't let anything here hurt you." "I will stay with you." "I understand how you feel." "This must be frightening for you."). Avoid using false reassurance (e.g., "Everything will be all right.").	
Touch client on arm, shoulder, or hand if rapport has been established. Otherwise do not touch him.	Client may be too stimulated or frightened to find touch reassuring.
Give antianxiety medications as ordered (preferably orally).	Oral medications such as diazepam have early peak action and decrease anxiety.
Assist the client to express his perception of what is happening. ("You're very distressed—can you talk about it?" "I'll stay with you.")	Gives the nurse an understanding of the client's perceptions and fears.
Encourage the patient to cry (e.g., "Sometimes it helps if you let yourself cry.").	Relieves tension.
Speak in short, simple sentences, giving only one direction at a time. Avoid lengthy explanations and many questions.	Client is so overwhelmed that he cannot follow lengthy or complicated processes.

TABLE 32-10 Intervention in Generalized Anxiety Disorder

Intervention	Rationale
Provide a calm, comfortable environment. Take client to room, pull curtain around bed, and so on.	Decrease environmental stimulation that may be stressful.
Identify the behavior you see with the client (e.g., "You seem to be uncomfortable now." "Are you feeling anxious now?" "Tell me how you are feeling now.").	Assists the client to gain awareness of anxiety.
Encourage the client to explore the situation. "Can you tell me when you started feeling anxious?" "What was happening when you started to feel anxious?" "Tell me what happened this morning."	The client will identify specific causes for the anxiety and clarify perceptions. Narrowed focus and selective inattentiveness can cause distortion in perception.
Accept and show understanding of the client's feelings. "That must be very uncomfortable for you."	Promotes trust and conveys concern and understanding.
Administer antianxiety medication as ordered, optimally before level of anxiety becomes severe.	Anxiolytic drugs provide relaxation of physical symptoms and allow client to focus on the situation, to problem-solve and learn.
Institute suicide precautions such as finding out if client feels suicidal, or has a plan to commit suicide. If so, check client frequently; if hospitalized, notify doctor. If at home, discuss with client possibility of staying with friends or relatives, or temporary hospitalization.	Recurrence of panic and/or anxiety becomes depressing and may cause the client to feel hopeless and wish to escape the pain.
Help the client to develop new coping mechanisms. Suggest other ways in which he might work out anxiety, for example, physical activity.	Anxiety must be endured in order to develop new coping mechanisms. This is a long-term process in anxiety disorders.
Help the patient explore previous coping mechanisms. "What have you done in the past when you felt this way?" "What do you usually do when you feel this way?"	Reinforces existing strengths and allows client to understand why some mechanisms are unhealthy.

sonal relationships, it is unlikely that treatment will be sought. The seriousness of the phobia is determined by its influence on the client's life-style.

2. Stressors. Recent trauma or stressful situations should be explored. The "traumatic" nature of the situation may not be readily apparent to the nurse. Listen to what the client says in order to understand his view of the stressful event. Certain themes, such as fear of failure, fear of closeness to others, and fears about sexuality may be covert, emerging only after many conversations. When a phobic episode occurs, assess the event that gave rise to it.

3. Secondary gain. The primary gain is a temporary decrease in anxiety due to avoidance of the phobic situation. Secondary gain may also be present in the form of new solicitousness on the part of family, friends, or employer.

The Nurse ☐ When working with the phobic client, it may be helpful to recall irrational fears in one's own life; although the feared object may have posed no threat, the response was that of avoidance. Remember that phobia is a coping mechanism and convey empathy about the intensity of the client's anxiety.

Environment □ The client's family or significant others may be helpful in contributing information about how the client's life-style has been affected. His environment may have become so restricted that his physical needs are unmet; or he may have turned to drugs or alcohol to relieve the anxiety.

PROBLEM IDENTIFICATION □ The first problem the nurse will diagnose in phobic behavior is a fear of situations, persons, or objects secondary to anxiety resulting in avoidance or withdrawal behaviors. The short-term goal is to assist the client to function in a safe, noncritical environment, while promoting healthier coping mechanisms for long-term functioning in his customary environment.

The second problem is the possibility that the client will engage in hazardous practices resulting from his anxiety and phobic defense. For example, fear of germs may cause him to avoid certain foods, with resulting poor nutrition. Protect the client from potentially hazardous behaviors and assist him to understand the phobia as a coping mechanism for which healthier coping skills can be substituted.

INTERVENTION □ Intervention in phobic behaviors is outlined in Table 32-11.

EVALUATION □ Successful intervention in phobic disorders is difficult. In therapy, a severe underlying personality disorder often becomes evident. A decrease in display of the symptom and the client's subjective feelings of comfort are a basic barometer. Increased ability to face the phobic situation, object, or person is a reliable measure of increased coping abilities.

CARE OF THE CLIENT DISPLAYING OBSESSIVE-COMPULSIVE BEHAVIORS

ASSESSMENT □

The Client □ Obsessive-compulsive behaviors are assessed through interviewing the client and taking note of recurring themes. Often the client will state his irritation or disgust with his "habit" and recognize it as irrational. He may feel hopeless about feeling better and helpless to control his behavior, even though he recognizes the harmfulness of his compulsion. Obsessive thoughts may be readily revealed because they are so disturbing to him. Questions such as "Do you think about this a lot?" or "How much trouble do these thoughts cause you?" may help to uncover obsessive thoughts that are not readily revealed.

Assess the client's ability to meet his physical and hygiene needs. Other compulsive behaviors

---

TABLE 32-11 Intervention in Phobic Behaviors

Intervention	Rationale
Do not belittle client's fears, no matter how ridiculous they appear.	The behavior is a coping mechanism and is used to decrease or avoid anxiety, which is increased by ridicule or "pep talks."
The client may say, "I know this is stupid" or "This is silly." Point out that the behavior achieves something. "You feel it's silly, but it helps you feel better."	Assists the client to recognize that the behavior is a way of coping with anxiety.
Provide activities that help the client to feel safe. Do not allow the client to totally withdraw. If at home, help the client make small steps to overcome fears with a supportive person.	Depending on the phobia, the client may totally withdraw. A gentle supportive atmosphere is important. Activities that do not increase anxiety will help the client remain involved and decrease avoidance of others.
Provide a noncritical environment with positive reinforcement.	In social phobia the client fears criticism.
Support treatment modalities such desensitization, reciprocal inhibition, antidepressants. *Do not force insight.*	Challenging the client's anxiety causes greater need for symptom which may cause panic.
Provide safety and comfort measures as necessary.	Certain phobias (e.g., about germs) may inhibit food or fluid intake, prevent proper hygiene and ability to rest.
Insure adequate fluid and food intake.	

may be more socially than physically destructive, such as the behavior of a husband who attempts to prove his masculinity by compulsively engaging in extramarital affairs.

The Nurse □ The client's rigidity of thought and behavior can be very disruptive to the nurse-client relationship. Statements and actions incessantly repeated can be very frustrating. The nurse may become aware of the urge to "push" the client onward, rather than accepting his behavior as expressing underlying fears and conflicts. "Commanding" the client to stop the behavior is fruitless, and serves only to increase frustration in both nurse and client.

Environment □ The client's family or employer may have become quite frustrated with the behavior by the time the client enters treatment. In fact, it may have been their insistence that the client seek help that prompted his entering therapy, especially in the case of compulsive behaviors. The client may already have lost his job because of his inability to finish a task and may find entrance into treatment an additional blow to his self-esteem. Financial or psychosocial stressors such as loss of a job, caring for an ailing and demanding parent, divorce, or death of a loved one may precipitate the behavior.

PROBLEM IDENTIFICATION □ Nursing diagnosis reveals two important problems. The first is alteration in thought process secondary to anxiety resulting in thoughts or behaviors potentially hazardous to health. The nurse's immediate goal is to help meet the client's needs for nutrition and safety. Through treatment, the goal is to help the client recognize the underlying anxiety which causes the unhealthy coping mechanism, and to decrease the anxiety in order to develop healthier coping behaviors.

The second problem is ineffective individual coping secondary to anxiety resulting in compulsive, ritualistic behavior. The short-term goal is a decrease in the amount of specific compulsive behavior. The long-term aim is to help the client relate anxiety to the performance of the rituals and to focus on expressing the anxiety.

INTERVENTION □ The overall goal of treatment is to help the client learn to confine or possibly eliminate the symptoms. A warm, supportive approach is needed, as well as time and patience. Accept and work with his behavior and allow him time to adopt healthier ways of coping. Table 32-12 lists interventions and their rationale.

EVALUATION □ Pay attention to both short- and long-term goals. Since the anxiety and conflicts that motivate the behavior developed early in life, long-term therapy is necessary for resolution. If a client requires temporary hospitalization, establishment of therapeutic relationships will promote client growth and accomplishment of short-term goals. Focus evaluation on specific behavioral changes, which can be noted through observation and through verbal interaction with the client.

CARE OF THE CLIENT DISPLAYING SOMATIC SYMPTOMS DUE TO PSYCHOLOGICAL DISORDERS

ASSESSMENT □

The Client □ Focus on the person rather than the symptom. Obtain a history of events prior to and at the time the impairment or symptoms occurred. For example, in conversion disorder, the nurse might ask "Tell me what was happening at home yesterday." or "Do you remember what you did that day?" "Tell me anything different that was happening for you, no matter how insignificant it seems." Since conversion is an unconscious process, the client will not be able to explain in direct terms why it has occurred.

A careful history, with observation of the client's behavioral response to stress, is necessary. Also note sources of primary and secondary gain related to the symptoms. Assess location, duration, and type of symptoms, review past medical history, note use of drugs or alcohol, and assess the level of depression and suicidal potential.

Potential for suicide can be assessed directly by asking such questions as "How much trouble are you having with thoughts of hurting yourself?" or "Are you feeling as though you want to hurt yourself?" Nurses often convey their idea of suicide as unacceptable by ignoring its possibility. If the client has had long-standing or intense suffering, death may seem to offer relief. A direct approach conveys understanding of the feelings and gives the client permission to discuss it.

The Nurse □ Anger and frustration are two very common responses to these somatization disorders. Lack of an organic basis for the client's

TABLE 32-12 Intervention in Obsessive-Compulsive Behavior

Intervention	Rationale
Provide for basic needs (grooming, food, rest).	The client becomes so involved in ritualistic thoughts and/or behaviors that basic needs may not be met.
Allow sufficient time for the patient to perform the ritual, (e.g., if he needs to remake his bed several times, awaken him early so the task can be completed before activities start).	Client needs this defense to reduce anxiety and, within limits, should be allowed to complete rituals.
Keep changes in the environment at a minimum and explain them. If possible, avoid changes in client's room.	Changes may heighten anxiety resulting in greater need for compulsive behaviors.
Use a warm, caring approach indicating acceptance of the client.	Forcing the client to give up the symptoms will increase his anxiety.
Indicate awareness and empathy for the client's behavior. "I notice you get up and straighten your chair each time someone sits by you. That must be very tiring for you." Further, help the client learn from the behavior by exploring the feelings. "Can you tell me how you are feeling?" "Tell me what you were thinking when Mary sat down."	Demonstrates empathy for the client's feelings and assists him to relate behavior to feelings.
Help provide a framework for the client's free time. Include structured, simple games or tasks that require concentration. Telling the client what will be done, rather than asking, can be helpful (e.g., "We are going to play cards now." "It's time for activity. I want you to paint this.").	This relieves the client of decision-making anxieties and gives him less time to focus on repetitive thoughts.
Help the client to explore ways of setting limits on his own behavior.	Provides alternatives for control of anxiety.
Show the client your interest and concern, reinforcing his self-worth. This can be done by recognizing his nonritualistic behavior (e.g., "I see you finished your picture. Can you tell me about it?").	Low self-esteem accompanies much of ritualistic behavior.

symptoms may cause the nurse to wonder if the discomfort felt is real. It is not uncommon to hear statements like "He's just faking it."

■ Point of Emphasis

The impairment is real to the client and a disbelieving attitude will only create a need for him to prove the validity of his complaint. Focus of care should be on attempting to understand the meaning and purpose of the physical symptoms in the client's life and to prevent injury due to the disability.

The nurse must realize the pain is real to the client and that it is unconsciously motivated. The client's anxiety and depression are symptoms that can benefit from nursing intervention.

Environment □ Often the client feels tremendous pressure from others to "perform" and his physical symptoms may give him the only acceptable excuse for failing to meet these expectations. (This is not a conscious decision.) An example is a teenage girl whose parents exert great pressure on her to excel scholastically and in extracurricular activities. Instead of turning to drugs or engaging in other activities that would invite parental rejection, she experiences some

TABLE 32-13 *Intervention in Somatic Symptoms Due to Psychological Disorders*

Conversion Disorder

Intervention	Rationale
Intervention for symptoms on a physical basis (e.g., range of motion, physical therapy) is required only if paralysis persists for a length of time. If required, it should be handled in a matter-of-fact manner and not emphasized.	The "sick" role and thus secondary gain is minimized by treating symptoms with a matter of fact, although caring approach.
Note times when symptoms are more pronounced and explore the feeling the client is experiencing. "Describe for me what is happening now." "Tell me how you are feeling inside."	All behavior has meaning and the affected functions may give clues to the underlying conflict.
Convey understanding and acceptance of negative feelings the client may have.	The need for physical symptoms will be decreased if client can verbalize negative feelings.
Statements that convey this acceptance are, for example, "Sometimes it's frightening to feel so angry." "It's hard to have feelings and not feel comfortable talking about them."	
Help patient to develop new ways to express feelings. "How do you think you might let him know you are angry?" "What would you like to do in this situation?"	Verbalization is healthier coping mechanism than physical illness.
Allow time for the patient to understand the symptoms. Don't push awareness of event and resulting symptoms prematurely.	The need for the symptoms has developed over time, and it will only cause increased anxiety if the nurse attempts to force insight.

Somatization

Intervention	Rationale
Provide care for symptoms matter-of-factly.	Decrease focus on physical complaints.
Spend a minimum of time discussing symptoms: "I understand you are having stomach pains and I have given you medication for that."	Decrease secondary gain.
Focus on the client as a person.	Helps understanding the client's anxiety and possible emotional problems.
Use a consistent, firm approach. Channel requests to one staff member.	Decreases secondary gain and manipulation.
Help the client verbalize anxiety.	Verbalization decreases need for somatic complaints.
Set limits on time spent with client.	The client's neediness may result in unreasonable demands. Express concern but needs to care for others.
Utilize biofeedback and relaxation techniques.	These help decrease the client's somatic symptoms due to anxiety and may afford temporary relief.
Intervene if suicide potential appears high. (Remove unsafe objects, place client near nursing station, do frequent checks, continue to assess client's suicidal feelings.)	Safety of client is immediate goal.

sort of "rare paralysis" of her legs which allow her, by "dragging her feet," to resist their pressure and gains attention and solicitude.

Marital, family, and social situations should be explored at the interview. The purpose (unconscious) served by the illness and effects on job and family responsibilities should be assessed.

Initially, significant others may be greatly concerned and worried, refusing to accept the diagnosis that no organic pathology exists. However, as it becomes evident there is no physical basis for the problem, they may become angry and reject the client. Working with family members helps them achieve greater understanding of the client's need for his defense. Often these families have learned patterns of somaticizing their distress and negative feelings into such disorders as "acid stomach," "migraines," and a "weak heart."

The most pronounced problem initially is a self-care deficit related to the body part involved. For example, conversion blindness would result in difficulties in walking, dressing, hygiene, eating, and so on. This self-care deficit is secondary to the anxiety-based physical impairment.

PROBLEM IDENTIFICATION □

Conversion Disorder □ The most pronounced problem initially is a self-care deficit (specific to problem, movement, feeding, others) secondary to anxiety-based physical impairment. The short-term goal is to meet the client's physical needs for care if he is unable to meet them.

The second problem is the disturbance in self-concept resulting in physical symptoms and difficulty in expressing feelings. The short-term goal is to assist the client to verbalize feelings and relate them to physical symptoms. Long-term goals for this client are to decrease his anxiety in order to reduce the physical symptoms and help the client recognize the anxiety underlying his symptoms so that healthier coping skills can be developed.

Somatization Disorder □ The major problem is ineffective coping secondary to intense anxiety, which is masked by somatic complaints. Other potential problems include substance abuse and suicide attempts. The short-term goal is to reduce the client's anxiety and eventually help him name his anxiety and express it, associating it with his somatic symptoms.

INTERVENTIONS □ Care of this client is difficult unless the nurse understands the unconscious nature of the symptoms and has empathy for the client's emotional pain, which may be evident only in somatic form. Table 32-13 outlines interventions in conversion and somatization disorder, many of which are also appropriate to other somatoform disorders.

EVALUATION □ Evaluation may be based on noting a decrease in physical symptoms along with an increased ability to express and deal with the anxiety and negative feelings. These disorders have developed gradually and are not easily and quickly resolved.

■ Enrichment Activities

DISCUSSION QUESTIONS

1. Discuss defense mechanisms commonly utilized in anxiety, somatoform, dissociative, and factitious disorders.

2. Identify two of the most common defense mechanisms you yourself use. At what point would these stop being helpful and become dysfunctional?

3. Identify ways in which a culture may reinforce certain personality traits (e.g., obsessive-compulsive personality) that may result in an unhealthy exaggeration of these traits.

4. Discuss the way in which a person's culture (society, community, family) may influence the development of certain defense mechanisms. For example, many families encourage competition and being "the best," and discourage the notion of failure. This results in a strong need to always be right, or perfect.

5. Discuss how excessive use of defense mechanisms can be detrimental to personal growth.

LEARNING ACTIVITIES

Think about a client in your clinical experience with an anxiety, somatoform, dissociative, or factitious disorder.

1. Assess the behaviors presented that signify dysfunctional coping.

2. Identify major defense mechanisms and the purpose they serve.

3. Identify why the defense mechanisms are unhealthy.

4. Formulate nursing diagnoses in these behaviors.

5. Develop interventions specific to your client that will reduce the need for the dysfunctional behaviors and will limit those behaviors.

6. Evalutate, over time, changes that have occurred in the behaviors.

■ Recommended Learning/ Reading Materials

Human Relations Media. *Psychological defenses.* Series B, Parts I,II,III. Filmstrips. Pleasantville, NY, 1980. Filmstrips explore the psychological defense mechanisms used by everyone in daily life, illustrating their usefulness and overuse.

Human Relations Media, Who's OK, Who's not OK: An introduction to abnormal psychology. Part II. *Neurotic behavior.* Filmstrips. Pleasantville, NY, 1980. Filmstrip explores disordered patterns of behavior related to anxiety or neurotic behavior. When an individual has consistently used defense mechanisms which interfere with daily life functioning, a neurotic pattern is developed. Various behavior forms and modes of treatment are presented.

The Psychiatry Learning System. 3d ed. II, No. 9, *Anxiety disorders* and No. 10, *Somatoform and dissociative disorders.* Chapel Hill, NC: Health Sciences Consortium, 1982. Videocassettes delineate signs, symptoms, and accompanying factors which characterize the anxiety, somatoform, and dissociative disorders.

Schreiber, Flora. *Sybil.* New York: Warner Paperback Library, 1973. A true story of a young woman with multiple personality disorder, this book traces Sybil's life from early childhood, exploring the causes, manifestations, and treatment of her disorder.

Horney, Karen. *Neurosis and human growth.* New York: Norton, 1950. A classic work on neurosis, this book presents Horney's theories on how a person develops certain attitudes of personality as a means of coping with early childhood emotional trauma.

May, Rollo. *The meaning of anxiety.* New York: The Ronald Press Company, 1950. May's classic work of human anxiety explores, on a philosophical, cultural, and psychological level, the origins, usefulness, and meaning of anxiety to human existence. It is an important work in order to understand anxiety as a pervasive feeling about society and an important component of individual human life.

■ References

American Psychiatric Association. *Diagnostic and statistical manual of mental disorders.* (3d ed.) Washington, D.C.: American Psychiatric Association, 1980.

Blacker, K.H., and Levitt, M. The differential diagnosis of obsessive compulsive symptoms. *Comprehensive psychiatry,* 20, 1979:532–547.

Bloch, A.M. Combat neurosis in inner city schools. *American journal of psychiatry,* 135, 1978:1189–1192.

Cavenar, J.O., Jr., and Werman, D.D. Origins of the fear of success. *American journal of psychiatryy,* 1338, 1981:95–98.

Chadoff, D. Diagnosis of hysteria. *American journal of psychiatry,* 131, 1974:1073–1078.

Clancy, J., Noyes, R. Jr., Hoenk, P.R., and Slymen, D.J. Secondary depression in anxiety neurosis. *Journal of Nervous and mental disorders,* 166, 1978:846–850.

Crowe, R.C.; Pauls, D.L.; Slymen, D.J.; and Noyes, R. A family study of anxiety neurosis morbidity risk in families of patients with and without mitral valve prolapse. *Archives of general psychiatry,* 37, 1980:77–79.

Engel, G.L. Conversion symptoms. In *Signs and symptoms: Applied pathologic physiology and clinical interpretation* (MacBride, C.M., and Blacklow, R.S., eds.). 5th ed. Philadelphia: J.B. Lippincott, 1970.

Freud, S. *The ego and the id.* rev. ed. New York: Norton, 1962. (Originally published 1932.)

———. *An outline of psychoanalysis.* rev. ed. New York: Norton, 1969. (Originally published 1940.)

Gross, M., and Huerta, E. Functional convulsions masked as epileptic disorders. *Journal of pediatric psychology,* 5, 1980:71–79.

Hagerty, B.K. Obsessive compulsive behavior: An overview of four psychological frameworks. *Journal of psychiatric nursing,* 19, 1981:37–39.

Henderson, S. The social network, support and neurosis. The function of attachment in adult life. *British journal of psychiatry,* 131, 1977:185–191.

Hollingsworth, C.E.; Tanguay, P.E.; Grossman, L.; and Pabst, P. Long term outcome of obsessive compulsive disorders in childhood. *Journal of the American Academy of Child Psychiatry,* 19, 1980:134–144.

Horney, K. *Our inner conflicts.* New York: Norton, 1972. (Originally published 1945.)

Horowitz, M.J.; Wilner, N.; Kaltreider, N.; and Alvarez, W. Signs and symptoms of post-traumatic stress disorder. *Archives of general psychiatry,* 37, 1980:85–92.

Hoyt, M.F. Therapist and patient actions in 'good' psychotherapy sessions. *Archives of general psychiatry,* 37, 1980:159–161.

Jones, M.M. Conversion reaction: Anachronism or evolutionary form? A review of the neurologic, behavioral and psychoanalytic literature. *Psychological bulletin*, 87, 1980:427–439.

Kerr, N. Anxiety: Theoretical considerations. *Perspectives in psychiatric care*, 17, 1978:36–46.

Kolb, L.C., and Brodie, H.K. *Modern clinical psychiatry*. 10th ed. Philadelphia: W.B. Saunders Co., 1982.

Lehmann, L.S. Depersonalization. *American journal of psychiatry*, 131, 1974:1221–1224.

Manchanda, R.; Sethi, B.B.; and Gupta, S.C. Hostility and guilt in obsessive-compulsive neurosis. *British journal of psychiatry*, 135, 1979:52–54.

Modai, I.; Sirota, P.; Cygielman, G.; and Wijsenbeek, H. Conversive hallucination. *Journal of nervous and mental disorders*, 168, 1980:564–565.

Murphy, J.M.; Sobol, A.M.; Neff, R.K.; Olivier, D.C.; and Leighton, A.H. Stability of prevalence. Depression and anxiety disorders. *Archives of general psychiatry*, 41, 1984:990–997.

Noyes, R., Jr.; Clancy, J.; Hoenk, P.R.; and Slymen, D.J. The prognosis of anxiety neuroses. *Archives of general psychiatry*, 37, 1980:172–178.

Putnam, F.W.; Loewenstein, R.J.; Silberman, E.J.; and Post, R.M. Multiple personality disorder in a hospital setting. *Journal of clinical psychiatry*, 45, 1984:172–175.

Rabins, P.V., and Slavney, P.R. Hysterical traits and variability of mood in normal men. *Psychological medicine*, 9, 1979:301–304.

Rainey, S.M.; Ettedgui, E.; Pohl, R.B.; and Bridges, M. Effect of acute beta-adrenergic blockage on lactate-induced panic. (Letter) *Archives of general psychiatry*, 42, 1985:104–105.

Reed, P.P. *Alive: The story of the Andes survivors*. Philadelphia: J.B. Lippincott, 1974.

Ries, R.K. DSM III differential diagnosis of Munchausen's syndrome. *Journal of nervous and mental disorders*, 168, 1980:629–632.

Roy, A. Obsessive compulsive neurosis: Phenomenology, outcome and a comparison with hysterical neurosis. *Comprehensive psychiatry*, 20, 1979:528–531.

———. Hysteria. *Journal of psychosomatic research*, 24, 1980:53–56.

Salzman, L., and Thaler, F. Obsessive compulsive disorders, A review of the literature. *American journal of psychiatry*, 138, 1981:286–296.

Schreiber, F.R. *Sybil*, Chicago: Regnery, 1973.

Sheehan, D.V.; Ballenger, J.; and Jacobsen, G. Treatment of endogenous anxiety with phobic, hysterical and hypochondriacal symptoms. *Archives of general psychiatry*, 37, 1980:51–59.

Slavney, P.R., and Rich, G. Variability of mood and the diagnosis of personality disorder. *British journal of psychiatry*, 136, 1980:402–404.

Snyder, S. Amitriptyline therapy of obsessive compulsive neurosis. *Journal of clinical psychiatry*, 41, 1980:286–289.

Steimer, M.; Welber, A.S.; Archer, R.; and Carroll, B.J. Multimodal treatment of a case of obsessive compulsive neurosis. *Journal of nervous and mental disorders*, 168, 1980:184–187.

Stern, T.A. Munchausen's syndrome revisited. *Psychosomatics*, 21, 1980:329–331, 335–336.

Sullivan, H.S. *The interpersonal theory of psychiatry*. New York: Norton, 1953.

———. *Clinical studies in psychiatry*. New York: Norton, 1956.

Thigpen, C.H., and Cleckley, H. *The three faces of Eve*. New York: McGraw-Hill, 1957.

Toone, B.K., and Roberts, J. Status epilepticus. An uncommon hysterical conversion syndrome. *Journal of nervous and mental disorders*, 167, 1979:548–552.

Torch, E.M. Review of the relationship between obsession and depersonalization. *Acta psychiatrica Scandinavia*, 58, 1978:191–198.

Weiss, K.J., and Rosenberg, D.J. Prevalence of anxiety disorders among alcoholics. *Journal of clinical psychiatry*, 46, 1985:3–5.

Zisook, S.; DeVaul, R.A.; and Gammon, E. The hysterical facade. *American journal of psychoanalysis*, 39, 1979:113–123.

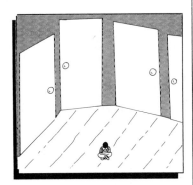

33

Affective Disorders and Suicide

David Anthony Forrester

Learning Objectives

Upon completion of this chapter, the reader will be able to:

1. Describe various etiological theories of affective disorders.

2. Apply the nursing process in planning care for clients experiencing affective disorders and/or suicidal ideation.

3. Identify a variety of physical, emotional, cognitive, and behavioral manifestations of affective disorders and suicide.

4. Identify appropriate nursing interventions for depressed and manic clients.

5. Identify appropriate nursing interventions for suicidal clients.

6. Evaluate nursing interventions.

The purpose of this chapter is to assist the reader in planning comprehensive nursing care for persons experiencing affective disorders and/or suicidal ideation. To accomplish this purpose, consideration will first be given to relevant terms and current theoretical explanations regarding the etiology and epidemiology of affective disorders and suicide. Next, attention will be given to currently used medical interventions and the implications these have for both client and nurse. Finally, the nursing process will be explored in an attempt to: (1) delineate the physical, emotional, cognitive, and behavioral manifestations of affective disorders and suicide; (2) formulate appropriate nursing diagnoses for clients experiencing affective disorders and/or suicide; (3) engage in the primary, secondary, and tertiary prevention of affective disorders and/or suicide; and (4) collaborate with the client to ensure meaningful evaluation of nursing care.

☐ *Affective Disorders*

As the term implies, the distinctive characteristic of affective disorders is an extreme disturbance in affect toward either depression or elation. Affective disorders comprise one of the most common psychiatric syndromes and are essentially of three types: depressive disorders, manic disorders, and bipolar affective disorders (characterised by alternating episodes of manic and depressive behavior). The following discussion regarding affective disorders includes: definitions of relevant terms, a description of the currently used classification system, and an epidemiological description of the occurrence of affective disorders. A number of theories pertaining to the etiology of affective disorders are also presented. These include psychodynamic and sociological theories, as well as a variety of biochemical theories.

DEFINITIONS

The term *affect* refers to the emotional feeling tone attached to an idea, object, event, or person. An individual's affect includes both the subjective internal experiences of inner feelings (mood) and the external behavioral manifestations of these feelings. The term is frequently heard in reference to clients in psychiatric settings. For example, if an individual experiences a dulling in the intensity of feeling, he is said to have a *blunted affect*. A *flat affect* means that an individual has a mark-

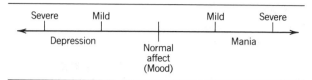

Figure 33-1 *Affective spectrum.*

edly dulled or blunted emotional tone attached to an object, idea, or thought. When a person's response to an event, situation, or interaction is inconsistent with the stimulus, he is said to have an *inappropriate affect*. A *labile affect* means that an individual's affect abruptly, rapidly, and repeatedly changes for no apparent reason. Finally, persons with *affective disorders* experience extreme disturbances in mood, toward either depression or mania. Figure 33-1 provides a representation of the affective spectrum.

The middle range of the affective spectrum is associated with mild changes in mood. These minor changes are generally considered "normal" in that they represent the routinely encountered highs and lows of day-to-day living. The two extremes of the spectrum, severe depression and mania, usually result in some degree of disruption in life-style and are considered pathological. Individuals with affective disorders experience episodes of severe depression or mania that are more prolonged and more intense than usual and interfere with activities of daily living.

Depression usually originates with the experience of some real or perceived loss and is nonpathological when it is proportionate to that loss. *Nonpathological depression* is a time-limited experience characterized by feelings of sadness, despair, and discouragement. *Pathological depression* has a longer duration and is characterised by exaggerated feelings of sadness, melancholy, dejection, worthlessness, emptiness, and hopelessness that are inappropriate and disproportionate with reality. Usually the depressed person will describe his mood as "depressed, sad, blue" or "down in the dumps."

Mania is always considered pathological and is characterised by an expansive emotional state. Mania may be manifest as extreme excitement, excessive elation, hyperactivity, agitation, pressure of speech, flight of ideas, increased psychomotor activity, fleeting attention, and sometimes violent, destructive, or self-destructive behavior. The elevated mood of the manic individual may

TABLE 33-1 Classification of Affective Disorders

Classification by	Type of Affective Disorder	
Etiology	Exogenous Depressive symptoms occur as a result of some external loss or event. Symptomatology is excessive in terms of degree and duration.	Endogenous Depressive symptoms occur without apparent external cause. Attributed to nutritional, hormonal, or chemical imbalance, or other pathological factors.
Symptomatology	Reactive Depressive symptoms occur as a reaction to bereavement. Client responds to psychotherapy.	Endogenous Depressive symptoms occur without apparent external cause. Client responds to somatic therapy (electroconvulsive therapy and pharmacotherapy).
Activity	Retarded Client exhibits decreased motor/cognitive activity.	Agitated Client exhibits psychomotor restlessness/agitation.
Mood changes	Unipolar Client exhibits one affective extreme, typically depression.	Bipolar Client exhibits cyclical affective extremes, typically mania alternating with depression.

Adapted from Murrary, R.B., and Huelskoepter, M.M. *Psychiatric/Mental Health Nursing: Giving emotional care.* Englewood Cliffs, NJ: Prentice-Hall, 1983

be described as euphoric and often has an infectious quality for the uninvolved observer. *Hypomania* is the term used to describe a pathological disturbance in mood which is similar to but not as severe as mania.

Persons with affective disorders variably experience feelings of extreme sadness, guilt, self-deprecatory thoughts or an elevated, expansive mood accompanied by inflated self-esteem, hyperactivity, overtalkativeness, and a perceived decreased need for sleep. These disturbances in mood may vary in intensity and duration and may occur alone, together, or in an alternating fashion.

CLASSIFICATION

A method of classification is necessary to understand affective disorders. Historically, attempts to do this have relied on the use of dichotomies to describe the etiology, symptoms, activity patterns, and mood changes associated with each disorder. This approach led to our understanding of affective disorders as: exogenous vs. endogenous, psychotic vs. neurotic, reactive vs. endogenous, retarded vs. agitated, mild vs. severe, unipolar vs. bipolar, and primary vs. secondary. Table 33-1 summarizes some of the terms used by various authors to describe affective disorders.

The *Diagnostic and Statistical Manual of Mental Disorders* (DSM-III, 1980) provides the most current and widely used classification system for affective disorders. Based on observed symptomatology, the DSM-III divides affective disorders into three main categories: major affective disorders, other specific affective disorders, and atypical affective disorders (see Table 33-2).

Major Affective Disorders

Major affective disorders include major depressive disorder and bipolar affective disorder. These disorders are distinguished by whether or not the

TABLE 33-2 DSM III Classification of Affective Disorders

Major affective disorders
  Major depression
  Bipolar affective disorder
Other specific affective disorders
  Cyclothymic disorder
  Dysthymic disorder
Atypical affective disorders
  Atypical depression
  Atypical bipolar disorder

client has experienced a manic episode. The client is diagnosed as having a major depression if he experiences only depressed episodes. If the client has had at least one manic episode with or without an episode of depression, then he is diagnosed as having a bipolar affective disorder (manic-depressive disorder). Clients diagnosed as having bipolar affective disorder are subclassified as manic if they are experiencing a manic episode; depressed if they are depressed, but have a history of at least one manic episode; or mixed if they display symptoms of mania and depression or marked lability of affect.

Other Specific Affective Disorders

Other specific affective disorders include cyclothymic disorder and dysthymic disorder. The symptoms of cyclothymic disorder are characteristic of both the depressive and manic syndromes, although they are not of sufficient severity and duration to meet the diagnostic criteria for major depressive or manic episodes. Similarly, the symptoms of dysthymic disorder are not of sufficient severity and duration to meet the criteria for a major depressive episode.

Atypical Affective Disorders

The residual category of atypical affective disorders includes atypical bipolar disorders and atypical depression. A client who displays manic features that are not severe enough or of sufficient duration to warrant a diagnosis of bipolar disorder or cyclothymic disorder would be diagnosed as having an atypical bipolar disorder. Likewise, an individual diagnosed as having an atypical depression displays depressive symptoms that are less severe than those seen in major depressive disorder or dysthymic disorder.

EPIDEMIOLOGY

Major Affective Disorders

Major Depressive Disorder. Studies indicate that the prevalence of major depression in industrialized countries is approximately 2.0 cases per 100 for men and between 2.0 and 9.3 cases per 100 for women. The incidence of major depression in men is about 82 per 100,000 per year and the incidence for women is between 247 and 7800 per 100,000 per year (Boyd and Weissman, 1982).

According to statistics reported in the DSM-III (1980), in the adult population of the United States, approximately 8 to 11 percent of the males and 18 to 23 percent of the females have at some time had a major depressive episode. It is estimated that 3 percent of the males and 6 percent of the females have experienced a major depression sufficiently severe to require hospitalization.

Depression has no apparent age limit. It can begin at any age, including infancy, and seems fairly evenly distributed throughout adult life. Although women appear to experience major depressions about twice as often as men, research studies indicate that there may be additional factors associated with major depressive disorder. Such factors include family experience, personality characteristics, and recent psychosocial stresses.

According to Orvaschel and colleagues (1980), hostile, chaotic, negative family environments are associated with an increased occurrence of depression in adults. Also, a family history that includes depression or alcohol dependence apparently predisposes family members to the development of depression. Certain personality characteristics have also been associated with depression. For example, individuals who are shy and somewhat passive have been found to experience depressive episodes more frequently than persons who are more assertive and self-assured. Recent psychosocial stresses may also predispose certain individuals to depression. Frequently these life events are associated with some form of loss. Death of a loved one, loss of one's job, retirement, dissolution of an affectional/intimate relationship, and financial difficulties may be contributing factors to the onset of depression.

Bipolar Affective Disorder. Approximately 1 in 10 clients diagnosed with a major affective disorder is bipolar. The incidence of affective bipolar disorder in the United States is about 9 to 15.2 new cases per 100,000 for men per year and about 7.4 to 32 new cases per 100,000 for women per year (Boyd and Weissman, 1982). According to the DSM-III (1980), it is estimated that between 0.4 and 1.2 percent of the adult population have had bipolar affective disorder.

Among the predisposing factors for bipolar disorder are age, social class, and family experience. The age of onset is around 30 years. The interval between manic and depressive episodes tends to decrease as the individual grows older while the length of each episode increases (Klerman and Barrett, 1973). Generally, individuals in the upper socioeconomic class who are highly creative and ambitious, and are high achievers and energetic are more at risk of developing bipolar disorder than those who do not fall into these categories (Krauthammer and Klerman, 1979). A family history of bipolar affective disorder is associated with an increased incidence of bipolar disorder in offspring (Nurnberger and Gershon, 1982). There is also evidence that bipolar affective disorder occurs more frequently among persons who are either single or divorced. However, it should be pointed out that because of the disruptive nature of bipolar illness, the disorder may actually be a contributing factor in divorce, rather than divorce being a precipitating factor in the disorder (Hagerty, 1984).

Other Specific Affective Disorders

According to the DSM-III (1980), both cyclothymic and dysthymic disorders usually begin early in adult life, although depressive episodes may begin in childhood or adolescence. Cyclothymic and dysthymic disorders are apparently more common in adult women while dysthymic disorder occurs with equal frequency for both genders in children. No information is currently available regarding predisposing factors for cyclothymic disorder. However, factors such as chronic physical disorders and psychosocial stressors have been linked to the occurrence of dysthymic disorder.

THEORIES OF ETIOLOGY

Psychodynamic Theory

In a classic paper, *Mourning and Melancholia*, Freud (1917) compared the conditions of mourning (grief) and melancholia (a major affective disorder). He described the cause of major depressions as a turning inward of angry, ambivalent feelings that are directed toward a lost love-object. In Freud's usage, the term "love-object" could refer to a tangible physical entity, such as a significant other person, or it could refer to an abstract idea such as freedom, liberty, or motherhood.

According to Freud, mourning is a normal process representing a temporary departure from a person's normal way of life while "working through" grief and resolving loss in a healthy manner. In contrast to mourning, melancholia is a pathological condition in which the individual responds to a loss with extreme feelings of dejection, apathy, and emptiness. The melancholic person experiences a decreased interest in the external world accompanied by an increased self-interest (narcissism). The hostile part of the individual's ambivalence for the lost love-object is experienced as anger which becomes self-directed and is internalized. Thus, the feature that is missing in mourning but usually present in melancholia is a loss of self-esteem.

Abraham (1927) described bipolar affective disorder when he compared normal grief with depression. Building upon Freud's psychosexual stages of psychological development, he maintained that adult depression was a reenactment of the strivings of the infantile loss during the oral phase. He believed that ungratified sexual desires stimulate feelings of hatred and hostility which diminish an individual's ability to give and receive love and affection. Thus, this repressed hostility results in emotional immaturity and predisposes the individual to feelings of emptiness and depression.

During World War II, Spitz and Wold (1946) studied the effects of maternal-infant separation and concluded that the infant behaviors they observed supported psychoanalytic theory. The infants' initial response to separation from their mothers was characterized by distress and weeping which were ultimately replaced by expressionless eyes and frozen, immobile faces. This syndrome was labeled *anaclitic depression* and manifested itself in despair, detachment, and failure to thrive.

Klein (1948) postulated that depression is a phase of development the child must resolve during the first year of life. An infant reacts to frustration with rage. When he becomes angry with his mother, he experiences fear that this anger will destroy the mother. Sadness, fear, and guilt result and eventually lead to a loss of self-esteem. According to Klein, children resolve these feelings when they feel assured of their mother's love. If that assurance never develops, there will always be a predisposition to feelings of sadness, helplessness, and guilt.

According to Bibring (1953), low self-esteem and helplessness are the vital elements of depression. He posits that depression is the result of residual needs that were not gratified during various stages of psychosocial development. These frustrated needs are reactivated later in life when the individual encounters a loss or lack of love and affection. The person feels helpless. Self-esteem is lost. Expectations and needs have not been met in the past and the person fears this will occur again. To avoid further loss or failure, the person isolates the self by adopting and defending depressive behaviors.

Sociological Theory

Currently, a number of social influences are thought to be contributing factors in the etiology of affective disorders. These social influences involve the interaction of a least two sets of variables: (1) stress factors, and (2) concomitant precipitating social factors. Recent literature indicates that this is particularly true for depressive disorders. Life stressors that tend to precipitate depressive episodes generally relate to a loss of something valuable, for example, divorce, death, or a threat to self-image. In general, the greater the number of stressors, the greater the likelihood of depression (Kerschner and Lancaster, 1984).

Marital stressors seem the most difficult for women, and job-related ones for men (Jacobsen, 1980). Unmarried women are at high risk for depression because of economic pressures, social isolation, and responsibilities for children. Poverty is the most difficult stressor. In fact, lower-class women are five times as likely to become depressed as middle-class women.

Social factors that appear to be of considerable influence in the etiology of affective disorders include familial environment and economic conditions. It is well known that early parenting behaviors contribute to a child's ability to develop an adequate level of self-esteem, personal belief system, and feelings of security and trust in others. Children who grow up in families that do not offer opportunities to develop these resources are at an increased risk of becoming depressed at some point later in their lives. Economic conditions can precipitate depression and feelings of inadequacy. The American life-style is often depicted as happy, carefree, and always smiling and purchasing things. However, many people are confronted with a variety of unpleasant and sometimes painful life stressors that dispute this image.

The role of women in our society also has implications for the development of affective disorders, especially depression. As mentioned previously, women are approximately twice as likely as men to become depressed. Despite numerous social forces to the contrary, women continue to

be stereotypically characterized as nurturant, caring, loving, and dependent. Many women are electing not to adhere to this image and are pursuing careers and more assertive, independent roles. The stress and ambivalence associated with these endeavors may contribute to depressive symptoms.

Biochemical Theory

Genetics. Data from studies of families, adopted persons, and twins indicate that approximately 20 percent of first-degree relatives of individuals with major affective disorders will exhibit symptoms of major depression or bipolar illness. Specifically, bipolar persons have been found to have both bipolar and unipolar first-degree relatives, although most exhibit symptoms consistent with bipolar illness. Unipolar persons typically show a high incidence of only unipolar depression in their family history. In spite of the limited number of cases available for study, the monozygotic twins of individuals with major affective disorders will demonstrate symptoms of major depression or bipolar illness at rates ranging from 33 to 92.6 percent (Allen, et al., 1974).

An additional association exists between major depressive disorder and alcoholism. There is a markedly higher prevalence of affective disorders and alcoholism among first-degree relatives of persons suffering from affective disorders than among the general population.

These data suggest that there is a predominance of affective illness in certain families. One explanation for this prevalence is that heredity determines the potential for affective disorders while biological and social forces influence onset and symptomatology.

Biogenic Amines. The biogenic amine hypothesis posits that there is a relationship between the occurrence of affective disorders and either excessive or insufficient availability of one or more neurotransmitter amines in the brain. In depression there is typically a deficit of one or more of the neurotransmitters, particularly norepinephrine (NE) and serotonin (5-HT). An imbalance of these transmitters has been associated with mania.

It is not possible to measure brain NE levels directly. However, a major metabolite of NE, 3-methoxy-4-hydroxyphenylglycol (MHPG), is excreted in urine and cerebrospinal fluid (CSF). MHPG is found in significantly lower levels in the urine of some depressed individuals. Clients with bipolar affective disorder tend to have the lowest 24-hour urinary MHPG excretion (Zis, 1982). Monitoring MHPG levels in CSF has not been found to yield reliable data related to affective disorders.

Tricyclic antidepressants, monoamine oxidase inhibitors (MAO inhibitors or MAOIs), and electroconvulsive therapy (ECT) have all been found to be effective in the medical management of affective disorders. These facts lend further credence to the biogenic amine hypothesis. The tricyclic antidepressants (such as phenelzine and tranylcypromine) interfere with the enzyme that assists in the breakdown of NE. ECT has been found to increase the level of brain NE. By restoring normal or near-normal levels of NE at brain receptor sites, these three medical treatments relieve the depressive symptoms associated with major affective disorders.

Electrolyte Metabolism. Electrolytes play an essential role in normal neurological functioning. They assist in the transmission, storage, and release of the key neurotransmitters associated with affective disorders. Depressed persons have been found to have a disturbance in the distribution of sodium and potassium across the cell membrane with an excess of sodium within the nerve cells. These electrolyte levels return to normal upon recovery (Frazier, 1977). It should be pointed out that lithium, a drug frequently used in the medical treatment of certain affective disorders, interferes with the cellular exchange of sodium and regulates the level according to whether the client is depressed or manic.

Neuroendocrine Abnormalities. Endocrine functioning has long been thought to play a role in depression and mania. Appetite, mood, sleep, libido, and autonomic activity are all functions that may be altered in clients experiencing affective disorders. These functions are regulated by the limbic system, which also regulates neuroendocrine activity. Abnormal levels of cortisol, human growth hormone (HGH), and thyroid-stimulating hormone (TSH) have all been documented in clients with major depressions.

Clients who are depressed have been found to exhibit an increased total cortisol secretion accompanied by a loss of their normal circadian pattern. Symptoms similar to depression are exhibited by clients with hypothyroidism. The available evidence suggests that clients with un-

ipolar (depressive) disorder are more susceptible to deficiencies of TSH than are clients with bipolar disorder (Gold, et al., 1979).

Controlled research investigations indicate that human growth hormone (HGH) responses to insulin-induced hypoglycemia are deficient in depressed clients (Carroll, 1978). Interestingly, the neurotransmitters norepinephrine (NE) and serotonin (5-HT) are thought to mediate the HGH response to hypoglycemia. It is therefore possible that affective disorders may be the result of disturbances in multiple biochemical networks. Thus, alterations in biogenic amines, hormones, and electrolytes may all be interrelated biogenic systems in the etiology of affective disorders.

☐ *Suicide*

Statistically, suicide ranks as the eleventh leading cause of death among the general population of the United States. These deaths, many of which are avoidable, result in inestimable loss in terms of the individual victim's life as well as the profound effects on survivor-victims (families and friends). These facts clearly indicate that suicide represents a major health problem in our society—however, the phenomenon of suicide continues to be fraught with mystery and is sometimes grossly misunderstood. The act of self-destruction continues to evoke many myths and misconceptions, some of which are compared with facts regarding suicide in Table 33-3.

Because of the intimate nature of the nurse-client relationship, the nurse is often the first member of the mental health team to become aware of a client's suicidal intent. This fact necessitates an intellectual awareness on the part of the nurse, if she is to provide meaningful care for the suicidal client. The following discussion consists of key terms regarding suicide and a description of the epidemiology of suicide in the United States, including a brief summary of social, demographic, and clinical variables thought to influence suicidal rates.

DEFINITIONS

Suicide is the taking of one's own life. It is considered destructive aggression directed inward. The term *suicide* is frequently used to describe an ideation, threat, potential gesture, attempt, or completed act. *Suicidal ideations* are thoughts about killing oneself. At various points in their

TABLE 33-3 Misconceptions and Facts About Suicide

Misconception	Fact
Women commit suicide more often than men.	Woman attempt suicide more frequently than men. However, men complete suicide more often than women.
Once a person is suicidal, he is always suicidal.	Suicidal behavior is time limited.
Suicide often occurs without warning.	Suicide attempts are generally preceded by a variety of physical, emotional, cognitive, and behavioral clues.
Suicide threats are merely a means of getting attention; they should not always be taken seriously.	All suicide threats should be interpreted as cries for help, which merit thorough risk assessment.
Suicide occurs more frequently among the rich (among the poor).	Suicide is not bound to any socioeconomic group.
Directly asking individuals about their suicidal thoughts and intentions will prompt suicide attempts.	The nurse must directly ask clients about suicide plans, in order to accurately assess the lethality of their intentions. Most suicidal clients experience relief that someone has acknowledged their distress.
Suicidal people are certain they want to die.	Suicidal people are ambivalent regarding their desire to live or die.
Employed, well-educated people with families do not attempt suicide.	Achievement of widely held criteria for success does not guarantee self-fulfillment or happiness. Suicide is related to a variety of social, demographic, and clinical variables.

lives, many people entertain thoughts of suicide. These ideations may never be verbally expressed or acted upon behaviorally. A *suicidal threat* is a verbal or behavioral indication from an individual that denotes suicidal intent. Not all suicide threats are acted upon, although the nurse must carefully assess the seriousness of any suicidal threat. *Suicide potential* is the degree of probability that an individual will attempt self-harm. A *suicidal gesture* is an apparent attempt by a person to cause self-injury without lethal conse-

quences and generally without actual intent to commit suicide. A suicidal gesture serves to attract attention to the person's disturbed emotional status, but is not as serious as a suicide attempt. A suicidal gesture is a cry for help and may be followed by a *suicide attempt*. An attempt occurs when individuals initiate behavior they believe will result in death. A suicide attempt is very serious as it involves risk to the person's health and life. *Completed suicide* results when individuals are successful in taking their own lives with conscious intent. *Suicidology* is the broad scientific study of the prevention and causes of suicide.

EPIDEMIOLOGY

Suicide accounts for more than 40,000 deaths per year in the United States. However, less than 30,000 suicides are reported annually. The remainder are classified and reported as accidental deaths, or even as deaths by natural causes. According to Miller (1982), suicide is the fourth leading cause of death for Americans under the age of 40, the third leading cause of death among adolescents, and the second leading cause of death among college students. In the United States, someone takes his life with conscious intent every 17½ minutes. Approximately 10 other Americans will attempt to end their lives in this same brief period of time.

Statistically, males are three times more likely to successfully commit suicide than females, although females attempt suicide more frequently than males at a rate of about 3 to 1. Men tend to use more lethal means to commit suicide, such as firearms or hanging. Women tend to attempt suicide by overdosing, poisoning, or cutting themselves.

Variables Influencing Suicide Rates

There are a number of social, demographic, and clinical variables that influence the occurrence of suicide.

Social Variables. High suicide rates are associated with industrialized, urban societies and areas that undergo extended periods of social unrest, internal governmental problems, and prolonged pessimism and apathy. Societies that value independence and have intense individual performance expectations, such as the United States, the Soviet Union, Japan, and Germany, also experience higher rates of suicide. High rates tend to occur in subcultural groups that are perceived as not caring about people as individuals, such as might be found in the complex inner-city, with its urban poor and homeless. Social roles, occupations, and professions that demand concern and nurturance for others, for example physicians, nurses, and police, are all associated with increased rates of suicide. American Indians also exhibit a very high rate of suicide.

In contrast, developing communities and groups that are family oriented and in which hope and optimism are high tend to experience lower rates of suicide. Cultures perceived as warm and nurturing (e.g., the Irish, Italians, and Norwegians) report lower suicide rates. Also, fewer suicides per capita occur in cultures that strongly disapprove of the act of suicide, such as the Italian, Spanish, and Irish cultures. The low suicide rates among Catholics and Jews are usually attributed to their cultural and religious emphasis on family.

Demographic Variables. The incidence of suicide is higher among single and married people without children, Protestant males, white people, adolescents, college students, and persons above the age of 40. It should be pointed out that the demographics of suicide are currently undergoing several dramatic changes. For example, suicide rates have increased 49 percent for white women and 80 percent for black women in the past 20 years (Kneisl and Wilson, 1984). This may be attributable to the many role transitions made by women during this period. Women have entered many new professional, occupational, and social positions. The stress encountered in these various new roles may be reflected, at least in part, by increasing suicide rates among women. Additionally, the current rate of suicide among young, urban black persons between the ages of 20 and 35 is twice that of white persons in the same age group.

Clinical Variables. Suicide rates tend to be higher among people who have attempted suicide before. In fact, of those individuals who attempt suicide, 12 percent will succeed in killing themselves within 2 years (Wenz, 1977). High rates of suicide are also associated with people who have physical illnesses resulting in alterations of body image or life-style. People who lost one or both parents early in life commit suicide more frequently than those who have not lost a parent. The loss or threat of loss of an individual's spouse,

job, money, or social position have also been identified as contributing factors to suicide. Such losses contribute to depression, and people who are depressed or are recovering from a depression are at much greater risk of committing suicide. People who abuse alcohol or drugs are also at risk of suicide, since these substances tend to impair one's insight and ability to control impulsive, self-destructive behavior.

The suicide rate in hospitals and institutions is much greater than that of the general population. In fact, hospitalized psychiatric clients have been found to be 30 times more likely to commit suicide than people in the general population (Farberow, 1981). Sixty-five percent of these suicides occur while clients are on pass or unauthorized absence. Thirty-five percent take place in the hospital. Psychotic clients are the most likely to kill themselves during hospitalization, while clients hospitalized for depression tend to be a greatest risk of committing suicide within the first several months following discharge. Suicide risk is the greatest among hospitalized clients during the first month of admission. Obviously, nurses should be aware of the potential for suicide among hospitalized and recently discharged clients.

☐ Medical Intervention

Medical interventions for clients experiencing affective disorders and/or suicidal ideations include both somatic therapies and individual and group psychotherapy. Somatic therapy consists of treating the body or *somea* of the client by a variety of biochemical or physical means. Common somatic therapies prescribed for clients who have affective disorders or who are suicidal include the administration of psychopharmaceuticals (antidepressant and antimanic medications) and electroconvulsive therapy (ECT). Obviously, both of these are medical interventions and can be initiated only by the physician. However, the nurse frequently has a functional role in the administration and evaluation of these therapeutic modalities. To ensure safety and maximum benefit to the client, the nurse must be cognizant of the indications, expected outcomes, potential side effects, and contraindications for these somatic therapies.

Traditionally, the practice of psychotherapy has fallen within the general domain of medical psychiatric practice. More recently, other members of the mental health team have assumed the role of psychotherapist. Among these is the clinical nurse specialist who holds specialized graduate-level academic credentials. Thus, individual and group psychotherapy are treatment modalities that may be initiated and administered by either a physician- or a nurse-therapist. Clearly, the nurse must have an understanding of the principles involved in psychotherapy, if she is to plan care that augments and supports the work accomplished by the client and psychotherapist.

PSYCHOPHARMACEUTICALS

Nurses often have a role in the administration of psychopharmaceutical agents. Currently, the medications of choice in treating clients with affective disorders include both the antidepressants (tricyclics, monoamine oxidase inhibitors, and tetracyclics) and the antimanics (lithium compounds). The nurse must be knowledgeable about each drug's actions, dosage, potential side effects, and contraindications. She must continually make astute observations in order to assess the drug's efficacy, monitor the client for the development of side effects, and participate in the education of the client and his family regarding the medication regimen.

Antidepressants

Antidepressants are used to treat major depressive disorders. This group of psychopharmaceuticals includes tricyclic antidepressants (TCAs), monoamine oxidase inhibitors (MAO inhibitors or MAOIs), and tetracyclic antidepressants. Table 33-4 provides a detailed list of each of these classifications of antidepressant medications, according to their generic and trade names, and summarizes their average adult daily dosages, interactions with other drugs, and the major side effects for each classification.

It should be stressed that the tricyclic compounds, the monoamine oxidase inhibitors, and the tetracyclic antidepressants provide relief for some of the symptoms related to depressive disorders. However, they do not treat the underlying causes of depression. Caution should be exercised to avoid using these drugs without a thorough assessment of causative factors involved in the client's depression.

Tricyclic Antidepressants (TCAs). TCAs were introduced in the United States in the late 1950s. Since that time, they have become the pharmacological treatment of choice for most

TABLE 33-4 Antidpressant Medications

Generic Name	Trade Names	Average Adult Daily Doses (mg)	Interaction with Other Drugs	Major Side Effects	
Tricyclic anti-depressants (TCAs)				Blood:	Agranulocytosis
Amltriptyline	Amavil Amitid Amitril Elavil Endep Rolavil	75–300	MAO inhibitors Thyroid Guanethidine	CNS:	Drowsiness, excitation, seizures, tremors, weakness, confusion, headache
				CV:	Orthostatic hypotension, tachycardia, EKG changes, hypertension, palpitations
Amoxapine	Asendin	50–300	MAO inhibitors	EENT:	Blurred vision, tinnitus, mydriasis, photosensitivity
Desipramine hydrochloride	Norpramin Pertofrane		MAO inhibitors CNS depressants Thiazide diuretics	GI:	Dry mouth, constipation, nausea, vomiting, anorexia, paralytic ileus, stomatitis, diarrhea
Doxepin hydrochloride	Adapin Sinequan	75–150	MAO inhibitors Thyroid Guanethidine	GU:	Urinary retention
				Skin:	Rash, urticaria, petechiae
				Other:	Sweating, weight gain, craving for sweets, allergy, edema
Imipramine hydrochloride	Antipress Imavate Janimine Presamine Ropramine SK-Promine Tofranil W.D.D.	75–300	MAO inhibitors Alcohol Barbiturates	Abrupt cessation after long-term therapy: Nausea, headache, malaise (does not indicate addiction)	

TABLE 33·4 *(continued)*

Generic Name	Trade Names	Average Adult Daily Doses (mg)	Interaction with Other Drugs	Major Side Effects	
Nortriptyline hydrochloride	Aventyl Pamelor	20–75	MAO inhibitors Vasodilators Anticholingergic agents		
Protriptyline hydrochloride	Vivactil	15–60	MAO inhibitors Thyroid Guanethidine		
Trimipramine	Surmontil	75–200	MAO inhibitors		
Monoamine oxidase inhibitors (MAO inhibitors, or MAOIs)				CNS:	Dizziness, vertigo, weakness, headache, overactivity, hyperreflexia, tremors, muscle twitching, mania, insomnia, confusion, memory impairment, fatigue
Isocarboxazid	Marplan	10–50	Other MAO inhibitors Other antidepressants	CV:	Orthostatic hypotension, arrhythmias, paradoxic hypertension
Nialamide	Niamid	75–100	Amphetamines Alcohol Barbiturates Morphinelike analgesics Cocaine Procaine Ether	EENT: GI: GU: Skin: Other:	Blurred vision Dry mouth, anorexia, nausea, diarrhea, constipation, abdominal pain Altered libido Rash Peripheral edema, sweating, weight changes
Phenelzine	Nardil	15–75	Phenothiazine compounds Methyldopa Dopamine Tryptophan Antihypertensives Antiparkinsonian drugs Insulin		
Tranylcypromine sulfate	Parnate	10–40	Thiazide diuretics Sympathomimetic amines— phenylephrine		
Tetracyclic antidepressants				Blood:	Agranulocytosis
Maprotiline hydrochloride	Ludiomil	75–300	MAO inhibitors	CNS:	Drowsiness, excitation, seizures, tremors, weakness, confusion, headache
				CV:	Orthostatic hypotension, tachycardia, EKG changes, hypertension
				EENT:	Blurred vision, tinnitus, mydriasis
				GI:	Dry mouth, constipation, nausea, vomiting, anorexia, paralytic ileus
				GU:	Urinary retention
				Skin:	Rash, urticaria
				Other:	Sweating, weight gain, craving for sweets, allergy
				Abrupt cessation after long-term therapy:	Nausea, headache, malaise (does not indicate addiction)

types of depression. Because of their effectiveness and relative lack of side effects, TCAs have completely replaced amphetamines and other psychomotor stimulants for the treatment of depression.

Tricyclic antidepressants are thought to increase the synaptic concentration of norepinephrine or serotonin, or both, in the central nervous system by blocking their reuptake by the presynaptic neurons. This action allows these neurotransmitters to accumulate, resulting in an antidepressant effect. TCAs produce sedative effects within a few hours following oral administration. Antidepressant effects occur 7 to 10 days after therapy is commenced. This delay is due to TCAs slow effect on the brain's neurotransmitter metabolism.

Because of the delayed effect of most of the TCAs in relieving suicidal ideations, the severely depressed client may be at greater risk of attempting suicide during the initial phase of drug therapy. The client may also be at risk of attempting suicide as TCAs begin to take effect and energy levels increase. Therefore, the nurse must be alert to the possibility of an impulsive ingestion of these substances. The physician should be reminded not to dispense large quantities of TCAs to the client for self-administration at home. Most authorities feel that these drugs should be used only in a closely supervised psychiatric hospital setting, for clients who are severely depressed and have serious suicidal tendencies.

The tricyclic compounds are often administered in a single evening dose at the hour of sleep to minimize their daytime side effects (e.g., sedation, anticholinergic effects) and may be beneficial for clients experiencing disturbances of sleep. It is important to note that TCAs should not be administered concomitantly with the monoamine oxidase inhibitors. The interaction between TCAs and MAO inhibitors sometimes results in severe excitation, hyperpyrexia, and/or convulsions.

Monoamine Oxidase Inhibitors (MAO Inhibitors, or MAOIs). MAO inhibitors are generally not used until two TCAs have been tried unsuccessfully, because they can cause more serious side effects than the TCAs. MAO inhibitors have been found to be effective in clients who are unresponsive to other antidepressant therapy for severe depression.

MAO inhibitors block the activity of the enzyme monoamine oxidase (MAO), which is involved in the metabolism of catecholamine neurotransmitters, such as epinephrine, norepinephrine, dopamine, and serotonin. The reduced MAO activity results in an increased concentration of these neurotransmitters in the central nervous system—a buildup that is thought to be responsible for the antidepressant action of MAO inhibitors.

Of the MAO inhibitors, isocarboxazid (Marplan) and phenelzine (Nardil) have a very slow onset of action, which may not occur for several weeks or months, and their effects may continue for up to 3 weeks after therapy has been discontinued. Tranylcypromine (Parnate) has a more rapid onset of action (usually several days), and MAO activity is restored 3 to 5 days after the drug is discontinued. The risk of suicide and precautions regarding continued administration and abrupt discontinuance of these drugs are the same as those for the tricyclic antidepressants.

A wide variety of side effects have been noted to occur following the administration of MAO inhibitors. This has been cause for concern among most authorities, since they have resulted in severe medical conditions and/or death (see Table 33-4).

The existence of hypertension is a contraindication for the use of MAO inhibitors, since paradoxic hypertension has been reported during treatment with these drugs. As a result of paradoxic hypertension, clients have been known to experience intracranial bleeding, sometimes accompanied by a severe occipital headache that may radiate frontally. Other symptoms that accompany this condition include stiffness or soreness of the neck, nausea, vomiting, diaphoresis, dilated pupils, photophobia, constricting chest pain, and tachycardia, bradycardia, or other arrhythmias. If any of these symtoms occur, the drug should be discontinued immediately.

Hypertensive crises have occurred as a result of the ingestion of certain foods and beverages by clients receiving MAO inhibitors. These offending foods are rich in amines (such as tyramine) or in amino acids (such as tyrosine) that may be decarboxylated in the body to form pressor amines normally inactivated by monoamine oxidase. Foods and beverages known to contain these amines are cheese (especially strong or aged varieties), bananas, avocados, beer, and Chianti wine. Drugs containing pressor agents (certain cold remedies, hay fever preparations, or anorexiants) should also be avoided. The nurse should provide continued reassurance, support, and reinforcement of these dietary and drug restrictions.

Tetracyclic Antidepressants. Tetracyclics are the most recent class of antidepressants to come on the market. Like TCAs, the tetracyclic antidepressants are thought to function by increasing the amount of norepinephrine and/or serotonin in the central nervous system, thus allowing these neurotransmitters to accumulate. The sedative and antidepressant effects of tetracyclic antidepressants are similar in onset and duration to the tricyclic antidepressants.

Antimanics

Antimanics are used to treat bipolar affective disorders (manic-depressive illness). This group of psychopharmaceuticals includes lithium carbonate and lithium citrate. The generic and trace names of these medications and a summary of their average adult daily dosages, interactions with other drugs, and their major side effects appear in Table 33-5.

Lithium Carbonate and Lithium Citrate. Lithium salts have been used in the United States since 1970 to combat bipolar affective disorders. Under proper supervision, lithium may prevent up to 80 percent of manic and depressive episodes. Episodes that do occur during lithium therapy are usually less severe and of shorter duration than those that might occur without such therapy.

The exact mechanism of action of lithium is not known. However, it is thought that lithium may alter certain chemical transmitters (NE) in the central nervous system, possibly affecting the exchange of sodium in brain cells. Lithium does not impair intellectual functioning, consciousness, or the range or quality of emotional life. It does effectively help clients to fully experience joy, sadness, tenderness, and sexual desire. Seven to 10 days are required for the drug to take effect after initiation of therapy.

Lithium's toxic level is very close to its therapeutic level. Consistent daily dietary sodium and

---

TABLE 33-5 Antimania Medications

Generic Name	Trade Names	Average Adult Daily Doses (mg)	Interactions with Other Drugs	Major Side Effects	
Lithium carbonate	Eskalith Lithane Lithobid Lithonate Lithotabs	600–1800	Diuretics Haloperidol Aminophylline Sodium bicarbonate Sodium chloride Probenecid	Blood:	Leukocytosis of 14,000 to 18,000 (reversible)
				CNS:	Tremors, drowsiness, headache, confusion, restlessness, dizziness, psychomotor retardation, stupor, lethargy, coma, blackouts, epileptiform seizures, EEG changes, impaired speech, ataxia, muscle weakness, incoordination, hyperexcitability
Lithium citrate	Lithonate-S	600–1800	Methyldopa		
				CV:	EKG changes (reversible), arrhythmias, hypotension, peripheral circulatory collapse, allergic vasculitis, ankle and wrist edema
				EENT:	Tinnitus, impaired vision
				GI:	Nausea, vomiting, anorexia, diarrhea, fecal incontinence, dry mouth, thirst, metallic taste
				GU:	Polyuria, glycosuria, incontinence, renal toxicity
				Metabolic:	Transient hyperglycemia, goiter, hypothyroidism (lowered T_3, T_4, and PBI, but elevated ^{131}I uptake), hyponatremia
				Skin:	Pruritus, rash, diminished or lost sensation, drying and thinning of hair

fluid intake is necessary to help prevent toxicity. Initially, lithium serum levels should be monitored weekly and monthly during maintenance therapy. Blood samples should be drawn 8 to 12 hours after the last dose. The level of serum lithium concentration should be maintained between 1 and 1.5 mEq per liter for acute symptoms and 0.6 to 1.2 mEq per liter after the acute attack subsides. This usually requires a dosage of 300 to 600 mg p.o. three times daily. If serum levels of lithium exceed 1.5 mEq per liter, the drug should be discontinued for 24 hours and then resumed at a lower dose.

Lithium toxicity may occur if serum levels of the drug are allowed to continue in excess of 1.5 mEq per liter. Signs and symptoms that might accompany lithium toxicity include nausea, vomiting, abdominal cramps, diarrhea, thirst, and polyuria. Promptly discontinuing the drug will reverse these toxic symptoms.

The client and members of his family should be warned to discontinue lithium therapy if signs of toxicity occur, and to notify the physician immediately. Because toxicity of lithium is increased when sodium intake is restricted, the client should maintain a normal diet and normal salt and water intake. He should be cautioned about driving a car or operating heavy equipment, since lithium may impair mental and physical activity.

Lithium is contraindicated during pregnancy since there exists a suspected relationship between lithium and congenital birth defects. This drug is also contraindicated in clients with cardiovascular or renal disease and in those with brain damage.

ELECTROCONVULSIVE THERAPY (ECT)

Electroconvulsive therapy (ECT) is a somatic treatment, in which a grand-mal seizure is artificially induced by briefly passing a low-voltage electrical current through the brain. Convulsive therapy began in 1927 with the use of Metrazol given intravenously to produce a seizure. This procedure, although somewhat effective, proved hazardous. Cerletti and Bini first used electrodes to induce convulsions in 1937 (Freedman, et al., 1975).

There has been much controversy concerning the use of ECT, which one time was widely used in the treatment of all psychotic disorders. More recently, the use of ECT has become limited almost entirely to those experiencing severe depres-

sions. It is also used to treat clients who have a poor response to psychopharmaceutical agents, or when clients are unable to take certain medications because of poor health, allergies, or severe side effects.

There are a number of symptoms that generally can be interpreted as predictors of a good response to ECT. They include: feelings of worthlessness, helplessness, and hopelessness; anorexia with recent weight loss; constipation; reduced libido; early morning awakening; and suicidal inclinations.

Clients are generally given a series of an average of 6 to 10 treatments. Many clients respond positively after 6 to 8 treatments given on alternating days, at a rate of three per week. Numerous theories have been proposed to account for this observed effectiveness, but none have been completely borne out by scientific research.

Prior to treatment with ECT, informed consent must be obtained from the client and a thorough physical examination must be done. This includes a complete blood count, urinalysis, electrocardiogram, and (in some agencies) x-ray films of the chest and lateral aspects of the spine. Clients should have an empty stomach and are generally not allowed to take anything orally (NPO) before treatment. They should be instructed to empty the bladder and assisted in removing hairpins and dentures (if any). The client should be dressed in loose-fitting clothing. Atropine sulfate may be given to decrease secretions and to interrupt the vagal stimulation effects of ECT. The nurse must give supportive care and verbal reassurance before and after the treatment to allay anxiety.

Once in the treatment room, the client lies in a supine position on a stretcher. A short-acting barbiturate, such as sodium pentothal or Brevital, and a muscle relaxant, usually succinylcholine (Anectine) are given intravenously in separate syringes. These medications reduce the severity of the muscular reaction. The client is preoxygenated with 95 to 100 percent oxygen and the chin is supported to ensure a more patent airway during the treatment. Following administration of the anesthestic, the electrodes are attached to the temporofrontal region of the scalp, the muscle relaxant is injected, and, just as paralysis is observed, the electrical stimulus is given.

The treatment consists of applying 70 to 130 volts of alternating current for 0.1 to 0.5 second. A convulsion occurs that is characterized by a tonic phase (facial twitching and curling of the toes) lasting approximately 10 seconds, and a clonic phase (slight tremor) of 30 to 40 seconds. These movements are so slight that they are sometimes almost imperceptible. If no movement at all is observed, the electrical stimulus is repeated. Subconvulsive treatments are ineffective.

During the paralysis and after the treatment, clients require artificial respiratory support. Oxygen is administered, and the client should be suctioned as necessary. His head should be turned to the side to prevent aspiration of saliva. The client usually sleeps for a short time following ECT. During this 15- to 30-minute period, pulse, respirations, and blood pressure are monitored until the client is conscious and breathing regularly.

Most clients become conscious in a few minutes, but may be extremely confused and lightheaded for an hour following ECT. Thus, they require very careful nursing supervision. The client should remain lying down for a least half an hour. During this time, it is important to provide reassurance and orientation to environmental surroundings. Close observation of the client is necessary both before and after return to the inpatient unit. Clients treated on an outpatient basis should be accompanied home and not left unattended.

One complication of ECT is memory impairment. Although this is generally experienced as a temporary problem of short duration, it often causes concern for many clients. Unilateral ECT has been shown to decrease memory impairment and confusion, but has not been found to be as effective as bilateral ECT. The nurse must be sensitive to the client's anxiety regarding any temporary memory loss and be supportive and reassuring during this time.

Clients who are known to have brain tumors or aneurysms should not receive ECT. An increase in intracranial pressure usually occurs during the convulsion induced by ECT. This can lead to brainstem herniation, causing death in a client with a preexisting elevation in intracranial pressure. This treatment can be used cautiously with clients who have cardiovascular disease (even recent myocardial infarctions), peptic ulcers, and glaucoma.

INDIVIDUAL AND GROUP PSYCHOTHERAPY

Individual and group psychotherapy alone has not been found to be particularly effective with severely depressed and manic clients. This is not surprising in view of the almost total lack of responsivity of depressed individuals and the exalted mood and pressure of activity experienced by manic persons. However, individual and group psychotherapy combined with psychopharmaceutical therapy seems to be useful in many cases.

Group psychotherapy is one means by which persons with affective disorders can gain new perspectives on themselves and others. Groups can range widely, from supportive types to analytic types. For constructive change to occur in any type of group, the nurse therapist must convey her belief in the unique human potential of each person in the group. To accomplish this objective, the nurse should try to gain an understanding of the client's personal situation, be sensitive to both verbal and nonverbal communication, and facilitate individual growth. The nurse understands that growth is facilitated by thoughtful interactions that foster independence and self-esteem.

☐ Nursing Process

Nurses may encounter clients experiencing affective disorders and/or suicidal ideation in virtually any setting. For example, nurses can observe and assess clients for symptoms of depression, mania and suicidal ideation in outpatient clinics, general medical/surgical units, the emergency department, inpatient psychiatric units, or during home visits in the community. Regardless of the setting in which these clients are encountered, the nurse engages in the orderly and systematic processes of assessment, problem identification (diagnosis), intervention, and evaluation.

ASSESSMENT ☐ The primary purpose of assessment is to collect data related to the client's mental health, in order to formulate a list of nursing care problems (nursing diagnoses). The nurse obtains data by: (1) observing and interacting with the client; (2) observing and interacting with the client's family and/or significant others, both with and without the client; and (3) interacting with other sources, such as community groups or agencies (Swanson, 1982).

For purposes of clarity, this section is organized to describe the symptomatology associated with major disorders (major depression and bipolar affective disorder) in terms of the symptoms of depression, mania, and suicide. Two major areas will be addressed: (1) client, family, and environmental assessment (including the physical, emotional, cognitive, and behavioral manifestations of depression, mania, and suicide) followed by (2) the nurse's self-assessment.

Client, Family, and Environmental Assessment □

Depression. Depressive symptoms tend to have an insidious onset. Frequently the client himself may be totally unaware of subtle changes in his own behavior and does not realize that something is wrong. Rather, it may be family members, friends, or coworkers who recognize and become concerned about changes in the client's mood and behavior. Thus, it is often significant others who confront clients about their behavior, instead of clients volunteering that they feel depressed.

Physical Manifestations. The physical or vegetative symptoms of depression include sleep disturbances and fatigue. Sleep disturbances usually take the form of both initial and middle insomnia and early morning awakening. Occasionally, a depressed client may complain of increased or too much sleep (hypersomnia). Regardless of how much sleep they get, people who are depressed never feel completely rested and often complain that they feel "exhausted" or "drained of energy."

Inquiring about the client's current sleep patterns is a safe, nonthreatening way for the nurse to begin assessing for suspected affective disorders. The nurse can obtain data regarding a client's sleeping patterns by asking questions such as:

Do you experience difficulty falling asleep at night?

Do you wake up during the night? If so, how often?

Are you able to go back to sleep?

What time do you wake up in the morning?

Do you feel rested upon waking up in the morning?

Among the earliest signs of depression is a decline in appetitive functions. Anorexia accompanied by weight loss (sometimes as much as 40 pounds in a few months) is reported by 75 percent of depressed clients (Hagerty, 1984). Depressed persons often experience a loss of interest in sexual activity (decreased libido). The nurse should inquire about any recent loss of appetite, weight loss, or decline in sexual desire or functioning.

Other physical manifestations of depression include: preoccupation with bodily functions or hypochondriasis, blurred vision, parasthesia, indigestion, nausea, vomiting, constipation or diarrhea, and menstrual irregularities.

Emotional Manifestations. Typically, depressed clients experience a diurnal variation in mood. Specifically, most of these clients feel most depressed upon waking in the morning and gradually less depressed as the day goes on. Depressed clients use words like "blue, sad, low, hopeless," and "helpless" to describe their feelings. They often report feelings of apathy, boredom, loneliness, emptiness, desperation, and profound unhappiness. These feelings permeate the depressed person's existence and are evident in the individual's blunted or flattened affect and decreased motivation. This depressive permeation accounts for these clients often reporting a diminished sense of pleasure in activities they formerly found enjoyable. For example, a client may volunteer that he no longer enjoys painting nor has the energy and patience for it anymore.

People who are depressed frequently have distorted perceptions of themselves and their environment. Their overall outlook is characterized by extreme pessimism and negativism. Depressed clients often express feelings of guilt, self-reproach, and self-criticism by reporting that they feel unattractive or worthless. Self-depreciating feelings are sometimes manifested by way of egocentric notions of causality. For example, the client may express feeling responsible for world hunger or some other crisis situation.

The egocentrism experienced by depressed individuals may also be manifest as preoccupations with bodily functions and self-image. They may worry and ruminate about past and present events, showing no apparent interest in or concern for the future. Depressed clients sometimes experience a sense of depersonalization, that is, they may feel set apart or different from others and estranged from their environment.

Cognitive Manifestations. Depressed persons experience distortions in cognitive processes as well as thought content. Such cognitive distortions include diminished quality and quantity of thoughts, difficulty concentrating, and memory impairment. The client may have suicidal or, less often, homicidal ideations. These may simply be passing thoughts or they may involve intricately detailed plans. Nurses should carefully assess clients' potential for self-destructive or otherwise violent behavior, by asking specific questions regarding the seriousness of their intent.

Depressed clients rarely experience hallucinations (false sensory perceptions). However, when hallucinations do occur, they usually take the form of voices telling them that they are bad, disgusting, or unworthy of life.

More commonly, severely depressed clients experience delusions (fixed false beliefs), frequently of a nihilistic nature. Nihilistic delusions are beliefs that the client lives in a shadow or limbo world, or that he is dead and that only his spirit really exists. Somatic delusions tend to be hypochondriacal in nature and involve false notions or beliefs concerning body image or body function. A client may report, for example, that he believes his heart is rotten or that he has some terminal illness.

Behavioral Manifestations. Pathognomonic expressions of depression include a sad expression, disheveled appearance, poor eye contact, stooped posture, slow speech, and either agitated or retarded motor behavior. Retarded behavior refers to the depressed client's slowed responses and movements. There is an overall lack of spontaneity and purposeful behavior is diminished. In the early phase of a depressive episode, clients may try to mask their despondency behind a cheerful facade. The client's sad feelings will become apparent, however, if the nurse is sensitive and uses a careful approach in inquiring as to his true feelings. This may require some measure of time, since it necessitates the development of a trust rapport between client and the nurse.

Depressed persons engage in isolating and withdrawn behavior. Their social relationships tend to be impoverished because they feel unworthy of friendship, love, and affection. They don't have enough energy to invest in others to establish meaningful relationships. Coupled with the tendency to withdraw in social situations is an increased desire for dependency. This need for dependency can be so pronounced that severely depressed clients may require assistance in performing the simplest activities of daily living, such as eating and bathing.

Mania. Manic symptoms are usually more pronounced and develop more rapidly than depressive symptoms. Manic individuals are unaware of the inappropriateness of their behavior and often make statements like: "I never felt better in my life!" Manic clients typically display symptoms of pressured speech, sleep disturbances (usually an inability to sleep well), and/or dangerous or grandiose behavior. They may present a bizarre or eccentric appearance by dressing flamboyantly, or using dramatic cosmetic applications. The nurse generally observes this behavior in a clinical setting after significant others or the police bring the manic client to the nurse's attention.

Physical Manifestations. Manic clients generally present a somewhat deteriorated, often eccentric physical appearance. Often they display an increased amount of energy and make statements to the effect that they feel "charged up." Manic episodes are frequently accompanied by an increase in sexual interest and activity, which may be extreme (hypersexuality). Sleep disturbances occur for manic individuals just as they do for depressed persons. Manic clients tend to report that they simply don't feel a need to sleep. Thus, manic individuals generally experience decreased sleep (hyposomnia) which contributes to their overall deteriorated appearance.

Again, as with the person suspected of being depressed, the nurse should inquire about sexual, sleep/rest, and activity patterns. It should be pointed out that manic individuals often deny that anything is different about their recent behavior. In this instance, the nurse must rely upon information obtained from significant others, such as the client's family members and friends. Objective assessment data obtained from persons who have known the client well and for an extended period of time can prove valuable in determining whether or not an individual is experiencing a manic episode.

Emotional Manifestations. Manic clients experience lability of mood that can be quite extreme. Generally they feel happy, carefree, and euphoric, although these moods can quickly change to feelings of irritability and hostility. Like depressed persons, manic individuals may also experience perceptual distortions. However, instead of feeling worthless, they experience feelings of grandiosity and an inflated sense of self-esteem, which is disproportionate to reality.

Cognitive Manifestations. Manic clients typically have difficulty concentrating, are easily distractible, and exhibit flights of ideas. They frequently experience delusions of grandeur. Like depressed individuals, manic persons rarely experience hallucinations; those that do occur generally tend to be of a sexual or religious nature.

Clients are generally not suicidal during a manic episode, but may have severely impaired judgment. Their expansive mood and feelings of grandiosity may result in an unrealistic appraisal of their personal abilities and power. For instance, a woman believing that she has supernatural powers may attempt to demonstrate her endurance by placing her hand into an open flame. Obviously, nurses should exercise extreme caution and provide a safe, protected environment for such severely impaired clients.

Behavioral Manifestations. Behavioral manifestations of mania include extreme lability of mood, pressured speech, hyperactivity, impulsiveness, increased social contacts, and hypersexuality. The manic client is often overly verbose. Speech is pressured and frequently accompanied by rhyming and punning. When the client is crossed, his otherwise cheerful and festive mood can quickly change to anger and hostility. Manic individuals have particularly poor impulse control. Their behavior is often uninhibited, reckless, and sometimes embarassing to those around them. Manic clients tend to be quite gregarious and often have increased numbers of social contacts. Their appearance is typically bizarre and eccentric. Women may wear excessive amounts of makeup and may dress provocatively. Interest in sexual activity is markedly increased.

Suicide. Seriously despondent individuals may express thoughts of committing suicide. The nurse must, therefore, be prepared to carry out a thorough suicide risk assessment. Specifically, this involves exploring, with clients, their suicide plans, methods, past suicide attempts, and the availability of means to carry out any self-destructive intent. This necessitates directly asking clients about their suicidal thoughts and intentions. In spite of misconceptions to the contrary, such inquiries do not prompt suicide attempts. In fact, most clients will express relief that someone has acknowledged their distress.

Physical Manifestations. There is a strong relationship between a diagnosis of depression and suicide. Nearly 75 percent of people who are successful in committing suicide had visited their physicians with a somatic complaint within 4 months prior to their deaths (Reubin, 1979). These complaints were often vague and nonspecific in nature. Headaches, chest pain, insomnia,

anorexia, gastrointestinal upsets, backache, loss of sexual drive, and general malaise are common examples of such somatic complaints. Many of these symptoms are the same as those associated with depression which further illustrates the close relationship between depression and suicide. Quite often, clients who present with such vague maladies are seen as "hypochondriacs" by physicians and nurses. Consequently no assessment is carried out regarding the client's emotional state, life stresses, or past and present coping patterns. It is important that nurses use a holistic approach when assessing such physical symptoms as anorexia and insomnia, which are quite often an expression of the emotional turmoil experienced by depressed and possibly suicidal clients. Clients may perceive physical symptoms as the most acceptable means by which they can get help in the health care system. Such symptomatology actually represents a cry for help and should be interpreted as such. Nurses in physicians' offices, clinics, hospitals, and community settings are in excellent positions to carefully assess the true nature of somatic complaints that may represent physical manifestations of depression and potential suicide.

Emotional Manifestations. The feeling most frequently reported by suicidal individuals is depression. Clients who express feelings of worthlessness, helplessness, hopelessness, and other feelings associated with depressive states are at an increased risk for suicide. Depressed persons see suicide as a means of escaping from anxiety-provoking and intensely frightening situations.

Suicidal persons experience profound ambivalence, anxiety, and fear. Their ambivalence revolves around both wanting to die (thus escaping an existence perceived as intolerable) and wanting to live. They are anxious about their inner torment and the plans they are making to resolve it. They are frightened by their overwhelming anxiety, isolation, hopelessness, and helplessness.

Clients considering suicide may also experience feelings of excessive guilt, self-blame, and frustration. Suicidal clients often experience severe anger. Their anger may be inwardly directed, "I'm worthless . . . I should be dead," or it may be outwardly directed, "I'll show them . . . they'll be sorry when I'm dead." Conversely, many suicidal individuals experience a sense of inner calm and tranquility. This emotional calmness may occur just prior to a suicide attempt, since it usually indicates that the individual has made a conscious decision to take his own life. Thus, the person may actually be experiencing a sense of relief from the inner conflict and psychogenic pain that accompanies depression and thoughts of suicide.

Nurses should be alert to sudden changes in mood and discuss these changes with the client. The client who seems to have suddenly recovered from a depressive episode may, in fact, have made the decision to kill himself. The nurse who observes such a mood change might ask the client, "Recently you've been so depressed and upset. Now you seem so cheerful and relaxed. Can you tell me what accounts for this sudden change?"

Cognitive Manifestations. As clients become more severely depressed, they may become preoccupied with thoughts of self-harm. These thoughts may range from considerations of self-mutilation with minimum actual suicide intent to meticulously thought-out plans to commit suicide. Often, depressed clients express suicidal ideation in terms of desperately wanting to die, but don't have a specific plan of action by which they intend to accomplish this.

The depressed client may view suicide as a way out of a life situation perceived as untenable. Insight and judgment are impaired. Suicidal clients often exhibit thought processes characterized by dichotomous thinking and semantic fallacies. For example, a client may make statements such as: "If I can't succeed in law school, then I can't do anything"; or, "If things don't improve, I'll kill myself." The first statement creates a dichotomous or double-bind situation for the client. Thus, the client doesn't cope with stress by considering alternatives or by engaging in constructive problem solving. The choice becomes success in law school or death. The second statement contains vague generalities that are open to semantic questioning. Words like "things" and "improve" are ambiguous and should lead the nurse to ask questions such as: "If what things don't improve?" and, "What kind of improvement do you mean?" When nurses hear this kind of statement, they should assist clients in identifying dichotomous thinking and constructive alternatives to suicide.

Behavioral Manifestations. Clients may exhibit a variety of verbal and nonverbal behaviors that nurses should associate with possible suicidal intent. For example, a previously depressed client whose behavior suddenly becomes remarkably improved and animated may actually be giving a signal that he has decided to commit suicide.

Clients considering suicide may also exhibit behaviors indicating that they are putting their final affairs in order (e.g., writing a will, buying a casket, or giving away personal possessions having some sentimental value). Suicidal intent my be indicated by certain types of statements taking the form of coded, indirect, direct, or written communication. For instance, the statement, "You don't have to worry about me; I won't be around much longer," is a coded communication which the nurse should associate with suicidal ideation. Indirect communications that the nurse should be concerned about are exemplified by statements such as, "Farewell." "I just can't go on any more." More direct communication of suicidal ideation might be as blatant as the client simply stating, "I'm going to kill myself." Written communication of suicidal intent may take the form of an actual suicide note. A thorough suicide risk assessment should be conducted whenever these types of behaviors and statements are observed.

Clients who are suspected of entertaining thoughts of suicide should be asked, "Have you been thinking of harming or killing yourself?" If the client responds affirmatively, the nurse should proceed with a thorough assessment of the specificity and lethality of the client's plan. The nurse should ask, "What are you thinking of doing to yourself?" A detailed plan that is very specific and organized, suggests an increased potential for suicide, as does a suicide plan that incorporates a highly lethal method. Individuals who attempt suicide by hanging, jumping, or with firearms have a higher rate of success than persons who overdose or lacerate their wrists.

The availability of suicidal means and any history of past suicide attempts should also be assessed. For example, the nurse may say, "You've indicated that you intend to shoot yourself. Do you own a gun?" A client who has previously attempted suicide by means of a highly lethal method of self-harm has an increased chance of eventually committing suicide. The nurse should thoroughly discuss any past history of suicide attempts with the client. "You said you attempted a drug overdose on four separate occasions in your life and that two of these took place within the last three months. Are you thinking of trying this again?" Frequent past attempts and more recent attempts indicate a greater current potential for suicide.

Clients who are taking antidepressant medications are at particular risk of attempting suicide. As therapeutic levels of these drugs are established and maintained in the bloodstream, outward behavior and energy levels improve. However, feelings of isolation, hopelessness, and helplessness still predominate and contribute to suicidal ideations. As the client's depressive symptoms begin to lift, he regains the energy to carry out his suicidal plan. Thus, clients receiving antidepressant drug therapy must be carefully and continually assessed for potentially suicidal behavior.

The strong association between alcohol abuse and suicide has long been recognized. This is especially true of depressed individuals, who tend to use alcohol in an attempt to cope with their inner turmoil and have a high rate of suicide. Alcohol acts as a depressant on the central nervous system—it not only impairs the senses, insight, and judgment, but masks inhibitions to impulsive behavior. The client who has a history of using alcohol to cope with stress is at an increased risk of attempting suicide. The client who is intoxicated has a high risk of immediately attempting suicide. It is therefore important to make a thorough assessment of the client's current and past patterns of alcohol intake when attempting to ascertain his potential for suicide.

Nurse's Self-Assessment □ The nurse must be cognizant of her own feelings and values that can influence interaction with individuals experiencing affective disorders and potentially suicidal persons. This is not an altogether easy objective to accomplish, particularly for the neophyte. However, when interacting with these clients, awareness of the origins and nature of one's feelings is of paramount importance to therapeutic intervention. Self-awareness results when the nurse engages in both self- and peer assessment.

The depressive and manic behaviors that are characteristic of affective disorders tend to have an infectious quality. These clients' voices, bodily postures, and movements all communicate subtle cues, reflecting their inner mood of depression or mania. These subtle expressions of mood often remain below the nurse's level of cognitive awareness, and she therefore sometimes perceives these feelings as originating within the self, rather than in the client. For example, it is not at all unusual for the nurse to experience feelings of sadness, frustration, and helplessness when interacting with a depressed client. Similarly, she might feel happy, cheerful, or even alienated when interacting with a manic client.

Nurses' therapeutic use of the self is sabotaged when they are unaware that they are confusing clients' feelings with their own. Such confusion results in naive efforts to be helpful. Efforts such as simply trying to cheer up the depressed person, or talking the manic individual out of feelings of grandiosity lead to failure and frustration for the nurse. Repeated experiences such as these may result in the nurse guarding against these unrewarding feelings by actually avoiding such clients.

Nurses who are self-aware engage in self-assessment by way of the processes of introspection and self-appraisal, in an effort to identify feelings that are potentially problematic when working with depressed or manic clients. Self-awareness is facilitated when the nurse asks herself questions such as, "How do I feel when I interact with this client? How do I handle my own feelings of sadness, depression or happiness?" Self-aware nurses use their feelings and the answers to these questions as data in the recognition of affective disorders. In fact, feelings that the nurse experiences within the self may be the first clues to depression or mania. Feelings evoked in the nurse often provide important clues for the identification of particular feeling states that the client may be unable to verbalize. Self-awareness increases learning about both the client and oneself, as well as growth in the therapeutic use of self.

Self-awareness is also an important component in successful therapeutic intervention with clients who are potentially suicidal. The act of self-murder is diametrically opposed to one of nursing's primary objectives, which is to support life. Thus, nurses sometimes find it is difficult to recognize or acknowledge the presence of suicidal clues. Nurses need to assess their own feelings and anxiety when caring for suicidal clients. This self-assessment is necessary if anxiety-laden, angry, or bewildered responses to potentially suicidal clients are to be avoided. The most important question of the suicide risk assessment is, "Have you ever had thoughts of hurting or killing yourself?" This is a difficult question to ask, even for experienced clinicians. It may be impossible for nurses who are unaware of their personal feelings regarding suicide to make such an inquiry.

Formalized working structures are needed to facilitate self-awareness in nurses who provide care for clients experiencing affective disorders and/or suicidal ideation. Nurses should be encouraged to share personal experiences and concerns about their responses to these clients.

Skilled clinical supervision and team meetings are examples of working structures that provide opportunities for nurses to validate their perceptions and feelings regarding their responses to clients. Self-awareness emerges not only as a tool for observation and assessment, but also as a means of personal and professional growth.

PROBLEM IDENTIFICATION □

Affective Disorders. Clients who have affective disorders may experience disturbances in any one or all of the 11 health pattern areas identified by Gordon (1982). The spectrum of affective symp-

toms ranges from mild to severe. These symptoms are manifested physically, emotionally, cognitively, and behaviorally. Many affective symptoms can have far-reaching effects on the client's/family's ability to function. A thorough nursing assessment provides both diagnostic and evaluative data about the client and family. Table 33-6 describes some of the major nursing diagnoses that may apply to clients experiencing affective disorders.

Each of these nursing diagnoses can be further delineated in more specific terms depending upon the nature and severity of each client's symptomatology. No attempt will be made here to offer a definitive list of all possible nursing diagnoses pertaining to depressed and manic indi-

---

TABLE 33-6 Taxonomy of Nursing Diagnoses for Clients Experiencing Affective Disorders

Clients who have affective disorders, either depression or mania, may experience any of the following:	Early morning waking
	Perceived lack of need
Disturbances in health perception-health management pattern	Disturbances in self-perception–self-concept pattern
Health management deficit	Anxiety: mild, moderate, severe (panic)
Potential for physical injury	Body image disturbance
Potential/actual noncompliance	Depression
Potential for poisoning	Fear
Potential for suffocation	Personal identity confusion
	Self-esteem disturbance
Disturbances in nutritional-metabolic pattern	Disturbances in role-relationship pattern
Potential/actual fluid volume deficit	Dysfunctional grieving
Alteration in nutrition: Nutritional deficit	Unresolved independence-dependence conflict
Disturbances in elimination pattern	Potential/actual alteration in parenting
Alteration in bowel elimination: Constipation/diarrhea	Social isolation
Alteration in urinary elimination: Retention/	Alterations in socialization
incontinence	Impaired verbal communication
	Potential for violence
Disturbances in activity-exercise pattern	Disturbances in sexuality-reproductive pattern
Decreased activity tolerance	Sexual dysfunction
Diversional activity deficit	Alteration in achieving perceived sex role
Impaired home maintenance management	Alteration in achieving sexual satisfaction
Self-care deficit	Inability to achieve desired sexual satisfaction
Self-bathing hygiene deficit	Alteration in relationship with significant other
Self-dressing grooming deficit	Change of interest in self and others
Self-feeding deficit	Disturbances in coping-stress tolerance patterns
Self-toileting deficit	Ineffective family coping
Disturbances in cognitive-perceptual pattern	Potential for growth
Potential/actual impaired cognitive ability	Disabling
Alteration in comfort: pain	Compromised
Impaired thought processes	Ineffective individual coping
Disturbances in sleep-rest pattern	Impaired problem-solving ability
Excessive sleep (hypersomnia)	Impaired social functioning
Inadequate sleep (hyposomnia)	Disturbance in value-belief pattern
Insomnia	Spiritual distress

Sources: Gordon, M. *Nursing diagnosis: Process and application.* New York: McGraw-Hill, 1982. Kim, M.J.; McFarland, G.K.; and McLane, A.M. (eds.). *Classification of nursing diagnoses: Proceedings of the fifth national conference.* St. Louis: Mosby Company, 1984.

viduals. The reader is referred to *Nursing Diagnosis Process and Application* by Gordon (1982) for additional diagnostic information.

Suicide. From a nursing perspective, suicidal ideation does not represent a specific diagnostic disorder, illness, or syndrome. Rather it is a description of a range of emotions, cognitions, behaviors, and physical manifestations that can potentially lead to self-murder. Table 33-7 identifies a number of nursing diagnoses that may apply to the client experiencing suicidal ideation. The nurse formulates specific diagnoses for each client, based upon a thorough suicide risk assessment and observations of the individual client's behavior.

TABLE 33-7 Taxonomy of Nursing Diagnoses for Clients Experiencing Suicidal Ideation

---

Clients who have suicidal ideation may experience any of the following:

Disturbances in health perception-health management pattern
Health management deficit
Potential for physical injury
Potential/actual noncompliance
Potential for poisoning
Potential for suffocation

Disturbances in nutritional-metabolic pattern
Potential/actual fluid volume deficit
Alteration in nutrition: nutritional deficit

Disturbances in cognitive-perceptual pattern
Potential/actual impaired cognitive ability
Alteration in comfort: pain
Impaired though processes

Disturbances in self-perception–self-concept pattern
Anxiety: mild, moderate, or severe (panic)
Depression
Fear
Personal identity confusion
Self-esteem disturbance

Disturbances in role-relationship pattern
Social isolation
Alterations in socialization
Potential for violence

Disturbances in coping-stress tolerance pattern
Ineffective individual coping
Impaired problem solving ability
Impaired social functioning

Disturbance in value-belief pattern
Spiritual distress

Sources: Gordon, M. *Nursing diagnosis: Process and application.* New York: McGraw-Hill, 1982. Kim, M.J.; McFarland, G.K.; and McLane, A.M. (eds.). *Classification of nursing diagnoses: Proceedings of the fifth national conference.* St. Louis: Mosby Company, 1984.

INTERVENTION □

Affective Disorders

Primary Prevention. □ The primary prevention of depression and mania is directed toward building adaptive strengths and coping resources in people, particularly those at high risk. Primary preventive measures for affective disorders include addressing broad social issues and initiating educational programs. Prior to encountering a crisis to self-esteem and personal worth, people need to learn more effective ways to cope with life events. Special attention should be given to high stress periods, such as the early child-rearing years when parents' sense of worth and competency may be threatened by children who do not conform to social expectations. Parents can become involved in educational programs for parenting or support groups to help them cope with family responsibilities more effectively. Genetic vulnerability also indicates a need for genetic counseling for families at risk.

Nurses can carry out group educational programs as well as individual counseling for people at risk of developing affective disorders. The nurse's primary objectives are to enrich the client's and family's self-esteem and to teach skills needed for successful coping. For example, classes in stress management, parenting, assertiveness, and coping with crises can all serve to decrease the tendency to become depressed.

Secondary and Tertiary Prevention. □ The goals of secondary prevention of affective disorders include early diagnosis and prompt treatment of depression and mania. Tertiary prevention is concerned with limiting the client's disability and facilitating reentry into the family unit and work place. The nurse functions both dependently and independently along with other members of the mental health team to accomplish the goals of secondary and tertiary prevention. She functions dependently by collaborating with the physician to see that appropriately prescribed medical interventions are carried out. For example, the nurse is frequently involved in the administration and evaluation of various somatic therapies, including psychopharmaceuticals and electroconvulsive therapy. The nurse functions independently by formulating a comprehensive plan to intervene in the specific nursing care problems experienced by clients with affective disorders. The following discussion of nursing interventions is organized according to the characteristic manifestations of depression and mania.

Depression. The essential features of a major depressive episode are a dysphoric mood, a disturbance in any appetitive function, psychomotor retardation or agitation, feelings of worthlessness and guilt, and suicidal ideation (DSM-III, 1980). These symptoms may be accompanied by a loss of interest in usual activities, and the client may or may not exhibit an impaired ability to think or concentrate. Abstracting from this clinical picture, it is clear that severely depressed individuals may potentially experience a wide variety of disturbances in a number of health pattern areas.

Severely depressed clients are often so preoccupied with feelings of self-doubt and sadness that they become stuporous and literally immobile. This immobilization may precipitate a number of disturbances in the depressed client's health perception–health management patterns. Although not by conscious choice, the depressed client is noncompliant with the health team's plan of care. He quite simply doesn't have enough energy to actively participate in his own recovery. Ultimately, the depressed client may be so impaired that he has an increased potential for physical injury.

As with all clients, the nurse is concerned with the depressed client's safety. The nurse must intervene on behalf of the severely depressed client to ensure his safety. The client should be provided with an environment with which he can easily cope. Noise and confusion should be kept to a minimum. By maintaining a calm, positive approach, the nurse is able to ease the depressed client's stress and lift his spirits. It is important to remember that the risk of suicide increases when the client's depression first begins to lift. Therefore, severely depressed clients should be closely supervised and frequently observed for behaviors indicating suicidal intent. Suicide risk assessment must be an ongoing process.

Disturbances in nutritional-metabolic patterns are common among depressed clients. These disturbances are generally manifest as nutritional and/or fluid volume deficits. The moderately depressed client may simply experience a loss of appetite, while the more severely depressed client may actually experience extreme repugnance and nausea at the thought of eating, or complain of being too tired to eat. Loss of energy and motivation (even to eat) are hallmark symptoms of depression.

The nurse should make careful observations of when, where, and how much the client eats. She may then wish to set aside some time to stay with the client during each meal in order to offer encouragement to the client to eat and to foster a more worthwhile self-concept. Collaborating with the dietician may be helpful to the nurse in planning meals that are both nutritious and appetizing. For example, the client may find fresh garden vegatables more palatable than steamed vegetables. Providing the client with small meals, snacks, and appetizing finger foods may also encourage his appetite. The client's family can participate in his plan of care by bringing his favorite foods from home. Ensuring that the client gets enough fluids and bulk may also be helpful in preventing problems of elimination. Frequent reassessment of the client's appetite and food tolerance is an indicator as to the necessity of the nurse staying with the client during the meals. Return of a hearty appetite can generally be taken as an indication that the client's depression is lifting.

As side effects of antidepressant medication(s), depressed clients may also experience disturbances in their patterns of elimination. These may involve alterations in bowel (e.g., constipation or diarrhea) and urinary (e.g., retention or incontinence) elimination. Encouraging the client to engage in physical activity and increasing the amount of fiber in the diet are often effective interventions. The nurse should collaborate with the physician concerning any additional medications or treatments needed to promote optimum bowel and urinary elimination. Accurate records of the client's elimination patterns are used to evaluate the severity of alterations and the effectiveness of nursing interventions, medications, or treatments.

The depressed client's apparent lack of motivation and apathetic attitude contribute to disturbances in activity-exercise patterns. Such disturbances may be manifest as a profound activity intolerance which may be so acute that the client appears to be totally lacking in any interest in his personal appearance. The client may not voluntarily engage in any routine self-care activities, such as bathing, dressing, grooming, feeding, or even self-toileting. It is important that the nurse accept him as he is and offer understanding and encouragement by matter-of-factly, but kindly pointing out the need to continue with routine hygienic activities.

A frequently used aid for the depressed client is a daily schedule which can be kept on hand at all times. Such a schedule should include every activity from getting up in the morning and brushing teeth, to exercise and rest periods, watching television, and eating. By using this schedule, the client is able to stay busy with activities that promote self-esteem and divert attention from rumination and inner suffering.

Depressed clients should be encouraged to participate in a variety of activities of daily living, such as self-care and household tasks, beginning with one simple activity (e.g., making the bed, folding linens) and adding other activities as capable. Activities related to grooming and personal appearance, such as hair care, shaving, or applying appropriate makeup are helpful to the client's self-concept and self-esteem. Activities related to nutrition are also beneficial—for example, the client may wish to participate in meal planning and cooking, beginning with simple recipes.

Diversional activities that generate self-esteem are appropriate for the depressed individual. Such activities should include stimulating, short-term individual or group projects, using brightly colored materials. Crafts such as collage, decoupage, needle work, clay molding, and rug hooking are examples. Activities designed to increase energy levels are also desirable. The client should begin with low-energy and move to high-energy activities. Walking, simple physical exercises, and indoor or outdoor gardening may be helpful in lifting the spirits.

Depressed individuals experience disturbances in their cognitive-perceptual patterns. Specifically, they tend to experience alterations in various thought processes which may be manifest as slowness of thought and as an inability to make decisions. Frequently, the depressed client finds long explanations upsetting. Therefore, it is essential that the nurse offer brief explanations about care procedures, approach client care in an unhurried manner, remain calm and pleasant, and demonstrate competence.

The depressed client often feels unworthy to make decisions and unable to respond correctly, even to simple questions. Forcing him to make decisions may result in agitation and self-conscious concern as to whether his decision was the right one. Therefore, the nurse should present the client with suggestions rather than choices. For example, she might suggest that the client have roast beef for dinner, rather than asking him to choose among roast beef, chicken, and salmon. As the depression lessens, however, the nurse should carefully assess the client's willingness and abil-

ity to make decisions. Encouraging the capable client to participate in decision making fosters self-esteem and independence.

A disturbance in sleep-rest patterns is another common problem experienced by depressed individuals, who commonly complain of initial or middle insomnia and/or early morning awakening. Here again, close observation and accurate record keeping are key factors in planning for effective nursing intervention. In addition to inquiring as to how the client is sleeping, the nurse should also observe him at frequent intervals, during the day and night, to assess how much sleep he is getting. These actions communicate concern and acceptance and may be comforting to the client. After thoroughly assessing the client's situation, the nurse may wish to employ such basic measures as back rubs, warm milk, hot showers, and soothing conversation while sitting at the bedside, to promote natural relaxation and sleep. Medications to induce sleep should be avoided, however, it may be necessary to collaborate with the physician concerning the client's need for medication if he is still unable to obtain adequate rest or sleep.

Depressed persons typically experience intense feelings of sadness, despair, and worthlessness. These feelings represent disturbances in the client's self-concept and role relationships. The nurse should make an effort to spend time during each shift with the depressed client, communicating acceptance by providing quiet, nonthreatening companionship. The positive regard thus demonstrated supplies encouragement and assists the client in regaining a higher sense of self-esteem. By listening carefully when the client speaks, the nurse conveys the feeling that someone does care and does recognize the client's distress. Listening also decreases the feelings of loneliness often experienced by depressed persons. Since the nurse is obviously not capable of spending every minute with one client, it may be advisable to have the depressed client write about his feelings throughout the day, so they can be discussed at a later time.

Self-esteem is further enhanced by involving the depressed client in activities in which success is possible. The nurse should first introduce the client into activities by working cooperatively on a one-to-one basis. Care must be taken not to suggest activities in which the client might do poorly and thereby reinforce feelings of inadequacy. As he becomes increasingly comfortable with activities on a one-to-one level, another client or staff member may be included in the nurse-client interaction. Gradually, the nurse may include a number of others in activities, providing valuable support and reassurance for the client through the group situation. Eventually the client should be able to tolerate activities and interactions with others without the nurse's presence, thus demonstrating an increase in independence and self-esteem.

Disturbances in the depressed client's self-concept and role relationships are also manifest in his social withdrawal which is sometimes due to his overwhelming feelings of worthlessness. This can be a difficult situation for the nurse to tolerate, since her time with the client may be characterized by little or no interaction. Although she may feel she is having little impact on the client's behavior, she must realize that he remains acutely sensitive to the environment, even though he may appear quite isolated. The client is influenced by the nurse's verbalizations and actions, and by sitting with him and accepting quiet behavior, the nurse helps the client to recognize that he is deemed worthwhile by at least one other person. Thus, through both verbal and nonverbal behavior, the nurse conveys an attitude of acceptance that eventually has an impact.

The nurse must not yield to the temptation of offering words of encouragement and support too frequently. The depressed client, who views himself as worthless, is likely to interpret such expressions as false assurances or sympathy. Thus, he may feel more dependent and worthless.

Consistency and dependability on the part of the nurse are important factors in dealing with depressed clients who feel worthless. The depressed client is likely to personalize inconsistencies and lack of dependability on the part of the nurse as signals that she doesn't care about him, because he isn't worth caring about. For example, if the nurse makes an appointment to meet with a client at a specified time, she should keep the appointment promptly as scheduled, thereby communicating that she does not share the client's view of himself as worthless. She is not only indicating that the client and his concerns are important and worthy of her time and energy, but that the therapeutic work accomplished between nurse and client is of value as well.

When working with depressed clients, it is important for the nurse to understand that it is impossible to force the client into therapeutic activities and relationships. She must be willing to move the relationship along at the client's own pace. This is often a frustrating process for the nurse, since the depressed individual tends to be withdrawn and moves quite slowly in establishing relationships. The nurse must constantly be alert for cues that the client can tolerate interaction. The depressed person may desperately desire contact with another but choose withdrawal as a means of coping with internal stress. Moreover, the withdrawn client may feel hopeless, and anticipate rejection and failure in forming a relationship. Thus, the depressed individual chooses social isolation rather than risking being misunderstood or rejected.

It is imperative that nurses exercise patience and tolerance with depressed clients who exhibit withdrawal behaviors such as silence or making hostile remarks. These behaviors are intended to protect the client by creating emotional distance between himself and others, and they may also elicit feelings of rejection, failure, hurt, disappointment, or hopelessness within the nurse. She may act on these feelings by avoiding future interactions with the depressed client. If this mutual withdrawal occurs, the nurse-client relationship reaches a stalemate and the nurse's actions actually reinforce the client's withdrawal and depression.

Depressed persons frequently experience difficulty in dealing with feelings of anger. They often feel guilty when verbally expressing anger and hostility. This guilt may stem from the fear that an expression of anger will open a floodgate of pent-up emotions, devastating the person to whom wrath is directed and resulting in a complete loss of self-control on the part of the client. The client needs to learn to express angry feelings both verbally and nonverbally and without guilt. Diversional activities, such as woodworking, hammering, kneading clay or dough, and participating in vigorous sport, may help the client vent anger in a constructive manner. Once the client is aware that it is acceptable to have and express angry feelings, he may slowly begin to verbalize these feelings as well as releasing them through physical activity. It is important that the nurse communicate acceptance when the depressed client expresses anger.

Mania. Manic clients are characterized by their expansive mood, increased activity, grandiose ideas, and bizarre or eccentric behavior and appearance. Like depressed individuals, these clients may or may not exhibit an accompanying thought disorder (DSM-III, 1980).

The hyperactivity experienced by manic clients can be so acute as to actually be life-threatening. These clients exhibit physical restlessness and unusual talkativeness (pressure of speech) which is often accompanied by inappropriate laughing, joking, and punning. Additionally, manic clients tend to become involved in activities without concern for the possible consequences. These hyperactive behaviors place the manic client at particular risk of physical injury. Therefore, the nurse must ensure that the client's immediate environment is made safe by removing any hazardous objects or substances and providing the client with surroundings that are as simple and calm as possible. Lighting and noise levels should also be kept low to promote a tranquil atmosphere.

The nurse should approach the manic client unhurriedly, demonstrating calmness so as not to contribute to his expansive mood. By providing an atmosphere of acceptance, the nurse encourages the client to express his feelings. She should talk with the client on an adult level, keeping comments and explanations short and concise. By listening attentively, the nurse is able to communicate acceptance and respect for the client as a person. However, indications that the nurse accepts manic or otherwise inappropriate behavior should be avoided. Similarly, arguing with the client or negatively criticizing him is counterproductive, since he may respond with hostility or violence. Instead, the nurse should serve as a role model for the client, by clearly communicating what is expected of him and holding him responsible for his behavior. By verbally identifying positive changes in the manic client's behavior on a daily basis, the nurse assists him in evaluating his successful progress.

Manic clients frequently experience disturbances in their nutritional-metabolic and elimination patterns. Because of the frenetic nature of manic behavior, these clients often don't take time to eat and defecate properly. Foods and drinks that are high in calories should be offered at frequent intervals throughout the day. To avoid constipation, the client should occasionally be reminded to use the rest room. Other disturbances in elimination may include polyuria and/or diarrhea, especially when the client is receiving lithium therapy. The client should be carefully monitored for these potential side effects of lithium therapy. They are usually managed by adjusting the medication dose, however, the physician may elect to intervene by administering additional medications to treat each side effect specifically. The nurse should ensure that an ongoing accurate assessment of nutritional and elimination patterns is carried out and properly documented.

Manic clients also experience severe disturbances in their activity-exercise patterns. These disturbances generally take the form of extreme hyperactivity, and therefore opportunities to engage in activities that decrease energy and tension should be provided. Examples of such activities include vigorous housekeeping chores, jogging, and athletic sports. Alterations in hygienic self-care activities may also be apparent. The manic client may need reminders to change clothes, bathe, shave, and brush his teeth.

Disturbances in sleep-rest patterns are typically experienced by the manic client as a perceived decreased need for sleep. A place to take short but frequent naps may encourage him to obtain adequate rest. Not unlike depressed clients, manic clients may benefit from a written schedule of prescribed daily activities. Specified periods of time can be set aside for the client to meet his basic human needs for nutrition, elimination, activity, and sleep-rest.

Disturbances in role relationships, sexuality (usually hypersexuality), and coping-stress tolerance patterns are also experienced by manic clients. The nurse should assist the client in identifying any pattern of behavior or sequence of events leading up to the manic episode. If there is an identifiable pattern preceding the onset of the manic state, nurse and client should seek to determine if that particular pattern can be changed. The nurse should also explore with the client the effects of his behavior on others. He must be made aware that he becomes an unstable force in others' lives when he behaves in an erratic and unpredictable manner. To gain insight into his behavior, the client should be encouraged to participate in therapeutic group interaction.

The importance of recognizing tension within oneself must be emphasized when intervening on behalf of the manic client. Diversional activities should be recommended for times when he begins to feel out of control. Such activities may include taking a long walk, cleaning, or listening to soothing music. The client should be taught the importance of remaining calm in conserving energy and reducing tension and anxiety. Additionally, he should be made aware that he may be placed on long-term lithium maintenance therapy and what actions and precautions this entails.

The major long-term objective that all manic

clients share is to learn more effective methods of coping. To this end, the client and family should work together, with the nurse's guidance, to set behavioral limits. What exactly constitutes acceptable versus unacceptable behavior should be clearly established and understood by all parties concerned. Family therapy may be a helpful adjunct in clearing up communications among significant others and in increasing the family's understanding of the client's problems and behavior.

Suicide

Primary Prevention. □ As with clients experiencing affective disorders, primary prevention of suicide entails identifying individual clients and groups at risk and assisting them in developing adaptive abilities that foster effective problem-solving and coping behaviors. Groups at particular risk of committing suicide include depressed individuals, people with no close family ties, Protestant males, people over the age of 40, single and married people without children, adolescents (especially college students), and people who have previously attempted suicide. Nurses can be instrumental in reaching out to these groups in various settings. For example, a student health nurse might start a social support group for college students on a university campus. Support groups for single adults often meet in local churches and community centers. The community health nurse can help make clients aware of the existence of various support groups and educational programs in the community. Whatever the context of the nurse's practice, she can, and should, be a motivating force for those who could benefit most from mutual support groups and activities.

Secondary and Tertiary Prevention. □ Unfortunately, it is only after an individual is successful in completing the act of suicide that one can be totally sure that he was seriously self-destructive. Protecting the client from self-destruction is an endeavor that must be shared by the entire mental health team. Because the nurse relates to the client on such a significant level, she is often the first member of the team to become aware of a potential suicide. The nurse must act responsibly in communicating any clues that indicate the client is considering suicide. No matter how insignificant the suicidal clues may seem, it is important to have a team meeting so that a coordinated therapeutic plan can be formulated to ensure the client's safety.

Once the nurse determines that a client *is* suicidal, a plan of care should be initiated immediately. This care plan is designed to meet two main objectives: (1) the client must be provided with a *safe environment*, and (2) most importantly, the client must be provided with a richly *therapeutic environment*.

The traditional approach to providing the suicidal client with a safe environment typically involves removing all potentially dangerous items from the immediate surroundings. Obviously, such objects as razor blades, ropes, and medications must be taken away. However, removal of personal possessions may be perceived by the client as proof of his worthlessness and may generate feelings of loss and rejection. The next important aspect of care and the most appropriate overall nursing intervention is to provide the client with a meaningful therapeutic environment.

The therapeutic relationship begins when the nurse conveys interest and an attitude of unconditional acceptance toward the client. If even one person is successful in establishing rapport with the suicidal client, he may be influenced to abandon his self-destructive plans. By spending time with the client, the nurse is able to provide constant watchful care and is available to listen. Her presence gives the client a sense of assurance that until he is able to control self-destructive impulses, control will be provided. Knowing that even one other person accepts him and is interested in his welfare may be the client's best protection against suicide.

Suicide is less likely when the client feels that someone knows, hears, and understands the intense painful feelings he is experiencing. Once he senses that the nurse is interested in him and accepts him, he may feel better able to ventilate his pain, hostility, or disgust. Encouraging statements such as, "What has been happening in your life lately?" may assist the suicidal client in sharing the source of his pain. By listening calmly and occasionally verifying that the client knows someone is listening, the nurse assists him in identifying and examining his feelings. Also, the nurse should ask if the client feels that there are others, perhaps family members, who do not listen to him. If his response is "Yes," assist him in finding constructive and appropriate ways to get them to listen. Family therapy may be indicated and is an excellent means of enhancing communication within the client's family.

Suicidal clients often experience a certain

amount of psychological relief after discussing their self-destructive ideas. The nurse should point out that suicide represents an unsatisfactory and permanent solution to a temporary problem. The nurse should secure a verbal behavioral contract with the client that he will not attempt suicide.

It is important that the nurse convey an attitude of hope and optimism when interacting with the suicidal client, who may be extremely ambivalent regarding life and death. That is, he may not be sure that he wants to live, but he does not want to live life as it presently is. He may not be able to see that life can be better. After allowing him to express how painful his life has been, the nurse should offer a message of optimism that life can be better. The client must be reassured that, although it may be difficult, his seemingly unsolvable problem can be worked out. It is essential that the nurse assist the client in identifying hopeful behavioral alternatives to suicide, without using an overly effervescent approach. By being overly hopeful and optimistic, the nurse risks seeming insincere to the suicidal client.

The suicidal client should be encouraged to participate in a variety of meaningful diversional activities. Sanding furniture, kneading dough, or playing an active sport are all opportunities to ventilate tension and hostility. By guiding the client's activities and encouraging him to eat, bathe, and take time to rest and sleep, the nurse assists him to again become involved in the interactions of living.

If suicidal clients are to survive, it is essential that they learn and practice principles of mental health. The client must be encouraged to report symptoms indicating a recurrence of suicidal ideation and its accompanying risk. Such symptoms include depression, feelings of hopelessness, and suicide planning. The long-term effects of suicide should also be described for the client. For example, the nurse could mention the long-term effects on the client's children, such as poor role modeling, being a one-parent child, and the child feeling abandoned.

Long-term goals for suicidal clients are individually determined. Individual or group psychotherapy is often indicated to assist the individual in developing a more realistic and positive self-concept. The client needs to learn new options for effective methods of coping, ways of expressing feelings to others, and behaviors to facilitate successful interpersonal relationships. Acceptance by others and a feeling of belonging are essential. Ultimately, the suicidal client must be provided with a continuing system of support, which involves both the ongoing therapeutic nurse-client relationship and a network comprised of immediate family, relatives, friends, and community groups.

EVALUATION □ The comprehensive nursing care plan contains the framework for evaluation. Since the nurse's interventions were designed to solve specific client problems, evaluative judgments about how these problems are being resolved should be obtained through nurse-client collaboration. Evaluative data are gathered in the form of both observed client behaviors and client self-reports. The nurse and client together determine if desired changes have occurred in his behavior. This determination is made not only by identifying which behaviors have been modified and which have disappeared, but also by identifying newly emerging behavioral patterns.

As mentioned earlier, the nurse should participate in formalized professional activities to develop self-awareness. Skilled clinical supervision and team meetings provide opportunities for the nurse to engage in self-evaluation. Such activities facilitate both personal and professional growth.

■ Enrichment Activities

DISCUSSION QUESTIONS

1. What epidemiological characteristics are associated with the occurrence of the major affective disorders, major depressive disorder, and bipolar affective disorder?

2. Discuss the various psychodynamic, sociological, and biochemical theories regarding the etiology of affective disorders.

3. What is the role of the nurse in administering and evaluating somatic therapies used in treating affective disorders (e.g., antidepressant/antimanic medications and electroconvulsive therapy)?

4. What are some of the physical, emotional, cognitive, and behavioral manifestations of depression and mania?

5. In the United States, which age, sex, occupational, and racial groups have the statistically highest rates of attempted and completed suicide?

6. What personal characteristics are associated with high risk suicide?

7. Of the many social, demographic, and clinical variables purported to influence the occurrence of suicide, which do you believe hold the most value as predictors of suicide? Discuss your choice.

8. Considering different cultural and religious beliefs, what do you think are the current attitudes in this country regarding suicide?

9. Is suicide, or its attempt, illegal in your state? Discuss your feelings regarding this.

10. Will your state's Blue Cross/Blue Shield and Medicare/Medicaid insurance plans pay for in- or outpatient care for suicidal clients? Discuss your feelings regarding this.

11. What are some of the physical, emotional, cognitive, and behavioral manifestations of suicide?

12. What factors should be considered when making a thorough suicide risk assessment?

13. What role does the nurse's self-assessment play in preparing her to provide care for clients experiencing affective disorders and/or suicidal ideation?

14. How does the process of self-assessment contribute to the nurse's personal and professional growth?

15. Formulate a number of tentative nursing diagnoses for clients experiencing affective disorders and/or suicidal ideation. How would you intervene to resolve these problems?

16. Discuss suicide as an individual health problem, a family health problem, and/or a community health problem.

17. Should the nurse use a different approach when intervening with a client who has had a less serious suicide attempt, than with a client who has made a serious attempt? Discuss your response.

18. What is the role of the nurse-client collaboration in the evaluation phase of the nursing process with clients experiencing affective disorders and/or suicidal ideation?

■ Learning Activities

1. Visit a local health-related facility and/or extended care facility and identify environmental factors that could be changed to help prevent depression.

2. Contact a variety of community agencies to determine the availability of support groups and educational programs that could help provide for the primary prevention of depression and suicide.

3. Visit the student health center on your campus to determine the availability of personnel and procedures to intervene with severely depressed and/or suicidal clients.

4. Interview a person who works for a suicide "hot line" to determine how he or she assesses suicide risk potential and intervenes via telephone.

5. Interview a member of the clergy to determine his interpretation of the meaning and implications of mental illness and suicide for his religion.

■ Recommended Readings

Busteed, E.L., and Johnstone, C. The development of suicide precautions for an inpatient psychiatric unit. *Journal of psychosocial nursing and mental health services*, 21, 5, 1983:15–19. This informative article provides an overview of suicide precautions used in inpatient psychiatric units, a demographic description of the clients who attempt suicide while admitted to psychiatric units, as well as a description of the process for developing a suicide precaution policy for a community psychiatric unit.

Capodanno, A.E., and Targum, S.D. Assessment of suicide risk: Some limitations in the prediction of infrequent events. *Journal of psychological nursing and mental health services*, 21, 5, 1983:11–14. A brief article highlighting potential predictor variables that may improve the nurse's efficiency in predicting suicidal risk. Among the variables considered are the social environment, feelings of hopelessness, previous suicide attempts, family history, and biological markers.

Fitzpatrick, J.J. Suicidology and suicide prevention: Historical perspectives from nursing literature. *Journal of psychosocial nursing and mental health services*, 21, 5, 1983:20–28. An in-depth article addressing nursing's concern for the broad areas of suicidology and suicide prevention. Both theoretical and historical elements are explored through a comprehensive review of existing nursing literature regarding suicide and suicidal behavior.

Hagerty, B.K. *Psychiatric-Mental Health Assessment*. St. Louis: Mosby Company, 1984. An excellent source for nurses and nursing students providing information about psychiatric-mental health function, dysfunction, current theories of psychopathology, and, most importantly, a diverse collection of instrumentation to access the clinical presentation of psychopathology.

Jones, S.L., and Pelikon, L. Nursing management of the depressed patient in the emergency room. *Psychiatric nursing forum*, 1, 2, 1984:6–14. An interesting case study approach is used to illustrate the clinical manifestations of the depressive syndrome, the emergency department nurse's role in suicide risk assessment, and principles of emergency nursing intervention.

■ *References*

Abraham, K. The first pregenital stage of the libido. *Selected papers on psychoanalysis*. London: Hogarth, 1927.

Allen, M.G., Cohen, S., Pollin, W., and Greenspan, S.I. Affective illness in veteran twins: A diagnostic review. *American journal of psychiatry*, 130, 1974:1234–1239.

American Psychiatric Association. *Diagnostic and statistical manual of mental disorders*. 3d ed. Washington, D.C.: American Psychiatric Association, 1980.

Bibring, E. The mechanism of depression. In *Affective disorders*. (Greenacre, P., ed.). New York: International Universities Press, 1953.

Boyd, J.H., and Weissman, M.M. Epidemiology. In *Handbook of affective disorders*. (Paykel, E.S., ed.). Edinburgh: Churchill Livingstone, 1982.

Carroll, B.J. Neuroendocrine function in psychiatric disorders. In *Psychopharmacology: A generation of progress*. (Lipton, M.A., et al. eds.). New York: Raven Press, 1978:487–497.

Farberow, N.L. Suicide prevention in the hospital. *Hospital and community psychiatry*. 32, 2, 1981:99–103.

Frazier, A. Biological aspects of mania and depression. In *Biological bases of psychiatric disorders*. (Frazier, A., and Winokur, A., eds.). New York: Spectrum, 1977:221–222.

Freedman, A.M., Kaplan, H.I., and Sadock, B.J. (eds.). *Comprehensive textbook of psychiatry*. 2nd ed, Baltimore: Williams and Wilkins, 1975.

Freud, S. Mourning and melancholia, 1917. In *The standard edition of the complete psychological works of Sigmund Freud*. Vol. 14. London: Hogarth, 1957.

Gold, M.S., Pottash, A.L.C., Davies, R.K., Ryan, N., Sweeney, D.R., and Martin, D.M. Distinguishing unipolar and bipolar depression by thyrotropin release test. *Lancet*, 2, 1979:411.

Gordon, M. *Nursing diagnosis: Process and application*. New York: McGraw-Hill, 1982

Hagerty, B.K. *Psychiatric mental-health assessment*. St. Louis: Mosby, 1984.

Jacobsen, A. Melancholy in the 20th century: Causes and prevention. *Journal of psychiatric nursing*, 7, 18, 1980:11–21.

Kerschner, D., and Lancaster, J. Community mental health: Problem identification, prevention and intervention. In *Community health nursing: Process and practice for promoting health*. (Stanhope, M., and Lancaster, J., eds.). New York: Mosby Company, 1984.

Kim, M.J.; McFarland, G.K.; and McLane, A.M. (eds.). *Classification of nursing diagnoses: Proceedings of the fifth national conference*. St. Louis: Mosby Company, 1984.

Klein, M.A. A contribution to the psychogenesis of manic-depressive states. In *Contributions to psychoanalysis*. London: Hogarth, 1948.

Klerman, G.L., and Barrett, J.E. The affective disorders: Clinical and epidemiological aspects. In *Lithium: Its role in psychiatric research and treatment*. (Gershon, S., and Shopsin, B., eds.). New York: Plenum Press, 1973:201–236.

Kneisl, C.R., and Wilson, H.S. *Handbook of psychosocial nursing care*. Menlo Park, CA: Addison-Wesley Publishing Company, 1984.

Krauthammer, C., and Klerman, G.L. The epidemiology of mania. In *Manic illness*. (Shopsin, B., ed.). New York: Raven Press, 1979:11–28.

Miller, M. Introduction to suicidology. In *Suicide intervention by nurses*. (Miller, M., ed.). New York: Springer, 1982, 3-27.

Murray, R.J., and Huelskoepter, M.M.W. *Psychiatric/mental health nursing*. Englewood Cliffs, NJ: Prentice-Hall, 1983.

Nurnberger, F.I., and Gershon, E.S. Genetics. In *The handbook of affective disorders*. (Paykel, E.S., ed.). Edinburgh: Churchill Livingstone, 1982:126–144.

Orvaschel, H., Weissman, M. M., and Kidd, K. K. Children and depression: The children of depressed parents, the childhood of depressed patients, depression in children. *Journal of affective disorders*, 2, 1980:1–16.

Reubin, R. Spotting and stopping the suicide patient. *Nursing '79*, 9, 4, 1979:82–85.

Spitz, R., and Wold, K.M. Anaclitic depression. In *The psychoanalytic study of the child*. Vol. 2. New York: International Universities Press, 1946.

Swanson, A.R. Depression. In *Comprehensive psychiatric nursing*. (Haber, J.; Leach, A.M.; Schudy, S.M.; and Sidelow, B.F., eds.). New York: McGraw-Hill, 1982:533–556.

Wenz, F. Effects of seasons and sociological variables on suicidal behavior. *Public health reports*, 92, 3, 1977:327.

Zis, A.P., and Goodwin, F.K. The amine hypothesis. In *The handbook of affective disorders*. (Paykel, E.S., ed.). Edinburgh: Churchill Livingstone, 1982:183.

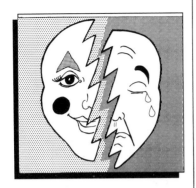

34

Schizophrenia and Schizophreniform Disorders

Joan Norris

Learning Objectives

Upon completion of this chapter, the reader will be able to:

1. Describe the concept of schizophrenia and discuss various theoretical formulations related to its course and treatment.

2. Distinguish among paranoid states, schizophreniform psychoses, and types of schizophrenia according to DSM-III guidelines.

3. Recognize barriers to nursing effectiveness, including mutual withdrawal, and plan approaches to enhance therapeutic interaction with withdrawn and autistic clients.

4. Use the nursing process with individuals experiencing autistic withdrawal and with their families to assess; identify problems and needs; plan individualized, theory-based intervention; and evaluate care.

5. Discuss mental health promotion activities appropriate to primary, secondary, and tertiary prevention for schizophrenia.

Schizophrenia is a descriptive concept for a group of psychiatric disorders that have been estimated to affect 0.85 to 1 percent of the world's population annually as new cases (Arieti, 1974; Rogers, 1982). Although the behavioral manifestations may vary widely, the most common and characteristic disturbance associated with schizophrenia is disordered thinking. Thoughts may be fragmented, disorganized, illogical, and bizarre. Perceptions may be distorted, motivation diminished, and affect blunted or inappropriately altered. Activity level may be drastically increased or decreased. Severe impairments are demonstrated in communication and interpersonal relationships. Identity, self-image, and functioning may be profoundly altered for extended time periods and, in many cases, for life.

Schizophreniform disorders are similar to schizophrenia in the symptoms and problems evidenced but are shorter in duration (two weeks to six months) and more likely to occur in response to severe stressors. For this reason, the expectation for full recovery and return to prior levels of functioning is optimistic.

Paranoid disorders are characterized by suspiciousness and grandiose or persecutory delusions (fixed, false belief systems which are not in accord with reality or culture). Individuals who are experiencing a paranoid disorder may vary widely in the degree to which their overall personality and ability to function are affected. Paranoia affects only a circumscribed component of one's life, that part relating to the delusional system, while a schizophrenic reaction, paranoid type, tends to leave the person impaired in several areas with much more severe and widespread debilitation.

In the past, schizophrenia (schizophreniform disorders were not delineated separately) was variously described as a disease, as an adaptational response to overwhelming stress, and as a lifestyle. Some writers insisted that a deteriorating course was inevitable while others held that schizophrenia could lead to reorganization at higher adaptive levels and in some cases, to greater creativity. An example of the latter viewpoint is *I Never Promised You A Rose Garden*, a first-person account of recovery by Green (1964). Because of this mixed outcome, efforts were made to distinguish between acute and "process" (chronic) schizophrenia in both Europe and America. The DSM III (1980) clearly differentiates schizophrenia (duration over six months) from brief reactive psychosis (duration of less than two weeks) and schizophreniform disorders (duration of two weeks to six months), although the behaviors of the clients may be similar.

When working with any of these clients who exhibit behaviors traditionally associated with schizophrenia, the nurse may feel overwhelmed by the severity of the client's disturbed behavior and also by the feelings of anxiety, frustration, and even hopelessness engendered in her. Considering the prevalence of the disorder as approximately one percent of Americans (Kolb, 1973) and the recent movement of previously institutionalized clients into the community, the nurse must be prepared to provide safe and effective care regardless of the practice setting. With patience and sensitivity, a therapeutic relationship can be developed, physical and emotional support provided, and the person assisted in what is a lonely and complex struggle for a meaningful life.

☐ *Theory*

EARLY DESCRIPTIONS

The term schizophrenia did not exist until the early twentieth century. Kraepelin described the condition in 1919 and called it "dementia praecox" meaning premature brain deterioration. Bleuler later renamed the disorder schizophrenia to reflect what he saw as a splitting of the psychic functions. He further categorized and named the disturbances experienced by clients as primary and secondary symptoms. Primary symptoms identified are often referred to as the 4 As: (1) associative looseness, (2) autism, (3) affect disturbance, and (4) ambivalence (Randels, 1982, 333–334). These symptoms were believed to be present in all cases. By associative looseness is meant the fragmentation and illogical connections that are present in thought and speech patterns. Autism is a term that describes the exclusion of reality and the tendency to focus on one's internal fantasies. Affect disturbances may include blunting (a flat, expressionless appearance) or inappropriateness (displaying a mood that does not fit the topic such as laughing while discussing the death of a loved one). Ambivalence is the simultaneous holding of opposing emotions about a person or object. This sets up an approach-avoidance conflict such as the need-fear dilemma in which a schizophrenic person is lonely and needs human relatedness but also fears rejection to the extent that efforts to make social contact are painfully threatening.

Bleuler also believed that the secondary symptoms such as delusions, hallucinations, and activity changes were individual responses to the primary problems (Arieti, 1974, 13–14). Freud's concepts of unconscious motivation were used to explain the nature of these other symptoms. For example, the defense mechanism of projection describes how one's self-accusations and hostility could become externalized into persecutory delusions. The repression of painful thoughts could explain the observed tendency of "blocking" in the speech pattern of schizophrenic clients. Kraepelin, Bleuler, and Freud all viewed schizophrenia as an organic disorder which produced a variety of behavioral symptoms based in the person's unique mental processes (Arieti, 1974, 9–31).

INTERPERSONAL THEORY

Harry Stack Sullivan did not exclude organic factors but believed the origin of schizophrenia to exist in painful early experiences such as the relationship to the mother figure. In his interpersonal viewpoint, the self ("me") is based in the reflected appraisals of significant others. Parental distress and anxiety communicates "bad me" feelings in the child which initiate attempts to decrease the discomfort. These attempts may involve dissociation, "not me," or parataxic disortion (an illogical or fantasy interpretation of the situation). In essence, Sullivan and his followers viewed the schizophrenic break with reality as occurring in response to a threat to self-esteem which resulted in overwhelming anxiety. In this panic state, the personality became disorganized, and primitive thinking and anxiety experiences emerged. One of Sullivan's major contributions was the viewpoint that schizophrenia could be treated with psychotherapy (Arieti, 1974, 24–29).

Carl Rogers, based on a 1967 study of the effects of therapists' degree of empathy in reducing pathological behavior in schizophrenia, describes accurate empathy as a potent force in bringing the client out of his social isolation and into personal relatedness. He quotes Jung in saying that the schizophrenic ceases to be schizophrenic when he meets someone by whom he feels understood (Rogers, 1975, 6).

Effects of the interpersonal milieu are further illustrated by Tudor's (1952, 1970) landmark nursing study which demonstrated the effect of mutual withdrawal (referring to the tendency of staff to avoid severely withdrawn clients) in main-taining pathological behavior. Peplau's interpersonal theory of nursing and many of her contributions to understanding and relating to schizophrenic clients are heavily influenced by Sullivan's interpersonal theory.

FAMILY THEORY

Lidz (1949, 1963, 1978) views schizophrenia as a severe disorganization in personality development and integration. In his view, healthy personality development occurs in a family context characterized by a parental coalition, appropriate generational boundaries, and adequate sex role socialization. Parents who have a complementary relationship promote this healthy socialization process by modeling sex roles, leadership, task accomplishment, and emotional competence. Unhealthy parental relationships lead to inconsistent and often irrational environments in which children may not learn appropriate social roles and reality testing. Two unhealthy patterns identified by Lidz (1957) are marital schism (chronic conflict and threat of separation) and skew (a relationship that maintains harmony through consistent domination of one partner by the other).

Most recently, Lidz (1978) addressed parental egocentrism and communication distortion as major influences that contribute to defective cognitive development and subsequent vulnerability to thought disorders. The egocentrism is described as an inability to distinguish boundaries between self and child and to differentiate between the person's own perceptions and needs and those of the child. The child is required to accommodate to reality based on the perceptions of others and becomes very parent centered. This distorts the developing sense of self and leads to disturbances in perceiving the degrees of control and influence that one person has over the thoughts and behavior of others. The developmental distortions are further reinforced by limited socialization outside the family.

In the 1950s, Bateson, Jackson, Haley, Satir, and others began to look at communication patterns in families of schizophrenic persons. Subsequently, faulty family communication was seen as contributing to, but not specifically causing, the ambivalence and interpersonal difficulties of these people.

Bateson and others described the double bind in which conflicting verbal and nonverbal messages by the sender leave the receiver of the mixed messages feeling confused and frustrated. A true double bind requires consistent repetition of this communication pattern and an underlying threat, such as loss of love, and must be an unavoidable situation (Bateson, 1956, 253–255). A case example of the double bind could be described as the relationship between Jason, age 6, and his widowed mother. To the casual observer, the mother seems very loving—always referring to Jason in endearing terms and frequently mentioning her constant love and sacrifice for her son. When Jason attempts to make physical contact by hugging her he is given the verbal message "You know how much Mommy loves her Jason" while being stiffly distanced by a gesture which holds him apart while superficially touching. The stiff posture and tight, cold tone of voice communicates a very different message from that of love. For the dependent member in this relationship (a child), the situation is inescapable. If it is a continuing behavior pattern on the mother's part and is perceived as threatening rejection, it has the components of a double bind.

Satir (1967, 186) describes a familial manner of handling conflict which she believes contributes to the disordered communication of the schizophrenic member. Rather than openly negotiating differences, one member may always strive to be agreeable despite his true feelings while another member excludes others' feelings by always disagreeing. The third role is that of the diverter (the schizophrenic role) who seeks to diffuse conflict by being irrelevant or by changing the subject. This irrelevant or "sick" communication is believed to help maintain the family system by defusing conflict.

Psychological impact in the family system is multigenerational and interactive. Children influence their siblings and parents and are influenced in turn by parents and siblings. These influences may be positive or negative, and the negative effects of one family member may be counteracted by the positive effects of another. Family roles must be flexible enough to accommodate the various needs and preferences of individual members who differ in age, sex, and physical and personality traits. Rigid or stereotyped roles tend to be maintained in families of schizophrenics (Singer, et al., 1978).

Whether or not family roles are a significant factor in the development of schizophrenia, the family as socialization and support system plays a vital role in the treatment plan for schizophrenic clients. At the very least, families require education, support, and coping strategies to promote

healthy development and to deal with the stresses of life for all of their members. The family with a schizophrenic member has additional needs and stresses which require thoughtful intervention if the family is to cope effectively and maximize personal growth in all members.

Wynne recommends that effective family intervention avoids blaming and psychodynamic interpretation and instead focuses on clear tasks for development of the social and communication skills of family members (Wynne, et al., 1978, 539–540).

PHYSICAL AND BIOLOGICAL ASPECTS

Organic and biological factors in the development of schizophrenia have been speculated upon since the disorder was first described. Since then research has been undertaken into the role of genetics, stress, abnormal metabolic processes, neurohormonal imbalance, and brain structure. This has resulted in many interesting findings, but the cause of schizophrenia remains a speculative blend of psychological and organic aspects. Mendel (1976, 76–77) discusses problems that affect such research, including lack of precise diagnosis, the question of including or excluding schizophreniform psychoses, and the need for greater replication of findings and better research designs.

Genetic research was summarized by Aultschuler (in Arieti, 1974) to calculate expectancies for the development of schizophrenia in the general population and in relatives of schizophrenics. The expectancy varies from 0.85 percent in the general population to 66 to 86 percent in monozygotic (identical) twins. The expectancy for siblings and dizygotic (fraternal) twins is similar, varying from 3 to 16 percent in different studies (Arieti, 1974, 446). These findings strongly suggest that although hereditary factors play a part in the development of schizophrenia, they cannot be the only, or in most cases, the primary factor involved. Since 14 to 34 percent of identical twins and 84 to 97 percent of siblings do not share the diagnosis, environmental influences must also be factors.

A neurohormonal model developed by Stern and Wise (in Mendel, 1976) is supported by some animal and human research. It is hypothesized that an enzyme deficiency involved in converting dopamine to norepinephrine may cause a buildup of toxic by-products which negatively affect the central nervous system (Mendel, 1976, 79). This model, like others that focus on the neurotransmitters nonepinephrine, dopamine, and serotonin, is consistent with the presumed mechanism of action of the antipsychotic drugs. These drugs make receptor sites less permeable to the neurotransmitters in four areas of the brain: (1) the reticular activating system, which monitors sensory input; (2) the limbic system and related areas concerned with emotion; (3) the hypothalamus, which affects response to sensory input; and (4) the areas producing extrapyramidal symptoms (Weiner, et al., 1979, 465). Additional attention has been focused on taraxein, a substance that Heath identified in the blood of schizophrenics (Rickelman, 1979, 30–31), deficient levels of the prostaglandin PGE1, and endorphins (Hopkins, 1980, 37). In the 1980s some experiments with hemodialysis to decrease schizophrenic symptoms are based on a toxin hypothesis. This research is currently inconclusive.

Stress as a factor in schizophrenia, with resulting central nervous system psychophysiological effects, has also been discussed by Jung and more recently by Arieti (1974, 485). Admission rates for schizophrenia vary widely according to particular social and demographic factors. In the United States, the highest rates of admission occur in industrialized areas (e.g., New York, Washington, D.C.) and the lowest rates in rural states (e.g., Kansas, Wyoming). This holds true in other countries as well. Widowed persons have three to five times the admission rates of married people. A majority of studies also indicate that immigration, migration, and membership in ethnic minority or socioeconomically disadvantaged groups increase expectancy rates (Arieti, 1974, 492–497). Changes in life-style, cultural traditions and values, the experience of poverty or discrimination, and loss of significant personal and social supports may all be considered significant stressors.

Multiple, complexly interrelated causes are most likely involved in the development of schizophrenia and schizophreniform disorders. A person may have a degree of genetic vulnerability and be confronted with stressors that exceed his adaptive capacity. The complex behavioral syndrome probably results from some common physiologically based occurrences and individualized psychodynamic responses. The current treatment approach to schizophrenia also addresses these various factors by combining long-term therapy with antipsychotic drugs, supportive psychother-apy, and client education in recognition and avoidance of unnecessary stress (Rogers, 1982).

DSM-III CATEGORIES

There is wide variation in the course and outcome of schizophrenia. Previous studies found that approximately a third of all clients have no personality deterioration or recurrence, another third have recurrences but function relatively well in remission, and a final third experience progressive deterioration and poor functioning (Pyke and Page, 1981, 39). Theorists have attempted to discriminate between the more acute or reactive form and the chronic or process form of schizophrenia. The former tends to have less hereditary association, a more highly functioning personality prior to onset of illness, and a better prognosis despite evidencing greater confusion and affective responses and very dramatic hallucinations (APA, 1980, 199). As previously mentioned, the distinction between schizophreniform psychosis and schizophrenia, which is important to researchers and to clinicians, is made on the basis of the duration of symptoms.

Further distinctions within the category of schizophrenic reactions are based on predominant behavior patterns. It is not unusual, however, for these diagnostic subtypes to vary in clients who have had several admissions over an extended period of time. To some extent this may reflect changes in dominant behaviors but may also reflect different emphases of diagnosticians. Table 34-1 enumerates the types of schizophrenic reactions and the behaviors associated with each type (APA, 1980, 190–193; Koontz, 1982).

Two additional categories of psychotic behavior were delineated. Schizoaffective psychosis describes affective symptoms existing in combination with other inconsistent features such as hallucinations and confusion. This term is used when behaviors and duration do not permit ready assignment to the designated schizophrenic types, to schizophreniform psychosis, or to the affective disorders. Paranoid disorders not categorized as schizophrenia include true paranoia and acute paranoid disorder. The prominent feature of these disorders is a fixed, well-organized delusional system with no related deterioration in thought processes or ability to function. These conditions are rare in relation to other mental disorders and much less commonly seen in hospitals. Severe stressors or onset of deafness may be related to the development of paranoid disorders (APA, 1980, 195, 202).

TABLE 34-1 Types of Schizophrenic Reactions

Types	Behaviors
Disorganized (formerly hebephrenic)	Incoherence Delusions, if present, are not systematized Affect is blunted, silly, or inappropriate
Catatonic	Severe changes in psychomotor activity (stupor or excitement) Negativism Posturing and stereotyped movements
Paranoid	Delusions of grandeur or persecution Related hallucinations may be present May have concerns about sexual identity or fears of homosexuality Angry, aloof, and argumentative behavior is common Later age of onset and more functional skills retained
Undifferentiated (formerly chronic undifferentiated)	Incoherent, disorganized behavior Delusions and/or hallucinations Does not fit other types or demonstrates a mixture of type behaviors
Residual	Continuation of symptoms such as flat affect, social withdrawal, and odd thought or behavior patterns following a schizophrenic episode Subcategory may indicate course of illness or absence of further symptoms (e.g., in remission)

Source: American Psychiatric Association *Diagnostic and statistical manual of mental disorders*, 3d ed. © 1980, A.P.A.

☐ Nursing Process

ASSESSMENT ☐ Components of comprehensive client assessment include: (1) current level of functioning in regard to physical and safety needs; (2) psychosocial needs and deficits; (3) prior levels of adjustment and functioning; (4) response to medical and nursing interventions; and (5) dis-missal planning needs. Related assessments which focus on the environmental system emphasize the family and social milieu of the client from a dual perspective: (1) as support system to the client and (2) as a distinct entity with dynamics, processes, and needs. Self-awareness dictates that the nurse assess her own attitudes, beliefs, and behaviors and their effects (or potential effects) on client care. Of special note is assessment of client strengths. Although this coverage may be assumed throughout the client assessment, it is easy for the nurse to be overwhelmed by immediate behavioral disturbances and overlook this vital component.

> ■ *Point of Emphasis*
>
> *To overlook the client's strengths is to omit vital keys in building an interpersonal bridge based on acceptance and empathy. Awareness of strengths helps the nurse avoid the destructive pattern of mutual withdrawal and provides access to real attributes that can be used to enhance client self-esteem.*

Client Assessment ☐ The individual who is experiencing a schizophrenic, schizophreniform, or paranoid disorder requires a comprehensive initial assessment in all dimensions of functioning, and continuous monitoring of any changes. Behaviors and areas of functional deficits vary widely among clients and may also change significantly in any given client over time.

Physical and safety needs are often priorities, particularly during psychotic episodes when perception and judgment are severely distorted. Side effects of pharmacotherapy are also important considerations. The ability of the client to maintain basic activities of daily living and meet bodily needs should be carefully monitored. The areas of general physical needs and related self-care deficits listed in Table 34-2 are useful for organizing assessments in this category.

Thought disorders are common problems that occur in schizophrenia and schizophreniform disorders. Table 34-3 lists common problems and the related behaviors as a guide to assessment and identification of thought disorders.

Psychosocial needs incorporate Maslow's (1970) higher order needs for self-esteem, love and belonging, and self-actualization. These needs are profoundly affected by developmental and socio-

TABLE 34-2 *Assessment of Self-Care Deficits in Physical and Safety Needs*

General needs	Observations
Oxygenation	Monitor vital signs for evidence of side effects of antipsychotic drug therapy: postural hypotension, tachycardia, and cardiac arrhythmias.
Fluid and nutrient intake	Is the client able to feed himself? Is mealtime behavior appropriate to social dining or should meals be served separately with staff supervision? Is fluid intake adequate to prevent dehydration (generally 2400 cc)? Is caloric intake appropriate to size and activity level? Suspiciousness or preoccupation may prevent adequate intake. Antipsychotic drugs may increase appetite, leading to obesity. Weekly weighing and daily recording of fluid and food intake are important for clients with potential or actual problems in this area.
Balance in rest and activity levels	Is the client achieving adequate rest and physical activity? In catatonic schizophrenia, activity may vary from none (in stupor) to exhaustive hyperactivity (in excitement). Is hyperactivity or suspiciousness impairing sleep? Motor activity may be affected by antipsychotic drugs.
Sensory and cognitive perception	Are thought or perceptual disturbances (e.g., hallucinations, delusions, looseness of associations) present? Orientation is generally intact although the client may believe himself to be a famous person. Is the client able to interpret and respond appropriately to environmental stimuli and reality? Does the client respond with distress to particular stimuli?
Urinary and bowel elimination	Elimination should be carefully recorded to observe for: (1) urinary retention (which may be related to catatonic negativism or to autonomic nervous system effects of antipsychotic drugs in clients with prostatic hypertrophy); (2) constipation (secondary to autonomic effects of drugs and/or diet and reduced activity). Is the client able to attend to elimination needs without supervision or assistance? Clients exhibiting feelings of depersonalization may hoard or conceal elimination products, and those with severely regressed behavior may be incontinent or involuntary, or may engage in fecal smearing.
Hygiene and appearance	Is the client capable of meeting own needs for personal hygiene, grooming, and dressing appropriately? Does the individual have particular beliefs or fears that interfere with bathing? Is supervision and tactful redirection needed to assure an acceptable appearance?
Sexuality	Does the client show any evidence of concerns or bizarre ideas related to sexual identity? Is the client experiencing any side effects of pharmacotherapy that alter sexual function or identity (e.g., altered libido, male gynecomastia and ejaculatory inhibition, female menstrual irregularities and lactation based on endocrine effects of antipsychotic drugs)?
Personal safety	Does the individual's view of reality or prior behavior indicate a potential for impulsive acts that might result in harm to self or others? Do "voices" accuse, threaten, or direct the client toward impulsive actions? Assess for adverse reactions and side effects of pharmacotherapy.

TABLE 34-3 Thought Disorders: Illustrative Problems

Thought Problem	Illustration
Concreteness	Literal meaning and inability to abstract. *Example*: In response to an inquiry about the meaning of the phrase "People in glass houses shouldn't throw stones," a concrete response might be "glass breaks."
Delusions (e.g., influence, control, grandeur, persecution, somatic)	Fixed false beliefs, not culturally based, which are not altered in response to facts or reasoning. *Example* (grandiose delusion): 23-YEAR-OLD CLIENT: I'm the master builder, I've built the local post office, the museum, and this hospital. Other: But this hospital is 50 years old—it's older than you are. Client: The master builder is ageless and timeless.
Blocking speech	Loss of train of thought in midsentence and inability to continue.
Poverty of speech (and ideas)	Vague speech with little real information conveyed.
Neologisms	"Made-up" words with meaning only to the individual.
Tangentiality	Thoughts or speech veer off on a "tangent" or sidetrack.
Stereotyped speech	Reverting to or persevering on the same idea over and over.

cultural aspects of life experience. Because these components are important in the development of ego strength they are related, in part, to psychodynamic issues in the development and expression of schizophrenia. On the other hand, the experience of a schizophrenic episode itself also creates the stigma of major mental illness and has an effect on self-esteem, self-concept, and the perceptions of others. Table 34-4 presents a guide for assessment of psychosocial needs.

Self-concept includes the sense of self and self-esteem. Both are affected in schizophrenia and schizophreniform psychoses. The sense of self is formed early in life as the infant learns to differentiate between inner perceptions and external persons and objects. The loss in some schizophrenics of this ability to differentiate is termed "loss of ego boundaries" and is believed to be related to severe regression (Randels, et al. 1982, 339). Development and level of self-esteem are based in large part on the reflected appraisals of significant others. This was discussed earlier as an assumption of Sullivan's interpersonal theory. The schizophrenic client, whom Jung described as generally introverted in personality, perceives social relationships as threatening and fears rejection. This further reinforces self-doubts, social isolation, and feelings of ineptness. Lack of motivation and difficulty in deriving pleasure from activities generally considered enjoyable are termed anhedonia (Randels, et al. 1982, 339).

Others have noted the tendency of many schizophrenics to have very high goals but to be unable to initiate the most basic activity toward accomplishing them. For example, a very bright young man who was diagnosed as having paranoid type schizophrenia talked often about his desire to become a lawyer and politician. He had dropped out of high school several years previously and had not yet followed through on the social worker's plan to help him pass a high school equivalency test. This gross disparity between ideal and reality is painfully devastating to self-esteem.

Although denial of mental illness is a common response to schizophrenia by clients, awareness of the fact of hospitalization and the thought disorders experienced must have an effect on self-esteem whether the client acknowledges mental illness or not. Low self-esteem and disturbances in self-perception are key issues in schizophrenia. Some clients are aware of their feelings of low self-esteem while others desperately defend against it via grandiosity and self-delusion.

Interpersonal relatedness is a basic human need. Maslow has described this as the need for love and belongingness. In schizophrenia, schizophreniform disorders, and paranoid states there is a tendency to withdraw interest and involvement from the external social world and to refocus inwardly on one's own fantasy preoccupations and view of the world. This is referred to as autistic or withdrawn behavior. Readiness for and level of social interaction should be carefully assessed. Is the client anxious and seclusive in any social setting? Can he tolerate one-to-one interaction but not that of a social group? Can the client initiate social interaction? Clients may passively avoid others by remaining alone in their room, seeking or pretending to engage in solitary pursuits such as napping, reading, TV viewing, or pacing. When others attempt to join them or engage them in conversation, they may respond only superficially and often find excuses to leave the social setting.

Some, most commonly those exhibiting paranoid characteristics, may actively distance others through adopting an aloof, superior manner and threatening the self-esteem or security of others. This may be through a forbidding or piercing look and haughty air, threats such as "He who approaches me will be struck down" or more sophisticated verbal insults. The latter form of distancing is illustrated by a situation in which two students, both new to the psychiatric setting, were attempting to socialize with a middle-aged client. He seemed a bit grandiose but generally sociable

---

TABLE 34-4 General Psychosocial Need Assessment

Need	Observations
Self-concept and esteem Sense of self	Is the client able to differentiate clearly between self and other and realistically evaluate limits of influence by self and other (e.g., absence of ideas of being controlled by external events or fears of losing self by giving up personal possessions or excretions)? How does the client perceive himself? (e.g., grandiosely, realistically, or grossly distorted—such as seeing self as an animal when looking in a mirror)?
Self-esteem	What is the view of self in relationship to goals vs. achievements? Is there evidence of defenses against low self-esteem (e.g., delusions of grandeur or projecting responsibility)? What is the client's perception of his illness and its effects (e.g., denial, resignation, feeling stigmatized, acceptance and coping)? What are the client's strengths (and does he perceive these strengths)?
Love and belonging Interpersonal relatedness	What is the client's level of social interaction (e.g., avoidance, superficiality, acceptance of a few trusted people)? How effectively does the client communicate? (Identified special assets and problem areas.) What is the client's social history (e.g., school, work, peer relationships)?
Family or social group support	Who is the client's identified family and/or group? What is the family attitude toward the client's illness? What are family strengths and liabilities? Are there supportive others able to lend assistance to the client and/or family?
Cultural impact	Are there significant socioeconomic or cultural variables likely to affect care and recovery (e.g., overall beliefs and attitudes toward mental illness, likelihood of seeking/complying with care, access to quality care)? What cultural values are significant in client and family coping attitudes? View of etiology (e.g., stress, "bad blood," a curse or trial from God, a disease to be cured by medication). Expectation for recovery (e.g., fatalism vs. active efforts, optimism vs. pessimism, realistic vs. unrealistic views). Culture/community acceptance. (Is the client and/or family to be stigmatized or supported? Is recovery and acceptance expected?) What community supports are needed by the client and family (e.g., aftercare, vocational training)?

until after a brief interaction, he rose, saying: "I see why you've come to me. You believe I'm a wizard. One of you has no body and the other no brain. I'll see what I can do for you." After leaving them like that, he had quite effectively created a reluctance in both to approach him again and risk further critique of their appearance or intelligence.

In addition to differing in the amount of social interaction engaged in, withdrawn clients vary in the depth of social interaction that can be readily developed. Because of their basic mistrust and the expectation of rejection, it is particularly difficult to build and terminate relationships with withdrawn clients. These clients engage in avoidance and testing manuevers to determine the nurse's sincerity and commitment to the relationship to a much greater extent than do other clients. The issue of termination in the therapeutic one-to-one relationship may be distorted into feelings of rejection and avoided in an attempt to deny painful feelings and any reawakening of related feelings of loss and rejection from the past. Friendships are commonly superficial or nonexistent. In assessing significant social relationships, the nurse needs to explore the nature of the reported friendship. The following exchanges illustrate how misleading a superficial assessment may be.

> NURSE A: Have you had any friends, Mark?
>
> MARK: Yeah, sure.
>
> NURSE A: Would you tell me a bit about them?
>
> MARK: A bunch of guys in high school and Joe from when I was in the Navy.
>
> NURSE A: And did you see a lot of them?
>
> MARK: Yeah, just about every day.

If Nurse A assumes on the basis of this exchange that Mark has had and maintains close social relationships, she would be mistaken and would fail to identify a significant problem of isolation. Consider the information elicited by Nurse B in exploring this topic.

> NURSE B: Can you describe any important friendships you've had, Mark?
>
> MARK: In high school and the Navy.
>
> NURSE B: Can you tell me about your high school friends?
>
> MARK: They were in my homeroom.
>
> NURSE B: Who was in your homeroom?
>
> MARK: The guys in my homeroom, they were friends.

> NURSE B: What kinds of things did you do with these friends?
>
> MARK: Oh . . . went to class. Sometimes I'd sit with them in the cafeteria.
>
> NURSE B: Did you go to school activities or parties with them?
>
> MARK: I didn't like parties. . . .
>
> NURSE B: You mentioned a friend in the Navy; who was that?
>
> MARK: His name was Joe.
>
> NURSE B: Tell me a little about Joe.
>
> MARK: He had the bunk next to mine. Sometimes we'd go on shore leave if he didn't have a girl with him.
>
> NURSE B: Have you kept in touch with Joe since you left the Navy five years ago?
>
> MARK: No.
>
> NURSE B: Would you say there are any people you're friendly with now?
>
> MARK: I'm friendly to anybody; I just don't go places much.
>
> NURSE B: Is there anyone you like to talk to?
>
> MARK: No, I'm not much of a talker—I guess you'd call me a loner.

Another problem in social relatedness is the tendency of withdrawn, autistic clients to communicate in vague, confusing, and symbolic terms. The client may use neologisms ("made-up" words) which have meaning only to him. The client may engage the nurse in highly abstract, often illogical discussions of obscure religious, philosophical, or political ideas. Delusional clients may describe elaborate plots or conspiracies by mysterious others complete with coincidences and loosely connected "proofs." These kinds of discussions leave the nurse confused and feeling that little was gained by the interaction, which suggests a need for attention to client communication patterns.

Assessment of developmental issues such as Erikson's (1963) core problems can provide valuable insights into client behavior. Table 34-5 illustrates use of core problems as an assessment framework.

The social history is best obtained from both the client and family. Significant elements that should be included are a description of the client's usual personality prior to any observable illness, major life events and client responses, significant stressors, and a description of the behavior and any known precipitants that led to the decision to seek psychiatric assistance. Major life events include birth (any unusual factors), siblings and

TABLE 34-5 Erikson's Core Issues and Relevant Problems of Schizophrenic Clients

Core Issues	Assess for Behavioral Indicators of
Trust vs. mistrust	Interpersonal anxiety and avoidance Expectation of rejection Paranoid ideas and delusions
Autonomy vs. shame and doubt	Low self-esteem Grandiosity as a defense against low self-esteem Loss of ego boundaries Delusions of controlling the fate of others Delusions of being controlled by others (e.g., via TV insertion of thoughts)
Initiative vs. guilt	Lack of realistic goals or goal-directed efforts
Industry vs. inferiority	Extreme gap between desired and real attainments due to lack of goal-directed activity
Identity vs. diffusion	Identity may be significantly influenced (stigmatized) by label of mental illness or schizophrenia. Goals and energies may be sporadic and diffuse. May select a pseudo or autistic identity rather than one based on reality.
Intimacy vs. isolation	Difficulties in trust and identity make true intimacy difficult or unattainable. May be a "loner." Narcissism, autism, and fear of rejection contribute to social isolation.
Generativity vs. stagnation and integrity vs. despair	Personality and ability to function may deteriorate. Even in remission, the client may live a flat, colorless, isolated existence.

cial skills; interests (for example leisure pursuits such as sports, reading, music) on which to build social contact and interaction; talents or achievements, such as artistic expression or the ability to hold a job, that provide opportunities for recognition and enhance self-esteem. Unless the nurse is able to recognize the person's strengths, it is highly unlikely that she will value the client as a unique individual—which is important in promoting the client's ability to recognize his own strengths and to value self.

> **■ Point of Emphasis**
>
> *Both client problems and client strengths are essential components of assessment.*

Family and Environment Assessment □ The immediate setting and the client's family and customary environment should be evaluated for potential stressors and opportunities to support therapeutic interaction and growth. The immediate environment may be a general hospital setting, a psychiatric unit, or an outpatient facility. (Refer to Chapter 14 on therapeutic milieu for a discussion of general assessment factors.) Specific aspects to consider for clients with schizophrenic, schizophreniform, and paranoid disorders include: (1) the fit between the environment and the client's needs for safety and security, social interaction, activity, and achievement; and (2) opportunities for developing coping skills. See Table 34-6 for a list of environmental assessments.

The family and home environment assessment begins with eliciting what constitutes family for the client. It may be the family of origin, a couple dyad, a nuclear family, an extended family, a community of voluntary members, residents of a halfway house, or some residents in a transient hotel. Once the client's definition of family is established, his opinion should be elicited as to how the family perceives him and perceives his illness, and how family members may be of assistance to him. Significant members of the client's family should be included in the family assessment.

The family assessment has a dual focus: family as a system and family as support system to the client. (See Chapter 12 on family dynamics for a discussion of assessment of the family as a system.) In assessing the family as client support system, one obtains members' perceptions of the

family position (including a description of relationships with siblings), school history (last grade completed, type of student, how the client felt about school), peer relationships (number and quality of friendships, dating, and sexual relationships), and work history (type of jobs, length of time held, relationship with employers, coworkers, feelings about work).

Client strengths should be assessed in a comprehensive way. They may include attributes such as intelligence, wit, sense of humor, and so-

TABLE 34.6 Immediate Hospital Environment or Setting Assessment Factors

Client Need	Setting Assessment Factors
Safety and protection (Is the client disorganized, impulsive, out of contact with reality?)	Is staffing adequate to provide one consistent person who can supervise, channel activities, and present reality? Are hazardous objects controlled and inaccessible? Is there a secluded or quiet area available if needed to reduce stimuli?
Meaningful activity (Is boredom or inactivity a problem?)	Is the environment dull, monotonous, and unstimulating? Are materials available to complete meaningful tasks (e.g., handicrafts, needlework, writing, drawing) to counteract the client's tendency to withdraw into fantasy?
Appropriate level of socialization	
Is the client anxious in all interactive situations?	Is sufficient time available to develop a one-to-one relationship?
Is one-to-one interaction tolerated with selected individuals?	Do trusted individuals use the environment therapeutically to assist the client to interact with a wider circle of people?
Is client behavior and level of social interaction appropriate to group placement?	Is a supportive group available to enhance the client's group tolerance and learning opportunities?
Coping skills (Has the client sufficient insight to recognize and confront common life problems to be faced on return to the community?)	Can the setting make available a variety of individualized and group approaches for coping with anxiety, stress recognition and management, social skill development, job training and support, medication monitoring, and situational crises?

sistance, coping strategies, and respite care (assistance in caring for the schizophrenic member during times of family crisis or to permit a vacation for the caretaker). Schizophrenia, by definition a chronic illness, will make long-term demands on families' physical and emotional resources. Community support can have a valuable role in assisting families to cope, but the type and availability of community assistance vary widely.

Self-Assessment □ Withdrawn and suspicious clients pose some very real challenges to the nurse. The avoidance and rejection of the nurse's attempts to form a relationship may be painful and frustrating. Nurses who have a need for either immediate results or personal acceptance may find this group of clients particularly difficult. On the other hand, nurses who can acknowledge the feelings engendered in the self by the client's rejection are in a better position to understand the threat posed to the client by the possibility of rejection. The need for patience is evident as one must slowly go about the task of winning the client's trust.

The nurse may experience real concerns about personal safety when confronted with an acutely psychotic and disorganized client. Discussion of these fears with the clinical instructor or other staff nurses will assist in evaluating the overall potential of the client for impulsive and assaultive behavior. Awareness of and adherence to safety procedures (as outlined in policy manuals) will help assure staff and client safety.

Additional painful feelings may be engendered if there are aspects of the client with which the nurse identifies such as significant age, interests, or experiences. These feelings may interfere with objectivity in viewing the client or may arouse specific fears of the illness in the nurse. These feelings may pose real barriers to therapeutic effectiveness; they suggest a need for consultation. The student should discuss these issues with the clinical instructor, while staff nurses may discuss them with a peer, the nursing supervisor, or another member of the mental health team.

Once a trusting relationship is established dependency needs of clients may pose a particular dilemma for the nurse. The goals of the therapeutic relationship include meeting dependency needs while promoting independence in the client. This is particularly important to the schizophrenic client who may interpret attempts to re-

client and his problems. How do members feel they may be of assistance to the client? What kinds of assistance does the family need in order to continue a supportive relationship with the client? For some families this may be a need for information and for opportunities to discuss their feelings. For others it may entail financial as-

duce dependency as rejection. Just as with the related problems presented in termination, the feelings and issues need to be recognized and discussed.

Mutual withdrawal was first identified by Tudor (1952, 1970) as a problem in working with withdrawn schizophrenic clients. The client's withdrawal was frequently reinforced by staff members' withdrawal from the client. This withdrawal tended to occur without staff awareness of their avoidance of significant interpersonal interactions with the client, and was frequently rationalized as being due to the client's hopelessness or preference for isolation. Marram (1969) discussed the sources of anxiety and related defenses associated with mutual withdrawal. Citing Menzies (1960), she delineated several sources of threat to nurses that led to avoidance. Those that commonly occur in relating to clients who demonstrate withdrawal and suspiciousness include contact with suffering, uncertain prognosis, arousal of strong or ambivalent feelings (e.g., guilt), identifying with stress in family members or colleagues, and fear of the disease itself. Defenses used include depersonalizing the client (responding to the "label," not the unique person), detaching and denying personal feelings, performing care in a ritualistic or routinized manner, avoiding accountability for client care by splitting up the one-to-one relationship, vagueness in terms of responsibilities and decision making, and reluctance to change.

■ *Point of Emphasis*

Mutual withdrawal is a nursing problem that can inhibit the building of relatedness to the client.

Self-awareness becomes essential for the nurse's professional growth and for monitoring the responses of nurses to individual clients. Clients who are most likely to experience avoidance or withdrawal by nurses are those most vulnerable to its effects—the withdrawn clients.

PROBLEM AND NEED IDENTIFICATION □

Client Problems □ Analysis of accumulated data results in identification of significant actual and potential client problems. Three aspects are basic to this analysis. First, it is important to recognize that even though the client's diagnosis is

a psychiatric condition, priority problems in an acute psychotic episode often relate to basic physical and safety needs. Second, the etiology of one problem may also constitute a separate problem in itself. For instance, communication difficulties such as mutism or vagueness are related to the client's social withdrawal and isolation (which in turn are caused by the underlying problem of low self-esteem). Third, not all problematic psychiatric behaviors (symptoms) are appropriately stated as individual problems. Although it is not wrong to define problems at a very specific level such as delusional thoughts or neglect of personal hygiene and appearance, it is preferable to group problems in related concepts. Several symptoms may be related to one overall problem. Grouping them permits a more comprehensive approach to goal formulation and intervention. In addition to delusional thinking, the problem of thought disorders may encompass related problems of reality distortion and loose associations. Similarly, the client with problems in appearance may also be experiencing self-care deficits in related areas such as nutrition and hygiene. This approach is suggested as a means of avoiding the confusion and fragmentation of dealing with twelve or more separate problems.

Physical problems are most commonly related to severely disorganized behavior, thought disturbances, and side effects of antipsychotic drug therapy. Table 34-2 lists physical needs and observations for common interferences.

In general, there are two basic, long-term problems associated with schizophrenia and schizophreniform disorders: (1) intolerance of and diminished capacity to cope with stress and anxiety; and (2) low self-esteem. From these overall problems flow the related problems of thought and perception, impulse control, social withdrawal and isolation, communication, and self-care. (Figure 34-1 depicts these problems and groups of related symptoms.) The stress and self-esteem problems are also interrelated, reinforcing each other.

Sedgewick (1975, 20–23) described several responses to stress, which include decreased clarity of thought, difficulties in task mastery, impaired decision-making and problem-solving ability, heightened focus on self, diminished environmental awareness, and decreased sense of personal competence. Low self-esteem both increases the degree of stress perceived and is an outcome of the stress responses described. Most people can identify with the experience of some of these identified stress responses. The schizophrenic client's vul-

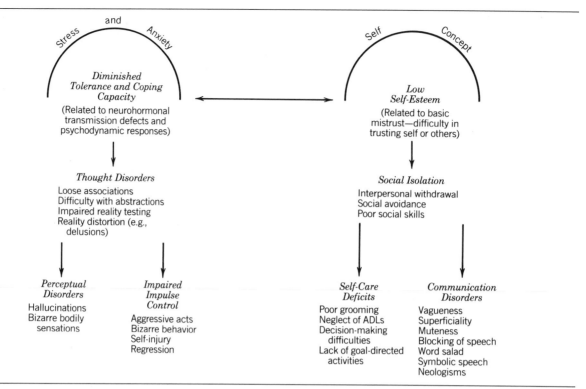

Figure 34-1 *Common problems occurring in schizophrenic clients.*

nerabilities in these areas exaggerate the general functional disorganization to crisis proportions.

Validation of the problem is not always directly possible by means of client acknowledgment or laboratory results. Sometimes the problem is identified on the basis of the absence of a generally accepted need. Maslow has identified basic needs of love and belonging and self-esteem. The schizophrenic client may deny that he has any interest or need for social acceptance and interaction, but knowledge of human needs validates that the absence of a supportive social group is a problem. Similarly, the client who believes himself to be a savior or superman would not initially recognize the problem of low self-esteem, yet to built one's identity on a fantasy is evidence of a negative self-concept. The nurse initially may need to rely heavily on observation, theory, and consensual validation from others such as family or nursing staff to verify the accuracy of nursing diagnosis.

Family Problems □ Family Problems and needs may be identified in the family system, in relationship to coping with the client's problems, or both of these areas. Problems in the family system are discussed in Chapter 12 on family dynamics and will not be repeated here, although the nurse will apply this knowledge in working with families who have a schizophrenic member. The emphasis in this chapter is on the family or social group which is coping with the experience of a schizophrenic or schizophreniform disorder. The problems of coping fall into the general areas of: (1) understanding the condition, client problems and need for support, and available resources; (2) acceptance of the client and diagnosis; and (3) role maintenance in a long-term or chronic situation.

Families may attempt to deny the client's illness, feeling that to acknowledge major mental illness brings shame. Some families may hold the client responsible for the illness while others may blame themselves. Feelings of hopelessness, anger, and fear for the client's future and the demands to be made on family members are common.

Knowledge is a basic need. The public's awareness of schizophrenia is limited and individuals may believe a variety of myths and misinformation. Families also need to understand how they can assist and support the client who is in remission, various treatment approaches and their importance to client well-being, and availability of support services in the community.

Emotional acceptance of the diagnosis may be difficult and requires time. The stigma of mental illness may create feelings of shame. Awareness of the possibility of genetic factors may increase fears and feelings of vulnerability about mental illness in family members. Parents, spouses, or children may blame themselves or each other for the client's emotional problems. The need to support the client and tolerate inappropriate or socially unacceptable behavior can cause resentment and subsequent guilt. The need to observe the client for deteriorating mental status and protect him from potential impulsive behavior while trying to retain a supportive and healthy family environment for all members can be difficult and emotionally draining.

Role maintenance issues need to be considered since hospitalizations, even in acute schizophreniform disorders, may be relatively lengthy (e.g., 30 days or more). In schizophrenia, there is also the likelihood of some residual effects and readmissions. Relationships between spouses or children may be disrupted by behavioral changes and period of hospitalization. Task roles ordinarily implemented by the hospitalized client will be neglected and must be assumed by others. If this happens often enough or for a prolonged time period, return of those roles to the client may be overlooked or difficult to accomplish. Significant role relinquishments such as those of breadwinner or parent may pose real burdens to other members who are assigned the tasks. It is also possible that tasks will be inappropriately redistributed (e.g., to members already overburdened or to those too immature to assume the needed degree of responsibility). A variety of needs in the family as a whole and in individual members may be disrupted by the client's illness.

> ■ *Point of Emphasis*
> *Families need information and emotional support.*

INTERVENTION □ Comprehensive nursing intervention involves establishing trust and relatedness through a therapeutic relationship, furthering the long-range treatment plan (generally supportive therapy and antipsychotic pharmaco-

therapy), and providing interdisciplinary and environmental assistance at all levels of prevention. These interventions involve focusing on the client's needs and problems, and coordinating the contributions of various disciplines (e.g., physicians, therapists, social workers). Although these approaches are discussed separately, it is important to note that they may and should be used concurrently and interactively depending on the client's needs and progress. Table 34-7 presents a sample nursing process for a schizophrenic client.

Client-Focused Intervention □ The key dilemma of the schizophrenic client involves an approach-avoidance conflict in which the human need for interpersonal warmth and relatedness is pitted against the fear and expectation of painful rejection. The symbolism of a campfire on a cold night is occasionally alluded to by clients who discuss their feelings of being cold and alone as they hold themselves back, knowing that going too close will mean "getting burned." This basic anxiety generated by interpersonal contacts must be kept in mind as the nurse or therapist attempts to build a relationship. Slow progress and frequent testing of the nurse's interest and sincerity are to be expected with these clients.

The primary instrument for establishing trust and interpersonal relatedness is the therapeutic relationship. Arieti, Sullivan, Fromm-Reichman, Tudor, and others have identified this as the first-priority psychosocial goal and approach. (Physical needs may, however, have temporary priority for survival and safety.)

Ruditis (1979) describes some key elements related to establishing trust: (1) one must show continuous interest and commitment to the client over a period of time (this may be prolonged in the case of schizophrenic client); (2) the nurse must be honest and trusting in self in order to generate confidence and credibility. This honesty or genuineness is related to the nurse's self-awareness and self-acceptance. The sense of credibility comes from the client's feeling that the work they do together will be of benefit. The nurse must consistently demonstrate through words and actions that she is trustworthy and truly cares about the client. Arieti (1974) also notes the importance of not being intrusive or making demands that further increase anxiety and withdrawal in the early, pretrust phase of the relationship. Several therapists (e.g., Rosen, Arieti) have used therapeutic assistants to build this kind of relationship, and the primary beneficial

TABLE 34-7 Sample Nursing Process Schizophrenic Reaction, Catatonic Type

Situation/Data Base:

Caroline Garr, age 22, was admitted to a locked psychiatric unit accompanied by her parents (with whom she lives) and a deputy sheriff. She was previously admitted two years ago following a broken engagement and was diagnosed as exhibiting schizophreniform disorder at that time.

She is disheveled; has significant body odor, and is wearing torn, mismatched, and soiled clothing. Speech is rapid and loosely associated, and echolalia is present. She assumes bizarre body poses and darts impulsively about, grasping at bystanders, spinning in a circle, and moving objects from place to place. Her parents state that she has been agitated for three days; eating and sleeping little, hearing "voices" and "harsh laughter." She is a part-time bookkeeping student at a community college and works part time as a grocery checker. Her mother describes her as shy and quiet and says she is generally alone when not working or in school. When the admitting nurse approaches Caroline, the latter laughs inappropriately and spins away from her.

The following care plan is appropriate to this immediate phase of illness and hospitalization. As these goals are met, the nursing process will refocus on intermediate and long-range goals prior to dismissal and aftercare in the community.

Problem:	Nutritional impairment (inadequate intake of nutrients and fluids) related to hyperactivity, behavioral disorganization, and self-care deficits.
Goal:	Caroline will improve her nutritional intake and hydration status.

Intervention	Rationale	Evaluation
Record intake and output and describe items eaten and amounts to measure caloric count. Record weight weekly.	Accurate records are essential for assessment and evaluation of adequacy and dietary balance.	Short-term criteria for adequate daily intake might include a minimum of 1800 calories representing Basic Four food groups and a fluid intake of 2400 cc.
Offer a variety of foods and fluids frequently and in small amounts. Include items that can be carried or eaten "on the run" (e.g., fresh fruits, sandwiches, malts); six small meals may be substituted for the usual three.	Short attention span and hyperactivity need to be considered in promoting intake.	Adequate hydration status is evidenced by good skin turgor and moist mucous membranes.
Incorporate client food preferences based on client and family report.	Food likes and dislikes must be taken into account to promote intake.	Long-range evidence of nutritional adequacy includes absence of both weight loss and signs of nutritional deficiency.

Problem:	Sleep and rest pattern impairment related to hyperactivity and excessive anxiety.
Goal:	Caroline will improve her rest and sleep pattern.

Intervention	Rationale	Evaluation
Plan restful, nonstimulating activities prior to retirement. Administer prn medication in early evening to control anxiety and activity level. Identify client preference for relaxing HS activities (e.g., warm bath, backrub, music) to enhance affects of HS sedation. Remove client to an environment that is less stimulating for rest periods and assess the effects of quietly remaining with the client with or without conversation and merely checking on her.	Hyperactivity and anxiety, if permitted to build, lead to further increases in activity. Interruption of the cycle promotes needed rest and prevents potential exhaustion. Interventions to promote rest and relaxation need to be individualized to the client.	Short-term criteria for adequate sleep would address client report and staff observation of client sleeping for her usual number of hours (generally 6–8). Observation of rest periods (sedentary or quiet activity) taken during the day would indicate interruption of hyperactivity and lessen the potential for exhaustion.

TABLE 34-7 (*continued*)

| Problem: | Cognitive process and sensory perception impairment (thought disorders and hallucinations) related to excessive anxiety and possibly neurohormonal transmission dysfunction under stress. |
| Goal: | Caroline will decrease anxiety level, hallucinations, and thought disorganization. |

Intervention	Rationale	Evaluation
Provide consistent reassurance and assistance in testing and interpreting reality and the environment via a consistent one-to-one staff assignment (e.g., "I don't hear voices and laughter" "The people in the corner of the room are enjoying a card game").	Anxiety distorts the perceptual field leading to misinterpretation of environmental cues. Misinterpretation may lead to fears, agitation, and impulsive actions. If the anxious person engages in seeking help from a variety of sources, the responses may be fragmented and inconsistent and may further increase client confusion and agitation.	Decreased anxiety level would be evidenced by self-report of fewer "voices" and staff observation of decreased episodes of hallucinating and agitation.
Communicate in clear, simple, concrete terms.	The nurse should not reinforce the client's distorted view of reality.	Criteria for improvement in disorder of thoughts would address a decrease in thought blocking and loose associations.
Promote simple, supervised, reality-based activities to focus client attention and activity (e.g., a walk with staff, crafts such as finger painting or clay sculpting, exercising to music, or occupational therapy tasks related to basic living skills).	Activities should be selected based on client interest and ability to focus attention.	

| Problem: | Communication impairment (use of symbolic, vague, and unusual terms) related to anxiety and autistic withdrawal. |
| Goal: | Caroline will improve her communication. |

Intervention	Rationale	Evaluation
Role-model effective communication. (Clarity, directness, use of consensual validation, sharing of thoughts and perceptions regarding the one to one relationship [e.g., "You seem very distant and quiet today. Have I done something to make you feel angry?"])	Effective nurse-client interaction involves exchange of information and empathic understanding.	Short-term criteria (individualized to client) would relate to ability to express needs in a comprehensible manner. This would include a decrease in symbolic or loosely associated speech.
If unsure of client message, do not assume or pretend to understand.		Long-term evidence would include more complex criteria such as (a) the ability to identify feelings and describe experiences and (2) use of consensual validation to verify own perception (as receiver) and check accuracy of other's understanding (as sender).
Use clarification techniques to encourage the client to communicate more clearly.	Clarification techniques assist the client to be more clear and descriptive. Assisting the client to clarify communication will enhance her ability to relate to others.	
Validate understanding of message by rephrasing it and asking client confirmation.		

(*continued*)

TABLE 34-7 (*continued*)

Problem:	Self-care deficit (poor hygiene and grooming) secondary to behavioral disorganization and regression.
Goal:	Caroline will improve self-care and appearance.

Intervention	Rationale	Evaluation
Assess for any additional causes for poor hygiene (e.g., fears related to showering, special significance of clothing choices).	Body image and sexual identity confusion may underlie hygiene and elimination problem.	Criteria for self-care would address increasing the number of self-care tasks that the client independently accomplishes from week to week (e.g., eat a meal, take a shower daily without reminders, maintain hair care and dress appropriately).
Assist and provide reassurance as needed to assure hygiene and appearance.	Poor hygiene and appearance tend to reinforce social isolation and low self-esteem.	Long-term goal would be independent performance of all activities of daily living at an acceptable level (specific to problem and need).
Positively reinforce self-care action to enhance personal hygiene and appearance.	Positive reinforcement increases the likelihood that self-care actions will increase.	

Problem:	Social isolation related to mistrust, fear of rejection, and subsequent social withdrawal behavior.
Goal:	Caroline will develop a beginning trust relationship with her primary nurse.

Intervention	Rationale	Evaluation
Primary nurse will seek out the client on a daily basis to indicate awareness, interest, and desire to be her nurse.	The nurse must consistently demonstrate interest and acceptance to win the client's trust. Client fear/expectation of rejection makes trust difficult and "testing" of nurse likely. Consistency of approach by staff can promote the relationship. Because of the anticipation of rejection, the nurse must avoid making initial demands on the client that would increase anxiety and possibly be misinterpreted as a rejection.	Criteria for trust relationships with the primary nurse would include acknowledging the primary nurse as "my nurse," initiating requests and conversation with the primary nurse, voluntarily spending time in daily activity with the primary nurse (30–60 minutes per day), and increased eye contact.
During episodes of disorganization and overactivity, other staff will channel questions and activities to the primary nurse for consistency and reassurance of approach.		
One-to-one approach will be warm, accepting, supportive, and undemanding.		
Client tolerance for interaction in both one-to-one and social activities on the unit will be carefully assessed and activities gradually increased as tolerance permits.		
The nurse will monitor own feelings and responses to avoid potential problem of mutual withdrawal.	Mutual withdrawal may occur because of nurse avoidance based on own discomfort with client behavior.	

characteristics appear to be warmth and nurturance.

Behaviors in the nurse or therapist that can promote trust are all-encompassing but can be illustrated by some basic examples. The nurse should not break a promise to the client since even the smallest breach of agreement may reinforce his distrust. If the nurse must be late for or miss a scheduled appointment, the client should be notified ahead of time and given an explanation. Extremely withdrawn clients who do not respond to verbal overtures may respond to nonverbal gestures such as offering to share food (an apple or a sweet) or to the use of touch. Touch, however, should be used with caution since the acutely guarded and suspicious person may perceive it as sexually or aggressively threatening. The withdrawn and silent person should not be pressured to speak or bombarded with probing questions. The sensitive nurse will remain with the client and assess his reaction to silent companionship and one-sided discussions by the nurse on neutral topics that do not demand responses. The client who is acutely uncomfortable in a structured social conversational setting may be less anxious and more open being with the nurse in an active setting such as taking a walk, preparing food or tables for a meal, or weeding a flower bed. Using simple, concise, direct statements (e.g., "I can see that you're frightened, I won't hurt you," or "I want to help") may also be helpful with extremely regressed, dissociated, or fearful clients.

Direct intervention for physical or safety needs should also be considered in terms of the overall effect on the relationship. The suspicious and delusional client who refuses food or drink can pose a challenge to the nurse to demonstrate trustworthiness. Communicating direct concern about the client's inadequate intake can be coupled with a matter-of-fact offer to explore ways in which the client would feel secure in eating. This might entail taking the client to the kitchen and having him supervise the selection of food from the general supply, "tasting," "sharing," the client's meal with him, or providing foods that are relatively tamperproof such as hard-boiled eggs in the shell, and unopened canned goods or containers of liquids. Restraining the client for his safety must be explained clearly as being for his benefit and protection. Intrusive or restraining interventions deemed necessary for client well-being (e.g., tube feeding, forced injection, or restraint) should be done by someone other than the staff member who is attempting to build the primary therapeutic relationship. (Clearly, these types of interventions, although necessary, will seriously impede establishing trust and relatedness.)

Hope is an additional factor in building the one-to-one relationship. Banes (1983) describes her experiences with institutionalization for a schizophrenic reaction, undifferentiated type. Despite being told she would likely be unable to leave the hospital, complete school, or hold a job, she has completed undergraduate work and a master's degree in social work, held a job for several years, and built a significant personal relationship. She attributes much of the progress to a "denial of hopelessness" by her parents and two nurses who worked with her, noting that to lose hope in the client's potential confirms the client's despair.

The effectiveness of empathic understanding and interpersonal interaction in a therapeutic relationship has been documented by research. Tudor (1952) demonstrated that severely regressed schizophrenic clients improved in behavior and social relatedness as a result of therapeutic interaction. This improvement disappeared when interaction was withdrawn. Carl Rogers (1975) has demonstrated the effectiveness of empathy in decreasing symptomatic behaviors of schizophrenia. It must be noted that the therapeutic relationship alone does not "cure" or demonstrate significantly better outcomes than other treatment approaches. It is, however, a vital tool in reaching the client, providing support, and altering the degree of dysfunctional behavior demonstrated.

■ Point of Emphasis

In general, establishing trust is the priority goal for withdrawn and/or suspicious clients.

Communication

The schizophrenic or schizophreniform client generally experiences problems with communication which can vary from vagueness to symbolic speech and incoherent "word salad." Cook (1971) describes the goals of the nurse as twofold: to decipher the client's unclear messages and to promote the client's awareness that he must learn to express himself more clearly. The client's difficulty in communication is related to autistic withdrawal and the characteristic thought disorders. These create a sense of disorganization and overload of incoming stimuli and lead to concreteness and misinterpretation of abstract ideas, autism, loose associations, and blocking of thought and speech patterns.

Simplicity, clarity, and concreteness are important tools for the nurse to use to avoid client confusion and misinterpretation. Clarification techniques are helpful in responding to symbolic or vague messages, obscure references, and sweepingly general use of pronouns (e.g., "They know all about us" or "Don't trifle with the King of Transylvania lest you be draculatized like me"). It requires patience and effort to listen to confusing speech. Although the temptations to "tune out" or to pretend understanding are strong, to do so would damage the potential for establishing trust. No matter how mysterious or garbled the communication, the careful listener can generally identify themes on which to focus in an effort to reach out to the client. Nonverbal communication such as giving an apple, a sweet, or one's time and attention can be a powerful means of conveying nurturance and security. Moser (1970) recommends this symbolic giving in addition to the need for decoding the client's verbalizations and attempting to share on a feeling level the schizophrenic's existence.

The following interaction illustrates the use of clarification by the nurse to attempt to decode the message and feelings of Bob, a suspicious client, who begins to look agitated.

BOB: They say you're trying to explode me.

NURSE: (puzzled) Who are they?

BOB: You know, the voices.

NURSE: I don't hear the voices, Bob. Are you telling me that you hear voices saying that I'm trying to explode you?

BOB: (angrily) Yes.

NURSE: I'm not sure I understand what you mean by that. Are you feeling like I've been pressuring you to talk?

BOB: You say 'What happened?' 'when was that?' 'who said so?' and your eyes look into me eternally until my head hurts.

NURSE: It sounds like you're feeling bombarded by my questions.

BOB: Yes too many—boom, boom.

NURSE: I'm glad you were able to tell me that so I won't ask so many questions anymore. For the rest of our time together today, I'd like to have you tell me what you'd like to do.

Reinforcing Reality

Autism and the disturbances of thought and perception common to schizophrenia and schizophreniform disorders may create profound distortions of reality. Whether the cause is related to social withdrawal into autistic fantasy, biochemically dysfunctional stress responses, or a combination of these factors, the result is frightening and isolating.

The acutely disorganized client may need to have one consistent person (on each shift) assigned to provide reassurance and reality interpretation. This is sometimes referred to as channeling or focusing. The aim is to provide one stable person for consistency during a period in which the client's perceptions are diffuse, disorganized, and distorted by excessive anxiety levels. During this time, the staff person will use principles of acute anxiety management to guide interventions such as brief, clear communication ("I will help you"), remaining with the person, and permitting short-term coping and tension relief activities as the client needs them to lower anxiety. Antipsychotic drugs are beneficial, and it may also be helpful to remove the client from the environment, if possible, if aspects of the environment appear to be causing or increasing anxiety and disorganization. Prevention of acute disorganization is also important. Careful observation and knowledge of client behavior patterns permits the alert nurse to identify increasing anxiety levels and intervene before the situation assumes crisis proportions.

Hallucinations and delusions are dynamically related to anxiety and to the client's internal needs. Although the primary nurse or therapist may choose to enter into an exploration of the meaning and feelings expressed by the client's autistic world, the overall milieu focus of therapy is on "here and now" experiences and feelings. Staff members should not engage in prolonged discussion or debate of vaguely abstract philosophical ideas (e.g., the interrelationships and hidden meanings in the writings of Zen Buddhism, the music of John Lennon, and the life of Pascal). They should indicate that they do not share or "go along with" the client's delusional beliefs or hallucinatory experiences. While presenting reality, it is well for staff to acknowledge that the client's autistic experiences are real to him and to attempt to identify real feelings and reality-based stresses related to them. The following illustration of this approach involves a nurse talking with a client who has persecutory (paranoid) delusions.

CLIENT: I first knew the FBI was involved in a plot to discredit me when I saw a government car drive into the warehouse on the corner near my home.

NURSE: When you began to have this feeling that you were being discredited, what other kinds of things were going on in your life?

CLIENT: I don't understand . . . you mean besides the FBI plot?

NURSE: Yes, how was work, school . . . those kinds of things?

CLIENT: Well, I quit work as a cab driver to go back to school and study accounting at the local college.

NURSE: And how was that going for you, John?

CLIENT: O.K. I guess. It's not easy to go back when you've been out of school for eight years.

NURSE: I'm sure it's not easy. Tell me what it was like for you.

CLIENT: I had to study a lot and the instructor didn't like me (he gave me Cs and Ds). I didn't know anybody else in the class—they were sort of snobbish and stuck together.

NURSE: And how were things for you at home when school wasn't going well?

CLIENT: Well, I moved back in with my Dad to save money when I quit my job. He was always on my back to study and do better. . . . It was just like being a kid in school again. My Dad lives down the street from the warehouse where the FBI car spies on me.

NURSE: So you quit your job and moved back in with your Dad so you could go back to school (responding to reality-based component of the message).

CLIENT: Yeah, I don't want to drive a cab all my life.

NURSE: But in school, you didn't know anyone to talk to and your grades were Cs and Ds. That must have been very disappointing for you.

CLIENT: Yes—it made me mad to sit there and get those tests back all marked up. My old man never did understand—he never went to college. Those FBI guys went to college though. They're lawyers and accountants . . . but look at them now . . . sneaking around trying to make somebody like me look bad.

NURSE: It seems to me this this must have been a really frustrating time in your life. You gave up a job and your own place to live so you could study accounting but you didn't get the grades you hoped for. You didn't know anybody in the class to talk to and your Dad didn't know how difficult it was. It must have seemed like nobody was giving you any credit for what you were trying to do.

Various terms have been used to describe the primitive schizophrenic thought process. Freud referred to primary process thinking and Sullivan spoke of parataxic disortion. Both were referring to the client's observable regression to early illogical and magical thinking patterns. The nurse assists the client by clearly and reassuringly reinforcing reality. It may be necessary to point out that although the client may visualize himself as turning into an animal or a member of the other sex, the nurse sees him as he is. Clients may need to be told that they cannot be controlled by others through the TV or they cannot cause a plane to crash by having angry thoughts.

With improved organization of thoughts and behavior, an active milieu can assist the client to focus on reality-based activities. Involvement in occupational and recreational therapy and social activities reduces the tendency to focus attention inward on fantasy. As the client's thinking becomes more reality based, and trust is established in the one-to-one relationship, it may be possible to assist the client in developing skill in consensual validation. Since reality is subjectively perceived, the way that most people determine the accuracy of their perceptions is through comparision with others' views (e.g., "Did you see what I saw? What do you think that means? What's going on here?"). The client who distorts reality by making invalid assumptions ("Nobody wants me around," "They're all laughing at me") can be encouraged to test some of these assumptions with the nurse's support. For example, the client may be encouraged to ask someone in the group if he might join their discussion or, in the case of laughter, to ask "What's so funny?"

The nurse uses consensual validation to test the accuracy of her perceptions of the client by comparing them with those of the client and with other staff and consultants. This is particularly important in checking out one's judgment of the stage of trust in the relationship, the degree of dependency appropriate for the client, and the unique meaning perceived by the client in relation to external events (among other subjective aspects of care).

Long-Term Goals. Low self-esteem has its origins and expressions in a wide variety of internalized perceptions of others' views. The withdrawn and autistic client may perceive himself to be physically awkward, socially inept, unattractive, sexually insecure, and personally dull and repugnant. These perceptions become reinforced by experiences in which the client's expectations and subsequent behavior elicit avoidance, rejection, or failure.

Interpersonal theory focuses on the importance of reality-based achievements and positive appraisals by significant others in enhancing self-esteem. Basic attitudes on the part of the nurse that convey respect, acceptance of the individual, and recognition of his potential for growth are essential in relating to all clients but are particularly important to these clients who are so vulnerable to any hint of rejection. Intervention to increase self-esteem begins with recognition and acknowledgment of client strengths. These assets should be used as building blocks to develop other areas and skills. For instance, a controlled and carefully organized suspicious client may be placed in charge of the checkout procedures for keeping track of recreational equipment on outings. This recognition of an ability not only builds self-esteem in regard to this strength but also provides a variety of superficial social interactions with staff and other clients which can be used to develop skills in another area.

Many withdrawn clients lack body coordination and a sense of pleasure in physical activity. Therapists and staff can plan a variety of physical activities aimed at improving coordination and enjoyment of bodily activities. Exercising to music, dancing as a form of expression, working with clay and wood, and numerous other activities provide opportunities to "get in touch" physically with the self. These can be individual or group focused. Group activities—such as keeping a parachute billowing afloat through the group's action, trust walks (walking while blindfolded, and dependent upon another person for guidance), or being cradled and rocked by members of the group, termination games in which the member going home must demonstrate strength by "breaking out" of the group's interlocked arms— all can have special meaning to the withdrawn client.

Difficulties with verbal expression and communicating feelings can often be overcome through nonverbal modes of expression. Painting, dance, music, and writing may provide both an expressive outlet and a means for attaining recognition and communication.

Social opportunities in the milieu include such things as meal planning and preparation, unit government, organizing field trips and outings, and being a "buddy" to another client who needs special assistance. The client can be involved at his present level of readiness and small incremental successes built up. The nurse can use the trust established on a one-to-one basis to gradually extend the client's social circle and feelings of competency.

School and occupational achievements may be minimal and characterized by a series of failures or interruptions. Occupational and vocational goals can be explored and realistically focused on attainable options. With long-term encouragement and support, it is possible to assist the person to actually obtain and keep a job or fully assume a productive role in the family. This kind of achievement truly builds self-esteem. However, it is not smoothly or easily accomplished because the client does not expect to succeed. Many setbacks are possible and require continued intervention and support.

Group discussions are helpful in planning ways of coping with the stigma of mental illness and hospitalization. Prior to dismissal all clients should have engaged in planning ways of handling questions about their illness, dealing with concerns of others, and knowing their rights in seeking employment. Self-help groups may be helpful for clients in the community.

Managing Stress and Anxiety

Anxiety has been described as a key component underlying many of the characteristic problems of schizophrenic clients such as ambivalence, thought disorders, hallucinations, and autism. These high levels of anxiety and the resulting difficulties in coping with the stress and anxiety of living are lifelong problems.

Long-term goals in relation to stress and anxiety management emphasize several approaches:

1. Teach the client to recognize problem levels of anxiety and manage them preventively to avoid disorganization and exacerbation of symptoms (e.g., Arieti describes how clients may be assisted to control hallucinations by recognizing the connection between a particular mood and the "listening attitude" in which the expectation of

the voices and their occurrence take place [1974, 574–575]).

2. Recognize situational and developmental milestones likely to induce stress and anxiety.

3. Teach individualized skills for managing anxiety.

4. Monitor long-term antipsychotic drug therapy to control excessive anxiety and related responses.

The first three approaches can be accomplished by supportive therapy and crisis intervention techniques on an outpatient basis whether the therapist is a psychiatrist, psychologist, social worker, or nurse. The fourth approach involves overall medical supervision and assessments of pharmacological effectiveness, compliance, and the drugs' side effects. These latter assessments may be accomplished by nurses or physicians. (Some of these assessments are incorporated in Table 34-2. See also Chapter 15 on psychotropic drugs.) Cohen and Andur (1981) described the use of group education and discussion techniques to improve client knowledge about and acceptance of medication. They noted that compliance is often impaired by the client's perception of the drug in relation to its side effects rather than its therapeutic effects. Both aspects need to be addressed and clients may be assisted in managing side effects with the physician's cooperation through dose reduction, antiparkinsonism drugs, and taking the medication at bedtime. Discussion of the benefits and limitations of medication and dealing with the issues of control engendered by long-term drug therapy were additional issues noted by the authors as valuable.

■ **Point of Emphasis**

Compliance in long-term antipsychotic therapy is more likely if the client views the drug as a means of enhancing his own behavior control.

Although suicide is not as prevalent in schizophrenia as in depression, Mendel notes that it is a serious risk because of the need to escape from the unbearable pain and exhaustion of severe anxiety (1976, 36). The nurse should be alert to this potential in both hospitalized clients and those who are reentering family and community living.

FAMILY INTERVENTION □

Family Support □ Family involvement is valuable in all phases of care from admission through aftercare in the community. Initial involvement generally takes place during the interview when data about family needs are also collected. Therapists in many treatment settings routinely conduct family conferences at intervals during treatment. The focus of these conferences may be client support, involving the family in the treatment and problem-solving process, and dismissal planning. Many family-oriented therapists may involve the family in the entire treatment process. Family education and coping groups are frequently established by nurses and other members of the mental health team. Bell (1975) found that families are less likely to discuss problems and concerns generated by mental illness than they would be if the illness were physical in nature. Thus questions may remain unasked and feelings unexpressed, and family members may feel separated from their customary sources of support in the extended family and community. In addition to possible feelings of shame, guilt, and anger, there may be elements of blame and confusion as family members question their own roles and vulnerability in the origins of the illness. If group supports are not available, home visits may be helpful and can be provided either by the psychiatric care staff or community health nurses.

Family as Client Support □ Discharge planning with families involves an examination of role changes in the family. What client roles were reassigned during his illness and how will the client's return affect this arrangement? If the client is returning to the parental home, very minimal expectations may be held for role functioning; if the client is a parent, there may be strong pressure exerted to resume customary roles even before he feels ready. Either of these situations is potentially a problem.

Shortened hospitalizations may result in clients returning home while still exhibiting dysfunctional behavior. Families need teaching and assistance in several areas, including:

1. Recognizing symptoms that indicate a need for medication readjustment or hospitalization.

2. Setting realistic expectations for client involvement at home.

3. Understanding and supporting long-term treatment goals such as medication compliance and vocational training.

4. Achieving awareness of community support systems and self-help groups, which in turn can provide help in coping with problem behaviors, family issues, and need for occasional respite from care.

5. Receiving education to assist in understanding the effects of stressors and techniques for reducing and managing stress.

LEVELS OF PREVENTION □

Primary Prevention □ Primary prevention is currently limited by the inadequate information available as to the cause of the disorder. Arieti (1974, 514–516) refers to the genetic potential and the early environment as significant factors for consideration. Since there is only a 10 percent probability that the child of a schizophrenic parent will also become schizophrenic, he suggests that genetic counseling and recommendation of birth control or sterilization be reserved for those people at higher risk (e.g., two spouses who have each been schizophrenic). The most effective form of primary prevention is promoting a mentally healthy family environment and positive parenting skills. This is even more important in the care of individuals who have a hereditary potential and are experiencing life stress. These interventions are generic in nature and not specific to schizophrenia. Intervention during significant life crises such as going away to college or childbirth may decrease stress and enhance coping skills.

Secondary Prevention □ Screening at-risk populations, early diagnosis, referral, and treatment can be facilitated by nurses and others in the community who are likely to come in contact with populations experiencing high levels of stress (e.g., social workers, teachers, clergy).

Community health nurses should be alert to early symptoms of autism and withdrawal as they interact with such high-risk groups as migrants, immigrants, minorities, and poor and unemployed people. School and student health nurses and obstetric nurses among others can stress the need for psychiatric referral when they recognize significant early symptoms. This is not always easily done. Families may deny any problems, particularly in the early stages. Vonnegut (1975)

describes the prolonged efforts of his friends to avoid having him hospitalized despite his hallucinations, suicide attempts, insomnia, and refusal to eat. Acute-care treatment appropriate to secondary prevention has been discussed throughout this chapter. Public education to decrease the stigma of mental illness could improve the likelihood of early treatment.

Tertiary Prevention □ In schizophreniform disorders, recovery should be complete and no residual symptoms should remain. Efforts directed at client understanding of how the disorder arose under stress and strengthening his ability to cope with stress enhance rehabilitation.

Schizophrenia is however, according to the DSM-III criteria, a chronic condition. This does not mean that the client cannot function; only that the potential and vulnerability for remission remain present throughout life. The degree of damage to the client's basic personality and level of functional deterioration depends on the severity of the condition itself and the nature of environmental support and stimulation. Early onset, a schizoid personality (introverted and passive), strong hereditary factors, and absence of significant stressors at onset are associated with residual symptoms. In the past, the effects of long-term institutionalization also had profound consequences for a client's social and mental deterioration. The community mental health movement was designed to combat this institutionalized social breakdown. However, the supportive services needed to rehabilitate and maintain clients in the community are not always present, with the result that former "back ward" clients are left in "back alleys" or placed in crowded institutional nursing home settings.

True tertiary prevention actively addresses the needed areas of rehabilitation: social, vocational, educational, and self-care. The settings may be group homes, day care, or outpatient. The approaches include individualized and/or group strategies to promote social skill development, remotivation, coping with the stresses of life (e.g., group living, job training or maintenance), and building leisure skills. The effectiveness of supportive group therapy in preventing relapse and enhancing autonomy and social interaction has been demonstrated in the findings of Alden (1979) and Parloff and Dies (1977) that group support may diminish both the need for rehospitalizations and the amount of antipsychotic medication required.

Butler (1979) and other authors have reported on the use of behavior modification techniques (specifically, token economy) in the psychiatric setting to improve social and self-care skills prior to dismissal. Kent (1970) notes the importance of eliciting family cooperation in controlling reinforcers and setting expectations. She further describes the effectiveness of this technique in shaping specific behaviors but warns that behavior is not generalized. Additional group strategies are used to motivate and involve clients in social planning and activities.

> ■ **Point of Emphasis**
>
> Tertiary prevention remains a vital but relatively neglected aspect of care. Nurses possess the comprehensive focus and emphasis on individual level of functioning that can best effect client improvement in this area.

EVALUATION □ Outcomes for clients experiencing schizophreniform psychoses are generally positive for full return to prior level of functioning. In schizophrenic reaction, residual type, however, it is realistic to anticipate that after acute psychotic disorganization subsides, several areas of diminished functional capacity will remain. This does not mean that it is inappropriate to target some of these residual deficits as goals, only that change will be slow and incremental.

The problems depicted in Figure 34-1 are shown from the general or long-range (stress/anxiety management and low self-esteem) to the more intermediate range with identification of specific problems such as thought disorders and social isolation. In the psychiatric setting nursing goals will be developed in reverse order with initial focus on short-term goals for physical needs, acute anxiety management, development of beginning trust, and reality testing. Long-range goals are then extended across hospital and community care and are facilitated by achievement of the short-term goals.

Establishing criteria for evaluation requires specificity and individualization. This is frequently confusing when one is dealing with subjective factors, as can be illustrated in the problem of social isolation. The social isolation itself is related to the client's avoidance and withdrawal from social interaction (which is in turn related to the underlying problems of anxiety and low

self-esteem). The short-term goal is to establish trust in a primary staff member. Evaluation criteria (individualized to unique client and behavior) might include the client's keeping scheduled appointments with the nurse, initiating topics of interest, and sharing personal thoughts and feelings spontaneously. For a more withdrawn client, the criteria might be remaining in the same room with the nurse for ten minutes and having occasional eye contact. Once trust is established on a one-to-one level, an intermediate goal of increased social interaction might be developed. Criterion measures might relate to time spent in social group situations on the unit and initiation of conversation with other clients. In the case of the more withdrawn client, a criterion for group involvement might initially involve participation in a group activity that does not require verbal social interaction, such as shuffleboard.

■ *Enrichment Activities*

DISCUSSION QUESTIONS

1. Discuss the relative merits of the diagnostic label "schizophrenia." For example, does the value of a medical diagnosis to treatment planning and research outweigh the stigma of the label to the patient?

2. Harry Stack Sullivan said "We are all more human than otherwise." Each of us has experiences that can assist our understanding and diminish our fear of characteristic schizophrenic behaviors.

   Discuss or individually consider some of the following human responses to stress from your own experiences as well as those observed in clients.

   a. Withdrawing or avoiding social contacts when feeling shy, vulnerable, or inferior.

   b. Blaming others and questioning their motives when not doing well in school, work, or personal relationships.

   c. Using fantasy to cope with feelings of loneliness, boredom, or low self-esteem.

   d. Experiencing difficulty with focusing on a problem and making a decision under stress.

3. Describe a variety of tertiary prevention approaches which nurses are well prepared to use in client rehabilitation.

4. Discuss relevant client teaching about antipsychotic drug therapy during hospitalization and discharge planning.

LEARNING ACTIVITIES

1. Listen to a recording of "Mr. Whisper" from the Dory Previn record album "On My Way to Where." Discuss how this song illustrates the need that hallucinations and delusions fulfill and the ambivalence that the schizophrenic client may feel about giving up autistic invention for reality.

2. Read a first-person experiential account of schizophrenia. All of the following are valuable in permitting the reader to glimpse the pain of the schizophrenic world and yet carry a sense of hope for recovery.

   Green, Hannah. *I Never Promised You A Rose Garden*. New York: Holt, Rinehart & Winston, 1964. Available in Signet Paperback.

   Vonnegut, Mark. *The Eden Express*. Praeger Publishing, 1975. Also condensed in *Book Digest*, December 1975.

   Previn, Dory. *Midnight Baby*. New York: Macmillan, 1976.

■ Recommended Readings

Wing, J. Social influences on the course of schizophrenia. In *The nature of schizophrenia—New approaches to research and treatment* (Wynne, L.C.; Cromwell R.; and Marrhysse, S. (eds.). New York: Wiley, 1978, 599–615. Focuses on the needs of clients and families in coping with this long-term illness. Secondary and tertiary prevention strategies are identified.

Carson, R.C. The schizophrenias. In *Comprehensive handbook of psychopathology* (Adams, H.E., and Sutker, P.B. (eds.). New York: Plenum Press, 1983. Contains a good discussion of genetic factors and effects.

Kanas, N., and Barr, M.A. Homogeneous group therapy for acutely psychotic schizophrenic inpatients. *Hospital and community psychiatry* 34, 3, 1984. Contains practical information specific to the needs of schizophrenic clients for supportive group therapy approaches.

■ References

Alden, A. et al. Group aftercare for chronic schizophrenia. *Journal of clinical psychiatry*, 40, 1979:249–252.

American Psychiatric Association. *Diagnostic and statistical manual of mental disorders*. 3d ed. Washington, D.C.: The American Psychiatric Association, 1980.

Arieti, S. *Interpretation of schizophrenia*. 2d ed. New York: Basic books, 1974.

Banes, J. An ex-patient's perspective of psychiatric treatment. *Journal of psychosocial nursing and mental health services* 21, 3 (March 1983):11–20.

Bateson, G., Jackson, D., Haley, J., et al. Toward a theory of schizophrenia. *Behavioral science*, 1, 1956:251–264.

Bell, R. The impact of illness on family roles. In *Contemporary community nursing* (Spradley, B., ed.). Boston: Little, Brown & Co., 1975.

Broad, J., and Trimbain, S. Family-focused nursing: Aftercare of the psychiatric patient. In *Family Health care* (Hymovich, D., and Barnard, M. (eds.). Vol. 2, 2d ed. New York: McGraw-Hill, 1979.

Butler, R. The evolution of a token economy program for female chronic schizophrenic patients. *Journal of advanced nursing* 4, 1979:307–318.

Carmack, B., and Corvin, T. Nursing care of the schizophrenic maternity patient during labor. *Maternal child nursing*, 5 (March/April 1980):107–111.

Cohen, M., and Andur, M. Medication group for psychiatric patients. *American journal of nursing* (February 1981):343–345.

Cook, J. Interpreting and decoding autistic communication. *Perspectives in psychiatric care*, 9, 1, 1971:24–28.

Edwards, M. Psychiatric day programs: A descriptive analysis. *Journal of psychosocial nursing and mental health services*, 20, 9 (September 1982):17–21.

Erikson, E. *Childhood and society*. New York: Norton, 1963.

Fenton, F., Tessier, L., and Stuening, E. A comparative trial of home and hospital psychiatric care. *Archives of general psychiatry*, 36, (September 1973):1073–1079.

Green, H. *I never promised you a rose garden*. New York: Signet, 1964.

Hopkins, S. The slow march of knowledge. *Nursing mirror*. 151, 5 (July 1980):37.

Kanas, N., and Barr, M.A. Homogeneous group therapy for acutely psychotic schizophrenic inpatients. *Hospital and community psychiatry*, 34, 3, 1983:257–258.

Kent, E. A token economy program for schizophrenic patients. *Perspectives in psychiatric care*, 4, 1970:174–185.

Kolb, L. Noyes' Modern clinical psychiatry, 7th ed. Philadelphia: W.B. Saunders Co., 1973.

Koontz, E. Schizophrenia: Current diagnostic concepts

and implications for nursing care. *Journal of psychosocial nursing and mental health services,* 20, 9, (September 1982):44–48.

Lidz, R.W., and Lidz, T. The family environment of schizophrenic patients. *American journal of psychiatry,* 106, 1949–50:332–345.

Lidz, T. Egocentric cognitive regression and the family setting of schizophrenic disorders. In *The nature of schizophrenia: New approaches to research and treatment* (Wynne, L.C.; Cromwell, R.; and Matthysse, S., eds.). New York: Wiley, 1978:526–532.

Lidz, T., Cornelison, A., Flick, S., and Alanen, Y. The intrafamilial environment of schizophrenic patients: II. Marital schism and marital skew. *American journal of psychiatry,* 114, 1957:241–248.

Lidz, T., Flick, S., Alanen, Y., and Cornelison, A. Schizophrenic patients and their siblings. *Psychiatry,* 26, 1963:1–18.

Maslow, A. *Motivation and personality,* 2d ed., New York: Harper & Row, 1970.

Marram, G. Toward a greater understanding of mutual withdrawal in a psychiatric setting. *Journal of psychiatric nursing and mental health services* (July–August 1969):160–163.

Mendel, W. *Schizophrenia—The experience and its treatment.* San Francisco: Jossey-Bass, 1976.

Menzies, I. A care-study in the functioning of social systems as a defense against anxiety: A report on a study of the nursing service of a general hospital. *Human relations* 13, 1960:95–121.

Moser, D.H. Communicating with a schizophrenic patient. *Perspectives in psychiatric care* 8, 1, 1970:36–45.

Parloff, M., and Dies, R. Group psychotherapy outcome research 1966–1975. *International journal of group psychotherapy,* 27, 1977:281–319.

Pyke, J., and Page, J. Schizophrenia. *The Canadian nurse* (May 1981):39–43.

Randels, P.; Villeponteaux, L.; et al. *Psychiatry learning system.* rev. ed. Chapel Hill, NC: Health Sciences Consortium, 1982.

Rickelman, B. Brain bio-amines and schizophrenia: A summary of research findings and implications for nursing. *Journal of psychiatric nursing and mental health services* (September 1979):28–33.

Rogers, C. Empathic: An unappreciated way of being. *The counseling psychologist* 5, 2, 1975:6.

Rogers, J. Roots of madness. *Science 82,* 3, 6 (July/August 1982):84–91.

Ruditis, S. Developing trust in nursing interpersonal relationships. *Journal of psychiatric nursing,* 17, 4 (April 1979):20–23.

Satir, V. *Conjoint family therapy.* Palo Alto, CA: Science and Behavior Books, 1967.

Schmidt, C. Withdrawal behavior of schizophrenics: Application of Roy's model. *Journal of psychosocial nursing and mental health services,* 19, 11 (November 1981):26–33.

Sechehaye, M. *Reality lost and regained: Autobiography of a schizophrenic girl.* New York: Grune & Stratton, 1951.

Sedgewick, R. Psychological responses to stress. *Journal of psychiatric nursing,* 13, 9 (September 1975):20–23.

Singer, M.; Wynne, L.; and Toohey, M. Communication disorders and the families of schizophrenics. In *The nature of shcizophrenia: New approaches to research and treatment* (Wynne, L.C.; Cromwell, R.; and Matthysse, S., eds.). New York: Wiley 1978:499–510.

Sullivan, H. S. The interpersonal theory of psychiatry. New York: Norton, 1968.

Tudor, G. A sociopsychiatric nursing approach to intervention in a problem of mutual withdrawal on a mental hospital ward. *Psychiatry,* The William Alanson White Psychiatric Foundation, Inc., 15, 2, 1952:193–217.

———. A sociopsychiatric nursing approach to intervention in a problem of mutual withdrawal on a mental hospital ward. *Perspective in psychiatric care,* 8, 1, 1970:11–35.

Vonnegut, M. *The Eden express.* New York: Praeger Publishing Co., 1975.

Weiner, M.; Pepper, G.; Kuhn-Weisman, G.; and Romano, J. *Clinical pharmacology and therapeutics in nursing.* New York: McGraw-Hill, 1979.

White, E., and Kahn, E.M. Use and modifications in group psychotherapy with chronic schizophrenic outpatients. *Journal of psychosocial nursing and mental health services,* 20, 2 (February 1982):14–20.

Wienckowski, Louis. Schizophrenia is there an answer? DHEW Publication no. HSM 73-9086, 1973.

Wynne, L.C.; Cromwell, R.; and Matthysse, S., (eds.) *The nature of schizophrenia: New approaches to research and treatment.* New York: Wiley, 1978.

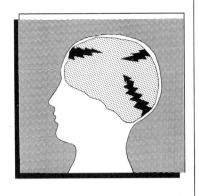

35

Organic Mental Disorders

Mary Ellen Kronberg

Learning Objectives

Upon completion of this chapter, the reader will be able to:

1. Define the types of organic mental disorders, emphasizing delirium and dementia.

2. Explain the behavioral manifestations of each of the above disorders.

3. Identify physical and psychosocial factors that contribute to organic dysfunction.

4. List tests used to diagnose organic mental disorders and their related nursing implications.

5. Examine personal feelings about organic mental disorders and the influence these feelings may have on effectiveness of client care.

6. Describe individualized care of the client with an organic mental disorder.

7. Incorporate the family and the environment in the nursing process when assisting clients with organic mental disorders.

The D.S.M.-III (1980) classification system identifies organic mental disorders and organic brain syndromes. Organic mental disorder is a more specific term indicating knowledge of the cause, while organic brain syndrome is more general. Both refer to psychobehavioral disturbances due to either temporary or permanent brain dysfunction.

Previous classification systems used the terms acute, chronic, reversible, and irreversible to distinguish the organic disorders. "Acute" and "chronic" are ambiguous terms. They are best used in their medical sense, for example, referring to the mode of onset and duration of a disorder. Reversibility is a criterion that is difficult to apply since it is generally established retrospectively, through research studies. Reversibility and irreversibility are more suitable for predicting likely outcomes of treatment, rather than classification of conditions. Although these terms may continue to be used, they are not included in the D.S.M.-III classification system.

One cannot use a single description to characterize all organic mental disorders. Symptoms assessed differ according to the affected brain area, type of onset, duration, progression, and cause. At times it is impossible to distinguish an organic from a functional mental disorder on the basis of behavioral manifestations. Neurologic and laboratory evidence of concurrent brain disorder (or at least a history of exposure to an identified organic factor such as head trauma, toxic poisoning, and so forth) is required for a diagnosis of organic mental disorder. The inferred causative organic factor will be medically investigated and identified, if possible, in individuals with this diagnosis. The organic factor may be a primary disease of the brain (e.g., cerebral tumor or cardiovascular accident), or a secondary process such as systemic illness, toxic disturbance, cerebral anoxia secondary to atherosclerosis, or cardiopulmonary problems.

☐ *Common Syndromes*

The D.S.M. III describes the most common organic brain syndromes as delirium, dementia, intoxication, and withdrawal. Other types of organic brain syndromes include amnestic (amensia) syndrome, organic hallucinosis, organic delusional syndrome, organic affective syndrome, organic personality syndrome, and atypical or mixed organic brain syndrome. Clients with organic men-

tal disorders are treated in medical and neurological as well as psychological settings. These disorders are not specific to any age group, although the elderly population is more susceptible to dementia. The symptoms may vary greatly among individuals.

DELIRIUM

Delirium (formerly called acute organic brain syndrome) represents a broad syndrome of disturbances in sensation, perception, memory, thought, and judgment. It is usually more severe at night. The sleep-wakefulness cycle is disturbed, causing restless sleep, drowsiness, insomnia, and interruption in the dream cycle. The client may be confused, he may have difficulty in thinking and attention; may display disordered memory and orientation; may have frequent misperceptions; and cannot concentrate on goal-directed activities. It has a rapid onset and is of brief duration. The disorder usually clears in a matter of days or weeks, rarely lasting longer than a month (Heller and Kornfeld, 1975). Sensory deprivation or overload, sleep and dream interruptions, immobilization, and overwhelming anxiety can cause delirium in the hospital setting. Physical factors causing delirium include medications, systemic infections, metabolic disturbances, nutritional defects, substance abuse, drug or alcohol withdrawal, general surgery, and brain trauma. Failure to find and treat the underlying physical cause of acute delirium may result in permanent brain damage. If no brain damage has occurred and the cause has been removed, the client will return to his previous level of functioning.

DEMENTIA

Dementia can be defined as a progressive loss of cognitive and other higher intellectual functions as a result of organic brain disease (Terry and Davies, 1980). Dementia was formerly called chronic organic brain syndrome. It interferes with social or occupational functioning. Memory for ongoing events, new learning, and past events is disrupted. Abstract reasoning, impulse control, and judgment are also impaired. The individual frequently displays personality and behavioral changes while the level of conscious wakefulness remains normal. It generally has a relatively gradual onset, yet it may occur suddenly when the cause is head trauma. The disorder has a prolonged duration which may extend over months or years. Dementia is frequently found in the elderly, although it can occur at almost any age in life depending on the cause (symptoms occurring before the age of 3 or 4 are usually diagnosed as mental retardation). Causative factors are similar to those of delirium with the addition of some aspects of aging.

Dementia is a lingering disease; it can be progressive, remain static, or fluctuate in intensity. Reversibility of the disease depends on the underlying condition and whether effective treatment is given in time (Adams, 1981). Generally, the progression of the disease may be halted but the client will not return to a previous level of function.

Alzheimer's Disease

The elderly population has grown over the past decades. Kolb and Brodie (1982) report that in 1900, one in 25 living persons was over the age of 65; in 1978, this ratio had increased to one in nine. Kolata (1981) states that one of every six persons over the age of 65 is at least moderately affected by dementia. The most common cause of dementia in the elderly is primary degenerative dementia or Alzheimer's disease. Spar (1982) found that Alzheimer's accounted for 40 to 60 percent of all cases of dementia in old age. The onset of Alzheimer's disease is usually between the ages of 50 and 60, although earlier cases have been noted. Prevalence of this disorder is higher in the eighth and ninth decades of life.

Postmortem brain studies have demonstrated characteristic changes that occur in Alzheimer's disease: (1) neurofibrillary tangles (filaments in the cytoplasm of neurons wrap around each other), (2) neuritic plaques (deposits that show neuron denervation), (3) granulovascular degeneration (fluid deposits and granulation in the neurons), and (4) reduced enzyme activity particularly of noradrenaline and of choline acetyltransferase, which is required in acetylcholine synthesis. Genetic factors remain unclear but there does appear to be an increased risk, approximately four times that of the general population, among close relatives of clients diagnosed as having Alzheimer's disease.

Women are more often affected by this disease than are men. Families in which Alzheimer's disease tends to develop also have a greater frequency of Down's syndrome, leukemia, and immune system disorders (Kolata, 1981; Wells, 1982). In persons with Down's syndrome, pathology typical of the disorder tends to develop if they live into early middle age. The course of the disease averages 10 years in younger persons, but only 3 years among older persons (Terry and Davies, 1980).

INTOXICATION AND WITHDRAWAL

Other common organic mental disorders are (1) intoxication and (2) withdrawal. These disorders are associated with (1) excessive ingestion of alcohol or drugs, and (2) stopping intake of a substance on which the client has become dependent. If the organic disorder is caused by the ingestion of a particular substance such as amphetamines, the disorder is named for that specific agent, in this case, amphetamine intoxication. Similarly, if the organic disorder is caused by a reduction in a particular substance, for example, alcohol, it is named for that specific agent, alcohol withdrawal delirium. For further information on substance use disorders and related problems, see Chapter 28.

OTHER CATEGORIES OF ORGANIC BRAIN DISORDERS

The following section focuses on the common organic brain disorders; the other disorders are briefly described. It is important for the nurse to be aware of all of these when providing care.

The amnestic syndrome occurs in the absence of symptoms of delirium or dementia. The person may display impairment in both short-term memory (anterograde amnesia) and long-term memory (retrograde amnesia). He has difficulty in incorporating memory into permanent storage or is unable to retrieve memory from storage. New information cannot be retained for longer than a brief period. These clients may occasionally use confabulation, for example, filling in memory gaps with inventions to save themselves from embarrassment. The amnestic syndrome is rare, generally resulting from lesions causing bilateral damage to the limbic system, the diencephalon, or both. The damage may be caused by head trauma, surgery, hypoxia, the herpes simplex virus, encephalitis, thiamine deficiency, or chronic alcoholism (DMS III, 1980).

Organic hallucinosis is characterized by recurrent or persistent hallucinations experienced when the person is in a state of clear awareness.

The hallucinations are attributable to a specific organic factor. The type of hallucination will vary with its etiology, the individual experiencing it, and the social setting. Causes include seizures, use of hallucinogens, prolonged use of alcohol, and sensory deprivation. The individual may firmly believe the hallucinations are real. A hallucination may be either pleasant or frightening and may last from hours to years depending on the causal agent.

The organic delusional syndrome resembles the paranoid schizophrenic disorder in some of its features. The delusions occur when the person's state of consciousness is normal, and are due to a specific organic factor. Other schizophrenialike manifestations may be mild cognitive impairment, pacing, rocking, speech incoherence, and some ritualistic behavior. These delusions are a direct consequence of a cerebral disorder such as temporal lobe epilepsy, encephalitis, or substance intoxication (e.g., cocaine, amphetamines or hallucinogens).

The essential feature in organic affective syndrome is an abnormal mood, either depressed or elated, that is a direct consequence of the organic disorder. The severity of this syndrome may range from a mild form to a severe or psychotic state. Examples of causative agents include toxic or metabolic factors, substances (hallucinogens, reserpine, methyldopa), acute viral infections, endocrine disorders (hypo- or hyperthyroidism, Cushing's syndrome), carcinoma of the pancreas, pernicious anemia, and brain trauma or tumor.

The personality is affected in the organic personality syndrome. There are disturbances of motivation, emotion, and impulse control. These changes are due to organic factors. In the frontal lobe syndrome, social judgment is impaired. The person may lose interest in his usual hobbies and be unconcerned about environmental events. The cause usually is structural damage to the brain, head trauma, tumor, vascular accident, or temporal epilepsy. Steroid drugs or an endocrine disorder may also be a causative factor.

The designation of atypical or mixed organic brain syndrome applies to syndromes that do not meet the criteria of the other organic brain syndromes. The term describes maladaptions noted during the waking state associated with evidence of an organic factor related to the cause of the disturbance. The D.S.M. III (1980) notes the neurasthenic syndrome associated with early Addison's disease as an example.

☐ *Causative Factors*

Organic mental disorders have many causes, including chemical and biologic disturbances (Table 35-1). There are also related conditions that interact with biochemical factors to exacerbate the signs and symptoms, among them decreased sensory adaptation secondary to the aging process (see Chapter 20), sensory deprivation and/or overload, underlying personality factors, and iatrogenic factors such as medication.

Quality and consistency of nursing care are vital in the client's progress and his adaptation to the situation. Nurses need to realize that elderly persons, whose number is increasing, are more likely to experience organic mental disorders. These persons are commonly cared for in the general hospital setting, where the nurse is readily available to clients and families. Because the nurse is accessible, she is frequently approached for information and assistance and is in a position to coordinate the client's care with other members of the health care team. She can assist in identifying the specific problems, explore options for supportive care, and assist with care in rehabilitation programs. As she observes changes in the client's condition, she can support and counsel both client and family. The nurse can function as a liaison between inpatient and community settings, perform home assessments, help the client and family establish a realistic care plan, and provide referrals to community agencies.

ASSESSMENT ☐ Assessment may be impaired if it is assumed that little or nothing can be done for the affected person. Treatable and reversible conditions may be overlooked, or not enough effort made to maintain the optimum functional level in the client whose condition is characterized by irreversible deteriorations. A holistic focus which incorporates physical and emotional aspects of client care while including family and environmental aspects is most likely to achieve the optimal level of functioning.

Client Assessment ☐ The symptoms of delirium and dementia are similar but there are significant differences in their onset. The onset in delirium is acute, the severity and symptoms fluctuating over a few hours to several days. Symptoms are often more pronounced at night. In dementia, there is gradual and progressive deterioration in mental abilities and obvious pro-

TABLE 35-1 Causal Factors in Organic Mental Disorders

General Category	Chemical and Biological Problems
Toxic and metabolic states	Medication toxicity, for example, bromide, barbiturates, ACTH, opiates, cortisone
	Metal/gas toxicity, for example, lead, mercury, manganese, carbon monoxide
	Porphyria
	Nutritional deficits, for example, vitamin deficiencies, Wernicke's Syndrome, Korsakoff's Syndrome, pernicious anemia
	Acid-base imbalance, for example, water intoxication or dehydration, hyper- and hypokalemia, hyper- and hyponatremia, acidosis
Endocrine disturbances	Thyroid (hypo- or hyperthyroidism, myxedema)
	Adrenal (Addison's disease, Cushing's syndrome)
	Parathyroid (hypo- or hyperparathyroidism)
	Pituitary (hypopituitarism)
	Pancreas, (carcinoma, hypoglycemia, acute pancreatitis)
Disorders of cerebral oxygenation	Atherosclerosis
	Cerebral embolism
	Intracerebral hemorrhage
	Cardiac insufficiency
	Pulmonary problems
Infections	Meningitis (e.g., tuberculosis)
	Encephalitis (e.g., acute viral infections)
	Fever (e.g., typhoid fever, rheumatic fever)
	Syphilitic meningeoencephalitis
	Pneumonia
Brain tumors	Benign or malignant tumors
	Intracranial neoplasm
Brain trauma	Concussion
	Contusion
	Lacerations
	Hematoma
Degenerative disorders	Alzheimer's disease
	Pick's disease
	Parkinson's disease
	Huntington's chorea
	Multiple Sclerosis

nounced difficulties related to recent memory. During initial assessment, the family's description of the duration and onset of symptoms, the client's previous adjustment and level of functioning, and any recent illnesses or events that may be associated with the present problems need to be carefully evaluated.

■ Point of Emphasis

Assessment of onset, duration, possible causative factors, and previous level of functioning will assist in differentiating between dementia and delirium.

Mental Status Changes. Common areas of impairment are reflected in the changes in mental status which are observable in both delirium and dementia (Table 35-2). The client loses awareness in one or more areas or orientation, that is, person, place, time. Most often awareness of time is first to be lost, and awareness of person is last. Orientation is assessed by asking the following questions: (1) What is today's date? What is the time right now? (2) What is the name of this place? (3) What is your name?

Because the questions are so simple, the nurse may feel uncomfortable asking them or may alter them so as to invalidate the responses: "You know this is a hospital, don't you?" or "What's the name of this hospital?" This type of questioning promotes confabulation by giving obvious cues; in the second example, the client could call upon remote memory, which would not test orientation. If either nurse or client is uncomfortable with the content of the questions, it is acceptable to preface them with an introductory comment such as "These questions may seem very simple, but they are important because illness can have an effect on your ability to respond to even such simple questions."

A hospitalized person's sense of time may be slightly blurred—the person may recognize general divisions such as morning, afternoon, night, month, and year yet not be able to name the specific day. "It's Tuesday or Wednesday in mid-June." Such a response is not necessarily an indication of a problem. Correctly orient the client and then recheck later. This may also be necessary in the case of the client who was admitted in an unconscious or confused state. Initially he

TABLE 35-2 Physical and Mental Alterations in Organic Mental Disorders

Motor coordination	May lose the ability to write simple phrases, to copy geometric designs, or to copy even simple shapes if there is background interference on the paper. Tremor or involuntary movements may be present.
Grooming	General appearance may reflect the client's confusion and altered activity level resulting in poor hygiene, dishevelment and/or inappropriate dress.
Speech	Comprehension and expression may be affected in either written or spoken form. Speech patterns may be incoherent, hesitant; jibberish may substitute for particular words or echolalia may be present.
State of consciousness	Sensorium may be clouded or hyperalert and may fluctuate from one extreme to another. Awareness of self and environment may be impaired.
Orientation	Disturbances of time, place, and person (ascending order of severity) may develop.
Attention span	One of the earliest and most prominent dysfunctions to occur, as attentiveness to external stimuli and stream of consciousness is impaired.
Memory	Immediate and recent recall is most seriously impaired; early memories may be accurately retained in dementia. Amnesia is memory loss for specific time frames or situations without impairment of consciousness/awareness.
Cognition	Ability to think abstractly is impaired, with difficulty in explaining proverbs, identifying similarities ("How are an apple and a pear alike?"), and difficulty in performing simple mathematical calculations.

needs to be oriented to the facts of hospitalization before it can be established whether he can retain this information.

Judgment impairment may be one of the earliest signs of organic mental disorders as decision-making and social skills diminish. It may be reflected in impulsive actions such as giving away one's money to a worthy cause without considering the necessity of retaining sufficient resources to meet one's own needs during retirement or becoming influenced by people who exploit the vulnerable elderly through various schemes to obtain their money. Dress may become bizarre; for instance, several outfits may be worn one over the other. Irritability and lability of emotions combined with poor judgment may result in actions that cut the person off from significant supports such as family or lifelong friends when the person isolates himself from others because of real or imagined slights. Judgment problems may also be manifested by ignoring social conventions such as refusing to bathe or wear clean clothing or urinating in the backyard rather than returning indoors to use the bathroom. Suspiciousness and delusional thinking may develop. The person may suddenly decide to retain all financial assets in cash at home or may collect uncashed checks while living in poverty.

Cognitive/reasoning impairments may range from mild to severe. Common difficulties include logical and mathematical thought processes (e.g., calculation) and the ability to acquire and retain new information (memory and recall). Progressive deterioration causes losses in the ability to think abstractly, and reasoning becomes concrete and egocentric. The client's world becomes narrowed so that personal control can be maintained. Reading comprehension is more impaired than auditory comprehension; reading for meaning is more impaired than ability to read aloud, and writing skills are more impaired than speaking ability (Wells, 1982). This suggests that use of written instructions to compensate for memory deficits in, for instance, teaching clients about a drug or dietary regimen will require further careful assessments.

Memory impairment is a prominent feature of organic mental disorders. Memory of recent events is lost first and may become very serious with the person unable to remember either simple tasks like shutting off the stove burners after cooking or significant events such as the death of a spouse and the marriages of children. Remote memory is more likely to be retained and the client may have fair to good recall of past events. An elderly person may comment that he can't remember where he went for lunch yesterday but can describe his third grade classroom and tell you who sat next to him.

Confabulation refers to the tendency to fill in memory gaps with likely fabrications in order to preserve one's self-esteem. In performing an assessment of memory, the nurse needs to corroborate the facts gathered with her own observations or the recall of other significant people. For instance, if recent memory is to be checked by the client's recall of what he ate for breakfast an hour ago, it is important to verify this information. It is possible for the client to describe a reasonable breakfast from general information and remote memory of customary habits despite having no memory of what was actually eaten this morning. It is generally preferable to ask the client to remember three unrelated words and/or numbers and then to check back later for actual recall. Remote memory for details such as date of birth, years when children were born, or first home as a newlywed can generally be tested by asking for this information and then verifying the accuracy of the responses with family members.

Affect and mood in organic mental disorders may fluctuate rapidly and range from anxiety to depression, irritability, apathy, or euphoria. Responses may be labile, unpredictable, or excessive in relation to the actual stimulus. Frequently, anxiety and lowered self-esteem are also present as clients recognize their own deterioration in mental capacities and their growing dependence on others for their survival.

On the other hand, a primary depression may imitate the dementias by presenting symptoms of cognitive impairment. In this case, the symptoms are referred to as pseudodementia. It is vital in cases of suspected dementia to obtain a full psychiatric evaluation; when in doubt, a trial course of antidepressant drug therapy may be prescribed. This helps to assure that a readily treatable condition, depression, is not overlooked and the assumption made that the client will be deteriorating progressively. Recent studies have also noted the concurrent presence of depression in both early and later stages of Alzheimer's disease. This coexisting depression can further contribute to functional disabilities. Antidepressants may also be prescribed on occasion if the physician believes this to be a factor (Aronson, 1984).

Perceptions may be distorted in individuals with organic mental disorders. Distortions may include illusions or hallucinations which are most commonly visual rather than auditory. Hallucinations are more likely in delirium as a result of toxic states associated with fever, drug reactions, or in withdrawal states such as delirium tremens. Initially, objects may be misinterpreted. Shadows may become exaggerated and appear menacing, sounds may become distorted by stress into personal images such as whispered insults or voices crying. Vivid hallucinations are very distressing to clients and may precipitate impulsive behavior in an effort to get away from menacing images such as grotesque insects or monsters. The Mental Status Questionnaire (see Table 35-3) is a brief evaluative tool to assess the degree of impairment as mild, moderate, or severe.

Self-Care Capacity. The deteriorations in mental status may seriously affect the client's self-care ability in regard to activities of daily living and meeting basic needs. See Table 35-4 for self care deficits in physical and safety needs.

Nutrition and fluid intake may be compromised by poor memory or judgment. Is the client capable of meal planning, shopping, cooking, and related activities? Is adequate self-care possible with specific modifications such as shopping assistance and replacing an old gas stove with a safer electric model? It is also important to recognize that provision of meals via a delivery service (e.g., Meals on Wheels) does not guarantee that they will be eaten. Meals may be forgotten,

---

TABLE 35-3 Mental Status Questionnaire

1. What is the name of this place?
2. Where is it located (address)?
3. What is today's date?
4. What is the month now?
5. What is the year?
6. How old are you?
7. When were you born (month)?
8. When were you born (year)?
9. Who is the president of the United States?
10. Who was the president before him?

Scoring: 9–10 correct, client is not confused

6–8 correct, client is slightly confused

3–5 correct, client is moderately confused

0–2 correct, client is severely confused

Adapted from: Kahn, R.L.; Goldfarb, A.I.; Pollack, M.; and Peck, A. Brief objective measures for the determination of mental status in the aged. *American Journal of psychiatry,* 117, 1960; 326–328.

TABLE 35-4 *Self-Care Deficits in Physical and Safety Needs in the Client with Organic Mental Disorder*

Oxygenation

Monitor vital signs and lung sounds. Observe circulatory status.	Oxygenation deficits in clients with marginal adaptive capacity in cardiopulmonary functions may be expressed by increased confusion if insufficient oxygen is available for brain functioning. Clients may be less able to communicate pain and other symptoms of compromised circulation.

Fluids and Nutrients

Record intake of fluids and calories. Monitor ability to select an adequate diet and eat unassisted. Observe for symptoms of dehydration or weight loss. Supplemental vitamins may be prescribed.	Memory deficits and confusion may leave the client too agitated, disorganized, or apathetic to eat adequately and ensure fluid status. Serving a well-balanced meal is no guarantee that it will not be spilled, forgotten, or ignored. Hyperactivity may greatly increase caloric needs.

Rest and Activity

Compare past and current patterns of activity and rest. What is the nighttime sleep pattern? Does the client become more restless and confused at night? Does apathy contribute to immobility and deprivation of social and environmental stimuli?	Apathy may significantly decrease and agitation will increase activity levels. Reduced stimuli at night contribute to higher levels of confusion at this time and decreased opportunities for validating and correcting perceptions.

Elimination

Observe for retention, adequacy of output, incontinence/involuntary stools, and ability to meet elimination needs unassisted.	Disorientation and confusion can alter the pattern of elimination and the ability to recall location of appropriate facilities and basic behaviors associated with urinary and bowel elimination.

Hygiene/Appearance

How much assistance is needed for bathing, grooming, and selection of appropriate attire? Observe condition of mouth, nails, and hair.	Client may neglect hygiene due to poor memory and disorientation. Clothing may be deficient or excessive (e.g., multiple layers of all items owned) in terms of the weather or situation.

Safety

Does the client wander? Is the gait steady enough for independent ambulation? Is orientation to person and place appropriate at all times of day? Is judgment adequate? Are hallucinations or delusions present which could lead to impulsive actions harmful to self or others? Is adequate supervision available to protect the client?	Disturbances of orientation and sensory perception can be very frightening resulting in "fight or flight" behavior. Confusion may precipitate wandering off or inappropriate behaviors and decisions. Family and staff members must supervise and limit client activities as necessary for client safety.

hoarded uneaten, or viewed with suspicion. Actual assessments will include regular observation and recording of client weight and hydration status.

Elimination patterns can be influenced by diet, activity, and presence of confusion. Incontinence may be caused by several factors: the urgency associated with urinary tract infections, weakening of muscles and sphincter control leading to stress incontinence, or confusion and the inability to recall and perform toileting activities accurately and independently.

TABLE 35-5 *Diagnostic Tests Associated with Organic Mental Disorders: Nursing Implications*

Test	Purpose	Nursing Implications
Skull x-ray films	To observe for fractures in the skull, calcifications, and shifting of structures due to space-occupying lesions.	Metal objects and dentures (if metallic) need to be removed. Inform the client that the procedure is painless.
Lumbar puncture	To examine cerebrospinal fluid for abnormal contents (e.g., pus, blood, protein, bacteria, abnormal glucose level) and to measure intracranial pressure.	A sterile procedure performed at the bedside by a physician, using local anesthetic, with the client in the lateral decubitus position for maximum flexion of the spine. The procedure is uncomfortable and the client may experience leg pain and pressure during the examination and a headache following it. Encourage fluid intake to replace the cerebrospinal fluid removed. Assist the client to remain motionless during the procedure and offer reassurance and support. This procedure is not used if increased intercranial pressure is suspected. Prior to the procedure, a consent form is signed. The client should void. Take specimens immediately to the laboratory.
Echoencephalogram/ ultrasound	A safe, rapidly performed visualization of brain structure to detect shifts caused by hemorrhages or tumors.	This is a painless procedure. A gel will be applied to several sites on the scalp to improve sound wave transmission.
Computerized axial tomography (CAT or CT Scan)	This scan provides a three-dimensional view of the cranium with or without use of dyes. A nonintrusive diagnosis of tumors, hemorrhages, malformations, and structural changes.	Wigs and hairpins should be removed and client must remain still for the 20–40 minutes of scanning. Check for allergy to iodine dye. Hold NPO for the preceding 4 hours since dye may cause nausea. The client will hear a clicking sound during the procedure but will experience no pain. The dye, if used, will be given IV and will cause a warm flushing sensation.
Pneumoencephalogram	Rarely used unless CAT scan is not available. CAT is more accurate, safer, and less painful for the same purposes.	The client is NPO after midnight and sedated. Air is injected into the lumbar subarachnoid space via lumbar puncture, with the client in a seated position. Nausea, headache, and sensations caused by the air moving about in the ventricles may be experienced. Vital signs are carefully monitored during and following the procedure. Bedrest for 24–48 hours following may be ordered with gradual elevation of the head of the bed. Fever and chills are possible. Serious complications such as brain herniation and seizures may occur. Written consent is generally required.
Cerebral angiogram/ arteriogram	A visualization via radioactive dye of the arterial structures to detect circulatory abnormalities of the brain.	Check for iodine dye allergy. The client is held NPO after midnight. Presedation and local anesthesia are used. Dye injection causes a short burning sensation. Written consent is required. Be prepared for anaphylactic reaction during and immediately following the procedure. Vital signs and neurological assessments are carefully monitored for the first 24 hours to check for hemorrhage or embolus. Assess the catheter insertion site for bleeding and inflammation and, if brachial or femoral insertion sites were used, check for peripheral circulation and function. Bedrest for 24 hours and local ice application to the site is generally ordered following the procedure.

(*continued*)

TABLE 35-5 (continued)

Test	Purpose	Nursing Implications
Electroencephalogram (EEG)	EEG graphically records the electrical activity generated by the brain. It is used to determine seizure foci in epilepsy, to note slowing of brain waves caused by brain lesions, and to determine brain death in comatose clients.	Sleep is generally limited the night prior to EEG. Hair should be freshly shampooed and dry. Do not give caffeine prior to the procedure. Electrode paste is applied and electrodes attached. The client, in a supine position with closed eyes, is recorded awake and sometimes sleeping. The client does not fast. During the EEG, the client should remain still and keep eyes closed. Paste should be shampooed out of hair following the EEG.

Hygiene and grooming should be assessed for adequacy. Is clothing appropriate for warmth and seasonal comfort? Are living conditions basically clean and free from pests and fire hazards? Are necessary aids such as dentures, glasses, and hearing aids maintained and functioning?

Mobility requires assessments of gait in relationship to the demands of the environment. Is stair climbing, for instance, hazardous but the only way to reach a second floor bathroom? Is the telephone readily accessible in times of emergency? Can the ambulatory client safely walk outdoors for exercise? Are there barriers that interfere with the mobility of the client dependent on a wheelchair?

Safety assessments include awareness of various factors that may pose hazards. Night wandering may predispose the person to overexposure in bad weather or to becoming lost. Is orientation sufficient for independent living or is supervision available for the confused client? It is particularly important to be alert to the possibility of impulsive behavior in hallucinating, emotionally labile, and severely depressed clients.

The problem of confusion is a general problem area characterized by disorientation; inability to follow directions; impairment of memory, thought, and perception; and agitation and restlessness which may be most evident at night (Wolanin and Phillips, 1981). Risk factors associated with the problems of confusion include age above 80 years, social isolation, abrupt relocation, pain, disruption of physical need patterns, use of central nervous system depressant drugs, and diminished or distorted cues for time and spatial perception. It should be noted that hospitalization and transfer to a nursing home are both likely to be associated with several of these risk factors.

Diagnostic Tests. When organic mental disorder is suspected, the physician generally does a complete medical workup including laboratory tests for blood count, blood chemistry, and urinalysis. Brain structures will be visualized by computerized axial tomography (CAT or CT) or ultrasound to detect tumors or hemorrhages. Cerebrovascular sufficiency may be examined via cerebral angiography. The electroencephalogram (EEG) may be used to evaluate functional patterns of brain activity. See Table 35-5 for a description of common diagnostic tests and nursing implications.

Family and Environmental Assessment □ Family assessments include the following areas: (1) the family as a secondary source of client information; (2) family ability to provide needed support to the organically mentally impaired client; and (3) family information and concerns about hereditary factors particularly in Alzheimer's disease and Huntington's chorea.

The family provides an excellent secondary source of data when the client is a confused or unreliable information source. A family tree or genogram is a vital component of assessment in organic mental disorders because many of the conditions categorized as dementia, for example, Alzheimer's disease and Huntington's chorea, have a strong hereditary correlation. Family members may also assist nurses to differentiate between the symptoms that led the client and family to seek help and those that occurred in response to the stress and relocation of hospitalization itself.

Family strengths and resources are vital aspects of client support during hospitalization and upon return to the community. Are some family members able to remain with the client during episodes of confusion to provide reassurance, reorientation, and safety without the necessity of restraints? Does the family have sufficient time and energy to sustain these efforts for as long as they are needed? Can the family provide the necessary support for the client on his return home? This may entail as little as making regular phone calls to him and running occasional errands or as much as constant supervision and care. Assessment of the family's capacity and willingness to undertake these efforts requires sensitivity and understanding on the part of the nurse. Many families cannot summon the physical and emotional resources to maintain a confused member in a home setting. Currently many families have two employed parents and dependent children, while single-parent families are stressed by the demands of work and child rearing. To further add to the guilt of these families is to do them a disservice and to predispose the client to potential neglect if the family cannot carry out the necessary tasks they may have reluctantly undertaken.

The family that is willing and able to provide the necessary assistance will require information and emotional support. The nursing assessment related to the family's ability to meet the client's needs in the community should address the following aspects.

1. Family perception of client need: Is the family aware of the degree of support needed by the client? Can they specifically describe the problem areas and identify potential solutions that are realistic in terms of the client's self-care and safety deficits?
2. Family values and feelings: Does the family have a strong commitment to maintaining the client in the family home or in a supportive independent living situation? Or is the family more concerned with what they "should do" in the eyes of others? The issue of negative feelings should be openly discussed. The decision to choose nursing home placement or maintain the client in the family home is a painful one for client and family regardless of the outcome. On the one hand lies the pain of increased separation from family and some loss of independence for the client in a nursing home. These aspects vary according to the degree of family involvement following placement. Families often feel regret and guilt about placement in a nursing home even if the client is accepting of the move. On the other hand, the difficulties of long-term maintenance of the client in the family home or a nearby residence should not be underestimated. Family members may have their schedules and life-styles disrupted. Resentments are likely if not inevitable. Also at issue is whether it is possible for the client to be treated as a valued and involved family member with reasonable socialization and independence. If remaining in a family setting necessitates cutting the client off from the social support of older friends and makes familiar pastimes difficult, it may be less satisfactory for the client than residential care.

3. Knowledge of available alternatives: Is the family aware of the variety of options available? Often the choices are not limited to overcrowding a son or daughter's growing family, or a nursing home placement. Independent residential settings may offer sufficient support services to maintain the client in an apartment with optional cafeteria, health care, and activity programs. Day-care programs may be available for clients whose families are away all day but would welcome them in the evening and on weekends. Respite care is a service that provides temporary caretakers to permit the family to take vacations or to assist in times of stress. These services, like nursing homes, should be visited by client and family during the decision-making process.

Environmental Assessment □ The environment is viewed from the time perspectives of past, present, and future. The past environment is assessed to obtain a history of exposure to etiologic factors such as those depicted in Table 35-1. The current environment needs to be assessed from the standpoint of client safety and conditions to promote optimum awareness and function. Questions concerning environmental safety include:

1. Is supervision or use of necessary siderails and restraints adequate and necessary to prevent injury of the confused client?
2. Are hazards removed to prevent accidents such as falling or stumbling over equipment or throw rugs?
3. Is the client's room appropriately placed for supervision if wandering behavior occurs? Clients who wander at night may walk out of a nearby entrance and become lost, injured in traffic, or victims of overexposure in bad weather.
4. Is lighting adequate to prevent injury to the client with poor vision and to avoid mis-

interpretation of shadows as objects with the subsequent agitation of clients experiencing illusions or hallucinations.

5. Is the client's response to medications and activity carefully evaluated for its effect on alertness and activity level? A client with marginal cardiac output may experience confusion related to deficient cerebral oxygenation following exertion. Many elderly clients experience confusion and agitation if barbiturates are administered as routine nighttime sedation.

Sensory input is an important component of maximizing the client's awareness and functioning, particularly in the strange environment of the hospital or extended care setting. The client's sensory deficits should be identified. The client or family should also be asked whether sensory assistive devices (glasses, contact lens, hearing aids) are used and if these are present and in working order. Does the client receive an appropriate amount of touch? The client's preferred level of sensory stimulation should be assessed as well as the level and variety of input available in the current environment. Is the client predisposed to either sensory deprivation or overload?

Attention to the future environment is an important component of discharge planning. Returning home, going to live with one's family, moving to a new apartment or a long-term care facility all require careful assessment of the client's unique needs, strengths, and self-care deficits in relationship to the specific environment's ability to provide for physical safety, security, and social needs. This may involve a home assessment visit by a community or home health care nurse or social worker.

Nurse's Self-Assessment □ Self-awareness by the nurse is a vital component of care for the client with an organic mental disorder because the beliefs, attitudes, and feelings of the nurse are likely to affect the quality of care provided.

Feelings of frustration, helplessness, and hopelessness frequently arise because of the long-term and debilitating nature of many of these conditions. Since brain cells do not regenerate and deficits may be significant and progressive, it is unrealistic to expect a cure in, for instance, the client with Alzheimer's disease. If this leads to "giving up" on the client, the effects on both him and his family can be very detrimental. On the other hand, awareness of these common responses

to any chronic illness can make the nurse more sensitive and understanding of the feelings of the family who must cope day to day with the problems. Although many dementias are irreversible, there is much that can be accomplished through excellent nursing care to slow deterioration in functioning and to increase the client's ability to adapt to and cope with deficits. Nurses who feel a need for immediate results or rapid, significant improvement in clients will have particular difficulty in this area.

Regressed and inappropriate behaviors such as self-exposure, repetitive and automatic verbalization (e.g., calls for help or cursing) may annoy and anger the nurse. The client's labile affect and unpredictable behavior may create anxiety and further stress on the part of caregivers. Frustration and anger may lead to guilt feelings and fears that the caregiver's irritability may result in poor care, neglect, or abusive actions. These feelings need to be openly addressed and dealt with. Working with the organically mentally impaired client can be very stressful. Long-term dependency and the demands of care may drain the energies of family and nurses alike, bringing related feelings of resentment and lack of appreciation since clients may resist the care needed and express little or no gratitude for caregivers' efforts. Peer reinforcement and support sources available to the nurse become an important area for assessment.

PROBLEM AND NEED IDENTIFICATION □ Based on the assessment factors previously discussed, the nurse will identify problems and needs of the client, the family, and herself that influence the client's level of functioning and adaptive capacity. The client may experience physical problems such as alterations in nutrition, elimination, sleep, and activity patterns. Disturbances of thought, memory, and perception are common in organic mental disorders. Behavioral and emotional changes may be organically based or may occur in response to the perceived deficits and loss experienced by the client. The client's knowledge of what is occurring and his ability to cope may range from adequate to highly ineffective. Recognition of client strengths, interests, and resources is as significant to an assessment as is identification of specific problems.

The family is likely to experience knowledge deficits regarding the course of the condition, the probable outcome, hereditary relationships, if any, and the availability of community resources.

Family coping may be effective, requiring only support and encouragement, or it may be ineffective, suggesting a need for nursing interventions to promote more adaptive coping. Steuer (1984) notes that many caregivers experience stress, anxiety, and depression.

Nurses too may be more or less effective in coping with the needs of these clients and their families. Ineffective coping may be limited to one or two individuals or may involve the entire nursing team working with the family and the client who has an organic mental disorder.

■ Point of Emphasis

Ineffective coping is a problem that may be identified in the client, the family, and/or the nursing staff.

NURSING INTERVENTION □ Rabins (1981) describes studies done in neurological hospitals, clinics, and consultation services which found that with proper care up to 30 percent of clients with a diagnosis of dementia could have improved health status. Even though little can be done to improve the intellectual functioning of persons with organic mental disorders, the quality of these individuals' lives can be maintained or significantly improved through thoughtful nursing intervention.

■ Point of Emphasis

One of the treatment objectives of nursing care for the organically impaired client is to maximize the level of functioning and the quality of life for both the client and the family.

Primary Prevention □ Clearly the most effective level of prevention is the primary level which reduces or eliminates exposure to the causative factors. A useful example is the increase in public awareness during the 1960s and 1970s of the effects of toxic metals such as lead. Occupational safety measures have since sought to reduce the exposure of workers to lead, mercury, and arsenicals. Public health information on the effects of lead on children has led to a ban on sale of lead-based interior paints, and significant efforts have been made to reduce lead pollutants in the air by setting standards to control lead emissions from cars and factories. Research that demonstrated higher lead levels in children exposed to the air in heavily trafficked areas was in part responsible for the shift to the use of unleaded gasoline.

Public awareness has increased in regard to the role of nutrition in specific organic mental syndromes such as those associated with pellagra, Wernicke's and Korsakoff's syndromes, as well as the generalized effects of malnutrition on the neurological developmental of the fetus, infant, and child. Nurses can demonstrate the continuing need for maternal-child nutrition programs for the needy and for public education for all prospective parents on the nutritional needs of pregnant women, growing infants, and children.

Further research is vital in determining the underlying causes of common and devastating dementias such as Alzheimer's disease, for which no method of prevention has yet been found. Nurses can support the public's awareness of the need for and the value of basic research in the etiology of the dementias.

Health educators, public safety advocates, and nurses share in the role of educating the public in health and safety behaviors which can significantly reduce the prevalence of organic mental disorders resulting from car accident trauma and substance abuse. The National Safety Council sponsors messages to promote the use of seat belts for both adults and children. Various alcohol and drug education programs advocate responsible drinking, the awareness that drugs create hazardous driving conditions, and ways to avoid situations conducive to drunk driving. All of these approaches reduce the number of organic mental disorders caused by the trauma of highway accidents.

The Food and Drug Administration is responsible for monitoring food additives and pharmaceuticals that pose potentials for toxic mental disorders. Formerly, bromides were a common over-the-counter medication to promote sedation and relieve gastrointestinal distress. Their role in causing a toxic organic mental syndrome was

---

■ Point of Emphasis

Primary prevention involves the effective interplay of research, public information and awareness, and political action to reduce potential exposures to agents and circumstances causing organic mental disorders.

identified, they are no longer permitted in over-the-counter remedies, and bromide poisoning has virtually disappeared.

Secondary Prevention □ Secondary prevention in organic mental disorders involves the screening of target groups at risk such as high-risk occupations, populations of chronic alcohol or drug abusers, and the elderly. Early recognition and treatment of the deliriums can avert permanent brain damage and chronic problems. Treatment initiated early in the course of the dementias can serve to maintain the highest level of independence and general functioning of which the client is capable and to support the family in caring for and making decisions that affect the client. Nurses in the fields of community health, occupational/industrial health, gerontology, medical-surgical hospitals, and psychiatric-mental health can all participate in efforts at early recognition of organic mental disorders and referral to physicians for diagnosis and prompt initiation of care.

Tertiary Prevention □ Tertiary prevention emphasizes rehabilitation and long-term efforts at maintaining the client's level of functioning. Nurses have a particularly valuable role in this area: they contribute to the physical and psychosocial rehabilitation of the client; coordinate the efforts of client, family, and health care personnel; and manage aspects of the environment to minimize barriers to client independence and support the client's needs, sense of security, and self-care capability on an individualized basis. Nursing care measures may be directed toward client problems, family problems, environmental problems, and/or nurse problems. Table 35-6 lists some current approaches to pharmacotherapy in Alzheimer's disease.

Client Care

Goals for clients must be realistic. Over- and underestimating client potential are both damaging since, on the one hand, stress and frustration will result and on the other, opportunity for improved functioning is overlooked. Regardless of the nature of the goals, the dignity of the client must be respected (Bartol, 1983). Nursing intervention appropriate to each of the designated problem areas is as follows.

Minor memory deficits that occur in a clear mental state can generally be managed by clients

TABLE 35-6 Pharmacotherapy in Alzheimer's Disease

Drug	Use	Effectiveness
Lecithin	Choline precursor to increase serum choline	Some memory improvement shown
Physostigmine	Slows breakdown of acetylcholine by enzyme	Given orally, often in combination with lecithin, to improve memory
Deanol	Increases cholinergic activity	No memory effects, some reduction in anxiety and depression
Hydergine, papaverine	Vasodilation to enhance cerebral circulation	Some maintenance or slight improvement in cognitive and emotional functioning
Methylphenidate, pentylenetetrazole (Metrazole)	Stimulate mood and attention	None demonstrated but frequently prescribed
Doxepin, trazodone (Desyrel)	Tricyclic antidepressant activity	Antidepressants with fewer anticholinergic side effects
Haloperidol (Haldol)	Antipsychotic	Reduces agitation and aggression with least hypotensive effect
Chloral hydrate	Sedative	Occasional use only to promote sleep
Oxazepam (Serax)	Tranquilizer	Reduces anxiety and agitation; fairly short-acting.

through a combination of relatively fixed habit patterns and written cues. "A place for everything and everything in its place" may provide needed stability and routine to minimize forgetfulness and misplacing objects. The tendency of many people to become rigid in their habit patterns may often be a means of compensating for memory deficits. A memo pad carried at all times permits written reminders and memory joggers to be noted throughout the day. Some of these items can be transferred to a "To Do" list or planning calendar for subsequent days. New learning is more apt to be retained if it is repeated in a variety of ways and paired to familiar concepts.

Disorientation and confusion are serious, commonly occurring problems in organic mental disorders whether of short or long duration. Reorientation should be attempted frequently. The client should be given orienting information in brief, clear terms repeatedly throughout the day following assessments of orientation. Informal opportunities for orientation should be incorporated consistently during care. For example, use statements such as "It's a beautiful May morning," "It's time for breakfast and then I'll help you with your morning bath," or "We'll play Bingo tonight at 7 right after supper." Cues to reinforce orientation should be extensively used in the environment, for example, large clocks, calendars, and brightly colored schedules and wall charts in rooms and hallways. Staff should wear extra-large name tags and reintroduce themselves until the client is able to recall their names and roles. It is vital to address the client clearly and respectfully by his correct name at all times. Terms such as "dearie" or "sweetie" are depersonalizing. In extended care facilities, it is often useful to use a buddy system in orienting new clients. This provides a sense of security and additional personal involvement for the client and an opportunity to increase the sense of usefulness and self-esteem of the client who serves as helper. Clients who become disoriented and agitated at night from delirium can generally be assisted by turning on sufficient light to provide visual cues and eliminate shadows. Familiar objects and furnishings such as favorite pictures, books, chair, or quilt may also provide a sense of comfort and familiarity.

> ■ **Point of Emphasis**
>
> *A consistently structured environment which provides numerous orienting cues, permits retention of familiar objects and provides adequate social input promotes orientation and reality contact.*

Inappropriate or impulsive behavior is best managed through gentle distraction and redirection. The client's short attention span permits the staff to tactfully and respectfully divert his attention toward other activities that are more likely to be productive and enjoyable. Close observation of clients who are impulsive or inappropriate is

essential to protect them from the ridicule or disapproval of others and to maintain their personal safety.

Perseveration, the tendency to repeat an action over and over, can be used to assist the client to perform simple activities that can promote a feeling of usefulness, such as dusting, sweeping, or raking.

Disturbances of thought and perception are not as detailed or based in symbolic needs as those of the schizophrenic client. Misperceptions tend to be transient and based on situational aspects such as (1) the need to explain the loss of a particular misplaced object by assuming it stolen; or (2) calling a staff member by a family member's name, an attempt to impose the comforting and familiar on a confusing world. Presenting reality in a gentle, reassuring way is the most effective way to deal with this problem. It is not helpful to "go along with" and reinforce the client's confusion. It is also not helpful to give the client more information than he can realistically assimilate at the time. For this reason, it is not particularly useful to explain that the sister for whom the nurse was mistaken has been dead for over 5 years. Simply stating "I'm not your sister, I'm your nurse, Helen Ames, and you are in the hospital," provides reality-based information. This, combined with an attitude of caring and an offer of any needed assistance, is most likely eventually to promote client orientation and security. Helping the client to look for lost objects is more helpful than discussing if they were stolen or by whom. Often they can be located, or the search may provide distractions.

Beam (1984) emphasizes that communication with the confused client should be carried on in a low tone; using simple, short words and brief phrases; and providing nonverbal reassurance.

If the client is experiencing vivid visual hallucinations, it is important to reassure him that the images are not really there, that the nurse does not see them and is not frightened. This information will need to be repeated over and over in a calm reassuring voice. Soothing touch and the physical presence of the nurse will also reduce agitation. Highly anxious and hallucinating clients should not be left alone.

Apathy may result from sensory deficits and deprivation. Clients who have visual or hearing problems, who must be on bedrest for several days or more, or who lack meaningful contacts with friends and family may respond with apathy. Later, because of the sensory and social deprivation, confusion or depression may result. Sensory aids should be maintained and used by the client. Note the need for glasses or a hearing aid on the care plan so that personnel assure the client's access to and use of these assistive devices. If sensory input is limited be certain to include compensatory input. For instance, the blind client needs additional and varied forms of auditory and tactile stimulation. Apathy may also result from grief or depression. (See Chapters 26 and 33 for related nursing care.)

Physical and safety need deficits must be carefully assessed and remedied because of the decreased capacity of organic mentally impaired clients to identify and communicate their needs. Physical needs such as oxygenation problems or fluid and electrolyte imbalances may be etiological factors in delirium. Other physical problems may result from long-term self-care deficits in the client with dementia who may experience problems in eating, sleeping, toileting, and grooming. Self-care capacity must be carefully assessed to permit the client to maintain the highest level of independence of which he is capable. This may require allowing much extra time to permit self-care and may necessitate changes in the environment in either the hospital or in the clients' home setting. Safety needs may become the priority if the client is acutely confused, impulsive, or agitated. Clients in withdrawal from alcohol or drugs are in acute physiological and psychological distress. They require continuous supervision, supportive care, and safety measures.

■ **Point of Emphasis**

Clients who are acutely confused and agitated require continuous supervision and support.

General supportive care measures include meeting physical, social, and developmental needs through exercise and diversional activities, remotivation and reminiscence groups for the older adult, and opportunities for interpersonal socialization. Touch can provide a powerful sense of interpersonal connectedness. Opportunities to use touch are numerous in both physical care and social situations in which one spontaneously reaches out to another.

Families of clients with hereditary disorders may require genetic counseling. In Huntington's chorea, for example, the age of onset is frequently in the 30s. By this time the person with the disorder may have already established a family. Recently there is hope for a test to identify which of the children has inherited this condition. Living with uncertain knowledge is a major stressor as is the decision to have or not have children of one's own. Appropriate referral for genetic counseling is a significant element of care for these families.

The family of the client with an organic mental disorder has specific needs for information, support during decision making, and emotional support. Informational needs include: (1) whether there is a hereditary component to the disorder and, if so, the sources for genetic counseling; (2) the potential duration and course of the illness, for instance if the client survives the acute symptoms whether he is likely to recover full functioning or is more likely to experience long-term mental deterioration; (3) informational and supportive agencies in the community such as self-help groups, adult day-care centers, and various levels of residential care available. Decision-making support involves gathering and coordinating (or referring the client to a social worker who will coordinate) information on resources, costs, and other alternative options to assist the family in making informed choices about client placement and care. A comprehensive approach would explore the wishes and feelings of both the client and family, their limitations and capacities, and the relative costs and benefits of the available facilities. Ideally, the client and family will visit the facilities before making a decision. Community or home health nurses can assess the client's current living situation in terms of suitability for his return to that environment. Too frequently, the decision about nursing home or extended care placement is made just prior to dismissal by the physician or social worker without adequate exploration with the family. Both client and family deserve better.

Emotional support involves actively listening to the feelings and concerns of client and family. Once placement is accomplished, in many cases there still remains the need for long-term support. The client who is returning to a relatively independent care setting may need a careful environmental assessment to support self-care and safety. For instance, are services accessible, is security adequate, and is emergency assistance readily obtainable? Daily monitoring of needs may be accomplished via family calls or friendly call-in services provided by agencies. Families require assistance in accepting and coping with concerns and negative feelings. Care of the organically impaired client can drain physical, financial, and emotional resources. The client may need to talk about feelings of being a burden to the family or resentments at feeling isolated and neglected. Ways to express caring and concern without nagging or accusing should be explored on both sides. Family coping should include marshaling the family's available resources to provide care. For instance, family councils can often brainstorm ways to provide the needed care in a consistent manner without unduly burdening a few members, despite the fact that individuals may vary widely in their ability to contribute. A teenager may become a regular errand runner and chauffeur, one family may provide room and board while the other contributes money for cleaning or sitting services to reduce the workload of housekeeping, older children can share time in walking, gardening, or listening to tales of the good old days with the client. Problem-solving and communication skills are key ingredients of effective family coping.

Self-help and coping groups are excellent sources of family support. These may be designed around the needs of families in relation to particular conditions such as head trauma, Alzheimer's disease or Huntington's chorea, or they may be designed around types of placement (e.g., home care or institutional care). Support groups provide information, opportunities to share feelings in an accepting atmosphere, and encouragement to members to use available services such as day care or respite care and handle their own needs. Hope and practical strategies for coping with problems are significant benefits. Steuer (1984) notes that although support groups have many benefits, there may be a risk of increasing anxiety and depression in some members if denial has been a strong defense and it is reduced by group involvement.

Practical suggestions which can be offered to families caring for clients with dementias include means of maintaining optimum level of independence through simplifying clothing fasteners and by encouraging the client to do as much as possible for himself even if it takes much longer than to do these things for him. Restlessness and agitation may be reduced by gentle touch or diversions such as playing favorite recordings of music from the person's younger days. Promoting relatedness between the client and family members may be accomplished by leafing through a picture book containing favorite items such as pictures of pets, hobbies, or nature scenes. Looking through old photo albums provides opportunities to reminisce for the client and for the family member to share in some moments of the client's life and the family history.

Nurse Focused Intervention □ Nurses, like family members who serve as caretakers for confused and dependent clients, can experience a range of negative feelings such as frustration in not meeting desired goals for client improvement, irritability at particular client behaviors or demands, and resentment at giving so much of self in physical and emotional care without, in many cases, a sense of recognition or gratitude from the client. Family guilt feelings at times may lead to avoidance of the client, criticism of the staff, or demanding behavior. The helpless client may manipulate family and staff attitudes against one another in an attempt to secure attention.

In addition to the interpersonal aspects of care mentioned, nurses may question the ethics and values related to quantity and quality of life issues when clients become physically ill and require medical intervention to survive. The nurse may question the value of her activities in circumstances in which the inevitable outcome is likely to be continued deterioration.

Recognizing that all of these issues may occur creates a vital need for self-awareness, monitoring the attitudes and feelings of other staff members, and openly identifying problems when they arise. Peer communication and support are crucial to the success of these efforts if problems are to be openly acknowledged and dealt with before they lead to potential abuses such as neglect, verbal hostility, or actual physically aggressive acts. Two points must be clearly communicated to all caregivers:

1. Negative feelings are common occurrences and can be dealt with in an open, supportive problem-solving atmosphere.
2. Neglect and abusive words or actions are intolerable and a cause for dismissal because clients deserve quality care and respect for their basic human dignity.

Problem-solving approaches that may be effectively tried include opportunities for ventilating feelings, a change of assignments, time off, stress-management activities, or a peer coping group instituted as part of the care team's approach to care. See Table 35-7 for a sample care

TABLE 35-7 :Sample Care Plan, Alzheimer's Disease

Assessment Data	Problem Identification	Goal	Intervention	Rationale	Evaluation
			First Problem		
Slow, shuffling broad-based gait. Reduced arm swing. Continuous aimless/purposeless and often repetitive activity. Paces restlessly and perseverates in repeating aimless movements. Awakens frequently at night and becomes very agitated and fearful—often believes she has been kidnapped and is held hostage. Enjoys walks outdoors, simple tasks, and listening to music.	Altered activity and rest patterns due to organic brain changes and confusion.	Maintain balance of activity and rest, including adequate sleep.	Provide simple, repetitious activities such as sweeping, dusting, or raking leaves. Schedule frequent rest periods during the day. Remain with her if needed to promote sedentary activity or social relaxation via listening to music, promoting rest by giving a back rub. At night, assure that physical needs are met before retiring. (Give light snack, limit fluids near bedtime, and promote elimination.) Provide adequate lighting in room to prevent shadows and distortions. Provide orientation and reassurance during night if awake.	Avoid complex tasks and make use of perseveration to provide sense of control and mastery. Scheduling and promoting rest is important because of client's distractibility and poor memory, may need to direct her back to restful activity. Frequent awakening can be aggravated by hunger or the need to void. Darkness and shadows may be distorted by the confused client. Reorientation and providing visual cues and reassurance tend to prevent agitation.	Record amount of sleep per night and number/duration of rest periods, for improvement. Goal criteria would be 6–7 hours/night of sleep and 3 or 4 rest periods of 30 minute or more during day.
			Second Problem		
Unable to identify place or time correctly. States her name is Anne Ellis (her maiden name). Fails to recognize family members.	Anxiety related to thought disorders (memory loss, confusion, delusions) associated with organic brain changes.	Promote sense of personal security and environmental awareness within limitations of disease process.	Communicate in clear, simple sentences and low, gentle voice tone. Reorient frequently in caring, respectful manner. Interpret	Harsh voices and complex situations increase agitation. Repetition and consistency of routine are basic to providing a predictable environment	Reduction in recorded numbers and intensity of episodes of agitation. Able to follow daily activity routine comfortably with

Behavior	Nursing Diagnosis	Goals	Intervention	Rationale	Evaluation
Speech is occasionally incoherent with episodes of clarity. Frequent echolalic. Becomes frustrated at difficulty in making needs known—yells or becomes angry. Becomes fearful and agitated in frustrating situations. Expresses fears that she is kidnapped, that her belongings have been stolen. Attention span is brief and memory is very poor, highly distractible.			reality and offer realistic reassurance (e.g., "You're not lost, Anne. You're in Valley Care Center. I'm a nurse.") Invite to remotivation and social reminiscing groups.	ronment. Habits, a buddy system, and varied environmental cues promote a sense of security. Anxiety can be communicated interpersonally. Distraction is a more effective means of coping with negative behavior because of the short attention span and memory problems. These groups meet special needs and provide appropriate social contact.	assistance of staff and other client.

Third and Fourth Problems

Behavior	Nursing Diagnosis	Goals	Intervention	Rationale	Evaluation
Eats large quantities of food. Neglects use of tableware and puts whole potatoes or servings of meat in mouth at one time. Occasionally puts inedible objects in mouth such as soap or pins. Weight loss of 5 pounds over past 2 or 3 months. Some days forgets to eat—becomes distracted and wanders off.	Nutrition alteration: caloric deficiency related to confusion and high activity level. Potential for injury (choking, aspiration, ingestion of foreign objects) due to confusion.	Maintain hydration and body weight. Maintain physical safety.	Supplement meals with between-meal nourishments. Provide finger foods and assistance in eating as needed (e.g., serve soup in a cup for drinking, cut foods into bite size pieces.) Supervise meals and promote pleasant atmosphere. Record intake of fluids and nutrients. Record weight weekly. Carefully remove wrappers and foreign objects from tray and room.	Continuous aimless activity increases caloric needs. Promote ease and attractiveness in meeting nutritional needs. Monitor adequacy of diet and fluid intake by recording actual amounts ingested periodically and regular graphic recording of weight. Supervision and assistance in food preparation and serving minimize hazards of choking or intake of inedibles.	Weekly weights remain stable with no further loss. No episodes of aspiration, asphyxia, or ingestion of foreign objects occur.

(continued)

TABLE 35-7 (continued)

Assessment Data	Problem Identification	Goal	Intervention	Rationale	Evaluation
			Fifth Problem		
Occasional episodes of incontinence occur more frequently at night. Resists showering and changing of clothing.	Altered toilet habits and hygiene due to confusion.	Maintain elimination and hygiene.	Assist to BR during day and during night when awake. Record voiding and defecation patterns. Observe for nonverbal cues indicating toileting need. Use persuasion and diversion to assure 2–3 baths/week and daily clothing changes.	Memory deficits necessitate monitoring and assistance in elimination and monitoring personal cleanliness and grooming.	Decrease in recorded episodes of incontinence.
			Sixth Problem		
Daughter and grandson visit weekly. Daughter frequently tearful and expresses sense of helplessness in response to her mother's deteriorating condition. "I try and I just can't get through to her—sometimes I think we'd be better off if I just quit coming to see her at all."	Potential for ineffective family coping related to chronic, deteriorating condition of client.	Maintain and promote family information and support needs.	Spend some time with the family during visits to promote interaction and role model effective approaches to engage their mother's attention. Spend time following each visit with the family. Actively listen to their concerns. Provide accurate information on the disease and its course. Refer to Alzheimer's support group in community. Share information on any particular approaches or needs of the client.	Personal contact and support of family is particularly important during long-term illness. Families have a need for expression and acceptance of feelings of discouragement, frustration, and helplessness. Accurate information and contact with others in similar circumstances can promote coping.	Family members will feel free to express concerns, questions, and feelings.

plan related to dementia, specifically Alzheimer's disease.

EVALUATION □ In delirium, the acute and time-limited nature of client problems permits establishing and attaining short-term goals for meeting physical needs, maintaining safety, and achieving orientation and behavior control. In discharge planning, it is important to ascertain whether the client accepts and understands the nature of the problem and any future preventive needs such as to avoid drinking, follow a therapeutic diet and medication regimen, or change occupations.

The client with dementia will require both short- and long-term goals. Short-term goals refer to maintaining physical needs and personal safety. Long-term goals to maximize the client's level of functioning will need to be specifically addressed with realistic criteria to monitor progress. For instance, the confused and disoriented client can be assisted to a higher level of orientation by means of structure and repetition. This may not involve the ability to correctly respond to a question about orientation but instead may demonstrate an improved ability to follow daily routines and meet personal needs.

Evaluation of family care should encompass several areas. Does the family:

1. Have an understanding of the client's condition and the general course and variations possible?
2. Experience a sense of trust and confidence in health care persons so that the members can ask questions and express their concerns and negative feelings?
3. Recognize options and alternatives available to provide support to clients and families in the community?
4. Demonstrate ability to cope with the various problems presented by the client's condition and their responses and needs in relationship to it?

Nursing self-evaluation would best be accomplished by seeking evidence that the quality of client care is high with open communication among staff to creatively solve problems of clients and of nursing staff. The work climate should be honest, supportive, and characterized by hopeful attempts at generating new solutions or means of coping.

■ *Enrichment Activities*

DISCUSSION QUESTIONS

1. Think about an older person in your life. Recall the life-style changes the individual experienced as aging took place. How did you feel when this person became forgetful or confused?

2. Recall an organically impaired individual you have cared for in the medical setting (e.g., a hospital or nursing home). What nursing interventions did you utilize? How did you feel about this client? Compare and contrast your feelings and interventions with this client to those with the personal acquaintance.

3. Your friend has just been informed that his mother has been diagnosed to have Alzheimer's disease. He asks you for information about the disorder. How would you inform him that this is a progressive degenerative disorder? To which community services would you refer him?

LEARNING ACTIVITIES

1. In small group discussion, compare the signs and symptoms of organic mental disorders to those of major depressive disorders. Compile a list of the distinguishing qualities and one of the similarities.

2. Practice the administration of the mental status questionnaire on a peer, then on a confused elderly individual. Compare the differences in response and administration for both individuals.

3. Role-play a community health nurse making a home visit to an organically mentally impaired individual who is confined to a wheelchair. The purpose of the visit is to assess the home environment (consider safety, barriers, and orientation). The nurse should explain the assessment and offer suggestions to the client and family members present.

■ *Additional Resources*

"Peege" (Phoenix films, D. Knapp and L. Berman, 1974). The central theme of this film is the breaking of communication barriers to reach individuals isolated by failing mental capacities. Peege is blind, unresponsive, and living in a nursing home. She is visited by her family who do not know how to deal with her unresponsiveness until the grandson utilizes touch and reminiscence to elicit a response.

Wolanin, M.O., and Phillips, L.R. *Confusion: Prevention & care,* St. Louis: Mosby Company, 1981. This excellent text emphasizes comprehensive nursing assessments and care for clients with confusion and those at risk.

Educational materials may be obtained from:

Alzheimer's Disease Association
360 N. Michigan Avenue, Suite 1102
Chicago, IL 60601
"The Dementias"
Office of Public Inquiries—National Institute of Neurological Communicative Disorders and Stroke
National Institutes of Health, Building 31, Room 8-A-16
Bethesda, MD 20205

■ *References*

Adams, H.E. *Abnormal psychology.* Dubuque, IA: Wm. C. Brown Company, Publishers, 1981.

Adams, M.; Hanson, R.; Norkool, D.; Beaulieu, A.; Bellville, E.; and Morss, K. Psychological responses in critical care units. *American journal of nursing,* 78, 1978:1504–1512.

Adolfsson, R.; Gottfries, C.G.; Roos, B.E.; and Winblad, B. Changes in the brain catecholamines in patients with dementia of Alzheimer type. *British journal of psychiatry,* 135, 1979:216–223.

Aronson, M.; Gaston, P.; and Merriam, A. Depression associated with dementia. *Generations* (Winter 1984).

Bartol, M. Reaching the patient. *Geriatric nursing* (July/August 1983).

Beam, M. Helping families survive. *American journal of nursing* (February 1984).

Cross, A.J.; Crow, T.J.; Perry, E.K.; Perry, R.H.; Blessed, G.; and Tomlinson, B.E. Reduced dopamine-beta-hydroxylase activity in Alzheimer's disease. *British medical journal* 282, 1981:93–94.

Diagnostic and statistical manual of mental disorders. 3d ed. Washington, D.C.: American Psychiatric Association, 1980.

Fink, M.; Green, M.; and Bender, M.B. The face-hand test as a diagnostic sign of organic mental syndrome. *Neurology,* 2, 1952:46–58.

Heller, S.S., and Kornfeld, D.S. Delirium and related problems. In *American handbook of psychiatry.* 2d ed., Vol. 4 (Reiser, M.F., ed.). New York: Basic Books, 1975.

Henker, F.O. Acute brain syndrome. *The journal of clinical psychiatry,* 40, 1979:117–120.

Holzer, M.L.; Stiassny, D.A.; Senner-Hurley, F.; and Lefkowitz, N.G. Brain trauma. In *Adult rehabilitation: A team approach for therapists.* (Logigian, M.K., ed.). Boston: Little, Brown & Co., 1982.

Jarvik, L.F.; Ruth, V.; and Matsuyama, S.S. Organic brain syndrome and aging: A six-year followup of surviving twins. *Archives of general psychiatry,* 37, 1980:280–286.

Kahn, R.L.; Goldfarb, A.I.; Pollack, M.; and Peck, A. Brief objective measures for the determination of mental status in the aged. *American journal of psychiatry,* 117, 1960:326–328.

Kolata, G.B. Clues to the cause of senile dementia. *Science,* 211, 1981:1032–1033.

Kolb, L.C., and Brodie, H.K.H. *Modern clinical psychiatry,* 10th ed. Philadelphia: W.B. Saunders Co., 1982.

Kraus, R. *Therapeutic recreation service: Principles and practices.* Philadelphia: W.B. Saunders Co., 1978.

Lazerus, L.W.; Stafford, B.; Cooper, K.; Cohler, B.; and Dysken, M. A pilot study of an Alzheimer patient's relatives' discussion group. *The gerontologist,* 21, 1981:353–358.

Lipowski, Z.J. A new look at organic brain syndromes. *The American journal of psychiatry,* 137, 1980:674–678.

Liston, E.H. Delirium in the aged. *Psychiatric clinics of North America,* 5, 1982:49–66.

Mace, N.L., and Rabins, P.V. *The 36-hour day: A family guide to caring for persons with Alzheimer's disease, related dementing illnesses, and memory loss in later life.* Baltimore: The John Hopkins University Press, 1981.

Mann, D.M.A.; Lincoln, J.; Yates, P.O.; Stamp, J.E.; and Toper, S. Changes in the monamine containing neurons of the human CNS in senile dementia. *British journal of psychiatry,* 136, 1980:533–541.

Pagana, D., and Pagana, T. *Diagnostic testing and nursing implications—A case study approach.* St. Louis: Mosby, 1982.

Pajk, M. Alzheimer's disease—Inpatient care. *American journal of nursing,* 84, 2, 1984:216–232.

Rabins, P.V. The prevalence of reversible dementia in a psychiatric hospital. *Hospital and community psychiatry,* 32, 1981:490–492.

Reisberg, B., and Ferris, S.H. Diagnosis and assessment of the older patients. *Hospital and community psychiatry,* 33, 1982:104–110.

Schneck, M.K.; Reisberg, B.; and Ferris, S.H. An overview of current concepts of Alzheimer's disease. *American journal of psychiatry,* 139, 1982:165–173.

Spar, J.E. Dementia in the aged. *Psychiatric clinics of North America,* 5, 1982:67–86.

Steuer, J. Caring for the caregiver. *Generations* (Winter 1984).

Terry, R.D., and Davies, P. Dementia of the Alzheimer type. *Annual review of neuroscience*, 3, 1980:77–95.

Torack, R.M. *The pathologic physiology of dementia.* New York: Springer-Verlag Berling Heidelberg, 1978.

Trockman, G. Caring for the confused or delirious patient. *American journal of nursing*, 78, 1978:1495–1499.

Wells, C. Chronic brain disease: An update on alcoholism, Parkinson's disease and dementia. *Hospital and community psychiatry,* 33, 1982:111–126.

Wilkinson, O. Out of touch with reality. *American journal of nursing*, 78, 1978:1492–1494.

Wolanin, M.O., and Phillips, L.R.F. *Confusion: Prevention and care.* St. Louis: Mosby, 1981.

Zarit, S.H. *Aging and mental disorders.* New York: Free Press, 1980.

PART SEVEN

Perspectives and Trends in Psychiatric-Mental Health Nursing

This section looks both to the past and to the future in discussing current needs for knowledge to improve the quality of care in psychiatric-mental health nursing. The need for research, utilization, and the role of quality assurance are the focus of the final chapter on research.

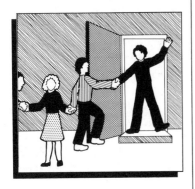

36

The Community Mental Health Movement

Amy Marie Haddad

Learning Objectives

Upon completion of this chapter, the reader will be able to:

1. Identify the impact of philosophy, politics, and scientific advances on the community mental health movement.

2. Compare the "moral treatment" of the nineteenth century to contemporary "therapeutic milieu."

3. Name three factors that encouraged the move to deinstitutionalization.

4. Define five of the essential services necessary for a community mental health center to qualify for federal funds.

5. Describe primary, secondary, and tertiary nursing interventions to be utilized on a local level in community mental health.

☐ *Influencing Factors*

Henry Ford once commented, "History is bunk." So, why look at the history of the community mental health movement when practicing nursing in today's community? An understanding of the numerous factors that have brought us to the present in the treatment of mental illness helps us appreciate the advances that have been made and explains why there was often a delay in progress. There are two important factors to remember when examining the history of the community mental health movement or history in general: (1) our "presentness" affects our interpretation of past events, i.e., we tend to see past events in a favorable light when they agree with our present beliefs and values, and (2) trends in the treatment of mental illness have not always been progressive. On the contrary, the path has been marked with highs and lows and more than one step backward. In fact, there have been times in the past when the quality of psychiatric treatment was better than it is today.

The relation that humankind bears to the total environment is influenced by factors of which we are not always aware. The possible influence that these factors had and still have on community mental health is interrelated and complex. Each individual in a community has a unique genetic background and interacts with the world in a unique way. Community mental health is concerned not only with each individual, but with the community as a whole.

A community is generally defined as a group of people living together and having interests, work, and values in common. The importance and impact of the interactive process between individuals, external systems, and the community is graphically illustrated in Figure 36-1. This is one type of model that examines the influence of factors on the well-being of the individual and the community as a whole.

CULTURAL INFLUENCE

Cultural influences in a community, often reflected in traditions and life-styles, give security and structure to daily living. Also, a self-concept grounded in the contributions and identities of past generations is developed in members of the culture. Culture influences the community's response to change, collective aspirations, and tolerance of deviation from the norm. Objective culture is the sign of a culture an outsider would notice, for example, the architecture, style of clothing, and mode of transportation. Subjective culture comprises the norms, standards of behavior, attitudes, and values of a community. For the purposes of this chapter, we are most interested in the cultural attitudes toward illness in general and mental illness in particular. The effect of culture on the individual's experience of a disease is especially marked in mental illness, as is true of many disease processes that do not have an identified objective cause.

RELIGIOUS INFLUENCE

The influence of religion on beliefs as to the cause of mental illness has been very strong in the past. The witch-hunts of the fifteenth century were carried on because the mentally ill were thought to be "possessed" or "bewitched" and were "cured" by being burned at the stake. Since religion gives comfort to its believers by explaining the unknown, it is understandable that religious leaders were called upon to explain the mystery of mental illness. The witch-hunts were not purely religious in origin. Social and political pressures of the time coupled with fear and superstition all made their contribution to this frenzy. Unusual or inappropriate behavior could only be explained as the work of the devil. The delusion of witchcraft died down after 1750 with the advent of the scientific method.

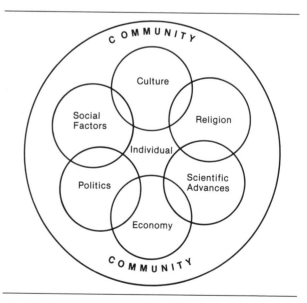

Figure 36.1 *Influence of selected environmental factors on individual and community mental health.*

SCIENTIFIC INFLUENCE

The works of René Descartes (1596–1650) inspired the development of a whole new world view for scientists and philosophers. Cartesian dualism or the "mind/body" split combined with reductionism led to the scientific method or materialism. By reducing the problem to its basic elements it was believed that the truth could be found. Great strides were made using the scientific method to solve the puzzle of many illnesses affecting human beings. For example, in the 1800s psychiatrists and neurologists looked for brain lesions by which they could identify specific mental diseases (Shryock, 1959, 263).

The scientific method led to the discovery of a connection between paresis, a neurological disorder, and tertiary syphilis. Salvarsan, an arsenical compound, was used to treat early and secondary syphilis before effective antimicrobial therapy was discovered. Salvarsan helped prevent some of the sequelae of syphilis, that is, damage to the central nervous system resulting in meningovascular syphilis, general paralysis, and tabes dorsalis. The scientific method provided a temporary solution (Salvarsan) to a disease process (secondary syphilis) that contributed to a large percentage of the "mentally ill" in the 1800s.

In addition to advances in health related areas, science was responsible for the rapid industrialization of many communities. The lifestyle changes brought about by technology continue to affect the community of today.

ECONOMIC INFLUENCE

The economy of a community sets priorities for survival. Basic human needs must be met first—adequate food, water, clothing, and shelter are essential. Interest in higher human needs and aspirations is directly related to the economic stability of a community. Social class is also related to economic security. Therefore, often the more economically sound social groups tend to the needs of the lower socioeconomic groups. The quality of treatment of the mentally ill has demonstrated this pattern repeatedly. Asylums, poorhouses, and the early state institutions are all examples of the efforts of financially secure groups to care for the impoverished mentally ill. The wealthy have generally been able to afford private care for their mentally ill in their homes or in exclusive retreats. The community mental health movement has traditionally dealt with the lower to middle socioeconomic groups. Distribution of quality care by competent providers to all individuals regardless of economic status is still a goal of the community mental health movement.

POLITICAL INFLUENCE

The involvement of government in the care of the mentally ill has coincided with its basic ideology. If the political power base is conservative and cautious, the impact on community mental health historically is maintenance of the status quo and little involvement on a local level. The more liberal political ideologies demonstrate greater government involvement and support of programs and treatment on a local level. Political disagreements that erupted into wars have had a profound effect on mental health on a local, national, and international level. Often in the aftermath of war, there have been improvements and reform in the care of the mentally ill. For example, the National Mental Health Act of 1946 was signed into law following World War II. Major factors influencing its passage were the "psychiatric" casualties of the war and the large number of draft deferments due to psychiatric problems. Politicians and the public wanted a better way to deliver mental health care.

SOCIAL INFLUENCE

Social standards are often reflected in the current jargon of a profession or group, for example, the use of the term "client" instead of "patient" in this text and other health related works. Why the shift from patient to client? The word patient is derived from Latin and means "to suffer"; it denotes calm acceptance of treatment and/or pain without complaining or losing self-control. Does this describe the role of those receiving services from our current health care system? Or does client better reflect the way we see our role as health care providers? Loosely defined, a client is a customer. Client has its origins in Latin and means "one leaning on another for protection." Patient or client. Either term carries with it the values and social expectations of the group or person using the term.

It is difficult to estimate the current impact of social standards and values on what we consider healthy or sick, sane or insane, and tolerable or intolerable behavior. We can, however, gauge the impact of social factors in the past identification and treatment of the mentally ill in the community. Social standards reflect the economy and technologic sophistication of the time. Dubos (1961, 172) noted a decrease in the tolerance of society for individuals with mental disease.

> But it is also a fact that the "village fool" who used to be an accepted member of any rural setting, the semisenile oldster who was expected to spend his last years rocking on the porch of the family homestead, and even the timid soul who escaped competition by retiring into a sheltered home atmosphere are likely now to become inmates of mental institutions because they cannot find a safe place in the crowded high-pressure environment of modern life (Dubos 1961, 172).

Florence Nightingale and Emily Dickinson are excellent examples of "timid souls" who retired from social contacts into the shelter and privacy of their homes. Florence Nightingale (1820–1910), hardly considered timid, retired to her bedroom after her return from the Crimean War. She remained there for the next 30 years, corresponding with the outside world from her bed. The cause of her illness remains a mystery. Her status and financial security allowed her to be productive and a social recluse. Emily Dickinson (1830–1886) is considered to be one of the most important female poets in the United States. Dickinson was shy and fastidious and retired from the world in 1854 to write poetry in her Amherst, Massachusetts, home until her death. Dickinson also had the financial security that allowed her to comfortably withdraw from society. Our hectic, rapidly changing world today would have little understanding or tolerance of a woman or man who chose this type of secluded life-style. There is also less and less tolerance in the traditional family setting for the needs and care of the "mentally ill" elderly, who find themselves in extended care facilities rather than the familiar surroundings of home and family. The "crowded high-pressure environment of modern life" noted by Dubos in the early 1960s is even more pertinent today.

Occupational diseases were often socially accepted as part of the job even if they led to mental illness. Lewis Carroll made reference to a common occupational disease in *Alice in Wonderland*. As Gardner (1974) comments:

> The phrases "mad as a hatter" and "mad as a March hare" were common at the time Carroll wrote, and of course that was why he created the two characters. "Mad as a hatter" may have been a corruption of the earlier "mad as an adder" but more likely owes its origin to the fact that until recently

hatters actually did go mad. The mercury used in curing felt was a common cause of mercury poisoning. Victims developed a tremor called "hatter's shakes," which affected their eyes and limbs and addled their speech. In advanced stages they developed hallucinations and other psychotic symptoms (Gardner 1974, 90, note 7).

A final example of the influence of social standards on community mental health is also an example of a gender stereotype. Society sets role expectations for its members, and those who do not comply are labeled as abnormal. Such was the case in the 1880s in the United States. A mysterious disorder was afflicting some women of the upper socioeconomic classes. Physicians called the disease "hysteria," as they assumed the origin of the disease was in the female reproductive organs. It should be noted that the rise of hysteria matched the rise in the custom of defining women strictly by their role as wives and mothers. Women in the upper class were expected to do nothing of any social or economic consequence (Veblen, 1934). The expert of the day on hysteria was Dr. S. Weir Mitchell and he prescribed the following treatment for those afflicted:

> Live as domestic a life as possible. Have your child with you all the time. Lie down an hour after each meal. Have but two hours intellectual life a day. And never touch pen, brush or pencil as long as you live (Gilman 1975, 96).

As might be expected, this forced inactivity did not alleviate the problems and often led to further invalidism and inability to cope with simple tasks of daily living.

INTERRELATIONSHIP OF FACTORS

The development of the community mental health movement bears the mark of all the external factors discussed (culture, religion, scientific advances, economy, politics, and social factors).

We cannot examine the individuals and events that represent turning points in the care of the mentally ill separately from the community fabric of which they were an integral part.

> ■ *Point of Emphasis*
>
> *Just as each human being is more than the sum of his or her parts, so is a community more than the sum of its parts.*

☐ Philosophical View of Mental Illness

Before the establishment of institutional care, the mentally ill were often allowed to wander about. Less humane practices included imprisonment, selling the insane, or quietly shipping them off to another community in the dead of night. Early hospitals in Europe dealt with a variety of ills and did not separate clients by disorder. One of the first institutions to deal exclusively with the care of the insane was St. Mary of Bethlehem Hospital in London (the infamous "Bedlam"). The word "bedlam" has become a part of our language and means any noisy, confused place or situation.

The earliest state-owned hospital in North America devoted entirely to mental illness was the "Lunatick Hospital" founded in 1770 in Williamsburg, Virginia. In colonial times the care of the insane was considered a local matter and was left to the vestry of the parish. When the vestry was unable to maintain an asylum, the insane were allowed to wander about or were put in prison.

In a petition to the House of Representatives of the province of Pennsylvania for a charter for a hospital to provide care for the insane, the wording indicates that many of the insane suffered from a disease that could be cured. The petition's rationale for the facility includes the following testimony:

> That some of them going at large are a terrour to their Neighbours, who are daily apprehensive of the Violences they may commit; and others are continually wasting their Substance; to the great injury of themselves and Families, ill disposed Persons wickedly taking Advantage of their unhappy Condition, and drawing them into unreasonable Bargains, and

> That few or none of them are so sensible of their Condition, as to submit voluntarily to the Treatment their respective Cases require, and therefore continue in the same deplorable State during their Lives, whereas it has been found, by the Experience of many years, that above two thirds of the Mad People received into Bethlehem Hospital, and there treated properly, have been perfectly cured.

Little concern was paid to the legal and ethical rights of these "Mad People" admitted to the Pennsylvania Hospital. For some years there was no fence or wall around the hospital until eventually, a wall had to be built—not to confine the patients, but to keep morbid curiosity seekers out.

☐ Pathologic Anatomy View of Mental Illness

Benjamin Rush (1746–1813) was elected a physician to the Pennsylvania Hospital in 1783 and served there until his death. Dr. Rush believed, as did his French contemporary Philippe Pinel, that insanity was a disease that could be cured with proper care and treatment. Dr. Rush encouraged improvements in the living environment of the mentally ill. He also encouraged what would now be called occupational therapy, that is, household tasks and chores to fill the patient's days. Unfortunately, Dr. Rush also strongly believed in liberal bleeding and purging of his patients with calomel, a mercury salt. He also proposed scaring patients back into their senses and humoring their delusions as a means to cure. Philippe Pinel (1745–1826) is noted for removing the chains from the mentally ill in France, is generally regarded as a great humanitarian, and indeed introduced more humane treatment methods. However, two factors are worth remembering: (1) Pinel was placed in charge of the Salpêtrière, a hospital for the insane, during the upheaval of the French Revolution. Many of the "patients" were political prisoners incarcerated in the insane asylum, and (2) Pinel was influenced by the scientific method and as a scientist wanted to observe his patients without the influence of restraint. The liberation of Pinel's patients allowed for better observation. Pinel was the first to record and classify patients by their symptoms and behavior, which was an important contribution to the treatment of mental illness.

At approximately the same time, William Tuke, a devout member of the Society of Friends, began a reform of the existing mental facilities in England. After a visit to Bedlam, Tuke worked to establish a treatment facility that reflected his humanistic world view. "The Retreat" established by Tuke and later supported by his grandson, Samuel Tuke, was a safe haven for the mentally ill known for its peaceful homelike atmosphere, good care, and low cost. It was known as "moral treatment," and the patients were treated with dignity and respect. Proponents of moral treatment, which was similar to contemporary milieu therapy, cited the torturous practices in other facilities as detrimental to any form of recovery.

As is often the case, social reform coincidentally occurs in several places at the same time. In the United States in the early 1800s, several significant social movements and their proponents were instrumental in bringing about reform in community mental health. A grass roots movement, known as the Popular Health Movement, espoused the principles of basic hygiene, a balanced diet, exercise, and self-care. People were encouraged to "be their own doctors." The movement even supported the scandalous suggestion that women would breathe better without wearing their corsets! The average uneducated laborer was drawn to the movement due in part to widespread mistrust of the "regular" or "heroic" physician of the day. Heroic medicine was so called because the physician did battle with disease and used the patient as the battlefield. Patients were bled and purged for any type of malady. Those healers who let nature take its course were labeled "irregulars" or "naturalists" by the medical establishment.

In the 1840s a schoolteacher began a campaign to reform the care of the mentally ill that spanned 20 years. Dorothea Dix (1802–1887) became aware of the living conditions of the mentally ill when she visited the East Cambridge jail in Massachusetts. In March 1841, Dix went to the jail to deliver Sunday school instruction to the female inmates. She was brought into contact with filth and overcrowding of criminals and the insane.

> She found among the prisoners a few insane persons, with whom she talked. She noticed there was no stove in their room, and no means of proper warmth. The jailer said that a fire for them was not needed, and would not be safe. Her repeated solicitations were without success. At that time the court was in session at East Cambridge, and she caused the case to be brought before it. Her request was granted. The cold rooms were warmed. Thus was her great work commenced" (Tiffany, 1918, 74).

The goals of Dix's work were twofold: (1) to provide care for the mentally ill separate from criminals and the poor, and (2) to provide quality care to the mentally ill based on the moral treatment model. The burden of reform on this broad scale became too much even for a woman of Dix's magnitude. The decline of moral treatment began in the 1860s as the cost of care in facilities that practiced this method continued to rise. Families became medically indigent paying for their mentally ill members. The client population was increasing, due in part to the increase in immigration, and there was a concurrent increase in the need for personnel to care for them.

The environment was fraught with ethnic and religious prejudice, while the Civil War and its drain on human and economic resources made the increasing cost of care of the mentally ill a political issue. State run facilities were built to deal with the increasing need for space on a local level. Also, the first formal nurse training programs were established in this decade. It was late in the 1800s before the first graduates began their practice, primarily in private duty. Graduate nurses practiced minimally in hospitals and rarely in facilities dealing with the mentally ill. There was only one training program for "mental nursing," which was established in 1881 at McLean Hospital in Massachusetts. An example of an attempt at community mental health a few years later reflects a very modern approach:

> . . . the first real outpatient clinic for mental cases in this country was established at the instance of Dr. John B. Chapin, in the outpatient department of the Pennsylvania General Hospital. It was opened November 1, 1885 for advice and treatment of mental diseases in their early or incipient stages occurring among the poor and indigent, when such diseases have not so far progressed as to require restraint within the walls of a hospital (Abbot, 1920, 218).

INVOLVEMENT OF HEALTH CARE PROVIDERS

Clifford W. Beers attempted suicide in 1890 by jumping from the top floor of his parents' house. His distraught family realized that he could not be safely cared for in the home and placed him in a mental institution. Upon his recovery 4 years later, he decided to publish the story of his experiences. *A Mind That Found Itself* by Clifford W. Beers was the first volume on insanity written for the lay public. The publication of this book allowed individuals and families affected by mental illness to discuss their problems more openly than ever before. The National Committee for Mental Hygiene was established by Beers in 1909. Supported by gifts and grants, the committee worked to bring about reform of mental facilities. The National Committee was the predecessor of the present-day National Institute of Mental Health (NIMH). Though Beers was an articulate and charismatic man, the task of national reform was too much for him. The complexity of the system had increased dramatically. The politics of state legislative bodies had to be dealt with on an individual basis if reforms were to occur. The National Committee for Mental Hygiene faced another problem that still limits the community mental health movement today.

■ **Point of Emphasis**

The mentally ill have never collectively fought for improvements in their treatment. Unlike other oppressed and ignored groups, they have never championed their own cause. It has been up to others to petition for changes, and the stigma of mental illness has limited this number to a brave handful.

The turn of the century brought with it the industrial revolution and an increase in the need for sanitation and hygiene. Lillian Wald (1867–1940), a public health nursing leader, toiled many years for improvements in child labor laws and preventive care on a community level. These were hard times economically, and the morale of the country was low. As the country grew, so did the number of poor and elderly. The average life expectancy in 1800 was 32 years. In 1900, the life expectancy had risen to 50 and by 1940 to 65 years of age. The shift in age affected the type of admission to mental facilities. It is estimated that the number of persons age 65 years and over increased from 3 million to 9 million from 1900–1940.

With the increase in client population, there was an increase in the need for caregivers. The superintendents of the state hospitals were politically appointed and were not necessarily in the medical profession. Since money was scarce, attendants of the lowest common denominator were hired to perform custodial care. Nurses were utilized only in the private facilities. The patient population was comprised of a large number of elderly. In the southern United States, many of the psychiatric beds were filled by individuals diagnosed as having pellagra. This disorder was so widespread that it seemed to be an epidemic. Dr. J.W. Babcock, superintendent of the State Hospital for the Insane in South Carolina noted that 15 percent of the admissions in 1911 were due to pellagra.

Pellagrins demonstrated behavior that ranged from confusion, memory loss, and disorientation to mania, depression, and psychosis. The medical leaders of the day could describe the disease but could not cure it. Many of these pa-

tients appeared doomed to live out their lives as chronic mental patients. The work of Tom Douglas Spies, M.D., and his associates in 1938 shed light on the cause of pellagra. Nicotinic acid was isolated and used in the treatment of pellagrins. The spontaneous recovery of even grossly psychotic individuals with a short course of treatment with nicotinic acid was almost miraculous. Once again, the scientific method lived up to its expectations and found a "cure" for mental illness.

Decades later nutritionists would discover that pellagra was not caused by a lack of nicotinic acid. Rather, the dietary habits of the southeastern United States were influenced by industrialization. Preground corn meal had replaced the traditional hominy, and when this made up the bulk of the diet, niacin was lost and pellagra was the result.

■ **Point of Emphasis**

The interaction of economic, social, and cultural factors profoundly affects the mental health of the community at large.

The medical community did not forget the lesson of pellagra and searched in renewed earnest for a cure for mental illness. The 1940s and early 1950s were characterized by custodial inpatient care and physical treatments of symptomatology. Ugo Cerletti (1877–1963) introduced electric shock therapy into psychiatry. Cerletti, a psychiatrist, had observed the use of electric shock in the slaughter of hogs, but it is not clear how he made the connection between its use to stun animals and its use on mental patients to alleviate depression and confusion. Other physical or somatic treatments included cold wet sheet packs, insulin shock therapy, and prefrontal lobotomy. Little reference was made to recovery and discharge planning. Physicians and nurses were becoming less and less optimistic of a cure for mental illness. A textbook for psychiatric nursing published in 1949 devoted only one-half page to nursing care aimed at recovery from mental illness. The vague instructions to the nurse reflect the lack of experience with patients who got well.

The patient should be encouraged to resume the direction of his own affairs insofar as his ability will permit. No one more greatly appreciates being treated as a reasonable and intelligent person than does a patient convalescing from a mental illness. To many patients the return to former associations and environment is accompanied by sensitiveness and suffering (Noyes and Haydon, 1949, 295).

The National Mental Health Act of 1946 provided for the establishment of the National Institute of Mental Health which was mandated to: (1) promote research in the area of diagnosis and treatment of mental illness; (2) support training and education of mental health workers; (3) provide grants to states in order to establish new treatment facilities; and (4) encourage studies and projects dealing with new treatment modalities, especially in the area of prevention.

These general objectives provided much needed organization in the area of mental health research. NIMH also provided financial support for continuing education for nurses in the form of traineeships. The increased need for psychiatric-mental health nurses was partially met through traineeship grants awarded to undergraduate and graduate programs. NIMH would also eventually support federally sponsored grants for the establishment of community mental health centers in a number of states.

OPENING THE DOOR TO DEINSTITUTIONALIZATION

A retrospective study by Eysenck (1952) reported the results of "outcome of therapy" comparing the improvement rates of patients receiving psycho-analysis (44 percent), psychotherapy (64 percent) and no treatment (77 percent). Subsequent studies have confirmed Eysenck's results. The different methods of counseling therapies seemed to have no greater impact than chance on recovery rates. Therefore, refinement of psychotherapeutic techniques was doing little to decrease the number of inpatients in overcrowded state facilities.

Three factors were instrumental in changing the way state facilities were run and opening the door to deinstitutionalization: (1) use of psychotropic drugs, (2) establishment of therapeutic communities within hospitals, and (3) geographic decentralization.

The advent of major tranquilizers and antidepressants in 1955 was directly responsible for a drop in census in mental hospitals the following year. Although not considered curative, these drugs were viewed in the same light that insulin was to the diabetic. Clients were able to be discharged and functioned in the community as long as they were maintained on medication. A new

phenomenon developed when clients discontinued taking medications—"revolving door" psychiatry. This is illustrated by the decrease in resident clients since 1955 and the steady increase in releases and admissions during the same period. Clients demonstrated repeated admissions interspersed with short periods out in the community.

The development of therapeutic communities within facilities drew on the curative capacity that the clients and staff possessed (see Chapter 14 on therapeutic milieu). The democratic atmosphere of the therapeutic community improved the effects of psychotherapy and indirectly enhanced self-esteem.

Admission procedures to state facilities were designed to identify those clients who would benefit from acute treatment services. The most qualified staff worked with those with potential for recovery. Less qualified staff worked in the "back wards" with the chronic mentally ill. When geographic decentralization changed this process, clients were admitted based on their home communities regardless of diagnosis—thus allowing them to share the familiar, positive aspects of the cultural and social environment from which they came and to which they would return.

Nursing became increasingly involved in direct client care in state facilities, private hospitals, and public health nursing. Social and political emphasis in the 1960s was on individual freedom, human rights and dignity, the promise of prosperity, and humanism. Community mental health theory and policy were developed on a national level and were supposed to filter down to the local level. Community mental health was viewed as the responsibility of the community as a whole. President John F. Kennedy promoted legislation that led to the passage of the Mental Retardation Facilities and Community Mental Health Centers Construction Act (CMHC) in 1963. A new treatment model was proposed to decrease the number of inpatients, increase community involvement in planning for mental health services, and extend services into the community. The CMHC Act was not promoting the mere transfer of psychiatric services from one building to another. Five essential services were necessary in order for a program to qualify for federal funds:

1. In-patient care: offers treatment to clients who require 24-hour care.
2. Out-patient care: offers treatment programs for adults, children, and families on an out-patient basis.

3. Partial hospitalization: offers day care or night care for clients who are able to return home evenings and weekends or who are able to work during the day.

4. Emergency care: twenty-four hour emergency service is available in one of the units named above.

5. Consultation and education: the center's staff offers consultation and education to community agencies and professional personnel (Burgess and Lazarre, 1976, 385).

The centers were encouraged to offer the following additional services as community need grew: diagnostic services, rehabilitation, pre- and aftercare, training, research, and evaluation. Funding for the CMHC Act proved to be a major problem. Money was appropriated at the federal level as seed money for the initial establishment of the center. It was never the intention of the CMHC Act to totally support local efforts. After 1963, there were numerous amendments and extensions of the original act. Table 36-1 compares and contrasts the original CMHC Act in 1963 and the most recent piece of legislation dealing with community mental health, the Mental Health Systems Act of 1980.

The critics of community mental health legislation and the service that has resulted from it point out its failure to meet its initial idealistic goals. Fundamentally, there has never been agreement that sevices based in the community are better than those in an institution. In the zealous first wave of the community mental health

TABLE 36-1 Changes in Community Mental Health Legislation 1963–1980

	Mental Retardation Facilities and Community Mental Health Centers Construction Act—1963	The Mental Health Systems Act—1980
Authorization of funds/aid to state and local programs	$150 million over a 3-year period 1965–1967	$711 million at approximately $237 million/year for 3 years
Key themes	Consolidation of services Comprehensive care Involvement of lay public in program development and supervision Change in operational and fiscal policy	More flexible delivery system Focus on underserved populations Development of federal/state/local partnerships Reaffirmation of importance of community mental health centers
Necessary services to qualify for funding	Inpatient services ER services Outpatient services Partial hospitalization Consultation and education Diagnostic service Rehabilitative service Precare and aftercare Training Research and evaluation	Inpatient service ER services Outpatient services Partial hospitalization Consultation and education Assistance to courts and public agencies in screening persons being referred to state mental health facilities Follow up care to the deinstitutionalized Transitional halfway house services Specialized services for children Specialized services for the elderly Drug and alcohol services, unless otherwise being provided in the area Care of chronic mentally ill

movement, many chronically ill mental clients were released into a world of which they had not been a part for many years. The very people that the legislation was trying to assist were being hurt the most.

An additional failing of the community mental health movement is the attempt to function with an acute care medical model in the community. Centers were set up with a traditional patriarchal model, the physician psychiatrist as director of the center, and the skill and greater expertise of nurses, psychologists, and social workers familiar with public health principles were underutilized.

☐ *Nursing Process*

ASSESSMENT AND PROBLEM IDENTIFICATION ☐

Client ☐

> ■ *Point of Emphasis*
>
> *The present population of clients requiring community mental health care is made up largely of the elderly and the chronic mentally ill.*

The Mental Health Systems Act utilized the term "chronic mentally ill" for the first time. This terminology suggests there are clients who will never recover and never be rehabilitated to function fully in the community. Client problem areas in community mental health settings include monitoring of medications, diet and nutritional status, and basic human needs. The lack of understanding of the illness process by clients and others in the community is an additional problem.

One point remains unchanged through all of the changes in CMHC legislation—each community needs to assess its own needs. The rapidly accelerated rate at which old habits and conventions disappear and new ones appear affects the community's ability to assess and plan for its needs. The present lack of community supports for aftercare in the form of housing, occupations, and social support dooms any attempt at reintegration. In the main, the location of care has indeed shifted from state facilities—but not necessarily to community settings. There has been a noticeable increase in nursing homes in the number of chronic mentally ill and elderly requiring psychiatric care. Nursing homes are no better equipped than community agencies to care for these clients, but reimbursement for services is available in this type of facility. Clearly, the quality of staffing in most nursing homes is not adequate to meet the needs of such a diverse population.

A social approach currently gaining momentum is a rebirth of the self-care and wellness movements of the past. One needs only to check the number of paperback books in popular literature supporting self-help and self-improvement to become aware of public interest in this area. The self-care movement could have a very positive effect on community mental health as healthier life-styles are encouraged.

Assessment of the environment for potentials for growth and mental health and for limiting factors should not be confined solely to the local level. The environment includes national and international concerns also. For example, adequate nutrition for childbearing women and infants is essential for normal growth and development and is a problem affecting the future mental health of communities on a local, national, and international level.

The nurse involved in community mental health work needs to continue to specialize in areas such as group therapy and crisis intervention. Nurses generally lack the political and economic understanding to be effective change agents on a community level. They must develop skills in long-range planning in order to communicate with those in political and key decision-making positions.

INTERVENTION ☐

Primary Prevention ☐

Public health principles that are helpful to the nurse in community health include the epidemiological model, which is based on the premise that deviations from health are the result of interactions among disease agents, human hosts, and environmental factors (Leavell and Clark, 1965). Application of this model to specific health problems is more useful than the medical model as it takes into account more than linear cause and effect. Early identification of risk factors to the host suggests appropriate levels of preventive intervention. Two other public health terms that are often utilized are prevalence (number of cases at a specified moment in time) and incidence (number of new cases during a specified period in time). The etiology of mental illness is unclear and so prevalence and incidence are difficult if not impossible to determine.

In examining nursing interventions on the primary level, it is important that the nurse recognize the dual role of provider and consumer of services. As a consumer of mental health services and a participant in their delivery, the nurse is in the unique position of evaluating services from two vantage points. Interventions at the primary level are designed to prevent mental illness from occurring. Community services that attempt to provide primary intervention include: parent assistance lines that help prevent child abuse; drug information groups to educate parents and teachers; and crisis intervention services provided by phone or in ambulatory settings. The nurse can participate in services such as these in a variety of roles ranging from direct care to educating small groups in anticipatory guidance and parenting.

Health promotion in one area of life-style always affects other areas in a positive fashion. The current interest of business and industry in cutting health care costs has opened the door to health promotion at the work site. An area that is of particular interest is the concept of stress management in the potential reduction of stress-related illnesses, both physical and emotional. Teaching stress management skills to employees at the work site assists them in identifying stressors and in learning and practicing coping skills; it also increases their awareness of their personal, social, and work environment. The nurse involved in health promotion in business and industry is in a key position to prevent mental illness from a perspective of the risk factors peculiar to the worker.

Nursing research in the areas of touch therapies and nontraditional healing modalities is another example of preventive intervention. The high-technology, fast pace of the contemporary community needs to be balanced by health care providers who consider phenomena that occur on a more fundamental level. The need for contact with other living beings is supported by the positive results gained by the presence of pets in extended care facilities. Nurse researchers are exploring the therapeutic effects of animals with clients who have difficulty communicating.

Finally, participating on a personal basis and as a skilled resource in the current self-care and self-help movement may do more to decrease the development of mental illness than any program dealing with its aftermath. Nurses might look to their own profession and examine how effectively the principles of wellness—self-responsibility, nutrition, fitness, and stress management—are practiced.

Secondary Prevention □ Secondary interventions are designed for early case identification so that treatment can be initiated promptly. Community services that the nurse might be involved with or refer clients to include Alcoholics Anonymous, rape counseling services, grief counseling services, and support groups. Nursing interventions at a secondary level are as broad as a nurse's skills. Settings and population groups can be identified by the nurse by an assessment of the needs of the community and how nursing services could meet those needs.

Central to effective intervention on the secondary level is the establishment of a network of colleagues and resources in the community to provide comprehensive service. The nurse might function as a member of a multidisciplinary team in a community mental health center, in a free-standing nursing clinic, in a traditional public health agency, or as a school nurse. It should be apparent that the nurse can practice community mental health regardless of the setting. Even traditional settings, such as acute care general hospitals, can benefit by the intervention of the community mental health nurse with clients and staff alike.

Tertiary Prevention □ Tertiary intervention involves limiting the disability associated with a particular disorder. Nursing interventions on this level should primarily focus on the needs of the chronic mentally ill. Issues that traditionally were out of nursing's domain are a part of tertiary treatment, such as adequate housing and employment for clients returning to the community. Development of a strong professional relationship with social workers is key as they are often able to find financial support for clients outside the hospital.

■ *Point of Emphasis*

A good collegial relationship with physicians is crucial to monitoring the physical health of clients in the community, particularly when the use of psychotherapeutic medications is involved.

The nurse has a responsibility to become involved as a member of planning boards in services dealing with the chronic mentally ill. Perhaps this level of intervention on a community basis is the most challenging as there is little immediate reinforcement for nursing efforts.

☐ *Future Perspectives*

Compared to their role in other areas of health care, nurses are relative newcomers to community mental health. In order to be part of the leading edge, nursing must draw upon its full complement of physical and social science background. The nurse of the future in community mental health must be concerned with reimbursement of service of comparable worth. Nursing agencies are already directly reimbursed for community health visits under Medicare. It is a small step, logically, to the establishment of private nursing practice to deliver some of the services previously mentioned.

Nurses will also be involved in health maintenance organizations that will comprise a more comprehensive delivery program to the community they serve. Nurses are also in an ideal position to embrace new models of health care delivery systems that are more concerned with process than the product of services, less concerned with cure and more concerned with care.

■ *Enrichment Activities*

DISCUSSION QUESTIONS

1. Utilize the epidemiological framework to identify agent, host, and environmental factors for adolescent suicide in your community.

2. Compare and contrast the role of the nurse in community mental health with the following disciplines: social work, psychology, and psychiatry.

3. Explore the services a nurse could offer to an emergency service that has no available inpatient or outpatient mental health services.

4. Discuss the benefits and pitfalls of institutional mental health services vs. community mental health services.

LEARNING ACTIVITIES

Upon completion of this learning activity the reader will be able to:
1. Identify at least two external factors that influenced the decision making of the group.
2. Discuss community concerns related to social and financial solutions to the problem posed in the role-play exercise.

Silver Hills, a southwestern community of approximately 40,000 people, has recently seen an influx of refugees from a densely forested Far Eastern country plagued by war and famine. The Heavenly Reward Church in Silver Hills sponsored the relocation of 50 refugee families and was in the process of matching the refugee families with sponsors in the congregation. Because of a lack of clear communication, the refugees arrived 3 weeks ahead of schedule.

The church hurriedly secures a local campground as temporary housing for the refugees. The relocation of the refugees into the Silver Hills community is more difficult than expected: unemployment is high owing to the closing of a local mine, and low income housing is scarce. Meanwhile, church volunteers at the camp site have noticed unusual behavior among several of the refugees who refuse to eat or perform basic hygiene and spend all day staring off into space or wandering about aimlessly. The refugee leaders do not seem to be overly concerned about these people and they ignore the behavior. The volunteers however, become increasingly concerned and take several of the afflicted refugees to the local hospital emergency room. The physicians at the hospital are reluctant to treat the refugees. One physician remarks, "They're not even citizens, yet!" The situation isn't getting any better so a community task force is set up to help deal with this multifaceted problem. You are a member of this task force representing community mental health nursing.

Instructions:

Place five chairs together. Assign members of the class to the following task force roles or request volunteers: (1) refugee leader, (2) camp volunteer, (3) member of the Silver Hills city council, (4) emergency room physician, and (5) community mental health nurse.

The task force will discuss the following questions as a group. Feel free to express your opinions about the situation:

1. Is there a problem? If so, what is it?

2. Who is responsible for the care of these refugees and their integration into the community?

3. How can this integration best be accomplished?

4. Who is going to pay for all of the refugees' needs?

5. The volunteers have identified "unusual" behavior by some of the refugees. Is this a problem?

After your discussion, come to a consensus on questions 1 and 2. What external factors influenced your decision? How did the values of the group members influence your decision? Who was most dominant in the group? Most passive?

■ Recommended Readings

Bloom, B. *Community mental health*, Monterey, CA: Brooks/Cole Publishers, 1977. Offers a thorough overview of the various aspects of community mental health including its place in legislative context. Also deals with the criticisms leveled at the community mental health movement and attempts to overcome them.

Capra, F. *The turning point—Science, society and the rising culture,* New York: Simon & Schuster, 1982. A thought-provoking examination of science and health care, theories in physics and the humanities, and the possible new path that is emerging away from the mechanistic, analytic mode of thinking.

Mechanic, D. Nursing and mental health care: Expanding future possibilities for nursing services. In *Nursing in the 1980's: Crises, opportunities, challenges* (Aiken, L.H., ed.). Philadelphia: J.B. Lippincott, 1982, 343–358. Emphasizes that nursing is in an advantageous position in community mental health because of its numerical superiority and experience. Encourages nurses to take a broader role and leadership positions in mental health.

Weisstein, N. Psychology constructs the female. In *Woman in sexist society* (Gornick, V., and Moran, B.K., eds.). New York: Basic Books, 1972, 207–224. Examines the "track record" of psychology in describing the true nature of women. Takes a critical look at developmental theory, clinical psychology, and biological theory that limit the human potential of both sexes.

Whall, A.L.; Engle, V.; Edwards, A.; Bobel, L.; and Haberland, C. Development of a screening program for tardive dyskinesia: Feasability issues. *Nursing research*, 32, 3, 1983:151–156. A feasibility study to develop a reliable method for screening of tardive dyskinesia in the community. Describes the role of the community mental health nurse in the aftercare setting in screening and monitoring for tardive dyskinesia.

■ References

Abbot, E.S. Outpatient or dispensary clinics for mental cases. *American journal of insanity*, 77, 1920:218.

Bachrach, L. A conceptual approach to deinstitutionalization. *Hospital and community psychiatry*, 29, 9, 1978:573–578.

Bassuk, E., and Gerson, S. Deinstitutionalization and mental health services. *Scientific American*, 238, 2, 1978:46–53.

Beers, C.W. *A Mind That Found Itself.* New York: Doubleday, 1908.

Burgess, A., and Lazarre, A. *Psychiatric nursing in the hospital and the community.* Englewood Cliffs, NJ: Prentice-Hall, 1976, 385.

Dubos, R. *Mirage of health.* New York: Doubleday, 1961, 172.

Eysenck, H. The effects of psychotherapy: An evaluation. *Journal of consulting psychology,* 16, 1952:319–324.

Gardner, M. *The annotated Alice: Alice's adventures in Wonderland and through the looking glass.* New York: The New American Library, Inc., 1974, 90.

Gilman, C.P. *The living of Charlotte Perkins Gilman: An autobiography.* New York: Harper Colophon Books, 1975, 96.

Leavell, H.R. and Clark, E.G. *Preventive Medicine for the doctor in his community: an epidemiological approach.* New York: McGraw-Hill, 1965.

Noyes, A., and Haydon, E. *Textbook of psychiatric nursing.* New York: Macmillan, 1949, 295.

Packard, F. *Some account of the Pennsylvania hospital.* Philadelphia: Pennsylvania Hospital, 1938, 46.

Shryock, R.H. *The history of nursing: An interpretation of the social and medical factors involved.* Philadelphia: J.B. Lippincott, 1959, 263.

Spies, T.; Aring, C.; Gelperin, J.; and Bean, W. The mental symptoms of pellagra. *The American journal of the medical sciences*, 196, 4, 1938:461–475.

Szasz, T. The myth of mental illness. *American psychologist*, 25, 1960:113–118.

Tiffany, F. *Life of Dorothea Lynde Dix.* Ann Arbor: Plutarch Press, 1918, 74.

Veblen, T. *Theory of the leisure class,* New York: Modern Library, 1934.

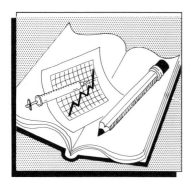

37

Clinical Application of Research in Psychiatric-Mental Health Nursing

Odessie G. Taylor

Learning Objectives:

Upon completion of this chapter, the reader will be able to:

1. Define nursing research.

2. List the purposes of research and the various responsibilities that are held for nurses prepared at each educational level in nursing.

3. Discuss the major research methods and then relate these to research purposes and to their use in projects for psychiatric nursing.

4. Identify researchable problems from the clinical setting.

5. Understand the barriers that interfere with the conduct and utilization of research.

6. Describe research utilization models and their use in the introduction of new knowledge into practice settings.

7. Foster the appropriate use of clinical research findings.

8. Discuss the components of a quality assurance program and the process for developing programs using criteria involving structure, process, and/or outcomes.

9. Participate in various aspects of formal quality assurance programs.

Research is a resource for nursing. Not only can it serve as a process but also as a product. As a process it can be utilized to discover new knowledge; as a product, its findings can help explain the world of nursing, solve specific problems of practice, and uncover new methods for nursing practice. Like all other disciplines, nursing possesses a specific body of knowledge and a particular view of the world. Consequently, nursing must be involved in the discovery and development of knowledge to be used in its practice to ensure that the new information meets the needs of the profession and its clients.

□ *General Factors About Research*

There is agreement that there is a difference between the definitions of the terms "research in nursing" and "nursing research." The first term refers to research about the profession, its characteristics, its practitioners or clinicians, how nurses actually practice, and how they are educated. This research focus is older, and related studies are more abundant in the literature since most of the early research in nursing addressed the socialization of student nurses, the attitudes of nurses about various topics, the best way to educate a nurse, the characteristics of graduates of different types of educational programs, and the professional or service orientation of staff nurses. Few efforts were made to define or describe the practice of nursing. During this time the practice of nursing was based on tradition or on authority of the nursing expert.

Nursing research refers to practice research and involves the nursing care process, nursing diagnoses, problems encountered in the provision of care, and the outcomes. This type of research has been with us since the time of Florence Nightingale, who was the first to advocate epidemiologic studies in nursing. However, only since the early 1970's have nurse researchers become committed to the nursing research type of scientific investigation. This focus for research must continue if theories of nursing are to be generated and tested in order to develop a science of nursing. This is not to say that studies involving research in nursing are not needed. Research in nursing and nursing research must both continue because we need not only a scientific basis for providing nursing care to our clients, but also knowledge

about our profession and its practitioners so that we can become more effective and efficient in providing health care.

Without a doubt, a scientific base for nursing practice is essential, and the development of this foundation will be accomplished only through the conduct of appropriate research. This, then, is the most important purpose in doing research. Other objectives related to the purpose are (1) to generate practice theories, (2) to verify nursing theories, and (3) to solve persistent practice problems. Ultimately, research will serve to improve the quality of nursing care. As this purpose and its four objectives are accomplished, two other related purposes become achievable. These are to enhance the professional status of nursing and to become scientifically accountable to the clients of nursing. All of these goals afford nursing a guide as to what must be done. Research must develop theories that identify and name the diagnoses with which nurses deal; theories that describe and categorize the diagnoses and the domains of nursing; theories that predict when certain conditions will occur; and theories that will allow nurses to intervene with expectations for success.

RESPONSIBILITY FOR RESEARCH

The responsibility for the achievement of those research goals rests with all members of the profession who must conduct or participate in basic, applied, and clinical research studies. Each type of research provides a different dimension, and all are needed so that a complete understanding of nursing and nursing practice is possible. For instance, basic research identifies relevant nursing concepts and identifies and describes nursing diagnoses while applied research helps determine whether sociological or psychological concepts are applicable to nursing practice. Clinical research will help us understand whether evolving descriptions of various nursing diagnoses are useful in assessing and recognizing nursing conditions.

Not all nurses are prepared to conduct research investigations, but each registered nurse has some responsibility for the research effort. The first level of involvement is the acknowledgment that research is valuable, important, and necessary for the discipline. In addition, the American Nurses' Association Commission on Nursing Practice (1981) has developed guidelines for research activities for nurses with various levels of educational preparation. From the present-

TABLE 37-1 *The Expected Research Activities According to the Educational Preparation of the Nurse*

Educational Preparation	Expected Research Activities			
	Use Research Findings	Identify Research Problems	Disseminate Research Findings	Conduct Research Studies
ADN	X	X		
BSN	X	X		
MSN	X	X	X	X
DNS	X	X	X	X
PhD	X	X	X	X

ation in Table 37-1, it can be noted that all registered nurses are expected to use research findings in practice and to identify areas in nursing needing to be studied by research.

It should be apparent that the capabilities of nurses for doing these activities will vary according to their educational preparation. In order to ensure research use and the identification of relevant research areas, nurses with both masters degrees and doctoral preparation should assist or provide consultative services in the retrieval of appropriate research studies and in clarifying research ideas into problem statements.

> ■ *Point of Emphasis*
>
> *Every nurse has a role and area of responsibility in nursing research-related activities.*

Conducting research investigations and disseminating their findings is done by nurses with masters and doctoral degrees. The expertise within this group varies, so differences in research activities may be noted. The masters' prepared nurse would facilitate the use of research; conduct quality assurance and clinical research studies; and disseminate research findings through presentations at professional meetings and by writing reports for publication. The nurse with the doctorate of science in nursing would generate nursing theories, develop the methods to be used in evaluating care, and conduct clinical research. The nurse with a doctor of philosophy degree would develop test, and define theory, and develop new methods of nursing research. From this description of responsibilities, it would ap-

pear that who does what is quite clear. However, this is not true in real life, since in certain situations nurses with other educational backgrounds may perform research activities. For example, in some situations, associate and baccalaureate prepared nurses may participate in planning studies and in data collection.

RESEARCH IN PSYCHIATRIC NURSING

Before one can describe what is and what is not psychiatric nursing research, one must define its parameters. A clear delineation is not possible since elements of past and present conceptualizations of psychiatric nursing are used by different members of the community of nurses. The development of psychiatric nursing followed a different course from other clinical specialties (Fagin, 1981; Martin, 1985). Important milestones during its development were (1) the incorporation of the idea of psychoanalysis as the most appropriate modality for treatment; (2) the union of public health nursing and psychiatry to produce a new area of specialization—psychiatric mental health nursing; (3) the acknowledgment that the origin of mental problems is not always within the individual but may be heavily influenced by the social system; (4) the development of a generalist practice of psychiatric-mental health nursing through the integration of psychosocial concepts throughout nursing curricula; (5) the rise of advanced nursing with the clinical nurse specialist functioning as a psychotherapist; (6) the advancement of the community mental health movement; (7) the development of drug therapy for various psychiatric conditions; and (8) the identification of specific neurochemical imbalances associated with neuropsychiatric conditions.

HISTORY OF NURSING RESEARCH

The definition and focus of psychiatric nursing changed as the above milestones occurred. Even now, this specialty area is in a state of flux; decisions need to be made about the role of the nurse as psychotherapist vs. combining the psychotherapy frame of reference with one clearly identified with nursing and mental health. The broader concept seems more helpful, since holism is primary to the definition and practice of nursing, that is, man as a biopsychosocial being interacting with his environments.

When Sills (1977) published her review of the psychiatric research literature, she noted that the 310 studies completed between 1952 and 1976 (see Table 37-2) had been done from one of three perspectives: within the person (153 studies), within the relationship (113 studies), and within the social system (44 studies). These perspectives seem to be related to specific milestones occurring during the development of the specialty. The table shows that (1) the number of studies using "within the person" increased from three in 1952–1956 to an all-time high of 56 studies in 1967–1971; (2) the number of studies using "within the relationship" varied from 18 in 1952–1956 and 1957–1961 to a high of 41 studies in 1967–1971; and (3) the number of studies involving the "within the social system" focus started with one study in 1952–1956 and reached a high of 16 studies in 1972–1976. Sills work seems to indicate that the interest and use of these frames of reference has not been consistent, and that since all are still used multiple definitions still exist.

A review of *Nursing Research, Advances in Nursing Science,* and *The Journal of Psychosocial and Mental Health Services* from 1981 through 1984 whose purpose was to pinpoint research studies completed by psychiatric and mental health nurses or/and research supported by the National Institute of Mental Health reveals some of the same trends and possibly one or two that are new in psychiatric nursing research. All of the earlier ideas continue to be used. However, the major emphasis in research seems to be on specific psychosocial concepts rather than on specific psychiatric conditions. Listed in rank order, the major concepts being studied are stress, social support, coping, death/bereavement, therapeutic touch, self-concept, compliance, mental health, and empathy. This change could indicate that psychiatric mental health nurses have a broader focus about their field and are accepting a more holistic stance about how they perceive their practice. Still another trend noted in the research studies was in the relationships of specific psychosocial concepts and various medical-surgical and maternal-child conditions such as stress and hypertension; loss of self-esteem, immaturity, and teenage pregnancy; or locus of control and cancer. The number of studies about specific psychiatric diseases/conditions was limited to six.

FUTURE NEEDS FOR RESEARCH IN PSYCHIATRIC NURSING

The need for research in psychiatric mental health nursing is acute. It is clear that the research should be multifocused with an approach that ensures study of all relevant areas. For those who focus on traditional psychiatric nursing, nursing authorities have noted these needs: (1) identifying risk and causal factors in discrete mental disorders; (2) determining how the practice of psychiatric nursing differs from that of others providing psychotherapy; (3) investigating the proper boundaries of nursing practice; (4) study-

TABLE 37-2 The Number of Studies Done Within 5-Year Periods from 1952 to 1976 Using Three Different Conceptualizations of Psychiatric Nursing

Type of Study	Number of Studies by 5-Year Intervals					
	1952–1956	1957–1961	1962–1966	1967–1971	1972–1976	Total
Within the person	3	26	42	56	26	153
Within the relationship	18	18	28	41	8	113
Within the social system	1	6	10	11	16	44
Totals	22	50	80	108	50	310

ing the high incidence of mental illness in the elderly with the intent of reducing it; (5) evaluating data on psychotherapeutic intervention to identify cost effective treatments; and (6) determining the linkages between nursing diagnoses and all psychiatric disorders (Fagin, 1981; Martin, 1985; Sills, 1977).

For those whose frame of reference encompasses community mental-health nursing and/or the integration of psychiatric concepts into other clinical specialties, other areas for research are identified. Nursing is considered by some as the diagnosis and treatment of human responses to health and disease. In other instances, nursing is said to deal with monitoring and intervening during various transitional stages or periods: normal growth and development; times when the integrity of the person's or family's wholeness is challenged (e.g., death, divorce, empty nest); and times when there is internal system instability (e.g., disease). Some of the concepts related to these transitional periods and needing further study are the following: stress and coping, compliance, chronicity, helplessness, parenting, perceptual/orientation dysfunction, self-concept, and social support. Another related area for study is the environment, since nurses may need to manipulate its components as a treatment modality as opposed to the manipulation of clients (e.g., does reduction of environmental stimuli reduce disorganized behavior in hyperactive clients?).

> ■ *Point of Emphasis*
>
> *There are numerous and varied needs for research in psychiatric-mental health nursing.*

☐ *The Research Process in Psychiatric-Mental Health Nursing*

Research is a systematic and cyclic process consisting of four phases: conceptual, empirical, interpretive, and communicative (Figure 37-1). Usually this scientific process proceeds from the starting point through all phases; but sometimes when new knowledge and/or understanding about the research variables are obtained from practice or literature, some steps or phases must be reconsidered and revised.

Then, when research is designed to generate new nursing theories, the starting point may be the second phase. In this instance, the purpose of research may be to develop a conceptual framework or new theoretical structure (Batey, 1971).

In experimental research, each phase is dependent upon the preceding phases, so the end points of each must be attained before the investigation moves forward. The conceptual phase is aptly named since it is during this time that the researcher thinks, reflects, and clarifies the ini-

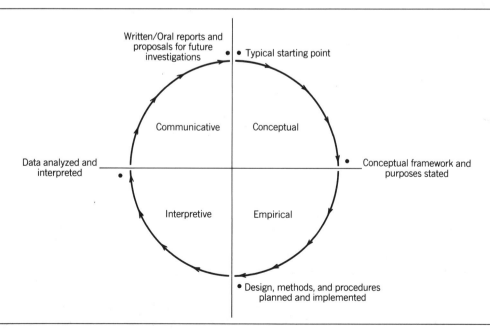

Figure 37.1 *The four phases of research with the end point of each phase.*

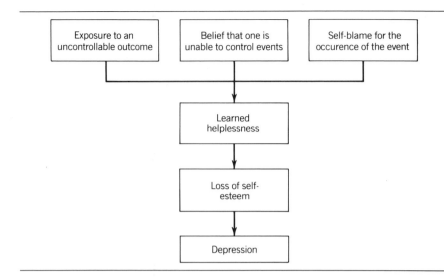

Figure 37.2 *A conceptual model depicting the development of helplessness and depression.*

tial research idea. This is an abstract stage in which the literature is reviewed to gain ideas on the research topic and to see if conclusive research has already been done. Ultimately, the thinking, reflecting, and reviewing leads to the development of a conceptual framework and to a specific statement of purposes for the research project. The conceptual framework is a description and discussion of how the variables are thought to interact with each other in the real world. For example, a part of a conceptual model that Murphy (1982) developed from a review of the literature about helplessness is presented in Figure 37-2.

The above conceptual framework indicates that a condition called "learned helplessness" occurs when a combination of three factors is present: (1) exposure to an uncontrollable outcome; (2) belief that one could not control this event; and (3) belief that one is responsible for that event. Without therapeutic intervention, learned helplessness could lead to a loss of self-esteem and possibly to depression. The concept of uncontrollable outcome is considered a broad term and could include such events as the death of a loved one, loss of a job, occurrence of a debilitating illness, and institutionalization of an elderly individual. Victims of repeated spouse or child abuse also fit this conceptual model.

Murphy indicated that specific relationships had not been verified by research. Several research purposes that could be derived from this conceptualization might include:

1. To identify events that may result in helplessness.

2. To determine the relationships between learned helplessness, the occurrence of an uncontrollable event, the belief that one has no control, and self-blame for the occurrence of the event (are these relationships nonexistent, positive, or negative?).

3. To ascertain in what situations learned helplessness leads to a loss of self-esteem or to depression.

When the specific research purposes have been stated, the investigator is able to move on to the empirical phase.

The first stage—the conceptual phase—provides a foundation and is the basis on which a plan or research design is developed whereby the purposes may be accomplished. If one wanted to base a study on the second listed purpose, one would have to find or develop a mechanism to determine when and if learned helplessness has occurred. An asessment instrument might be one means. In addition, a questionnaire or rating scale would be needed to identify the three variables thought to be important in the development and occurrence of learned helplessness. Other plans and decisions that would have to be made as the research design, instruments, and procedures are developed are: (1) the appropriate sample and its selection; (2) how to protect the rights of subjects; (3) how to assure that the data are reliable and valid; (4) how to organize data; and (5) the appropriate statistical procedure for the study. At the close of the empirical phase the data have been collected and statistical procedures have been done.

Interpretation is the third phase and it is here that the investigator attempts to make sense of the data. The findings are studied to learn if any of the statistics are significant. The conceptual framework is reviewed in light of these findings to learn whether the initial speculations held about the relationships between the research variables are true, or whether the framework needs to be modified in light of the findings.

One of the most important activities occurs during the communicative phase. It is here that the research findings are shared with other members of the discipline through written or spoken communications. In order for research to accomplish its stated purposes, the sharing of knowledge is essential so that others may use the facts in practice or in other research projects. All researchers are responsible for obtaining a critical review of their work, and for identifying gaps in the knowledge base so that future areas for research can be addressed.

MOST USEFUL TYPE OF RESEARCH

From the foregoing presentation, it would seem that research in nursing is a straightforward process. Unfortunately, this is not true. Research in nursing as well as in some of the psychosocial disciplines is in a period of transition. The process depicted here describes research mainly as experimental or quantitative researchers see it, yet there is a question whether quantitative or qualitative methods or their combination would be more useful in the conduct of nursing research.

Some researchers regard qualitative and quantitative methods as extremes, in that the philosophical foundation for each type of research differs, and consequently it is inappropriate to use them together. Various terms come into play with quantitative methods identified as hard, objective, measurable, focused, casual, controlled, manipulative, reductionistic, and masculine; while qualitive methods are described as soft, subjective, descriptive, broad, naturalistic, empirically grounded, developmental, interpretive, holistic, and feminine.

Traditionally, quantitative methods have been preferred because they have had a longer period of use. They are seen as more credible (objective) and controlled (not contaminated by intervening variables). The experimental design is the preferred model for all research of this type but other methods include quasi-experimental, quantitative, descriptive, correlational, and some

survey procedures. Some emerging professions tend to accept this mode of operation in order to become more credible and acceptable to other more established disciplines.

The main argument for the exclusive use of qualitative methods is that it fits one of the major beliefs held by the nursing community. That belief is holism! No one can deny that nursing as a group speaks of biopsychosocial man as the sum of those attributes, which cannot be separated. Further, nurses claim a humanistic frame of reference as a basis for practice. Since quantitative research strips the context from the research findings, it does not fit situations as experienced by humanistic biopsychosocial man. Qualitative research is felt to preserve situations and provide holistic findings. Research studies using qualitative methods are grounded theory, phenomenology, ethnography, action research, and case studies (Murphy, 1985).

The position that both methods are valuable is supported by a growing number of nurses, some of whom believe that both methods are needed because four levels of nursing theories must be generated and/or tested as the science of nursing develops. In ascending order, these levels are naming, describing, predicting, and prescribing. When there is limited knowledge about a phenomenon or limited evidence of its existence, qualitative research is thought to be useful. Consequently it should be used to develop the first two levels of theory. Let us assume that no one had recognized or described the condition called "learned helplessness" but that someone had noticed that following particular crisis situations, some individuals seemed less able to make decisions and to provide for their ongoing needs. Using qualitative means, it would be possible to identify and name this disorder. This would be a first level theory—naming. In order to do this, records of patients might be reviewed to identify the occurrence of the disorder; or, nurses and others providing care could be interviewed to learn if additional information could be gained about its prevalence. This process could also be used to identify additional nursing diagnoses.

After evidence is found that "learned helplessness" does exist, the same or other qualitative procedures can be followed to describe it. If this is a condition that nurses must deal with in practice, they must be able to identify it. What are its signs and symptoms? What are the assessment parameters, indicators, and boundaries? How will nurses recognize it so that interventions can be implemented? Qualitative methods are useful in this process.

Finally, quantitative methods would be followed in the next two levels of theory development because the groundwork for more definitive studies would have been obtained by qualitative methodology. Quantitative research or the experimental design is seen as the method most appropriate when information about cause and effect is to be developed and when one wants to prove which therapeutic modalities are most effective. Causal (predictive) and prescriptive (intervention) theories are at the third and fourth levels of theory develpment.

There is still another position about the need to use both quantitative and qualitative research methods in addition to its value in developing the various levels of research, and that is that arguing about this issue is too time consuming and nursing does not have time for arguing. Nursing needs to move quickly to develop its science; since both methods are productive, both should be used until such time as the issues about research methodology become clearer and a better methodology evolves.

Until recently texts on nursing research discussed descriptive research sparingly; now, however, articles on qualitative research are common, and in 1985 several books on this type of research were written by nurses. It would appear that both methods should continue to be used.

☐ *Responsibilities for All Nurses: Problem Identification and Use of Research*

According to the American Nurses' Association Commission on Nursing Practice (1981), all professional nurses should be research consumers and should help to identify relevant problems for research studies. First, however, the barriers related to the conduct of research studies and the use of research must be discussed, because without an understanding of these factors, one might be reluctant to participate in or use research findings.

BARRIERS TO RESEARCH

In the past the major barrier to research in nursing was the fact that nurses were not prepared to

do it. This problem is being alleviated, as the number of nurses receiving masters and doctoral degrees increases. At the baccalaureate level, the nurse is expected to participate in research projects and to read and use research findings in practice, though there are practicing nurses who have not had this preparation. Over time, continuing and inservice educational programs will address these needs. Other barriers to research can be categorized as related to research itself, the profession, or a given situation (Table 37-3).

Research barriers include problems that deal with the research report. Probably the most common comments are that the report is not easily read, that it's difficult to understand, and that the findings are not useful in practice. Other complaints include: (1) relevant clinical problems are not studied; (2) researchers are isolated from practice; (3) research studies are not replicated; (4) research reports are not readily available; and (5) general knowledge about completed research is lacking. Some nurses feel that doing research is not really work so the researcher doesn't need to be paid. Still others perceive that the interval between the point of discovery and the implementation of the finding is too long (Lancaster, 1984; Mercer, 1984).

The professional problems are of a more serious nature, the overriding issue being the professional socialization of nurses. Nurses have traditionally been oriented to acting and doing. Scientific efforts have not been supported by the entire profession, and "knowing" on the basis of

TABLE 37-3 Barriers to Doing and Using Research in Nursing	
Broad Categories of Barriers	**Factors Related to Each Category**
Research	Studies difficult to read and understand
	Finding not useful in practice
	Studies not relevant to nursing practice
	Studies not replicated
	Research reports not readily available
Professional	Socialization of nurses
	Professional orientation to doing rather than thinking
Situational	Limited administrative support for research
	Limited support for change
	Lack of peer support for researcher

tradition or authority has had more emphasis than the scientific method. Consequently, nurses would rather act than think, were not committed to science or research, and had difficulty in dealing with scientific criticism.

Situational problems vary from institution to institution but some trends are common. Much of the criticism has been directed toward the nursing service administration, though part of the problem may be related to the fact that the nursing staff "did not want to change" and placed blame for lack of research and utilization of its findings on others, rather than accept individual responsibility. Criticism is also directed toward schools or colleges of nursing for inadequate preparation of students. In addition, nursing service administrators are accused of placing limited value on research, providing few rewards when research is done, and providing limited or no support for research. Support consists of allowing time for conduct/utilization of research, giving approval, and providing financial aid. Still another problem is that a lone researcher in an institution needs ongoing peer support in order to generate research ideas and designs, and to remain productive.

IDENTIFYING PROBLEMS FOR RESEARCH

Is it necessary that all professional nurses identify problems for research? The answer is Yes. The criticism that much research is irrelevant and unrelated to clinical practice could thereby be resolved. Traditionally, researchers have been based in academic settings with limited contacts in practice so that their research findings may not have been relevant to clinical problems. Few nursing clinicians were involved in research. Changes are underway, however. Undergraduate nurses are being taught how to identify problems, clinicians are becoming involved in research projects, and faculties in academia are becoming involved in practice. The combination of these efforts should produce more relevant research. Without a doubt, research in a practice discipline must come from the practice settings, for ultimately the findings from research return to those settings in order to resolve practice problems. Clinicians need to be made aware that research does not invariably have immediate application. Some research is basic; it identifies and describes aspects of practice rather than providing a prediction of occurrence/incidence of disorders or a prescription of therapeutic measures.

Definition of a Researchable Problem

The selection, statement, and clarification of the research problem may be the most important action in research as the ultimate outcomes of research are dependent upon this process. Not all problems are researchable. Some already have answers, and some that do not have apparent answers can be solved in a practical manner.

What is a researchable problem? It is an irritation encountered in practice; a felt difficulty; a gripe; a discrepancy between the way things are and the way they should be; a situation needing solution, improvement, or alteration; a condition that needs to be solved, something that seems wrong; a question that needs to be answered; a discrepancy between what is known and what needs to be known in order to solve a practice problem.

Any of them could produce a problem for study. Some factors could interfere with, prevent, or delay the identification of problems. Possibly the most important factor is an ignorance of the field being studied. One cannot formulate relevant and important problems in any field without having knowledge of that field. Next, one must have an open and questioning mind in order to see that what has always been considered "right" in a clinical setting may not necessarily produce appropriate results. Being overly familiar with a field or being tradition bound can be blinding. Finally, if one feels that only one research methodology is correct, this could limit the number of problems developed for investigation (Artinian and Anderson, 1980; Valiga and Mermel, 1985).

The criteria for the selection of research problems include feasibility, value/importance of the problem, availability of instruments and methods, investigator characteristics, problem controlled by the discipline of nursing (e.g., rehabilitation of chronically ill), and personal interest. A determination of feasibility involves looking at the project costs related to time, energy, and money and whether there is administrative and peer support for the study. Are the costs and support such that conditions are adequate to allow the researcher to proceed? The value or importance of the project is an assessment made to ascertain whether the problem (1) is recognized by others; (2) creates serious deficits in care; or (3) would lessen cost and service needs if it were solved. One problem for many researchers is the relative lack of instruments, techniques, or procedures available for use in a study. For instance, tools to measure nursing variables and/or diagnoses are not yet available. The investigator's characteristics are important in any study. What is the educational and experience level of the researcher? Does she possess the necessary skills to conduct the study? Are assistants needed, and what are their qualifications? If consultants must be used, are they available? What is the cost? Can these questions be answered and resolved, or should the project be postponed until more of the people/resources are available? Studies done in nursing should be relevant to and under the control of nursing. If not, they are inappropriate. For example, why should nurses attempt to find out what drugs are therapeutic, when it is more appropriate that they learn about the effectiveness of a structured and consistent environment as a treatment modality for confusion? Last, research takes considerable time and extends over months, even years. The study must be capable of sustaining the investigator's interest over time.

Nursing is in the beginning stages in developing its science, so there are any number of potential problems for study. However, identifying the problems may be difficult. Where and how can a nurse do this? Sources of problems are either external, or internal to the nurse. External sources are those found in books or reports and therefore available to anyone. Internal sources are those ideas that occur and are developed by individual nurses (Valiga and Mermel, 1985).

External sources might be most useful to nurses who lack original ideas, because the areas for research have already been identified. For example, research studies frequently report implications for nursing and what additional research is needed. Some difficulties arise when these external sources are used. First, one has to take at face value that the identified area is indeed one needing research and one that is within the domain of nursing. In addition, the nurse researcher must consider whether this is a topic that will sustain her interest over time. The external sources include (1) contracts for specific projects funded by government or by a foundation; (2) priorities identified by professional organizations or health care agencies; (3) recommendations made on the basis of previous research projects. Several areas for research in psychiatric nursing were identified at the beginning of this chapter and were developed on the basis of a review of the psychiatric literature.

Internal sources for research ideas arise within the individual nurse, such as questions about specific clinical situations. Possibly more research problems are identified as clinicians consider recurring irritations experienced in practice. An idea that may arise as a passing impression ultimately grows to become a clear enunciation of a problem area through further experience, reading, listening, and reflecting. The "what if," "why not," and "this ought to work" become attached to a clinical problem for which a solution is needed (Fuller, 1982; Valiga and Mermel, 1985).

■ Point of Emphasis

Researchable problems may arise from areas where information is lacking, but other techniques can be used. All nurses should become sympathetic to the idea that helping to identify research problems is a responsibility; as they read records and professional journals, make rounds, and listen to co-workers, clients, and their families, they become aware that these are sources for research ideas. Nurses should become expert observers and listeners as they contemplate the concerns of clients and families, the responses of clients in similar situations, and the similarities and differences found among individuals with the same health problems. It is through the active involvement of nurses in clinical situations and their reflections on the meaning of those events that important and relevant research problems originate.

CLINICAL SITUATIONS

Two clinical situations are described to demonstrate how research ideas evolve and how research purposes and methods are derived from those ideas. In the first situation, the nurse uses the following means to identify her area of concern and potential research problem: focused observation, talking with peers, reading records, reading relevant literature, and reflecting.

The nurse's decisions indicate that she feels that the clients demonstrate symptoms of low self-esteem, and there are indications that certain activities may be therapeutic in increasing self-esteem. For example, could support groups or assertiveness and job training be effective? The intent of her study would be to determine the effectiveness of these two types of treatment.

Research purposes could be stated as hypotheses in this manner:

1. Abused women will have increased self-esteem after participation in a structured support group for 3 months.
2. Abused women will have increased self-esteem following the completion of a program for assertiveness and job training.
3. The increase in self-esteem will be greater for abused women who participate in support groups than for those who complete an assertiveness and job training program.
4. The increase in self-esteem will be greater for abused women who complete an assertiveness and job-training program than for those who participate only in support groups for 3 months.

The design of the research study would be quasi-experimental, with random assignment to one of three groups: job training, support group, control group. Self-esteem would be measured before and after the treatments for all individuals included in the study. The intent of the project would be to confirm or deny the stated hypotheses.

The second situation involves a nurse who is working in a community clinical setting and has been observing specific situations, has noted patient and family interactions, and has observed unusual intrafamily responses. The references she consults are not helpful. She decides that the problem should be studied.

In this situation, background information is limited. The intent of the study, therefore, might be to describe the characteristics of the clients and families who seem to adjust successfully to physical illness/disability, and the characteristics of clients and families who do not make a good adjustment. The research purposes may be stated as follows:

1. What are the characteristics of patients and families in both successful and unsuccessful adjustment to physical illness/disability?
2. What are the processes/activities in which clients and their families participate during either successful or unsuccessful adjustment to physical illness/disability?
3. What antecedent factors are found in situations where clients become dependent, depressed, and indecisive following physical illness/disability?

In order to conduct this study, the nurse would use qualitative methods. She could select family units from successful and unsuccessful families and then administer structured open-ended interviews to obtain the information needed. The data collected would be coded and analyzed so that the characteristics, activities, and antecedents could be identified. Future research might be done to determine what treatments would alter the characteristics, activities, or antecedents so that adjustment would improve.

Any clinical area will provide rich resources for research ideas. Through focused observation, listening, talking, and reflecting, identification of important research ideas is possible.

☐ *Utilizing Research in Nursing Practice*

As a group, nurses feel that they are out of step with or behind other disciplines in various aspects of practice. This is not so, however; what is true is that nurses as a group have had only limited experience in making use of research. The reasons for this include the following: (1) available information is not being used; (2) current explosive growth in both quantity and quality of information will exacerbate the problem if action is not taken; (3) all the available resources are needed in order to deal effectively with existing problems; and (4) information needed for decision-making is not always available (Glaser, et al., 1983). In the United States the lag between discovery and use of knowledge is 7.4 years; in Japan, however, the lag is only 3.4 years.

Some terms related to utilization need to be clarified. (1) Utilization refers to application of new or available knowledge in a new way or by a new user. (2) Dissemination and diffusion are related to the extent to which knowledge has been dispersed, the former term referring to a wide dispersal of knowledge, the latter, to the limited and deliberate spread of information. (3) Change is involved whenever new knowledge/information is introduced.

In the 1970s, nurses began to be concerned with utilization of research and its findings. It may have been that until that time they had believed that as research was completed and reported, it would be read and used by practitioners to improve the quality of nursing care. This did not happen—something needed to be done. Three organizations were responsible for the development of projects that were subsequently funded by the Division of Nursing in the Department of

Health, Education, and Welfare (now HHS) and the National Foundation/March of Dimes: The Western Interstate Commission for Higher Education (WICHE), Michigan Nurses Association, and the University of Washington, College of Nursing (Table 37-4).

When WICHE began the Clinical Nursing Research Utilization Program in 1974, its broad purpose was to develop a model for research utilization programs. Sixty-eight pairs of practicing nurses were selected from 68 settings and assigned to one of three regional workshops where they were to develop knowledge and skills in initiating utilization projects in their assigned practice settings. These dyads provided an ongoing peer support system. The approaches were a problem-solving focus, a social interaction orientation, and a diffusion model.

At the end of the project there were significant contributions: 68 demonstration projects; a utilization model for continuing educational programs; and recommendations for future projects in this area (Krueger, et al., 1978). Sixty-six percent of the demonstration projects were successful and most often involved a problem-solving utilization model. The final recommendations were (1) to provide research findings in a usable form; (2) to make the profession responsible for collating research findings; (3) to disseminate research findings through publications; (4) to conduct continuing education courses to update the knowledge base of practicing nurses; and (5) to incorporate into undergraduate curricula the content and experiences needed to help a nurse become a research consumer.

The response to the recommendations was quick: research skills for undergraduates in nursing were included in *Criteria for the Evaluation of Baccalaureate and Higher Degree Programs in Nusing* (NLN) in 1977, with the result that baccalaureate programs became responsible for including research content in order to comply with accreditation standards. In addition, the Conduct and Utilization of Research in Nursing (CURN) project begun by the Michigan Nurses Association in 1975 at the University of Michigan was a response to the first three recommendations from the WICHE project. Two purposes were identified for the CURN project: (1) to develop and test a model in order to facilitate the use of scientific knowledge; and (2) to begin the process of delegating responsibility for utilization of research to nursing departments rather than the individual nurse. Two major products were developed by this

TABLE 37-4 Characteristics of Three Projects to Develop Utilization Models

Major Utilization Projects	Specific Characteristics of Each Project		
	Sponsor	Purposes	Product
Clinical Nursing Research Utilization Program (1974–77)	Western Interstate Commission for Higher Education (WICHE)	Development of a model for research utilization	68 small utilization projects Multiple publications Utilization model to use in continuing education Recommendation regarding research utilization
Conduct and Utilization of Research in Nursing Project (CURN 1975–81)	Michigan Nurses Association at University of Michigan	To develop and test a model to facilitate use of scientific nursing knowledge To delegate responsbility for research utilization to nursing department	Ten research-based protocols related to specific nursing problems Problem-driven utilization model
Nursing Child Assessment Satellite Training Project (NCAST–1976–78)	Division of Nursing National Foundation/March of Dimes University of Washington	To determine whether the use of satellite communication would be a more efficient method for introduction of new research knowledge than old standard methods To determine whether an interactive communication facility provides a viable system to ensure effective application of new assessment techniques	New assessment techniques Evidence to support use of a satellite

project; one is a series of 10 research-based protocols about 10 specific nursing problems, the other is a problem-driven model which nursing departments can use in developing and organizing utilization programs. The 10 protocols have been published in booklet form, and are available to all nurses. Among the topics are *Distress Reduction Through Sensory Preparation, Mutual Goal Setting in Patient Care*, and *Pain: Deliberative Nursing Intervention*. In addition, the model for utilization and its components has been compiled and published (Horsley, et al., 1983). All of the WICHE's recommendations have been addressed by either the National League for Nursing's Accrediting Service or the CURN project.

The most recent major utilization project was done at the University of Washington by Barnard and Hoehn (1978). This study followed the WICHE recommendations in addressing the possibility that a new delivery system would be effective and efficient in introducing advanced health care assessment techniques. The findings were ultimately disseminated by satellite. The end products were new assessment techniques in

children, and evidence to support the use of satellites in research utilization programs.

PRACTITIONER UTILIZATION MODEL

Several models have been developed to facilitate research or knowledge utilization. Four major ones are the practitioner model, the problem-driven model, the knowledge-driven model, and the linkage model. All of these have been or could be used; one may be more appropriate for group use than another. For example, the individual nurse would find the practitioner model developed by Stetler (1985) most helpful.

The model has three phases: validation, comparative evaluation, and decision-making. During the first phase, the practicing nurse must do a critique of the research study and determine whether the reported findings are weak or strong. If the findings are weak, the process is stopped because questionable findings should not be implemented into practice. With strong findings, the nurse would proceed to the second phase in which a comparative evaluation is done to determine whether any use can be made of the study's findings. Areas evaluated are the comparability between the study setting and practice setting; other research substantiating the new findings; the effectiveness of current practice procedures; and the feasibility of changing procedure at that time. In the final phase a decision is made as to the use of the findings: no use, direct use, or indirect use. If the findings are inappropriate for the setting, too costly, or potentially harmful, a decision not to use would be made. If the research results could clarify an identified problem, they would be used directly to resolve the problem. Indirect application is cognitive and could be used by the nurse to enhance understanding of situations and the dynamics of practice, and to develop new ways for thinking, perceiving, or observing a situation.

> ### ■ *Point of Emphasis*
>
> *The practitioner model demonstrates how the nurse might close the gap between research and practice, and it could ultimately become an integral component in her decision-making.*

THE CHANGE PROCESS

Whenever an agency utilizes research findings, change must occur if the process is to be successful. All other models for utilization involve group use, therefore change is a factor as the models are considered (Figure 37-3).

Whether or not change will occur depends on determinants which may be either facilitating or restraining. Determinants include the characteristics of the innovation; the willingness and ability of the agency to adopt the innovation; the availability and type of change facilitator; communication with participants; the fit between innovation and setting; the timing of the implementation; and quick identification and resolution of resistance. Any of the first six determinants may be facilitative or restraining (Glaser, et al., 1983).

Characteristics of an innovation that may facilitate change are the perception that the innovation is worthwhile, credible, easily understood, and compatible with the users' norms. Restraining characteristics include complexity, abstractness, and the process as opposed to a product (a process is more easily altered than a product). The availability of personnel and other resources will also facilitate, whereas lack of sufficient funding

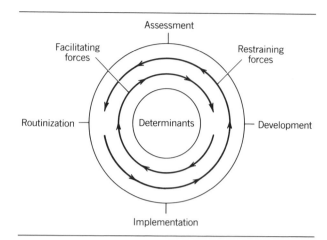

Figure 37.3 *Change process and its determinants.*

will restrain. Facilitating factors would be the appointment of a knowledgeable person to direct the change process and a communication system that keeps all innovation participants informed of programming and progress. Their absence would be restraining. There should be a fit between the innovation and the setting, just as timing of implementation is important. For example, if there is general dissatisfaction with current procedures, the staff are more open to change. The person who is responsible for change should be ever mindful of resistance and deal with it quickly so that the innovation can be successfully implemented.

THE PROBLEM-DRIVEN MODEL

The problem-driven model might be described as a problem in search of a solution. It is considered by some authorities to be the best model for planned change because of its longer history, and its user orientation and involvement is thought to lead to a greater commitment and potential for innovation survival (Glaser, et al., 1983; Crane, 1985). See Figure 37-4.

The problem-driven model is the one that the CURN project has proposed for institutional or agency use. The needs as expressed by the users or agency are paramount in driving or directing activities. During the diagnostic phase this need is clarified so that the specific problem perceived by the agency is clearly defined and stated. For example, the problem might be *the number of elderly clients who become confused after undergoing major surgical procedures.* These clients enter the hospital fully rational and oriented, only to manifest acute confusion in the immediate post-

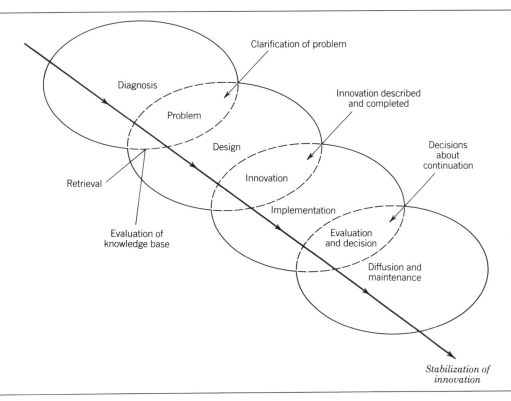

Figure 37.4 *Problem-driven utilization model for nursing.*

operative period. What can be done to minimize or prevent such confusion?

References must be studied, evaluated, and synthesized so that summarizing statements can be made about them. Evaluation criteria focus on the scientific merit of each study, whether findings are replicated and appropriate for nursing practice, and whether it will be possible to evaluate the implementation of the new care protocol (Haller, et al., 1979). Questions such as the following should be addressed: How often have researchers reached the same conclusions? Were the findings valid and reliable? Are there any risks associated with the use of the findings? Does nursing have control over the use of the findings? Do benefits exceed the cost of implementation? Are resources (people, material) available to implement the findings? Can the effectiveness of implementing the findings be evaluated?

Let us use, for our example, the problem of confusion in elderly postoperative clients. A group of nurses in 1979 initiated an investigation of such confusion. They were able to identify activities that helped to prevent and control confusion during the postoperative period following hip surgery (Williams, et al., 1979). The studies continued until 1985 when the researchers identified (1)

probable causes of confusion in the postsurgical elderly; (2) deliberate goal-directed interventions to prevent confusion; and (3) responsive nursing interventions after early symptoms of confusion (Campbell, et al., 1986; Williams, et al., 1985a,b). The conceptual framework showing how confusion develops and how nurses should intervene is presented in Figure 37-5.

Nursing approaches were related to six factors resulting from hospitalization: strange environment, alteration in sensory input, loss of control and independence, disruption in life patterns, immobility and pain, and disruption in elimination patterns (Williams, et al., 1985). The treatment consisted of having the interventions incorporated into the customary plan of care, with a clinical nurse specialist making a daily visit to those patients who had had repairs of hip fractures. Techniques included environmental manipulation and interpersonal intervention. Specific activities included: (1) providing continuity of care; (2) providing clues such as a clock and a calendar, keeping drapes open during the day; (3) anticipating and preventing pain; (4) weaving orienting information into the conversation; (5) keeping clients informed about and explaining the rationale for treatment; (6) correcting sensory deficits

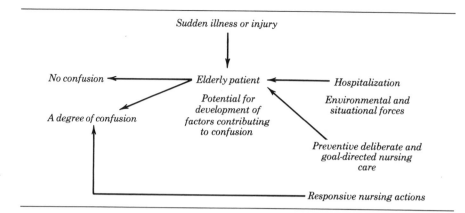

Figure 37.5 *The development and prevention of confusion in sick or injured elderly.*

(e.g., having glasses and hearing aid in place; (7) keeping the number of hospital personnel who interact with clients to a minimum; (8) encouraging family members to visit; (9) assisting clients to gain a sense of control over events; (10) explaining settings, routines, and the role of personnel; (11) turning the client and changing his position periodically; (12) building on the client's strengths and abilities; (13) making eye contact at the client's level; (14) encouraging family and friends to bring in familiar objects; (15) assessing the client's usual habits and/or difficulties and planning accordingly.

The new information would be considered in terms of current hospital procedures and practices and any other available options. A decision would be made about whether to adopt the findings as an innovation, not to adopt, or to modify the findings. If a decision for adoption was made, the findings as reported would be developed into a specific protocol or innovation for use in that agency. Implementation would involve introducing the innovation to personnel on one or more units of the agency through inservice education. Group work might allow for role playing to give the staff experience in handling the activities and receiving feedback about their performances. Once the personnel have become comfortable, the protocol could be implemented relative to the elderly surgical clients on one unit. Just before the identified behavior occurs, it would be necessary to measure the client's confusion and continue to do this throughout the hospitalization. It might be helpful to have available a control group of patients who do not receive any special treatment. After a specified period an evaluation could be done to see if the clients receiving the special treatment manifest less confusion than the others.

If the evaluation was positive, a decision might be made to continue with the innovation. If problems had developed during the initial implementation, modifications might be needed before continuing. Diffusion would be accomplished by introducing the innovation to other units of the hospital so that all who could benefit from the innovation had access to it. Maintenance involves activities that incorporate the innovation into the institution's procedures through written policies, obtaining the equipment needed, teaching staff what they need to know about innovation, periodically monitoring the staff, and developing quality control measures. When the innovation is done routinely, stabilization has occurred.

■ *Point of Emphasis*

The problem-solving model is most useful in a field where there is a well-developed knowledge base. This is the utilization model that the CURN project recommended for institutional use.

THE KNOWLEDGE-DRIVEN UTILIZATION MODEL

The knowledge-driven model promotes research-based change, and is used most often in technological change. It is based on the assumption that if an innovation is well developed and presented in a proper manner and at the right time, the user will accept and use it. The user is passive and his needs are not the motivating force in the use of knowledge. The innovation is developed and packaged and ready for use, a process that may be time consuming and costly. This model was used in the

CURN project when the 10 protocols were developed and packaged. As shown in Figure 37-6, the phases of this model do not differ significantly from those of the problem-driven model.

Differences may be noted between the two models. for instance, in the first phase of the knowledge-driven model, the initiating and driving force is the new knowledge base rather than a felt need. However, the same processes are used in both to secure, evaluate, and synthesize research findings so that summarizing generalizations can be made about the replicated and valid findings. It is in the design phase that the innovation is developed and packaged in the knowledge-driven model and in which it is somewhat similar to the problem-solving model. During implementation, the protocol or innovation is tested for the first time, evaluated, and then modified as necessary. In the final phase of the knowledge-driven model, the innovation is evaluated and a continuation decision is made. Diffusion, maintenance, and stabilization processes are the same for both models.

LINKAGE-UTILIZATION MODEL

The linkage model integrates the most useful features of the other models, providing ongoing interaction between systems that previously were separate: the user system which has been a problem-solving system and a research resource system. The former might be any health-care agency while the latter might be a university or research organization. There would be a reciprocal relationship between these two problem-solving structures in that each would be concerned with its capabilities in resolving the problems of the other systems. Consequently, the user system would appreciate the innovation and solution-formulation of the resource system; but the resource system would understand the other's problem-solving capabilities and begin to anticipate the knowledge needs of the user system. In order to be able to meet all of the needs of a user agency, the resource center might need a linkage to a larger knowledge or resource system (Crane, 1985; Loomis, 1985).

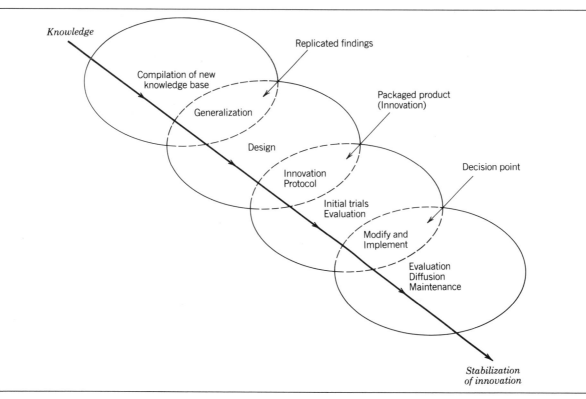

Figure 37.6 *Knowledge-driven utilization model for nursing.*

There are four components in the linkage model that attach the practice system to the knowledge-generating system. First, the user (practice) system has its own specific needs, its own problem-solving system, and a need and desire to use new information from outside resources. Second, the knowledge-generating system originates and develops new information, skills, and products but is also able to identify or develop solutions that are relevant to and useful for the practice system's problems. Third, a mechanism must be available to transmit information and feedback between the two systems about problems needing solution, and feedback about the effectiveness of solutions that are provided. Finally, a mechanism is needed that allows for transmission of new knowledge to the user system. The use of the system allows for individual formulation of problems and expert help in obtaining relevant solutions to the identified problem.

A change in how nurse practitioners and nurse researchers interact perhaps would be even more helpful in the research utilization process. If practicing nurses were involved with the researcher in developing and conducting clinical research studies, these nurses would have an ongoing familiarity with current research and would know which findings were available for utilization. The researcher would know the specific problem areas in practice. This would be a linkage of practice and research and might be more viable than any utilization model.

☐ Evaluation of Nursing Care

The need to evaluate nursing and health care has been recognized since the time of Nightingale. When nursing care was first evaluated and was noted to be lacking in some way, the problem was frequently attributed to either a deficiency in or defective preparation of the nurse, and educational programs were modified to remove these deficiencies/defects. Over the years, the delivery system in nursing has been considered inadequate or inefficient, so the system has gone from individualized nursing to functional nursing to team nursing and finally to primary nursing. It seems that we have come full circle and there may still be those who question whether quality nursing care exists.

The health care system has also gone through various phases wherein various components have been considered as health care has been assessed. Prior to the 1960s, the great concern was whether everyone had a right to health care and consequently had access to care. After the introduction of Medicare, the concern became the quality of the care being provided. During the late 1970s and 1980s, health care workers, federal legislators, and citizens have become concerned about the federal deficit and its strong relationship to health care cost. The cry of the 1980s has become cost containment with less emphasis on quality of health care.

FACTORS INFLUENCING QUALITY OF CARE

Anticipated and unanticipated changes are now occurring in the health care system so that one cannot predict with certainty what the structure will be within a few years. It seems, however, that changes will be closely related to efforts toward cost containment. Other factors that have affected quality in the past and will continue to have an influence include third-party payers, licensing of health professionals, consumerism, accreditation, and professional accountability.

Third-Party Payers

Some say that there have been two revolutions in health care since 1965: the first one followed the legislation establishing Medicare and Medicaid, the second followed the legislation establishing prospective payment systems for Medicare recipients. The first revolution resulted in a massive increase in numbers of hospitals, nursing homes, and health care professionals; the second one will result in changes in the structure of and kinds of health care facilities, with more community-based care and increasing personal health/illness responsibility on the part of all individuals.

Third-party payers have influenced the quality of care. With the inception of Medicare/Medicaid, there was initial institutional responsibility for utilization review of all client admissions to assure appropriate use of hospitals that were being reimbursed for care. Soon the focus was changed to Professional Standard Review Organizations (PSRO) which were local organizations designed to monitor utilization reviews and evaluate medical care in hospitals and in some ambulatory centers. Since prospective payment through the diagnosis related groups (DRGs) has evolved, legislation has mandated a statewide system called Peer Review Organization (PRO). This organization is primarily concerned with cost containment as reflected in five objectives: (1) reduce readmissions due to substandard care; (2) ensure the provision of medical services that reduce potential for complications; (3) reduce avoidable deaths; (4) reduce unnecessary surgery; and (5) reduce complications, postoperative and otherwise. At this writing, certain health care units and facilities (such as non-Medicare clients, psychiatric clients, rehabilitation clients, and nursing home clients) are not yet covered by prospective payment and are exempt from PRO evaluation and control. Nevertheless, changes have been noticed in these care situations with shortened length of stays and a greater acuity of illness during institutionalization (Dans, et al., 1985; Mattson, 1984).

Some of the federal regulations specifically affecting the provision of care in community mental health centers (CMHC) were developed and discontinued during the 1970s and 1980s. For example, federal legislation in 1975 and 1980 provided that all federally funded centers had to develop and participate in quality assurance activities, but these pieces of legislation were later repealed. Block grants for CMHCs are now available to the states; thus the state rather than the federal government is responsible for evaluating care (Mattson, 1984).

One might wonder if psychiatric and other long-term care will come under the prospective payment system. Many people feel that if this payment system is able to reduce or contain the cost of health care, other components such as physician fees paid by Medicare and insurance companies will also adopt this system. Then too, corporations and industry now paying employee health insurance premiums will also insist on cost-saving mechanisms. It appears that every component of the health care system will be subjected to cost containment and possible prospective payment. However, psychiatric nursing may remain exempt because this care still receives only limited coverage by insurance companies, and block grants provide diminishing support for community mental health centers. So the general sense may be that costs in psychiatric care are already contained.

Licensing of Health Professionals

The overriding purpose in licensing most health care professionals has been to ensure the quality of care for all citizens. There has always been the assumption that licensing laws are necessary because the public does not have sufficient information to judge the competence of any health care professional.

There is limited evidence to determine whether licensure accomplishes this purpose, but the reason for this might be related more to the fact that it is difficult to define and assess quality. Questions about the need for licensure are being discussed: If the initial licensure ensured competence of the practitioner, shouldn't there be periodic reevaluations to determine continuing competence? Doesn't licensure merely restrict professional entry rather than ensure quality? One point that should be made about most licenses for health professionals is that the professional who holds the license is held accountable for her practice (Hemenway, 1983).

Consumerism

While there may have been an assumption that the typical consumer of health care was relatively uninformed about health care and its professionals, some trends predict that health consumers may be expected to assume increasing responsibility for their health care. These trends and changes are multifaceted and include (1) a shift from acute to chronic illness with control of disease possible only with life-style modifications; (2) decreased length of stay in all acute hospitals with expectation for self-care following discharge; (3) hospitalizations limited to extreme acute illness and/or surgery; (4) increased management of illness/injury on an ambulatory basis; and (5) some health care costs shifting from the insurance company to the recipient of care or his family.

If these trends and changes become solidified, then the consumer will need to become more sophisticated so he can manage not only the care associated with relatively simple physical activities of living but also that associated with skills now considered within the professional domain.

> ■ *Point of Emphasis*
>
> *As the consumer pays more for his care, he may hold the professional more heavily accountable.*

Accreditation of Agencies

In order for agencies to operate in a state, they must be accredited by the state and sometimes by a national agency. In most instances the state regulations deal with minimal standards while national and sometimes voluntary accreditation standards have more to do with quality. The Joint Commission on Accreditation of Hospitals (JCAH), accrediting arm of the American Hospital Association, is responsible for accrediting all types of hospitals and nursing homes. Even though the focus of federal agencies is shifting from quality assurance to cost containment, the JCAH still mandates specific criteria dealing with quality assurance (Mattson, 1984; Egelston, 1980).

When quality assurance was first addressed by the JCAH, the criteria and standards were somewhat rigid, and some agencies had difficulty complying with them. Since 1979 the standard for quality assurance has been more flexible, and allows for differences among institutions. The new standard allows for integration of all institutional activities related to quality assessment and assurance, and encourages methods that are pertinent and appropriate to their particular situation.

Professional Accountability

Each professional group working in a health care agency is responsible for developing standards of practice and ensuring that quality is maintained. During the 1980s the number of malpractice suits increased dramatically, and health care consumers are dissatisfied with the fragmentation and depersonalization of care. Thus there seems to be a even greater need for voluntary self-regulation by professionals if they want to maintain autonomy and not be controlled by others. Hospitals and other health care facilities are becoming increasingly concerned about the competence of professional practitioners and stand ready to assure peer review in the practice setting, so that the hospital is not held liable for malpractice.

At one time all forces seemed to be focused on quality assurance in health care. With the recognition that costs need to be contained, only consumers, professionals, and accrediting bodies continue to emphasize quality. In other instances the attainment of quality care may be limited to the extent that such care can be provided within health-care budgets, which are being reduced yearly.

Quality Assurance Programs

Quality assurance programs should be comprehensive so that all units providing direct care to clients can be evaluated periodically. But what is meant by quality assurance? What are its purposes? Who is responsible for it? Schmadl (1979) developed the following definition as it applies to nursing: Quality assurance involves assuring the consumer of a specified degree of excellence through continuous measurement and evaluation of structural components, goal-directed nursing process, and/or consumer outcome, using preestablished criteria, standards, and available norms, followed by appropriate alteration with the purpose of improvement.

The purposes of quality assurance can be derived from that definition. First, quality of care is assured by ongoing and systematic evaluations. Second, if the evaluation so indicates, appropriate action must be taken to obtain the necessary improvements in nursing care. The two purposes are to evaluate and to change activities so as to improve care.

Various types of quality assurance programs have been developed since their introduction in the 1970s. Some have had only three phases such as problem identification, surveillance, and corrective action. A five-stage model proposed by Williams, et al., (1982) includes the two concepts of quality and cost containment, and seems more appropriate to current concerns in health care. The stages shown in Figure 37-7 include problem identification, problem verification, problem cause/resolution planning, problem resolution, and problem resolution documentation. In Stage One, the problems are identified and priorities are established on the basis of: (1) the importance of the problem in terms of its occurrence and all costs associated with it such as staff requirements and usual complications; (2) treatment modalities that are known to be effective and safe; and (3) the present treatment patterns and the potential for improvement in treatment.

A group of knowledgeable professional practitioners would make the decision about what the problems are and their ranking.

■ **Point of Emphasis**

The most important fact may be that care is being evaluated rather than that any specific program is being followed. Quality assurance programs must be cost effective if their use is to be supported and continued.

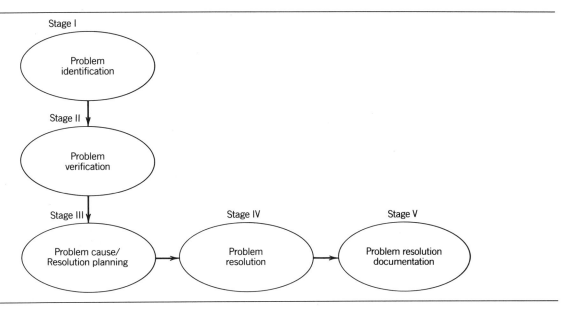

Figure 37.7 *Five-stage approach to quality assurance.*

After the problem to be studied has been identified in the first stage, the quality assurance team would then verify that the highest-priority problem was actually present in the clinical setting. They would identify the timing, frequency, and the conditions of its occurrence. During the third stage the quality assurers would analyze their data, collect additional information, and do a literature review. The intent of this process is to clarify the problem, to look at its possible causes, and to determine strategies for its alleviation. The plan of action to resolve the problem would be put in place in Stage Four. After the plan had been in place for a specified period of time, documentation would be obtained to determine the results.

Measurement in Quality Assurance

One of the most important elements in quality assurance is measurement. Without it, it would be impossible to determine the presence or absence of quality. However, measurement of the concept is difficult. In the early days of quality assurance, *how* to measure was the first concern; next there was a movement that looked at relationships between structure, process, criteria, and frameworks; more systematic evaluations now examine not only quality but the relationship of quality to cost, and may establish norms for care in relation to specific DRGs.

Terms that need to be defined are described below. They include evaluation, measurement, criterion, standard, norm, structure, process, and outcome.

Measurement and evaluation are related: measurement is an objective process whereby the dimensions, qualities, quantities, and/or capacities are determined; evaluation involves a subjective generalization following a judgment made on the basis of the measurement (Schmadl, 1979). The relationship of the terms criterion, standard, and norm is depicted in Figure 37-8.

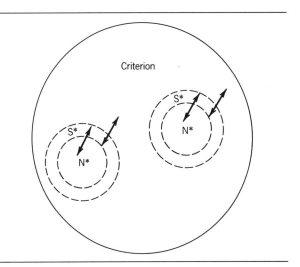

Figure 37.8 *Probable relationship between three related entities.*

S = standard
N = norm

A criterion is a variable indicator of some other concept such as quality, and the criteria can be listed. A standard is established; it represents a value assumed or assigned to a criterion. The value assigned is usually a desired or achievable level of performance and may be the same as or different from a norm. Norms are current levels or ranges of performance for the criterion and are determined on the basis of empirical data. (For example, the norm for temperature in humans is 98.6°F.) Standards are also based on clinical evidence but frequently the quality of knowledge that is available prevents the development of appropriate and measurable standards. Norms and standards may or may not have the same value depending on each specific criterion. In some instances the standard is measured against the norm in the evaluation process. Both norms and standards are also subject to change in value as new facts and knowledge are discovered. In the process of developing a quality assurance program, therefore, one would need to determine the problem area, list criteria, develop standards, and determine norms (Bloch, 1977; Schmadl, 1979).

Some examples of these three concepts are provided:

Example 1

Criterion	Standards	Norms
Orientation	Oriented to time, place, and person	Same as standard

Example 2

Criterion	Standards	Norms
Mental health	Increase in self-esteem	—
	Active coping strategies	
	Life satisfaction	

In the first example, it is easy to see that the criterion of orientation can be measured by the standard and the norm. This is somewhat simplistic, but it shows that the standard and the norm can be the same. In the second example, mental health is shown with three standards to use in its measurement. At the present time we would have difficulty dealing with norms because accurate means for measurement of self-esteem, coping strategies, and life satisfaction are unavailable, so norms or ranges for scores cannot be established. As assessment in these areas improves, it should be possible to determine an adequate self-esteem or coping score.

Criteria may be of three types in health care: structure, process, or outcome. There is no clear consensus about whether one is better than the others or which two of the three are the best. The current focus is on outcome criteria or at least on process-outcome criteria, however nurses have felt that all three should be used in some instances. Structural criteria refer to the agencies' resources—human and nonhuman. They focus on the prerequisites for client care and are related to the simplest and oldest form of evaluation, assuming that when adequate and appropriate staff and facilities are provided, the end result will be quality care. This form of evaluation may have elements of validity since it is usually accepted that a safe environment and an adequate staff will lead to quality in care. Standards for these criteria are easy to measure, but the emphasis is not on giving care nor on the outcomes of care. Some criticize structural criteria as being rigid because the situational givens have been accepted as appropriate and correct even though other factors may be more important (Bloch, 1977; Schmadl, 1979). Some examples of structural criteria are (1) number of registered nurses needed to provide safe care on an acute locked ward; (2) the ratio of staff to clients on an adolescent unit for drug abusers; (3) presence of a small conference room for conducting psychotherapy.

Process criteria are those related to what the nurse or other health care providers do with and for clients. This includes nursing process but is not limited to it. The domain is represented by all that is done and should be done as well as those activities not done whether needed or not. It is thought that evaluation of process measures (1) is cheaper than outcome measures; (2) provides clues necessary for corrective action; and (3) is more useful when done in conjunction with related outcome measures. In addition, in order for process measures to have any degree of validity, one must be able to prove that the process is necessary and important in correcting a nursing problem (Bloch, 1977; Mattson, 1984; Schmadl, 1979).

Process might well include the delivery method of care. For example, was care provided in a task-oriented fashion or was it individualized to meet specific client needs? Process could also include one-to-one therapeutic interactions, groups used as therapy, or groups used as support.

Any interaction or activity designed to accomplish some treatment goal could be included under process.

The use of outcome criteria is favored by many nurses because this type concentrates on client welfare as the ultimate outcome of care. At a given point in time, the client's functional level is examined in terms of impact of medical or nursing intervention. While some nurses prefer to set limitations in specifying outcomes, it seems reasonable that outcome criteria could and should include not only physiological and anatomical changes but also cognitive, psychosocial, and behavioral changes. Two major problems related to using these criteria are apparent. First, the development of nursing has not progressed to a point where relevant and valid outcome criteria and standards can be developed for many important care situations. Second, because many disciplines function together in providing care, it is not possible to always determine which health care worker's activity produced the effect (Bloch, 1977; Mattson, 1984; Schmadl, 1979).

Documentation Records

The client's medical record serves many functions. It is useful in keeping all members of the health team informed about treatment and responses to care. Records are necessary in conducting quality assurance programs because they become a source to identify/document clinical problems, they are a resource so one can determine the therapeutic interventions used in each episode of care, and they should contain all outcomes of care. When outcomes and process standards of care are evaluated, the record is paramount. Without careful and deliberate documentation, assessment of care is not possible. Poorly kept records also impede other aspects of the overall quality assurance program such as risk management and utilization review. In fact, developing the means to improve medical records might be one of the first activities in a quality assurance program.

■ **Point of Emphasis**

In any client situation, all professionals should accept their responsibility for keeping accurate and complete records.

Quality Assurance in Psychiatric Nursing

The forces that have the potential for facilitating quality assurance are accreditation agencies, consumer interest and concern, and increased peer review by professionals. Difficulties that may be peculiar to the field of psychiatry are the need to preserve client confidentiality, and relatively unstandardized records that lack a degree of precision. Precision in diagnosis and treatment has been improved since the introduction of DSM-III (Mattson, 1984).

In order to show how a quality assurance program involving a mental health problem could be carried out, the same research-based knowledge about prevention and control of confusion can be used (see conceptual framework in this chapter). Using the five-stage quality assurance and cost containment model, the quality assurance nurse team would need to identify and verify the problem, identify its causes and intervention strategies, implement plans to resolve the problem, and evaluate and document plan effectiveness. From a list of identified problems occurring on a surgical unit the quality assurance team identified confusion in the elderly postoperative client as a serious problem because it increases the length of stay in the hospital and it occurs in many clients. On the basis of this information, this problem was assigned a high priority. The team of nurses then did an onsite observation and chart review to verify that this was a serious ongoing problem. These observations and review verified that confusion developed in 60 percent or more of older postsurgical patients who were not confused when admitted.

Since these nurses were primarily experienced in medical-surgical nursing they asked a psychiatric nurse clinician to help identify possible causes for this confusion. The clinician was aware of the studies by Williams (1979, 1985a, b) and her group. The results of this study formed the basis of a plan for intervention to prevent confusion or to limit its progression. The plan to resolve the problem was implemented; after it had been in place for 3 months, an assessment was done to determine if the planned interventions had been successful in reducing the occurrence or progression of confusion.

Criteria along with standards and norms were also developed so that this quality assurance program could be evaluated. Table 37-5 presents the criteria with specific standards and norms.

TABLE 37-5 Criteria to be Used in a Quality Assurance Program to Prevent or Reduce Confusion

Criteria[a]	Measurement Parameters	
	Standard	Norm
Staff (S)	Sufficient and consistent nursing staff to monitor clients and provide protective interventions	Nursing staff should be such that continuity in care and individual client needs are met.
Environment (S)	The environment is controlled so that normal clues about time and place are available to clients.	Same as above
Nurse intervention (P)	There is documentation in the record that preventive and responsive interventions were provided.	The nurse is responsible for maintenance of health and the prevention of complications.
Client orientation (O)	The client will remain oriented to time, place, and person.	Same as standard
Client memory (O)	The client will retain recent and remote memory.	Same as standard
Client interpretation of sensory stimuli (O)	The client will not experience illusions or hallucinations.	Same as standard

[a] S = structure; P = process; O = outcome.

While only six criteria are listed, others might be important to an evaluation of this sort. The criteria included are staff, environment, nurse intervention, client orientation, client memory, and client interpretation of sensory stimuli. The criteria included at least one example of structural, process, or outcome criteria. The standard provides the means to determine if quality can be assured. If, for instance, the number of staff were inadequate for implementing the interventions in a consistent fashion, they would not have met this standard or approached the norm of ensured continuity in meeting client needs. In regard to client orientation, the standard would not be met unless the client remained oriented to time, place, and person throughout the postoperative period. The evaluation of program success would depend on the extent to which the record or observations substantiated the standards as presented in Table 37-5. Did the program reduce the occurrence and progression of confusion in the selected population? If for some reason the program was unsuccessful, modifications in the interventions with another trial would be appropriate. This quality assurance program is similar to a utilization project as both are designed to produce change.

COST CONTAINMENT

Cost containment is a concern shared by all persons associated with health care agencies and those who pay for these services directly and indirectly. The DRGs with prospective payment have been the major method to date in cost containment with regard to Medicare, while a state prospective payment system was already in place for most Medicaid charges. It is expected that if the prospective payment system effectively contains costs, it will be applied to all components of health care including psychiatric and rehabilitative care. Insurance companies may also institute a comparable system to reduce their costs.

Nursing service departments and others have felt that the DRG system does not reflect the total cost of providing care because of client variations in degree/intensity of illness. Consequently several institutions have developed classification systems to indicate how much nursing care is needed by clients who fall within each DRG classification. For instance, a Class I category might indicate clients who have minimal nursing care needs, while a Class IV category might be appropriate for clients in intensive care units who need constant care and supervision. Most of the classification systems apply to nonpsychiatric facilities, but some have already been developed for use with psychiatric clients (Reitz, 1985; Schroder and Washington, 1982; Sovie, et al., 1985). When these classifications are combined with the DRG system, it will be possible to determine the actual cost of nursing care by each DRG. When psychiatric care is ultimately covered by a prospective system, nursing departments will be able to predict the cost of care if classification systems are accurate.

Cost containment is a factor to be dealt with, but it is important to include quality in any consideration of cost. At some future time we may be able to state the minimum cost of providing safe and effective care. We know that as cost of care increases, quality does not necessarily increase in proportion to cost. Two other mechanisms are also used in quality assurance and cost containment programs: utilization review and risk management.

Utilization Review

The utilization review method has a longer history than any other component of a quality assurance program. Its purpose is to determine on a periodic basis whether clients who have been admitted to an agency for care still need that level of care, or whether they should be transferred to a different level, or discharged. Utilization review has been used in ambulatory settings, in hospitals, and in nursing homes.

The same focus is extremely important since the prospective payment system has been incorporated into care facilities. Someone needs to monitor admissions in terms of diagnosis, the number of days allowed for that DRG, and how many days remain in the DRG scheme. If clients stay for a longer period than Medicare will cover, then the agency must pick up those costs. If the client stays for a shorter period, then the agency may earn a profit. There is concern, however, that the client may be discharged before he is able to care for himself. If this were to occur, the quality of care would be questioned.

Risk Management

Risk management is a recent element in quality assurance. It may have come about because of the increase in malpractice suits. Risk management programs minimize the risk to clients and also minimize the risk of lawsuits to the institution. Areas of possible risk in psychiatric care include client safety, specific treatments and procedures, client assessment, competence of the professional staff, and ensuring client rights. Risk management should be integrated with quality assurance activities so that the former does not receive greater emphasis.

The activities of a program to manage risk are varied. First, each professional discipline would be involved in identifying client problems and implementing procedures to resolve the problems on an ongoing basis. Second, accident and incident reports should be reviewed so as to identify new problems and institute remedies before the problems become serious. Third, medical records should be reviewed as to their accuracy and adequacy. Finally, educational programs should be developed and made available to the staff so that they remain competent and aware of potential risks to clients (Mattson, 1984).

■ Enrichment Activities

DISCUSSION QUESTIONS

1. What are the purposes of research?
2. What responsibility do all nurses have for research activities?
3. What types of knowledge are needed in nursing?
4. Describe the four phases used in conducting research.
5. Are the levels of theory development important in planning research? How?
6. How can utilization of research in nursing be facilitated?
7. Describe two types of models that have been developed for utilization of research.
8. Describe three types of criteria used in quality assurance programs.
9. Differentiate between criteria, standard, and norm.

10. Why are outcome criteria difficult to use in evaluation of care in hospitals?

11. How would you develop a quality assurance program in a clinical setting?

12. What changes can be anticipated in quality assurance programs in the next few years?

LEARNING ACTIVITIES

Matching Questions—Match the Terms in Column A with the Phrases in Column B as Indicated

A. *Terms*

1. Criterion
2. Theory
3. Innovation

B. *Definitions*

a. That which may be tested or generated by research
b. A concept or variable known to be an indicator of quality
c. That which is collected during a research study
d. That which is discovered in research and packaged for use
e. Knowledge developed only by qualitative methods

A. *Terms*

4. Conceptual framework
5. Utilization model
6. Standard

B. *Uses*

a. The end product of theory development and research
b. A structure important in explanation of how to use knowledge in practice
c. The structure that leads to purpose identification and design of a research study
d. A measure of either the desired or achievable level of performance
e. The mean score of a variable commonly found in practice

A. *Level of Preparation*

7. BSN
8. MSN
9. PhD

B. *Expected Research Activities*

a. Can develop new research methods
b. Can help others in using research and conduct evaluation studies
c. Can identify research problems and use findings in practice
d. Can only collect data in structured situations

A. *Phase of Research*

10. Conceptual
11. Empirical
12. Interpretive

B. *End Product*

a. Research idea
b. Purpose of the study
c. Problems for future studies
d. Research design, procedures, and plan for analysis
e. Findings and their meaning

A. *Type of Criteria*

13. Structure
14. Process
15. Outcome

B. *Major Disadvantage for Use*

a. Contributions of all health professionals cannot be separated and measured
b. Records may not be accurate so that related treatment activities are not valid
c. The method is too expensive in terms of needed time for evaluation
d. Inputs are assumed to be the most important determinants of quality
e. The activity occurs too fast to be measured

A. *Components of Quality Assurance Program*	B. *Uses*
16. Utilization review	a. To assure appropriate admissions to a health care facility
17. Documentation	
18. Risk management	b. To prevent lawsuits by early recognition and resolution of problems
	c. To assure accountability of health professionals
	d. To provide the resources needed in assessment of quality care
	e. To assure that the appropriate structural components are in place

Answers

1. b	10. b
2. a	11. d
3. d	12. e
4. c	13. d
5. b	14. b
6. d	15. a
7. c	16. a
8. b	17. d
9. a	18. b

■ Recommended Readings

HOW TO EVALUATE RESEARCH STUDIES

Binder, D.M. Critique: Experimental study. In *Readings for nursing research* (Kampitz, S.D., and Pavovich, N., eds.). St. Louis: Mosby Company, 1981:152–160.

Downs, F.S. *A source book of nursing research.* Philadelphia: F.A. Davis, 1984:1–17.

Duffy, M.E. A research appraisal checklist for evaluating nursing research reports. *Nursing and health care,* 6, 10, 1985:539–547.

Horsley, J.A.; Crane, J.; Crabtree, M.K.; and Wood, D.J. *Using research to improve nursing practice: A guide.* New York: Grune & Stratton, 1983:130–134.

Knafl, K.A.; and Howard, M.J. Interpreting and reporting qualitative research. *Research in nursing and health,* 7, 1984:17–24.

Kommenich, P.; and Noack, J.A. The process of critiquing. In *Readings for nursing research* (Krampitz, S.D., and Pavlovich, N., eds.). St. Louis: Mosby Company, 1981:145–151.

Miles, M.B.; and Huberman, A.M. Drawing valid meaning from qualitative data: Toward a shared craft. *Educational researcher,* 13, 5, 1984:20–30.

Parse, R.R.; Coyne, A.B.; and Smith, M.J. *Nursing research: Qualitative methods.* Bowie, MD: Brady Communication Company, 1985:113–117.

Sherman, K.M.; and Kirsch, A.K. Research Q & A. *Nursing research,* 27, 1, 1978:69–70.

Ward, M.J.; and Fetler, M.E. Research Q & A. *Nursing research,* 28, 2, 1979:120–126.

TEN UTILIZATION PROTOCOLS DEVELOPED BY THE CURN PROJECT

Structured preoperative teaching

Reducing diarrhea in tube-fed patients

Preoperative sensory preparation to promote recovery

Preventing decubitus ulcers

Intravenous cannula change

Distress reduction through sensory preparation

Mutual goal setting in patient care

Clean intermittent catheterization

Pain: Deliverative nursing interventions

Closed urinary drainage systems

OTHER REFERENCES ON UTILIZATION

Knowledge: Creation, diffusion and utilization. Published by Sage Publishers.

Phillips, L.R.F. *A clinician's guide to the critique and utilization of nursing research.* Norwalk, CT: Appleton-Century-Crofts, 1986

Rogers, E.M. *Diffusion of innovvations.* New York: Free Press, 1983

■ References

American Nurses' Association Commission on Nursing Practice. Guidelines for the investigative function of nurses. Kansas City, MO, 1981.

Artinian, B.M., and Anderson, N. Guidelines for identification of researchable problems. *Journal of nursing education,* 19, 4, 1980:54–58.

Barnard, K.E., and Hoehn, R.E. Nursing child assessment satellite training: Final report. Hyattsville, MD: DHEW, PHS, HRA, Division of Nursing. Contract No. HRA 231-77-002, 1978.

Batey, M.V. Conceptualizing the research process. *Nursing research,* 20, 4, 1971:296–301.

Bloch, D. Evaluation of nursing care in terms of process and outcome: Issues in research and quality assurance. *Nursing research,* 24, 4, 1975:256–263.

———. Criteria, standards, norms—Crucial terms in quality assurance. *Journal of nursing administration,* 7, 7, 1977:20–80.

Campbell, E.B.; Williams, M.A.; and Mlynarczyk, S.M. After the fall: Confusion. *American journal of nursing,* 76, 2, 1986:151–154.

Crane, J. Research utilization: Theoretical perspectives. *Western journal of nursing research,* 7, 2, 1985:261–268.

Dans, P.E.; Weiner, J.P.; and Olter, S. Peer review organizations: Promises and potential pitfalls. *New England journal of medicine,* 313, 18, 1985:1131–1137.

Egelson, E.M. JCAH standards on quality assurance. *Nursing Research,* 29, 2, 1980:113–114.

Fagin, C.M. Psychiatric nursing at the crossroads: Quo vadis. *Perspectives in psychiatric care,* 19, 1981:99–106.

Fuller, E.O. Selecting a clinical problem for research. *Image: The journal of nursing scholarship,* 14, 2, 1982:60–62.

Glaser, E.M.; Abelson, H.H.; and Garrison, K.N. Putting knowledge to use. San Francisco: Jossey-Bass Inc., 1983.

Haller, K.B.; Reynolds, M.A.; and Horsley, J.A. Developing research-based innovation protocols: Process, criteria, and issues. *Research in nursing and health,* 2, 1979:45–51.

Hemenway, D. Thinking about quality: An economic perspective. *Quality Review Bulletin,* 9, 1, 1983:321–327.

Horsley, J.A.; Crane, J.; Crabtree, M.K.; and Wood, D.J. *Using research to improve nursing practice: A guide.* New York: Grune & Stratton, 1983.

Krueger, J.C.; Nelson, A.H.; and Wolanin, M.O. *Nursing research: Development, collaboration, and utilization.* Germantown, MD: Aspen System Corporation, 1978.

Lancaster, J. Bonding of nursing practice and education research. *Nursing and health care,* 5, 7, 1984:379–382.

Loomis, M.E. Knowledge utilization and research utilization in nursing. *Image: The journal of nursing scholarship,* 17, 2, 1985:35–39.

Martin, E.J. A speciality in decline? Psychiatric-mental health nursing, past, present, and future. *Journal of professional nursing,* 1, 1985:48–53.

Mattson, M.R. Quality assurance: A literature review of a changing field. *Hospital and Community Psychiatry,* 35, 6, 1984:605–615.

Mercer, R.T. Nursing research: The bridge to excellence in practice. *Image: The journal of nursing scholarship,* 16, 2, 1984:47–51.

Murphy, M.E. Designing nursing research: The qualitative-quantitative debate. *Journal of advanced nursing,* 10, 1985:225–232.

Murphy, S.A. Learned helplessness: From concept to comprehension. *Perspectives in psychiatric care,* 20, 1, 1982:27–31.

National League for Nursing Department of Baccalaureate and Higher Degree Programs. Criteria for the appraisal of baccalaureate and higher degree programs in nursing (Fourth Edition). New York, NY, 1977.

Reitz, J.A. Toward a comprehensive nursing intensity index. Part I, development. *Nursing management,* 16, 8, 1985:21–30.

Schmadl, J.C. Quality assurance: Examination of a concept. *Nursing outlook,* 7, 7, 1979:462–465.

Schroder, P.J., and Washington, W.P. Administrative decision making: Staff-patient ratios. *Perspectives in psychiatric care,* 20, 3, 1982:111–123.

Sills, G.M. Research in the field of psychiatric nursing 1952–1977. *Nursing research,* 26, 3, 1977:201–207.

Sovie, M.D.; Tarcinale, M.A.; Vanputee, A.W.; and Stunden, A.E. Amalgam of nursing acuity, DRGs and costs. *Nursing management,* 16, 3, 1985:22–42.

Stetler, C.B. Research utilization: Defining the concept. *Image: The journal of nursing scholarship,* 17, 2, 1985:40–44.

Valiga, T.M., and Mermel, V.M. Formulating the researchable question. *Topics in clinical nursing,* 7, 2, 1985:1–14.

Williams, J.W.; Hudson, J.I.; and Nevins, M.M. *Principles of quality assurance and cost containment in health care.* San Francisco: Jossey-Bass, 1982.

Williams, M.A.; Holloway, J.R.; Winn, M.C.; Wolanin, M.O.; Lawler, M.L.; Westwick, C.R.; and Chen, M.H. Nursing activities and acute confusional states in elderly hip-fractured patients. *Nursing research,* 28, 1, 1979:25–35.

Williams, M.A.; Campbell, E.B.; Raynor, W.J.; Musholt, M.A.; Mlynarczyk, S.M.; and Crane, L.F. Predictors of acute confusional states in hospitalized elderly. *Research in nursing and health,* 8, 1, 1985a:31–40.

Williams, M.A.; Campbell, E.B.; Raynor, W.J.; Mlynarczyk, S.M.; and Ward, S.E. Reducing acute confusional states in elderly patients with hip fractures. *Research in nursing and health,* 8, 3, 1985b:329–337.

APPENDIX A *

Standards of Psychiatric-Mental Health Nursing Practice

☐ **PROFESSIONAL PRACTICE STANDARDS**

The eleven standards statements that follow are reprinted with the permission of the American Nurses' Association. The narrative discussion which follows each standard is adapted from the accompanying discussion of rationale and criteria appropriate to structural, process, and outcome evaluation of each statement. The interested reader is encouraged to read the full document which is available from the American Nurses' Association–Division on Psychiatric and Mental Health Nursing Practice.

STANDARD I. THEORY

The Nurse Applies Appropriate Theory that is Scientifically Sound as a Basis for Decisions Regarding Nursing Practice.

* The Standards of practice are reprinted and the criteria and rationale are adapted with permission of the American Nurses' Association.

The steps of nursing process must be firmly grounded in theory and research from the nursing literature and that of the related social and biological sciences. This can be facilitated in the practice setting through maintaining a resource library and providing educational programs that focus on theoretical aspects of human behavior and related nursing implications. Nurses need to examine their beliefs about humans and use theory appropriately to improve nursing practice and quality of care.

STANDARD II. DATA COLLECTION

The Nurse Continuously Collects Data That Are Comprehensive, Accurate, And Systematic.

An accurate, comprehensive data base rests upon nursing skills of observing, interviewing, and recording. The nurse involves the client in the process of data collection for assessment of physiological and psychosocial status. This includes aspects such as client development, mentation, mood, spiritual values and beliefs, social systems and supports, life-style and coping patterns, socioeconomic factors, cultural values, health beliefs, strengths, knowledge of personal rights, and contributory data from significant others such as family and involved health care professionals. If the client's illness interferes with participation in data collection, the nurse seeks affirmation of the content and quality of the data base from the client's significant others and involved health care workers. The client record should be organized according to a standardized and systematic format to promote retrieval of pertinent data.

STANDARD III. DIAGNOSIS

The Nurse Utilizes Nursing Diagnoses and/or Standard Classification of Mental Disorders to Express Conclusions Supported by Recorded Assessment Data and Current Scientific Premises.

The nurse uses the data base and nursing judgment to diagnose actual or potential problems of the client that are within the domain of nursing practice. Validation of the problems identified should be accomplished with the client when appropriate, with the client's family, and with nursing peers. These problems may reflect limitations in the client's self-care ability based on stress; stress or crisis related to illnesses; development or self-concept changes; altered thought or perceptual processes; emotional distress; impaired communication or relatedness; and physical symptoms resulting from psychological factors. These nursing diagnoses are firmly grounded in an adequate client data base and nursing knowledge. They are subject to modification on the basis of new data as the client's status changes. Nursing diagnoses should be recorded accurately and in terms that promote nursing care planning and research activities.

STANDARD IV. PLANNING

The Nurse Develops a Nursing Care Plan with Specific Goals and Interventions Delineating Nursing Actions Unique to Each Client's Needs.

The plan of care is developed on a collaborative basis, recorded and communicated to others. It is based on appropriate participation of the client, family, and members of the interdiscipli-nary health team and is revised on an ongoing basis as needed. The plan identifies realistic goals of care with measurable outcome criteria, sets priorities, and targets dates for goal attainment. Interventions are developed around mutual goal setting and responsibility appropriate to the client's ability level and are based in theoretical rationale. Designated areas of responsibility among the health team members are identified for specific aspects of the plan of care and the plan includes guidance for actions to be performed by staff members under nursing supervision.

STANDARD V. INTERVENTION

The Nurse Intervenes as Guided by the Nursing Care Plan to Implement Nursing Actions that Promote, Maintain, or Restore Physical and Mental Health, Prevent Illness, and Effect Rehabilitation.

Nursing intervention is directed toward all aspects of health and well-being for the client. This includes mental and physical health promotion, health restoration, prevention of illness, and rehabilitation efforts following illness. The health care agency is responsible for assuring adequate nurse-client ratios to implement the standards of care. The nurse appreciates the hierarchical nature of human needs in planning interventions and serves as client advocate in situations that call for it. Interventions are validated with the client and with peers and are recorded.

STANDARD V-A. INTERVENTION: PSYCHOTHERAPEUTIC INTERVENTIONS

The Nurse Uses Psychotherapeutic Interventions to Assist Clients in Regaining or Improving their Previous Coping Abilities and to Prevent Further Disability.

The generalist nurse identifies client responses to health problems in order to reinforce healthy behavior, functional adaptation, and client strengths and to modify or eliminate dysfunctional behaviors. Skills of interviewing, communication, crisis intervention, and problem solving are used to intervene with clients in order to promote expression of feelings and processes of coping, adaptation, and growth.

STANDARD V-B. INTERVENTION: HEALTH TEACHING

The Nurse Assists Clients, Families, and Groups to Achieve Satisfying and Productive Patterns of Living through Health Teaching.

Health education of clients, families, groups, and communities is a vital role of the nurse. Various teaching strategies are used including experiential learning in the care environment in order to apply principles of teaching and learning to promote social skills and physical and mental health. Client educational approaches used and the knowledge acquired are recorded.

STANDARD V-C. INTERVENTION: ACTIVITIES OF DAILY LIVING

The Nurse Uses the Activities of Daily Living in a Goal-Directed Way to Foster Adequate Self-Care and Physical and Mental Well-Being of Clients.

The nurse uses knowledge of human growth and development and awareness of the client's ability to function on a daily basis in the tasks of living to promote behavioral changes that enhance the client's level of functioning. This requires careful appraisal and consistent intervention to promote self-care ability. The nurse respects client rights, encourages client participation in care planning, and uses limit setting in the least restrictive and most humane way possible. Self-care activities include, but are not restricted to, maintenance of basic human needs, attention to personal hygiene and grooming, appropriate behavioral control, ability to engage in brief social interactions, and identification of stressful events and reactions prior to the need for care. This awareness of client functional ability is important by the end of the acute phase of care as is the ability to monitor client progress toward goals.

Rehabilitation-phase goals include independent responsibility for self-care of physical needs, social interaction, impulse control, appropriate behavior, and use of resources to assist in coping. The client should be aware of the purpose, dose, schedule of administration, side effects, and related actions to be taken for all prescribed medications. If the client is unable to meet this goal, a parent or significant other person should be knowledgeable in this respect to assure the client's safe compliance. Severely, chronically ill clients should be assisted to participate in developing a plan to use available community supports to maintain themselves in the community.

STANDARD V-D. INTERVENTION: SOMATIC THERAPIES

The Nurse Uses Knowledge of Somatic Therapies and Applies Related Clinical Skills in Working with Clients.

The nurse uses knowledge of client rights and nursing responsibilities in addition to specific knowledge of pharmacological and somatic therapies to guide nursing actions. Observations of client responses are guided by appropriate knowledge, recorded, and evaluated in terms of treatment goals. The nurse collaborates with the physician and others to supervise the treatment regimen in terms of client safety, provides health education and opportunities for expression of feelings and concerns about somatic therapies to clients and their families, and implements the plan of care in compliance with the state nurse practice act.

STANDARD V-E. INTERVENTION: THERAPEUTIC ENVIRONMENT

The Nurse Provides, Structures, and Maintains a Therapeutic Environment in Collaboration with the Client and Other Health Care Providers.

The nurse assures a clean, safe, humane, and attractive milieu for treatment in conjunction with the agency responsible for the setting. The nurse orients the client to the setting and assesses the influence of various environmental factors on the client's functional status and behavior, collaborates to provide milieu activities pertinent to client's therapeutic goals, and uses the therapeutic potential of the environment and daily living activities to promote skill development and personal growth in clients. Any use of restraint or limits is justified in terms of client's goals and safety and discussed with client and staff including the conditions necessary to remove the restrictions. Milieu evaluation focuses on both the client's home environment and the ongoing evaluation of the health care setting.

STANDARD V-F. INTERVENTION: PSYCHOTHERAPY

The Nurse Utilizes Advanced Clinical Expertise in Individual, Group, and Family Psychotherapy, Child Psychotherapy, and Other Treatment Modalities to Function as a Psychotherapist, and Recognizes Professional Accountability for Nursing Practice.

The nurse who functions as a psychotherapist is qualified as a *specialist* in psychiatric-mental health nursing. (This requires graduate preparation and supervised practice.)

STANDARD VI. EVALUATION

The Nurse Evaluates Client Responses to Nursing Actions in Order to Revise the Database, Nursing Diagnoses, and Nursing Care Plan.

The nurse recognizes that nursing care is dynamic and subject to alterations in client status, nursing diagnoses, and subsequent interventions needed. Evaluation of care should include consultation with the client or those acting on behalf of the client as well as with peers or consultants within psychiatric-mental health nursing. Evaluation of care is recorded and nursing care plans revised on the basis of evaluation.

☐ PROFESSIONAL PERFORMANCE STANDARDS

STANDARD VII. PEER REVIEW

The Nurse Participates in Peer Review and Other Means of Evaluation to Assure Quality of Nursing Care Provided for Clients.

Nurses participate in peer review and quality assurance activities for their own professional growth and for the improvement of client care.

STANDARD VIII. CONTINUING EDUCATION

The Nurse Assumes Responsibility for Continuing Education and Professional Development and Contributes to the Professional Growth of Others.

The nurse identifies personal learning needs to order to update or increase nursing knowledge and skills by attending inservice and continuing education programs and professional workshops or meetings, and by assisting in promoting the learning needs of other nurses through informal and formal modes of communication.

STANDARD IX. INTERDISCIPLINARY COLLABORATION

The Nurse Collaborates with Other Health Care Providers in Assessing, Planning, Implementing, and Evaluating Programs and Other Mental Health Activities.

Interdisciplinary collaboration is used to plan and implement quality mental health care to clients. Nursing participates along with the client and health team in problem solving and decision making in the clinical setting as well as in activities such as teaching, supervision, and research.

STANDARD X. UTILIZATION OF COMMUNITY HEALTH SYSTEMS

The Nurse Participates with Other Members of the Community in Assessing, Planning, Implementing, and Evaluating Mental Health Services and Community Systems that Include the Promotion of the Broad Continuum of Primary, Secondary, and Tertiary Prevention of Mental Illness.

The nurse who plans and evaluates psychiatric and mental health services or programs in community health systems is qualified as a *specialist* in psychiatric-mental health nursing.

STANDARD XI. RESEARCH

The Nurse Contributes to Nursing and the Mental Health Field Through Innovations in Theory and Practice and Participation in Research.

All nurses are responsible for the development of nursing knowledge in the psychiatric-mental health field. The generalist nurse can assure the protection of rights of subjects, approach practice with an open mind, and utilize research findings in practice. Participation in research studies is determined by level of education.

APPENDIX B

*DSM-III Diagnostic Classification Categories**

The *Diagnostic and Statistical Manual* of the American Psychiatric Association (3d edition) was published in 1980 to provide approved diagnostic terms and numerical codings for classification. Five axes are included for the evaluation of any client. Axes one and two refer to psychiatric conditions, syndromes, or disorders. These diagnostic classifications are listed below. Axis three pertains to physical diagnoses or conditions. Axes four and five provide a means of rating contributing stressors and highest level of patient functioning achieved over the past year. The numerical codes, criteria for diagnosis, and other vital information are not reprinted here, and the interested reader is referred to the manual itself. (See also related content in this text.)

Disorders Usually First Evident in Infancy, Childhood, or Adolescence

☐ Intellectual
　　Mental retardation (mild, moderate, severe, profound)

* Reprinted with the permission of the American Psychiatric Association from the *Diagnostic and Statistical Manual of Mental Disorders*. 3d ed., © 1980.

☐ Behavioral
　　Attention deficit disorder
　　　　With hyperactivity
　　　　Without hyperactivity
　　　　Residual type
　　Conduct disorder
　　　　Undersocialized aggressive
　　　　Undersocialized nonaggressive
　　　　Socialized aggressive
　　　　Socialized nonaggressive
　　　　Atypical
☐ Emotional
　　Anxiety disorders of childhood or adolescence
　　　　Separation anxiety disorder
　　　　Avoidant disorder of childhood or adolescence
　　　　Overanxious disorder
　　Other disorders of infancy, childhood, and adolescence
　　　　Reactive attachment disorder of infancy
　　　　Schizoid disorder of childhood or adolescence

Elective mutism

Oppositional disorder

Identity disorder

☐ Physical

Eating disorders

Anorexia nervosa

Bulimia

Pica

Rumination disorder of infancy

Atypical eating disorder

Stereotyped movement disorders

Transient tic disorder

Chronic motor tic disorder

Tourette's disorder

Atypical tic disorder

Atypical stereotyped movement disorder

☐ Other

Stuttering

Functional enuresis

Functional encopresis

Sleepwalking disorder

Sleep terror disorder

☐ Developmental

Pervasive developmental disorders

Infantile autism

Infantile autism, residual state

Childhood onset, pervasive developmental disorder

Childhood onset, pervasive developmental residual state

Atypical pervasive developmental disorder

Specific developmental disorders

Developmental reading disorder

Developmental arithmetic disorder

Developmental language disorder, receptive type

Developmental articulation disorder

Mixed specific developmental disorder

Atypical specific developmental disorder

Organic Mental Disorders

☐ Organic mental disorders arising in the senium and presenium. Primary degenerative dementia (note senile or presenile onset)

With delirium

With delusions

With depression

Uncomplicated

Multi infarct dementia

☐ Substance induced

Alcohol

Intoxication

Idiosyncratic intoxication

Withdrawal

Withdrawal delirium

Hallucinosis

Amnestic disorder

Dementia associated with alcoholism

Barbiturate or similarly acting sedative hypnotic

Intoxication

Withdrawal

Withdrawal delirium

Amnestic disorder

Opioid

Intoxication

Withdrawal

Cocaine

Intoxication

Amphetamine or similarly acting sympathomimetic

Intoxication

Delirium

Delusional disorder

Withdrawal

Phencyclidine (PCP) or similarly acting (e.g., TCP)

Intoxication

Delirium

Mixed

Hallucinogen

Hallucinosis

Delusional disorder

Affective disorder

Cannabis

Intoxication

Delusional disorder

Tobacco

Withdrawal

Caffeine
  Intoxication
Other/unspecified substance
  Intoxication
  Withdrawal
  Delirium
  Dementia
  Amnestic disorder
  Hallucinosis
  Delusional disorder
  Affective disorder
  Personality disorder
  Atypical or mixed disorder

Organic Brain Syndromes

(Etiology unknown or outside the mental disorders section of ICD-9)
  ☐ Delirium
  ☐ Dementia
  ☐ Amnestic syndrome
  ☐ Organic delusional syndrome
  ☐ Organic hallucinosis
  ☐ Organic affective syndrome
  ☐ Organic personality syndrome
  ☐ Atypical or mixed organic brain syndrome

Substance Use Disorders

☐ Substance abuse or dependence
  Alcohol
    Abuse
    Dependence
  Barbiturate or similarly acting sedative-hypnotic
    Abuse
    Dependence
  Opioid
    Abuse
    Dependence
  Cocaine abuse
  Amphetamine or similarly acting sympathomimetic
    Abuse
    Dependence
  Phencyclidine (PCP) abuse
  Hallucinogen abuse
  Cannabis
    Abuse
    Dependence

Tobacco dependence
Other–mixed or unspecified
Combined dependence

Schizophrenic disorders

☐ Schizophrenia
    Disorganized
    Catatonic
    Paranoid
    Undifferentiated
    Residual

Paranoid Disorders

☐ Paranoia
☐ Shared paranoid disorder
☐ Acute paranoid disorder
☐ Atypical paranoid disorder

Psychotic Disorders not Elsewhere Classified

☐ Schizophreniform disorder
☐ Brief reactive psychosis
☐ Schizoaffective disorder
☐ Atypical psychosis

Affective Disorders

☐ Major affective disorders
    Bipolar disorder
      Mixed
      Manic
      Depressed
    Major depression
      Single episode
      Recurrent
    Cyclothymic disorder
    Dysthymic disorder (or depressive neurosis)
☐ Atypical affective disorders
    Atypical bipolar disorder
    Atypical depression

Anxiety Disorders

☐ Phobic disorders (or phobic neuroses)
    Agoraphobia
      With panic attacks
      Without panic attacks

Social phobia

Simple phobia

☐ Anxiety states (or anxiety neuroses)

Panic disorder

Generalized anxiety disorder

Obsessive compulsive disorder (or neurosis)

Post-traumatic stress disorder

Acute

Chronic

Delayed

Somatoform Disorders

☐ Somatization disorder

☐ Conversion disorder (hysterical neurosis, conversion type)

☐ Psychogenic pain disorder

☐ Hypochondriasis (or hypochondriacal neurosis)

☐ Atypical somatiform disorder

Dissociative Disorders or Hysterical Neuroses–Dissociative Type

☐ Psychogenic amnesia

☐ Psychogenic fugue

☐ Multiple personality

☐ Depersonalization disorder

☐ Atypical dissociative disorder

Psychosexual Disorders

☐ Gender identity disorders

Transsexualism

Gender identity disorder of childhood

Atypical gender identity disorder

☐ Paraphilias

Fetishism

Transvestism

Zoophilia

Pedophilia

Exhibitionism

Voyeurism

Sexual masochism

Sexual sadism

Atypical paraphilia

☐ Psychosexual dysfunctions

Inhibited sexual desire

Inhibited sexual excitement

Inhibited female orgasm

Inhibited male orgasm

Premature ejaculation

Functional dyspareunia

Functional vaginismus

Atypical psychosexual dysfunction

☐ Other psychosexual disorders

Ego-dystonic homosexuality

Psychosexual disorder not classified elsewhere

Factitious Disorders

☐ Factitious disorders with psychological symptoms

☐ Factitious disorders with physical symptoms

☐ Chronic factitious disorders with physical symptoms

☐ Atypical factitious disorder

Disorders of Impulse Control Not Elsewhere Classified

☐ Pathological gambling

☐ Kleptomania

☐ Pyromania

☐ Intermittent explosive disorder

☐ Isolated explosive disorder

☐ Atypical impulse control disorder

Adjustment Disorder

☐ With depressed mood

☐ With anxious mood

☐ With mixed emotional features

☐ With disturbance of conduct

☐ With mixed disturbance of emotions and conduct

☐ With work inhibition

☐ With academic inhibition

☐ With withdrawal

☐ With atypical features

Psychological Factors Affecting Physical Condition

Personality Disorders

- ☐ Paranoid
- ☐ Schizoid
- ☐ Schizotypal
- ☐ Histrionic
- ☐ Narcissistic
- ☐ Antisocial
- ☐ Borderline
- ☐ Avoidant
- ☐ Dependent
- ☐ Compulsive
- ☐ Passive-aggressive
- ☐ Atypical
- ☐ Mixed
- ☐ Other

Conditions Not Attributable to Mental Disorder that are a Focus of Attention or Treatment

- ☐ Malingering
- ☐ Borderline intellectual functioning
- ☐ Adult antisocial behavior
- ☐ Child or adolescent antisocial behavior
- ☐ Academic problem
- ☐ Occupational problem
- ☐ Uncomplicated bereavement
- ☐ Noncompliance with medical treatment
- ☐ Phase of life or other life circumstance problem
- ☐ Marital problem
- ☐ Parent-child problem
- ☐ Other (specify) family circumstances
- ☐ Other interpersonal problem

Glossary

Abandonment–The act of physically or emotionally leaving someone (usually a child) to manage for himself without the support or guidance of a caring adult.

Abuse–To injure another human being (e.g., child, spouse, mate, elderly person) physically, verbally, or emotionally.

Abuser profile–A short outline describing the behaviors of an abusive person that helps to identify the severity of a situation during a crisis assessment.

Acting out–Behaviors that discharge (unconsciously) inner tensions by displacing behavioral responses from one situation to another; may result from transference.

Active listening–Process of focusing one's attention on the verbal and nonverbal components of another's message, paraphrasing it for validation, and summarizing the content and feeling conveyed.

Adaptation–An organism's response to its environment.

Adolescence–A period of growth in which the ego responds to the physiological, cognitive, and emotional demands placed on it in an attempt to develop a clear, coherent sense of self capable of meeting the challenges of adulthood.

Adult protective services–A branch of public welfare which responds to reports of abuse of adults and the elderly. This service offers counseling to the family and makes appropriate referrals in crisis situations.

Advice giving–A barrier to a therapeutic relationship in which the nurse decides upon the client's goals for him and does not give the client choices or responsibility for his own behavior.

Affect–Feeling tone or mood.

Aggression–Offensive behavior that may be physical or verbal.

Akathisia–Motor restlessness and need to keep moving, an extrapyramidal side effect of antipsychotic drug therapy.

Alexithymia–A condition characterized by a marked difficulty in expressing feelings in words or in fantasies.

891

Alienation–Withdrawal or detachment from one's society.

Alternative nuclear family forms–A fundamental grouping of people, other than the traditional parent-child family, consisting of one or more generations who live together in order to achieve common social goals.

Alzheimer's disease–An organic mental disorder characterized by a progressive deterioration in mental and psychological functions.

Ambivalence–Simultaneous but opposite emotions directed toward a person or object.

Amnesia–Inability to recall important personal information; may be localized, selective, generalized, or continuous.

Anaclitic depression–A withdrawn and apathetic emotional state found in infants who have been institutionalized and/or deprived in some way of consistent, loving care.

Anorexia nervosa–Eating disorder characterized by starvation.

Anticipatory grief–Grief work that is done prior to the actual death; it usually occurs following the news of a terminal illness.

Anticipatory planning/guidance–That part of crisis intervention in which the focus is the solidification of changes made by the client to reinforce growth. Also a preventive measure for potential crisis events which focuses on planning alternative coping strategies for anticipated problems.

Antisocial personality–A personality disorder wherein the person exhibits behaviors and attitudes that persistently disregard the feelings/rights of others; also known in the past as sociopathic or psychopathic personality.

Anxiety–A nonspecific feeling of dread accompanied by symptoms of physiological stress such as rapid heart rate, difficult breathing, nausea, tremors, and muscle tension. Similar to fear, but anxiety lacks a specific object causing the perception of threat.

Assertiveness–Behavior that allows a person to express honest feelings comfortably, to be direct and straightforward, and to exercise personal rights without denying the rights of others and without experiencing undue anxiety of guilt.

Attachment–An interactive process of bonding, initially occurring between infant and parent and forming the basis for lifetime attachments.

Attention deficit disorder–A disorder of childhood characterized by inattention and impulsive behavior which is not appropriate to expected level of development; formerly referred to as hyperactivity or minimal brain dysfunction.

Attitude–An opinion, disposition, or mental set toward a particular idea, concept, person, or object.

Autism–Highly subjective thought processes such as fantasies, daydreams, delusions, or hallucinations which originate from the internal and generally unconscious self; an emotional disorder of infancy and childhood in which there are serious impairments of communication, relationship, motor expression and development (infantile autism).

Autoeroticism (masturbation)–Self-stimulation of the genitalia for sexual gratification.

Autonomy–A developmental task of Erik Erikson's theory in which the child (approximately 18 months to 3 years) is concerned with achieving a sense of independence and separateness from the mother or primary caretaker; failure to achieve this task leads to self-doubt.

Aversion therapy–A behavioral technique in which undesirable behavior is paired with a painful stimulus in order to suppress the undesirable behavior (e.g., administering emetics or electroshocks with alcohol ingestion to treat alcoholism).

Aware–Knowing or realizing; conscious of.

Belief–An idea, issue, concept that the person accepts as true.

Blaming–A communication pattern in the family in which an individual changes the situation by increasing tension (temporarily) to force other family members into submission.

Blended or reconstituted family–A two-generational family resulting from the joining of two adults and the children of one or both of them.

Blunted affect–Dulling of intensity of feeling.

Borderline personality–Personality disorder characterized by an inability to develop appropriate object relationships and the use of defense mechanisms (projection, splitting, devaluation, and idealization) when confronted with anxiety from perceived/real changes in relationships.

Briquet's syndrome–*See* somatization disorder.

Bulimia–Eating disorder characterized by episodes of bingeing and purging (through vomiting, laxatives, diuretics, and fasting).

Burnout–Emotional and mental exhaustion in professionals; for example, the nurse exhibits loss of concern for the client, dehumanizing of clients, negativism, derogatory labeling, griping, and complaining.

Care-eliciting behaviors–Behaviors that cause responses of attachment and care giving; for example, when an infant cries, he elicits the love and care of the parent.

Categorical imperative–Kant's principle that all persons must be respected as rational creatures.

Clarify–To make or become easier to understand.

Cognitive deprivation–Lack of reasonable and understandable feedback and structure in the child's environment which prevents the child from understanding the environment and himself.

Coitus–Vaginal-penile intercourse.

Commune–A group of people with intertwining types of relationships who choose to live together in one household or closely adjoining structures; a sense of commitment to the others in the group exists.

Compulsion–Persistent, ritualized behavior that a person performs according to a personal set of rules or stereotypes; the person feels compelled or forced to carry out this activity, although he may wish to avoid it.

Computing–A communication pattern in the family in which an individual attempts to use logic and reasoning to handle all problems, rejecting the importance of feelings.

Conduct disorders–Behavioral disorder of children and adolescents characterized by repetitive and persistent patterns of behavior incongruent with societal or age-appropriate norms.

Confabulation–Filling gaps of memory loss by fabrication of details.

Confidant–A person with whom self-disclosures are made and are reciprocated in an atmosphere of trust.

Confrontation–Positively viewed, confrontation means objectively pointing out incongruencies or sources of confusion in the client's verbal or nonverbal behavior; misused confrontation may be a guise for venting anger at a client.

Congruence–Communication of unity, or similar messages in one's verbal and nonverbal behavior.

Consequentialism–Ethical focus on the consequences of an act in judging rightness or wrongness of the act itself.

Conversion–A defense mechanism used unconsciously, in which the person converts an emotional conflict or need into a physical symptom.

Conversion disorder–A somatoform disorder characterized by disturbances of motor or sensory activity which are psychogenic in origin.

Conversion reaction–Outdated term for conversion disorder.

Coping–An organism's response to its environment.

Counterphobic–Seeking out situations that are or were previously feared and avoided phobically.

Countertransference–An emotional response of the nurse in which anger, irritation, sadness, or withdrawal is usually experienced toward the client; the nurse experiences these irrational responses toward the client based on people in her own life; this initially is unconscious but the nurse must strive to examine the meaning of such feelings, become aware of the countertransference, and eliminate it.

Crisis–A temporary state in which a threat is felt and the individual's usual problem-solving methods fail; the resulting disequilibrium is transient (approximately 6 weeks) and can be a stimulus for growth.

Crisis intervention–Treatment that is focused on resolving immediate problems, assuming health and normal adjustment of the client prior to the crisis event.

Cunnilingus–Using the mouth and lips to lick or suck a woman's clitoris, labia, vulva, and introitus.

Cycle of Violence–Abused children often become abusive to their parents, to their spouses, and/or to their elderly parents (and original role models) later in life.

Defense mechanism–Mental maneuver that unconsciously or subconsciously serves to protect the person from threatening impulses or feelings (e.g., rationalization, sublimation, denial, projection).

Delirium–Broad syndrome of disturbances in sensation, perception, memory, thought, and judgment; acute rapid onset and brief duration.

Delusions–Fixed false beliefs (not culturally based) which are not amenable to reason or proofs.

> **Grandiose**–Characterized by excessive ideas of self-importance (e.g. "I am the redeemer").
>
> **Nihilistic**–The belief that parts of the self or external world do not exist.
>
> **Persecutory**–Characterized by the belief that others are plotting against one.

Dementia–Progressive loss of cognitive and other higher intellectual functions as a result of organic brain disease; slow, insidious onset.

Deontology(also called formalism)–An ethical perspective focusing on duties and obligations derived from rules and principles such as autonomy, beneficence (doing good), nonmalificence (not doing harm), and justice.

Dependence(e.g., on drugs or alcohol)–Includes psychological and/or physiological craving and the development of tolerance; greater amounts are required for desired effects and/ or withdrawal (physical) symptoms occur when use of the substance is stopped or severely decreased.

Depersonalization–Episode in which feelings of unreality, estrangement, and separateness from one's self and one's actions occur.

Derealization–A situation in which the person experiences a sense of unreality of the environment.

Desensitization–Exposure of a phobic person to a predetermined list of anxiety-provoking situations which are on a continuum from least to most severe. Relaxation techniques are used at each level to decrease and eliminate the anxiety response.

Desexualization–The result of attitudes, beliefs, and behaviors that are insensitive to or deny the complexity and reality of human sexuality; desexualization often occurs in health care settings.

Detoxification–The time period in treatment of substance abuse problems in which the client is supervised and supported though the process of becoming free of the abused substance and any withdrawal symptoms associated with being drug or alcohol free; this may vary from 2 days to 2 weeks and may be accomplished in either a medical or nonmedical setting; medical settings are preferred if serious withdrawal symptoms such as delirium tremens or seizures are anticipated.

Developmental (maturational) crisis–Expected, internally generated crisis occurring in response to a stress that is related to growth problems encountered in moving from one stage of development to the next.

Developmental task–Usually, the typical "work" of a particular stage of development. For example, school work/performance is what a schoolage child is struggling to master, while a young adult is facing work/marriage/ childbearing decisions and responsibilities.

Disassociation–An unconscious defense mechanism used to control or block out anxiety from feelings that threaten the person's sense of self.

Disengagement–A gradual, emotional process in which a person moves away from a relationship or situation in which he had invested significant emotional energy.

Distracting–A communication pattern used by a family member to avoid conflict by shifting the focus from the immediate problem to something that is irrelevant.

Double bind–Two conflicting communications from someone seen as essential to another person; often one message is verbal while the other is nonverbal.

Dysfunctional grief–Grief that does not follow the normal course; examples are delayed grief and absence of grief; may also be termed morbid, pathological, or complicated grief.

Dystonia–Acute, involuntary contractures of skeletal muscles induced by neuroleptic drug therapy; varies from tics and difficulty swallowing through spasms of major muscle groups (e.g., oculogyric crisis, trunk flexion).

Echolalia–Pathological repetition or parroting of another's speech.

Ego–The abstract mental structure which mediates between the person and reality and between the demands of the instinctual drives and the social conscience; ego functions include those of perception, reality testing, action, secondary process thought, and synthesis of thinking and emotion.

Ego states–The Parent, Adult, and Child are mental contructs of Transactional Analysis.

Egodystonic–Thoughts, attitudes, and behaviors that disrupt the individual's identity or sense of self.

Egosyntonic–Thoughts, attitudes, and behaviors that are congruent with an individual's identity or sense of self.

Empathy–Process whereby one person perceives and experiences the current feelings and experiences of another person from the perspective of the other.

Encopresis–An emotional disorder of childhood in which the child repeatedly soils his pants with feces past the age when fecal continence would be expected; primary encopresis occurs from lack of any toilet training; secondary encopresis is a stress symptom occurring after inadequate or inconsistent training; reflective of environmental changes or conflict.

Enuresis–An emotional disorder of childhood, also known as bedwetting, in which a child experiences urinary incontinence past the age (3) when toilet training would be expected; primary enuresis results from lack of any training, while secondary enuresis occurs after bladder control has been achieved.

Erectile dysfunction–The inability to achieve an erection firm enough to accomplish vaginal intromission, or to maintain one long enough to achieve orgasm.

> **Primary**–A serious condition in which a man has never been able to maintain an erection to orgasm.
>
> **Secondary**–A condition in which a man who has been able to maintain erections in the past can no longer do so; may have physiological, psychological, or situational causes.

Exhibitionism–A repeated and preferred method of obtaining sexual gratification by exposing the genitals to unsuspecting and unwilling victims.

Exploitation (of own age or disability)–Refers to the use of one's advanced years or problems to gain special favors or dispensations.

> **Of others**–Using a child (or another adult) to fulfill unconscious or conscious desires in a way that is detrimental to his growth and development.

Extended family–Multigenerational family which includes all relatives by marriage, birth, or adoption into the nuclear family.

External crisis–*See* situational crisis.

Family Boundaries–The lines or limits that specify the members of a family and the roles the members will take; boundaries may be rigid (closed, allowing no interaction with others outside of the family), diffuse (lacking clarity, with relationships that are overly involved or dependent), or clear (allowing for open, honest communication while promoting individual identity).

Family crisis counseling–Therapy involving the entire family and its response to the crisis event.

Family myths–A series of well-integrated beliefs, shared by all family members, concerning characteristics and positions of each person in the family that go unchallenged in spite of reality distortions.

Family roles–The "part to play" for each family member to ensure that the family functions in its typical manner; the role is a pattern of behavior or sequence of acts directed toward a goal.

Family rules–The limits that define what roles family members will play within the family; rules are overt (clearly defined and readily apparent) or covert (not stated or poorly defined).

Family system–A group of interrelated people or "parts" which interact and form a family; the family system contains subsystems and is also a subsystem of the community.

Family themes–Expectations of how the family is to function that perpetuate both positive and negative aspects of the family's interactions.

Family therapy–Therapy that is focused on the family as the client rather than the individual; all or most of the family members will be treated as a group.

Fellatio–The act of stimulating the penis and scrotal area with the lips, tongue, or mouth.

Fetishism–A condition in which the use of nonliving objects (fetishes) is a repeatedly preferred or exclusive method of achieving sexual excitement; fetishes are not limited to articles of female clothing used in crossdressing or to objects designed to be used for the purpose of sexual stimulation (e.g., vibrator).

Fictitious–Not genuine, real, or natural.

Flashbacks–A reexperiencing of an event or situation, usually of significant emotional content, in which the person may see, hear, or feel the same sensations of that past event; the person is conscious and remembers having the experience after it is over.

Flat affect–Markedly dull or blunted emotional tone.

Fugue–Traveling around aimlessly without recall of personal identity or information.

Gay household–A family that is constructed of two or more homosexual individuals with or without children.

Gender role–Everything that one says and does, including sexual arousal, to indicate to others or to the self the degree to which one is male or female.

Generic crisis intervention–An approach based on the belief that there are common psychological tasks and problem-solving behaviors that must be achieved to resolve a crisis; the focus is on these rather than on the individual and his response.

Grief–A characteristic response to the loss of a valued object, be it person, body part, possession, job status, or ideal.

Grief response–The process by which an individual begins to adjust to the loss of something or someone important to him.

Grief work–Readjustment to loss that involves emancipation from the deceased, readjustment to the environment, and the formation of new relationships.

Hallucination–A sensory perception that occurs in the absence of a real sensory stimulus (hearing voices when no one is speaking).

Histrionic–A trait characterized by overly dramatic, colorful, intensely reactional, and excitable behavior.

Histrionic personality disorder–An inflexible life pattern in which the person melodramatically seeks attention and responds intensely to stimuli, seemingly craves excitement, and focuses attention on self.

Homeostasis–A concept related to an individual's or a system's efforts to adapt in response to stress in order to keep tension low and maintain functioning.

Homosexuality–Sexual life-style in which a person prefers, or exclusively requires, sexual interactions with someone of the same sex; homosexuality is considered a psychiatric disorder (DSM III) only if it is ego dystonic, that is, a source of distress for the client.

Hospice–Philosophy of care or programs designed to relieve the physical and emotional suffering of terminally ill clients.

Hyperactivity–Excessive or unusual amounts of activity.

Hyperkinesis–Excessive amounts of movement.

Hypochondriasis–A preoccupation with the fear or belief of having a serious illness and interpretation of all physical signs and symptoms as abnormal; the physical disease is not present, but another disease may be present (e.g., a person with an ulcer may believe it is cancer).

Hysteria–An outdated, Freudian term for the loss of or alienation in a physical function due to an emotional conflict; *see* conversion disorder.

Hysterical neurosis–Same as hysteria, now known as conversion disorder.

Id–The abstract mental structure, as described by psychoanalytic psychology, which represents unconscious drives and impulses; it is characterized by primary process thought.

Idealization–A process by which all negative feelings regarding a deceased person are buried, leaving only positive thoughts; also the transfer of an excessive amount of psychic energy to a love object which is then overvalued.

Ideas of reference–The erroneous belief that external events relate to the individual, for example a person may believe (based on his own insecurity and suspiciousness) that a group of people laughing across the room are laughing at him or that TV programs are specifically addressed to him on a personal meaning level.

Illusions–Misinterpretation of actual sensory stimuli (e.g., the wind blowing is "the presence of spirits").

Inappropriate affect–Response to an event, situation, or interaction that is inconsistent with the stimulus.

Individual crisis intervention–Focus of the intervention is on the individual and his unique response to a crisis event.

Industry–The developmental task of the child of 6 through 12 years, according to Erik Erikson, in which the child rapidly develops motor coordination, greater independence, and exploration of the world around him; the child's sense of self-worth is increased and grows at this time; failure to achieve industry results in feelings of inferiority.

Inhibited sexual desire–Persistent and pervasive inhibition of sexual desire.

Initiative–A developmental task in which, according to Erik Erikson, the preschool child begins to become more aware of feelings and values of others and begins to develop a conscience and value system; failure to achieve this task results in feelings of guilt.

Insight–Ability to perceive self and problems realistically.

Intellectualization–A defense mechanism used to protect the self from painful emotions; the person may analyze situations or offer facts and information, but exhibits little or no emotional tone or affect.

Internal crisis–*See* developmental crisis.

Intoxication–A state of mental impairment resulting from excess intake of alcohol or other mood-altering substance; technically, an acute organic brain syndrome secondary to alcohol or drug ingestion.

Introductory phase–The second stage (after preinteraction phase) of the one-to-one relationship in which nurse and client begin face-to-face interaction; a contract is set with the client, and assessment and identification of problems begins with the client; this phase varies in length until the client trusts the nurse and enters the middle or working phase.

Joint custody–An arrangement between divorced parents in which the child or children live part of the week with one parent and the remainder with the other parent.

Judge–To form an idea, opinion, or estimate about any matter; to criticize or censure.

Kleptomania–A recurring irresistible urge to steal items that are not useful or monetarily valuable; tension increases before the act and relief or pleasure is experienced.

La belle indifference–A French term for the frequently observed attitude of seeming indifference about loss or alteration in physical functioning due to conversion disorder.

Labeling–A barrier to a therapeutic relationship in which the client is dehumanized by viewing him as a diagnosis ("he's a schizophrenic") or by describing him in slang or jargon (e.g., a turkey or manipulator).

Labile affect–mood abruptly, rapidly, and repeatedly changes for no apparent reason.

Latch key children–Those children who are alone at home for several hours after school dismissal.

Libido–The Freudian term for the "life force" which is found in every individual including drives for hunger, thirst, and sex.

Life structure–Daniel Levinson coined this term to describe his concept of a person's life pattern or design based on some present and past life decisions; this life structure is constructed, stabilized, then modified or changed drastically over the adult years.

Loose associations–Abrupt shifts and disruptions in train of thought manifested in disconnected speech.

Maintenance role–Behaviors as a group member which serve to foster group cohesiveness and caring.

Mania–Pathological condition characterized by an expansive emotional state of extreme excitement; hyperactivity; agitated, pressured speech; flight of ideas; fleeting ideas; increased psychomotor activity, and sometimes violent behavior.

Manipulation–Behavior that is designed to influence or control situations so that one's needs are met. All persons use manipulation to some extent; examples of negative forms of manipulation include flattery, threats, verbal abuse, feigned helplessness, provocative behavior, pitting clients and staff against each other, breaking rules, and starting rumors.

Marasmus–A generalized listlessness that includes physical wasting and illness; not due to organic illness. Occurs in infants who are part of a severely disturbed mother-infant relationship.

Material abuse–The use of another person's income or property without permission.

Maturational crisis–*See* developmental crisis.

Middle (working) phase–In this phase of the one-to-one relationship, both client and nurse have developed rapport and work to identify goals collaboratively; problem solving, experimenting with new behaviors, and more effective communication on the client's part are seen in this phase, which lasts until the nurse and client begin to terminate it.

Milieu–French term for environment.

Milieu therapy–An ideology based on social learning theory involving the deliberate planning and structuring of the client's environment in an attempt to modify maladaptive behavioral responses while promoting positive insights and responses.

Minimal brain dysfunction–A term sometimes used to describe a complex of behaviors such as inattention, impulsivity, hyperactivity, and often, learning disabilities; sometimes used interchangeably with the term attention deficit disorder.

Mutism–Absence of speech; may be physically capable of speaking (elective mutism).

Narcissism–Love of the idealized self.

Narcissistic personality disorder–An inflexible life pattern in which the person holds a grandiose and overinflated view of personal achievements or talents and demands constant admiration and attention to himself.

Negative reinforcement–The removal of an undesirable stimulus or condition as a reward following a behavioral response.

Negativism–An attitude usually found in toddlers (but often in adults) who are struggling to be independent and to remain in control; the attitude is characterized by lack of cooperation and refusal to consider ideas or alternatives even though they might be helpful or pleasant.

Neglect–A disorder in the parent-child relationship wherein the parent fails to endow the child with personal value; neglect is a subjective situation but denial of food, shelter, and clothing is obvious neglect.

Neologism–Words created by a person which have meaning only to that person.

Nuclear dyad–A married woman and man without children.

Nuclear family–Traditionally defined as two-generational, consisting of two parents (male and female) with their children by birth or adoption.

Nurse patient/client relationship–Also the one-to-one or therapeutic relationship; a process of communication and relationship building designed to identify the client's values, needs, and goals and to engage in planning actions to meet those goals.

Objectivity–The quality of being without bias or prejudice.

Omnipotence–The belief that one is better able to solve another's problems, or always has the "right answer" for someone else.

Omniscience–The belief that one knows more about a person's thoughts or feelings than he himself knows.

Oppositional disorder of childhood–Negative, uncooperative, and self-defeating behavior pattern.

Organic mental disorder–Newer terminology for organic brain syndrome; psychobehavioral disturbances due to temporary or permanent brain dysfunction.

Orgasmic dysfunction–The inability of a woman to reach orgasm; may have a physiological cause, but usually has a psychological cause; often reversible with learning through self-exploration or by a caring, gentle, skilled partner.

Overidentification–A process in which the nurse views the client's problems and feelings as being like her own and loses the ability to view the client as a separate individual.

Panic–A state in which a person feels tremendous fear or terror; physical feelings such as a sense of choking, trembling, a racing heart, and a feeling as though he is "out of control" or "falling apart"; during panic states the person's awareness and perception are severely impaired.

Paradox–An interaction with two conflicting messages.

Paranoia–A chronic type of paranoid disorder in which the person believes he is somehow being persecuted; this persecutory delusion is fixed and of a thematic nature for at least 6 weeks; no hallucinations are present.

Paranoid–A term used to describe behavior that is hyperalert, suspicious, guarded, and secretive, or wherein a person sees hidden meanings and motives in another's behavior.

Paranoid disorder–A state, lasting at least 1 week, in which the person believes he is being persecuted.

Paranoid personality disorder–An inflexible life pattern in which the person is always distrustful and suspicious, guarded and secretive, and hypersensitive to other's behavior.

Paraphilia–A sexual behavior preference that relies upon unusual, atypical experiences or fantasies for sexual gratification; paraphilias may center around an inappropriate object (child, animal, leather gloves) or particular act (inflicting or receiving pain).

Paternalism–Governing others as a father does his children, making decisions for their welfare rather than permitting them to decide for themselves.

Pavor Nocturnus–Sleep terror disorder; abrupt awakening from sleep preceded by a piercing scream 30 minutes to 3-½ hours after onset of sleep; episodes last 1–10 minutes with associated symptoms of anxiety, agitation, perspiration, and hyperventilation.

Permission giving–A basic level of intervention in the area of sexuality wherein the nurse simply lets the client know both verbally and nonverbally that sexuality is an acceptable topic of concern.

Perseveration–Involuntary repetition of the response to a previous question when introduced to a new question; also, repetition of an activity or inability to shift from one activity to a new one.

Personal comfort level–A multifaceted characteristic determined by self-awareness, accurate information, effective communication skill, acknowledgment, and acceptance of personal and professional limitations and of the rights of clients (e.g., for sexual health care).

Pervasive developmental disorder–A state in which multiple developmental areas in a child are affected, such as language, reality testing, social skills, and motor development.

Phobia–An irrational fear of a person, object, or situation which causes an individual to use any method possible to avoid such persons, objects, or situations.

Pica–Consumption of non-nutritive substance such as dirt, clay, sand, hair, paint chips, and bugs.

Preinteraction phase–The initial stage of the one-to-one relationship in which the nurse assesses available information about the client and her own thoughts, feelings, and behaviors in regard to the client.

Premature ejaculation–A condition wherein ejaculation occurs before the individual wishes it because of recurrent and persistent absence of reasonable voluntary control of ejaculation and orgasm during sexual activity.

Projection–Unconscious attempt to put onto others or the environment what the individual perceives as unacceptable or bad in the self.

Pseudohostility–A state of chronic conflict and alienation among family members which is effectively denied through minimization.

Pseudomutuality–A condition of false closeness within a family.

Psychogenic–Originating in the mind.

Psychological factors affecting physical condition–DSM III classification for any physical condition in which psychological factors are significant in the initiation or exacerbation of an illness, or as a reaction to it.

Psychopath–An outdated term for a person with antisocial personality disorder.

Psychophysiologic–Physical symptoms caused by emotional factors.

Psychosocial assessment–The process involving gathering information from and about the individual and comparing these data to some standards or norms of psychosocial development; briefly, an assessment is a judgment of one's emotional needs and resources as an individual, and within a family and a community.

Psychosocial crisis–Intense emotional dilemmas between two opposing personality characteristics; for example, an infant's psychosocial crisis is trust vs. mistrust—the infant struggles with trusting and its consequences and mistrusting and its consequences. Erikson's stages are based on psychosocial crises.

Psychosocial stages–Stages constructed by several theorists (Erikson, Buhler) that are based on psycho (internal) and social (external) forces prompting one toward further growth and development.

Psychosomatic–Constant interaction of the mind (*psyche*) and body (*soma*).

Pyromania–A recurring irresistible urge to set fires in which tension mounts before setting the fire and is relieved after the fire is set.

Rapport–A sense of emotional harmony, which includes mutual trust and understanding, that develops between two people.

Reactive attachment disorder–Often known as nonorganic failure to thrive, this disorder is seen in infants, and is characterized by lack of social responsiveness, smiling, reciprocal gazing, and visual tracking; physical characteristics include weak cry, poor muscle tone, weak rooting response, and low activity level unrelated to organic factors.

Reality testing–Ability to understand a situation, the variety of actions that one could perform in a particular situation, and the consequences of the actions.

Reciprocal gazing–A behavior seen in early infancy in which the infant looks at the person looking and/or speaking to him; this is a social behavior that contributes to the bonding/attachment process.

Reciprocal inhibition—A treatment technique in which anxiety-provoking situations are paired with pleasant stimuli which may decrease the anxiety (e.g., biofeedback, meditation, relaxation).

Reframing—Consciously perceiving an event or a situation in a different way from the way in which it was originally perceived.

Repression—An unconscious mechanism, used as a defense, in which painful feelings such as anger, sadness, and fear are not allowed into consciousness because the person fears what might happen if these feelings are expressed.

Respite care—Care that relieves another of his demanding care-giving role for a short period of time.

Review statement—A therapeutic communication approach that assumes that the client already has some information, and whose purpose is to bring that information to the client's awareness; for example, "As you know, the cervix sits at the opening of the vagina and expands when the baby is ready to be born."

Rites of passage—Arnold Gennep's term for rituals surrounding universal events that signify important transitions throughout a life span.

Role—A set of behavioral norms and expectations applied to the occupant of a particular status (position) in society.

> **Achieved role**—A role developed over time through competition and individual effort; an achieved role is earned and can be controlled (e.g., parent, nurse, professor).

> **Ascribed role**—A role over which an individual has no control; an assigned role (e.g., gender, ethnicity, age).

> **Role conception**—The understanding that a person has of a particular role.

> **Role enactments**—Actual conduct or behaviors of a person who is assigned to, or elects to enter, a given social status.

> **Role expectations**—A set of beliefs and cognitions that certain persons hold regarding what behaviors are appropriate for a specific social status.

Rumination—A situation in which a person thinks endlessly about a subject, turning it over and over and replaying it in his mind constantly with no resolution or outcome.

Rumination disorder—An emotional disturbance of the infant-mother dyad in which the child regurgitates food, resulting in weight loss or failure to gain weight.

Scapegoating—The process by which one member is blamed for the problems or misfortunes experienced by a family, group, or organization.

Schizoid—A term applied to behavior in which the person demonstrates emotional aloofness and indifference to others and seems withdrawn and cold.

Schizotypal—A term applied to behavior in which the person demonstrates social isolation, ideas of reference, magical thinking, suspiciousness, social anxiety, or illusions.

School phobia—An anxiety-based behavior in which a child fears the school situation whether or not the significant person is nearby.

School refusal—A situation in which the child (usually age 11 or 12) will not attend school, despite all consequences, due to the panic generated at separation from the significant person.

Secondary gain—Increased attention, interest, or solicitousness from others which a person may receive when he has an emotional illness or symptoms of illness.

Selective memory and perception—Refers to a tendency to perceive or recall only that which reinforces a particular viewpoint (e.g., only the "good" or the "bad" associated with persons or events).

Self—The identity, characteristics, or essential qualities of any person; the totality of an individual at any given moment, including both conscious and unconscious attributes.

Self-awareness—Having conscious knowledge of the self.

Self-concept—An individual's perception of himself as distinguished from other people and objects in the external world.

Self-esteem—A view of oneself as being worthwhile, capable, and lovable.

Self-serving roles (in group)—Roles that meet individual members' unconscious needs in groups but serve to divert the attention and progress of the members as a whole from the group's goals.

Separation anxiety–A phenomenon in which the infant or toddler, deprived of his significant caretaker, perceives a threat to his security and protests (screaming, crying), despairs (preoccupied with the caretaker's return), and detaches (becomes uninterested in parent to defend against painful feelings); this is a normal response to separations around age 18 months to 2-1/2 years but is normally not prolonged or extreme under usual situations.

Simple phobia–Particular phobias related to a specific object or situation, e.g., claustrophobia, a fear of closed places.

Single-parent family–A two-generational family consisting of a father or mother and his or her children.

Situational crisis–A crisis event that occurs in response to either expected or unexpected external events.

Social clock–Bernice Neugarten's term referring to one's sense of mastering adult achievements about the same time as other adults in the same culture and age group.

Social deprivation–Inadequate or absent social experiences that impair a child's ability to function in a larger social arena.

Social learning theory–A theory based on the premise that man's behavioral responses are influenced by the variables in the physical and interpersonal environment.

Social phobia–An irrational fear of situations in which one may be criticized or humiliated; the individual attempts to avoid such situations yet recognizes the fear as being out of proportion to the event.

Socialization–A lifelong process by which individuals learn the ways of a given society or social group so that they can function within it.

Socialized conduct disorder–A term applied to a child with a conduct disorder in which the child evidences attachment to selected others but may appear callous and manipulative toward those to whom he is not attached.

Sociopath–An outdated term for a person with antisocial personality disorder.

Somatization disorder–A complex of frequent and multiple somatic complaints in which the client seeks medical attention for vague, unexplained symptoms; no actual physical findings are present but depression, anxiety, marital and interpersonal difficulties, unnecessary surgeries and substance abuse are frequently seen.

Somatoform disorders–A category of diagnoses that feature physical symptoms suggestive of organic disorders; however, no organic findings or physiological sources are found for the symptoms.

Splitting–Unconscious attempt to separate the "good" and "bad" in both self and others based on inability to accept that the personality can have both a "good" and a "bad" self.

Statement of universality–A therapeutic communication approach that assumes that human beings have common experiences yet allows for the uniqueness of each individual within an experience; for example, "Many people wonder if they will be able to have erections after prostate surgery; have you wondered that about yourself?"

Status epilepticus–Uninterrupted recurrences of grand mal seizures which may occur in an epileptic client or in response to abrupt withdrawal of barbiturates or antianxiety agents.

Stimulus deprivation–In early life, the child is deprived of sensory and motor stimulation.

Stress–The constant interaction between individual and environment; always present in all organisms and varies in response to stressors.

Stressors–Events that affect an individual and which may be pleasant or unpleasant, internal or external, physiologic or psychosocial.

Substance abuse–Excessive use, tendency to use on a daily basis or during the day, and inability to cut down or stop using a substance consistently; impairment of social and occupational functions due to use of drugs and/or alcohol.

Suicidal gesture–Apparent attempt by a person to cause self-injury with lethal consequences.

Suicidal ideation–Thoughts about killing oneself.

Suicidal threat–Verbal or behavioral indication from an individual that denotes suicidal intent.

Suicide–Destructive aggression turned inward; taking one's own life.

Suicide attempt–Initiation of behavior that the person believes will result in his death.

Suicide potential–Degree of probability that an individual will attempt self-harm.

Suicidology–Scientific study of the prevention and causes of suicide.

Superego–The abstract mental structure, described by psychoanalytic psychology, that represents social learning and ideal aspirations—the "shoulds" of society; it is primarily unconscious and evaluates the actions of the ego.

Suppression–A defense mechanism wherein the person consciously strives to forget or not express a certain feeling or thought.

T group–A training group in which the purpose is interpersonal learning.

Tardive dyskinesia–A slowly developing and irreversible extrapyramidal complication of neuroleptic drug therapy characterized by uncontrollable movements of the muscles of the mouth and face.

Task group–A group whose primary purpose is the achievement of a specific task (e.g., planning, policy making, evaluating).

Teleological–Goal-oriented focus, as in an ethical theory that emphasizes the outcomes of an act.

Telephone crisis lines–"Hot lines" to provide immediate response to individuals when they are experiencing crises; emphasizes the initial phase of management of a crisis.

Temperament–The developmental and behavioral styles exhibited by a person that are evident at birth.

Termination phase–The last phase of the one-to-one relationship in which the client and the nurse work through the experience of loss as the relationship draws to an end.

Therapeutic community–Application of milieu therapy in the hospital environment promoting an atmosphere of self-examination, problem solving, and changing behaviors.

Therapeutic community meeting–Daily meeting of all clients and staff working and living in a defined area; the purpose of the meeting is to provide a climate for free expression of feelings between members, role examination, and discussion of conflicts regarding everyday living activities among the members.

Therapeutic use of self–The nurse as a person, with knowledge and skills, thoughts, feelings, and behaviors, utilizes who she is in order to facilitate the client's emotional growth.

Thought broadcasting–The belief that a person's thoughts can be heard by others; a symptom of schizophrenia.

Thought stopping–The conscious effort of interrupting an unwanted thought and replacing it with a wanted or more desirable thought.

Tolerance–Increasing levels of resistance to the physiological and psychological effects of alcohol or drugs; results in the necessity of ingesting gradually larger doses in order to maintain the effects.

Transactional analysis–A therapy approach devised by Eric Berne which focuses on analysis of communication transactions, life scripts, ego states, and "games."

Transference (in psychoanalytic therapy)–Positive or negative feelings and wishes directed toward significant others from the past are projected onto the therapist, reactivating strivings from early life; an unconscious phenomenon in which the client views another as similar to someone in his past and relates to the person as if he were that person.

Transsexualism–A condition (continuous for at least 2 years) wherein a person desires a gender identity opposite to his or her sexual anatomy.

Triangulation–The inclusion of a third person or thing in a dyad relation as a mechanism to relieve stress.

Undersocialized–A term applied to a child with a conduct disorder in which the child, failing to experience a significant attachment and bonding, has difficulty bonding with others in later life; behavior characterized by lack of concern for others, lack of guilt or remorse, and lack of altruistic behavior.

Unloading the question–A therapeutic communication approach used to get and to give information about variations in sexual experiences; for example, "Some women have an orgasm in dreams, some when masturbating, some when having intercourse and other sexual activities, and some women report not having orgasms at all; in general, when do you have an orgasm?"

Utilitarian theory–An ethical perspective that emphasizes the consequences of an act and focuses on the principle of providing the greatest good for the greatest number.

Vaginismus–Involuntary muscular contractions and spasms around any object at the vaginal entrance; the condition may make intercourse painful or impossible.

Validate–To confirm the existence of.

Value–To place an estimate of worth on a particular thing; to think of as important and desirable; ideas or issues that are rated or ranked in importance.

Victim crisis–A situation in which an individual has suffered from aggression by another person or by the environment; the aggression can be physical or emotional.

Vigilance–An overly attentive watchfulness of the environment, usually found in anxiety states.

Voyeurism–Spying on unsuspecting people, usually strangers, who are disrobing, nude, or engaging in sexual activities; the behavior is preferred or essential for sexual gratification and no sexual activity with the observed people is sought.

Working phase–*See* middle phase.

Zoophila–The use of animals as a repeatedly preferred or exclusive method of achieving sexual excitement.

Index